Congenital Heart Disease
Textbook of Angiocardiography

Volume I

by

Robert M. Freedom, MD, FRCP(C)

John B. Mawson, MB, CHB, (NZ), FRCAR, FRCP(C)
Shi-Joon Yoo, MD
Leland N. Benson, MD, FRCP(C)

With contributions by

J.A.G. Culham, MD, FRCP(C)
Cathy MacDonald, MD, FRCP(C)
C.A.F. Moes, MD, FRCP(C)
David Nykanen, MD, FRCP(C)

Foreword by

G.A. Trusler, MD

With 2703 illustrations

Congenital Heart Disease
Textbook of Angiocardiography

Volume I

by

Robert M. Freedom, MD, FRCP(C)

Professor of Paediatrics and Pathology
The University of Toronto Faculty of Medicine
Head, Division of Cardiology
Department of Paediatrics
Medical Director, Cardiac Program
The Hospital for Sick Children
Toronto, Ontario, Canada

John B. Mawson, MB, CHB, (NZ), FRCAR, FRCP(C)

Assistant Professor of Radiology
The University of Toronto Faculty of Medicine
Head, Section of Cardiovascular Radiology
Department of Diagnostic Imaging
The Hospital for Sick Children
Toronto, Ontario, Canada

Shi-Joon Yoo, MD

Specialist in Cardiac and Fetal Imaging
Department of Radiology
Sejong Heart Institute
Puchon, Korea

Leland N. Benson, MD, FRCP(C)

Professor of Paediatrics
The University of Toronto Faculty of Medicine
Director, Variety Club Cardiac Catheterization
Laboratories
Division of Cardiology, Department of Paediatrics
The Hospital for Sick Children
Toronto, Ontario, Canada

With contributions by

J.A.G. Culham, MD, FRCP(C)

Professor of Radiology
The University of British Columbia Faculty of Medicine
Senior Staff Radiologist
The Children's Hospital of British Columbia
Vancouver, British Columbia

Cathy MacDonald, MD, FRCP(C)

Assistant Professor of Radiology
The University of Toronto Faculty of Medicine
Staff Radiologist, Section of Cardiovascular Radiology
Department of Diagnostic Imaging
The Hospital for Sick Children
Toronto, Ontario, Canada

C.A.F. Moes, MD, FRCP(C)

Professor of Radiology Emeritus
The University of Toronto Faculty of Medicine
Former Head, Section of Cardiovascular Radiology
Department of Diagnostic Imaging
The Hospital for Sick Children
Toronto, Ontario, Canada

David Nykanen, MD, FRCP(C)

Assistant Professor of Paediatrics
The University of Toronto Faculty of Medicine
Associate Director, Variety Club Cardiac
Catheterization Laboratories
Division of Cardiology, Department of Paediatrics
The Hospital for Sick Children
Toronto, Ontario, Canada

FUTURA

Futura Publishing Company, Inc.
Armonk, NY

Library of Congress Cataloging-in-Publication Data

Congenital heart disease: textbook of angiocardiography / Robert M. Freedom ... [et al.].
    p.   cm.
   Includes bibliographical references and index.
   ISBN 0-87993-656-8 (set)
   1. Congenital heart disease—Diagnosis.   2. Angiocardiography.
I. Freedom, Robert M.
   [DNLM: 1. Heart Diseases—in infancy & childhood.   2. Heart
Diseases—radiography.   3. Angiocardiography—in infancy &
childhood.   WS 290 T355 1997]
RJ423.5.A52T49   1997
618.92′1207572—dc20
DNLM/DLC
for Library of Congress

96-42295
CIP

Copyright © 1997
Futura Publishing Company, Inc.

Published by
Futura Publishing Company, Inc.
135 Bedford Road
Armonk, NY 10504

Every effort has been made to ensure that the information in this book is as up to date and accurate as possible at the time of publication. However, due to the constant developments in medicine, neither the author, nor the editor, nor the publisher can accept any legal or any other responsibility for any errors or omissions that may occur.

Printed in the United States of America on acid-free paper.

For those whose lives are affected

by congenital heart disease

Foreword

I am privileged to write a brief foreword for this magnificent work, *Congenital Heart Disease: Textbook of Angiocardiography.* It is fitting that it should emanate from the Hospital for Sick Children in Toronto where cardiac angiography has been an art form in the diagnosis of congenital heart disease for so many years, and from which so many publications on the angiocardiography of congenital heart disease have emanated. This started with John Keith, the first head of cardiology, and continued with Dick Rowe (both now deceased) and reached a pinnacle with the redoubtable Bob Freedom, Head of the Division of Cardiology for more than the past decade. *Congenital Heart Disease: Textbook of Angiocardiography* emphasizes morphological descriptions of each anomaly and its many anatomic variations. The natural history of each condition is clearly depicted and is extensively portrayed by a beautiful compilation of angiocardiography. The great usefulness of the interventional catheter, which has developed so much over the past 10 years, and its symbiosis with angiocardiography is well described by Lee Benson. The careful details of catheter and angiographic techniques and their indications provide the science of angiocardiographic imaging, but the art of this text comes from the extensive experience of the authors.

My relationship with cardiology extends back over 35 years when John Keith was the head of cardiology and Bill Mustard, head of cardiac surgery. In those early years every child and every operation was potentially new and different. It was a great learning experience. Happily, there was a feeling of mutual help and trust between cardiologists and surgeons. That feeling was carried forward by Dick Rowe and subsequently by Bob Freedom. Conferences continue to be maintained with a refreshingly friendly spirit of collegiality where the prime interest is the long-term welfare of the child. As surgeons we were and continue to be aware of our good fortune in having the support of an outstanding cardiology team.

The present leader of the team, Bob Freedom, a dear friend and colleague over many years, is and has been a tremendous strength and resource with a prodigious memory and a great knowledge of both morphology and angiography, combined with excellent skills with a catheter. I suspect that Bob sometimes wishes he had become a cardiac surgeon, but perhaps he has the best of both worlds. Despite a heavy clinical and administrative load, he remains extraordinarily productive. As witness herein, Bob and his co-authors, John Mawson, Shi-Joon Yoo, and Lee Benson have produced a text on angiocardiographic imaging destined to become a classic.

George A. Trusler, MD, FRCS(C)

Professor of Surgery Emeritus
The University of Toronto Faculty of Medicine
Former Head, Division of Cardiovascular Surgery
The Hospital for Sick Children
Toronto, Ontario, Canada

Preface

When one of us (RMF) was asked: Why write an entirely new book dedicated almost entirely to angiocardiography? Has the subject changed that dramatically? The answer was an unhalting **yes.** Congenital heart disease seemingly is becoming more complex; we are becoming aware of profound changes in cardiac form and function as we seek to treat all different expressions of congenitally malformed hearts in patients, many of whom were once considered inoperable and condemned to an early death. One can list operations that weren't routinely being conducted 10 to 15 years ago: the bidirectional cavopulmonary connection to stage toward the Fontan; the palliative arterial switch procedure for some forms of univentricular atrioventricular connection; the double switch procedure for some forms of hearts with discordant atrioventricular and ventriculoarterial connections; arterial switch operation for the patient treated with a previous atrial repair for transposition of the great arteries and now with either a failing right ventricle or pulmonary hypertension from pulmonary venous obstruction, etc. Cross-sectional echocardiography, with Doppler and color flow imaging has rightly assumed its mantle of importance in our field, but echocardiographic imaging hasn't supplanted angiocardiographic imaging. Indeed, for many kinds of congenitally malformed hearts, these imaging modalities are not mutually exclusive; rather they are complementary.

Once I had decided to take on this task, I asked Lee Benson, colleague, friend, and Director of the Hospital for Sick Children's Variety Club Cardiac Catheterization Laboratories, to share with me the 'ownership' of the book. I asked Lee to contribute sections on intervention and the angiographic aftermath of those activities. While this work will have a Toronto flavor, it is enhanced by the contributions of John Mawson and Shi-Joon Yoo. John is the Senior Cardiovascular Radiologist at the Hospital for Sick Children, and it is worth noting that he received much of his initial training in pediatric cardiovascular radiology from the late Peter Brandt—one of the pioneers in this arena—in Auckland, New Zealand, with subsequent training from a dear friend and former colleague, Gordon Culham, in Vancouver, British Columbia. Some years ago when in Singapore on a speaking engagement, I had the good fortune of meeting Shi-Joon Yoo. We chatted briefly, and he presented me with a small gift. Back at the hotel, I opened the package ot find his wonderful textbook, *Angiocardiograms in Congenital Heart Disease. Teaching File of Sejong Heart Institute* (Yoo S-J, Choi Y-H. Oxford Medical Publications, Oxford, 1991). This is a book of remarkable clarity with beautiful illustrations. A year later, Joon was taking a sabbatical here at the Hospital for Sick Children, and it was at that time I asked him to become involved with this project. For those around the world who know Shi-Joon Yoo, they understand why I asked him to join in this cooperative effort. Both John, here, and Joon, now back in Korea, have added so much to the clarity and comprehensive character of this work.

From the perspective of angiocardiography, this textbook is meant to be complete, and while we could not show examples of every image, we hope that we have provided angiocardiographic and clinical references to most forms of congenitally malformed hearts, both common and rare. This is obviously an unenviable task, and clearly there will be errors of omission. Most of the angiocardiograms used in this work are from patients studied at the Hospital for Sick Children, with some from New Zealand and Korea (the latter contributed by our co-authors). Our colleagues and friends from around the world have given us permission to use some of their material as well. These specific contributions are, of course, acknowledged in the figure legends, but we would like to express our gratitude to them here for their generosity. Because of limitations of space, we could not dedicate as much space to those changes in form and function that result from surgical intervention. There is, however, much in this work addressing these important changes, but in a more focused format. This effort is more, however, than an atlas. It is not just a 'show' but rather a 'show-and-tell'. We have tried to put into a clinical perspective those images that we have portrayed. What management issue(s) should be considered from the images that you see, and what angiocardiographic information you should seek to best enhance patient care. Furthermore, the narrative in the text is not just directed toward the art and science of angiocardiography. Rather we have tried to place certain issues of morphology and image into management and outcome, and thus the essence of this 'show-and-tell'. As the senior author, I will share with my colleagues any praise for this work. However, I alone will shoulder any fault for error.

Robert M. Freedom, MD
Toronto, Ontario, and Granville Ferry,
Nova Scotia, Canada

Acknowledgments

This herculean effort could not have been completed without contributions and support from many sources. Dr. Robert H.A. Haslam, Professor and Chair of Paediatrics of the University of Toronto Faculty of Medicine, and Paediatrician-in-Chief of the Hospital for Sick Children, provides the academic milieu for clinical research. With his nurturing and mentoring style, his academic leadership and with his wisdom gleaned from years of pediatric leadership, he understands and appreciates clinical and outcome research. The former Chair of the Department of Pathology of the Hospital for Sick Children, Dr. M.J. Phillips, and the current Chair, Dr. Larry Becker, have provided access to pathological material and resources for display and photography. In this regard, Dr. Don Perrin (Pathologists' Assistant) and Michael Starr, Staff Photographer, both of the Department of Pathology have been so helpful to RMF over the years, lending their art and skill to the dissection and photography of congenitally malformed hearts.

We have been privileged to work on a daily basis with a superb group of cardiovascular surgeons. We all benefited from the pioneering work, dedication, and great humor of the later William T. Mustard, the first Director of Paediatric Cardiovascular Surgery at the Hospital for Sick Children. Dr. Mustard's successor, George A. Trusler, just retired in December, 1994, after a long and distinguished career. George, a dear friend and colleague provided for all of us an academic, meticulous, and nurturing career, and his patients benefited tremendously from his skill. His successor, Dr. William G. Williams is currently joined in surgical endeavors by Drs. John Coles, Glen Van Arsdell, Michael Black and Ivan Rebeyka, now in Alberta, Canada.

The collaboration with our cardiovascular radiology colleagues has meant so very much to our patients and to us. Dr. J.A.G. Culham, a cardiovascular radiologist, now at the British Columbia's Children's Hospital was a co-author of the first textbook of angiocardiography emanating from this institution. Dr. C.A.F. Moes, Professor of Radiology Emeritus of the University of Toronto Faculty of Medicine, contributed to the present textbook and also was a co-author of our earlier textbook of angiocardiography. Dr. Cathy MacDonald joined the Department of Radiology some years ago and has contributed several chapters to this effort. We appreciate the leadership of Dr. Derek Harwood-Nash (now deceased) and Dr. Alan Daneman, former Chairs of the Department of Radiology of the Hospital for Sick Children who both foster and support such academic collaboration. Dr. David Nykanen who joined the staff of the Division of Cardiology several years ago with a focus on interventional cardiac catheterization procedures contributed a number of chapters and specific sections on intervention, and this effort is all the better for his contributions.

The overwhelming number of angiocardiograms used in this textbook were performed at the Hospital for Sick Children in Toronto, and the majority of those used for this textbook were performed in the past decade. We must acknowledge the contributions of our colleagues within the Division of Cardiology who along with RMF and Lee Benson performed these studies. These colleagues include Drs. Ian Adatia, Christine Boutin, Robert Gow, Robert Hamilton, Teruo Izukawa (now retired), Brian McCrindle, and Jeffrey Smallhorn. We have used some angiocardiograms performed prior to 1985 by colleagues who have left the Hospital for Sick Children, including Drs. John Dyck, Peter Hesslein, B.S.L. Kidd, Peter Olley, and the late Richard D. Rowe. The Variety Club Cardiac Catheterization laboratories have been staffed with nurses and technicians of extraordinary dedication. These include Kathy Hunter, Sandra Bogdon, Susan Hoey, Angie Basciano, and Frank Hamilton, and we thank them for their talent.

The authors are particularly indebted to those friends and colleagues throughout the world who at our request made available their own material for inclusion in this textbook. Some of these materials were figures from their publications, while other material was in the form of color 35-mm slides or black-and-white prints of angiograms. We have reformatted much of this material to be consistent with the graphic format of most of the angiograms reproduced herein.

The ability to define cineangiocardiograms of consistent textbook quality necessitates knowledge of congenital heart disease, axial angiocardiography, film processing, contrast agents, catheter size, and flow rates, etc. The authors must acknowledge the unique contributions of Mr. Haverj Mikailian to this effort, the senior radiology technician who has worked with the Division of Cardiology in the catheterization laboratories for more than two decades. a bright and dedicated individual, Haverj's greatest delight is producing angiocardiograms of world-class quality. Totally professional and motivated only by the desire for excellence, Haverj was central to the review of all angiocardiograms used in this textbook. He and RMF reviewed the overwhelming number of angiocardiograms performed since 1983, to this date, marking the completion of a comprehensive angiocardiographic review for *Angiocardiography of Congenital Heart Disease* (R.M. Freedom, J.A.G. Culham, C.A.F Moes. MacMillan Publishing, New York, 1984). Haverj's radiology technical staff includes or has included Marie Craven-Turner, Marlene Baily, Albert Aziza, Gayle Nystrom, Deidre Milne, and Ellen Charcot.

A tremendous effort to provide consistency in the photographic reproduction of the 35-mm cine films was provided by Tiiu Kask, director of the Graphics Centre, and her staff. This staff includes Diogenes Baena and Ian Douglas, both photographers in the Graphics Centre, and Philip Dakin, graphic artist. Without their dedication to this seemingly never-ending task and consummate professionalism, we would not have been able to complete this work. We must single out Phil Dakin for his unending dedication to the completion of this work. His skill and knowledge, tempered by a great sense of humor and understanding, proved invaluable. This work could not have been accomplished without his tremendous input.

Much of the hard- and software used in the production of this textbook from the perspective of the Division of Cardiology, the Hospital for Sick Children, is based on MacIntosh format. In this regard, for a number of years, Mr. Don Klees and his Avanet Data Corporation has served as computer consultants to the authors and to the Division of Cardiology. Mr. Klees and his colleague, Mr. Ian Free, have worked tirelessly on our behalf, and we are deeply appreciative of their efforts.

Funding for completion of this work has been derived from several sources. Supportive of Divisional Clinical Research activities over many years are Mr. and Mrs. Dov. Lidor and the Bestbuy Corporation. This family and their corporate family and friends have been very important to the funding of these textbook activities. In addition, The Hospital for Sick Children Foundation was most generous in providing financial support for this effort and we are most appreciative of the time and interest the Foundation president, Dianne Lister, and her predecessor, Claus Wirsig have taken in this project.

For many years, the Division of Cardiology of the Hospital for Sick Children has utilized Siemens angiocardiographic imaging technology. This has been so important to the acquisition of the excellent images displayed in this textbook. We acknowledge the generosity of the Siemens Company in supporting some of the cost of this project. Specifically, we are indebted to both Mr. Don Ramsay, technical sales representative of the Diagnostic Imaging Products, and Mr. Gerd Baer, Vice President of the Medical Systems Division who both endorsed and supported this effort. The authors also would like to acknowledge the support of Mr. Ravi Anand, the senior technical representative from Siemens who has worked with us for more than 8 years. On those occasions when technical problems occur, Ravi is always available, providing us with his technical excellence and knowledge.

The former President and CEO of the Hospital for Sick Children, Mr. David Martin, and the current President and CEO, Mr. Michael Strofolino were and continue to be supportive of those activities that support and endorse patient care. While neither physicians nor scientists, they value basic and clinical research as the lifeblood of any institution dedicated to patient care, education, and research. We appreciate their ongoing efforts to provide an environment to conduct these activities.

The authors must acknowledge the important roles of all the trainees in the Division of Cardiology who over the years have participated in clinical care and research and who daily stimulate and motivate us as their teachers. We know soon the 'student' will become the teacher and caregiver, and indeed, this is the 'genetics' of what we do.

The authors must acknowledge the contributions of their secretaries, those unflappable individuals who provide day-to-day direction to our professional activities. Drs. Benson and Nykanen's lives are put into order by Sandra Gretto, and Dr. Freedom by Mrs. Lisa Berejiklian-Cullen, Ms. Therese Benoit, Administrative Coordinator for the Division of Cardiology, Tiziani Lolli, his secretary for patient activities and Teresa Tota.

The authors are most indebted to their editor, Ann Kerr of Futura. She provided tremendous professionalism, laced with great humor and collegiality. We all found it just a delight to work with Ann. And what about Steven Korn, President of Futura Publishing Company? With his knowledge, charm, wit, and dedication, who would not want to to do a book with him, or even a second book? Futura is devoted to the production of excellent textbooks, figure-heavy, and we appreciate their dedication to this educational forum.

The Authors

Individual Acknowledgments

More than 30 years ago when as a medical student at the UCLA School of Medicine, I had the good fortune, indeed privilege to meet and work with Drs. Arthur Moss, Forrest Adams, George Emmanouilides, Herbert Ruttenberg, Leonard Linde, Sam Sapin, Stan Goldberg, Bill Vincent, and Harrison Latta. They encouraged a then young, impetuous medical student to pursue his interest in pediatric cardiology and cardiac morphology. During a year devoted to cardiac morphology, I wrote to and received advice and encouragement from Dr. Jesse Edwards. In those early years, his two red volumes became my 'bible'. I will always remember the generosity and kindness that Jesse showed me, and I am honored that Jesse and I became and have remained friends and collaborators. The faculty at UCLA next supported me in my desire to take an elective with Richard Van Praagh shortly after he had moved from Chicago to Boston. The time spent with Dick, a Toronto native and alumnus of the University of Toronto School of Medicine and the Hospital for Sick Children and Stella at the Cardiac Registry at the Boston Children's Hospital was one of the most exhilarating times of my life, solidifying my desire to become a pediatric cardiologist. Finishing medical school, I journeyed to Boston, completing my pediatric training at the Children's Hospital and was fortunate to be selected into the cardiology training program headed by Dr. Alexander S. Nadas.

Those were exciting years and Alex Nadas, Don Fyler, Curt Ellison, Bill Plauth, and Amnon Rosenthal proved to be wonderful role models, demonstrating on a daily basis, the best in patient care, teaching, and clinical research. While a senior fellow in Boston, I had the good fortune of meeting Richard Rowe, then director of the Division of Cardiology at Johns Hopkins, and Dick recruited me when I completed my training to come to Baltimore to become head of the diagnostic cardiac catheterization laboratory. While in Baltimore, I forged friendships with Catherine Neill, Bob Gingell, Dan Pieroni, Glenn Rosenquist, Bob White, Donald Harrington, and Jerry Krovetz, and those years 'under the dome' proved maturing and stimulating. I was only in Baltimore several years when Dick Rowe was recruited back to the Hospital for Sick Children in Toronto to succeed John Keith (now deceased) as the Director of Pediatric Cardiology. How excited I was when Dick asked me to join him in Toronto and I accepted a staff position here in December, 1973, officially landing on Canadian soil in August, 1974. The more than two decades here at the Hospital for Sick Children have been wonderful and productive years. Dick Rowe of Christchurch, New Zealand meant so much to his family and friends, to his academic community, to pediatric cardiology and to me, that perhaps one of my deepest personal sadnesses was the untimely death of Dick Rowe in January, 1988, just weeks before his planned retirement.

The massive efforts to produce these kinds of textbooks require extraordinary dedication, not just of the authors, but of their families. I appreciate the humor, dedication, and absolute professionalism of my co-authors. However, the solace necessary to conceive and complete this work could not have been accomplished without the love and understanding of Penny and Jonathan. They ask so little, but give so much. Finally, for my twin brother, Gary, we know about that special bond between twins.

Robert M. Freedom, MD
Granville Ferry, Nova Scotia & Cheju Island,
South Korea

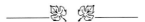

I was privileged to begin my Cardiac Radiology training at Green Lane Hospital in Auckland, New Zealand working with Drs. Peter Brandt and John Ormiston, (Cardiac Radiologists), and Drs. Louise Calder and John Neutze, (Paediatric Cardiologists). Dr. Brandt was one of the pioneers of cineangiocardiography, particularly in his application of a "projections" approach to imaging and "segmental approach" to interpretation. To him I owe a particular debt for his patience, encouragement and teaching. Mr. Darren Brown is thanked for photographing the Green Lane Hospital angiocardiograms that have been used in this book.

It has been a pleasure working with Dr. Gordon Culham, (Paediatric Radiologist) both at B.C. Children's Hospital in Vancouver, and since then, collaborating at long distance. Dr. Robert Freedom (Paediatric Cardiologist) has been a stimulating colleague at the Hospital for Sick Children in Toronto. Both he and Mr. Haverj Mikailian, have been particularly supportive.

In the Department of Diagnostic Imaging at the Hospital for Sick Children, Toronto, Dr. Alan Daneman, former Chief, and Dr. David Gilday, Chief, have supported this project. Mrs. Lori Fearon has with great patience typed and retyped manuscripts.

My wife Claudia's support and love during this endeavour has been of the utmost importance.

John B. Mawson, MD
Toronto, Ontario, Canada

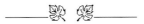

I would like to express my gratitude to Professors Man Chung Han and Kyung Mo Yeon who taught me cardiac radiology when I was a resident at the Seoul National University from 1978 until 1982. Special thanks must be given to Dr. Young Kwan Park, the President of the Sejong General Hospital in Pucheon, Korea, late Dr. Yung Kyoon Lee, the former Chief of the Sejong Heart Institute, and Dr. Yong Ho Auh, the Chief of the Department of Diagnostic Radiology, the Asan Medical Center/the University of Ulsan in Seoul, Korea for their constant advice, encouragement, and enthusiasm.

Also, I would like to express may sincere gratitude to Dr. Alan Daneman, the former head of the Department of Diagnostic Imaging, the Hospital for Sick Children, Dr. Patricia E. Burrows, the former chief of the Cardiovascular Radiology Division and Dr. C. A. Fred Moes, the former senior cardiovascular radiologist of the same division, for providing me an opportunity to study pediatric cardiac imaging at The Hospital for Sick Children in 1991 and 1992 and for their teaching. It was my great fortune to have a chance to work with Dr. Robert M. Freedom, the first author of this book, and his colleagues. During my stay in the Hospital for Sick Chil-

dren and thereafter, Dr. Freedom played a key role in upgrading my academic career as a cardiac radiologist.

Dr. Heung Jae Lee, the Chief of the Department of Pediatrics at the Samsung Medical Center in Seoul, and Dr. Jeong-Wook Seo, the Chief of the Department of Pathology at the Seoul National University Children's Hospital, are my brother-like friends. Without their encouragement and friendship, I would not be so much interested in pediatric cardiology. I am very much proud of having such friends.

I would like to thank Mrs. Young-Lan Kim of the MI Production for her painstaking effort in drawing most of the diagrams in this book.

Finally, I would like to thank my wife and daughters for their patience and consideration. I would like to dedicate this book to my mother and father.

Shi-Joon Yoo, MD
Seoul, Korea

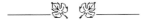

The lineage of a textbook is varied and represents not only the collective knowledge of its authors, but a quilt work of their experiences. Throughout my academic life, it has been my medical colleagues, particularly at the Hospital for Sick Children, who have had and continue to have, the greatest influence on my work, direction and goals, and for their collective support, each is acknowledged. However, there have been three individuals in particular, who have had a unique impact on the direction I have taken. Appreciation goes to Dr. Robert M. Freedom, senior cardiologist, professor and head of the division of pediatric cardiology at the Hospital for Sick Children, Toronto. Bob was (and remains) my teacher and mentor. He conceived of this project, having created the environment which allowed its realization, and was the driving force who saw it to completion. He is selfless in this generosity, and the ultimate clinician. In this era of 'high-tech' diagnosis, there is lost at times the perspective of clinical relevance and the understanding of the pathologic anatomy of pediatric cardiovascular disorders. Bob is the master teacher of these critical skills which are the foundation of our profession, and I am honored to call him my friend. Dr. Richard D. Rowe, was associated with the Hospital for Sick Children throughout his career until his untimely death in 1988. He will be remembered as a gentle and thoughtful clinician whose contributions to pediatric cardiology remain with us today, not only through his clinical skills and research, but in the hundreds of trainees who had the opportunity to work with him and learn from him. Dick Rowe supported and encouraged my early sojourn into the little known field of interventional cardiology, which is the focus of my career to this day. Dr. William F. Friedman, professor and former head of pediatrics at the University of California, Los Angeles, introduced me to the scientific footings of pediatric cardiovascular medicine, emphasizing the relevance of basic research to clinical practice, and the reliance of one on the other. For this important prospective on clinical medicine I will always be grateful.

This textbook could not have become the reality it is, without the dedication and support of the technical staff in the Variety Club Cardiac Catheterization Laboratories. Appreciation goes to Mr. Haverj Mikailian, and his coworkers, Ms. Marie Craven-Truner, Ms. Marlene Bailey, and Mr. Albert Aziz. Haverj and his team are master movie makers, for which without their technical radiological skills, these beautiful images would not have materialized. The same can be said of the nurse-technicians in the Variety Club Cardiac Catheterization Laboratories, where the performance of pediatric cardiac catheterization requires a dedicated, caring and compassionate staff. Without such support from Ms. Kathy Hunter—head nurse, Ms. Sandra Bogdon, Mrs. Susan Hoey, Ms. Angie Basciano, Mr. Frank Hamilton, Mr. Kurt Kruger and Mrs. Geogina Gonzales, these procedures could not have been performed. A special thanks goes to Ms. Sandra Greto, who labored ceaselessly over the preparation of this material.

Finally, and most dear to me, is the encouragement and support I have always received from my family, my Mom and Dad, and from Kathy, Leah and Aaron, who put up with an absent husband and father during the preparation and writing of this text.

Leland N. Benson, MD
Toronto, Ontario, Canada

The Onsite Production of *Congenital Heart Disease: Textbook of Angiocardiography*

Philip Dakin

This discussion outlines some of the methodologies used by the authors in conjunction with the Graphic Centre of the Hospital for Sick Children in Toronto to produce the *Congenital Heart Disease: Textbook of Angiocardiography*. There were striking departures in the onsite technical 'production' of this textbook when compared with others authored or co-authored by one or more of the present writers.[1-3] The text and references were formatted on MacIntosh equipment networked throughout the Division of Cardiology and Department of Radiology. Reference manager software such as Endnote and Endlink (Niles and Associates, Berkeley, CA) provided the capability to deal with the many thousands of references. All written material was eventually focussed through the office of RMF. But it was the large number of images and the desire of the authors to provide images of striking clarity with consistent labeling, that provided the biggest challenge.

This text contains more than 2700 figures, the vast majority obtained from 35-mm cineangiocardiograms performed from 1975 to 1996 at the Hospital for Sick Children in Toronto. Early in the formulation of the size, scope and format of *Congenital Heart Disease: Textbook of Angiocardiography,* we decided that virtually all the images used would be manipulated and stored digitally (Fig. 1). This step into the computer age was taken initially to replace the labeling system "Letraset" (Letraset International Ltd., England), a sheet of adhesive letters and symbols that are transferred onto a photograph by rubbing with an instrument such as a pencil. Labeling each figure, in duplicate, in this manner is a time consuming and expensive process that in the past produced acceptable, albeit inconsistent results at best. The Letraset technique had been used by the authors to label the images for their previous publications.[1-3] However, an image editing program such as

Adobe PhotoShop (Adobe Systems Incorporated, Mountain View, CA) allows the labeling of images, as well as the removal of any existing Letraset (or other adhesive) labels when photographing the original cine film was impractical (or impossible). Apart from time management, there are many additional benefits to handling the images digitally including consistency and clarity of labeling, image cropping, manipulation of density and contrast, removal of scratches and dust. Once the image is stored in a digital form, it is available for teaching and talks using slides, and can be married to electronic text, CD-ROM, real-time video sequences, etc.

Ideally, one would be able to transport a digitally-acquired angiographic image directly to a database and thence to a document such as a book chapter or paper or presentation. (Fig. 1D). However, current technology cannot yet produce digital images comparable to the resolution and tonal range of photographic film. Additionally, the vast majority of the more than 20,000 angiograms reviewed for this text were acquired prior to digital catheter laboratories being available and thus are stored as 35-mm cine film; only a fraction of the images used have been selected from digital angiocardiograms.

Traditionally, as many as seven photographic steps are needed to take an image from the original cine film to the pages of this book (Fig. 1A). Just as an old story becomes distorted (or enhanced) as it gets passed from generation to generation so too are photographic images. Every time a different form of image is needed another generation of film must tell the story of the image subject to variables such as exposure and lens quality. Most of the originals were submitted for digitizing in the form of 5 × 7 in. black and white prints and had therefore already gone through at least three photographic stages as described above. Digitizing the images at this stage will only produce results as good as the print itself. Because scanning the analogue images into digital format would have been done during the final production phases for their placement in the book, we were not adding another stage but merely moving the digitizing to an earlier point in the production process (Fig. 1B and 1C). Only after the cine film is processed and developed can the assessment of angiographic quality and both diagnostic and 'artistic' excellence be determined. Frames of interest are marked by the authors and the cineangiocardiogram is then sent to the Graphics Centre to have negatives and the prints made of the frames. Modifications were made to a slide duplicating machine (Charles Beseler Co., Florham Park, NJ) enabling it to advance through the hundreds of feet of cine film to expose specific frames onto 35-mm negative film. A 5 × 7 print is made from the negative that would be labeled by hand.

Before the tremendous task of digitizing, labeling, and storing the images could begin, testing was needed to calculate the amount of data that would be generated by 2700 images and the kind of computer system needed to effectively process this amount of data. We realized that we would probably scan and label more images than we would eventually use. Our existing equipment, consisting of a 33-megahertz, Macintosh Quadra 950 (Apple Computer, Inc, Cupertino, CA) with 64 megabytes of RAM and a 1-gigabyte hard drive was used for the testing along with an Agfa Arcus II scanner (Agfa-Gevaert, NV, Germany). By scanning 50 images @ 400 dpi amd five line drawings @ 1000 dpi with this system, we were able to calculate the average image size at around four megabytes requiring a hard drive with a storage capacity of 12 gigabytes. It was decided that four Quantum Grand Prix hard drives of 4.3 gigabytes each would be used. This configuration provided some data security and most importantly, allowed us to perform multitasking using up to four computers simultaneously.

The Quadra 950's 33-megahertz co-processor chip was adequate for scanning, but proved to be much too slow to process images efficiently. A Macintosh PowerPC 9500 with a fast 132-megahertz co-processer and 32 megabytes of RAM was added to the team and provided the main image processing work station. Both computers were set up side by side and connected via an Ethernet network to the output devices. One of the drives was SCSI connected to the Quadra 950 for use with the scanner, and the remaining three to the PowerPC 9500 for processing and storage. Computer hardware comprises only half of the system's functionality, software being the main interface which dictates the equipment's intelligence and usability. Batch scanning of 5 × 7 prints was an option offered by Agfa Fotolook (Agfa-Gevaert, NV, Germany). Two or three images could be placed on the scanning bed at one time, each image scanned at the operator's preset specifications, saved in a choice of image formats, and placed into a designated folder. Unfortunately, the choice of formats was limited and an extra step was needed to save each image using an Adobe PhotoShop format in order to be able to use a layering function crucial to our process. The use of a text layer allowed us to annotate figures without permanantly embedding the labels into the background image.

PhotoShop was the software tool around which the imaging system was built. The intuitive interface and vast arsenal of image processing tools provided by this software gave us complete control over every aspect of the images. A "Dust and Scratches" filter would sweep each image automatically removing specks of a predetermined size. Seamless removal of old Letraset labelling and blemishes as well as manipulation of density and contrast are just a few more of its tangible assets. Many of the steps needed to process an image in PhotoShop such as format change, adding layers, and filter applications were repetitive and time consuming. A 'finicky' program called PhotoMatic (Daystar Digital, Flowery Branch, GA) alleviated some of the repetitive tasks. It uses a scripting language (AppleScript) in conjunction with PhotoShop to record specific functions and then perform them on any given number of images. This allowed the computer to work unsupervised on hundreds of images overnight leaving a folder of processed images waiting to be cropped and labeled in the morning. The conditions under which these scripts would run needed to be precise and therefore required extensive testing and consultation with the manufacturer to get it up and running. The important job of cataloging all the figures was given to a program called Aldus Fetch (Aldus Corporation, Seattle, WA). Fetch enabled us to view each of the figures in catalog form and print them four to a page along with its reference number and location.

Horror stories of data loss and system crashes are told and retold wherever computers are used; this production was not immune from these difficulties. Early in the process we would open 10 to 20 images at a time to collect opening and saving times into 5-minute breaks. The most significant and by far the most bizarre data loss came in the form of partial text disappearance. An image would be labeled, saved, and then brought into a catalog to be printed. There are four ways in which each of the images can be viewed: 1) as an icon in the finder; 2) as a 'thumbnail' in the catalog; 3) in PhotoShop; 4) on a printed page. The labels applied in the text layer or at least some of them, were not apparent on some of the images when opened in PhotoShop but were still visible in the other three viewing options. Even after consulting local experts and Adobe Systems, the problem remains unresolved but it has not reoccurred since a software patch was installed and the drives were defragmented.

Once the images have been digitized, labeled, cata-

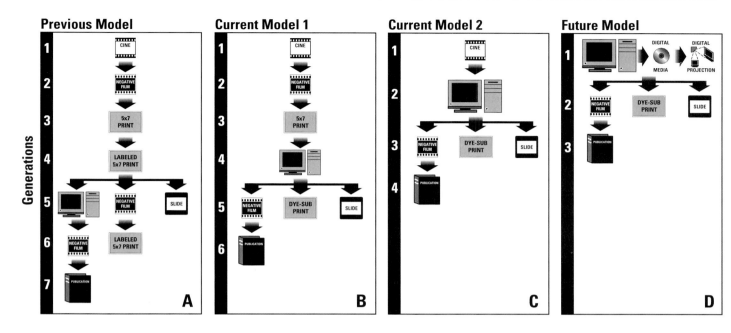

Fig. 1. A: This flow sheet shows the earlier flow of a 35-mm cine film and its conversion to a 5 × 7 print, labeled with Letraset, rephotographed, and submitted to the publisher for incorporation into the text. At least seven generations were required before incorporation of the figure into the completed text. **B:** This flow sheet demonstrates the handling of cine film used in the production of *Congenital Heart Disease: Textbook of Angiocardiography* with digital labeling of all scanned images. The Letraset-step was obviated by this technique. Cine film still had to be processed to prints as in A. **C:** Some information could be scanned directly for digital labeling without first producing a 5 × 7 black and white print. These materials included chest radiographic, magnetic resonance images, and images acquired from digital subtraction techniques. **D:** This flow sheet indicates that future productions will not require any film processing, but rather all data will be directly acquired and processed digitally.

logued, and stored, they can be output as required. High-quality glossies were printed on a 300 dpi Kodak 8600 dye-sublimation printer (Eastman Kodak Company, Rochester, NY). All catalogs were printed on a 400 dpi Canon 800 laser printer with a Silicon Graphics Indy (Silicon Graphics, Inc, Mountain View, CA) server running Cyclone queue management software (Colorbus, Irvine, CA); this allowed for checking of images against legends and text as well as cross-referencing. A Lasergraphics Personal Plus high resolution film recorder (Lasergraphics, Irvine, CA) was also available for slide output.

These notes, we hope, will provide some understanding of how the authors and Graphic Centre staff worked together to produce *Congenital Heart Disease: Textbook of Angiocardiography.* These comments should not be interpreted as a "how-to" manual; rather, it is "how we did it". On reflection we now appreciate what we can do differently the next time to improve the quality of image collection, collation, and reproduction. Indeed, already we have the capability to dig-

itize frames directly from the cine film, thus eliminating the need for a 5 × 7 print (Fig. 1C). Eventually, when digital catheter laboratories completely replace cine film, we hope to achieve a seamless transfer of digitally acquired data directly to a presentation format (Fig. 1D).

During the many hours the authors and I worked together, a sense of mutual understanding, respect, and affection developed. What better testimony to this work that consumed us all for more than a year, on days, nights, and weekends?

References

1. Freedom RM, Culham JAG, Moes CAF. *Angiocardiography of Congenital Heart Disease.* New York: Macmillan Publishing; 1984, 691 pages.
2. Freedom RM. *Pulmonary Atresia and Intact Ventricular Septum.* Mount Kisco, NY: Futura Publishing Company, Inc; 1989, 262 pages.
3. Freedom RM, Benson L, Smallhorn JF. *Neonatal Heart Disease.* London: Springer-Verlag; 1992, 881 pages.

Contents

Volume I

Section I: General Principles

Section II. Specific Conditions

Part 1. Malformations with Left-to-Right Shunt

Part 2. Malformations of Atrioventricular or Ventriculoarterial Connection

Section III: Acquired and Metabolic Disorders

Section IV: Miscellaneous

Glossary of Abbreviations

A, aorta
AA, aortic arch
AB, anterior or superior bridging leaflet
ALSA, aberrant left subclavian artery
Aneur, aneurysm
AO, aorta
AOV, aortic valve
APC, aortopulmonary collateral artery
APP, atrial appendage
ARSA, aberrant right subclavian artery
ARV, atrialized right ventricle
AS, anterosuperior or dextrodorsal leaflet
ASA, anomalous systemic artery
ASC, anteroseptal commissure
ASD, atrial septal defect
ATL, anterior tricuspid leaflet
ATR, atrium
ATR RV, atrialized portion of right ventricle
AV, atrioventricular valve, aortic valve
AZY, azygous vein
BAL, balloon
BAV, bicuspid aortic valve
BCV, brachiocephalic vein
BDCPC, bidirectional cavopulmonary connection
BT, BTS, Blalock-Taussig shunt
CA, common atrium
CAVO, common atrioventricular orifice
CB, conal branch of coronary artery
COR, coronary artery
CoS, COS, CS, coronary sinus
CPV, common pulmonary vein
CS, crista supraventricularis
CT, dividing left atrial membrane
Cx, circumflex coronary artery
D, defect
DAO, descending thoracic aorta
Diag, diagonal branch
DIV, cardiac diverticulum

DORV, double-outlet right ventricle
DV, descending pulmonary vein
DV, ductus venosus
E, esophagus
ECA, external carotid artery
EFF, effusion
HA, hemiazygous vein
HEP, hepatic artery
HV, hepatic vein
IC, inferior chamber
ICA, internal carotid artery
IE, inlet extension
IMA, internal mammary or thoracic artery
INF, inferior surface coronary artery
INF, infundibulum
INLET, inlet zone of right ventricle
INN, innominate artery or vein
INT, intermediate coronary artery
IRSA, isolated right subclavian artery
IS, infundibular septum
IVC, inferior caval vein
JA, juxta-arterial
JT, juxta-tricuspid
LA, left atrium
LAA, left atrial appendage, left aortic arch
LACV, levoatrial cardinal vein
LAD, left anterior descending coronary artery
LAD, left atrial diverticulum
LAP, left atrial appendage
LAVO, left atrioventricular orifice
LBCV, left brachiocephalic vein
LC, lower chamber
LCA, left coronary artery
LCC, LCCA, left common carotid artery
LF, left-facing sinus
LIA, left innominate artery
LIVC, left-sided inferior vena cava
LLPV, left lower pulmonary vein
LM, left lateral mural leaflet

LMB, left main bronchus
LPA, left pulmonary artery
LPV, left pulmonary vein
LSA, left subclavian artery
LSVC, left superior caval vein
LV, left ventricle
LVD, left ventricular diverticulum
LVOT, left ventricular outflow tract
MI, muscular inlet
MO, muscular outlet
MPA, main pulmonary artery
MPM, medial papillary muscle
MT, muscular trabecular
MV, mitral valve
MYO, myocardium
NF, nonfacing sinus
OE, outlet extension
OM, obtuse marginal coronary artery
OS, outlet septum
OSl, ostium primum atrial septal defect
P, pulmonary artery
PA, pulmonary artery
PAB, pulmonary artery band
PB, posterior or inferior bridging leaflet
PD, posterior descending coronary artery
PDA, patent arterial duct
PM, papillary muscle
PM-JA, perimembranous juxta-arterial
PV, pulmonary valve; pulmonary vein
PVV, pulmonary vein varix
RA, right atrium
RAA, right aortic arch
RAA, right atrial appendage
RAD, right atrial diverticulum
RAP, right atrial appendage
RBT, right Blalock-Taussig shunt
RC, right coronary artery
RCA, right coronary artery
RCCA, right common carotid artery
RF, right-facing sinus
RIVC, right inferior caval vein

RLPV, right lower pulmonary vein
RM, right lateral mural leaflet
RMB, right main bronchus
RPA, right pulmonary artery
RPV, right pulmonary vein
RRA, right renal artery
RSA, right subclavian artery
RSVC, right superior caval vein
RUL, right upper lobe pulmonary artery
RUPV, right upper pulmonary vein
RV, right ventricle
RVD, right ventricular diverticulum
RVOT, right ventricular outflow tract
SBL, superior bridging leaflet
SC, superior chamber
Sinu, sinusoid
SMA, superior mesenteric artery
SPL, splenic artery
SS, straight sinus
ST, stenosis
STL, superior tricuspid leaflet
SVC, superior caval vein
SVMR, supravalvular stenosing mitral ring
T, transverse aortic arch, trachea, tunnel
TGA, transposition of the great arteries
Trab, trabecular zone of right ventricle
TR, common arterial trunk
Tri Inflow, tricuspid valve inflow
TRU, truncus arteriosus
TS, transverse sinus
TSM, trabecular septomarginalis
TU, tunnel
TV, tricuspid valve
UC, upper chamber
VA, vertebral artery
V-C, ventriculocoronary connection
VENT, ventricle
VIF, ventriculoinfundibular fold
VS, ventricular septum
VSD, ventricular septal defect
VV, vertical vein

Section I

General Principles

Chapter 1

Imaging Modalities in Pediatric Cardiovascular Disorders

With Cathy MacDonald, MD, FRCP(C)

This textbook is dedicated primarily to a comprehensive overview of angiocardiography in congenital heart disease and the clinical and management implications based on these images. But the precise definition of congenital heart malformations is predicated on far more than one imaging modality. The clinical recognition of congenital heart disease necessitates a broad understanding of normal and abnormal cardiac physiology, the tremendous anatomic scope of the congenitally malformed heart, and the integration of clinical, noninvasive, and invasive imaging technologies to provide with absolute clarity and with nonambiguity the anatomic cardiac diagnosis or diagnoses. Before one takes a patient to the angiocardiography suite, a detailed history, general physical, and cardiac examination may provide considerable information important to the development of the investigatory and imaging algorithms. The plain chest radiograph provides information about heart position, the disposition of the major bronchi, and the abdominal situs (see Chapter 3). The chest x-ray provides important information about heart size and contour, the state of the pulmonary arterial vasculature, and pulmonary venous markings, whether normal or abnormal, symmetrical or asymmetrical. The contour of the heart may suggest left juxtaposition of the atrial appendages (see Chapter 13). The recognition of an abnormally symmetric and horizontal hepatic shadow may be one of the earliest clues that one is dealing with a patient with incompletely lateralized viscera, and the patient with right or left atrial isomerism (see Chapter 41). The appearance of a heart in the right chest on the chest x-ray, a small volume right hemithorax, and an abnormal vascular silhouette may be indicative of the so-called scimitar syndrome (see Chapter 19). These are but a few instances to remind us that the plain chest x-ray is not a tool of the distant past, but one that retains its role as an important imaging instrument. We need not be reminded that the scalar electrocardiogram is still important for providing information about heart rate and rhythm, frontal P-wave and QRS axis, and chamber enlargement. An abnormal leftward and superior P-wave axis may provide a clue that one is dealing with a patient with left atrial isomerism and poorly developed sinoatrial nodes (see Chapters 3 and 41). The leftward and superior frontal QRS axis may provide evidence that one is perhaps dealing with a patient with an atrioventricular septal defect. And so on.

The past 20 years are witness to an ever-evolving and increasingly sophisticated technology that is able to image the heart with striking clarity, and also provide physiologic, hemodynamic, and metabolic information about the patient without resorting to invasive methodologies. There are now a number of different imaging modalities available to evaluate congenital heart malformations, each having advantages and limitations. Imaging the heart and great vessels not only requires details of cardiac anatomy, but also physiologic assessment of cardiac function, hemodynamics, and metabolism. The optimal imaging modality is one that is inexpensive, portable, noninvasive, and risk-free. Images should be high quality and data collection

From: Freedom RM, Mawson JB, Yoo SJ, Benson LN: *Congenital Heart Disease: Textbook of Angiocardiography.* Armonk NY, Futura Publishing Co., Inc. ©1997.

should be rapid with computer capabilities available for pertinent calculations and repeat measurements during exercise or after intervention. Currently, no single imaging system exists for structural and functional cardiovascular assessment. Complementary modalities are usually necessary. This chapter highlights a variety of modalities, stressing their practical and potential applications in imaging congenital heart lesions, with a more detailed discussion on the newer technique of magnetic resonance imaging (MRI).[1]

Echocardiographic Imaging

This book is dedicated to the angiocardiographic assessment of congenital malformations of the heart; however, additional modalities of cardiac imaging have evolved that have complemented, and in many situations, replaced the requirement for invasive study. Echocardiography is one such modality that can represent and detail complex anatomic lesions, and in many instances, better delineate anatomic and hemodynamic alterations to the cardiovascular circulation (eg, atrioventricular valve morphology and function). Echocardiography combines a number of techniques and approaches (Table 1-1) that can be applied depending on the hemodynamic or morphological question. Developed over 30 years ago, echocardiography has earned an extremely prominent place in clinical cardiology. These echocardiographic methods permit evaluation of atrial, ventricular and great artery size and function, intracardiac morphology and blood flow patterns, identification of intracardiac masses, valvular abnormalities (thickening, fibrosis, calcification, vegetations) pericardial effusions, and congenital morphological abnormalities, and can be applied *in utero*.

Table 1-1

Echocardiographic Techniques and Approaches

Techniques

    M-mode echocardiography
    Two-dimensional echocardiography
    Doppler echocardiography:
        Pulsed-wave Doppler
        Continuous-wave Doppler
        Color-Doppler flow mapping
    Tissue characterization
    Three-dimensional echocardiography

Approaches

    Transthoracic echocardiography
    Transesophageal echocardiography
    Transabdominal echocardiography (*in utero* imaging)
    Transvaginal echocardiography (*in utero* imaging)

As is the case with all clinically applied diagnostic ultrasound, echocardiography has inherent advantages including safety, portability, patient comfort, repeatability, ease of application, and relative cost effectiveness. However, the technique is highly operator dependent. Image quality is dependent not only on patient characteristics (position and size), but the examination requires operator adjustments to signal gain (amplification), time-gain amplification, and gray scale mapping. These adjustments may significantly effect image presentation and diagnostic quality.[2] Patient size (body habitus) may also effect image quality. Although less of a problem in the young child, echocardiographic imaging can be limited by hyperexpansion and certain thoracic musculoskeletal deformities, due to alteration of the ultrasound by air or adipose tissue. Additionally, the tomographic images from the echocardiographic examination are truly not parallel to each other, but acquired with some angulation. This angulation between images is due to the restraint of the acoustic window, requiring intercostal, subcostal, and suprasternal imaging.

Despite these caveats, echocardiography has developed into a significant imaging modality for noninvasive diagnosis. The fact that many lesions can be well characterized and treatment algorithms outlined based on ultrasound evaluation is without question.[3,4] Cardiac catheterization has also evolved from a modality used to obtain a comprehensive diagnosis to one where specific anatomic-hemodynamic questions and therapeutic interventions complement information already available from various noninvasive studies. There will remain those unique complex anomalies that continue to pose difficulties not only with anatomic definition, but patient care planning[5]; for these, angiographic definition is required. The application of any diagnostic modality must be applied with the knowledge of its limitations, the specific questions that must be answered for patient care, and the complementary information that can be obtained from other forms of imaging.

Magnetic Resonance Imgaging

MRI has become an important tool for defining cardiovascular anatomy, physiology, and pathology in a wide spectrum of congenital abnormalities, and has had significant impact on the management of children with heart disease.[6–17] Noninvasive techniques are in some instances replacing and in other instances complementing catheterization and angiography for the diagnosis of cardiac diseases. MRI is generally a supplementary noninvasive technique greatly influenced by the information achieved with echocardiography, which remains the mainstay in the evaluation of most patients suspected of having cardiac disease. The development of flow-sensitive and faster sequences has expanded the diagnostic role of MRI, allowing for dynamic studies and improved quantitative analysis of cardiac function. Compared with echocardiography, MRI has the advantage of being able to image distant structures, image through air or bone, have minimal artifact from most prosthetic materials, and to display images in exact reproducible planes with a wide field of view and three-dimensional reconstruction.

MRI has several unique features that make it an attractive imaging modality—high natural contrast between flowing blood and the cardiovascular structures allowing for imaging without intravenous contrast and the ability to display large fields of view in any angled plane without ionizing radiation.

The main clinical application of MRI has been in morphological diagnoses. The role of MRI in cardiac imaging is, however, evolving with the evaluation of ventricular function, volumes, and mass proving to be highly accurate and reproducible. The areas where MRI has been most useful with regard to congenital cardiovascular disease include: central pulmonary artery anomalies, aortic anomalies, complex disease, pulmonary venous anomalies, cardiac masses, and postoperative assessment.[18]

Technique

A cardiac MRI examination must be tailored to answer a particular question. The results of previous diagnostic tests and any surgical intervention should be known.[19] MRI is now capable of imaging even the sickest patients with the availability of nonferromagnetic life-support equipment. Safe diagnostic studies may be performed in patients with sternal wires, vascular access ports, and most prosthetic valves.[6] The exception is the old Starr-Edwards valve, which contains a metal ball.[20] Surgical clips, embolization coils, and ferromagnetic cardiac occluders may be safely imaged 6 weeks after placement, which appears to be appropriate time for adequate tissue growth, to ensure stable positioning of the implant. Although imaging patients with these metallic devices has been shown to be safe, the amount of artifact these implants produce may hinder examination quality, especially if the region of concern is in the immediate area of the device. The degree of artifact produced depends on the type and amount of metal used in the device and the pulse sequence.[21,22] Pacemakers and intracranial clips are absolute contraindications to MRI exposure.

MRI for cardiac imaging is performed using ECG-gating. Patients with marked arrhythmias are therefore not good candidates for MRI studies. Respiratory compensation or gating are options used to reduce chest motion artifacts. Diagnostic quality studies can generally be obtained in more than 90% of patients.[6] Nondi-

agnostic studies are usually a result of patient motion, anxiety, exaggerated respiratory motion, or arrhythmias.

Several imaging techniques have been used.[23] For cardiovascular morphology, the multislice spin-echo technique is most often used. This sequence displays flowing blood as a signal void in contrast to higher signal intensity of the adjacent vessel wall or myocardium. In general, only T1-weighted, first-echo images (time to echo [TE] <30 ms) are necessary, which typically requires <10 minutes to acquire a set of tomograms at 8 to 12 anatomic levels. T2-weighted, second-echo images (TE >30 ms) are often impractical in children due to their long acquisition times and are usually reserved for tissue characterization of a cardiac mass, thrombus, or abnormal myocardium.

For evaluation of cardiac dimensions and function, the gradient-echo (GRE) sequences have become the MRI technique of choice having both high temporal and spatial resolution. The images are obtained at multiple phases of the cardiac cycle and displayed in a cine "movie" mode allowing for evaluation of ventricular wall motion, wall thickness, chamber volume, and mass without geometric assumptions. In addition, valve motion and blood flow patterns may be assessed. A feature of cine GRE is the bright signal produced by flowing blood. Variations in signal intensity relate to abnormal flow patterns rather than to differences in relaxation times. Signal loss is due to local dephasing of spin signal as a result of high-velocity and turbulent flow seen with valvular disease, obstructive lesions and shunts. The high intensity blood pool of cine GRE compliments spin-echo studies, it allows differentiation of solid masses from flow artifacts as well as easier detection of some intraluminal masses, differentiation of vascular from air containing structures, evaluation of abnormalities in cardiac function, visualization of shunts and abnormal communications, detection of flow alterations in valvular heart disease and obstructive lesions and postoperative follow-up of chamber and vessel growth and function.[24–32]

GRE sequences may also be used in velocity-encoded cine MRI that allows for measurement of blood flow velocity and volume flow by subtracting the velocity-encoded sensitized image from a nonencoded compensated image. This technique can quantify shunts and measure flow and pulsatility separately in the individual vascular structures.[33,34]

It is now possible to perform three-dimensional reconstruction from either thin spin-echo or GRE images. Advantages of three-dimensional display include definition of intracardiac and great vessel anatomy in a format consistent with the gross intraoperative appearance, demonstration of small vascular structures and anatomic structures without superimposition, and simultaneous display of structure and function.[16,19,35,36]

Ultrafast sequences further broaden the role of MRI in both clinical and research imaging of the cardiovascular system. Ultrafast MRI requires no gating because each image is a snapshot acquired within a single heartbeat and single breathhold. This technique offers the potential to acquire rapid anatomic and functional measurements with greater resolution and reproducibility with each image free of cardiorespiratory motion artifact. Ultrafast sequences may therefore be used in patients with high respiratory rates, high heart rates, and cardiac arrhythmias. The range of measurable parameters broadens from simple chamber measurements in end systole and end diastole to quantitating estimates of complex indices such as cardiac muscle perfusion and myocardial wall stress. Flow volumes and patterns within the great arteries have been studied, allowing stroke volumes, systolic and diastolic function, and pulmonary : systemic flow ratios to be calculated. There is the prospect of studying the coronary artery circulation.[37,38]

Children who are younger than 7 years of age generally require sedation. Effective sedation can usually be achieved with either oral chloral hydrate (50 to 100 mg/kg) or with Nembutal® (Abbott Laboratories, Abbott Park, IL, USA) (5–6 mg/kg) given intravenously just prior to entry into the magnet. During the procedure the ECG signal is monitored, respiration is observed, and oxygen saturation is monitored transcutaneously. In addition, a capnometer with nasal cannula may be used to monitor expiratory Pco_2.

MRI may be performed in any desired plane to optimally depict the anatomy. High-quality images can be obtained in planes orthogonal to the natural cardiac axis, which allows for more accurate definition of myocardial borders.[8] The slice thickness used for most studies is 5 mm. Thin 3-mm sections are used when studying small infants and assessing small structures. Although decreasing slice thickness minimizes partial volume errors, it also results in noisier images and requires more images to cover the region of interest.

Vascular Imaging

Central Pulmonary Artery Anomalies

Magnetic resonance images provide information regarding the status of the main and central pulmonary arteries, which is essential in the management of children with congenital cyanotic heart disease and right outflow tract obstruction. The presence, caliber, and confluence of the pulmonary arteries is important in planning corrective or palliative surgery. There is good correlation between MRI and angiography in defining the proximal pulmonary arteries.[39–42] It is not necessary to opacify the pulmonary arteries for visualization; this enables MRI to determine the presence of central pulmonary arteries and central conflu-ence (Figs. 1-1 through 1-4). MRI, however, is unable to assess the peripheral vessels distal to the hila accurately.

MRI is able to detect systemic-to-pulmonary artery collateral vessels. The collateral vessels are usually located posteriorly, in contrast to pulmonary arteries, which are situated anterior to the bronchi.[39,40] It is not possible to determine single or dual supply to all lung segments or to assess the presence of stenosis (Fig. 1-5).

After a palliative systemic-pulmonary arterial shunt, MRI studies are ideal for following pulmonary arterial growth and for identifying distortion or stenosis of the pulmonary arteries caused by construction of the shunt (Fig. 1-6).[40,43]

In conditions that dilate the pulmonary arteries, MRI not only shows the degree of vessel enlargement but also the degree of airway compression. MRI is also capable of demonstrating much of the intracardiac pathoanatomy associated with pulmonary artery obstruction. The length of the atresia may be shown to be extensive or focal. In particular cases of pulmonary artery atresia with an intact ventricular septum MRI is effective for determining the size of the right ventricle.

MRI has been used to image congenital abnormalities of pulmonary artery origin such as the pulmonary artery sling. MRI clearly displays the relationship of the anomalous left pulmonary artery to the airway, as well as demonstrating associated congenital tracheal or bronchial anomalies.[14]

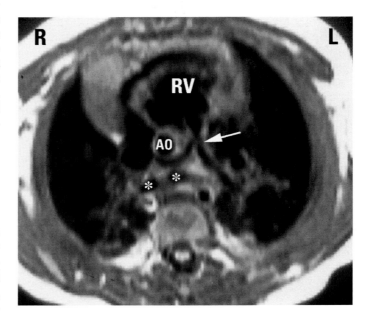

Fig. 1-1: Pulmonary artery hypoplasia.
Transverse T1 spin-echo image at the level of the tracheal bifurcation (✳) demonstrates marked diffuse pulmonary artery hypoplasia with a central confluence between the right and left pulmonary arteries (arrow). No discrete proximal pulmonary artery stenosis is identified. Note the nearly sagittal orientation of the proximal pulmonary arteries.

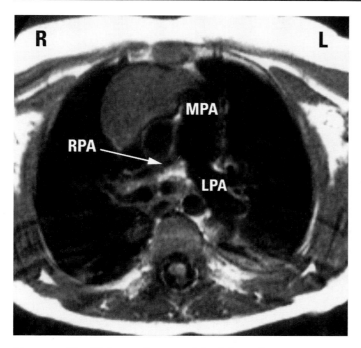

Fig. 1-2: Alagille's syndrome with right pulmonary artery hypoplasia.
Transverse T1 spin-echo image through the central pulmonary arteries demonstrates diffuse right pulmonary artery hypoplasia without a discrete stenosis. The left pulmonary artery is of normal size.

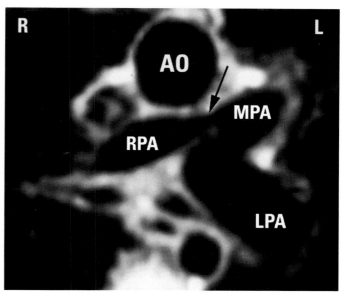

Fig. 1-4: Tetralogy of Fallot with proximal right pulmonary artery stenosis.
Transverse T1 spin-echo image through the central pulmonary arteries demonstrates a discrete proximal right pulmonary artery stenosis (arrow). There is hypoplasia of the main pulmonary artery with a normal caliber left pulmonary artery. Note the nearly sagittal orientation of the proximal left pulmonary artery.

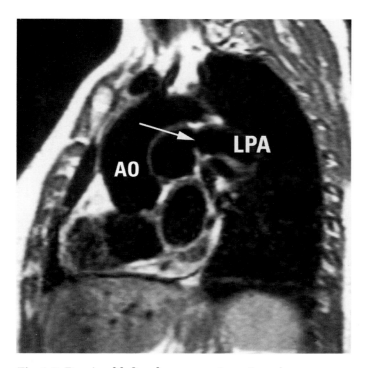

Fig. 1-3: Proximal left pulmonary artery stenosis.
Sagittal T1 spin-echo image through the left pulmonary artery identifies a discrete proximal left pulmonary artery stenosis (arrow).

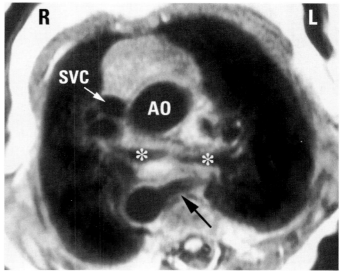

Fig. 1-5: Pulmonary atresia with ventricular septal defect. Nonconfluent central pulmonary arteries and multiple aortopulmonary collaterals.
Transverse T1 spin-echo image just below the level of the tracheal bifurcation (✱). Nonconfluent central pulmonary arteries with the hilar left and right pulmonary arteries identified anterior to their respective main stem bronchi (✱). The aortic arch is right sided with a right-sided proximal descending aorta. A large systemic collateral artery (arrow) originates from the descending aorta coursing towards the left lung.

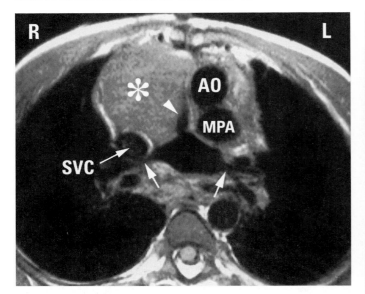

Fig. 1-6: Bilateral distal pulmonary artery stenoses.
Transverse T1 spin-echo image through the central pulmonary arteries. Complex congenital heart disease with tricuspid atresia, discordant ventriculoarterial connections, hypoplastic right ventricle, and subaortic stenosis managed with bilateral Blalock-Taussig shunts. Postoperative Damus-Kaye-Stansel anastomosis and central shunt from ascending aorta to the pulmonary artery confluence. The central shunt (arrowhead) is patent surrounded by a large seroma (✱). The central pulmonary artery confluence is of good size, with bilateral severe stenosis of the pulmonary arteries at the hilum (arrows) related to the previous Blalock-Taussig shunts.

MRI can accurately illustrate the detailed anatomy of an aortopulmonary window, including the exact site of origin of the right pulmonary artery that may arise from the ascending aorta in cases of distal communication (Fig. 1-7).[44]

MRI offers a unique noninvasive method of evaluating pulmonary arterial hypertension. In patients with pulmonary hypertension and an increase in pulmonary vascular resistance, spin-echo images have shown good correlation between increased intensity of the MRI signal within the proximal pulmonary arteries and elevated pulmonary vascular resistance. MRI, however, seems to be unreliable in detecting mild elevations in pulmonary vascular resistance.[6,12,45] Velocity mapping shows distinct changes in pulmonary artery distensibility and blood flow patterns in patients with pulmonary artery hypertension.[19,46]

Thoracic Aortic Anomalies

Thoracic aortic abnormalities are well outlined by MRI. In the majority of cases it provides diagnostic information at least as good as angiography. The most common pediatric aortic lesions studied include coarctation of the descending aorta and its posttreatment complications and vascular rings. Other causes of aor-

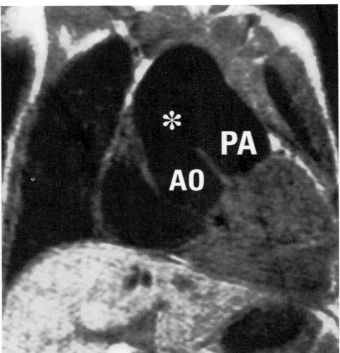

A

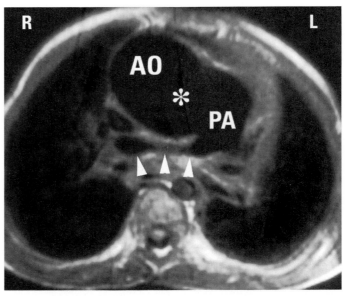

B

Fig. 1-7: Aortopulmonary window with right pulmonary artery hypoplasia.
A: Right anterior oblique coronal T1 spin-echo image through the great arteries demonstrating a large defect (✱) in the distal aortopulmonary septum with the presence of separate aortic and pulmonary valves. **B**: Transverse T1 spin-echo image demonstrates the distal aortopulmonary communication (✱) involving the right pulmonary artery (arrowheads), which is diffusely hypoplastic.

tic obstruction, aortic dilatation, and positional anomalies can be accurately assessed.

MRI is the imaging modality of choice for confirming and characterizing these lesions.[47–51] MRI identifies the site and extent of the coarctation, involvement of the arch vessels, dilated collateral vessels, and additional obstructive lesions. MRI can reliably distinguish between coarctation and hypoplasia of the isthmus or transverse arch. A discrete coarctation may appear as a circumferential narrowing, a prominent posterolateral shelf or as a long tapered narrowing. Cine MRI provides additional information about flow velocity and severity of obstruction, the length of lucent jets through and distal to the coarctation site have been shown to correlate with angiographic severity. The lucent flow jets seen on cine MRI also allow for separation and analysis of ductal flow, which may cause confusion in neonates with coarctation evaluated by spectral Doppler Figs. 1-8 through 1-10).[52,53]

After treatment, MRI is able to assess for coarctation restenosis, residual transverse arch hypoplasia, and repair site false aneurysms with dissection and rupture. MRI can also show the severity of left ventricular hypertrophy (Figs. 1-11 through 1-13).

Congenital supravalvar aortic stenosis is classically associated with Williams syndrome, but may also be seen in rubella syndrome or multiple left-sided obstructive lesions (Shone's syndrome). MRI

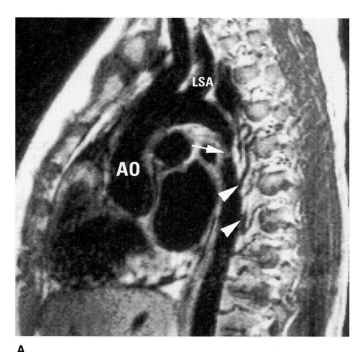

A

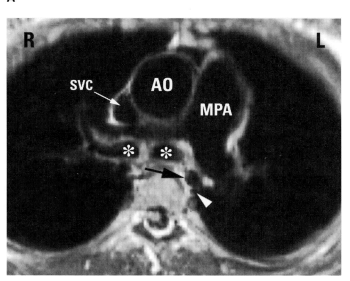

B

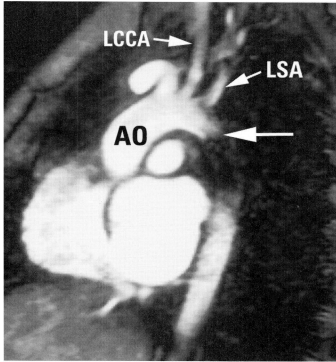

C

Fig. 1-8: Discrete coarctation of the descending aorta with extensive collaterals.
A: Oblique sagittal T1 spin-echo image demonstrates the discrete circumferential narrowing (arrow) distal to the origin of the left subclavian artery without associated transverse aortic arch hypoplasia. There are multiple dilated collateral vessels (arrowheads) identified. **B**: Transverse T1 spin-echo image at the level of the carina (✱) demonstrates the severe obstruction of the descending aorta (arrow) and the dilated collateral vessels (arrowhead). **C**: Oblique sagittal cine GRE image of the aorta obtained during systole demonstrates a flow void (arrows) at the site of the coarctation due to high-velocity turbulent flow across the obstruction.

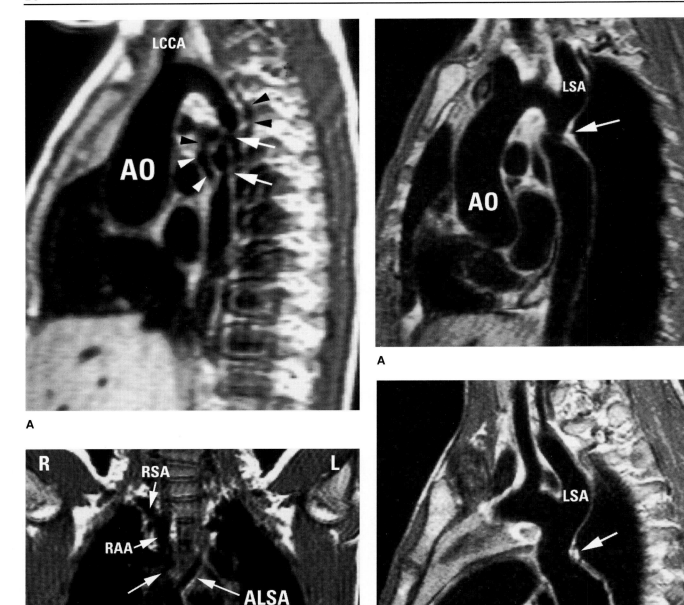

Fig. 1-9: Right aortic arch with aberrant left subclavian artery and a severe long segment coarctation with extensive collaterals.

A: Oblique sagittal T1 spin-echo image of a right aortic arch with an elongated irregular stenosis of the proximal descending aorta (arrows). There are multiple dilated collateral vessels (arrowheads) surrounding the aortic obstruction. **B:** Coronal T1 spin-echo image of the right-sided descending aorta with a long segment irregular coarctation (arrow) proximal to the origin of the aberrant left subclavian artery.

Fig. 1-10: Discrete coarctation of the descending aorta pre- and postballoon dilatation angioplasty.

A: Predilation oblique sagittal T1 spin-echo image of the thoracic aorta demonstrating a discrete obstruction of the descending aorta with a focal posterior shelf (arrow). The left subclavian artery is enlarged and there is post-stenotic aortic dilatation. The transverse arch is unobstructed and no significant dilated collateral vessels are identified. **B:** After balloon dilatation of the native coarctation, there is significant improvement in the caliber of the aortic lumen (arrow).

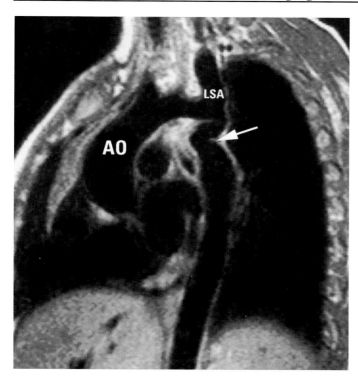

Fig. 1-11: Postrepair discrete recoarctation.
Oblique sagittal T1 spin-echo image of the thoracic aorta demonstrates a discrete obstruction (arrow) of the descending aorta caused by a residual posterior indentation. Mild hypoplasia of the transverse arch is present.

clearly shows the aortic obstruction as well as evaluating the proximal pulmonary arteries for areas of stenosis.[51]

The thoracic aorta may be abnormally enlarged in a variety of congenital conditions. Dilatation of the ascending aorta typically at the level of the sinuses of Valsalva, aneurysm formation, dissection and rupture occur in association with Marfan syndrome, bicuspid aortic valve, Turner syndrome, Ehlers- Danlos syndrome, and Noonan syndrome. In patients with Marfan and Turner syndrome, yearly MR screening is recommended to follow aortic size. Measurements of the aorta are generally performed in the axial plane, a ratio of the aortic root to the descending aorta above 1.5 is considered to be abnormal (Figs.1-14 and 1-15).[51,54]

Focal congenital aneurysms of the sinuses of Valsalva occur with high ventricular septal defects or high flow lesions of the coronary arteries. MRI has been used to study a coronary-cameral fistula.[55]

MRI accurately characterizes anomalies in the position and branching pattern of the thoracic aorta and defines the critical relationship between the vascular

ring and airway clearly localizing the site of associated airway obstruction.[56–58] MRI has been shown to demonstrate a variety of aortic arch anomalies, including double aortic arch and right aortic arch with retroesophageal left subclavian artery. Direct imaging of the vascular anomaly with MRI permits more accurate preoperative surgical planning (Fig. 1-16).[57]

The innominate artery syndrome relates to anterior tracheal compression by the innominate artery origin. MRI clearly shows the severity of the tracheal obstruction and the relationship of the aortic arch branches to the trachea.[51,59,60]

Pulmonary Venous Abnormalities

Recognition of normal pulmonary venous connections is possible in nearly all individuals. The lower lobe and right upper lobe veins are directly recognized in nearly all cases. The left upper lobe pulmonary vein is the most difficult to detect because of its proximity to the left atrial appendage. The proximal segment of the vein seen ventral to the bifurcation of the left bronchus can usually be followed to the roof of the left atrium;

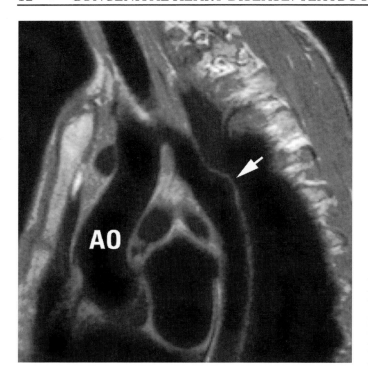

Fig. 1-12: After left subclavian flap repair of coarctation with persistent transverse arch hypoplasia.
Oblique sagittal T1 spin-echo image of the thoracic aorta demonstrates mild transverse aortic arch and isthmus hypoplasia without a discrete recoarctation. There is dilatation of the proximal descending aortic lumen with a prominent posterior convexity (arrow) related to the subclavian flap angioplasty repair.

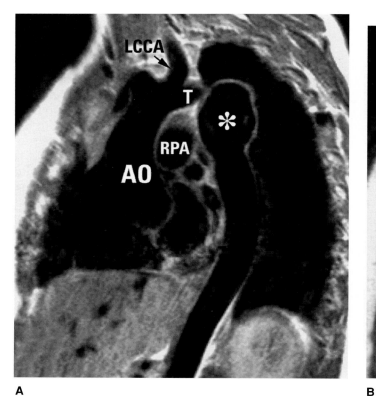

A

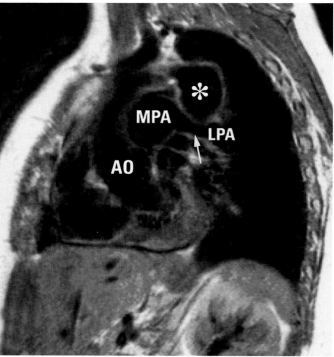

B

Fig. 1-13: After left subclavian repair of coarctation: Aneurysm at the repair site resulting in left pulmonary artery stenosis.
A: Oblique sagittal T1 spin-echo image of the thoracic aorta after left subclavian flap arterioplasty repair. The descending aorta shows a focal dilatation at the coarctation repair site (✱) that progressively enlarged over a series of examinations. The transverse arch is hypoplastic. **B**: Adjacent oblique sagittal T1 spin-echo image through the left pulmonary artery. The focal aneurysm of the descending aorta (✱) results in extrinsic compression and stenosis of the proximal left pulmonary artery (arrow).

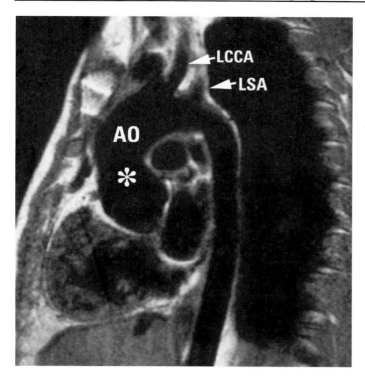

Fig. 1-14: Marfan syndrome with dilatation of the ascending aorta.
Oblique sagittal T1 spin-echo image of the thoracic aorta demonstrates moderate dilatation of the sinuses of Valsalva and proximal ascending aorta (✳), with a normal caliber descending aorta.

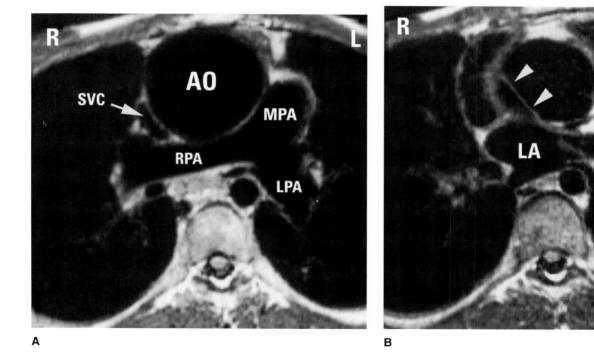

A

B

Fig. 1-15: Marfan syndrome with aortic dissection.
A: Transverse T1 spin-echo image at the level of the pulmonary artery bifurcation demonstrates marked dilatation of the ascending aorta resulting in extrinsic compression of the superior vena cava and trivial narrowing of the right pulmonary artery. **B:** Transverse T1 spin-echo image through the aortic root. There is marked dilatation of the aortic root with an intimal flap (arrowheads) identified across the lumen. The intimal flap is delineated due to high-velocity flow producing signal void within both the true and false channels.

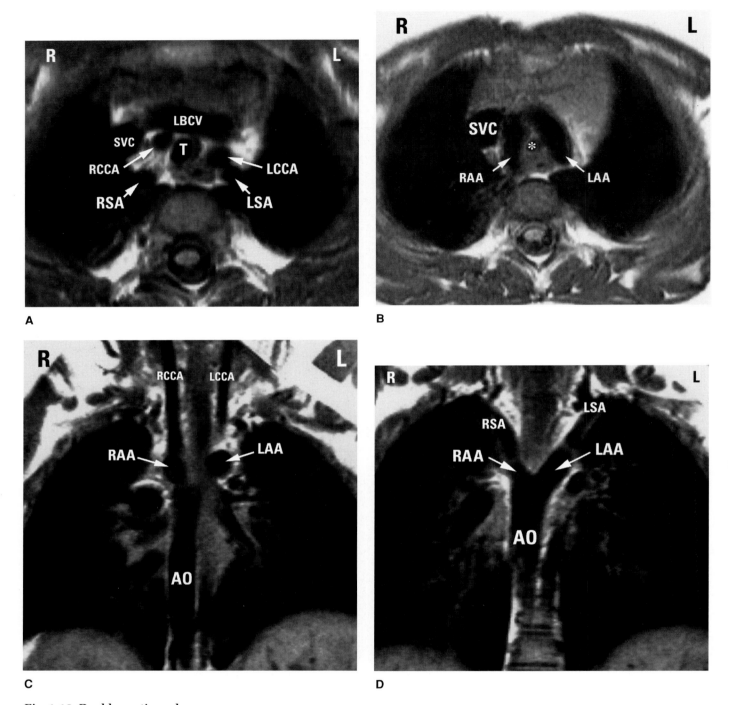

Fig. 1-16: Double aortic arch.
Transverse **(A,B)** and coronal **(C,D)** T1 spin-echo images demonstrate the vascular ring surrounding and compressing the trachea (T). Both right and left arches (a,c,d) are patent, each giving rise to their respective common carotid and subclavian arteries. Note the right-sided descending aorta. See also Chapter 34, Fig. 34–9.

this can be regarded as normal even if the actual atrial connection is not directly seen (Fig. 1-17).[6,13,39,61,62]

MRI has been shown to be highly accuracte in diagnosing both partial and total anomalous pulmonary venous connections. Partial anomalous pulmonary venous connections are nearly always defined on transverse or coronal magnetic resonance images. MRI is ca-

pable of directly demonstrating the complete course of anomalous pulmonary venous connections including the pulmonary veins, pulmonary venous confluences, vertical vein, and entrances of the anomalous vein. MRI may also indicate the precise location of pulmonary vein stenosis before and after surgical correction (Figs. 1-18 and 1-19).[39,61–64]

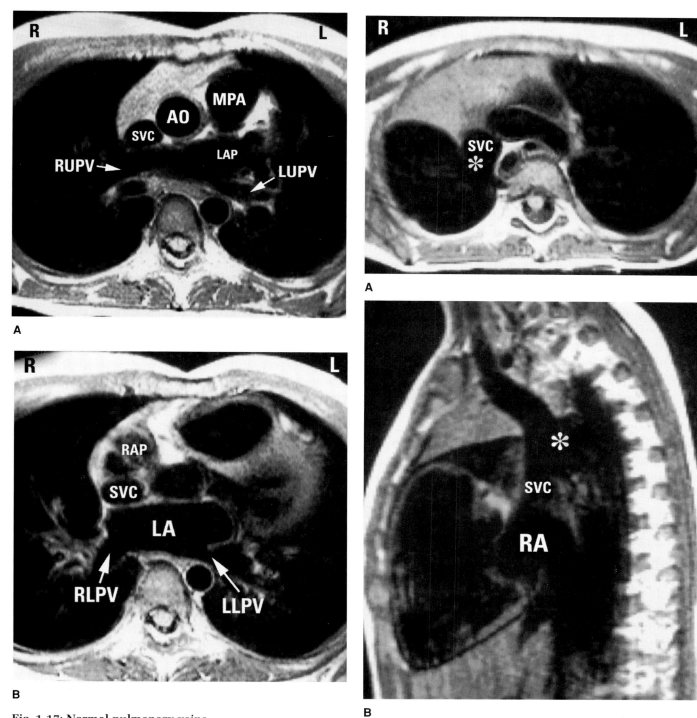

Fig. 1-17: Normal pulmonary veins.
A: Transverse T1 spin-echo image obtained at the level of the left atrial appendage identifies both left and right upper pulmonary veins draining normally to left atrium. **B**: Transverse T1 spin-echo image obtained at the level of the superior vena cava-right atrial junction demonstrates a normal connection of the right and left lower pulmonary veins to the left atrium.

Fig. 1-18: Unilateral partial anomalous pulmonary venous connection.
Transverse **(A)** and sagittal **(B)** T1 spin-echo images demonstrate the anomalous right upper pulmonary vein (✱) entering the dilated superior vena cava.

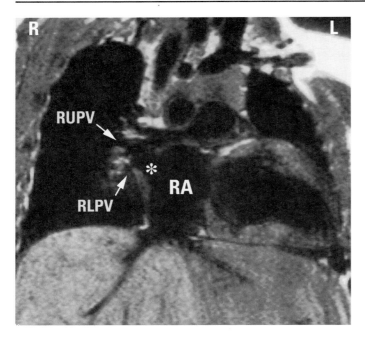

Fig. 1-19: Right atrial isomerism with unilateral total anomalous pulmonary venous drainage.
Coronal T1 spin-echo image at the level of the inferior vena cava-right atrial junction. There is a confluence of the right upper and lower pulmonary veins forming a common pulmonary vein that connects to the roof of the right-sided atrium (✱).

MRI has been shown to be a useful tool in assessing left inflow obstructive lesions. In cor triatriatum, the intra-atrial membrane and the anomalous posterior chamber have been demonstrated.[65] Absent or stenotic pulmonary veins may be clearly defined.

Systemic Venous Abnormalities

Anomalies of the systemic venous system have been depicted by MRI (Fig. 1-20).[66] Drainage of the left superior vena cava into the left atrium is commonly observed with the asplenia syndrome. Azygous continuation of an interrupted inferior vena cava can also be demonstrated. This may be an isolated anomaly or associated with complex anomalies, and is characteristically seen in polysplenia syndrome (Fig. 1-21).[67]

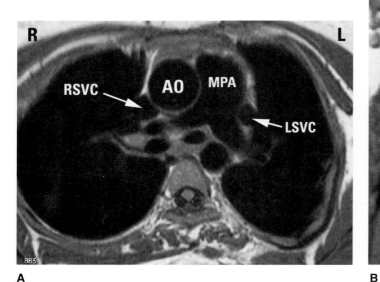

A   B

Fig. 1-20: Bilateral superior vena cavae.
A: Transverse T1 spin-echo image at the level of the pulmonary artery bifurcation demonstrates bilateral superior vena cavae.
B: Coronal T1 spin-echo image demonstrates the persistent left superior vena cava draining into a slightly enlarged coronary sinus.

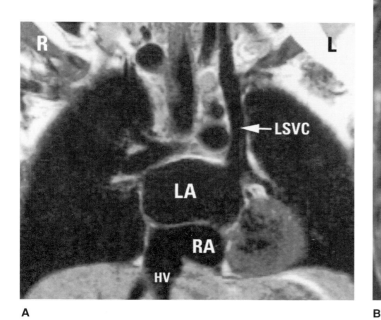

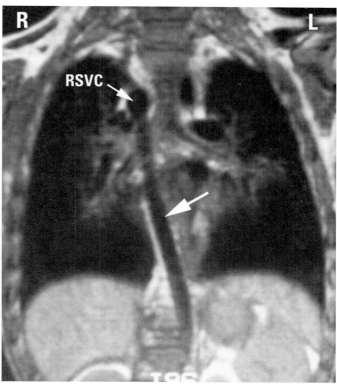

A **B**

Fig. 1-21: Left atrial isomerism with bilateral superior vena cavae and interruption of the inferior vena cava with azygous continuation.
A: Coronal T1 spin-echo image demonstrates the persistent left superior vena cava draining directly into the roof of the left atrium. There is absence of the intrahepatic portion of the inferior vena with the hepatic veins draining directly into the right atrium. **B**: Coronal T1 spin-echo image demonstrates an enlarged azygous vein (arrow) draining into the right superior vena cava.

Cardiac Imaging

Simple Cardiac Defects

Although reports show comparable sensitivity and specificity of MRI to echocardiography in the detection of atrial and ventricular septal defects, echocardiography is the study of choice because of its lower cost and convenience.[6]

The various portions of the atrial and ventricular septa are clearly shown on transverse images. Multisectional imaging in coronal and sagittal planes may provide supplementary information.[68–70]

Magnetic resonance images can separate the sinus venosus, secundum, and primum portions of the atrial septum. Atrial septal defects are clearly shown in more than 90% of cases.[68–70] There may be some difficulty in detecting an atrial septal defect because of the thinness of the interatrial septum and its curved shape, which does not allow for displaying the entire septum on a single plane.[6] The thinned region at the fossa ovalis may be mistaken for a secundum septal defect. A true defect should result in a signal void on two adjacent levels and have sharp, thick margins.[39] Cine MRI or ve-locity-encoded sequences can be used to demonstrate abnormal flow across a true defect.

Primum defects are shown in the images adjacent to the atrioventricular valves. In the evaluation of atrioventricular septal defects, MRI may be more accurate than echocardiography in predicting the size of the ventricular defect and is superior to either echocardiography or angiography in identifying the presence of ventricular hypoplasia (Fig. 1-22).[71,72]

The interventricular septum is for the most part a thick, muscular structure and easily seen via MRI. MRI has been shown to be more than 90% accurate in diagnosing ventricular septal defects.[39,73] The ability to image in different planes allows for precise definition of location and size of the defect and its relation to the atrioventricular and arterial valves (Fig. 1-23).[74,75]

Complex Congenital Heart Disease

The ability of MRI to display multiplanar global anatomy with a large field of view allows for definition of segmental cardiovascular anatomy in patients with complex anomalies.[76,77]

Transverse images extending from the base of the

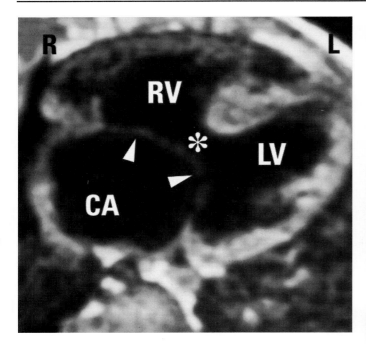

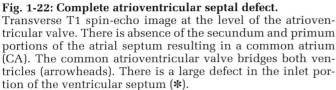

Fig. 1-22: Complete atrioventricular septal defect.
Transverse T1 spin-echo image at the level of the atrioventricular valve. There is absence of the secundum and primum portions of the atrial septum resulting in a common atrium (CA). The common atrioventricular valve bridges both ventricles (arrowheads). There is a large defect in the inlet portion of the ventricular septum (*).

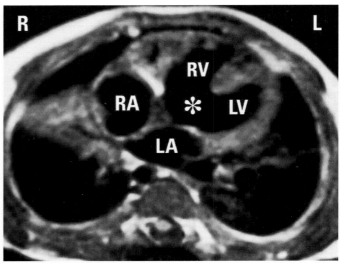

A

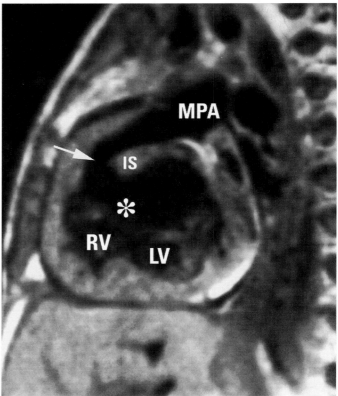

B

Fig. 1-23: Tetralogy of Fallot.
A: Transverse T1 spin-echo image demonstrates a large perimembranous ventricular septal defect (*). **B:** Sagittal T1 spin-echo image shows the anterior malaligned infundibular septum with moderate infundibular stenosis (arrow) and the large ventricular septal defect with outlet extension (*).

heart to the cardiac apex allow for a sequential analysis of the central cardiovascular anatomy, which is most important in completely defining the components of complex anomalies. Studies have shown that MRI is at least as accurate as angiography in defining atrial and ventricular morphology, the orientation of the ventricular septum, and the position of the great arteries. MRI is well suited for evaluating ventricular size because cardiac structures are not superimposed and is more effective in diagnosing viscerobronchial anatomy and venoatrial connections (Fig. 1-24). MRI, however, is not as effective as angiography in diagnosing semilunar valve anomalies.[39,78–83]

The images at the base of the heart clearly demonstrate the anatomic relationship of the great vessels and the ventriculoarterial connections. Disparity in size of the great vessels, characteristic of some cardiac anomalies is clearly evident.

The anatomic features of a double outlet right ventricle on MRI have been reported.[39,84–86] There is a characteristic side-by-side relationship of the great vessels at the level of the arterial valves. A complete circle of muscle is seen separating the arterial valves from the

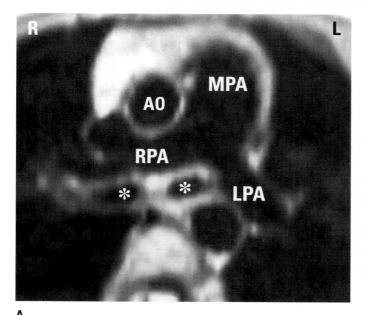

A

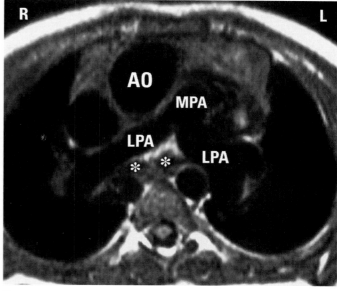

C

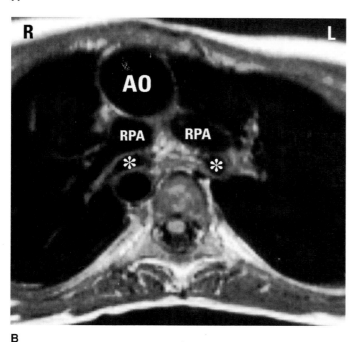

B

Fig. 1-24: Pulmonary Artery Morphology Defining the Visceroatrial situs. Three separate patients.
A: Transverse T1 spin-echo image at the level of the tracheal bifurcation (✳) demonstrates normal central pulmonary arteries. The morphological right pulmonary artery courses anterior to the right main bronchus. The morphologically left pulmonary artery courses over the left main bronchus. **B: C:** Transverse T1 spin-echo image at the level of the tracheal bifurcation (✳). Right atrial isomerism with bilateral morphological right pulmonary arteries. Transverse T1 spin-echo image at the level of the tracheal bifurcation (✳). Left atrial isomerism with bilateral morphologically left pulmonary arteries.

anterior leaflet of the mitral valve. MRI has been shown to be excellent in characterizing the ventricular septal defect and its relation to the arterial valves and outlet septum. Associated ventricular hypoplasia and outlet obstruction can be accurately determined. MRI has been able to define the anatomy of a double outlet left ventricle.[87]

In truncus arteriosus, MRI at the base of the heart can demonstrate a single large trunk connected to the ventricles arising above a ventricular septal defect. The relative sizes of the two ventricles can be defined. Sagittal images are useful for demonstrating the origin of the pulmonary arteries from the truncus. Thin (3 mm) im-

ages optimally assess the size and the presence of any focal stenosis of the central pulmonary arteries.[39]

Images through the middle of the ventricular chambers define the ventricular loop and permit analysis of ventricular dimension, configuration, internal trabecular pattern, muscle thickness, and position of the atrioventricular valves. The ability of MRI to define ventricular morphology is effective in recognizing the various types of single ventricles.[39,79–81] The presence and connections of the atrioventricular valves, the bulboventricular foramen, the remnant of the ventricular septum and the rudimentary ventricular chamber can also be accurately assessed (Figs. 1-25 and 1-26).[6]

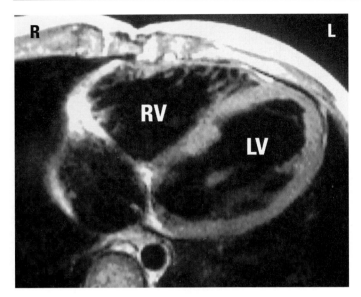

Fig. 1-25: Normal ventricular morphology.
Transverse T1 spin-echo image through the middle of the ventricles demonstrates normal ventricular anatomy. The morphologically right ventricle demonstrates a coarsely trabeculed endocardial surface, whereas the morphologically left ventricle demonstrates a smooth pattern.

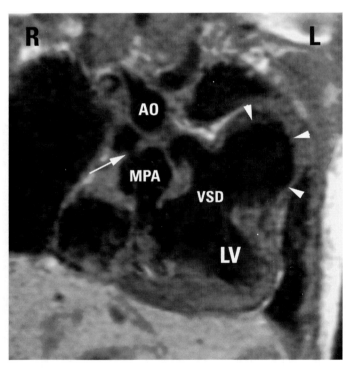

Fig. 1-26: Univentricular heart of left ventricular morphology.
Coronal T1 spin-echo image demonstrates the left ventricular type of single ventricle with a leftwards rudimentary right ventricle and discordant ventriculoarterial connections with subaortic stenosis (✳). There is aneurysmal dilatation of the patched free wall of the subaortic right ventricle (arrowheads). The pulmonary artery originating from the dominant left ventricle has been banded (arrow). The ventricular septal defect is unrestrictive.

Abnormalities of atrioventricular connections are frequently a component of complex anomalies. In the crisscross heart and the heart with superoinferior ventricles MRI has been shown to be superior to echocardiography in demonstrating the twisted atrioventricular connections, abnormal relationship of the cardiac chambers and the presence of unusual cardiac recesses (Figs. 1-27 and 1-28).[88,89]

The morphology of the atrioventricular valves is almost exclusively evaluated with echocardiography. MRI, however, may provide complementary information in defining the anatomical features of Ebstein's anomaly of the tricuspid valve, demonstrating associated anomalies involving the conotruncal region and the central pulmonary arteries, and in defining cardiac chamber size.[90–92] MRI is well suited to imaging the atrioventricular sulcus, which may be important in differentiating an absent atrioventricular connection from an imperforate valve. The atrioventricular sulcus has been shown to contain muscle and fat when an atrioventricular valve is atretic (Fig. 1-29).[93,94]

Cardiac Masses

Although tumors are infrequently congenital, MRI is probably the most effective technique for evaluating the precise location and extent of myocardial masses and distinguishing them from pericardial or paracardiac masses (Figs. 1-30 and 1-31).[24,95,96]

Tissue characterization on the basis of magnetic relaxation times has the added benefit of improved specificity to the MRI diagnosis. Short T1 relaxation times result in a characteristic high signal intensity of myocardial lipomas (Fig. 1-31). A fibroma is often suggested by a decrease in relative signal intensity on T2-weighted sequences. Other cardiac lesions, however, have less specific tissue-intensity characteristics (Fig. 1-31).[97–101] GRE imaging is most helpful in distinguishing between tumor and thrombi; in most cases clots are of low signal intensity with tumors producing a medium signal intensity compared to flowing blood.[102]

MRI is helpful in following a tumor's response to therapy. It provides an accurate assessment of remaining tumor volume and extracardiac extension, as well as showing changing tissue characteristics with the tumor decreasing in signal intensity as it is replaced with fibrous tissue.[103]

In the assessment of cardiac tumors, there may be a role for contrast enhancement with gadolinium DTPA. Contrast media has been shown to aid in the detection and characterization of mass lesions. After the administration of contrast, vital tissue within a tumor can be differentiated from nonvascularized, necrotic, or cystic areas. In addition, contrast media may also help in differentiating tumor from nonvascularized thrombus.[102,104]

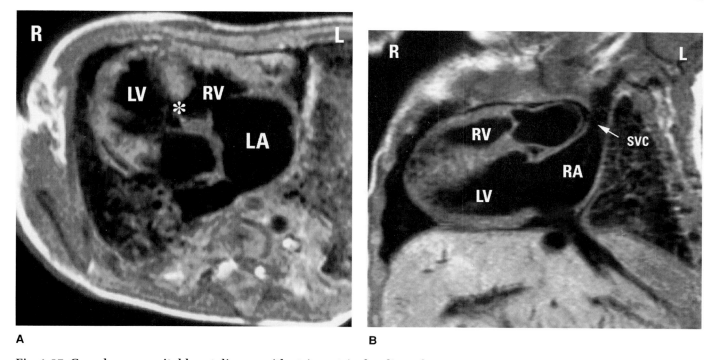

A

B

Fig. 1-27: Complex congenital heart disease with atrioventricular discordance.
Transverse **(A)** and coronal **(B)** T1 spin-echo images through the ventricles confirm discordant atrioventricular connections and dextrocardia. The morphologically right ventricle, which is mildly hypoplastic, is positioned superior and slightly to the left of the morphologically left ventricle. A perimembranous ventricular septal defect is present (✱).

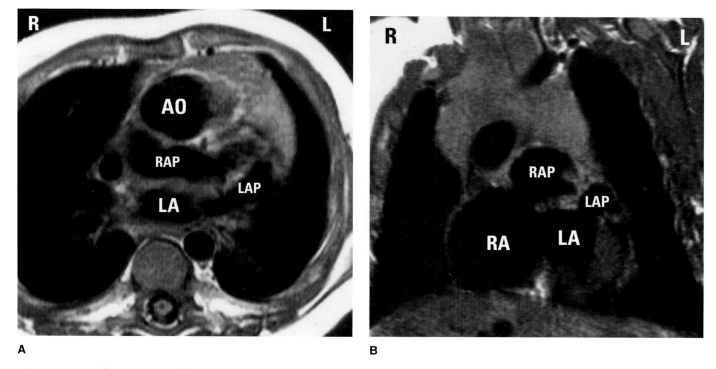

A

B

Fig. 1-28: Complex congenital heart disease with juxtaposed atrial appendages.
Transverse **(A)** and coronal **(B)** T1 spin-echo images demonstrate left juxtaposition of the right and left atrial appendages.

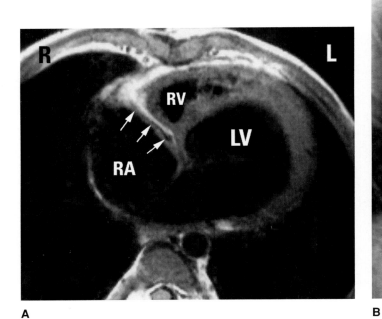

A

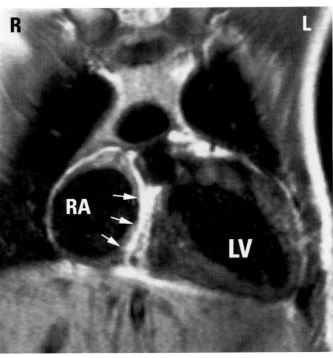

B

Fig. 1-29: Tricuspid atresia.
Transverse **(A)** and coronal **(B)** T1 spin-echo images demonstrate an atretic tricuspid valve with high-intensity fat tissue (arrows) extending across the atrioventricular groove. The right ventricular chamber is hypoplastic with a dominant left ventricle.

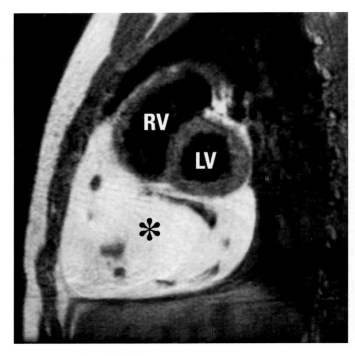

Fig. 1-30: Epicardial lipoma.
Sagittal T1 spin-echo image through the ventricles demonstrates a large high signal intensity mass (✳) characteristic of fatty tissue. The mass arose within the epicardial fat adjacent to the pericardium (arrow) resulting in significant superior displacement of the heart. There were no signs of intramural or intracardiac tumor extension.

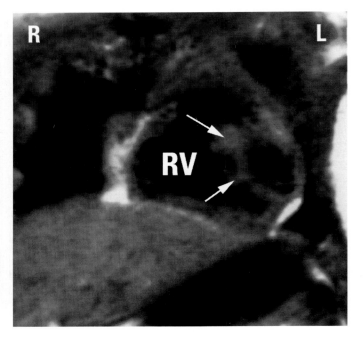

Fig. 1-31: Cardiac rhabdomyomas.
Coronal T1 spin-echo image through the right ventricle demonstrates multiple focal small masses (arrows) arising from the right ventricular margin of the ventricular septum that are isointense with the myocardium. The patient was known to have tuberous sclerosis.

Right Ventricular Dysplasia

Right ventricular dysplasia is defined as either complete or localized replacement of the right ventricular myocardium with fat or fibrous tissue. MRI has become part of the diagnostic work-up in the evaluation of patients with ventricular arrhythmias where a diagnosis of right ventricular dysplasia is considered. MRI is able to establish a diagnosis of right ventricular dysplasia by demonstrating transmural fat in the free wall of the right ventricle on T1-weighted images. Cine GRE studies may support the diagnosis by demonstrating focal contraction abnormalities of the right ventricle.[105]

Postoperative Evaluation

MRI is very effective in postoperative evaluation. Repeat studies may be performed without the use of radiation or contrast and both intra- and extracardiac anatomy are well demonstrated. MRI has been shown to be effective in evaluating complex surgical procedures for cyanotic heart disease. Specific operations which involve supracardiac anastomoses have been well demonstrated.[39,106]

MRI can reliably evaluate conduits, anastomoses, and the status of the central pulmonary arteries. Doppler echocardiography is useful in assessing the degree of obstruction, but is often unclear in defining the level of obstruction. The location and severity of a conduit obstruction may be accurately diagnosed on spin-echo magnetic resonance images as a region of severe narrowing measuring <50% the diameter of the conduit when implanted. Cine MRI velocity mapping has been shown to have excellent correlation with gradients measured by cardiac catheterization and Doppler techniques. MRI with velocity mapping if available has been recommended as the study of choice in routine annual assessment of ventriculopulmonary conduits (Fig. 1-32).[106–108]

MRI is useful in the pre- and postoperative evaluation of Fontan surgery candidates. MRI provides accurate depictions of the extracardiac vascular anatomy, which is important information in patients being considered for Fontan surgery. MRI has been used to study the function of the heart at all stages of the Fontan procedure. MRI is ideal for ventricular volumetric and mass assessment in complex cardiac lesions.[109,110]

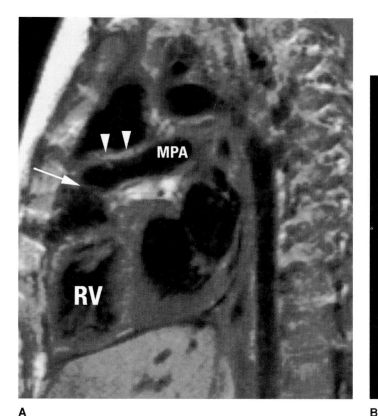

A

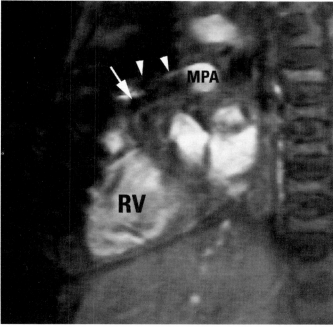

B

Fig. 1-32: After repair of severe tetralogy of Fallot with a right ventricle-pulmonary artery conduit.
A: Sagittal T1 spin-echo image demonstrates the conduit (arrowheads) and graft valve (arrow) between the right ventricle and pulmonary artery. The conduit is narrow without a defined focal obstruction. There is right ventricular hypertrophy with increased trabeculation. **B:** Sagittal cine GRE image through the conduit (arrowheads) during systole demonstrates a signal void at the level of the graft valve (arrow) indicating obstruction with high-velocity turbulent flow beginning at the valve level.

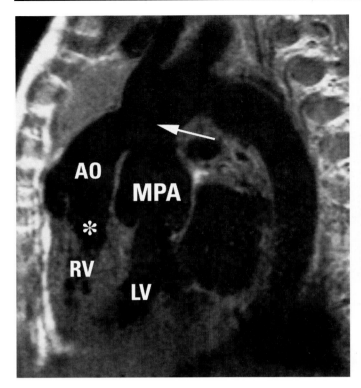

Fig. 1-33: Damus-Kaye-Stansel procedure.
Sagittal T1 spin-echo image demonstrates a Damus-Kaye-Stansel procedure with end-to-side anastomosis of the proximal main pulmonary artery to the ascending aorta (arrow) performed in a patient with tricuspid atresia, discordant ventriculoarterial connections, hypoplastic right ventricle and subaortic stenosis (✻).

After a palliative Damus-Kaye-Stansel or Norwood procedure, MRI has been shown to be equivalent to angiography in demonstrating the anatomy of the neoaorta, the central pulmonary arteries, the patency of the surgical shunts, and the size of the interatrial communication (Figs. 1-33 and 1-34).[111]

After the arterial switch operation for transposition of the great arteries, the central pulmonary arteries are often stretched and compressed as they pass around the proximal ascending aorta. MRI is very effective in evaluating the proximal pulmonary arteries for stenosis as well as examining the anastomosis of the switched great vessels (Fig. 1-35).[106,112]

The morphology and patency of shunts and any distortion of the pulmonary artery at the anastomotic site is well demonstrated. In addition, MRI is an excellent method for serial assessment of pulmonary artery growth following a palliative systemic-pulmonary artery shunt. However, it is somewhat limited in diagnosing areas of stenosis within small shunts (Fig. 1-36).[106,113,114]

MRI has also been shown to be an effective method for assessing cardiac function and anatomy after in-

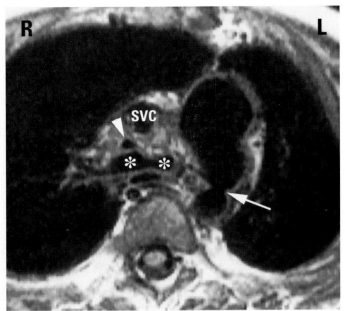

A

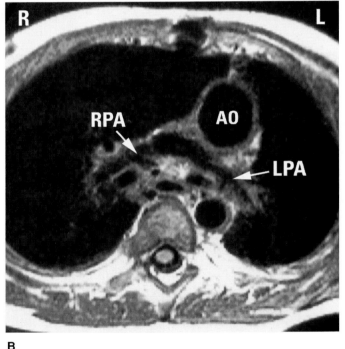

B

Fig. 1-34: Norwood procedure for hypoplastic left heart syndrome.
Sequences of transverse T1 spin-echo images. **A:** At the level of the tracheal bifurcation (✻) there is enlargement of the reconstructed transverse arch with a residual coarctation at the distal patch anastomosis (arrow). The right Blalock-Taussig shunt is patent (arrowhead). **B:** At a level through the central pulmonary arteries there are hypoplastic confluent pulmonary arteries without discrete stenosis. *(continued on next page)*

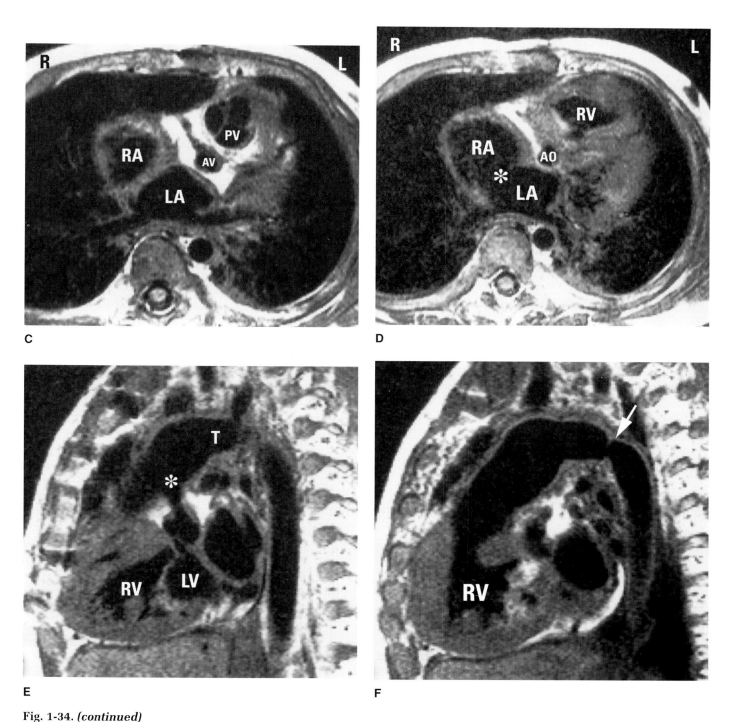

Fig. 1-34. *(continued)*
C: At the level of the arterial valves the diminutive aortic valve with a normal appearing pulmonary annulus is seen. **D:** Transverse image through the atria demonstrates a large atrial communication (✳). Sequential sagittal T_1 spin-echo images **(E,F)** through the thoracic aorta demonstrates the end to side aorto-pulmonary anastomosis (✳) and patch augmentation of the ascending aorta and transverse arch with residual coarctation at the distal patch anastomosis (arrow). The hypertrophied and enlarged right ventricle is identified, as well as the diminutive left heart structures.

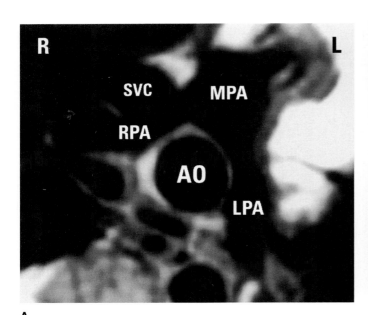

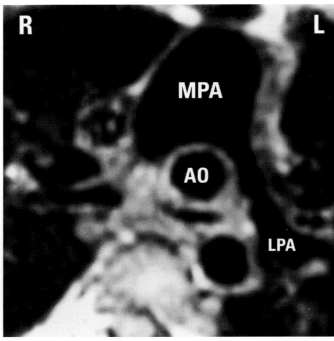

A   B

Fig. 1-35: Arterial switch procedure for complete transposition.
A: Transverse T1 spin-echo image postarterial switch procedure demonstrates the characteristic appearance of the pulmonary artery bifurcation with the pulmonary arteries astride the ascending aorta. **B:** Transverse T1 spin-echo image demonstrates diffuse narrowing of the left pulmonary artery as it is stretched around the ascending aorta.

tracardiac reconstructions such as the Mustard and Senning procedures. It compares favorably with echocardiography and radionuclide angiography in assessing right ventricular dysfunction and tricuspid re-

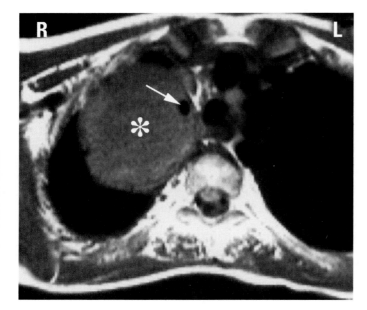

Fig. 1-36: Complication of Blalock-Taussig shunt.
Transverse T1 spin-echo image of a patent right Blalock-Taussig shunt (arrow) that is surrounded by a large seroma (✱). See also Fig. 1–6.

gurgitation. MRI and echocardiography are comparable in diagnosing a residual ventricular septal defect and left ventricular outflow tract obstruction. MRI is superior for defining the anatomy of the great arteries. In combination with echocardiography, MRI was found to have a higher sensitivity in diagnosing systemic or pulmonary venous obstruction than either method alone. The baffle anatomy is often difficult to follow on contiguous MRI because of its oblique course through the atrial cavity, making echocardiography a better imaging technique in assessing intra-atrial baffle obstruction and residual baffle leaks.[106,115–117]

MRI is also useful in detecting complications after complete repair of tetralogy of Fallot including residual pulmonary artery stenosis, incomplete closure of the ventricular septal defect and aneurysmal dilatation of the outflow tract patch (Fig. 1-37).[43]

Cine MRI and color Doppler flow mapping are complementary in the assessment of pulmonary artery banding in difficult cases where there is uncertainty about the position of the band, the quality of the central pulmonary arteries, and the degree of obstruction. The narrowest flow diameter on cine MRI and the length of the proximal signal loss closely relate to the pressure gradient across the pulmonary artery band. MRI is able to provide excellent definition of the position of the band in relation to the main and branch pulmonary arteries.[118]

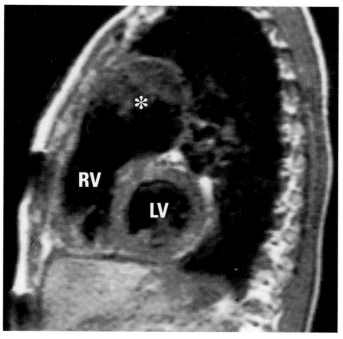

A

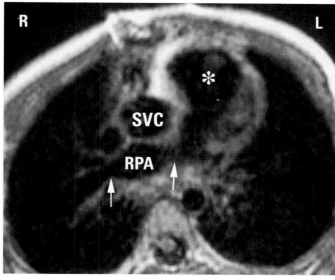

B

Fig. 1-37: After repair of tetralogy of Fallot aneurysm with distal pulmonary artery stenosis.
Sagittal **(A)** and coronal **(B)** T1 spin-echo images demonstrate discrete right pulmonary artery stenosis (arrows) and aneurysmal dilatation (✳) of the right ventricular outflow tract patch.

Functional Evaluation

To completely evaluate the child with congenital heart disease, physiologic information is necessary. MRI currently is unable to measure absolute pressures within cardiovascular structures, although gradients can be estimated as in Doppler techniques. MRI is, however, more accurate than echocardiography and angiography in the assessment of ventricular volumes, mass, and function. MRI acquires contiguous images through the entire ventricular mass and provides a three-dimensional data set from which accurate measurements can be calculated without the need of assumed geometric models important with complex anatomy.

GRE cine MRI segments the cardiac cycle and is performed at a rate sufficient to produce 15 to 30 images per cardiac cycle. This technique provides dynamic information of flow in combination with structural anatomy, allowing for evaluation of valvular stenosis and regurgitation, cardiovascular shunts, ventricular volumes, myocardial mass, cardiac output, and ejection fractions. The images however are not acquired in real time and therefore represent the average of multiple beats.[16,119–123]

In normal subjects, stroke volume is the same in both ventricles. When the stroke volume is greater in one of the ventricles this indicates a volume overload lesion, such as valvular regurgitation or a shunt. In isolated lesions the regurgitant fraction or shunt size can be measured as the difference between the two stroke volumes divided by the larger stroke volume.[14,29,123,124]

Velocity-encoded cine MRI sequences allow for measurement of blood flow velocity and volume in the central circulation and can be used to assess ventricular function. The velocity image can discriminate between forward and retrograde blood flow. This technique measures the volume of blood ejected from the ventricles, and therefore, the effective forward flow from each ventricle can be measured if the aortic or pulmonary valves are competent. The volume flow in the aorta and pulmonary artery are nearly equivalent in normal individuals. A difference in stroke volume can be used to measure the volume of shunt flow or regurgitation. This technique has the advantage of being able to quantify flow separately in the right and left pulmonary arteries.[33,34,39] This technique has been used to estimate peak gradients across obstructions by measuring the peak velocity. Studies have shown successful assessment of gradients across coarctations of the aorta and across Rastelli conduits.

Conclusion

Current MRI provides high-resolution depiction of cardiovascular anatomy in children with congenital heart disease and is the imaging modality of choice for showing abnormalities of the aorta and pulmonary arteries, venous connections in heterotaxia syndromes, complex cardiac lesions, cardiac masses, and postoperative anatomy. The combination of anatomic and quantitative functional information makes MRI an increasingly attractive tool. In the future, MRI will be helpful in assessments of flow and perfusion, faster imaging sequences to allow for real-time functional evaluation, myocardial tagging offering a unique way to study cardiac biomechanics, and spectroscopic capabilities for tissue characterization.[16,125]

Ultrafast Computed Tomography

Computed tomography (CT) has a limited role in the evaluation of patients with congenital heart disease. The slow acquisition time of conventional CT scanning results in degraded images caused by cardiac and respiratory motion. Also there may be suboptimal contrast because of difficulty in synchronizing image acquisition to peak ventricular opacification. These fundamental problems are largely resolved with the development of the ultrafast computed tomography scanning that uses several technical innovations, providing rapid image acquisition speeds, and high-resolution multislice cross-sectional scanning. Ultrafast scanning utilizes an electron beam that is focused and deflected by electromagnetic coils, striking multiple target rings that produce x-rays that are detected above the patient. This results in faster image acquisition, greater number of acquisitions in a given time, and multiple level acquisition without patient or scanner movement. Each sweep of a target ring takes 50 ms or less with each target ring producing two images. The images have a resolution of 0.25 to 0.5 mm and are 3.0 to 10.0 mm thick. Imaging can be prescribed in axial, short-axis, and long-axis planes.[126–133]

Ultrafast computed tomographic scanning is operable in three distinct scan programs providing high-resolution morphological studies, quantitative functional data, and flow dynamics. Cross-sectional imaging overcomes the problem of superimposition of overlapping structures and with a high spatial, temporal, and contrast resolution there is very accurate delineation of endocardial and epicardial contours. Evaluation and quantitation of regional and global systolic and diastolic function in right and left ventricles with calculations of wall thickness, ventricular volume, and mass are reliably performed. Ultrafast computed tomography can provide quantitative measurements of cardiac output, ejection fraction, and stroke volumes. The potential exists for rapid, accurate, and reproducible measurements of cardiac function with technology becoming more automated. The outstanding spatial resolution of the images makes it possible to obtain precise information about segmental anatomy of congenital heart lesions. In addition, ultrafast computed tomography provides a precise technique for simultaneously measuring shunt lesions and providing anatomic information.[134–140]

The cine or movie mode consists of electrocardiographically triggered scanning with images displayed in a closed loop format. This mode may be used to evaluate a variety of physiologic parameters including global and regional right and left ventricular function, ejection fractions, cardiac wall thickening, and valvular motion.[126,127,135]

The flow mode uses a bolus of intravenous contrast, imaging the contrast bolus as it traverses blood vessels, cardiac chambers, and myocardium. Electrocardiographic gating can be used so that scans are generated at the same phase of the cardiac cycle. A region of interest can be place and time-density curve created reflecting changes in contrast density over time. Analysis of the curve permits calculation of cardiac output, quantitation of shunts and regional myocardial blood flow.[126,135]

The volume mode is analogous to conventional CT, however, short scan times minimize motion artifact providing high-resolution anatomical information.[126,127]

The ability to produce three-dimensional images from the tomographic images enhances resolution and wall motion analysis. This furthers the information on cardiac physiology and morphology in patients with cardiovascular disease.[134]

Ultrafast computed tomography may be advantageous for evaluating regional systolic function because of clearer endocardial-cavity edge detection, absence of overlapping structures, and visualization of the entire ventricle. Ultrafast computed tomography has been shown to be superior to biplane ventriculography for the evaluation of segmental and subsegmental wall motion.[126,135,141–143]

The ejection fraction measured by ultrafast computed tomography is obtained using myocardial outlines to determine the cavity areas at end systole and end diastole. Precise and rapid measurements of both right and left ventricular volumes are possible. Ejection fraction calculations correlated well with biplane ventriculography. The calculated ejection fractions permit both global and regional evaluation of ventricular systolic function.[126,127,135,144–149]

The cardiac output is an important parameter for assessing cardiovascular function. Ultrafast computed tomography accurately measured cardiac output and showed good correlation with thermodilution and radioactive microspheres. Cardiac output can be quantified by ultrafast computed tomography either by multiplying ventricular stroke volume by mean heart rate or using a flow-mode acquisition with a time-density curve. The first method involves calculating the ventricular stroke volume, which is the difference between the summed end-diastolic and end-systolic volume of the tomographic slices of the ventricle. The flow method demonstrates a wash-in phase, concentration peak, washout slope, and a recirculation peak. The mean CT number is proportional to the contrast concentration with the cardiac output quantified from the time-density curve.[126,135,136,150,151]

Ultrafast computed tomography can obtain accurate measurements of myocardial mass independent of geometric assumptions. Ultrafast computed tomography has been demonstrated to be useful for measurement of both left and right ventricular mass. Ultrafast computed tomography can accurately determine the presence of ventricular hypertrophy.[126,135,136,152–156]

Conventional CT images anomalies of the great vessels. Its slow scan speed limits its use for evaluating intracardiac pathology. Ultrafast scanning using the high-resolution volume mode and three-dimensional imaging provides precise anatomic definition of a wide variety of congenital cardiovascular defects. Ultrafast computed tomography has demonstrated precise anatomic definition of congenital abnormalities of the great vessels, complex congenital anomalies, fistulas involving the coronary arteries, valvular anomalies and a case of cor triatriatum. CT excels in evaluation of visceroatrial situs and in defining the intrinsic structure and positional relations of the great arteries. Postoperative repair of congenital anomalies, serial examination, and follow-up with Ultrafast computed tomography may be of use with certain disorders.[126,135,157–170] The precise location of an atrial and ventricular septal defect can be obtained with the cine mode. The dynamic flow-mode technique is useful in determining the location of an intracardiac shunt and in quantitation of the shunt size. Time-density curves are obtained over the chambers or vessels of interest, these flow curves plot contrast density over time providing a graphic representation of contrast movement. Ultrafast computed tomography can quantitate shunts at moderate levels and is more sensitive than oximetry in demonstrating small shunts.[126,135,152,171–173]

The high temporal and spatial resolution of ultrafast computed tomography is ideal for evaluating cardiac masses. The tumor size, site of attachment, involvement of valvular structures, and extracardiac extent can be accurately characterized.[135]

Ultrafast computed tomography scanning is a useful imaging procedure with high spatial resolution, high-density resolution, and tomographic capabilities providing quality evaluation of cardiac structure and function. There are however, a number of persisting limitations of ultrafast computed tomography for cardiac imaging. Although ultrafast computed tomographic scanning is less influenced by patient motion, image acquisition time may be prolonged when multi-

ple images at multiple levels are acquired resulting in total breath-holding times approaching 30 to 45 seconds. Respiratory movement results in movement of the heart affecting quantitative accuracy. Irregular heart rhythms will result in acquisition of different slices at different levels which affects the accuracy of quantitative data. Artifact from metallic objects results in distortion of nearby structures. Images require injection of contrast agents to obtain quantitative information about cardiac function as well as anatomic information. It is necessary to accurately time the contrast bolus to the circulation time. Up to 5% of scans are nondiagnostic due to mistiming of contrast. Although radiation exposure is relatively small, this is a potential disadvantage. In addition, ultrafast scanning has the disadvantage of nonportability and expense.[126,152]

Nuclear Cardiology

Radionuclide techniques assume an important complementary role in the diagnosis and assessment of pediatric cardiac disorders. The major applications of radionuclide imaging in children with cardiac disease include: gated blood pool ventriculography, first-pass radionuclide angiocardiography, myocardial perfusion imaging of coronary blood flow, pulmonary scintigraphy, myocardial infarction and myocardial inflammation detection. Standardized techniques have been developed and with increasing reliability of these techniques defined roles in providing both diagnostic and prognostic information have been established.[174–176]

Assessment of Ventricular Function

Radionuclide angiography is useful in quantitating ventricular function in complex heart disease both pre- and postoperatively when standard imaging by two-dimensional echocardiography may be unreliable. In addition, radionuclide angiography may be helpful when echocardiography is unobtainable due to overlying lung or abnormal physiology. The two most commonly used techniques to assess ventricular function are the equilibrium radionuclide angiogram and the first-pass radionuclide angiocardiogram. Both techniques have their own limitations and advantages. The most important parameters obtained are the right and left ventricular ejection fractions, wall motion analysis, ventricular volumes, intracardiac shunts, and diastolic function. Radionuclide ventricular function analysis can provide useful information in managing patients with a variety of congenital heart disorders.[174,177–188]

Gated blood pool scintigraphy acquires imaging data while the radionuclide is still confined to the vascular space and permits an evaluation of both global and regional ventricular function. The technique usually uses technetium 99m (99mTc) attached to red blood cells or serum albumin with images acquired as an equilibrium electrocardiographically gated angiogram. To perform radionuclide angiography there must be a regular heart rate and rhythm, patient inertia, minimal diaphragmatic motion, intravascular tracer, and sufficient count density. This method is able to evaluate ventricular function and focal wall motion abnormalities at rest and during peak exercise. Several measurements can be obtained with radionuclide angiography including ventricular ejection fraction, stroke and end-diastolic volume, cardiac output, and regurgitant fractions.[189]

A second method is the first-pass technique that images the radionuclide as it circulates through the cardiac chambers and great vessels in its first transit. This method can provide information on right ventricular function and shunt detection as well as analysis of tracer flow patterns. Recent advances in gamma cameras and computer technology have made first-pass radionuclide angiography faster and more accurate. Commonly used 99mTc has limitations as a tracer for first-pass angiography due to radiation dose constraints limiting the injected dose and to persistent background interference with repeated injections. A group of ultrashort radionuclides are available that have a short half-life and low radiation dose allowing multiple studies to be performed within a short time. This method is accurate in the assessment of ventricular ejection fractions and is ideally suited for children as it can be performed in just a few seconds.[174,190,191]

The most important measurement obtained from radionuclide angiography is the left ventricular ejection fraction obtained at rest and during exercise. The calculated ejection fraction uses quantifying ventricular counts rather than a geometric assumption. The counts are proportional to ventricular volumes providing accurate measurements of ejection fraction.[179,192,193]

An evaluation of regional wall motion is generally a subjective analysis, although a more quantitative assessment of wall motion can be obtained with regional ejection fraction measurements. Focal or global myocardial wall motion abnormalities in children may be seen with anomalous coronary origins, myocardial involvement in Kawasaki syndrome, cardiomyopathies, cardiac tumors, and in various congenital heart diseases pre- and post surgery.[179,192,193]

Ventricular volume calculations can be performed using a count-based technique or the geometric method.[179]

Radionuclide angiocardiography is helpful in diagnosing and assessing the magnitude of left-to-right shunting in certain congenital lesions. It is a helpful tool in assessing the indications for operation as well as assessing the success of the surgical repair. Qualitative analysis of a left-to-right shunt is done through

monitoring the flow of tracer through the cardiac chambers. A more quantitative approach uses time-activity curves plotting the passage of the tracer bolus through the pulmonary circulation. Radionuclide angiography has been compared to oximetric measurements in the assessment of left-to-right shunts. The radionuclide method is more precise and less invasive. It is preferred when accurate measurement of a left-to-right shunt is required. In addition radionuclide angiography provides a valid measurement of the right ventricular ejection fraction and delayed contraction phase analysis that may be a sensitive indicator of early right ventricular dysfunction in patients with left-to-right shunt lesions.[179,194–201] Radionuclide angiocardiography may also be used to detect and quantify right-to-left shunts.

Myocardial Perfusion

Myocardial planar scintigraphy and single photon emission computed tomography (SPECT) in children is performed with either technetium-99m MIBI (hexakis (2-methoxyisobutylisonitrile) technetium (I), Sestamibi, Cardiolite, DuPont Merck Pharmaceutical Co, Billerica, MA, USA) or thallium-201, which are actively taken up by myocardial muscle proportional to regional blood flow. In children, technetium-99m MIBI is preferred, with sharper images requiring a shorter recording time and less radiation to the patient. Images can be acquired during physiologic or pharmacological stress and after resting redistribution, enabling stress-induced myocardial ischemia to be detected. Clinical indications include assessing myocardial perfusion in children with coronary artery abnormalities such as anomalous coronary arteries and Kawasaki disease, pulmonary atresia with intact ventricular septum, and in transposition of the great arteries following the arterial switch operation (Fig. 1-38). In addition, the ratio of right ventricular-to-left ventricular counts using thallium-201 has been shown to be a good predictor of right ventricular overload in a variety of congenital heart lesions.[175,202–206]

Pulmonary Perfusion

Pulmonary perfusion imaging uses 99mTc-labeled macroaggregated albumin (99mTc-MAA). This technique provides information on relative pulmonary and systemic perfusion, qualifying right-to-left shunts, patency of surgical systemic-to-pulmonary shunts, and an assessment of regional distribution of total pulmonary blood flow in children with pulmonary artery malformations or stenosis. The quantitative perfusion radionuclide method is a sensitive, relatively noninvasive test that demonstrates lung perfusion abnormalities and enables appropriate planning for further invasive studies. It is useful for pre- and postcatheter or

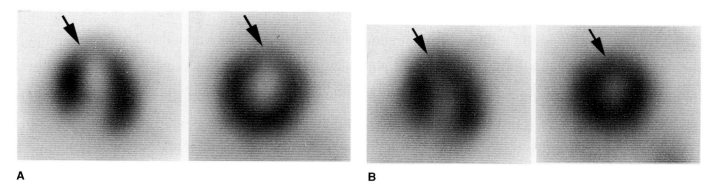

A **B**

Fig. 1-38: Anomalous left coronary artery with myocardial ischemia.
A: Thallium-201 myocardial scintigraphy with vertical and short-axis images demonstrating a focal myocardial perfusion defect within the anterior wall of the left ventricle (arrow). **B:** After reimplantation of the anomalous left coronary artery, there is reperfusion of the myocardium (arrow).

surgical arterioplasty, stent placement, and coil occlusion of systemic collaterals (Fig. 1-39).[174,175,207,208]

Myocardial Infarction

Myocardial infarction imaging in children may be used in a variety of congenital or acquired coronary artery diseases including anomalous coronary artery origins, familial hypercholesterolemia, and Kawasaki disease (see also Chapter 30).[174]

Myocardial Inflammation

Inflammation imaging radionuclides include 67 gallium (^{67}Ga) and 111 indium (^{111}In) and are occasionally useful in Kawasaki disease, myocarditis and pericarditis.[174]

Miscellaneous

Radionuclide splenic scanning in heterotaxy syndromes is performed using ^{99m}Tc-labeled denatured red blood cells. Documentation of the absence of the spleen is more difficult than confirming its presence. There are pitfalls in the accuracy and reliability in the diagnosis of asplenia using radionuclide splenic scanning due to overlapping signals from the blood pool of the symmetrical large midline liver. There are other more reliable techniques such as ultrasonography and computerized tomography in determining asplenia.[209]

Radionuclide venography can be used to evaluate venous drainage in patients with central venous lines and in patients suspected of central venous obstruction. Defining the presence of a left superior vena cava is easily done with a left hand injection.[174]

Cardiac Positron Emission Tomography

Conventional imaging techniques will allow precise characterization of cardiac anatomy and function.

However, there remains a number of unique questions of physiologic significance that cannot be addressed by such imaging techniques, including myocardial viability and metabolic activity. Positron emission tomography (PET) imaging allows a window for the assessment of regional myocardial flow, and cardiac metabolism, *in vivo*, critical for determination of effective treatment regimens. Although PET scanning has been considered mainly a research tool, lower prices for instrumentation and automation of some techniques have led several institutions to apply the imaging technique to routine clinical evaluation.

By creating a positron-emitting radionuclide (from a cyclotron, a generator, or by radiosynthesis) from a nonradioactive molecule the tracer can be imaged as it

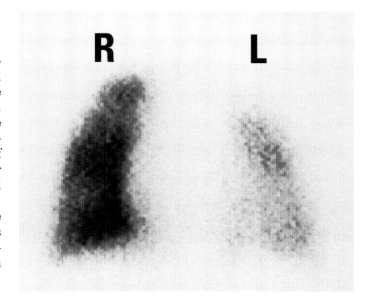

Fig. 1-39: Left pulmonary artery hypoplasia.
Pulmonary scintigraphy demonstrating hypoperfusion of the left lung in a patient with diffuse hypoplasia of the left pulmonary artery.

is utilized within the myocardium. Fatty acid metabolism (the tracer-^{11}C palmitate), tricarboxylic acid metabolism (the tracer-^{11}C acetate), exogenous glucose uptake (^{18}F fluorodeoxyglucose (FDG)) and myocardial blood flow (tracers—[82]rubidium, [15]O water, and ^{13}N ammonia) can be assessed as these tracers decay. With decay of the positrons (as the element becomes stable), they travel a short distance and combine with an electron, creating through annihilation, the formation of electromagnetic energy (two gamma rays or photons) that are emitted 180° from one another. The photons that are emitted are detected by pairs of sensors placed around the patient, through coincidence detection. Static tomographic images can then be computer reconstructed or the acquisition gated to the cardiac cycle for dynamic reconstruction.

A number of cardiological problems can be evaluated by taking advantage of the metabolic activity of the myocardium. A normal heart is able to utilize many different substrates for generation of energy. While the heart will preferentially utilize fatty acids as its energy source (particularly during a fast), after a glucose level, the heart will use glucose as a substrate. Infarcted heart muscle is characterized by decreased myocardial blood flow and decreased uptake of a metabolic tracer. During ischemia, due to lack of sufficient oxygen, fatty acids cannot be effectively metabolized by β-oxidation. Therefore, the heart switches to anaerobic glycolysis. The increase in glucose utilization in ischemic myocardium compared with normal heart muscle can be imaged by fluorin-18-labeled deoxyglucose (FDG). Fatty acid activity can be characterized with the tracer ^{11}C palmitate, when it is taken up by the myocyte and undergoes b-oxidation with release of the ^{11}C as [11]C0$_2$. In ischemia, b-oxidation does not occur and the ^{11}C does not leave the myocyte. Thus, in the normal myocardium the ^{11}C enters and leaves the heart, while in ischemia, it accumulates in the tissue. As for glucose, the glucose analog FDG is also taken up by the myocytes and undergoes phosphorylation, but does not undergo further glycolysis. It does not readily diffuse from the myocyte; and is effectively trapped. Thus, the FDG becomes an excellent tracer for exogenous glucose uptake. [11]C acetate similarly traces the tricarboxylic acid (TCA) cycle, as it is not readily oxidized in the TCA cycle, or any other major metabolic pathway in the heart. Measurement of TCA cycle activity is thought to assess overall oxidative myocardial metabolism, as all essential oxidative substrates pass through the TCA pathway. Acetate kinetics can be also used to estimate myocardial oxygen consumption.

These traces allow evaluation of coronary artery disease (evaluation of blood flow and metabolism) during ischemia and reperfusion and during hypoxia (FDG), infarction and thrombolysis. PET studies have further supplemented other myocardial perfusion studies in the evaluation of viable myocardium before and after bypass graft surgery.

Finally, and perhaps more pertinent to the patient with congenital heart disease, PET imaging has been applied to the evaluation of the hypertrophic cardiomyopathy,[210] dilated cardiomyopathy,[211] and in a unique population with Duchenne's muscular dystrophy.[212] The reader interested in a more detail of PET is referenced to more in-depth discussion.[213,214]

References

1. Graham TP. Noninvasive assessment of cardiovascular disease in the young: A clinical overview. *J Am Coll Cardiol* 1985;5(1):4S-11S.
2. Feigenbaum H. *Echocardiography.* 4th edition. Philadelphia: Lea & Febiger; 1986, pp. 1–49.
3. Huhta JC, Glasow P, Murphy DJ Jr, Gutgesell HP, Ott DA, McNamara DG, Smith EO. Surgery without catheterization for congenital heart defects: Management of 100 patients. *J Am Coll Cardiol* 1987;9:823–829.
4. Krabell KA, Ring S, Foker JE, Braunlin EA, Einzig S, Berry JM, Bass LF. Echocardiographic versus cardiac catheterization diagnosis of infants with congenital heart disease requiring cardiac surgery. *Am J Cardiol* 1987;60:351–354.
5. Musewe NN, Dyck JD, Smallhorn JF. Echocardiography and the neonate with real or suspected heart disease. In: *Neonatal Heart Disease.* Freedom RM, Benson LN, Smallhorn JF, eds. London: Springer-Verlag; 1992, pp. 135–148.
6. Didier D, Higgins CB, Fisher M, Osaki L, Silverman N, Cheitlin M. Congenital heart disease: Gated MR imaging in 72 patients. *Radiology* 1986;158:227–235.
7. Fletcher BD, Jacobstein MD, Nelson AD, Riemenschneider TA, Alfidi RJ. Gated magnetic resonance imaging of congenital cardiac malformations. *Radiology* 1984;150:137–140.
8. Higgins CB, Byrd BF, Farmer DW, Osaki L, Silverman NH, Cheitlin MD. Magnetic resonance imaging in patients with congenital heart disease. *Circulation* 1984;70:851–860.
9. Jacobstein MD, Fletcher BD, Nelson AD, Goldstein S, Alfidi RF, Riemenschneider TA. ECG-gated nuclear magnetic resonance imaging: Appearance of the congenitally malformed heart. *Am Heart J* 1984;107:1014–1020.
10. Higgins CB, Byrd BF, McNamara MT, Lanzer P, Lipton MJ, Botvinich, E, Schiller NB, Crooks LE, Kaufman L. Magnetic resonance imaging of the heart: A review of the experience in 172 subjects. *Radiology* 1985;155:671–679.
11. Lanzer P, Botvinick EH, Schuller NB, Crooks LE, Arakawa M, Kaugman L, Davis PL, Herfken R, Lipton MJ, Higgins CB. Cardiac imaging using gated magnetic resonance. *Radiology* 1984;150:121-127.
12. Higgins CB. Overview of MR of the heart—1986. *AJR* 1986;146:907–918.

12a.Donnelly LF, Higgins CB. MR imaging of conotruncal anomalies. *AJR* 1996; 166:925–928.

12b.Higgins CB, Sakuma H. Heart disease: Functional evaluation with MR imaging. *Radiology* 1996;199: 307–315.

12c.Ho VB, Kinney JB, Sahn DJ. Contributions of newer MR imaging strategies for congenital heart disease. *Radiographics* 1996;16:43–60.

13. Sieverding L, Klose U, Apitz J. Morphological diagnosis of congenital and acquired heart disease by magnetic resonance imaging. *Pediatr Radiol* 1990;20:311–319.

14. Schlesinger AE, Hernandez RJ. Congenital heart disease: Applications of computed tomography and magnetic resonance imaging. *Semin Ultrasound CT MR* 1991;12:11–29.

15. Bisset GS. Magnetic resonance imaging of congenital heart disease in the pediatric patient. *Radiol Clin North Am* 1991;29:279–291.

16. Fellows KE, Weinberg PM, Jeanne MB, Hoffman EA. Evaluation of congenital heart disease with MR imaging: Current and coming attractions. *AJR* 1992;159: 925–931.

17. Dinsmore RE, Wisner GL, Levine RA, Okada RD, Brady TJ. Magnetic resonance imaging of the heart: Positioning and gradient angle selection for optimal imaging planes. *AJR* 1984;143:1135-1142.

18. Higgins CB, Caputo GR. Role of MR imaging in acquired and congenital cardiovascular disease. *AJR* 1993;161: 13–22.

19. Bank ER. Magnetic resonance of congenital cardiovascular disease. *Radiol Clin North Am* 1993;31:553–572.

20. Soulen RL, Budinger TF, Higgins CB. Magnetic resonance imaging of prosthetic heart valves. *Radiology* 1985;154:705–707.

21. Shellock FG, Curtis JS. MR imaging and biomedical implants, materials, and devices: An updated review. *Radiology* 1991;180:541–550.

22. Shellock FG, Morisoil, SM. Ex vivo evaluation of ferromagnetism and artifacts of cardiac occluders exposed to a 1.5-T MR system. *J Magn Reson Imaging* 1994;4: 213–215.

23. McNamara MT, Higgins CB. Cardiovascular applications of magnetic resonance imaging. *Magn Reson Imaging* 1984;2:167–186.

24. Soulen RL. Magnetic resonance imaging of great vessel, myocardial, and pericardial disease. *Circulation* 1991;84(suppl I):I-311-I-321.

25. Sechtem U, Pflugfelder P, Higgins DB. Quantification of cardiac function by conventional and cine magnetic resonance imaging. *Cardiovasc Intervent Radiol* 1987;10: 365–373.

26. Pettigrew RI. Dynamic cardiac MR imaging: Techniques and application. *Radiol Clin North Am* 1989;27: 1183–1203.

27. Buser PT, Auffermann W, Holt WW, Wagner S, Kircher B, Dircher B, Wolfe C, Higgins CB. Noninvasive evaluation of global left ventricular function with use of cine nuclear magnetic resonance. *J Am Coll Cardiol* 1989;13: 1294–1300.

28. Sechtem U, Pflugfelder PW, White RD, Gould RG, Holt W, Lipton JMJ, Higgins CB. Cine MRI: Potential for the evaluation of cardiovascular function. *AJR* 1987;148: 239–246.

29. Sechtem U, Pflugfelder P, Cassidy MC, Holt W, Wolfe C, Higgins CB. Ventricular septal defect: Visualization of shunt flow and determination of shunt size by cine magnetic resonance imaging. *AJR* 1987;149:689–691.

30. Wood AM, Hoffmann KR, Lipton MJ. Cardiac function. Quantification with magnetic resonance and computed tomography. *Radiol Clin North Am* 1994;32(3):553–579.

31. Didier D, Ratib O, Friedli B, Oberhaensli I, Chatellain P, Faidutti B, Rutishauser W, Terrier F. Cine gradient-echo MR imaging in the evaluation of cardiovascular diseases. *Radiographics* 1993;13:561–573.

32. Chung KJ, Simpson IA, Newman R, Sahn DJ, Sherman FS, Hesselink JR. Cine magnetic resonance imaging for evaluation of congenital heart disease: Role in pediatric cardiology compared with echocardiography and angiography. *J Pediatr* 1988;113:1028-1035.

33. Kondo C, Caputo GR, Semelka R, Foster E, Shimakawa S, Higgins CB. Right and left ventricular stroke volume measurements with velocity encoded cine MR imaging: In vitro and in vivo validation. *AJR* 1991;157:9–16.

34. Naylor GL, Fermin DN, Congmore DB. Blood flow imaging by cine MR. *J Comput Assist Tomogr* 1986;10: 715–722.

35. Laschinger JC, Vannier MW, Guiterrez F, Gronemeyer S, Weldon CS, Spray TL, Cox JL. Preoperative three-dimensional reconstruction of the heart and great vessels in patients with congenital heart disease. *J Thorac Cardiovasc Surg* 1988;96:464-473.

36. Laschinger JC, Vannier MW, Gronemeyer S, Gutierrez F, Rosenbloom M, Cox JL. Noninvasive l l reconstruction of the heart and great vessels by ECG-gated magnetic resonance imaging: A new diagnostic modality. *Ann Thorac Surg* 1988;45:505–514.

37. Pearlman JD, Edelman RR. Ultrafast magnetic resonance imaging. Segmented Turboflash, echo-planar, and real-time nuclear magnetic resonance. *Radiol Clin North Am* 1994;32(3):593–612.

38. Chrispin A, Small P, Rutter N, Coupland RE, Doyle M, Chapman B, Coxon R, Guilfoyle D, Cawley M, Mansfield P. Echo planar imaging of normal and abnormal connections of the heart and great arteries. *Pediatr Radiol* 1986;16:289–292.

39. Higgins CB, Hricak H, Helms CA. *Magnetic Resonance Imaging of the Body.* New York: Raven Press; 1992, pp. 567–616.

40. Gomes AS, Lois JF, Williams RG. Pulmonary arteries: MR imaging in patients with congenital obstruction of the right ventricular outflow tract. *Radiology* 1990;174: 51–57.

41. Fletcher BD, Jacobstein MD. MRI of congenital abnormalities of the great arteries. *AJR* 1986;146:941–948.

42. Kersting-Sommerhoff BA, Sechtem U, Higgins CB. Evaluation of pulmonary blood supply by nuclear magnetic resonance imaging in patients with pulmonary atresia. *J Am Coll Cardiol* 1988;11:166-171.

43. Mirowitz, SA, Gutierrez FR, Canter CE, Vannier MW. Tetralogy of Fallot: MR findings. *Radiology* 1989;171: 207–212.

44. Yoo SJ, Choi HY, Park IS, Hong CY, Song MG, Kim SH. Distal aortopulmonary window with aortic origin of the right pulmonary artery and interruption of the aortic arch (Berry syndrome): Diagnosis by MR imaging. *AJR* 1991;157(4):835–836.

45. Didier D, Higgins CB. Estimation of pulmonary vascular resistance by MRI in patients with congenital cardiovascular shunt lesions. *AJR* 1986;146:919–924.

46. Bogren HG, Klipstein RH, Mohiaddin RH, Firmin DN, Underwood SR, Rees RSO, Longmore DB. Pulmonary

artery distensibility and blood flow patterns: A magnetic resonance study of normal subjects and of patients with pulmonary arterial hypertension. *Am Heart J* 1989;118:990–999.

47. Rees S, Somerville J, Warad C, Martinez J, Mohiaddin RH, Underwood R, Longmore DB. Coarctation of the aorta: MR imaging in late postoperative assessment. *Radiology* 1989;173:499–502.

48. von Schulthess GK, Higashino SM, Higgins SS, Didier D, Fisher MR, Higgins CB. Coarctation of the aorta: MR imaging. *Radiology* 1986;158:469–474.

49. Fletcher BD, Jacobstein MD. MRI of congenital abnormalities of the great arteries. *AJR* 1986;146:941–948.

50. Amparo EG, Higgins CB, Shafton EP. Demonstration of coarctation of the aorta by magnetic resonance imaging. *AJR* 1984;143:1192–1194.

51. Burrows RE, MacDonald CE. Magnetic resonance imaging of the pediatric thoracic aorta. *Semin Ultrasound CT MR* 1993;14:129–144.

52. Simpson IA, Chung KJ, Glass RF, Sahn DJ, Sherman FS, Hesselink J. Cine magnetic resonance imaging for evaluation of anatomy and flow relations in infants and children with coarctation of the aorta. *Circulation* 1988;78:142–148.

53. Mohiaddin RH, Kilner PJ, Rees S, Longmore DB. Magnetic resonance volume flow and jet velocity mapping in aortic coarctation. *J Am Coll Cardiol* 1993;22:1515–1521.

54. Kersting-Sommerhoff BA, Sechtem UP, Schiller NB, Lipton MJ, Higgins CB. MRI of the thoracic aorta in Marfan patients. *J Comput Assist Tomogr* 1987;149:9–13.

55. Kubota S, Suzuki T, Murata K. Cine magnetic resonance imaging for diagnosis of right coronary arterial-ventricular fistula. *Chest* 1991;100:735–737.

56. Kersting-Sommerhoff BA, Sechtem UP, Fisher MR, Higgins CB. MR imaging of congenital anomalies of the aortic arch. *AJR* 1987;149:9–13.

57. Bisset GS, Strife JL, Kirks DR, Bailey WW. Vascular rings: MR imaging. *AJR* 1987;149:251–256.

58. Jaffe RB. Magnetic resonance imaging of vascular rings. *Semin Ultrasound CT MR* 1991;11:206–220.

59. Fletcher BD, Cohn RC. Tracheal compression and the innominate artery: MR evaluation in infants. *Radiology* 1989;170:103–107.

60. Vogl T, Wilimzig C, Hofmann U, Hofmann D, Dresel S, Lissner J. MRI in tracheal stenosis by innominate artery in children. *Pediatr Radiol* 1991;21:89–93.

61. Hsu YH, Chien CT, Hwang M, Chiu IS. Magnetic resonance imaging of total anomalous pulmonary venous drainage. *Am Heart J* 1991;121(5):1560–1565.

62. Masui T, Seelos KC, Kersting-Sommerhoff BA, Higgins CB. Abnormalities of the pulmonary veins: Evaluation with MR imaging and comparison with cardiac angiography and echocardiography. *Radiology* 1991;181:645–649.

63. Livolsi A, Kastler B, Marcellin L, Casanova R, Bintner M, Haddad J. MR diagnosis of subdiaphragmatic anomalous pulmonary venous drainage in a newborn. *J Comput Assist Tomogr* 1991;15(6):1051–1053.

64. Seelos KC, Masui T, Kersting-Sommerhoff BA, Higgins CB. Depiction of anomalies of the pulmonary venous return by means of MR imaging, angiography, and echocardiography. *Radiology* 1990;177P:99.

65. Rumancik WM, Hernanz-Schulman M, Rutkowski MM, Kiely B, Ambrosino M, Genieser NG, Naidich DP. Mag-

netic resonance imaging of cor triatriatum. *Pediatr Cardiol* 1988;9:149–151.

66. Fisher MR, Hricak H, Higgins CB. Magnetic resonance imaging of developmental venous anomalies. *AJR* 1985;145:705–709.

67. Jelinek JS, Stuart PL, Done SL, Ghaed N, Rudd SA. MRI of polysplenia syndrome. *Magn Reson Imaging* 1989;7:681–686.

68. Lowell DG, Turner DA, Smith SM, Bucheleres GH, Santucci BA, Gresick RJ, Monson DO. The detection of atrial and ventricular septal defects with electrocardiographically synchronized magnetic resonance imaging. *Circulation* 1986;73:89–94.

69. Dinsmore RE, Wismer GL, Guyer D, Thompson R, Liu P, Stratemeier E, Miller S, Okada R, Brady T. Magnetic resonance imaging of the interatrial septum and atrial septal defects. *AJR* 1985;145:697–703.

70. Diethelm L, Dery R, Lipton MJ, Higgins CB. Atrial-level shunts: Sensitivity and specificity of MR in diagnosis. *Radiology* 1987;162:181–186.

71. Jacobstein MD, Fletcher BD, Goldstein S, Riemenschneider TA. Evaluation of atrioventricular septal defect by magnetic resonance imaging. *Am J Cardiol* 1985;55:1158–1161.

72. Parsons JM, Baker EJ, Anderson RH, Ladusans EJ, Hayes A, Quereshi SA, Deverall PB, Fagg N, Cook A, Maisey MN, Tynan M. Morphological evaluation of atrioventricular septal defects by magnetic resonance imaging. *Br Heart J* 1990;64(2):138–145.

73. Didier D, Higgins CB. Identification and localization of ventricular septal defect by gated magnetic resonance imaging. *Am J Cardiol* 1986;57:1363–1368.

74. Yoo SJ, Lim TH, Park IS, Hong CY, Song MG, Kim SH. Defects of the interventricular septum of the heart: En face MR imaging in the oblique coronal plane. *AJR* 1991;157:943–946.

75. Sechtem U, Pflugfelder P, Cassidy MC, Holt W, Wolfe C, Higgins CB. Ventricular septal defect: Visualization of shunt flow and determination of shunt size by cine MR imaging. *AJR* 1987;149:689–692.

76. Higgins CB, Silverman N, Kersting-Sommerhoff B, Schmidt K. *Echocardiography and MRI of Congenital Heart Disease.* New York: Raven Press; 1990.

77. Kersting-Sommerhoff BA, Diethelm L, Teitel DF, Sommerhoff CB, Higgins SS, Higashimo SS, Higgins CB. Magnetic resonance imaging of congenital heart disease: Sensitivity and specificity using receiver operating characteristic curve analysis. *Am Heart J* 1989;118:155–162.

78. Higgins CB, Holt W, Pflugfelder P, Sechtem U. Functional evaluation of the heart with magnetic resonance imaging. *Magn Reson Med* 1988;6:121–139.

79. Peshock RM, Parrish M, Fixler D, Parkey RW. Magnetic resonance imaging of single ventricle. *Circulation* 1985;72(suppl III):III-29.

80. Jacobstein MD, Portman MA, Fletcher BD. Magnetic resonance imaging in univentricular atrioventricular connection. *Am J Cardiac Imaging* 1987;1:221–226.

81. Kersting-Sommerhoff, Diethelm L, Stanger P, Dery, R, Higashino SM, Higgins SS, Higgins CB. Evaluation of complex congenital ventricular anomalies with magnetic resonance imaging. *Am Heart J* 1990;120:133–142.

82. Niwa K, Uchishiba M, Aotsuka H, Tateno S, Tashima K, Fujiwara T, Matsuo K. Magnetic resonance imaging of heterotaxia in infants. *J Am Coll Cardiol* 1994;23(1):177–183.

83. Guit GL, Bluemm R, Rohmer J, Wenink AC, Chin JG, Doornbos J, van Voorthuisen E. Levotransposition of the aorta: Identification of segmental cardiac anatomy using MR imaging. *Radiology* 1986;161:673–679.

84. Mayo JR, Roberson D, Sommerhoff B, Higgins CB. MRI of double outlet right ventricle. *J Comput Assist Tomogr* 1990;14:336–339.

85. Parsons JM, Baker EJ, Anderson RH, Ladusans EJ, Hayes A, Fagg N, Cook A, Qureshi SA, Deverall PB, Maisey MN, Tynan M. Double-outlet right ventricle: Morphologic demonstration using nuclear magnetic resonance imaging. *J Am Coll Cardiol* 1991;18:168–178.

86. Yoo SJ, Lim TH, Park IS, Hong CY, Song MG, Kim SH, Lee HJ. MR anatomy of ventricular septal defect in double-outlet right ventricle with situs solitus and atrioventricular concordance. *Radiology* 1991;181:501–505.

87. Rebergen SA, Guit GL, de Roos A. Double outlet left ventricle: Diagnosis with magnetic resonance imaging. *Br Heart J* 1991;66:381–383.

88. Yoo SJ, Seo JW, Lim TH, Park IS, Hong CY, Song MG, Kim SH, Choe KO, Cho BK, Lee HJ. Hearts with twisted atrioventricular connections: Findings at MR Imaging. *Radiology* 1993;188:109–113.

89. Igarashi H, Kuramatsu T, Shiraishi H, Yanagisawa M. Criss-cross heart evaluated by colour Doppler echocardiography and magnetic resonance imaging. *Eur J Pediatr* 1990;149:523–525.

90. Link KM, Herrera MA, D'Souza VJ, Formanek AG. MR imaging of Ebstein anomaly: Results in four cases. *AJR* 1988;150:363–367.

91. Kastler B, Livolsi A, Zhu H, Roy E, Zollner G, Dietemann JL. Potential role of MR imaging in the diagnostic management of Ebstein anomaly in a newborn. *J Comput Assist Tomogr* 1990;14(5):825–827.

92. Choi YH, Park JH, Choe YH, Yoo SJ. MR imaging of Ebstein's Anomaly of the Tricuspid Valve. *AJR* 1994;163: 539–543.

93. Fletcher BD, Jacobstein MD, Abramowsky CR, Anderson RH. Right atrioventricular valve atresia: Anatomic evaluation with MR imaging. *AJR* 1987;148:671–674.

94. Huggon IC, Baker EJ, Maisey MN, Kakadekar AP, Graves P, Qureshi SA, Tynan M. Magnetic resonance imaging of hearts with atrioventricular valve atresia or double inlet ventricle. *Br Heart J* 1992;68:313–319.

95. Freedberg RS, Kronzon I, Rumancik WM, Liebeskind D. The contribution of magnetic resonance imaging to the evaluation of intracardiac tumors diagnosed by echocardiography. *Circulation* 1988;77:96–103.

96. Go RT, O'Donnell JK, Underwood DA, Feiglin DH, Salcedo EE, Pantoja M, MacIntyre WJ, Meaney TF. Comparison of gated cardiac MRI and 2D echocardiography of intracardiac neoplasms. *AJR* 1985;145:21–25.

97. Lund JT, Ehman RL, Julsrud PR, Sinak LJ, Tajik AJ. Cardiac masses: Assessment by MR imaging. *AJR* 1989;152: 469–473.

98. Amparo EG, Higgins CB, Farmer D, Gamsu G, McNamara M. Gated MRI of cardiac and paracardiac masses: Initial experience. *AJR* 1984;143:1151–1156.

99. Dooms GC, Higgins CB. MR imaging of cardiac thrombi. *J Comput Assist Tomogr* 1986;10:415–420.

100. Gomes AS, Lois JF, Child JS, Brown K, Batra P. Cardiac tumors and thrombus: Evaluation with MR imaging. *AJR* 1987;149:895–899.

101. Winkler M, Higgins CB. Suspected intracardiac masses: Evaluation with MR imaging. *Radiology* 1987;165: 117–122.

102. Funari M, Fujita N, Peck WW, Higgins CB. Cardiac tumors: Assessment with Gd-DTPA enhanced MR imaging. *J Comput Assist Tomogr* 1991;15:953–958.

103. Szucs RA, Rehr RB, Yanovich S, Tatum JL. Magnetic resonance imaging of cardiac rhabdomyosarcoma—Quantifying the response to chemotherapy. *Cancer* 1991;67:2066–2070.

104. Niwa K, Tashima K, Terai M, Okajima Y, Nakajima H. Contrast-enhanced magnetic resonance imaging of cardiac tumors in children. *Am Heart J* 1989;118(2): 424–425.

105. Ricci C, Longo R, Pagnan L, Dalla Palma L, Pinamonti B, Camerini F, Bussani R, Silvestri F. Magnetric resonance imaging in right ventricular dysplasia. *Am J Cardiol* 1992;70:1589–1595.

106. Kersting-Sommerhoff BA, Seelos KC, Hardy C, Kondo C, Higgins SS, Higgins CB. Evaluation of surgical procedures for cyanotic congenital heart disease by using MR imaging. *AJR* 1990;155:259- 266.

107. Canter CE, Gutierrez FR, Molina P, Hartmann AF, Spray TL. Noninvasive diagnosis of right-sided extracardiac conduit obstruction by combined magnetic resonance imaging and continuous-wave Doppler echocardiography. *J Thorac Cardiovasc Surg* 1991;101:724–731.

108. Martinez JE, Mohiaddin RH, Kilner PJ, Khaw K, Rees S, Somerville J, Longmore DB. Obstruction in extracardiac ventriculopulmonary conduits: Value of nuclear magnetic resonance imaging with velocity mapping and Doppler echocardiography. *J Am Coll Cardiol* 1992;20: 338–344.

109. Julsrud PR, Ehman RL, Hagler DJ, Ilstrup DM. Extracardiac vasculature in candidates for Fontan surgery: MR imaging. *Radiology* 1989;173:503–506.

110. Fogel MA, Weinberg PM, Fellows KE, Hoffman EA. Magnetic resonance imaging of constant total heart volume and center of mass in patients with functional single ventricle before and after staged Fontan procedure. *Am J Cardiol* 1993;72:1435–1443.

111. Kondo C, Hardy C, Higgins SS, Young JN, Higgins CB. Nuclear magnetic resonance imaging of the palliative operation for hypoplastic left heart syndrome. *J Am Coll Cardiol* 1991;18:817-823.

112. Beek FJA, Beekman RP, Dillon EH, Mali WPTM, Meiners LC, Kramer PPG, Meyboom EJ. MRI of the pulmonary artery after arterial switch operation for transposition of the great arteries. *Pediatr Radiol* 1993;23: 335–340.

113. Katz ME, Glazer HS, Siegel MJ, Gutierrez F, Levitt RG, Lee JKT. Mediastinal vessels: Postoperative evaluation with MR imaging. *Radiology* 1986;161:647–651.

114. Jacobstein MD, Fletcher BD, Nelson D, Clampitt RT, Alfidi RJ, Riemenschneider TA. Magnetic resonance imaging: Evaluation of palliative systemic-pulmonary artery shunts. *Circulation* 1984;70:650–656.

115. Chung KJ, Simpson IA, Glass RF, Sahn DJ, Hesselink JR. Cine magnetic resonance imaging after surgical repair in patients with transposition of the great arteries. *Circulation* 1988;77:104–109.

116. Rees S, Somerville J, Warnes C, Underwood R, Firmin D, Klipstein R, Longmore D. Comparison of magnetic resonance imaging with echocardiography and radionuclide angiography in assessing cardiac function and anatomy following Mustard's operation for transposition of the great arteries. *Am J Cardiol* 1988;61:1316-1322.

117. Campbell RM, Moreau GA, Johns JA, Burger JD, Maser

M, Graham TP, Kulkarni MV. Detection of caval obstruction by magnetic resonance imaging after intraatrial repair of transposition of the great arteries. *Am J Cardiol* 1987;60:688–691.

118. Simpson IA, Valdes-Cruz LM, Berthoty DP, Powell JB, Hesselink JR, Chung KJ, Sahn DJ. Cine magnetic resonance imaging and color Doppler flow mapping in infants and children with pulmonary artery bands. *Am J Cardiol* 1993;71:1419–1426.

119. Semelka RC, Tomei E, Wagner S, Mayo J, Kondo C, Suzuke JI, Caputo GR, Higgins CB. Normal left ventricular dimensions and function: Interstudy reproducibility of measurements with cine MR imaging. *Radiology* 1990;174:763–768.

120. Benjelloun H, Cranney GB, Kirk KA, Blackwell GG, Lotan CS, Pohost GM. Interstudy reproducibility of biplane cine nuclear magnetic resonance measurements of left ventricular function. *Am J Cardiol* 1991;67:1413–1420.

121. MacMillan RM, Murphy JL, Kresh JY, Chandrasekaran K, Muhr WF, Haskin ME. Left ventricular volumes using cine-MRI: Validation by catheterization ventriculography. *Am J Card Imaging* 1990;4:79–85.

122. Sechtem U, Pflugfelder PW, Gould RG, Cassidy MM, Higgins CB. Measurement of right and left ventricular volumes in healthy individuals with cine MR imaging. *Radiology* 1987;163:697–702.

123. Sieverding L, Jung WI, Klose U, Apitz J. Noninvasive blood flow measurement and quantification of shunt volume by cine magnetic resonance in congenital heart disease. *Pediatr Radiol* 1992;22:48–54.

124. Sechtem U, Pflugfelder PW, Cassidy MM, White RD, Cheitlin MD, Schiller NB, Higgins CB. Mitral or aortic regurgitation: Quantification of regurgitant volumes with cine MR imaging. *Radiology* 1988;167:425–430.

125. Peshock RM. Clinical cardiovascular magnetic resonance imaging. *Am J Cardiol* 1990;66:41F-44F.

126. Bateman TM. X-ray computed tomography of the cardiovascular system. *Curr Probl Cardiol* 1991;16(12):767–829.

127. Flicker S, Naidech HJ, Altin RS, Eldredge WJ, Carr KF. Ultrafast computed tomography techniques in cardiac disease. *J Thorac Imaging* 1989;4(3):42–49.

128. Stanford W, Galvin JR, Weiss RM, Hajduczok ZD, Skorton DJ. Ultrafast computed tomography in cardiac imaging: A review. *Semin Ultrasound CT MR* 1991;12:45–60.

129. Lipton MJ, Higgins CB, Boyd DP. Computed tomography of the heart. Evaluation of anatomy and function. *J Am Coll Cardiol* 1985;5:55S-59S.

130. Sethna DH, Bateman TM, Whiting JS, Mahony L, Brown J, King H. Comprehensive and quantitative cardiac assessment using cine- CT: Description of a new clinical diagnostic modality. *Am J Card Imaging* 1987;1:18–28.

131. Peschmann KR, Napel S, Cough JL, et al: High-speed computed tomography: Systems and performance. *Appl Optics* 1985;24:4052-4060.

132. Rumberger JA, Lipton MJ. Ultrafast cardiac CT scanning. *Cardiol Clin* 1989;7:713–734.

133. Georgiou D, Brundage BH. Conventional and ultrafast cine-computed tomography in cardiac imaging. *Curr Opin Cardiol* 1990;5:817–824.

134. Mousseaux E, Gaux JC. Ultrafast computed tomography of the heart. *Curr Opin Radiol* 1992;4(IV):34–40.

135. Bleiweis MS, Georgiou D, Brundage BH. Ultrafast CT and the cardiovascular system. *Int J Card Imaging* 1992;8:289–302.

136. Marcus ML, Stanford W, Hajduczok ZD, Weiss RM. Ultrafast computed tomography in the diagnosis of cardiac disease. *Am J Cardiol* 1989;64:54E-59E.

137. Wood AM, Hoffmann KR, Lipton MJ. Cardiac function: Quantification with magnetic resonance and computed tomography. *Radiol Clin North Am* 1994;32(3):553–579.

138. Lipton MJ. Quantitation of cardiac function by cine-CT. *Radiol Clin North Am* 1985;23:613–626.

139. Sethna DH, Bateman TM, Whiting JS, et al: Comprehensive and quantitative cardiac assessment using cine-CT: Description of a new clinical diagnostic modality. *Am J Card Imaging* 1987;1:18–28.

140. Ritman EL. Fast computed tomography for quantitative cardiac analysis—State of the art and future perspectives. *Mayo Clin Proc* 1990;65:1336–1349.

141. Rumberger JA, Weiss RM, Feiring AJ, et al: Patterns of regional diastolic function in the normal human left ventricle: An ultrafast computed tomographic study. *J Am Coll Cardiol* 1989;14:119–126.

142. MacMillan RM, Rees MR. Measurement of right and left ventricular volumes in humans by cine computed tomography: comparison to biplane cineangiography. *Am J Card Imaging* 1988;2:214–219.

143. Marzullo P, L'Abbate A, Marcus ML. Patterns of global and regional systolic and diastolic function in the normal right ventricle assessed by ultrafast computed tomography. *J Am Coll Cardiol* 1991;17:1318–1325.

144. Reiter SJ, Rumberger JA, Feiring AJ, Stanford W, Marcus ML. Precision of measurements of right and left ventricular volume by cine computed tomography. *Circulation* 1986;74:890–900.

145. Pietras RJ, Wolfkiel CJ, Velesik K, Roig E, Chomka EV, Brundage BH. Validation of ultrafast computed tomographic left ventricular volume measurement. *Invest Radiol* 1991;26:28–34.

146. MacMillan RM, Rees MR, Maranhao V, Clark DL. Comparison of left ventricular ejection fraction by cine computed tomography and single plane right anterior oblique ventriculography. *Angiology* 1986;36:299–305.

147. Rich S, Chomka EV, Stagl R, Shanes JG, Kondos GT, Brundage BH. Determination of left ventricular ejection fraction using ultrafast computed tomography. *Am Heart J* 1986;112:392–396.

148. Roig E, Georgiou D, Chomka V, Wolfkiel C, LoGalboZek C, Rich S, Brundage BH. Reproducibility of left ventricular myocardial volume and mass measurements by ultrafast computed tomography. *J Am Coll Cardiol* 1991;18:990–996.

149. MacMillan RM, Rees MR. Measurement of right and left ventricular volumes in humans by cine computed tomography comparison to biplane cine radiology. *Am J Card Imaging* 1988;2:214–219.

150. Garrett JS, Lanzer P, Jaschke W, et al: Measurement of cardiac output by cine computed tomography. *Am J Cardiol* 1985;56:657–661.

151. Wolfkiel CJ, Ferguson JL, Chomka EV, Law WR, Brundage BH. Determination of cardiac output by ultrafast computed tomography. *Am J Physiol Imaging* 1986;1:117–123.

152. MacMillan RM. Magnetic resonance imaging vs. ultrafast computed tomography for cardiac diagnosis. *Int J Card Imaging* 1992;8:217–227.

153. Rumberger JA, Feiring AJ, Lipton MJ, et al: Use of ultrasfast computed tomography to quantitate regional myocardial perfusion: A preliminary report. *J Am Coll Cardiol* 1987;9(1):59-69.

154. Roig E, Georgiou D, Chomka EV, et al: Reproducibility of left ventricular myocardial volume and mass measurements by ultrafast computed tomography. *J Am Coll Cardiol* 1991;18:990–996.

155. Marcus ML, Rumberger JA, Stark CA, Weiss RM, Reiter SJ, Feiring AJ, Stanford W. Cardiac applications of ultrafast computed tomography. *Am J Card Imaging* 1988;2:116–121.

156. MacMillan RM. Ultrafast CT in cardiovascular disease. *Practical Cardiol* 1990;16:67–79.

157. Takasugi JE, Godwin JD, Chen JTT. CT in congenitally-corrected transposition of the great vessels. *Comput Radiol* 1987;11(5/6):215–221.

158. Tanaka F, Itoh M, Esaki H, Isobe J, Inoue R. Asymptomatic cor triatriatum incidentally revealed by computed tomography. *Chest* 1991;100:272–274.

159. Yamada T, Harada J, Tada S. Complex congenital cardiovascular anomalies evaluated by continuous-rotation computed tomography in children. *Pediatr Cardiol* 1989;10:65–74.

160. Predey TA, McDonald D, Demos TC, et al: CT of congenital anomalies of the aortic arch. *Semin Roentgenol* 1989;24:96–113.

161. Eldredge WJ, Flicker S. Evaluation of congenital heart disease using Cine-CT. *Am J Card Imaging* 1987;1:38–50.

162. Frey EE, Sato Y, Smith WL, Franken EA Jr. Cine-CT of the mediastinum in pediatric patients. *Radiology* 1987;165:19–23.

163. McCray P, Grandgeorge S, Smith W, Wagener J, Frey E. Cine-CT diagnosis of pulmonary artery sling. *Pediatr Radiol* 1986;16:508-510.

164. MacMillan RM, Shahriari A, Sumithisena S, Fender BK, Maranhao V, Clark D. Contrast-enhanced cine computed tomography for diagnosis of right coronary artery to coronary sinus arteriovenous fistula. *Am J Cardiol* 1985;56:997–998.

165. Marshall J, Eldredge WJ, Kurnik PB. Coronary artery-to-left ventricle communication with abnormal regional coronary flow demonstrated by ultrafast computed tomography. *Am Heart J* 1990;119:677–679.

166. Garrett JS, Schiller NB, Botvinick EH, Higgins CB, Lipton MJ. Cine-computed tomography of Ebstein anomaly. *J Comput Assist Tomogr* 1986;10:664–666.

167. MacMillan RM, Rees MR, Maranhao V, Clark DL. Cine-computed tomography of cor triatriatum. *J Comput Assist Tomogr* 1986;10:124–125.

168. MacMillan RM. Magnetic resonance imaging vs. ultrafast computed tomography for cardiac diagnosis. *Int J Card Imaging* 1992;8:217–227.

169. White RD, Lipton MJ, Higgins CB, Federle MP, Pogany AC, Kerlain RK Jr, Thaxton TS, Turley K. Noninvasive evaluation of suspected thoracic aortic disease by contrast-enhanced computed tomography. *Am J Cardiol* 1986;57:282–290.

170. Farmer DW, Lipton MJ, Webb WR, Ringertz H, Higgins CB. Computed tomography in congenital heart disease. *J Comput Assist Tomogr* 1984;8:677–687.

171. Garrett JS, Jaschke W, Aherne T, Botvinick EH, Higgins CB, Lipton MJ. Quantitation of intracardiac shunts by cine-CT. *J Comput Assist Tomogr* 1988;12(1):82–87.

172. Jaschke W, Gould, RG, Assimakopoulos P, Lipton MJ. Flow measurements with a high-speed computed tomography scanner. *Med Phys* 1987;14:238–243.

173. MacMillan RM, Rees MR, Eldredge WJ, Maranhao V, Clark DL. Quantitation of shunting at the atrial level using rapid acquisition CT with comparison with cardiac catheterization. *J Am Coll Cardiol* 1986;7:946–948.

174. Treves ST. *Pediatric Nuclear Medicine.* Second Edition, New York: Springer-Verlag; 1985, pp. 198–232.

175. Covitz W, Eubig C. Radionuclide imaging in congenital heart disease. *Med Assoc Ga* 1986;75(1):40–43.

176. Watson NE Jr, Cowan RJ, Ball JD. Conventional radionuclide cardiac imaging. *Radiol Clin North Am* 1994;32(3):477–500.

177. Felipe RF, Prpic H, Arndt JW, van der Wall EE, Pauwels EK. Role of radionuclide ventriculography in evaluating cardiac function. *Eur J Radiol* 1991;12(1):20–29.

178. Hannon DW, Gelfand MJ, Bailey WW, Hall JW, Kaplan S. Pin hole radionuclide ventriculography in small infants. *Am Heart J* 1986;111(2):316–321.

179. Borges-Neto S, Coleman RE. Radionuclide ventricular function analysis. *Radiol Clin North Am* 1993;31(4):817–830.

180. Corbett JR, Jansen DE, Willerson JT. Radionuclide ventriculography. Technical aspects. *Am J Physiol Imaging* 1987;2(1):33–43.

181. Akagi T, Benson LN, Green M, De Souza M, Harder JR, Gilday DL, Freedom RM. Ventricular function during supine bicycle exercise in univentricular connection with absent right atrioventricular connection. *Am J Cardiol* 1991;67(15):1273–1278.

182. Ogata H, Nakata T, Endoh A, Tsuchihashi Y, Yonkura S, Tanaka S, Tsuda T, Kubota M, Iimura O. Scintigraphic imaging of a case of congenitally corrected transposition of the great vessels and an adult case of single atrium and single ventricle. *Ann Nucl Med* 1989;3(2):89–93.

183. Gal R, Port SC. Radionuclide angiography in congenitally corrected transposition of the great vessels in an adult. *J Nucl Med* 1987;28(1):116–118.

184. Peterson RJ, Franch RH, Fajman WA, Jones RH. Comparison of cardiac function in surgically corrected and congenitally corrected transposition of the great arteries. *J Thorac Cardiovasc Surg* 1988;96(2):227–236.

185. Benson LN, Burns R, Schwaiger M, Schelbert HR, Lewis AB, Freedom RM, Olley PM, McLaughlin P, Rowe RD. Radionuclide angiographic evaluation of ventricular function in isolated congenitally corrected transposition of the great arteries. *Am J Cardiol* 1986;58(3):319–324.

186. Akagi T, Benson LN, Green M, et al. Ventricular performance before and after Fontan repair for univentricular atrioventricular connection: Angiographic and radionuclide assessment. *J Am Coll Cardiol* 1992;20:920–926.

187. Hurwitz RA, Caldwell Rl, Girod DA, et al. Ventricular function in transposition of the great arteries: Evaluation by radionuclide angiocardiography. *Am Heart J* 1985;110:600–604.

188. Treves ST, Newburger JW, Hurwitz RA. Radionuclide angiocardiography in children. *J Am Coll Cardiol* 1985;5:120S–127S.

189. Hurwitz RA, Siddiqui A, Caldwell RL, Weetman RM, Girod DA. Assessment of ventricular function infants and children. Response to doubutamine infusion. *Clin Nucl Med* 1990;15(8):556–559.

190. Port SC. Recent advances in first-pass radionuclide angiography. *Cardiol Clin* 1994;12(2):359–372.

191. Hurwitz RA, Treves S, Kuruc A. Right ventricular and left ventricular ejection fraction in pediatric patients

with normal hearts: First-pass radionuclide angiocardiography. *Am Heart J* 1984;107:726–732.

192. Kurtz D, Ahnberg DA, Freed M, La Farge CG, Treves S. Quantitative radionuclide angiocardiography: Determination of left ventricular ejection fraction in children. *Br Heart J* 1976;38:966–973.

193. Parrish MD, Graham TP, Bender HW, Jones JP, Patton J, Partain CL. Radionuclide angiographic evaluation of right and left ventricular function during exercise after repair of transposition of the great arteries. *Circulation* 1983;67:178–183.

194. Baker EJ, Ellam SV, Lorber A, Jones OD, Tynan MJ, Maisey MN. Superiority of radionuclide over osimetric measurement of left to right shunts. *Br Heart J* 1985;53(5):535–540.

195. Kim OH. Radionuclide detection and differential diagnosis of left-to-right cardiac shunts by analysis of time-activity curves. *Osaka City Med J* 1986;32(2):65–88.

196. Baker EJ, Shubao C, Clarke SE, Fogelman I, Maisey MN, Tynan M. Radionuclide measurement of right ventricular function in atrial septal defect: Ventricular septal defect and complete transposition of the great arteries. *Am J Cardiol* 1986;57(13):1142–1146.

197. Ito T, Maeda H, Takeda K, Nakagawa T. Factor analysis of gated cardiac blood pool data: Application to patients with congenital heart disease. *Nucl Med Commun* 1991;12(10):865–873.

198. Bourgignon MH, Links JM, Douglass KH, et al. Quantitation of left-to-right shunts by multiple deconvolution analysis. *Am J Cardiol* 1981;48:1086–1092.

199. Ham HR, Dobbeleir A, Viart P, Piepz A, Lenaers A. Radionuclide quantitation of left-to-right cardiac shunts using deconvolution analysis: Concise communication. *J Nucl Med* 1981;22:688–692.

200. Hurwitz RA, Treves S, Keane JF, Girod DA, Caldwell RL. Current value of radionuclide angiocardiography for shunt quantification and management in patients with secundum atrial septal defect. *Am Heart J* 1982;103:421–425.

201. Madsen MT, Argenyi E, Preslar J, Grover-McKay M, Kirchner PT. An improved method for the quantification of left-to-right cardiac shunts. *J Nucl Med* 1991;32:1808–1812.

202. Nakajima K, Taki J, Ohno T, Taniguchi M, Taniguchi M, Bunko H, Hisada K. Assessment of right ventricular overload by a thallium-201 SPECT study in children with congenital heart disease. *J Nucl Med* 1991;32(12):2215–2220.

203. Flynn B, Wernovsky G, Summerville DA, Castaneda AR, Treves ST. Comparison of technetium-99m MIBI and thallium-201 chloride myocardial scintigraphy in infants. *J Nucl Med* 1989;30:1171–1181.

204. Kondo C, Nakanishi T, Sonobe T, Tatara K, Momma K, Kusakabe K. Scintigraphic monitoring of coronary artery occlusion due to Kawasaki disease. *Am J Cardiol* 1993;71:681–685.

205. Kondo M, Kubo A, Yamazaki H, et al. Thallium-201 myocardial imaging for evaluation of right ventricular overloading. *J Nucl Med* 1978;19:1197–1203.

206. Vogel M, Smallhorn JF, Gilday D, et al. Assessment of myocardial perfusion in patients after the arterial switch operation. *J Nucl Med* 1991;32:237–241.

207. Tamir A, Melloul M, Berant M, Horev G, Lubin E, Blieden LC, Zeevi B. Lung Perfusion Scans in Patients with Congenital Heart Defects. *J Am Coll Cardiol* 1992;19(2):383–388.

208. Del Torso S, Milanesi O, Bui P, Benetti E, Stellin G, Mazzucco A, Daliento L, Svaluto Moreolo G, Pellegrino PA. Radionuclide evaluation of lung perfusion after the Fontan procedure. *Int J Cardiol* 1988;20(1):107–116.

209. Bakir M, Bilgic A, Ozmen M, Caglar M. The value of radionuclide splenic scanning in evaluation of aspenia in patients with heterotaxy. *Pediatr Radiol* 1994;24(1):25–28.

210. Grover-McKay, Schwaiger M, Krivokapich J, Perlogg JK, Phelps ME, Schelbert HR. Regional myocardial blood flow and metabolism at rest in mildly symptomatic patients with hypertrophic cardiomyopathy. *J Am Coll Cardiol* 1989;13:317–324.

211. Geltman EM, Smith JL, Beecher D, Ludbrook PA, Ter-Pogossian MM, Sobel BE. Altered regional myocardial metabolism in congestive myopathy detected by position tomography. *Am J Med* 1983;74:773–785.

212. Perloff JK, Werye E, Schelbert HR. Alterations in regional myocardial metabolism, perfusion and wall motion in Duchenne's muscular dystrophy studied by radionuclide imaging. *Circulation* 1984;69:33–42.

213. Phelps ME, Mazziotta JC, Schlebert HR, (eds). *Positron Emission Tomography and Autoradiography*. New York: Raven Press, 1986.

214. Reivich M, Alvai A, (eds). *Positron Emission Tomography*. New York: Alan R Liss, 1985.

Chapter 2

Physical Principles of Image Formation and Projections in Angiocardiography

With J.A.G. Culham, MD, FRCP(C)

Introduction

Safe and effective angiocardiography first requires understanding of the physical principles relating to catheters and contrast agents used, imaging equipment, and image formation. Second, it requires an understanding of anatomic and physical principles related to angiocardiographic projections. Part I of this chapter initially summarizes the physical principles associated with contrast media use and delivery by catheter. Following this, the physical principles of the imaging chain are discussed, including image processing and measurement. Where relevant, quality control and radiation safety issues are addressed and emphasized. Part II of this chapter addresses the selection of angiographic projections to acquire the relevant information about a patient's segmental anatomy and malformations. A flexible and inventive approach is emphasized.

It cannot be emphasized enough, however, how important it is to have a clear idea of the information required from the catheterization procedure and as much as is possible, to plan the procedure in detail beforehand. This includes the expected sites of contrast injections, the choice of projections, and the filming parameters. Guidelines covering cardiac catheterization and the catheterization laboratory are available and reference should be made to this document.[1]

Part I. Image Formation

Contrast Media

Contrast media are agents that enhance the natural contrast between tissues. While "positive" contrast media—iodine based in the vascular system—are the best known, "negative" contrast media should not be forgotten. Carbon dioxide (CO_2) is occasionally used,[2–4] however, the negative contrast of unopacified blood is important in association with iodine-based media. A discussion of contrast selection, relative and absolute contraindications to its use, adverse effects, and the treatment of these (including anaphylactic reactions) is beyond the scope of this chapter, but is extensively discussed in articles and reviews[5–13] and in texts dealing with catheterization technique.[14,15] Furthermore, multiple reviews[5,8,12,15–19] are available covering the chemistry, physiologic and pharmacological effects of iodine-based intravascular contrast media.

The iodine based media are tri-iodinated benzoic acid derivatives.[19] The various commercially available products have, for convenience, been divided in the literature in two ways: *ionics* and *nonionics*, or *high-osmolar* or *low-osmolar agents*. However, Powe[20] and Brismar[21] have suggested that these be more accurately referred to as *ionic monomers, ionic dimers, nonionic monomers*, or *nonionic dimers*. All are derivatives of benzoic acid.

From: Freedom RM, Mawson JB, Yoo SJ, Benson LN: *Congenital Heart Disease: Textbook of Angiocardiography*. Armonk NY, Futura Publishing Co., Inc. ©1997.

Ionic monomers are sodium and meglumine salts of diatrizoic acid that, in solution, dissociate to form a cation and an anion. As the initial molecule contains three iodine atoms, in solution, the iodine:particle ratio is 3:2. This group includes iothalmic acid (Conray® [Mallinckrodt, St. Louis, MO) and metrizoic acid (Isopaque® [Nycomed, England]), with anions iothalamate and metrizoate, respectively. *Ionic dimers (monoacid dimers)* are based around a double-ring benzoic acid derivative containing six iodine atoms that dissociates in solution to give an iodine:particle ratio of 3:1. The group includes the anion ioxaglate (hexabrix). The *nonionic monomers* are single-ring structures that do not dissociate in solution and thus have an iodine:particle ratio of 3:1. The first-generation agent, metrizamide, is no longer commercially available. More recent derivatives, some of which are the mainstays for current vascular imaging, include iopamidol, iohexol, iopromide, iopental, ioversol, and ioxilan.[18] The qualitative and quantitative effects of these agents are similar.[22] The *nonionic dimers* with an iodine:particle ratio of 6:1 are currently under evaluation. Iodixanol (Visipaque®, Sanofi-Winthrop) is commercially available. The physiochemical aspects of each of these groups of iodinated contrast media relate to their clinical/toxic effects as well as to the physical principles of their use.

Iodine Content

The degree to which these agents enhance normal contrast between tissues (radiopacity) is proportional to the iodine concentration.[12] All other components of the molecule act as a carrier for the iodine in a form that can be injected safely in large volume and high concentration.[8] The required iodine concentrations for angiography vary according to the modality used. Morris[23] has suggested that for cineangiography, 180 to 290 mg iodine per milliliter be used and for digital subtraction angiography, 15 to 65 mg of iodine per milliliter; however, we routinely use higher concentrations of contrast media for cineangiography both in children and in adults, preferring 300 to 350 mg of iodine per milliter of the nonionic monomers in order to achieve high-density contrast during injections.

Solubility

The solubility of the contrast agent in solution (including blood) depends either on its ability to dissociate and form a salt (as with ionizing monomers and dimers) or on its hydrophilic properties where hydrophilic groups have been incorporated to the molecule (as with nonionic monomers, dimers).[8] The formation of sodium and meglumine salts of the various benzoic acid derivatives contribute to the toxicity. The overall solubility of the agents contributes to layering effects (see below).

Osmolality

Osmolality is a measure of the number of dissociated particles (ions, molecules, aggregates) in each liter of solution[8] and correlates with physiologic effects.[24] Ionic monomers and dimers have 5 to 8 times the normal physiologic osmolality of blood of 300 mOsm/kg of water.[8] The nonionic monomers and dimers are considerably closer in their osmolality to that of blood.

Viscosity

Viscosity reflects the resistance of a solution to deformation during flow .[23] This depends on the shape, number, and charge of the particles as well as the iodine concentration, but is largely controlled by the side chains of the molecule.[8] The lower the viscosity, the more rapid the potential injection, particularly via small catheters, and potentially, the better the opacification of small vessels.[25] We routinely warm the contrast to blood temperature prior to injection to decrease the viscosity and thus improve the potential flow rate that can be achieved within a catheter. This also decreases vasospasm, helps to maintain body temperature (particularly important with neonates where keeping the infant warm during a prolonged catheterization requires thought and planning), and improves contrast-blood mixing.

Viscosity and solubility contribute to layering and streaming effects seen during angiocardiography. Paulin[26] discussed the layering of contrast, which even at that time was a well-recognized phenomenon.[27,28] There is a paucity of literature relating to layering and streaming effects, reflected in Paulin's comment that " . . . the phenomenon is widely recognized but apparently one doesn't talk—or at least write—that much about it."[29]

Paulin[26] discussed the factors contributing to layering and streaming as being speed of injection, viscosity (noting the decrease with lower viscosity), the caliber and course of the vessel and the velocity of the blood stream. Within a vessel, streaming effects are seen at the margins of vessels due to the profile of flow across a vessel, slow at the margins and highest centrally, due to sheer forces. Streaming is more likely to occur with high concentrations of contrast media. Slow injection into an area of laminar flow is more likely to bring out layering and streaming effects compared with a fast injection into turbulent flow where complete mixing will result.[29] "Take a sample of blood-contrast mixture and it will not separate in any container as seen on horizontal X-ray exposures. If you add the contrast slowly into a blood sample, it will layer nicely underneath the blood, similar to vinegar and oil"[29] (Figs. 2-1 through 2-3). Once complete mixing has been achieved, sedimentation will not occur quickly and thus does not play any practical role in cineangiography.

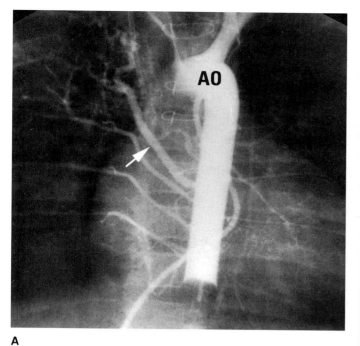

A

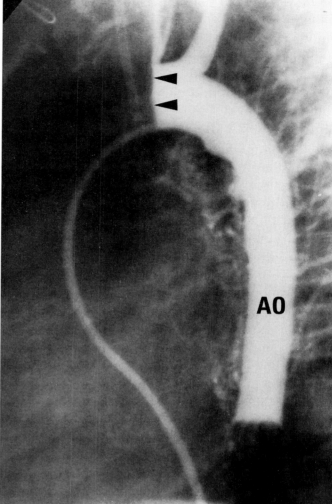

B

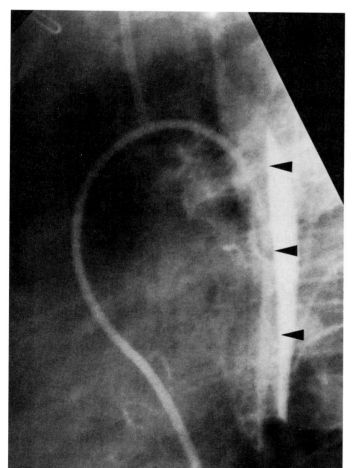

C

Fig. 2-1: Layering of blood and contrast.
Balloon occlusion descending thoracic aortogram via an antegrade approach. **A**: The frontal projection demonstrates a well-opacified descending thoracic aorta with a hypertrophied intercostal (arrow) contributing to right upper lobe pulmonary blood flow. **B**: Lateral projection. After delivery of all the contrast, the blood-contrast interface is apparent (arrowheads) with the horizontal x-ray beam. **C**: Late in the sequence, unopacified blood washes over the top of the contrast column, but the interface with the remaining dependent contrast is apparent (arrowheads).

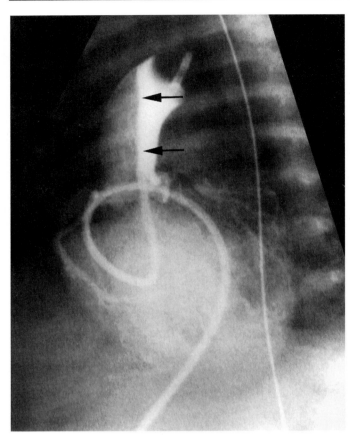

Fig. 2-2: Layering of blood and contrast.
Balloon occlusion ascending aortogram filmed in lateral projection in a patient with complete TGA. The layering effects (arrows) are well seen with contrast being dependent.

In the early 1960s when these physical effects were well recognized, Paulin[26] advocated the use of a horizontal x-ray beam so as to confirm that contrast and blood are well mixed prior to evaluating vessel patency and width, or alternatively, turning the patient, as in a Sones patient cradle (with a fixed image intensifier tube arrangement). In the left anterior oblique (LAO) position, a graft from ascending aorta to left anterior descending (LAD) initially takes an anterior course (upward with the patient supine) to get around the pulmonary trunk, so contrast may layer proximally with nonopaque blood streaming over the top. Thus, the LAD may not opacify and the observer may think that the LAD graft is occluded. However, when the patient is turned into a right anterior oblique (RAO) position, the contrast will flow downhill and opacify the graft and LAD. This streaming into a dependent vessel is also seen in aortography in children, for instance, in patients with complete transposition of the great arteries (TGA), whether using a barrel and lateral projection combination, or an RAO-LAO combination. With the child supine, a rightward anterior aorta has the right posterior facing coronary sinus dependent, with the right coronary artery at a lower level than the left coro-

nary artery. Thus, the right coronary artery may fill before the left or if there is insufficient contrast or poor mixing, the left may not fill at all. This phenomenon of differential filling may in fact be very helpful in discriminating overlapping vessels. This effect of gravity can be used to advantage elsewhere, as in pulmonary venous wedge angiography. Contrast is well mixed by the stage that a retrograde wedge venous injection has traversed the capillaries and entered the proximal pulmonary artery (PA). If the patient is positioned prior to wedge injection with the contralateral side down, the contrast-blood mixture has the opportunity to run downhill into the most dependent portion of the central pulmonary artery, the most proximal patent portion.

Streaming effects are well recognized in a number of situations, some of which are of diagnostic importance. In tetralogy patients, contrast in the overriding ascending aorta is "washed out" by the unopacified blood streaming through the ventricular septal defect (VSD) (*see* Fig. 2-29). Unopacified blood entering a contrast-filled chamber or vessel may identify the site of a VSD (Fig. 2-4) or confirm the presence of a patent

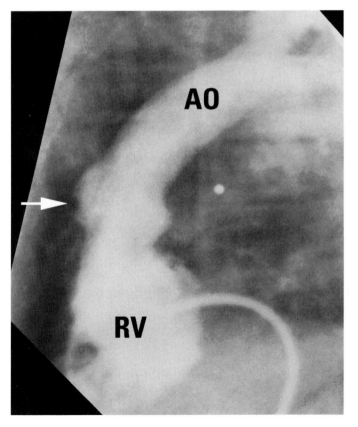

Fig. 2-3: Layering of contrast and air.
Venous approach to RV in a patient with complete TGA. The lateral projection with the patient supine demonstrates how an air bubble introduced during the injection has layered on top of the contrast in the least dependent sinus, the right anterior facing sinus (rightward anterior aorta).

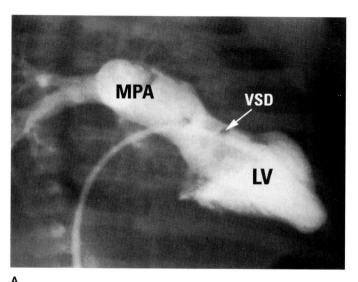

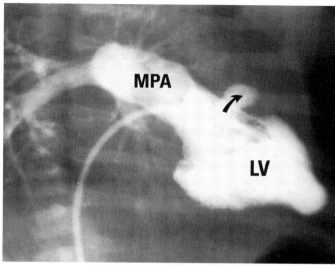

A   B

Fig. 2-4: Contrast washout.
Left ventriculogram performed via a venous approach across the atrial septum in a patient with complete TGA. **A**: Early in the injection, a black hole is apparent high in the perimembranous region, representing streaming of unopacified blood from the higher pressure (systemic) RV into the lower pressure LV. **B**: Slightly later in the injection, an ectopic beat favored left to right shunting from LV to RV with a small amount of contrast in this projection entering RVOT (arrow). (Courtesy of Dr. J. M. Ormiston, Green Lane Hospital, Auckland, New Zealand).

arterial duct (Fig. 2-5). In cyanotic patients, particularly those who have had sternotomies and/or thoracotomies, competitive pulmonary flow from transpleural collaterals can be seen either as reversal of contrast flow in branch vessels during pulmonary arteriography or as small black holes in branch pulmonary arteries both reflecting contrast "washout" by unopacified blood. Similar effects can be seen during balloon occlusion angiography (Fig. 2-6). Such streaming effects are probably most useful in patients with tetralogy-type pulmonary atresia and major aortopulmonary collateral arteries (MAPCAs). Selective injection of major aorto-pulmonary collateral arteries or true pulmonary arteries relies heavily on identification of "washout" to indicate the location and degree of interconnection between vessels in each lobe or bronchopulmonary segment (see Chapter 21, Figs. 21-51 through 21-53).

Catheters

The physical properties of angiographic catheters have been reviewed by Amplatz and Moller.[30] Of the physical properties of the various plastics (polyolefins [polyethylene and polypropolene], fluorocarbons [Teflon], vinyls, urethanes and polyamides [nylons]), the two of most importance to the physical principles of angiocardiography are the coefficient of friction, relevant to contrast passage through the catheter, and the tensile strength, relevant to injection pressure and flow rates.

Catheters are constructed in one of two methods. The plastic may be woven or braided and incorporate a stainless steel braid, the surface coated with multiple applications, usually of polyurethane. Sideholes are woven into the catheter. Alternatively, an extrusion technique may be used with several layers of extruded plastic surrounding a steel braid. The nonbraided catheter tip is welded into position with sideholes being punched in this tip. The standard torque catheters are relatively thick, with relatively small internal diameters. High-flow versions of these catheters with larger internal diameters achieve better flow rates, but have decreased torque characteristics.

The excellent discussion of flow dynamics by Amplatz and Moller[30] is summarized here. Flow depends on injection pressure, internal catheter diameter and catheter length (both usually determined by a patient's size); smoothness of the bore (reflecting the coefficient of friction of the catheter material); number, size, and arrangement of the various sideholes and endholes;, and the chosen contrast's viscosity and density. Flow is inversely proportional to the catheter length and directly proportional to the fourth power of the radius (according to Poiseiulle's law) if laminar catheter flow is achieved. Relatively minor modifications to this law have been proposed to allow for the effects of the tapering of the ends of the catheters and various endhole and sidehole configurations. While these approximate calculations are no longer required on a day-to-day basis if flow-controlled contrast injectors are used during

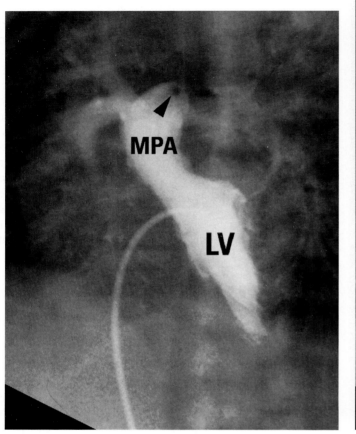

A

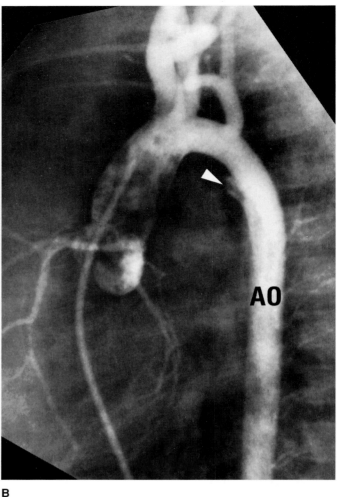

B

Fig. 2-5: Contrast washout.
A: Left ventriculogram, shallow LAO projection with cranial tilt in a patient with complete TGA and a PDA. Left-to-right shunting through the ductus is evident as washout in the MPA. **B**: Antegrade aortogram. Steep LAO projection. Note how the unopacified blood has not yet mixed with the contrast column in proximal descending thoracic aorta (arrowhead) during right-to-left shunting.

angiocardiography, an appreciation of the factors affecting the pressure and flow characteristics of the various catheters is important. Angiographers are continually surprised that an increase in catheter length is associated with a decrease in the maximum contrast flow rate! Usually, the maximum flow rates and pressures for individual catheters are printed on the catheter packaging. We try not to exceed 80% to 90% of these stated values, partly to accommodate the viscosity of the contrast agent, but more importantly, to accommodate the variability in characteristics between catheters of the same type. Intuitively, LePage[31] demonstrated that the wire reinforced catheters were more likely to rupture near their tip, viz: within the patient. Commonly, catheters now have a specially designed weak point close to the hub so that if the pressure and flow characteristics of the catheter are

exceeded during injection, then the catheter will rupture outside the patient.

Sideholes serve a number of roles in a catheter[30,32]: to increase mixing of blood and contrast, to decrease the resistance to flow, to decrease velocity of the contrast jet, and to stabilize the catheter so as to reduce recoil (Fig. 2-7). In a report on the effects of the number and arrangement of sideholes on contrast delivery, Susman and Diboll[33] found that by adding sideholes of large caliber, flow increased up to a maximum of 3 sideholes. Whereas this number permits maximum flow within the catheter, additional sideholes will decrease the jet velocity, a factor in the induction of cardiac arrhythmias[34] and wall injury.

During catheter use, a stable position is required to decrease recoil, particularly if there are few or no sideholes. For ventriculography, the catheter may be stabi-

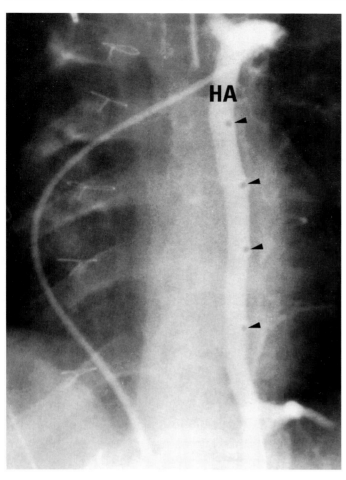

Fig. 2-6: Contrast washout.
Balloon occlusion hemiazygous injection, frontal projection. Unopacified blood from intercostal veins washes into the column of contrast in the hemiazygous vein, seen end-on as black holes (arrowheads).

lized against the atrial wall if a transvenous approach is used. During aortography, a stable position is achieved by advancing the catheter to its final position in the ascending aorta so that it is stabilized against the greater curve. With the use of a pigtail catheter, some straightening of the curl is well recognized during contrast injection at high pressure/flow (Fig. 2-8). While this effect has been reduced with high-flow catheters, the potential remains for straightening to occur such that a jet may be directed from the endhole at a coronary artery or at the aortic valve, or more importantly, the straightened tip may engage a coronary artery, more likely the left.

For both ventriculography and aortography, whether using flow-directed (balloon) catheters, or steerable catheters (pigtail, National Institutes of Health) the tip of the catheter *must* be in the desired location and free before contrast is injected. If not, with ventriculography, myocardial stain, and perforation may occur (Fig. 2-9), and during injection in a great

artery, dissection either of the aortic wall or of a coronary artery may occur. Before injecting, fluoroscopy of the catheter in two projections is imperative to assess the position of the tip and its relative motion. Also, a test injection is mandatory to confirm the desired catheter position (Figs. 2-10 and Fig. 2-11), to confirm that appropriate projections have been chosen (*see* Figs. 2-19 through 2-21), and to confirm that appropriate contrast volumes and flow rates have been selected. A summary of contrast injection factors is provided in Table 2-1. Note that on principle, one aims to inject the contrast as fast as is reasonably possible so as to achieve the best opacification. With ventricular injections, this may result in ectopics. Only when looking specifically at ventricular function do we aim to avoid ectopics by using a slower injection rate; otherwise, the transient alterations in pressure and flow resulting from ectopic beats can be of such use for diagnosis when analyzing the angiogram that it has been said that one is "favored by ectopics."[35]

Contrast Injectors

Both manual and power injections can be used during cineangiography. Manual injections are used for test injections during selective coronary angiography, for wedge injections (as for pulmonary venous or pulmonary arterial wedge angiography), injection of small chambers (hypertensive right ventricle [RV] and pulmonary atresia-intact ventricular septum [PAT-IVS]), or selective injections of vessels such as MAP-CAs. As pointed out by Amplatz and Moller,[30] larger pressures (and thus higher flow rates) can be achieved by using syringes of smaller diameter. Recently, Krieger et al,[36] citing the difficulties of achieving constant, adequate injection of contrast during selective coronary angiography, have reported the use of a CO_2 power-assisted hand-held syringe that delivers a constant pressure.

The delivery of large volumes of contrast media in a short period of time to achieve adequate opacification of cardiac chambers and great vessels, prompted the development of various power injectors, lever or spring-driven, pneumatic or electrical.[37,38]

Power injectors are of two basic types, pressure-controlled and flow-controlled, and have been well reviewed by Amplatz and Moller.[30] Using mechanical, pneumatic or hydraulic power, the pressure-controlled injectors deliver a constant pressure. The settings have to be determined from charts based on catheter lumen and length and viscosity of contrast medium. Conversely, flow-controlled injectors deliver contrast at a constant rate that is independent of resistance and is adjusted automatically within the pressure range of the device. With all these injectors however, it is still mandatory that the operator appreciate the contrast

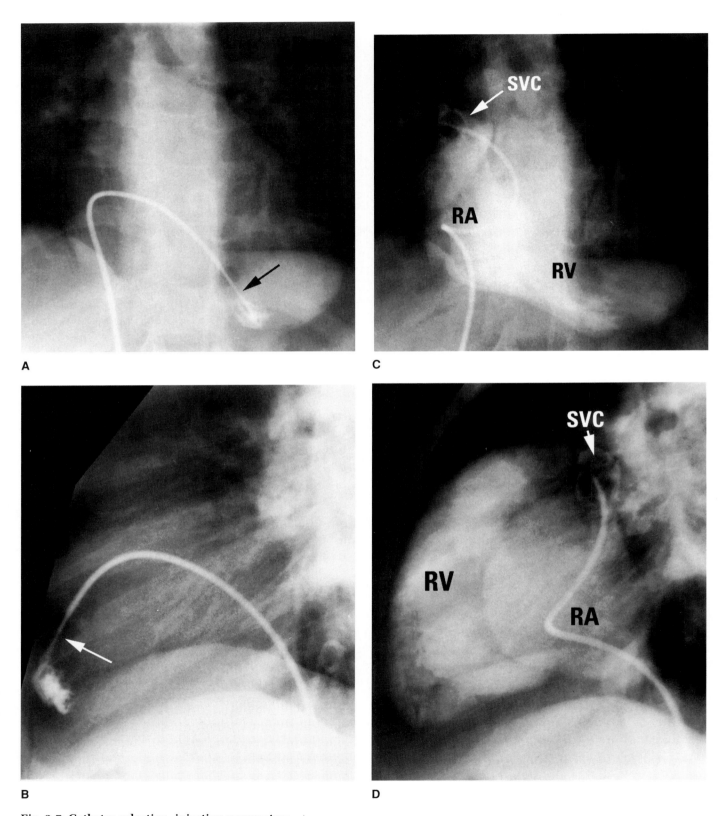

Fig. 2-7: Catheter selection, injection parameters.
Attempted right ventriculogram using a Berman balloon catheter with a single endhole. Frontal (**A**) and lateral (**B**) projections early in the injection show the jet of contrast from the endhole (arrow). Frontal (**C**) and lateral (**D**) projections after catheter recoil show that this has ended up in the SVC. Flow rate and pressure were too high for the catheter choice and positioning.

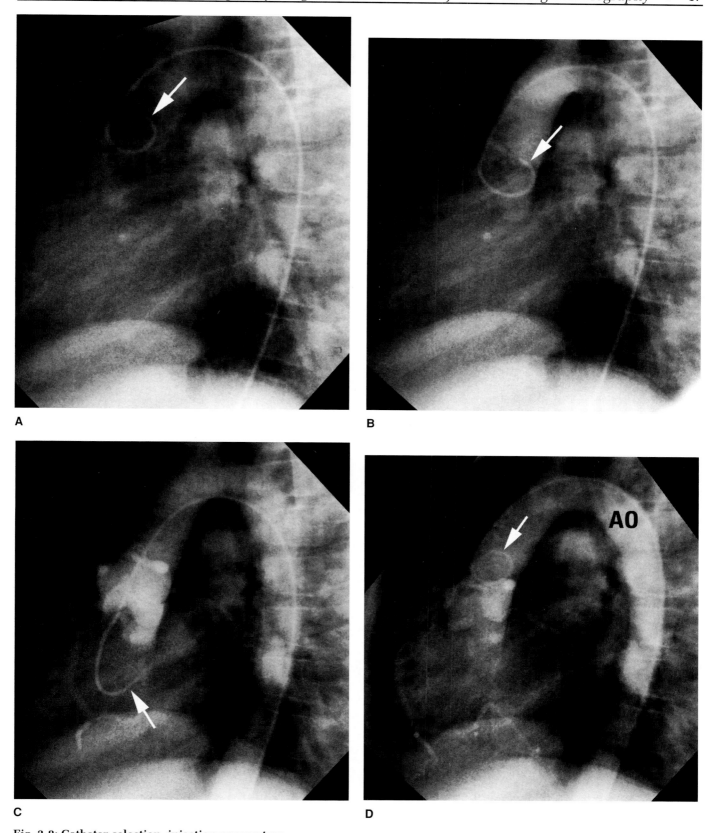

Fig. 2-8: Catheter selection, injection parameters.
Attempted retrograde aortogram (LAO projections) in a patient with VSD and cusp prolapse. **A**: Initially the pigtail catheter is stabilized against the greater curve of the aorta (having been advanced to its final position), but is beginning to unwind with the initial injection. **B**: The catheter unwinds through aortic valve to LV (**C**) before recoiling back to the aorta after the injection is complete (**D**).

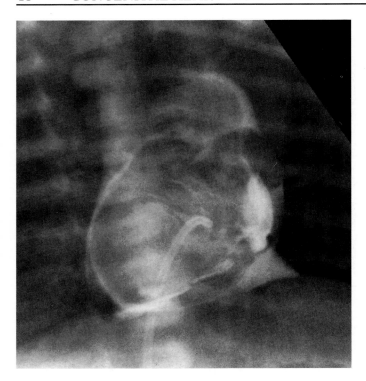

Fig. 2-9: Value of a test injection.
Frontal projection in a child after ventriculography demonstrates contrast outlining the pericardial cavity, reflecting the myocardial perforation that occurred during the ventricular injection. A test injection had not been performed prior to ventriculography, and the restricted motion of the catheter tip as it was buried in the myocardium had not been appreciated. (Courtesy of Dr. J.M. Ormiston, Green Lane Hospital, Auckland, New Zealand).

volume, flow rate, and pressure limitations of the individual catheters being used.

Various settings are available on these mechanical injectors:

Pressure: The injector should be set to operate at the maximal pressure that the catheter will tolerate (higher for a nonballoon than for a balloon catheter) relative to the flow rate chosen. With a flow-controlled injector, the maximum pressure setting should be selected.

Rise Time: Theoretically, this allows a more gradual onset of contrast injection so as to reduce catheter recoil or tip-straightening, a concern with pigtail and endhole catheters particularly. Amplatz and Moller[30] point out that " . . . all injections have a very gradual onset because of the compliance of the plastic syringe, which expands, and the compression of the rubber piston, which obviates the need for an additional set rise time. Thus this setting should be zero."

Phasic Contrast Injection: We do not believe there is any value in an injection timed with the cardiac cycle in children. Indeed, a "square-wave" injection as achieved with a power injector, offers information from the flow characteristics of contrast within a vessel or chamber as well as from the washout characteristics due to unopacified blood, information that could be lost with a phasic contrast injection.

Flow Rate: This can safely be set close to the flow limit for the individual catheter being used. The best opacification is usually achieved with injection of the desired contrast volume in the shortest period of time, but modifications to this principle are discussed in the chapters on individual lesions.

Contrast Volume: It is rare that more than 2–3 mL/kg of contrast is required for any given injection. The "mechanical stop" available on modern injectors prevents more than the desired amount being delivered. See Table 2-1 for a summary of injection volumes used in various situations, and the relevant chapters for more detailed information.

There are a number of complications associated with the use of power injectors to deliver contrast media, which have been reviewed by Amplatz and Moller[30] who also offer some points on their prevention.

It should be noted that these power injectors usually are mounted on their own mobile stand. Recently, ceiling-mounted injectors have become available for space saving and ease of use.[39]

Radiographic Image

Differences in the ability of a patient's tissues to attenuate an x-ray beam, accentuated by the addition of (usually) iodine-based contrast media, are the basis for cardiac angiography. These differences in the x-ray beam emerging from the patient cause differences in the fluorescence of image intensifier screens. This fluorescence, or emitted visible light, is used to create the image, either analog (as on cine film) or digital.

Numerous reviews deal with the formation of the radiographic image and the equipment used.[40–44] Of these, Moore[42] discusses aspects of the physics of cardiac angiography in detail. A basic understanding is imperative in the rational and safe performance of cardiac catheterization and angiography.

Image Characteristics

A radiographic image has a number of characteristics, all of which are interrelated. Changes in one are usually reflected in concomitant changes in the others. The *density* of the image refers to the degree of blackening. Point-to-point variations in the density of the image are referred to as image *contrast*. Random fluctuations in density of the image, which may or may not be perceptible to the eye, are the image *noise*. While there are a number of contributors to noise, by far the largest is "quantum mottle."

Before evaluating other characteristics of a radiographic image, the perceived density of the angio-

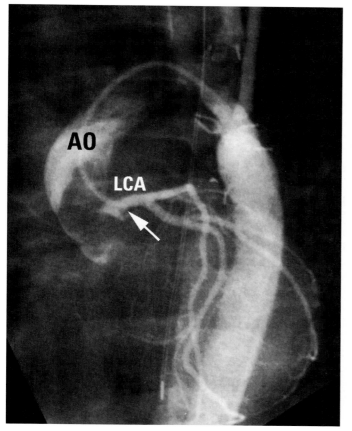

A

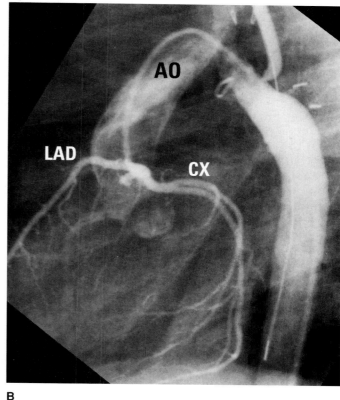

B

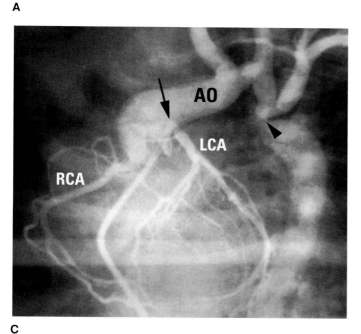

C

Fig. 2-10: Value of a test injection.
Two separate patients. **A:** Shallow LAO projection of an attempted ascending aortogram designed to show a recoarctation. The catheter has inadvertently entered proximal LCA (arrow). **B:** Lateral projection of the same injection. **C:** Another patient. An attempted antegrade aortogram in a mid-LAO projection designed to demonstrate the arch hypoplasia and coarctation (arrowhead). Inadvertently, the catheter has entered proximal LCA (arrow).

graphic image should be adjusted so that it is acceptable: not so black that opacified small vessels become "burned out"; not so white that soft tissues and opacified chambers or vessels merge. After this, attention can be paid to such characteristics as contrast. The smaller the object, the more contrast it must have in or-

der to be visualized. The visibility of an object is proportional to the relationship between its contrast and the surrounding noise. Thus, in order to increase the visibility of a small object, one needs either to increase the contrast of that object or to decrease the noise. This is of special importance in cardiac angiography where

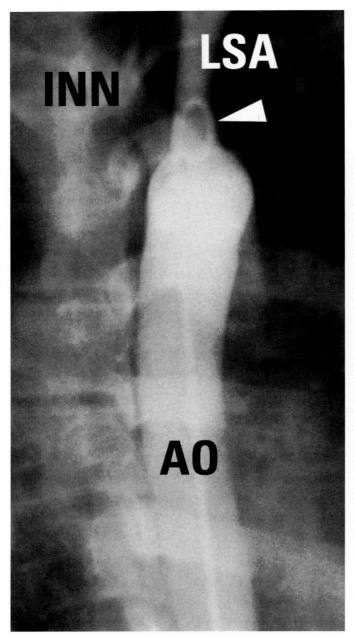

A

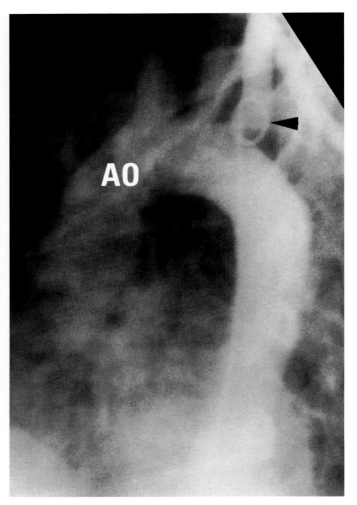

B

Fig. 2-11: Malpositioning of catheters.
Two separate patients. **A:** Retrograde aortogram in shallow RAO and steep LAO **B:** projections show that the pigtail catheter is in the base of LSA rather than in the aorta.

(continued on next page)

one is often attempting to make visible either for fluoroscopy or for hardcopy, small objects such as catheters, guidewires and anatomic structures such as coronary arteries and sinusoids.

Two other characteristics of an image need to be considered. An image usually has *magnification* reflecting distances between the source (focal spot), object (patient) and receptor (image intensifier). In addition, the margins of an object will exhibit some degree of loss of definition, or *blur* (unsharpness). "Total image blur" reflects blur due to focal spot size, motion, image receptor characteristics (scatter of light emitted during fluorescence as well as grain size) and translu-

cency. Of these, focal spot and motion blur are by far the most important. The focal spot is the area on the anode of the x-ray tube while x-rays are produced when bombarded by a stream of electrons. A small focal spot is used when a limited number of x-ray photons are required.

Whether a small or large focal spot are used, the focal spot is not a point source, and thus an object will exhibit a "penumbra" or halo. Thus, increasing the focal spot size will increase blur or alternatively, in order to maintain the same blur or contrast (depending on whether the object is large or small) as the magnification is increased (for instance with an air gap tech-

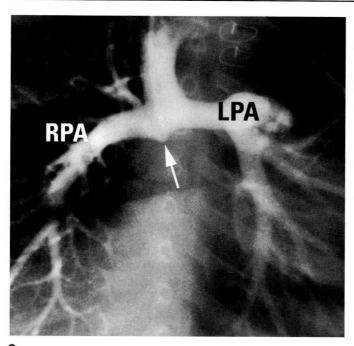

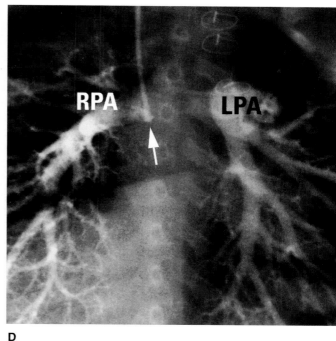

C

D

Fig. 2-11: *(continued).*
C: Another patient. PA injection via the cavopulmonary anastomosis filmed in RAO projection with caudal tilt. Early in the injection, a nipple is appreciated on the inferior margin of RPA (arrow). **D:** As contrast clears, it is evident that this nipple is due to the catheter having been advanced firmly against the wall of the vessel. The malposition of catheters in both patients could potentially have been avoided with test injections.

nique), one needs to use a smaller focal spot size. Motion blur reflects motion of an object during the time of the radiographic exposure. As motion blur is more apparent with increasing magnification and increasing object speed, the blur of, for instance, a coronary artery or a guidewire during systole, will increase as the heart rate increases, if an air-gap or other magnification technique is used, or if the exposure time increases. In the-

ory, to minimize focal spot blur, the object (for instance, the heart) should be as close to the receptor (the image intensifier) as possible to minimize magnification. This in turn, will also minimize motion blur. It is of interest however, that the practicality may be slightly different. Moore[42] points out that heart wall speed has been estimated in adults to be approximately 100 mm/s such that in order to "stop motion," an ex-

Table 2-1

Summary of Contrast Injections

Catheter Location	Contrast Volume* (mL/kg)	Injection Time (seconds)	Notes
Ventricle (for function)	1.0	1.5–2	Injection over 2–3 cycles to avoid ectopics Increase contrast volume if dilated chamber, AV value regurgitation
Ventricle (for shunt)	1.5–2.0	0.5–1	
MPA	1.0	1.0	Use balloon occlusion technique or increase contrast volume if looking at pulmonary veins
Aorta	1.0	1.0	Increase contrast volume if AI or shunt such as PDA
Aorta (balloon occlusion for coronaries)	0.7	1.0	

* Nonionic monomer (eg, Isovue [Squibb Diagnostics, Montreal, Canada]) 300 mg Iodine/mL.
MPA indicates main pulmonary artery; AV, atrioventricular; AI, aortic insufficiency; PDA, patent arterial duct.

posure should have a maximum time of 8 ms. In children, the smaller anatomy and higher wall speeds are reflected in a "stop motion" time of 2 to 3 ms for an exposure. A small focal spot is, however, a less intense radiation source and thus in children, there may be a longer exposure time required in order to achieve an appropriate film blackening. Thus overall, a larger focal spot with a shorter exposure time may give the best combination of focal spot and motion blur!

Moore[42] demonstrates elegantly one of the most important relationships between these various image characteristics for the angiographer, viz: blurring and contrast being dependent on object size. The basic overall principle is that image blur (unsharpness) manifests as blurring of the margins of large objects (such as well-opacified left ventricle or aorta), but as loss of contrast of small objects (such as guidewires and coronary arteries), where large and small are relative to the size of a focal spot.

Image Production

An understanding of the interaction between the patient and the individual components of the radiographic equipment (power supply and x-ray tube, image intensifier, image processor, and cine projector), and how these relate to image "quality" (density, contrast, noise, blur, magnification), require some consideration.

Just as the angiographic image has characteristics of density, contrast, noise, blur, and magnification, any image can also be characterized by the three physical characteristics of the beam. *Tube voltage* refers to the voltage across the x-ray tube, usually specified as kilovolts (kV). *Tube current* refers to the rate of flow of electrons from tube filament to the target (anode) and is usually specified as milliamperes (mA). The *time of exposure* is specified by the time in milliseconds (ms). Current and exposure time are usually grouped together as milliamper per second (mA/s).

An increase in any of the three factors will give a resultant increase in the number of x-ray quanta produced by the x-ray tube, by increasing the efficiency of production if the voltage is increased, or by increasing the number of electrons striking the anode if the current or exposure time is increased.

Increasing the tube voltage results in an increase in the ability of the x-ray beam to penetrate the patient, and thus results in an increase in film blackening or density. For a small change in kilovolts, there is a relatively large change in density such that between about 70 to 90 kV, the rule of thumb is that every increase of 10 kV results in roughly a doubling of the film density. The higher kilovolt beam can penetrate the thicker tissues of the subject without overpenetrating the thinner tissues, but the reverse of this is not the case. Thus, an increase in kilovolts will result in a decrease in image contrast although this effect is not as dramatic as the perceived change in density. With current and exposure time increases, density will slowly increase.

In order to maintain the constant density of the angiographic image, any change in one factor must be offset by a reduction in the others. The "10 kV" rule is a useful rule of thumb and indicates that a doubling of mA/s needs to be offset by a decrease of 10 kV in the 70 to 90 kV range. This concept is of importance with the changing thickness of a patient's mediastinum, through which the x-ray beam travels, either a change in patient or a change in projection. An increase of approximately 4 cm of soft tissue thickness doubles the attenuation of the x-ray beam, referred to as the "tissue half value thickness,"[42] or expressed another way, halves the number of x-ray quanta penetrating the patient, thus giving a decrease in film density. In order to maintain the average density of the radiographic image, the mA/s would need to be doubled or the killivolt potential (kVp) increased by 10.

One does, however, need to consider the trade-offs when manipulating factors to achieve constant image quality as patients and projections change. In the situation described above, an increase in x-ray quanta to compensate for the increased patient thickness achieved by increasing mA/s may increase motion blur, whereas changing from a small to a large focal spot size so as to maintain a constant exposure time may increase the focal spot blur. Such beam manipulation is relatively infrequent in the adult population where the demands on the image system are relatively constant: patient size will usually fall in the range of 50 to 120 kg (a variation of 140%) and imaging will usually involve LV, aorta, and coronaries unless there is a large adult population with congenital heart disease where imaging will likely include RV, PAs, and venous anatomy. In contradistinction, the typical pediatric catheterization laboratory handles patients between 3 and 40 kg (a variation of over 1300%) and imaging is as often designed to show peripheral mediastinal structures (such as shunts and SVC) and branch PAs, as heart and great vessels. No wonder it is so tremendously difficult to maintain a high quality of image in the pediatric laboratory with such variable requirements!

Of the energy of the electrons striking the anode, 99% are converted to heat. Heat production at the anode determines the maximum mA/s, and thus limits how low the kilovolt can be set; in turn, this limits the maximum image contrast that can be achieved. The tube's "power rating" specified in watts (at a standard exposure time of 0.1 seconds by convention) specifies the maximum power ($P = IxV$) that can be applied to the tube to avoid melting the anode target surface. While the type of electrical power, target material, angle and rotational speed, and the focal spot all effect the power rating of the tube, in the pediatric population, for practical purposes, only two factors are of interest: the rotational speed and the focal spot size.

When a small focal spot is selected in order to decrease focal spot blur, heat is deposited in a smaller area of the anode than with a large focal spot, so that power rating will be lower which will limit its use with thicker tissues. Rotation of the anode significantly increases the ability of the tube to dissipate heat and is an absolute requirement during cine filming. High rotational speeds increase the life of the anode, but also contribute to wear of the bearings. During fluoroscopy, a low-speed rotation or even a static tube can be specified, which will potentially reduce the wear on the bearings and potentially extend the tube life. As patient's size increases, the amount of heat produced increases. Delays while the anode cools are rarely, if ever, seen in the pediatric arena. A detailed discussion of all issues related to power rating and heat production can be found in Moore.[42]

Image Receptors

X-rays used to image the patient strike the primary image receptor, the image intensifier. This intensifier may be coupled to television for fluoroscopy and for the making of a digital record ("filmless cine") or coupled to radiographic film to form a cine record.

All these receptor systems have characteristics of speed and blur, which are determined primarily by the image intensifier, and contrast, which is determined primarily by cine film and its processing. *Speed* refers to the sensitivity of the receptor to x-rays, such that an increase in sensitivity requires fewer x-rays to produce an image of a standard optical density. Image intensifier speed can be increased by increasing the size of the phosphor crystals, making the phosphor layer thicker, or by adding a chemical additive that enhances light emission. Speed of film can be increased by increasing the emulsion thickness or by using larger silver halide grains. However, if the receptor is too "fast," the number of x-ray quanta required to achieve an image of appropriate optical density becomes so small that statistical fluctuations ("quantum mottle") become relatively large and the resulting random density variations in the image result in a loss of contrast of small objects, and thus a loss of visibility (resolution).

The characteristic of receptor *blur* refers to the diffusion of light after its emission by the phosphor crystals, either within the phosphor layer of the image intensifier or within the emulsion of the cine film. In essence, blur is equivalent to spatial resolution of the image intensifier and/or film, and is measured by a line pair test pattern of which various types are available. As the spatial resolution of cine film is so much greater than that of the image intensifier, a line pair test pattern

will measure the resolution of the image intensifier (but note that by itself, this measurement is unlikely to reflect the resolution of the imaging chain under usual working conditions, as other sources of image blur may be greater than blur within the receptors). Moore[42] discusses in detail issues of resolution.

Speed and blur are intimately related. Reducing receptor blur, for instance by reducing phosphor crystal size or phosphor layer thickness, will result in a reduction of the number of x-ray quanta absorbed and thus a reduction in "speed." This in turn necessitates an increase in imaging factors such as mA/s in order to achieve the required image optical density or blackening. If this in turn is achieved by increasing the time of exposure then motion blur will increase and if it is achieved by switching from a small to a large focal spot, then focal spot blur will increase. Additionally, patient dose will increase.

As discussed previously, *contrast* refers to the relative point-to-point changes in image density. For cine film, this can be measured under standard conditions by exposing an aluminum step wedge, and measuring the change in image density from step to step of the wedge. This is usually displayed in graphical form plotting optical density against the logarithm of exposure, the Hurter and Driffield curve. Contrast then is the slope of this curve whereas speed is the relative position of the curve along the x-axis. Given the range of densities in the chest, the cine film should be of medium contrast (gamma = 2–2.5) with a long straight line segment covering the range of useful optical densities (the dynamic range). Image intensifiers are so contrast sensitive that it is the cine film that usually determines the contrast of the imaging system. The noise due to quantum mottle with fast systems may so degrade the image that it is necessary to select either a slower receptor system (image intensifier or film) or select a lower contrast film such that the density variations are not so obvious.

The image intensifier is the key receptor in the system. X-rays transmitted through the patients strike the input phosphor of the image intensifier and are converted to visible light. The adjacent photocathode layer absorbs this light, and in turn, releases electrons in direct proportion to the intensity of light absorbed. These electrons are accelerated across the image intensifier tube and focused to the output phosphor that emits a green light. The wavelengths of this output emission must be matched to the cine film if this is being used as the recording medium.

If the magnification mode of the image intensifier is being used, then a smaller area in the center of the input phosphor of the image intensifier is used, but the electrons released are focused onto the same size of output phosphor to achieve the magnification (usually accompanied by an automatic decrease in x-ray beam area). *Conversion factor* refers to the amount of light from the output phosphor relative to the amount of radiation striking the input phosphor. For electronic magnification, the conversion factor is halved, or in practical terms, the radiation needs to be doubled to achieve the same light output (equivalent to image density). With interventional packages now available with fluoroscopic units, high quantum detection efficiency (high QDE) image intensifiers are available. This high QDE is usually achieved by increasing the phosphor thickness so that there is an increase in the conversion factor, but this is at the expense of receptor blur that may be noticeable on the cine film.

Radiation degrades the input phosphor with time, resulting in a loss of conversion factor manifested as an increase in the amount of radiation required to achieve the same image optical density.

Image intensifier resolution (blur) is limited by the scatter of light in the phosphor layer. Resolution is maximal as the center of the image intensifier, with off-axis loss of resolution of up to about 10% that may be noticeable on cine film. This scatter of light will decrease the contrast inherent in the x-ray beam transmitted from the patient by about 5% with a new tube. As the phosphor degrades with time, so the loss of contrast will increase. It is impractical to measure this contrast loss directly, but the percent-of-contrast technique[42] can be incorporated into the quality assurance program.

The location of the image intensifier relative to both the x-ray tube and patient is of relevance to image quality and to imaging factors. One characteristic of the x-ray beam from the "point" source of the focal spot is its divergence. This property is manifest as magnification that is proportional to the distance ratio between the focal spot and patient and between the focal spot and image intensifier. As this ratio increases, magnification increases due to beam divergence, which increases the focal spot and motion components of blur as previously discussed. However, in addition, the intensity of the beam falls off according to the inverse square law so that a doubling of magnification requires a quadrupling of beam intensity to achieve the same image optical density. If this is achieved by increasing mA/s by increasing exposure time, motion blur will further increase and if this is achieved by switching from a small to a large focal spot, then focal spot blur will increase; if this is achieved by increasing the kilovolts, then there will be a reduction in image contrast. Overall, an increase in the amount of radiation required is equivalent to an increase in patient dose.

The image intensifier incorporates a grid on its face so that scatter radiation exiting the patient is absorbed by the lead strips of the grid, and thus will not reach the phosphor of the intensifier where it would contribute to blur. However, this scatter reduction technique comes at a cost to patient irradiation: more x-ray quanta are required if the desired film blackening is to be achieved, thus patient dose increases. If the image intensifier is not placed as close to the patient as practical, then the patient takes a second "hit" in terms of dose as, by the inverse square law, an increase in x-ray quantum is required. (Most cardiac catheterization laboratories are not able to afford the luxury of dedicated small-size, pediatric image intesifiers, so that when imaging children, particularly infants, using a biplane configuration, the image intensifiers cannot be brought close to the patient's chest, thus, an airgap results). If a grid is fixed in place, magnification can only be achieved electronically. If, however, the grid can be removed, magnification can be achieved geometrically using an air-gap technique. The image intensifier is moved away from the patient so that the ratio of focal spot:patient distance and focal spot:intensifier distance is increased, thus the image is magnified. Scatter radiation is absorbed in the air-gap between patient and image intensifier. The cost is in terms of patient dose based on the inverse square law. But the number of x-ray quanta, and thus patient dose required to achieve standard film blackening, is only slightly less with electronic magnification with the intensifier close to the patient and a grid in place than with geometric magnification with an air-gap technique.

Processing of Cine Film

The final recording medium for many pediatric labs remains cine film. The processing requirements of cine film are such that there is, without doubt, a need for a dedicated processor. Processing of the cine film exposed by the light output from the image intensifier magnifies the latent image contained within the silver halide grains of the emulsion by reducing exposed silver halide grains to metallic silver. The image is then fixed. Washing and drying steps are included in the processing.

The developing solution contains developing agents, alkali to adjust the pH, preservatives, and restrainers to prevent fogging of the film (the developing of unexposed silver grains). The complex developing solution must be "replenished" with the various agents at a rate that is appropriate for the amount of cine film being developed. Image degradation can occur with under-replenishment, over-replenishment, or solution that is appropriately replenished but oxidized. Over-replenishment is equivalent to increasing the temperature of the developer, whereas under-replenishment is equivalent to decreasing the temperature. Overall, replenishment problems affect contrast, density, and film fog.

The length of time that the film is in the developing solution and the developing temperature are of critical importance to film density and contrast. The longer the developing time and the higher the temperature, the greater the film density becomes, ie, the H and D curve is shifted to the left. With increasing temperature, the contrast increases, ie, the slope (gamma) of the curve increases. Variations in the temperature of the developer of more than ± 0.25°C are unacceptable (note that variations within other components of the processing system of ±1°C, may be acceptable). Speed variations of greater than ±5% are similarly unacceptable if maintenance of optimum processing conditions is being attempted. Agitation of the developing solution should be even so that there is an even development of the film frame to frame.

Fixing is the process of removing unexposed silver halide grains from the emulsion. In addition to agents to achieve this, the solution contains buffer, stabilizers, and a chemical to harden the film emulsion so as to prevent or minimize shrinkage of the emulsion.

Washing removes the developing and fixing chemicals (browning of the film over time indicates retained fixer). After the washing step, the film must be dried at carefully selected temperatures and humidity. If too hot, the film will become brittle and curl. Too low a temperature or too high a humidity level and the film will become soft and sticky. At various stages of the process, filtration of the chemical solutions removes sediment that would otherwise cling to the film. Some of these processor problems may not manifest for months or years after the fact: an improperly "fixed" image will eventually brown; a slightly sticky film may be stuck together when reviewed weeks or months later; a hard film will eventually begin to break. Thus, processor quality control is an extremely important part of the ongoing quality assurance program. Daily sensitometry should be undertaken. Light from the sensitometer will usually be green so as to match the output phosphor emission of the image intensifier. While a 21-step sensitometer allows a plot of the entire H and D curve, for daily quality assurance, an 11-step sensitometer is adequate. Background and fog, optical density at the speed step, and the difference in contrast between the speed step and the next highest step (contrast index), should all be measured.[45]

Acceptable limits of variation should be set and these parameters then plotted daily. If parameters vary outside the acceptable limits, cine films should not be developed until the variance is corrected. Note that with a change in the batch of film being used, there may be a variation in parameters, especially film speed. Moore[42] describes how to measure these changes and to change the diaphragm (f-stop) of the cine camera lenses so as to maintain on-frame optical density.

Cine Projectors

Cine projectors have developed from the editing projectors used by the motion picture industry. Various models are available, but all are able to accept any 35-mm cine film for projection, thus making cine film the universal language of communication for angiography of the heart and coronary arteries.

There are two types of projector: an intermittent film advance type where a frame of film is briefly stationed and light is projected through this stationary frame, or a rotating prism-type where the films moves continuously over a rotating multifaceted prism through which light is projected. The former gives a sharper image, but is limited in the frame rates that it can achieve. The latter, with its variable speed control, is more user-friendly for both diagnosis and film review.

All projectors require three components: a transport system with variable speed forward and reverse modes; condenser optics to focus the light source into the aperture (modern projectors have a heat-absorbing glass and a fan so that the halogen source will not burn the film); imaging optics to project and focus a bright image onto the screen with brightness, focus, and diaphragm controls.

The projector should not be the limiting step in the imaging chain. The on-frame resolution[42] of the test strip viewed with projector both stationary and running, should be the same as that of the test strip viewed through a magnifying glass. In other words, all the information on the cine frame should be displayed on the projected image. Once this is confirmed, weekly testing of the projector image quality can be done by viewing the resolution charts of the SMPTE test film frames.[42] The projectors should be cleaned weekly to remove dust from the flat surfaces, the condenser glass, and the lens. With the older projector models, the bulb must be centered each time it is changed. With the newer models, replacement, cleaning and positioning of the halogen light source is best left to the company during preventative maintenance. Note that the current through the halogen source should be adjusted to maximize brightness, the source should be centered both up-down and left-right for the projector screen, and the source should be focused so that geometric magnification by moving the projector screen in and out, will maintain the image in focus. Of course, via the inverse square principle, there will be a marked difference in brightness of the image on the small screen compared with a projected image in a conference setting.

Filmless Cine (Digital Imaging)

The exposure of cine film during angiocardiography is achieved by emitted light from the output phosphor of the image intensifier. If, however, digital acquisition and display is desired, the light from this output phosphor can coupled to a matrix of photo cells and displayed on a video display unit (VDU), usually in a matrix of 1024×1024, although higher matrix configurations are now available. Although the advantages of cine film are well known to cardiologists and radiologists, cine film does, however, have a number of disadvantages. Given the increasing shift of the cardiac catheterization laboratory workload from diagnostic to interventional procedures, one of these disadvantages, the lack of postprocessing capability, has become increasingly important.[46] Digital display during the catheterization procedure offers instant replay, postprocessing including measurement, subtraction capabilities, and a contrast sensitivity (at full bit depth) that aids in the assessment of small dimension, low-contrast structures such as guidewires or coronary arteries. Biplane frame rates in a pediatric cardiac laboratory are usually limited to 30 frames per second due to the

enormous volume of data being acquired and processed. These frame rates may be achieved by interleaving data rather than progressive scanning and by decreasing the image matrix, both of which result in a decrease in resolution. Additionally, the gray scale bit depth may be reduced, which reduces contrast and thus visibility of small structures at low contrast. Even with all the factors optimized, the resolution remains rather less than that of cine film.

Two further issues require comment. First, the volume of data required to be stored is enormous and retrieval of archival data may not be easy. This is of particular importance in facilities dealing with congenital heart disease where multiple studies obtained over many years may need to be reviewed. A second issue of

Fig. 2-12: Measurements.
Four separate patients. **A:** A catheter method of correction has been used to measure dimensions in this patient with multiple levels of stenosis after arch reconstruction. **B:** A grid method of correction has been used to measures MAPCA size and stenosis in a patient with tetralogy-type pulmonary atresia. A check using a catheter method of correction indicates that the correct grids have been used, but demonstrates the potential error introduced with the catheter method.
(continued on next page)

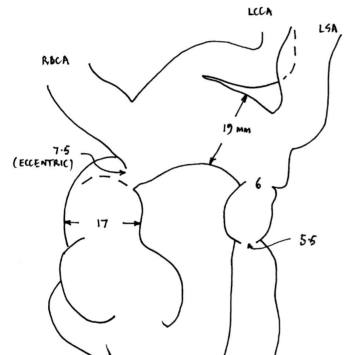

LAO Projection   L. Arch
(Composite Measurements)

Cath method of correction

A

Descending Aortogram (PA)

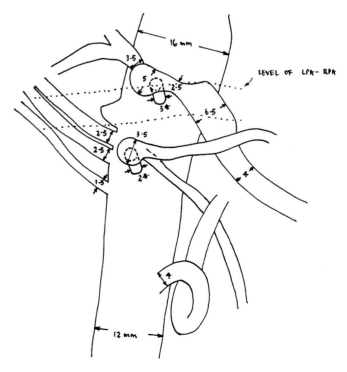

Grid Correction	40/120 = 0.33	PA	40/142 = 0.28	LAT*
Cath Correction	1.67/4 = 0.37		2.1/7 = 0.30	

B

equal importance reflects data portability. Currently, cine film is the universal language of communication for cardiac catheterization studies. Currently, the accepted format for a transport medium is DICOM-3 with the physical format being CD-ROM.[46] Numerous issues must still be resolved, including the issue of data compression.[47]

There is no doubt that in the long term, digital acquisition and storage will become the bench mark, particularly as the resolution of the system improves to come close to, or match, that of cine films. In the meantime however, systems which have both cine and digital acquisition capabilities remain a good compromise.

Measurements

Measuring the dimensions of structures is an important feature in diagnostic studies and in interventional procedures. Whereas the measurement of many structures such as atrial septal defects (ASDs), valve annulus and stenosis, ventricular dimensions, and aortic and patent arterial duct (PDA) dimensions are increasingly the domain of echocardiography, measure-

ments from angiocardiography remains important. PA dimensions and stenoses, aortic dimensions and coarctation, and measurement of MAPCAs and their stenoses are still required. In the interventional arena, measurement of stenoses and surrounding vessels or valve annulus dimensions are done prior to balloon angioplasty or stent placement as well as prior to coil placement during embolization (Fig. 2-12). With the advent of quantitative coronary angiography using edge detection algorithms to estimate coronary artery stenoses, there has been a renewed interest in measurement techniques and accuracy.[48–50] If one wants a true dimension, rather than just a comparative size between two objects on the same cine frame, then the measurement requires correction for magnification by comparison of the measured dimension with a known reference. Thus, various techniques have been developed to estimate a correction factor for magnification using either the injection catheter, grids, spheres of known size, or isocentric techniques.

The renewed interest in measurement technique and accuracy has refocused attention on a number of

TCPC

(Composite Measurements from Multiple Views)

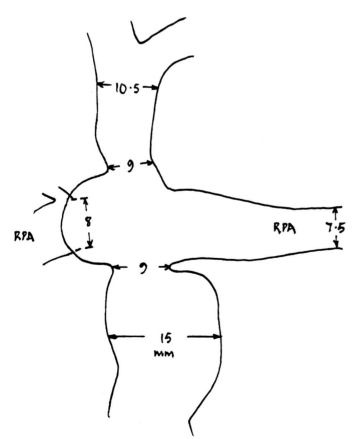

Fig. 2-12: *(continued)*
C: Dimensions of a modified Fontan circuit using a catheter method of correction, reported to the nearest half millimeter. **D:** Dimensions of LPA branches before and after angioplasty. The diagram is traced from the viewing screen but dimensions are measured from the screen, not from the paper tracing.

LPA Branch Dilation
(Composite Dimensions from PA, LAT Projections)

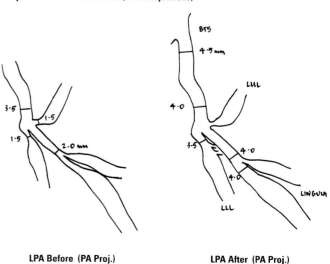

LPA Before (PA Proj.)   LPA After (PA Proj.)

C   D

previously well-known phenomena related to these measurement techniques: there is a large potential error in using a small object of known size (such as a catheter) as a correction factor for measuring objects of large dimension[51,52]; if a catheter is used as a correction factor, measurement of the contrast-filled segment significantly underestimates the catheter diameter compared with the measuring edges of the unopacified catheter,[52,53] as does measurement of the diameter close to the tip where there may be a taper; the edges of a catheter, which are of relatively low inherent contrast, may not be sharp, thus introducing an error reflecting uncertain end points.[54,55] There has been some concern in the literature that the catheter diameters may vary significantly from those stated on the outside of the packet by the manufacturer, however, for a number of standard catheters, this has not been found to be the case.[56]

If not using an isocentric technique for digital measurement, then on principle, we prefer to use a large object such as a grid, to assess a correction factor, recognizing that there is some inherent distortion due to image intensifier geometry at the periphery of the field. There is no doubt that it is cumbersome to film a standard grid at the right distance from the image intensifier for each patient in each projection used, so many catheter laboratories now hold a standard set of grids filmed at varying distances from the image intensifiers (these must be filmed so that the plane of the grid is parallel to the face of the image intensifier). As patients of different sizes are imaged in different projections, a few frames can be clipped from the roll of film containing grids, and spliced to the patient's cine film. To decrease distortion at the edge of the grids, we measure five squares of the standard 1-cm grid in the same area of the cine frame where the object to be measured is present. So as not to claim an accuracy that is not present in the system, we express the measurements to the nearest millimeter or half-millimeter. As an additional check, we also do a rough calculation using the catheter as a correction factor just to confirm that the correct grid has been used for measurement!

Quality Control

Quality control of the imaging chain in the cardiac catheterization laboratory has been extensively discussed,[42] and summarized.[30,44,57,58] Regular planned testing (daily, weekly, or monthly) of the various components of the imaging chain by catheter laboratory staff has been described. By far, the most important of these are quality control of the processor and quality control of the viewing conditions. Testing by catheterization laboratory staff and service-level testing is discussed in detail by Moore.[42]

Apart from planned quality control , however, the ability to optimize image quality and to recognize problems as they arise, is not easy, but is of extreme importance and is a test of one's fundamental understanding of factors affecting the imaging chain. The following summarizes information from various sources.[30,42,44]

1. Image Density: the image is too dark or too light.
   a. The centering of the region of interest within the image intensifier field is incorrect: as the automatic brightness control is based on an average optical density of the image, too much lung or too much soft tissue (such as chin or liver) in the image may contribute to the region of interest being burned out or underpenetrated.
   b. Where possible, tight coning of the image should be achieved. Filters can be used to even out some changes in density, or lead strips can be applied directly to the under-couch tube to exclude air outside the chest wall as in an RAO projection of a left ventriculogram or a lateral projection of a right ventriculogram. If the cones are too wide, scatter will contribute to a decrease in image contrast.
   c. Processing factors are extremely important in achieving the desired optical density: incorrect temperature or processing time will contribute not only to a change in image density, but to a change in contrast.
   d. The film characteristics may be incorrect, either too fast or too slow.
   e. The diaphragm (iris) may be open too wide or closed too tightly.
2. Image Contrast: Operator error and patient characteristics contribute to most of the problems of image contrast.
   a. Large patient size requires an increase in kVp, and additionally, there is increase in scatter radiation, both of which contribute to a decrease in image contrast.
   b. The iodinated contrast medium injection is a major operator variable contributing to image contrast. The higher the iodine concentration of the contrast selected, the better the opacification will be. Larger volumes of contrast injected at faster rates result in increased opacification, and thus, increased contrast of the image.
   c. kVp selection: If this is selected manually, too high a kVp for the size of the pediatric patient will result in a decrease in image contrast. Additionally, there will be a reduction in mAS reflected in an increase in noise due to quantum mottle and thus a decrease in image contrast, particularly where one is attempting to see small objects.

d. The imaging factors need to be appropriate for the grid or gridless technique; if the grid is in place, this needs to be properly oriented.

e. A frame rate of 60 frames per second is often desirable for pediatric studies, but there is less time for anode cooling and thus a higher kVp is selected that decreases image contrast.

f. Processing factors are of great importance and if the contrast is too "flat" or too "contrasty" one needs to confirm that the daily sensotometric measurement falls within the limits that have been set. A change in temperature or in processing time can contribute to a change in image contrast, as can a change in chemistry.

g. The film gradient itself may have been incorrectly selected, either too fast or too slow.

h. A gradual change in image contrast may reflect an old or dirty projector bulb that will adversely affect beam strength and cast a brownish light.

i. A gradual decrease in contrast of the angiographic image may also reflect degradation of the image intensifier phosphors or pickup tube reflected in a decreased gain of the system.

3. Image Noise:
a. For a patient of a given size, selection of an increasingly high kVp results in a concomitant reduction in mAS; if mAS is reduced to a sufficiently low level, then quantum mottle, the major contributor to noise, will be evident.

b. The dose per frame can be set both for fluoroscopy and for cine filming and will vary with the image intensifier mode in use. Whereas the lowest possible setting is desirable to reduce patient dose, too low a setting will result in quantum mottle.

c. If a fast cine film has been selected (large grain size or thicker emulsion), this will be reflected in noise of the image.

4. Image Blur (unsharpness):
a. The resolution of the imaging chain most often reflects patient and operator issues. As blur increases, large structures are perceived as having unsharp margins. Conversely, structures of small inherent contrast such as small vessels or guidewires, are seen as losing resolution.

b. Resolution of the imaging chain (without the patient) is evaluated by various tests, including a line pair test. Assuming that the projector is not at fault (see below), then a reduction in line pair resolution may reflect a change in the image intensifier phosphor, focus, or gain of the pick-up tube, all of which fall within the domain of the servicing representative.

c. Line pair resolution viewed with a magnifying glass should be the same as when the line pair test pattern on a cine film strip is viewed on the projector. If not, then strength of the light beam and focus of the projector optics need to be checked.

d. Selection of the focal spot needs to be appropriate to the patient size as the focal spot geometry contributes to penumbra (but see the comments above concerning the interplay between focal spot size and imaging time).

e. If the image intensifier is not brought as close to the chest of the patient as possible, then the beam geometry is reflected in some magnification of the image and the resulting increase in penumbra contributes to unsharpness.

f. Motion unsharpness, particularly evident with the heart rates of pediatric patients, reflects the pulse width of the beam.

Radiation Protection

Radiation protection issues are important not just for the patient but for laboratory personnel as well. Additionally, a dose of x-radiation has an impact on the life of the imaging chain, particularly the image intensifier.

Numerous reviews of radiation protection in the cardiac catheterization laboratory are available.[40,59–63] On a more general note, the ICRP principles for protection of the patient in diagnostic radiology have been summarized.[64]

The genetic and somatic risks of ionizing radiation have been well discussed[42,64] with recent work suggesting that children are more sensitive to ionizing radiation than adults. While the unit of radiation exposure is the roentgen (R), the absorbed dose, in units of gray, is more relevant for patient and operator dose discussions.

The most important factors in patient and operator dose are the fluoroscopy dose and dose per cine frame chosen for the imaging chain in any particular catheterization laboratory. Patient dose reflects not only the amount of tissue irradiated, but also secondary radiation due to scatter within the patient's soft tissues. Assuming that the fluoroscopy and cine frame doses have been set as low as reasonably possible and that progressive pulse fluoroscopy rather than continuous flouroscopy is used, patient dose can be reduced by coning individual images as tightly as possible, by using additional filters and lead bars, by keeping the image intensifier as close to the patient's chest as is possible (unless an air-gap technique is used), by using an appropriate grid for the patient's size, and by avoiding unnecessary fluoroscopy and angiography.

The primary beam leaving the patient is detected by the image intensifier unless it is absorbed either in air or by the operator's fingers or hand in the primary beam. Secondary radiation due to scatter can contribute to image intensifier exposure, although this can be reduced somewhat by use of a grid or an air-gap technique. It is this secondary radiation, however, that is of special importance to the operator, assuming he or she does not place a body part in the primary beam.

The operator can reduce dose due to scatter radiation in a number of ways. During fluoroscopy, standing as far away from the patient (and thus the beam) as possible reduces the amount of scatter radiation reaching the operator. This is particularly important with cranially or caudally angled projections and with large patients. Apart from standard apron shielding, additional shielding can be gained with a thyroid shield and leaded eye glasses. Additionally, a movable shield can be placed between the operator and the patient. During cineangiography, there is usually no need for any personnel to remain in the laboratory, as long as the patient and monitors can be viewed from the control room. Overall, fast efficient catheterization with a minimum of fluoroscopy/angiography, with appropriate fluoroscopy/angiography image doses, and meticulous attention to techniques of radiation protection, are the most important contributors to minimizing both the patient's and the operator's absorbed dose.

Part II. Angiographic Projections

Part II of this chapter encompasses a discussion of standard angiographic approaches, how to achieve them and how to apply these projections in a segmental approach to identifying chamber morphology, and the tracing of the atrioventricular (AV) and ventriculoarterial (VA) connections. This discussion emphasizes modification of these standard projections to achieve a flexible approach to imaging complex malformations or abnormalities of position. A detailed discussion of the imaging of specific lesions can be found in the appropriate chapters.

In the management of patients with congenital heart disease, the spatial orientation and the morphology of the heart of the cardiac connections and malformations are of critical importance. The anatomy of the systemic and pulmonary veins, the cardiac chambers and the great arteries, as well as the connections between them and their relationships to each other, all need to be clearly identified. Any abnormal communications or obstructions need to be localized and evaluated. In each patient, the segmental approach[65–69] is logical in order to correctly identify the connections and morphology; this approach becomes especially important in evaluating children with complex congenital heart disease (see also Chapters 3, 35, 36, and 44).

The overall understanding of an individual patient's cardiac anatomy will be based on a synthesis of data from numerous imaging techniques including chest x-ray, magnetic resonance imaging (MRI), echocardiography, and cardiac angiography. In spite of advances in echocardiography and more recently, MRI, plain film radiography and cardiac catheterization and angiography still play important roles. Good quality cineangiography based on the principles discussed in Part I, and correctly interpreted, provides pivotal morphological data that influences management decisions.

Selective angiocardiography was described by Chavez[70] after the introduction of clinical cardiac catheterization in 1941 by Cournand and Ranges.[71] Modifications to the techniques for cineangiocardiography developed rapidly.[72] The standard approach had been frontal and lateral projections for virtually all angiocardiograms, but a landmark paper[73] introduced the concept of imaging along anatomic planes that incorporated tilting of the image intensifier cranially to help with the profiling of specific cardiac structures. This axial approach to angiocardiography was popularized by Bargeron and Soto,[74,75] although their summary paper[75] implied that most projections needed to incorporate cranial-tilt. Brandt and Calder[67,76,77] advocated a more flexible approach to the imaging of children with congenital heart disease using a wider range of angiographic projections.

In most patients, the heart is oriented obliquely to all three body planes with the left ventricular apex being rather more leftward, anterior, and inferior than the base of the heart (Fig. 2-13). In young children, this axis is a little more horizontal; as the child grows, the inferior direction of the apex becomes more pronounced, and is particularly so in those with a tall, narrow physique. Similarly, those who have a narrow anteroposterior diameter intuitively will have a rather more coronal orientation of the heart within the chest than those who have a deeper anteroposterior diameter.

The interventricular septum is a complex geometric structure describing an "S" from apex to base (Fig. 2-14), often referred to as the sigmoid septum (see also Chapter 6).[78] From its caudal to cranial aspect, the interventricular septum curves through an arc of approximately 100° to 120°. The right ventricle (RV) essentially forms an appliqué of the LV.[79] Whether using movement of the patient beneath fixed equipment, or less patient movement beneath mobile equipment (the usual situation currently) angiocardiography has now matured and uses a wide range of projections, often in-

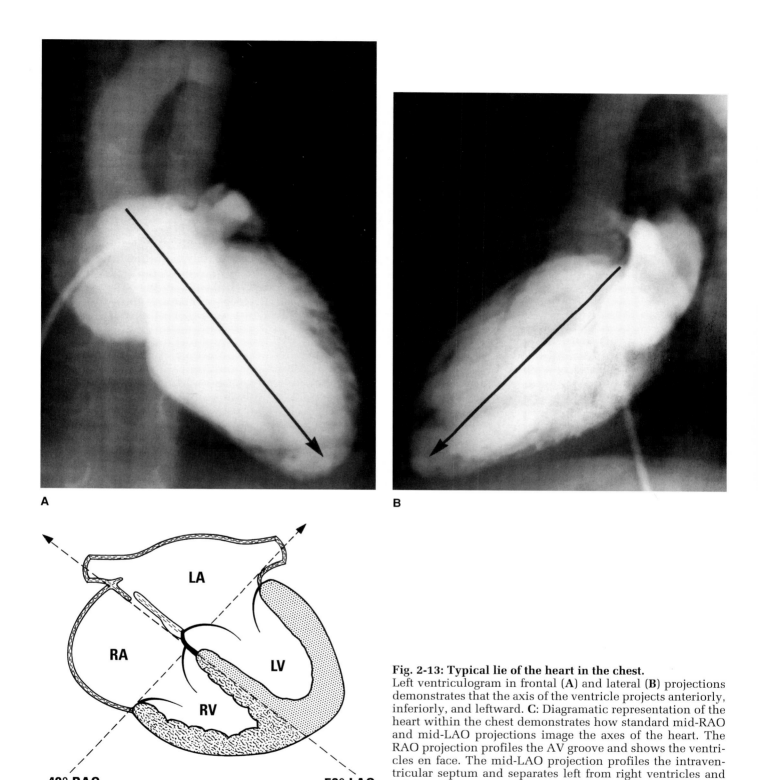

A

B

C

40° RAO

50° LAO

LA

RA

LV

RV

Fig. 2-13: Typical lie of the heart in the chest.
Left ventriculogram in frontal (**A**) and lateral (**B**) projections demonstrates that the axis of the ventricle projects anteriorly, inferiorly, and leftward. **C**: Diagramatic representation of the heart within the chest demonstrates how standard mid-RAO and mid-LAO projections image the axes of the heart. The RAO projection profiles the AV groove and shows the ventricles en face. The mid-LAO projection profiles the intraventricular septum and separates left from right ventricles and left from right atria.

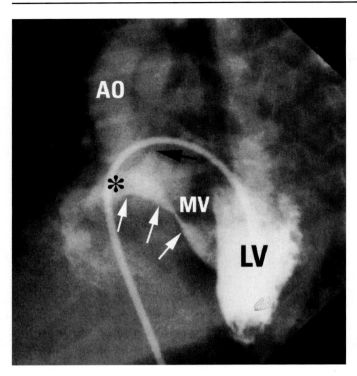

Fig. 2-14: Sigmoid septum.
Antegrade approach via atrial septum and mitral valve to LV filmed in long-axial oblique projection. Aortic-mitral continuity is evident (black arrow). The extreme sigmoid sweep of this patient's septum is well seen (white arrows). Contrast mixes from left to right across the VSD (✱).

corporating caudocranial (CaCr) or craniocaudal (CrCa) angulation of the x-ray beam as part of a compound projection to outline or profile specific structures. Angiographic imaging is enhanced by the selection of projections which image along anatomic planes (often with two projections at right angles) and with the selection of projections that minimize overlapping and foreshortening of structures.

Terminology

Angiographic projections are designated according to standard radiographic convention either using the position of the recording device as the reference, or using the direction of the x-ray beam toward the recording device (usually the image intensifier), as the reference.[80] When the image intensifier is directly above the supine patient, the x-ray beam travels from posterior to anterior, thus the projection is designated postero-anterior (PA) or based on intensifier position, frontal. This image intensifier position by convention is designated 0°. When the intensifier is moved through 90° to a position beside the patient, usually the left side, a lateral projection results. Between these two positions of 0° and 90°, there are a multitude of projections termed LAO. With the intensifier moving to the right of the patient's midline, RAO and right lateral projections are

achieved, and again, there are a multitude of RAO projections between these two standard positions. When the intensifier travels through an arc that is posterior to the patient (x-ray tube becomes anterior), right posterior oblique (RPO), antero-posterior (AP) and left posterior oblique (LPO) projections are achieved (Fig. 2-15), although are rarely, if ever, required.

Standard angiographic imaging equipment not only allows the image intensifier-x-ray tube C-arm to be rotated around the transverse axis of the supine patient, but also allows the tube to angled toward the patient's feet or head. Again, using the direction of the x-ray beam toward the recording device as the standard, CaCr and CrCa projections respectively are achieved (Fig. 2-16).

In summarizing the above projections, it becomes apparent that the convenient terms RAO, LAO, PA, and lateral (left) designate the position of the recording device. As the lateral projection usually has the image intensifier to the left of the patient, this position will be implied by use of the term lateral unless otherwise specified. Additionally, in order to simplify the terminology as much as possible, a cranial image intensifier

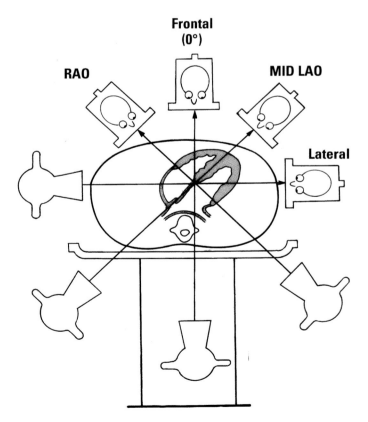

Fig. 2-15: Naming of standard projections with an under-couch x-ray tube.
The thorax of the supine patient is viewed as if the observer were standing at the feet. The standard projections are designated according to the position of the image intensifier.

position will be referred to as cranially-tilted or simply cranial rather than the more cumbersome CaCr projection, designating the direction of the x-ray beam. Similarly, caudally-tilted or simply caudal will be used to refer to the image intensifier position in a CrCa projection. Even with these simplifications, two of the compound LAO projections, cranially-tilted shallow LAO and cranially-tilted mid-LAO, are something of a mouthful and may be used interchangeably with four-chamber and LAO projections, respectively.

While by definition, the term projection refers to the course of the x-ray beam, to make things as simple as possible, the term projection will be used to refer to the image intensifier position, and will be used interchangeably with the term view.

The common projections used in cineangiography are listed in Table 2-2, together with any alternative terminology used in the literature. The angle(s) denote the position of the image intensifier using the frontal projection in a supine patient as the reference projection of 0°. Examples of fluoroscopy equipment positions for these common projections are outlined in Fig. 2-17.

Biplane Angiography

Dedicated pediatric cardiac catheter laboratories often incorporate a biplane imaging unit. Biplane angiography has the advantages of reducing the contrast load to the patient, of special importance in neonates and infants. Additionally, this allows an assessment of motion of structures and contrast flow in two projections recorded simultaneously. There is, however, a cost. Given the size of image intensifiers used currently in biplane equipment, this cost is usually a compro-

Table 2-2	
Summary of Projections	
Projection	*Angles*
Conventional RAO	40° RAO
Mid-RAO	
Frontal	0°
PA	
Shallow LAO	1°–30° LAO
Straight LAO	31°–60° LAO
Mid-LAO	
Steep-LAO	61°–89° LAO
Left Lateral	90° Left
Cranially tilted RAO	30° RAO + 30° Cr
Elongated RAO	
Cranially tilted Frontal	0° + 30°–45° Cr
Sitting up	
Cranially tilted shallow LAO	25° LAO + 30° Cr
Hepatoclavicular four-chamber	
Cranially tilted mid LAO	50° LAO + 30° Cr
Long axial oblique	
Cranially tilted steep LAO	70° LAO + 30° Cr
Caudally tilted frontal	0° + 45° Ca
Barrel	(May need shallow LAO
Orifice	or RAO; May need to
Laid-Back	place bolster under hips
	to achieve required
	caudal tilt)

mise in the projections that can be achieved simultaneously, usually less than ideal. For very small children, this large size of intensifier means that they cannot both be brought close to the patient. Thus, an air-gap technique results that of necessity increases the patient dose, especially if the grids cannot be removed. If the grids can be removed, this air-gap can be used to advantage to achieve magnification, to allow small structures to be visualized as discussed above.

The choice of simultaneous projections will depend not only on the information required and on intensifier size but also on equipment capability (mobile or fixed), patient size, and the ability to manipulate patient position. Standard biplane configurations include RAO/LAO (together with cranial or caudal tilt of the image intensifier for compound projections) and frontal/lateral (again, potentially with cranial and caudal tilt). However, the possible combinations are almost endless and some approaches incorporate a double-LAO combination (25° LAO with 40° cranial tilt, 70° LAO with 50° cranial tilt) (Fig. 2-18), useful for profiling for example, both the inlet and outlet extensions of perimembranous VSDs (*see* Fig. 2-40).

The Cranial—LAO Projections: The Key Group of Angiographic Projections

We consider a working understanding of this key group of projections to be of critical importance in the

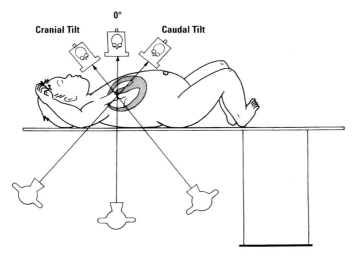

Fig. 2-16: Naming of standard projections with an under-couch x-ray tube.
Convention is that the terms, cranial tilt and caudal tilt refer to the position of the image intensifier.

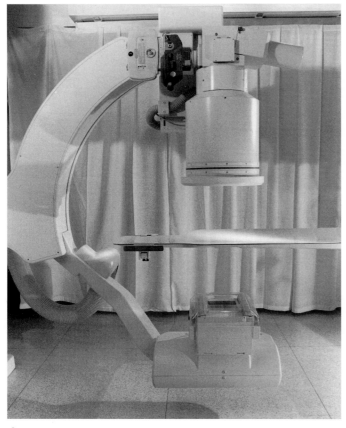

A

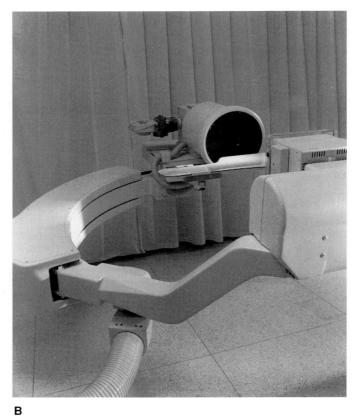

B

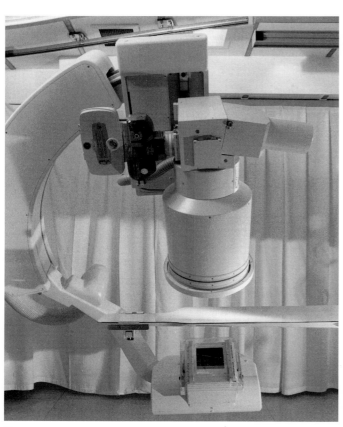

C

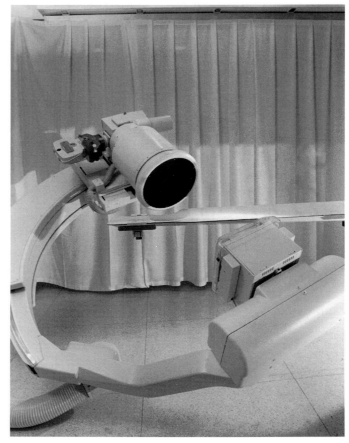

D

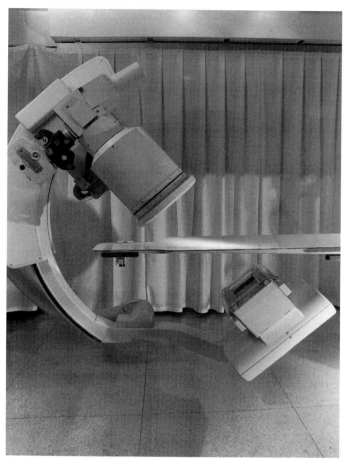

E

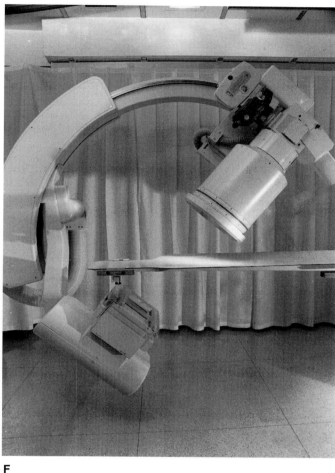

F

Fig. 2-17: Standard projections.
A: Frontal (PA). **B**: Lateral. **C**: RAO. **D**: Mid-LAO with cranial tilt (long-axial oblique). **E**: Cranially-tilted frontal (sitting up). (**F**) Caudally-tilted frontal.

use of a flexible approach to the filming of congenital heart disease. Indeed, a cookbook approach to imaging, where standard projections at fixed angles are used to image every child with congenital heart disease, produces passable angiography in most situations (although often testing the operator's skill in image interpretation!). However, a working understanding of the complexities of normal cardiac anatomy, particularly the interventricular septum, and the imaging of that septum with different projections, allows one to adjust the projection (or the patient position) based on the fluoroscopic image, thus profiling angiographically specific regions of interest to maximize the information obtained. Additionally, such an understanding allows a flexible approach to the imaging of complex lesions in a manner which could be termed "designer angiography."

There are a number of rules of thumb that allow the operator to judge the steep or shallow nature of an LAO projection. Of importance are the relationship of

the cardiac silhouette to the spine, and the position of the venous catheter and ventricular apex.

In order to profile the mid-point of the membranous component of the ventricular septum (and thus the majority of perimembranous VSDs), aim to have approximately two-thirds of the cardiac silhouette to the right of the vertebral bodies, thus one-third of the silhouette projected over and to the left of the vertebral bodies (Figs. 2-19 and 2-20). This will usually result in a cranially tilted left ventriculogram showing the LV septal margin, with the apex and the LV component of a venous catheter (via atrial septum and mitral valve) pointing directly to the bottom of the image. A shallower projection will have more of the cardiac silhouette projected over and to the left of the spine and will profile the more infero-basal aspect of the septum, ideal for inlet or basal VSDs. Additionally, this allows an evaluation of AV valve relationships (such as in AV septal defects or criss-cross heart), inlet extension of perimembranous VSDs down between the two AV

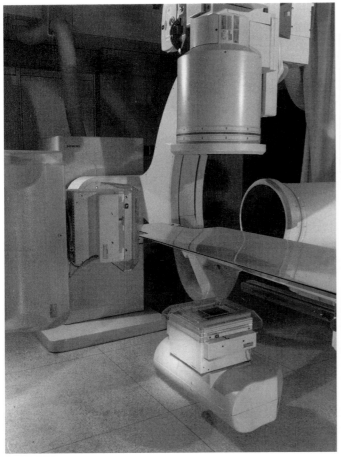

A

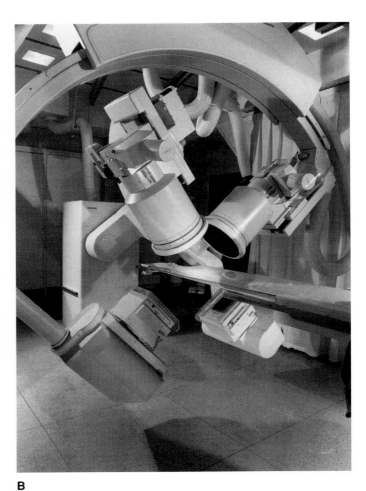

B

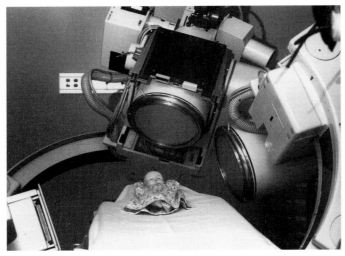

C

Fig. 2-18: Biplane configurations.
A: Frontal and lateral. **B**: RAO and LAO. **C**: Shallow LAO with cranial tilt and steep LAO with cranial tilt (double LAO).

valves, and posterior muscular VSDs. In this situation, the ventricular apex, the catheter through the mitral valve and the LV septal margin, will all point more to the (operator's) right side of the image (Figs. 2-19 and 2-20). A steeper projection, coming more around toward a left lateral position, will have less of the silhouette across the spine or will in fact separate the spine and the cardiac silhouette completely, the closer the projection is toward a true lateral. In this situation, the LV septal margin, the ventricular apex and the venous catheter through the mitral valve, will all point toward the (operator's) left side of the image (Fig. 2-19). This steep cranial-LAO projection can be used to profile the outlet extension of perimembranous VSDs, sometimes the lower margin of a conal/infundibular VSD, and defects in the anterior muscular or apical region. However, the lateral shoulder of the left ventricle may hide the outflow tract if adequate cranial tilt is not achieved.

The use of the catheter to indicate the position of the ventricular apex, is not reliable if the venous catheter has been advanced to the left ventricle via a VSD, or an arterial catheter is used via a retrograde approach. In both cases, the catheter tip tends to be rather more basal and postero-left lateral in position.

Three major factors may require the cranially-tilted LAO projection to be modified in order to achieve an adequate image of the chosen anatomy. If previous imaging such as with echocardiography or the test injection with contrast, show a significant discrepancy in sizes of the two ventricles (such as tetralogy with an enlarged and heavily trabeculated right ventricle, or in left or right ventricular hypoplasia), the septum may be rotated accordingly and the LAO projection may need to be steepened or made more shallow in order to profile the appropriate part of the septum. Second, turning the patient's head to the right to avoid irradiation during the cranially-tilted LAO projection, will also turn the patient's thorax, and thus steepen the LAO projection. In this case, the clue often is in the amount of heart over the spine, and one usually needs to make the projection more shallow to compensate. Third, cardiac position may vary as with meso or dextrocardia or the position may reflect thoracic shape as with scoliosis or pectus excavatum.

When setting up a cranially-tilted LAO projection for a left ventriculogram, the first step is to achieve the desired steep or shallow LAO projection; after that, one needs to be sure that a good amount of cranial tilt has been achieved so as to open out the apical-basal dimension of the septum. This can be estimated in the LAO projection by how much of this cardiac silhouette is projected over the hemidiaphragms, with more superimposition as more cranial tilt is achieved (as a result, it is useful in intubated patients to have the anaesthetist suspend respirations at full inspiration or in cooperative patients, to have them hold their breath in

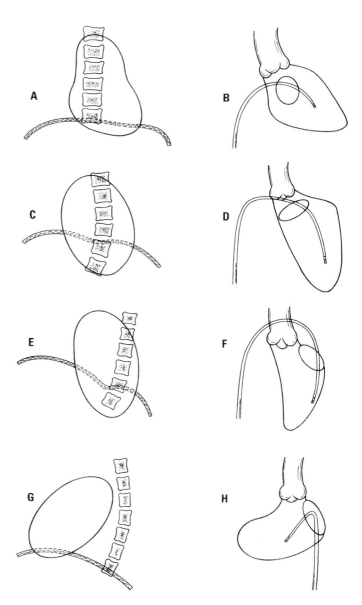

Fig. 2-19: Setting up the standard LAO projections.
The reference projection is the LAO. On fluoroscopy of the patient's chest, aim for approximately a third of the cardiac silhouette to be overlying or to the left of the spine as is in **E**. A venous catheter via the mitral valve will point straight down toward the floor **F** and on a test injection and ventriculogram, the interventricular septal margin should point straight down toward the floor. To achieve a four-chamber position, we initially aim to have approximately half of the cardiac silhouette across or to the left of the spine as in **C**. The catheter via the mitral valve will then point toward the bottom left aspect of the fluoroscopy image as in **D** as will the ventricular axis during contrast injection. For a steep LAO projection, we aim to initially separate the cardiac silhouette from the spine as in **G**. A catheter via the mitral valve will point toward the bottom right aspect of the fluoroscopy image **H** as will the ventricular axis during contrast injection. **A** and **B** show frontal projections.

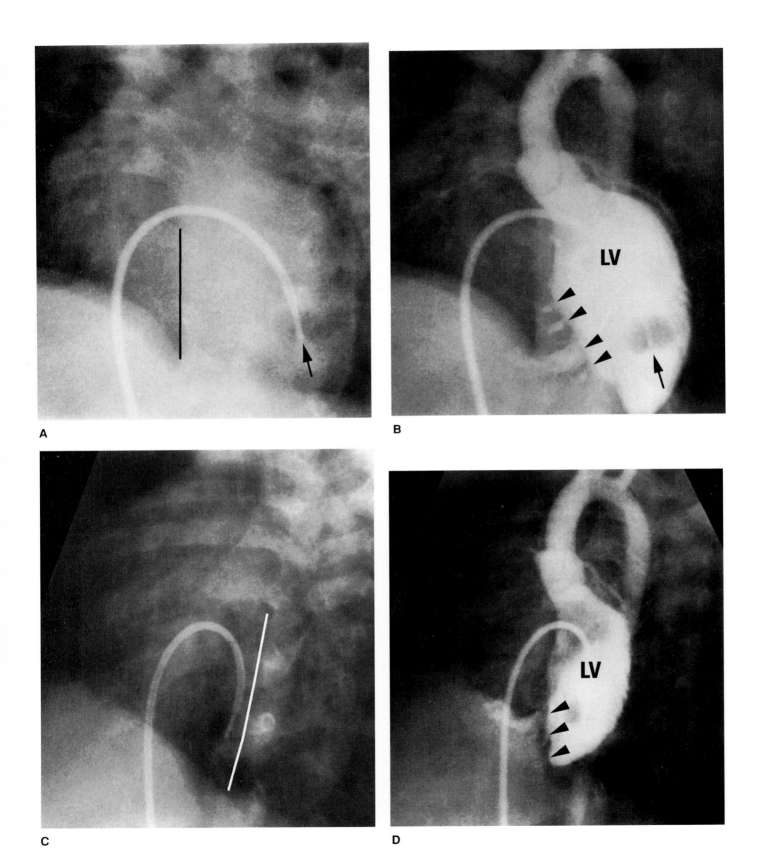

deep inspiration, so as to minimize the superimposition of the abdominal structures on the ventriculogram). Additionally, the amount of cranial tilt can be judged based on the course of the venous catheter via the mitral valve to left ventricle: with a good amount of cranial tilt, the catheter will have a long course down to the apex at the lower aspect of the image, but with lesser° of cranial tilt, the catheter will have an apparent shorter course such that with a straight LAO projection, it will appear to come straight toward the viewer (Fig. 2-21).

Usually the left ventricular apex is directed caudally but in some children there is an upturned apex such as in tetralogy or in those with a marked lumbar lordosis. In these situations, an attempted cranial projection may look like a straight LAO (Fig. 2-21). Thus in order to open out the apex to base dimension of the interventricular septum, a caudally-tilted LAO projection can be considered. Note that the upturned apex may result from padding under the child's hips (to elevate the pelvis for vessel puncture at the groin) so, as a matter of principle, this padding should be removed to reduce the natural lumbar lordosis and thus maximize the amount of cranial tilt that can be achieved.

Venoatrial Connections

The first step in applying a segmental approach to the identification of cardiac connections is to identify and localize the atria, usually based on electrocardiogram (ECG)[69] and echocardiography,[69] with plain chest and abdominal films sometimes providing useful clues.[66,79] Based on the rule of visceroatrial concordance,[65,66] abdominal visceral situs and bronchial anatomy offer clues,[81] although bronchial anatomy particularly is very often difficult to be confident of on neonatal films. More reliable is the rule of venoatrial concordance[65,66] whereby the atrium receiving the hepatic portion of the IVC is almost exclusively the morphologically right atrium (see Chapters 3 and 41). By exclusion, the contralateral atrium is the morphologically left atrium, a useful practical rule of thumb except where heterotaxy syndromes are suspected; in these situations, the morphology cannot be assumed (see Chapters 3 and 41).

If not already established by noninvasive means or by assessment of the catheter course during cardiac

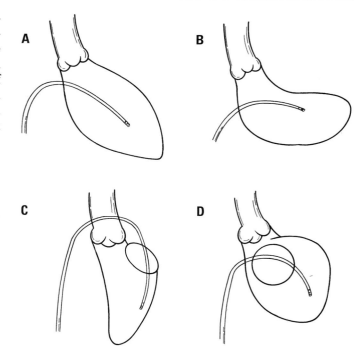

Fig. 2-21: Achieving cranial tilt.
Usually, the left ventricular axis, as seen from an RAO projection (**A**) points caudally and to the patient's left. Thus, a LAO projection, will open out the dimension between the aortic valve and the ventricular apex as in (**C**). If the child has an upturned apex as in tetralogy of Fallot, or if the bolster remains under the child's hips, the RAO projection will look like (**B**). Adding the usual amount of cranial tilt to a mid-LAO projection will not adequately open out the apex to base dimension of the left ventricle but rather, will look down the barrel of the ventricles as in (**D**). This can be corrected either by adding more cranial tilt, or by removing the bolster from under the child's hips.

catheterization, demonstration of systemic venoatrial connections and atrial morphology is best performed by inferior vena cava (IVC) and/or superior vena cava (SVC) injections in frontal and lateral projections (see Chapter 12) or by atrial injections filmed in RAO and cranially-tilted shallow LAO projections; the shallow LAO projection usually profiles the interatrial septum while the addition of cranial tilt not only improves the information about atrial septal morphology (Figs. 2-22 and 2-23), but also gives information as to AV connections (Fig. 2-24).[67]

Fig. 2-20: Achieving standard LAO projections.
A: For a four-chamber projection, note that approximately half the cardiac silhouette is across or to the left of the spine and the catheter points toward the bottom left-hand aspect of the image. During ventriculogram (**B**), the ventricular apex and catheter (arrow) point toward the bottom left aspect of the image. The basal aspect of the interventricular septum is profiled and is intact. The multiple mid-muscular VSDs (arrowheads) are not well profiled. For a LAO projection, about a third of the cardiac silhouette is over or to the left of the spine and the catheter points down toward the bottom of the frame. **C:** During ventriculography (**D**), the ventricular apex points toward the bottom of the frame and a number of the mid-muscular VSDs are now profiled (arrowheads).

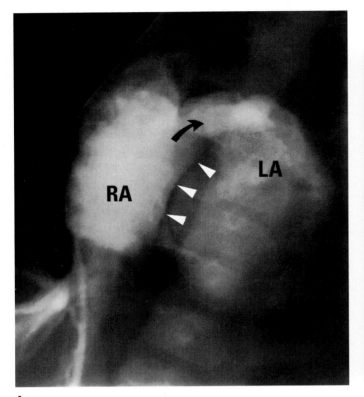

A

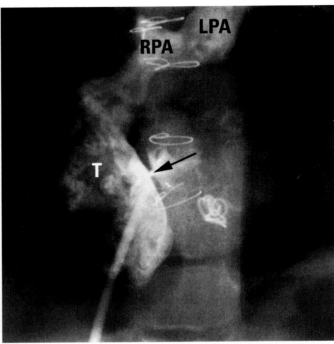

B

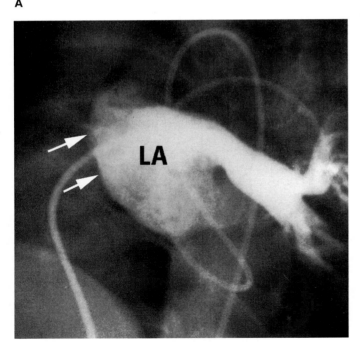

C

Fig. 2-22: Atrial septal profile.
Three separate patients. **A**: Shallow LAO projection of RA injection. The ASD is well profiled (curved arrow) and as contrast fills the left atrium, the atrial septum is apparent (arrowheads). **B**: Injection in lateral tunnel of a Fontan circuit filmed in frontal projection. After closure of the tunnel fenestration with an umbrella device, some residual right-to-left mixing is apparent. The density of the central aspect of the umbrella device (arrow) and the wall of the tunnel, are beautifully profiled. **C**: Pulmonary vein injection filmed in a shallow LAO projection with cranial tilt. The atrial septum is well profiled (arrows) and contrast is just beginning to shunt left to right in this patient with left AV valve atresia.

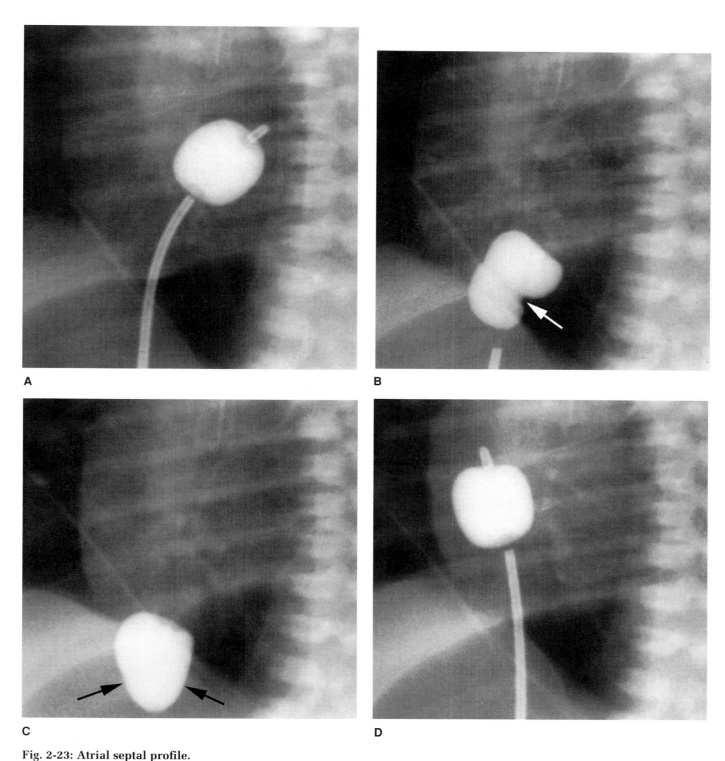

Fig. 2-23: Atrial septal profile.
Mid-LAO projections during balloon atrial septostomy separating the expected positions of RA and LA. **A**: Initially, the catheter is in the LA and does not project beyond the cardiac contour, thus is not in the LAA. An RAO projection prior to balloon inflation indicated that the catheter was neither directed posteriorly into a pulmonary vein nor anteriorly through the mitral valve. **B**: During withdrawal of the catheter, the indentation due to the atrial septal margin (arrow) immediately prior to tearing is apparent. **C**: As the catheter is withdrawn into the IVC, the typical tapering is seen (arrows). **D**: The catheter is advanced to the RA. (Courtesy of Dr. J. M. Ormiston, Green Lane Hospital, Auckland, New Zealand).

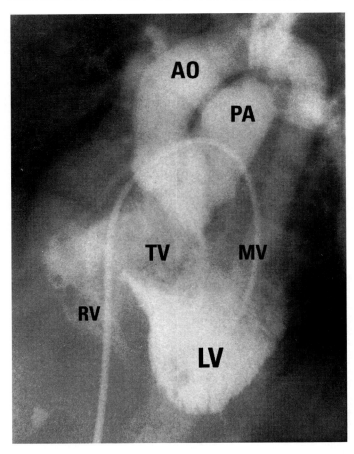

Fig. 2-24: Atrioventricular connection.
Ventriculogram filmed in four-chamber projection. Projecting the expected plane of the interventricular septum back to the level of the AV valves indicates how the right AV valve overrides the septum.

Pulmonary Venoatrial Connections

The pulmonary venous connections to the atria are so variable that they can never be assumed (see also Chapters 24 and 41). If the echocardiac information is not confirmed on the levophase of pulmonary or ventricular angiography, balloon occlusion pulmonary angiography (using a large contrast bolus and a long cine run at a slower frame rate) or direct injection into each of the pulmonary veins (Fig. 2-22c), can be undertaken. Usually, a projection that profiles the interatrial septum, usually a cranially-tilted shallow LAO projection, gives adequate information as to which side of the atrial septum the pulmonary veins return to. If specific information about each of the pulmonary veins and particularly their ostia needs to be obtained, then normally positioned right and left pulmonary veins can be demonstrated by shallow RAO and LAO projections respectively. The lower pulmonary veins enter the left atrium in a plane that is slightly posterior to the upper pulmonary veins, so the addition of a modest amount of caudal tilt can be used to separate the upper and lower veins on each side.

The presence of anomalous pulmonary venous drainage requires some flexibility in filming the angiography not only to demonstrate the course and site of venous drainage but also to identify any sites of stenosis. Initially, frontal and lateral projections with a wide field of view should be obtained. Following that, further injections may need to be performed with flexible projections designed to show sites of specific interest (see Chapter 24).

Atrioventricular Connections

The designation of a ventricle as morphologically right or left is extensively discussed in Chapter 3; suffice it to say that this rests mainly on the nature and distribution of the mural trabeculations. Ventriculography usually allows the ventricular morphology to be clearly identified, especially when both ventricles have been examined. While the AV connections can be well shown by atrial or venous injections as discussed above, ventriculography usually gives the required information as well as information on the ventriculoarterial connections (see below). In children with normal heart position and normal ventricular development, a 40° RAO projection parallel to the AV groove, combined with a shallow cranially-tilted LAO projection parallel to the basal sinus septum, will give this information. However, with abnormal heart position or asymmetry in the development and typography of ventricles, these views may need to be modified. The chest x-ray, echocardiography, MRI, previous cineangiograms, or test injections during catheterization, can all contribute to an informed guess as to which projections will best profile the AV groove and the basal sinus septum. The normal anatomy and assessment of AV connections seen with these projections, is well summarized elsewhere.[67]

The assessment of concordance or discordance of AV connections in the presence of a basal VSD or AV septal defect where the interventricular ridge is difficult to identify (or lacking), can be very difficult. In the cranially-tilted shallow LAO projection, the septal margin of LV can be projected back to the plane of the AV valves (Fig. 2-24) in order to identify the overriding AV valve (especially with a hypoplastic ventricle) or double inlet ventricle; this projection also allows an assessment of connection in the presence of crossed AV connections and with imperforate valves. The presence of straddle of the interventricular septum by valve chordae, can occasionally be identified directly with chordae seen as filling defects, but more usually, is suspected once the presence of valve override has been established; echocardiography will best assess the AV valve morphology and attachments.

Ventriculoarterial Connections

Ventriculoarterial connections are determined by the relationship of the semilunar valves and their respective outflow tracts to the interventricular septum and ventricular free wall.[67] In a normal heart with normal great arterial relationships (aortic valve rightward and posterior to the pulmonary valve), the atrial septal and septal leaflet tricuspid valve relationships to the aortic valved ring (beneath the nonfacing sinus) delineate the atrial portion of the membranous septum.[67] The infundibular (conal) septum attaches beneath the parts of the facing sinuses adjacent to the facing commissure, while the parietal band after it has run over the top of the tricuspid valve and before it contributes to the infundibular septum, attaches around the adjacent parts of non- and right-facing sinuses, as part of the interventricular septum. The LV free wall attaches around the remainder of the adjacent parts of non and left facing sinuses. Beneath the pulmonary valve ring, that component that is not infundibular septum, is all RV free wall.

With an intact ventricular septum, injections in either ventricle filmed in virtually any projection will demonstrate the ventriculoarterial connections. In the presence of a VSD however, projections that allow assessment of the relationship of the superior aspect of the interventricular septum to the semilunar valves, are crucial. If the infundibular septum is profiled and seen en face in two projections at right angles, then by implication, the semilunar valve relationship to the ventricular free wall should be visible. With left ventriculography in children having concordant connections, projections that will give this information are mid-RAO and mid-LAO (usually with cranial tilt) although as previously discussed, flexibility is required to achieve comparable projections in those whose chamber orientation is variant. The relationship between semilunar valves and infundibular anatomy are variables and do not accurately predict the connections. In particular, aortic-mitral separation can be seen in the absence of a VSD such that a concordant connection is preserved. Similarly, aortic-mitral continuity may be preserved in the presence of a VSD but there may be sufficient override of the aortic valve above a VSD that the connection is deemed to be double outlet right ventricle, usually an issue in tetralogy.

With left ventriculography in the presence of a VSD, the interventricular septal margin needs to be carefully traced after the expected curve of the septum, either perimembranous in a cranially-tilted mid-LAO projection or infundibular septum in an RAO projection. Given that even the expected curve of the septum can vary widely,[78] such tracing at least allows an estimate of override of a great artery (Figs. 2-25 through 2-27) if a diastolic frame is used (Fig. 2-28) (note that contrast flow patterns, either positive or negative, in complex cases cannot be relied upon to predict the connections) (Fig. 2-29). By convention, override of approximately 50% in two projections at right angles indicates an ambiguous ventriculo-arter-

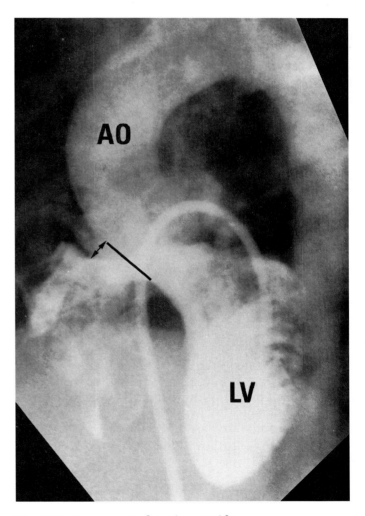

Fig. 2-25: Assessment of aortic override.
Venous approach via mitral valve for a left ventriculogram in a tetralogy patient, filmed in LAO projection. Projecting the expected plane of the interventricular septum across the VSD toward the aortic root does not coincide with the right anterior-facing sinus. The discrepancy (arrow) reflects the override.

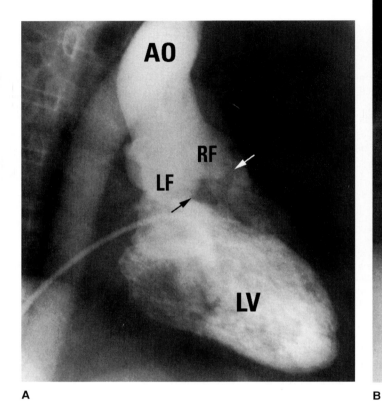

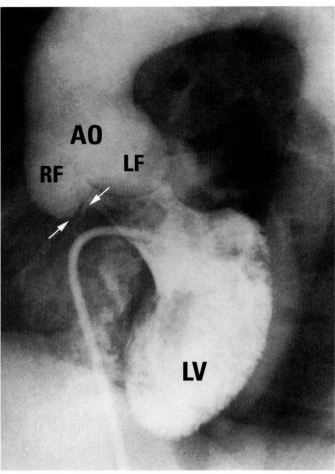

A   B

Fig. 2-26: Assessment of override.
Left ventriculogram in a tetralogy patient with the catheter via the VSD. **A**: RAO projection shows a discrepancy between the left ventricular margin and the aortic root (arrows) reflecting aortic override. Note the apex of the catheter course is in the base of the ventricle indicating its passage through VSD rather than via mitral valve. **B**: While an LAO projection would have been preferred for assessment of override, this somewhat steep cranially tilted LAO projection clearly shows the discrepancy between the interventricular septum and the aortic root reflecting the override (arrows).

Fig. 2-28: Assessment of override.
Retrograde left ventriculograms in a patient with tetralogy filmed in long-axial oblique projection. **A**: Projecting the expected plane of the interventricular septum across the VSD toward the aortic root shows a discrepancy on this diastolic frame, reflecting the aortic override. **B**: The systolic frame, however, overemphasizes the degree of override.

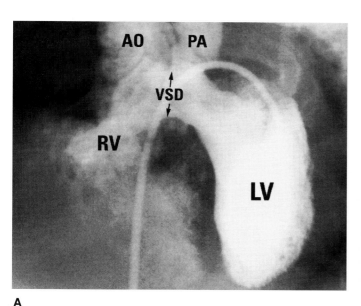

A

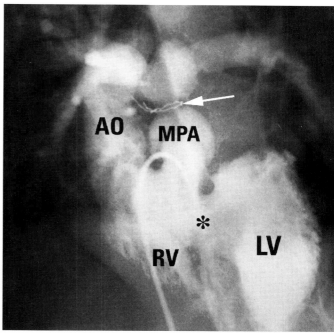

B

Fig. 2-27: Assessment of aortic override.
Two separate patients. **A**: Venous approach via mitral valve for left ventriculogram filmed in LAO projection. Pulmonary-mitral continuity (arrow) as well as an assessment of the expected sweep of the interventricular septum indicate that the MPA is more committed to the LV, and thus, the malformation represents complete TGA rather than DORV. (Courtesy of Dr. J. M. Ormiston, Greenlane Hospital, Greenlane, Auckland, New Zealand). **B**: Another patient. Venous approach via mitral valve to LV filmed in long-axial oblique projection. Projecting the expected sweep of the interventricular septum across the VSD (✱) toward the pulmonary valve, strongly suggests that the MPA is more closely related to the RV than to the LV, thus the malformation represents DORV. Note the PA band (arrow).

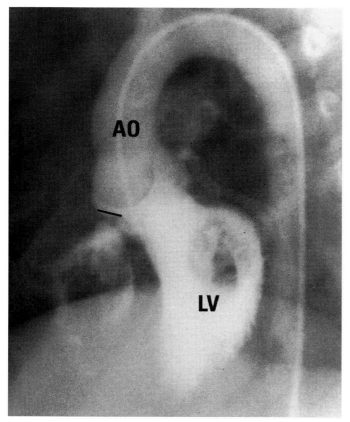

A

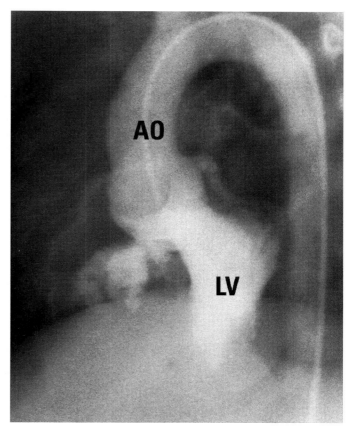

B

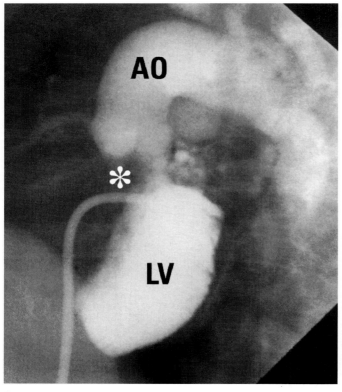

A

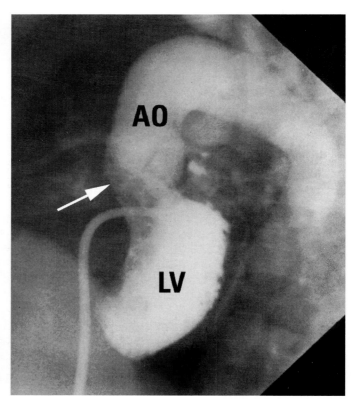

B

Fig. 2-29: Assessment of override.
Venous approach via mitral valve for left ventriculogram
filmed in steep LAO projection with cranial tilt. **A:** Mid-way
through the injection, unopacified contrast from RV via the
VSD (✳) suggests gross override. **B:** With slightly better filling, the interventricular septal margin is outlined (arrow) and
shows minimal, if any, discontinuity in this projection. **C:**
Later in the sequence, the washout of the aortic root via unopacified blood from the RV is clearly evident (arrow).

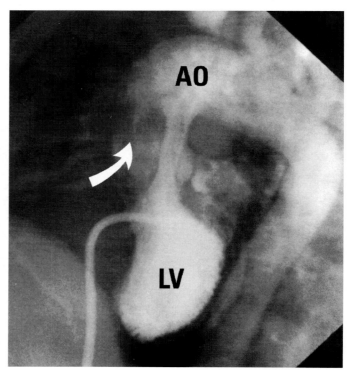

C

ial connection while override of greater than 50% in two projections at right angles indicates a double outlet ventricle. In the presence of a very large VSD, the greater the extensions of the septum that need to be estimated, the more imprecise becomes this designation of override.

Ventricular Septal Defects

The imaging of specific VSDs is commented on in Chapter 6; however, the principles of imaging of the ventricular septum, particularly a VSD, are such key issues in the whole angiographic approach to congenital heart disease, that they are dealt with conceptually here.

The complex three-dimensional nature of interventricular septum in the normal heart, has already been commented on (see above). To identify the position of a VSD in the septum and to localize its margins, imaging carves the septum until the silhouette is lost. The key injection is in the high-pressure chamber, usually the LV chamber. Two views at right angles will give the best chance of localizing a defect, but the operator should be prepared to do a second injection if the margins have not been well localized initially. The key projection is the mid-LAO of about 50°-60°, with as much cranial tilt as possible (long-axial oblique projection); this should profile the perimembranous region, open out the apex to base dimension of the ventricle and show characteristics of contrast flow from high- to low-pressure ventricles. Additional projections include the shallow LAO with cranial tilt (four-chamber projection) to show basal defects or basal extension of a perimembranous VSD, RAO to

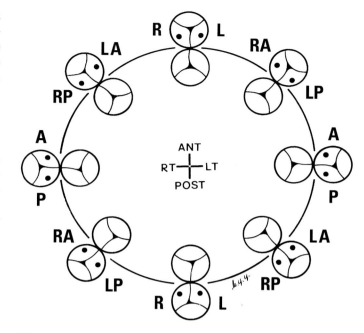

Fig. 2-30: Diagramatic representation of great artery positions and sinus terminology.
Great artery positions are displayed as viewed either on a caudally tilted balloon occlusion aortogram, or with echocardiography (see Chapter 35). Sinuses are labeled descriptively as facing or nonfacing rather than using a numerical system, as discussed in Chapter 35. A indicates anterior; P, posterior; L, left, R, right.

show the high anterior and infundibular defects, and mid-LAO (sometimes with *caudal*-tilt) to show the superior-inferior extent of a defect. These projections and their interpretation have been well reviewed elsewhere.[77,82]

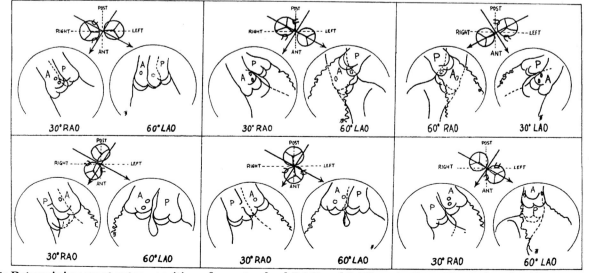

Fig. 2-31: Determining great artery positions from standard RAO and LAO projections (Reproduced with permission from Reference 66.)

Great Artery Relationships

The relationship of the great arteries is of importance particularly in evaluation of patients with discordant VA connections. Not only does this influence anatomy of the infundibular channel and VSD, but is crucial in working out coronary artery anatomy (see Chapter 30). The degree of overlap or separation of the great arteries on two views at right angles to each other allows an assessment of the relationship of the great arteries (Figs. 2-30 and 2-31).

Coronary Arteries

The projections used for imaging of the coronary arteries are discussed in detail in Chapter 30.

Aortography in Coarctation

Aortography for specific lesions is discussed in the relevant chapters. However, the filming of coarctations is a key area that illustrates the projections for aortography and the need for a flexible approach to imaging (see also Chapter 32).

Biplane projections will usually show the site of an isthmus coarctation well, whether the combination is RAO and LAO, PA and lateral, or shallow and steep LAO; appropriate modifications will need to be made to minimize superimposition of opacified structures, usually ascending on descending aorta or aorta on the spine (Fig. 2-32). Additionally, modifications will need to be made to accommodate a right aortic arch as opposed to the standard left arch; essentially, the projec-

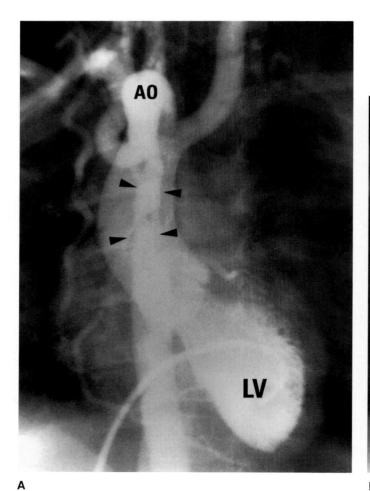

A

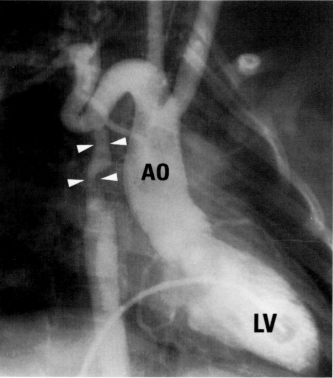

B

Fig. 2-32: Coarctation.
Left ventriculograms in a patient with right-sided cervical aorta, aberrant left subclavian artery, and extensive coarctation. **A:** The initial frontal projection superimposes ascending on descending aorta, although the coarctation (arrowheads) is suspected by looking through the dilute contrast in the ascending aorta. **B:** An RAO projection better opens out the arch anatomy and demonstrates the coarctation (arrowheads). The aberrant left subclavian artery is not seen as it was acting as a collateral channel with its reversed flow washing out into the descending aorta below the coarctation.

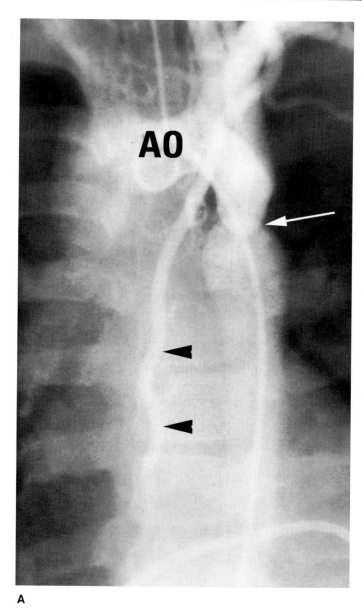

A

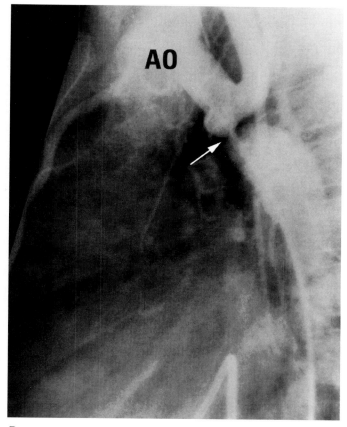

B

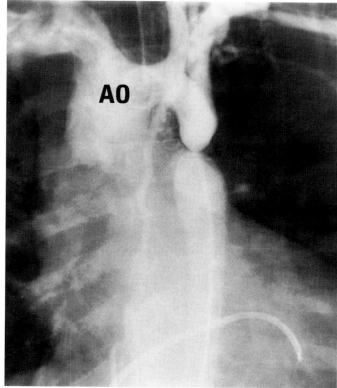

C

Fig. 2-33: Coarctation.
Retrograde aortograms. **A**: Frontal projection does not profile the coarctation well (arrow). Note the prominent chest wall collaterals from left subclavian (arrowheads). **B**: The reciprocal lateral projection shows the plane of the coarctation and suggests that to profile this adequately, a caudally tilted frontal projection would be required. **C**: Caudally tilted frontal projection now profiles the coarctation.

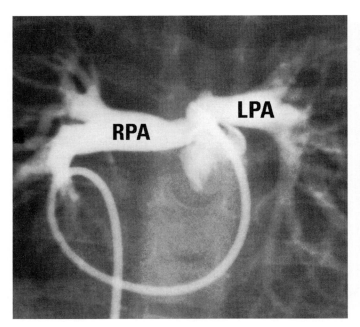
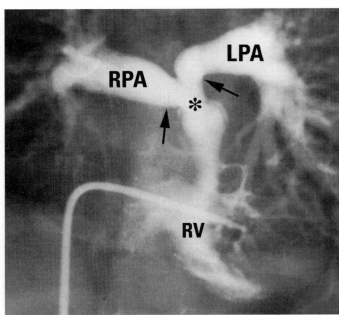

A   B

Fig. 2-34: Pulmonary arteries.
A: Selective MPA injection in a frontal projection superimposes MPA on the origins of both branch PAs. **B:** A right ventriculogram filmed in a cranially-tilted frontal projection opens out well the central PAs and shows the MPA stenosis (✱) as well as the mild narrowing at the origin of both branch PAs (arrows).

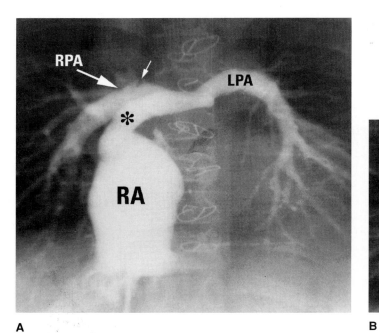
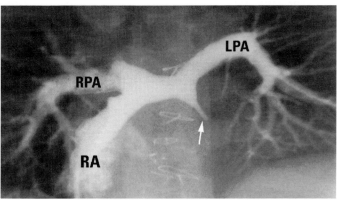

A   B

Fig. 2-35: Pulmonary arteries.
A: Postoperative lateral tunnel modified Fontan, a frontal projection in the tunnel does not ideally show the PA interconnection across the mid-line or the tunnel connection to RPA. **B:** Tunnel injection filmed in cranially tilted frontal projection. The tunnel connection to RPA is well seen (✱) as is the interconnection between the two PAs. The atretic MPA is clearly identified (arrow).

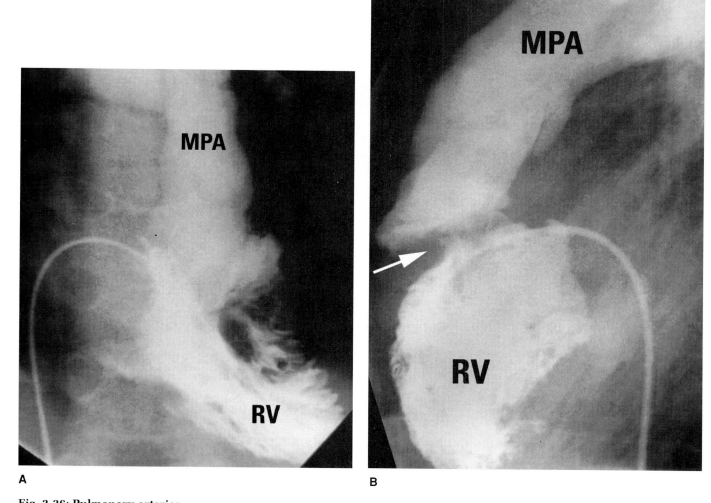

Fig. 2-36: Pulmonary arteries.
A: Right ventriculogram filmed in cranially-tilted frontal projection shows the hypertrophied RV and demonstrates the MPA. However, the cranial tilt masks the striking subvalve narrowing due to an anomalous muscle bundle clearly seen in the lateral projection (**B**). The axis of this bar (arrow) suggests that a frontal projection with caudal tilt would have been needed.

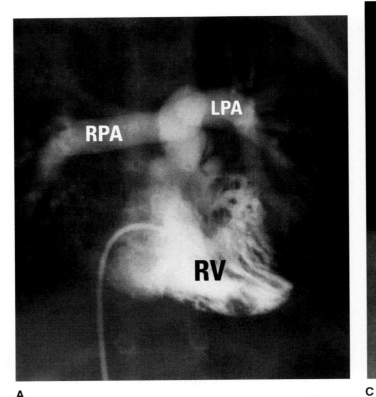

A

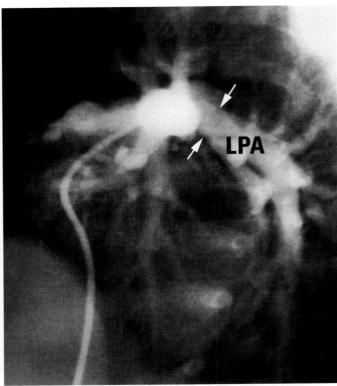

C

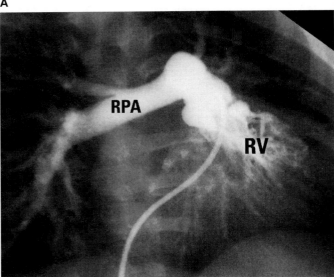

B

Fig. 2-37: Pulmonary arteries.
A: Right ventriculogram filmed in frontal projection clearly shows how the origins of both PAs are not well profiled. **B**: Selective MPA injection in RAO projection opens out the RPA and shows a normal caliber origin. **C**: The reciprocal LAO projection with a small amount of cranial tilt profiles the origin of LPA (arrows) and shows a mild stenosis.

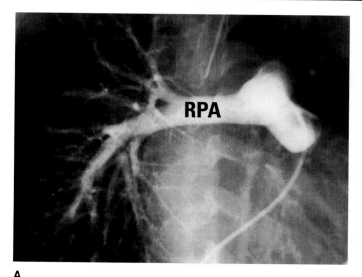

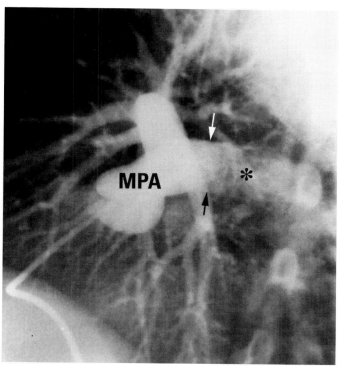

Fig. 2-38: Pulmonary arteries.
MPA injection in a tetralogy patient in RAO (**A**) and mid-LAO with cranial tilt (**B**) projections shows the origins of both PAs. Mid-LPA is not well seen (✳) due to unopacified blood entering via the Blalock-Taussig shunt.

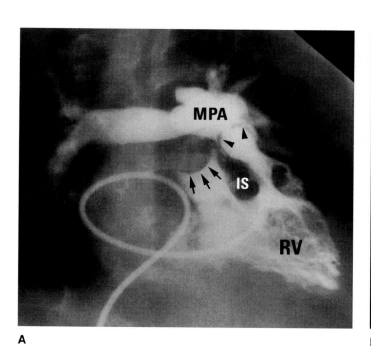

Fig. 2-39: Pulmonary arteries.
Right ventriculogram in a tetralogy patient. **A**: RAO projection demonstrates the tetralogy anatomy with a prominent infundibular septum, reversal of contrast through the VSD to outline the aortic valve (arrows) and the narrowed infundibular channel leading to the pulmonary valve stenosis (arrowheads). The RPA origin is mildly narrowed. **B**: A steep LAO projection during diastole shows the dimension of the infundibular channel (✳) and the stenosis of the short MPA. The LPA origin is, however, not profiled.

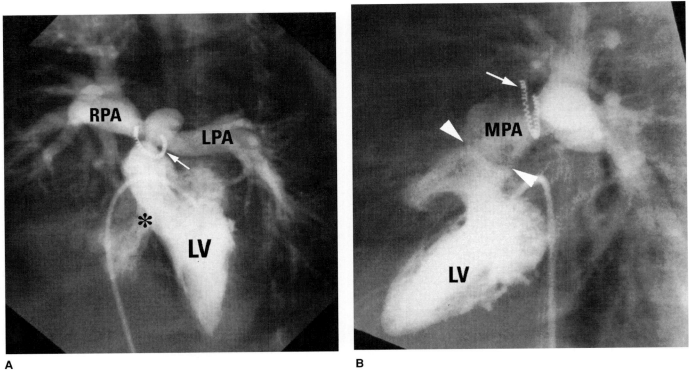

Fig. 2-40: Pulmonary artery band.
Left ventriculogram via venous approach through mitral valve. **A:** Four-chamber projection shows that the adjustable (Vince) band is adequately tight (arrow), but compromises the origins of both pulmonary arteries. **B:** Steep LAO projection profiles the band (arrow) and suggests that it is sufficiently distal to the plane of the pulmonary annulus (arrowheads) to be free of the pulmonary valve leaflets.

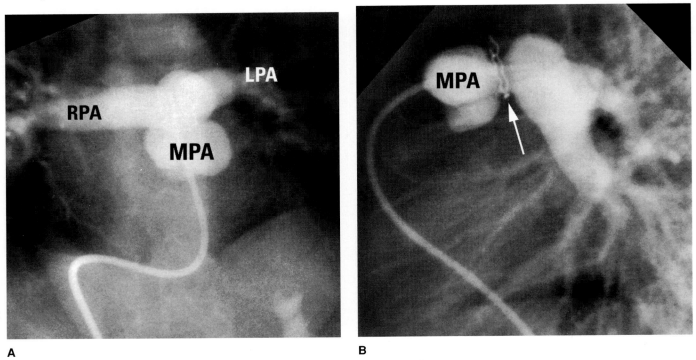

Fig. 2-41: Pulmonary artery band.
Selective MPA injection. **A:** Cranially tilted frontal projection does not profile the band or the LPA origin, but suggests that the RPA origin is uncompromised. **B:** Lateral projection profiles the band (arrow) and suggests that it is just free of the pulmonary valve leaflets. The LPA origin is not well assessed in either of these projections; a mid- or steep LAO and/or cranial tilt, would have been required.

tions chosen to film a right aortic arch should be mirror images of those chosen to film a left arch and coarctation.

However, from time to time, there is quite marked tortuosity of the aorta in the vicinity of the coarctation shelf or overlapping structures (such as an aberrant subclavian artery, patent ductus or ductal diverticulum, post-stenotic dilatation of descending aorta), which will make it difficult to adequately profile the narrowest section. At these times, flexibility and an innovative approach is required. Steep or shallow RAO or LAO projections may give the required result, often with added cranial or caudal tilt (Fig. 2-33). It is important to keep the cones relatively wide initially and to maintain a fairly long cine run so as to look for collateral pathways and particularly, steal phenomena involving vertebrals, subclavians and often, aberrant vessels.

Pulmonary Arteries

Cranially-tilted frontal together with lateral projections (Figs. 2-34 through 2-36)[83,84] and RAO/LAO projections (Figs. 2-37 through 2-39)[66] have been used to image the proximal and hilar sections of pulmonary arteries, whether the contrast injection is in the ventricle or selectively in the PA. Often, overlapping structures obscure the origins of the branch PAs such as with pulmonary valve stenosis and post stenotic dilatation of MPA (often extending into a pulmonary ductal diverticulum) or a horizontally oriented or caudally oriented MPA as in tetralogy. In these situations, the standard projections can be modified by increasing or decreasing the RAO or LAO component or by adding cranial or caudal tilt. After the placement of a PA band, the marked dilatation of the sinuses proximal to the

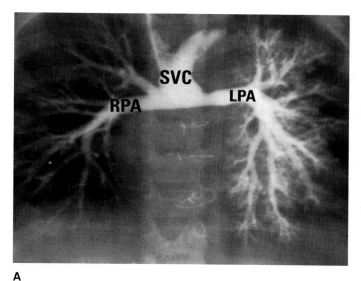

A

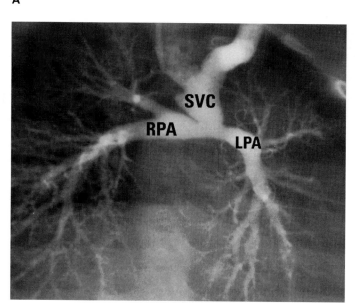

C

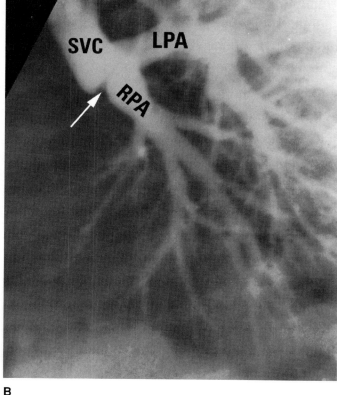

B

Fig. 2-42: Cavopulmonary anastomosis.
Selective SVC injections. **A:** The initial frontal projection does not profile the SVC anastomosis with RPA. **B:** The reciprocal lateral projection shows the orientation of the SVC and suggests that to adequately profile the anastomosis with RPA, a caudally tilted frontal projection would be required. **C:** RAO projection with caudal tilt now profiles the anastomosis and the SVC.

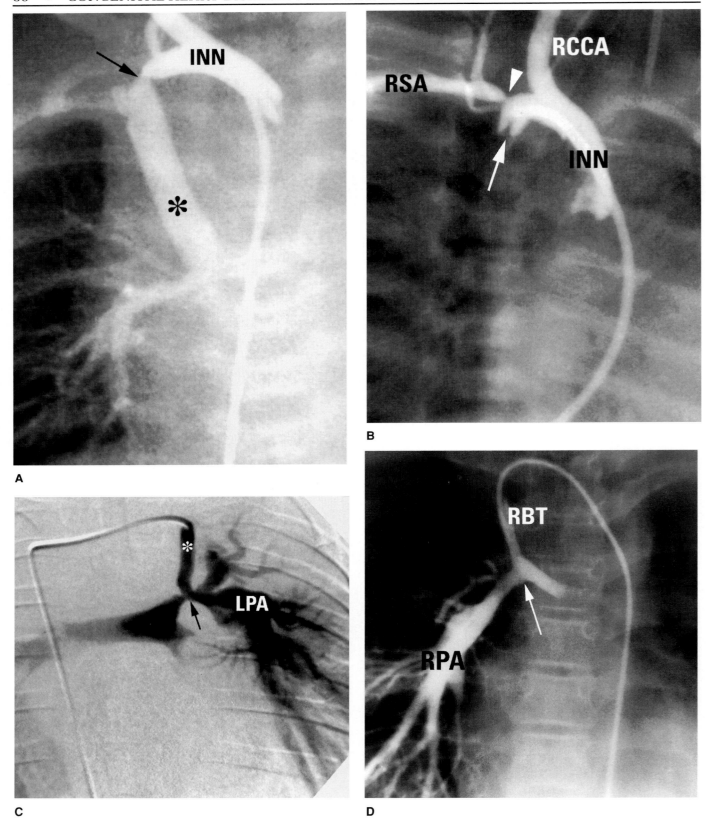

Fig. 2-43: Block-Taussig shunt.
Four separate patients. **A**: Selective innominate injection filmed in frontal projection shows the shunt well (✷) and the proximal stenosis (arrow). **B**: Selective innominate injection in shallow RAO projection shows the stenosis of RSA at the proximal anastomotic site (arrowhead) and the shunt occluded by clot (arrow). **C**: Selective shunt projection in frontal projection (DSA technique). The shunt (✷) has severely compromised LPA (arrow). **D**: Selective shunt injection in frontal projection shows compromise of the hilar RPA and the tenting of the vessel (arrow).

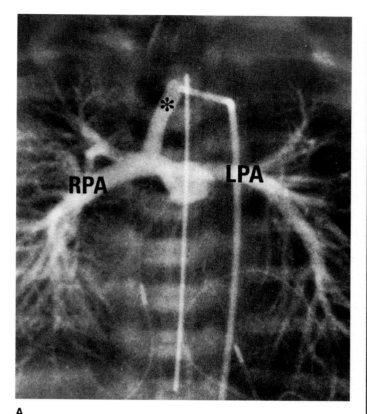

A

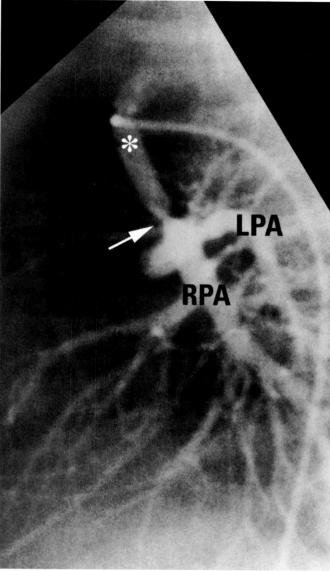

B

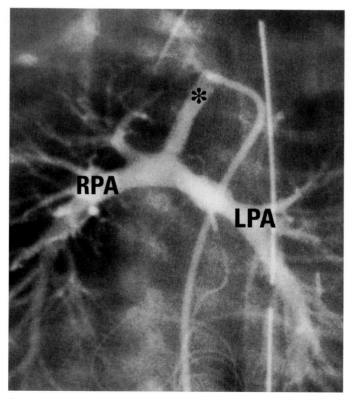

C

Fig. 2-44: Blalock-Taussig shunt.
Selective Blalock-Taussig shunt injection. **A:** Frontal projection shows the shunt (✱) but does not show any stenosis of the distal anastomosis with RPA. **B:** The reciprocal lateral projection, however, suggests significant stenosis distally. The plane of the anastomosis indicates that a caudally tilted projection (arrow) would be required to profile this. **C:** A caudally tilted shallow RAO projection better profiles the anastomosis with the stenosis being seen as a lucent line (arrows).

band together with the post-stenotic dilatation, make not only the origins of the PAs difficult to evaluate (compromised by band slippage), but a steeper LAO or even lateral projection may be required to profile the band itself to assess the tightness (Figs. 2-40 and 2-41) (see also Chapter 19).

After shunt procedures, either Blalock-Taussig, or cavopulmonary anastomosis (classic or bidirectional)

whether on the right or left, these shunts often travel a course from superoanterior to posteroinferior. Additionally, they may be anastomosed to the posterosuperior or anterosuperior aspect of the pulmonary artery, rather than directly superior. The steep LAO lateral projection during a test injection can be used to assess this course and may indicate that caudal tilt on the frontal, RAO or LAO projection may be necessary in or-

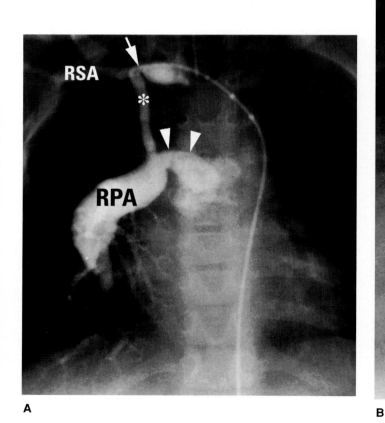

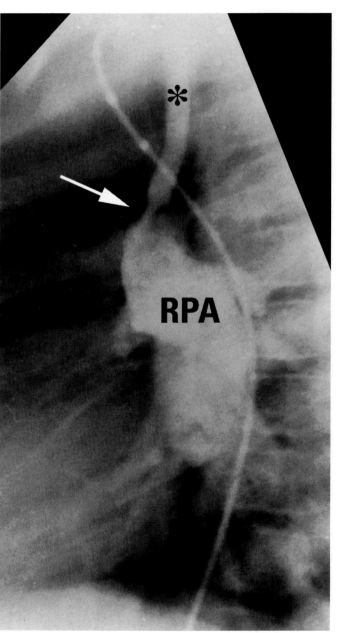

A

B

Fig. 2-45: Blalock-Taussig shunt.
Selective Blalock-Taussig shunt injection. **A**: Frontal projection shows the shunt (✱) and identifies a stenosis of the subclavian immediately proximal to the shunt (arrow). The shunt has compromised distally and tented the RPA (arrowheads). **B**: The reciprocal lateral projection shows jetting through a stenosis and suggests that in order to better profile this, a frontal projection should have cranial tilt added to it as indicated (arrow).

(continued on next page)

der to profile the anastomosis with the PA to exclude narrowing (Fig. 2-42).

Imaging of the lobar branch PAs is becoming increasingly important with the capabilities of intervention, particularly in addressing stenoses after shunt procedures or peripheral pulmonary stenoses such as in tetralogy or Noonan's syndrome. The proximal as-

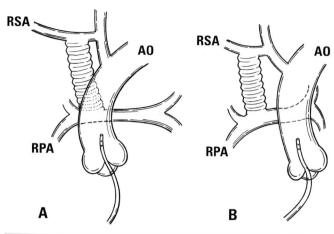

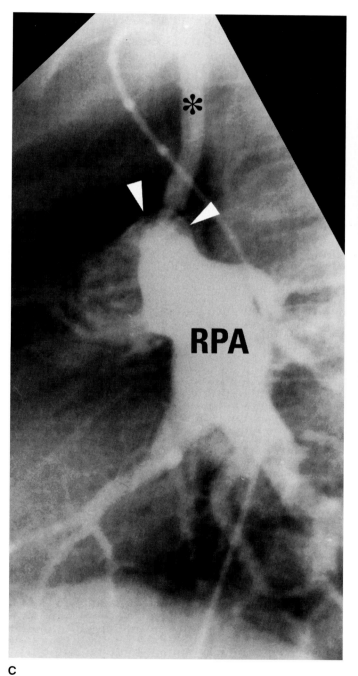

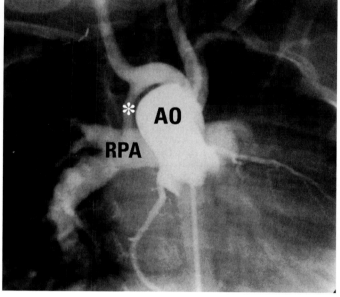

C

Fig. 2-46: Blalock-Taussig shunt.
If a selective innominate or Blalock-Taussig shunt injection cannot be achieved and an aortic root injection is performed, a frontal projection (**A**) will usually superimpose the ascending aorta on the distal shunt and anastomosis. An RAO projection (**B**) will, however, separate these. **C**: Aortic root injection in shallow RAO projection in a patient with complete TGA, VSD, and PS. The classic Blalock-Taussig shunt (✳) is well seen, separated from the ascending aorta. (Courtesy of Dr. J. M. Ormiston, Green Lane Hospital, Auckland, New Zealand).

pects of these vessels are often overlapped in frontal or shallow projections but may be well seen in lateral projections (sometimes with the addition of caudal or cranial tilt).

Blalock-Taussig Shunt

For both classic and modified right-sided Blalock-Taussig shunts, frontal and lateral projections usually show the shunt and its anastomoses (although note the

C

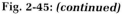

Fig. 2-45: *(continued)*
C: Slightly later in the injection, the tented-up aspect of RPA (arrowhead) immediately proximal to the shunt anastomosis, overlaps the distal shunt and masks the stenosis.

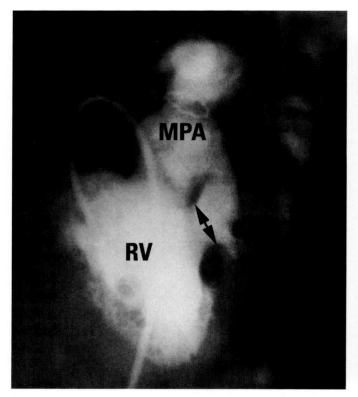

A

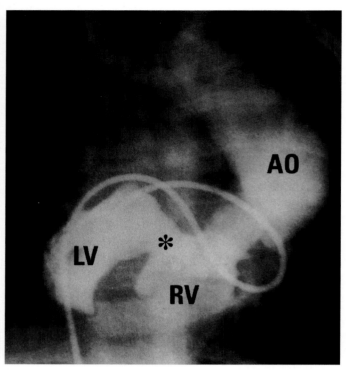

B

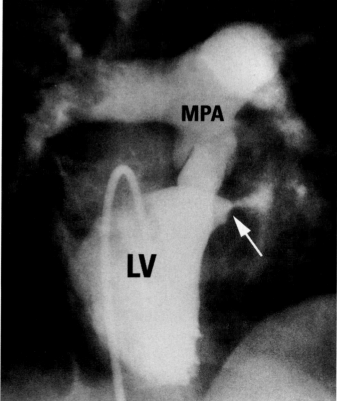

C

Fig. 2-47: Profiling VSDs with unusual cardiac malformations or orientation.

Three separate patients. **A**: Right ventriculogram in a patient with dominant RV and a leftward superiorly oriented LV. A LAO projection profiles the VSD (arrows) well. **B**: Another patient. Left ventriculogram in a patient with mesocardia and corrected transposition filmed in a frontal projection. The VSD (✳) is well profiled as is the infundibular channel leading from RV to aorta. **C**: Another patient with corrected transposition and mesocardia. Left ventriculogram filmed in a cranially tilted shallow RAO projection profiles the interventricular septum and the VSD, which is restrictive (arrow).

comments above about profiling the distal anastomosis) and project MPA clear of the RPA as long as the catheter is positioned within the Blalock-Taussig shunt or in the innominate or subclavian (the latter two sites usually give better information about the upper anastomosis and assess the quality of the native vessel both proximal and distal to the shunt) (Figs. 2-43 through Fig. 2-45). However, if the native vessel or shunt itself cannot be selectively entered and the catheter is in the ascending aorta, a shallow RAO projection should separate the shunt from the ascending aorta (Fig. 2-46); if the shunt has been placed very proximally on a PA, the degree of RAO required to separate it from the ascending aorta will of necessity need to be increased.

If a left-sided shunt has been placed, whether with a right or left arch, a frontal projection will usually show the shunt whether or not an aortogram or selective injection is performed.

Profiling the Ventricular Septum with Unusual Heart Positions or Discrepancy in Ventricular Sizes

From time to time, information from chest x-ray, echocardiography, MRI, previous cineangiocardiograms, or test injections during cardiac catheterization, may indicate that the interventricular septum lies in an unusual position. In this situation, the operator may need to search for projections that profile the basal sinus septum and infundibular septum together with the ventricular free walls in order to profile VSDs as well as to confirm AV and VA connections.

If the chest x-ray demonstrates mesocardia or dextrocardia, frontal or RAO projections with cranial tilt may give the equivalent information to the standard cranially-tilted LAO projections (Fig. 2-47). The flattened septum of corrected transposition of the great arteries (TGA) or complete TGA in an older child in whom an arterial switch operation has not been performed, may be profiled with a more shallow LAO projection than usual. In such cases, the septum usually lacks the 100°-120° concavity from anterior to posterior and thus cannot be carved into 30° sections with the usual projections. If so, the cranially-tilted LAO projection can be followed by a straight LAO or even a caudally-tilted LAO projection to localize defects.

With suprasystemic pressure in the RV, the septum shows the reverse of the usual curve and frontal or shallow LAO projections should profile the perimembranous region, while steeper projections will show both basal sinus septum and the outlet septum.

With a discrepancy in the size between the ventricles, the relatively larger chamber will rotate the contralateral ventricle, thus the significant RV hypertrophy seen in tetralogy results in the plane of the interventricular septum being rather steeper or even directly coronal, necessitating a much steeper LAO projection than usual in order to profile the perimembranous region. In contradistinction, with RV hypoplasia such as in an unbalanced AV septal defect or tricuspid atresia, the interventricular septum will lie in a shallower orientation and thus a perimembranous or posterior muscular VSD can be profiled by a shallower LAO projection than usual.

Very occasionally, a chest wall deformity, or a child with a very narrow AP diameter, will result in an unusual lie of the heart and in these situations, projections will again need to be searched for which profile the relevant anatomy.

References

1. Pepine CJ, Allen HD, Bashore TM, Brinker JA, Cohn LH, Dillon JC. ACC/AHA Guidelines for cardiac catheterization and cardiac catheterization laboratories. *Circulation* 1991;84:2213–2247.
2. Zwaan M. Angiography and angioscopy with injector-applied carbon-dioxide. *Eur Radiol* 1994;4:389–394.
3. Kerns SR, Hawkins IF Jr. Carbon dioxide digital subtraction angiography: Expanding applications and technical evolution. *AJR* 1995;164:735–741.
4. Kerns SR, Hawkins IF Jr, Sabatelli FW. Current Status of Carbon Dioxide Angiography. *Vasc Imaging* 1995;33(1): 15–29.
5. Bettman MA, Buenger RE, Gelfand DW, Lasser EC, McClennan BL. Manual on iodinated contrast media. *Am Coll Radiol* 1991:38.
6. Cooper MW, Reed PJ. Comparison of ionic and non-ionic contrast agents in cardiac catheterization: The effects of ventriculography and coronary artiography on hemodynamics, electrocardiography, and serum creatinine. *Cathet Cardiovasc Diagn* 1991;22:267–277.
7. Matthai WH Jr, Hirshfeld JW. Choice of contrast agents for cardiac angiography: Review of recommendations based on clinically important distinctions. *Cathet Cardiovasc Diagn* 1991;22:278–289.
8. Stolberg HO, McClennan BL. Ionic versus nonionic contrast use. *Curr Probl Diagn Radiol* 1991;20:51–88.
9. Barrett BJ, Parfrey PS, Vavasour HM, O'Dea F, Kent G, Stone E. A comparison of nonionic, low-osmolality radiocontrast agents with ionic, high-osmolality agents during cardiac catheterization. *N Engl J Med* 1992;326(7): 431–436.
10. Steinberg EP, Moore RD, Powe NR, et al. Safety and cost effectiveness of high-osmolality as compared with low-osmolality contrast material in patients undergoing cardiac angiography. *N Engl J Med* 1992;326(1):425–430.
11. Matthai WH Jr, Kussmaul WG III, Krol J, Goin JE, Schwartz JS, Hirshfeld JW Jr. A comparison of low- with high-osmolality contrast agents in cardiac angiography.

Identification of Criteria for selective use. *Circulation* 1994;89(1):291–301.

12. Stolberg HO, ed. *The Use of Iodinated Contrast Media in Diagnostic Imaging.* Toronto: Ontario Association of Radiologists; 1994, p. 112.

13. Goss JE, Chambers CE, Heupler FA. Systemic anaphylactoid reactions to iodinated contrast media during cardiac catheterization procedures: Guidelines for prevention, diagnosis, and treatment. *Cathet Cardiovasc Diagn* 1995;34:99–104. 14. Abrams HL, ed. *Coronary Arteriography. A Practical Approach.* Boston: Little, Brown and Company; 1983, p. 338.

15. Baim DS, Paulin S. Intravascular contrast agents. In: Grossman W, Baim DS, eds. *Cardiac Catheterization, Angiography, and Intervention.* Fourth edition. Philadelphia: Lea & Febiger; 1991, pp. 25–27.

16. Higgins CB. Contrast media in the cardiovascular system. In: Sovak M, ed. *Radiocontrast Agents.* Berlin: Springer-Verlag; 1984, pp. 194–251.

17. Hoey GB, Smith KR. Chemistry of x-ray contrast media. In: Sovak M, ed. *Radiocontrast Agents.* Berlin: Springer-Verlag; 1984, pp. 21–125.

18. Sovak M. Introduction: State of the art and design principles of contrast media. In: Sovak M, ed. *Radiocontrast Agents.* Berlin: Springer-Verlag; 1984, pp. 1–22.

19. McClennan BL. Low-osmolality contrast media: Premises and Promises. *Radiology* 1987;162:1–8.

20. Powe NR, Kinnison ML, Steinberg EP. Results of randomized controlled trial of low versus high osmolar contrast media. *Radiology* 1989;170:381–389.

21. Brismar J, Jackobson BF, Jorulf H. Miscellaneous adverse effects of low versus high osmolality contrast media: A study revised. *Radiology* 1991;179:19–23.

22. Almen T. Experience from 10 years of development of water-soluble nonionic contrast media. *Invest Radiol* 1980;15:S283-S288.

23. Morris TW. Intravascular contrast media and their properties. In: Skucas J, ed. *Radiographic Contrast Agents.* Second edition. Rockville, MD: Aspen; 1989, pp. 119–129.

24. Grainger RG. Osmolality of intravascular radiological contrast media. *Br J Radiol* 1980;53(632):739–746.

25. Roth R, Akin M, Deligonul U, Kern MJ. Influence of radiographic contrast media viscosity to flow through coronary angiographic catheters. *Cathet Cardiovasc Diagn* 1991;22:290–294.

26. Paulin S. Coronary arteriography: A technical, anatomic and clinical study. *Acta Radiologica* 1964;Suppl 233.

27. Dotter CT, Veatch W, Wishart D, Dotter P. The effects of specific gravity upon the distribution of intravascular contrast agents. *Circulation* 1960;22:1144–1148.

28. Fox JA, Hugh AE. Some physical factors in arteriography. *Clin Radiol* 1964;15:183–195.

29. Paulin S. *Personal communication.* 1991.

30. Amplatz K, Moller JH. *Radiology of Congenital Heart Disease.* St. Louis: Mosby Year Book; 1993, p. 1207.

31. LePage JR, Prast AD, Sorondo I. Intravascular catheter rupture. *Angiology* 1973;24:62–67.

32. De Bruyne B, Stockbroeckx J, Demoor D, Heymdrickx GR, Kern MJ. Interventional physiology. Role of side holes in guide catheters: Observations on coronary pressure and flow. *Cathet Cardiovasc Diagn* 1994;33: 145–152.

33. Susman N, Diboll WB. Fluid dynamics in the tip of the multiholed angiographic catheter. *Radiology* 1969;92: 843–858.

34. Rodriguez-Alvarez A, Martinez de Rodriguez G. Studies in angiography. The problems involved in the rapid, selective, and safe injections of radiopaque materials. Development of a special catheter for selective angiocardiography. *Am Heart J* 1957;53(6):841–853.

35. Brandt PWT. *Personal communication.* 1990.

36. Krieger RA, Furst AE, Hildner FJ, Midwall J, Kieval J. CO_2 power-assisted hand-held syringe: Better vizualization during diagnostic and interventional angiography. *Cathet Cardiovasc Diagn* 1990;19:123–128.

37. Baum S. Catheters and injectors. In: Abrams HL, ed. *Abrams' Angiography.* Third edition. Boston: Little, Brown and Company; 1983, pp. 187–204.

38. Amplatz K, Moller JH. Angiographic Equipment. In: Leib DBK, ed. *Radiology of Congenital Heart Disease.* St. Louis: Mosby Year Book; 1993, pp. 155–156.

39. Roth R. Triple mount for ceiling suspended power injectors: A real space saver. *Cathet Cardiovasc Diagn* 1991;24:72–73.

40. Judkins MP. Angiographic equipment: The cardiac catheterization angiography laboratory. In: Abrams HL, ed. *Coronary Arteriography. A Practical Approach.* Boston: Little, Brown and Company; 1983, pp. 1–50.

41. Curry TS, Dowdey JE, Murry RC. *Physics of Diagnostic Radiology.* Fourth edition. Philadelphia: Lea and Febiger; 1990, p. 522.

42. Moore RJ. *Imaging Principles of Cardiac Angiography.* Rockville, MD: Aspen; 1990, pp. 256.

43. Wolbarst AB. *Physics of Radiology.* Norwalk, CT: Appleton and Lange; 1993, p. 461.

44. Green CE. *Coronary Cinematography.* Philadelphia: Lippincott-Raven; 1996, p. 132.

45. Lawrence DJ. A simple method of processor control. *Med Radiography Photography* 1973;49:2–28.

46. Holmes DR Jr. President's page. *Cathet Cardiovasc Diagn* 1995;36:293.

47. Holmes DR Jr. To compress or not, that is the question. *Cathet Cardiovasc Diagn* 1995;36:382.

48. Hermiller JB, Cusma JT, Spero LA, Fortin DF, Harding MB, Bashore TM. Quantitative and Qualitative coronary angiographic analysis: Review of methods, utility, and limitations. *Cathet Cardiovasc Diagn* 1992;25:110–131.

49. Foley DP, Escaned J, Strauss H, et al. Quantitative coronary angiography (QCA) in interventional cardiology: Clinical application of QCA measurements. *Prog Cardiovasc Dis* 1994;36(5):363–384.

50. Strauss BH, Escaned J, Foley DP, et al. Technologic Considerations and practical limitations in the use of quantitative angiography during percutaneous coronary recanalization. *Prog Cardiovasc Dis* 1994;36(5):343–362.

51. Jacobs JH, Bove AA, Smith HC, Chesebro JH. Use of a metal ring-marked catheter for geometric calibration in quantitative coronary angiography. *Cathet Cardiovasc Diagn* 1988;15:121–124.

52. Leung W-H, Demopulos PA, Alderman EL, Sanders W, Stadius ML. Evaluation of catheters and metallic catheter markers as calibration standard for measurement of coronary dimension. *Cathet Cardiovasc Diagn* 1990;21: 148–153.

53. Herrman J-PR, Deane D, Ozaki Y, den Boer A, Serruys PW. Technical notes. Radiological quality of coronary: Guiding catheters. A quantitative analysis. *Cathet Cardiovasc Diagn* 1994;33:55–60.

54. Reiber JHC, Kooijman CJ, Boer AD, Serruys PW. Assessment of dimensions and image quality of coronary con-

trast catheters from cineangiograms. *Cathet Cardiovasc Diagn* 1985;11:521–531.

55. Koning G, van der Zwet PMJ, von Land CD, Reiber JHC. Angiographic assessment of dimensions of 6F and 7F Mallinckrodt Softouch coronary contrast catheters from digital and cine arteriograms. *Int J Card Imaging* 1992;8:153–161.

56. Reiber JHC, Jukema W, van Boven A, van Houdt RM, Lie KI, Bruschke AVG. Technical Notes. Catheter sizes for quantitative coronary arteriography. *Cathet Cardiovasc Diagn* 1994;33:153–155.

57. Heupler FA Jr, Al-Hani AJ, Dear WE. Guidelines for continuous quality improvement in the cardiac catheterization laboratory. *Cathet Cardiovasc Diagn* 1993;30:191–200.

58. Page HL, Cameron AAC, Heupler FA, Hildner FJ, Tommaso CL, ed. *Quality Management in the Cardiac Catheterization Laboratory. Policies and Guidelines Established by the Society for Cardiac Angiography and Interventions.* Breckenbridge, CO: Society for Cardiac Angiography and Interventions; 1994, p. 172.

59. Judkins MP. Guidelines for radiation protection in the cardiac catheterization laboratory. *Cathet Cardiovasc Diagn* 1984;10:87–92.

60. Baim DS, Paulin S. Angiography: Principles Underlying proper utilization of cineangiographic equipment and contrast agents. In: Grossman W, Baim DS, ed. *Cardiac Catheterization, Angiography, and Intervention.* Fourth edition. Philadelphia: Lea and Febiger; 1991, pp. 15–26.

61. Johnson LW, Moore RJ, Baiter S. Review of radiation safety in the cardiac catheterization laboratory. *Cathet Cardiovasc Diagn* 1992;25:186–194.

62. Balter S. Guidelines for personnel radiation monitoring in the cardiac catheterization laboratory. *Cathet Cardiovasc Diagn* 1993;30:277–279.

63. Schueler BA, Julsrud PR, Gray JE, Stears JG, Wu KY. Radiation exposure and efficacy of exposure-reduction techniques during cardiac catheterization in children. *AJR* 1994;162:173–177.

64. International Commission on Radiological Protection. *Summary of the Current ICRP Principles for Protection of the Patient in Diagnostic Radiology.* Tarrytown, NY: Pergamon Press; 1993, p. 24.

65. Van Praagh R. The segmental approach to diagnosis in congenital heart disease. *Birth Defects: Original Article Series* 1972;8:4–23.

66. Brandt PWT, Calder AL. Cardiac connections: The segmental approach to radiologic diagnosis in congenital heart disease. *Curr Probl Diagn Radiol* 1977;7:1–35.

67. Brandt PWT. Cineangiocardiography of atrioventricular and ventriculo-arterial connexions. In: Godman MJ, ed.

Pediatric Cardiology. Volume 4. Edinburgh: Churchill Livingstone; 1980, pp. 191–210.

68. Anderson RH, Becker AE, Freedom RH, Macartney FJ. Sequential segmental analysis of congenital heart disease. *Pediatr Cardiol* 1984;5:281–288.

69. Freedom RM, Smallhorn JF. The segmental approach to congenital heart disease. In: Freedom RM, Benson LN, Smallhorn JF, ed. *Neonatal Heart Disease.* London: Springer-Verlag; 1992, pp. 119–133.

70. Chavez I, Dorbecker N, Celis A. Direct intracardiac angiocardiography: Its diagnostic value. *Am Heart J* 1947;33:560.

71. Cournand A, Ranges HA. Catheterization of the right auricle in man. *Proc Soc Exp Biol Med* 1941;46:452.

72. Kjellberg SR, Mannheimer E, Rudhe U, Jonsson B. *Diagnosis of Congenital Heart Disease.* Second edition. Chicago: Year Book Publishers Inc.; 1959, p. 866.

73. Puyau FA, Burko H. The tilted left anterior oblique position in the study of congenital cardiac anomolies. *Radiology* 1966;87:1069–1073.

74. Bargeron LM, Elliot LM, Soto B, Bream PR, Curry GC. Axial angiography in congenital heart disease. *Circulation* 1977;56:1075–1083.

75. Soto B, Bargeron LM. Present status of axially angled angiocardiography. *Cardiovasc Intervent Radiol* 1984;7:156–165.

76. Brandt PWT, Partridge JB, Wattie WJ. Coronary arteriography; Method of presentation of the arteriogram report and a scoring system. *Clin Radiol* 1977;28:361–365.

77. Brandt PWT. Commentary: Axially angled angiocardiography. *Cardiovasc Intervent Radiol* 1984;7:166–169.

78. Goor D, Lillehei CW, Edwards JE. The sigmoid septum. Variation in the contour of the left ventricular outlet. *AJR* 1969;107(2):366–376.

79. Freedom RM, Culham JAG, Moes CAF. *Angiocardiography of Congenital Heart Disease.* New York: Macmillan; 1984, p. 691.

80. Grainger RG. Terminology for radiographic projections. *Br Heart J* 1981;45:109–111.

81. Freedom RM, Fellows KE. Radiographic visceral patterns in the asplenia syndrome. *Radiology* 1973;106:387–391.

82. Kirklin JW, Barratt-Boyes BG. *Cardiac Surgery.* Second edition. New York: Churchill Livingstone; 1993, p. 1778.

83. Kattan KR. Angled view in pulmonary angiography. *Radiology* 1970;94:79–82.

84. Freedom RM, Olley PM. Pulmonary arteriography in congenital heart disease. *Cathet Cardiovasc Diagn* 1976;2:309–312.

Chapter 3

The Segmental and Sequential Approach to Congenital Heart Disease

How does one bring an overall consistency to the nomenclature applied to the infinite variety of complex cardiac anomalies? The answer lies in the development of a nomenclature based on cardiac morphology-anatomy and cardiac connections. This system would appeal to a wide constituency because it would promote communication and understanding with unambiguity and would facilitate the appreciation of how a heart functions (Fig. 3-1).[1-45] The development by Richard Van Praagh of a segmental approach in order to provide understanding of congenital heart disease more than 30 years ago set the stage for a more universal language for those caring for children with congenitally malformed hearts. Beginning with publications in 1963 and 1964 on the anatomic types of dextrocardia and single or common ventricle, Van Praagh and colleagues explored a series of complex cardiac malformations and provided a depth of understanding of the cardiac anatomy of these diverse cardiac malformations. But the importance, and indeed theme, of these early contributions was not just the description and categorization of certain forms of complex congenital heart malformations, but rather the development and application of a systematic and segmental approach that could be applied to virtually any form of congenitally malformed heart.[1,3,4,6-15]

The benchmark contribution of Van Praagh was to conceptualize the heart in terms of specific morphological building blocks that could be connected into a single anatomic and functional unit.[1,3,4,9,13-15] These building blocks consisted of the atria, the ventricles, and the great arteries and their connecting units (Figs. 3-2 through Fig. 3-13). The building blocks were defined by their specific morphological characteristics, not their right/left orientation in space. In the initial application of the segmental approach, the spatial relation between the atria and ventricles and ventricles and the great arteries was used to deduce the type of atrioventricular and ventriculoarterial connections. These considerations matured into the 1972 publication summarizing Van Praagh's segmental approach to the diagnosis of congenital heart disease.[1] Van Praagh's vision and implementation of his morphological-anatomic approach continues to evolve, and through a series of publications he has advocated and disseminated his segmental approach.[1-15,20,21]

Other investigators using the same anatomic cardiac building blocks have stressed the connections between the various segments. Instrumental in espousing the connections approach was Robert H. Anderson of the United Kingdom. Through a series of publications and presentations beginning in the early 1970s that used the same building blocks, Anderson and colleagues (who were then primarily but not exclusively from the United Kingdom and Europe) advocated the role of connections (atrioventricular and ventriculoarterial) as an important enhancement to the sequential and segmental approach as initially advocated by Van Praagh, eschewing the deductive approach to cardiac connections.[16,17,25,26,30,32-43] The sustained emphasis by the United Kingdom group on cardiac connections gained considerable support once the segments were

From: Freedom RM, Mawson JB, Yoo SJ, Benson LN: *Congenital Heart Disease: Textbook of Angiocardiography.* Armonk NY, Futura Publishing Co., Inc. ©1997.

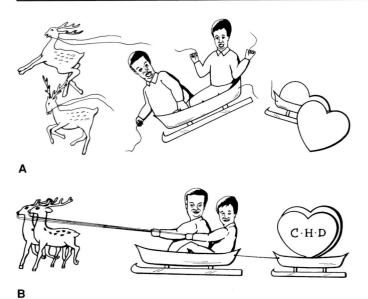

A

B

Fig. 3-1: Whether a sleigh or train, a sequential and segmental approach is essential in the nosology of congenital heart disease.
A: Without a system and a sequence, there is chaos. **B:** Less chaos.

identified. The dialogues between Anderson and Van Praagh initially seemed quite polarized, yet despite this perceived polarity, today their views are similar.[21] Van Praagh created the template, indeed the very foundation of today's systematic, sequential, and segmental approach to the diagnosis of congenital heart disease. For all of us, Van Praagh developed the *Esperanto* of congenital heart disease. In a summary of his application, Van Praagh stated in 1984: "The morphologic-anatomic approach to the diagnosis of congenital heart disease (CHD) is based on the situs, alignments, connections, and associated malformations of the cardiac segments (anatomic and developmental components which together make up all human hearts)."[4]

The Cardiac Segments

The three cardiac segments are the atria, the ventricles, and the great arteries (Figs. 3-2 through 3-13). The atria and ventricles are connected by or at the atrioventricular junction, and the ventricles and great arteries are connected by the infundibulum or conus.

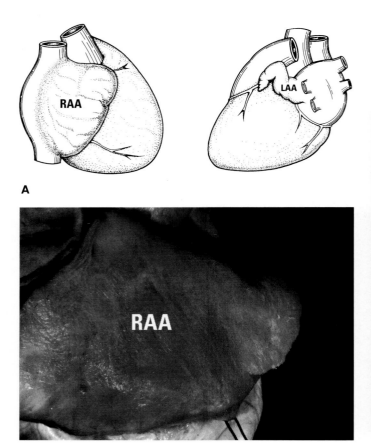

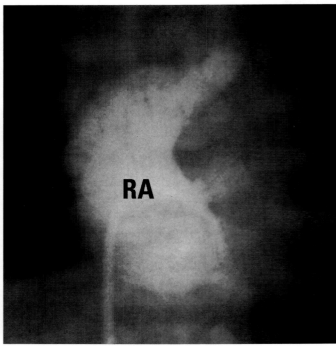

A

B

C

Fig. 3-2: The fundamental building blocks of a segmental and sequential approach to congenital heart disease: The atria.
A: Schematic diagrams of the morphologically right and left atria. **B:** Morphologically right atrium with its broad appendage.
C through E: Angiographic appearance of morphologically right atrial appendage.

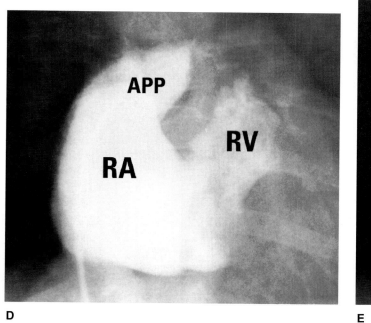

D

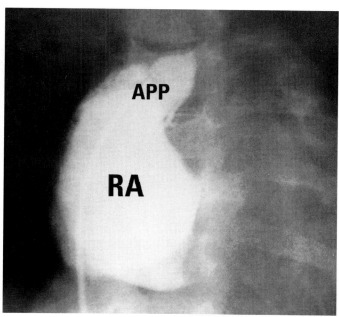

E

Fig. 3-2 (Continued)

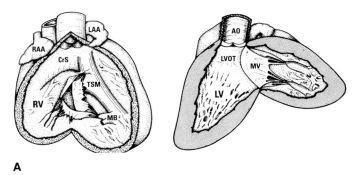

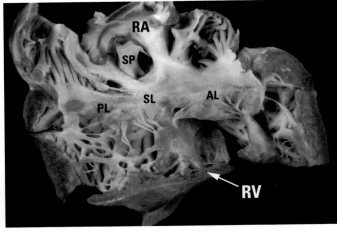

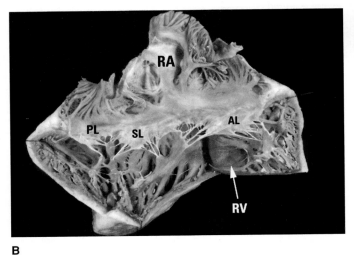

Fig. 3-3: The morphologically right ventricle: The tricuspid valve and right ventricular inlet.
A: Diagrams of the morphologically right and left ventricle. **B** and **C:** View of the inlet of the right ventricle in two specimens. The right atrium connects through a tricuspid atrioventricular valve with the coarsely trabeculated right ventricle.

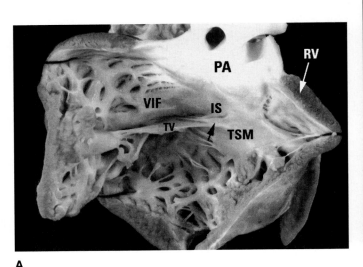

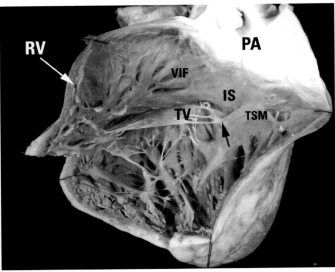

Fig. 3-4: The morphologically right ventricle: Its trabecular and infundibular components.
A and **B:** View of the trabecular and infundibular components of the right ventricle in two specimens. The morphologically right ventricle is characterized by the coarsely trabeculated mural myocardium. The infundibulum of the right ventricle is composed in part of the fusion of the ventriculoinfundibular fold, the infundibular septum, and the trabecula septomarginalis. These structures in the normal heart comprise in large part the crista supraventricularis, or supraventricular crest, with its parietal and septal components. Note that it is the right-sided ventriculoinfundibular fold that separates the pulmonary valve from the tricuspid valve. The infundibular septum separates the arterial outlets; and the trabecula septomarginalis is a septal right ventricular structure. The anteroseptal leaflet of the tricuspid valve is attached (arrow) to the papillary muscle of the conus or Lancisi, thus having attachment to the interventricular septum.

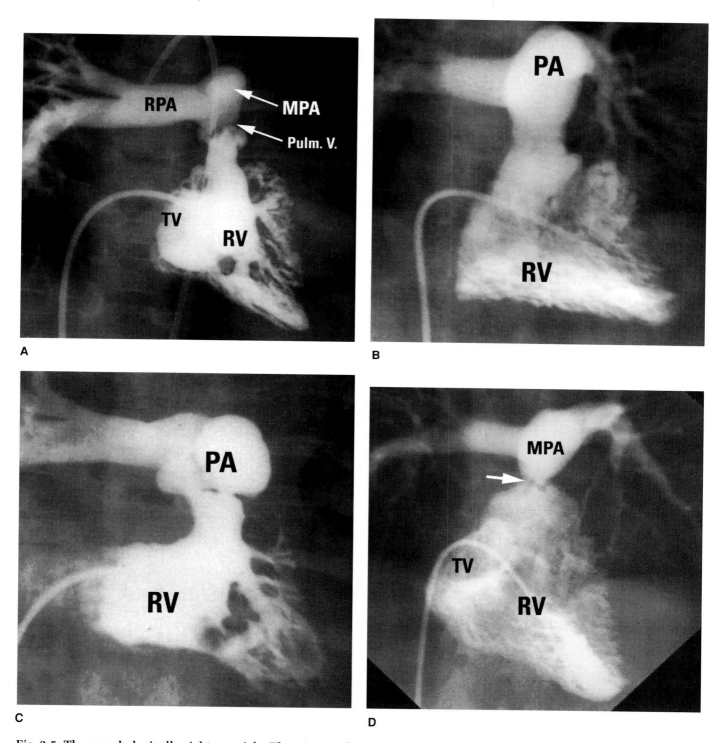

Fig. 3-5: The morphologically right ventricle: The angiocardiographic appearance.
A: Frontal right ventriculogram shows a relatively smooth inlet component receiving the tricuspid valve; the coarse mural trabecular pattern that is pathognomonic for a ventricle of right ventricular morphology; the relatively smooth subpulmonary infundibulum, separating the tricuspid from the pulmonary valve. **B and C:** The angiographic appearances of other right ventricles, again with their characteristic coarse septal trabecular pattern. **D:** The morphologically right ventricle of a patient with some dysplasia of the pulmonary valve (arrow) from a diastolic frame.

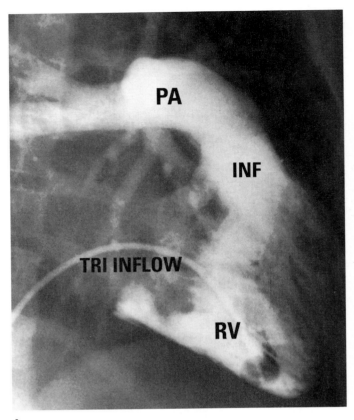

A

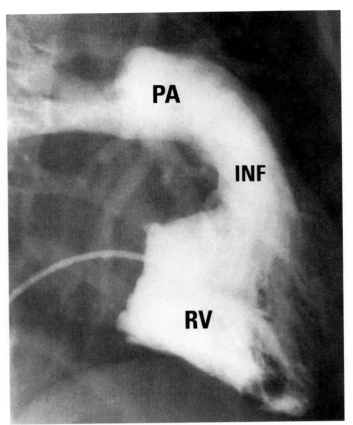

B

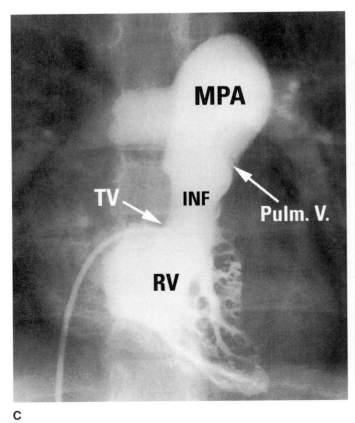

C

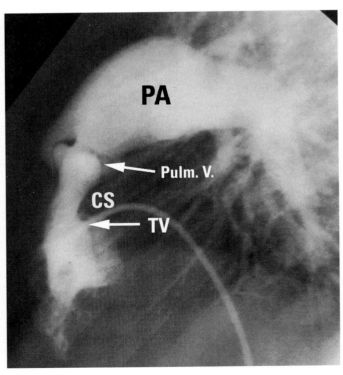

D

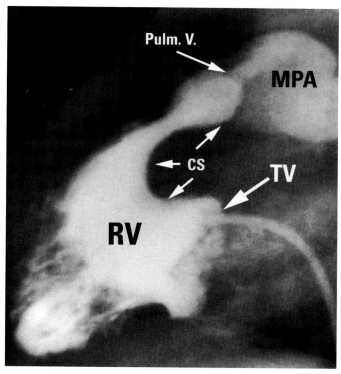

E

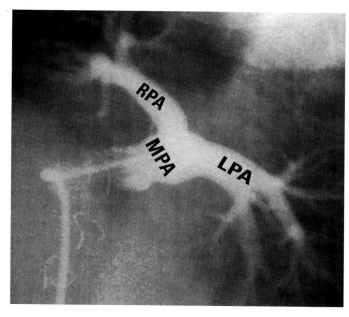

Fig. 3-7: The main, right, and left pulmonary arteries as demonstrated by cranially-angled pulmonary artery angiogram.

Fig. 3-6: Shallow right anterior oblique right ventriculogram shows the right ventricular inlet and outlet zones or components of the morphologically right ventricle.
A: Ventricular diastole with open tricuspid valve. B: systole with closed tricuspid valve. C through E: Various expressions of the right ventricular infundibulum. C and D: Frontal and lateral right ventriculogram from a different patient with pulmonary valvular stenosis. The designation crista supraventricularis has been used to note that muscle separating pulmonary from tricuspid valve in the normal heart. E: Lateral right ventriculogram showing the profound separation between pulmonary and tricuspid valves.

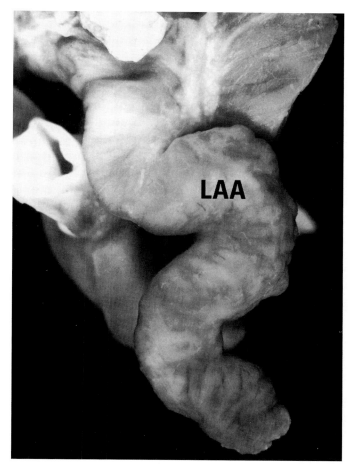

Fig. 3-8: The morphologically left atrium with its long finger-like atrial appendage and relatively narrow os.

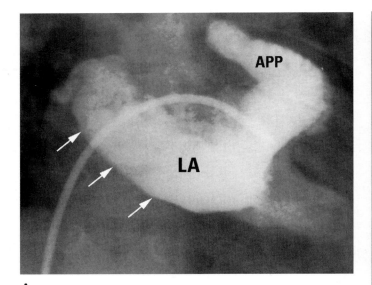

A

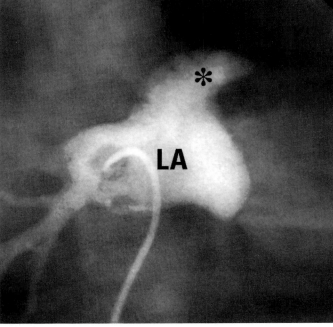

C

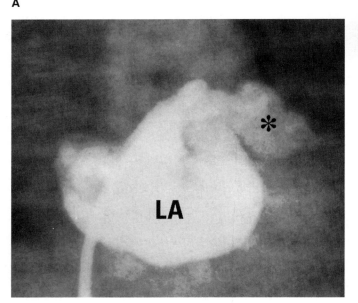

B

Fig. 3-9: The angiocardiographic appearances of the morphologically left atrium.
A: The venous catheter has been advanced through a patent ovale foramen into the left atrium. The plane of the atrial septal is shown in white arrows; the finger-like atrial appendage is evident. **B:** Another left atriogram shows a somewhat smaller atrial appendage (✳). **C:** In this patient with mitral stenosis, the left atrial appendage (✳) is still somewhat small.

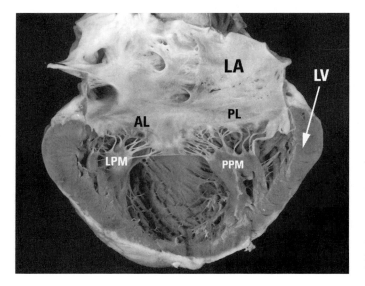

Fig. 3-10: Left atrium and left ventricular inlet.
The left atrium receives the four pulmonary veins and connects through a bicuspid atrioventricular valve to a morphologically left ventricle. That feature uniting all ventricles of left ventricular morphology is the relatively smooth left ventricular septal surface. The mitral valve with its miter-like morphology attaches to papillary muscles that do not attach to the ventricular septal surface.

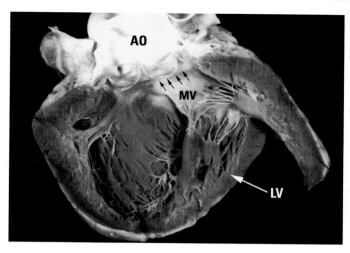

Fig. 3-11: The left ventricular septal surface, its outlet, and the aorta.
The relatively smoother left ventricular surface is seen without septal attachments of the mitral valve (see also Fig. 3-3A). The normal pattern of mitral valve-aortic valve fibrous continuity is seen (arrows), indicative of the markedly attenuated left-sided ventriculoinfundibular fold. The septal surface of the morphologically left ventricle does not have a trabecula septomarginalis.

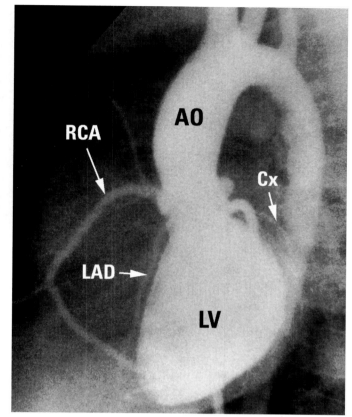

B

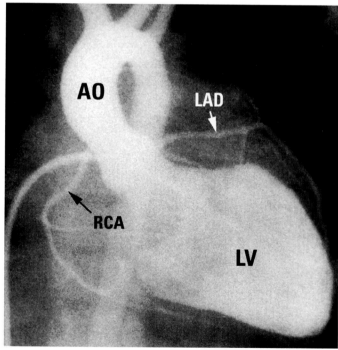

A

Fig. 3-12: The angiocardiographic appearance of the morphologically left ventricle.
A: Frontal and (**B**) lateral left ventriculogram. Note the smooth septal surface and the aortic-mitral fibrous continuity. **C:** Long axial oblique left ventriculogram with the smooth septal surface, and the aortic valve-mitral valve continuity.

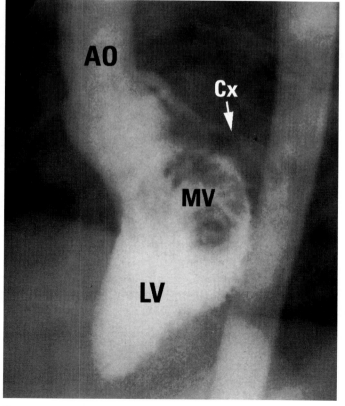

C

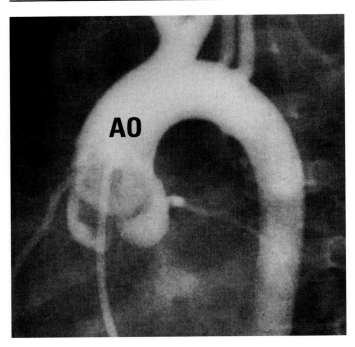

Fig. 3-13: The aorta with normal coronary arteries and brachiocephalic arch vessels.

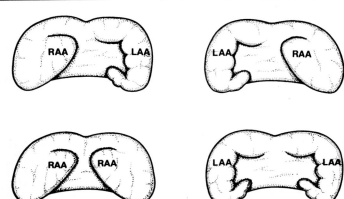

Fig. 3-14: Patterns of atrial arrangement in congenital heart disease.
Top, left: Atrial situs solitus or the normal atrial arrangement. **Top, right:** Atrial situs inversus, or inverse normal. The bottom two patterns depict so-called atrial isomerism patterns: right atrial isomerism with bilateral right atrial appendages or left atrial isomerism with bilaterally left atrial apendages.

The Atria

The normal atrial arrangement is characterized by a morphologically right atrium to the right and a morphologically left atrium to the left (Fig. 3-14). [1,3,4,9,13–15,25,26,30,32,37,42,44–52] In the normal heart, the right-sided morphologically right atrium has a broad, triangular atrial appendage with a wide connection at its junction with the smooth-walled atrium (Fig. 3-2). The morphologically right atrium has a conspicuous crista terminalis, and the right atrium normally receives the superior and inferior caval veins, and the coronary sinus. In contrast, the left atrial appendage is thin, hooked, and often crenellated, with a narrow junction with the morphologically left atrium (Figs. 3-8 and 3-9). The normal right atrial appendage is remarkably consistent in position. In one patient operated on for a secundum atrial septal defect, median sternotomy revealed that the right atrial appendage lay at the acute margin of the heart. Surgical atriotomy also revealed that the crista terminalis was displaced clockwise, extending from the left of the superior vena caval orifice anteriorly along the interatrial septum, to the left border of the inferior vena cava; the musculi pectinati radiated forward and to the right. This highly unusual anomaly is likely caused by a clockwise rotation of the atrial portion in relation to the normally positioned sinus venarum portion of the atrium, which resulted in sinoatrial malfusion.[52a] The normal left-sided, morphologically left atrium receives the pulmonary veins and

its atrial appendage is not guarded by a terminal crest. Atrial situs inversus is the inverse arrangement of the above. Because of the many anomalies of systemic and pulmonary venous connections and because of the large defects of the atrial septum so common to many complex forms of congenital heart disease, most inestigators agree that the character of the atrial appendage is the final clinical arbiter of the atrium as morphologically right or left, not atrial septal morphology, nor the specific systemic nor pulmonary venous connections.[22]

There are a group of hearts, often exhibiting complex anomalies, in which the atria are morphologically incompletely lateralized (Fig. 3-14).[24–26,32,37,38,47–63] Such hearts with incompletely lateralized atria frequently coexist with splenic anomalies, and the atrial appendages tend each to resemble either a morphologically right or left atrial appendage (see Chapter 41). Hearts with bilaterally right atrial appendages are considered by some to exhibit right atrial isomerism, an interesting, though not entirely appropriate description. Patients with nonlateralized, bilaterally right-appearing atrial appendages tend to have the complex cardiac malformations associated with asplenia (see Chapter 41), whereas those patients with bilaterally left-appearing atrial appendages tend to have the heart malformations seen in patients with polysplenia (Fig. 3-15). However, a number of departures from these general guidelines have been published (see Chapter 41).[64–69] Patients with incompletely lateralized atria usually have varying degrees of visceral symmetry, with bronchopulmonary symmetry or isomerism as well. Some do not adhere to the concept of atrial isomerism, and a vigorous debate continues (see also Chapter 41).[70–75]

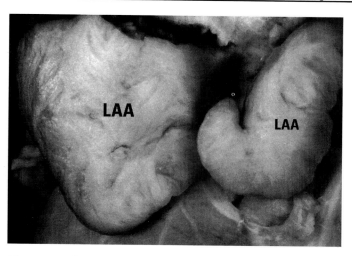

Fig. 3-15: The morphology of bilaterally left atrial appendages-left atrial isomerism.

The Anatomic Identification of Atrial Situs

Three types of atrial situs must be considered: 1) atrial situs solitus or the normal atrial relationship; 2) atrial situs inversus or the inverse normal or mirror-image of the normal atrial relationship; or 3) ambiguous or isomeric atria, typically found in patients with visceral symmetry (Fig. 3-14).[3,4,9,13,15,25,26,30,32,42,45–47,49,59–64,70–81] Splenic anomalies including asplenia or polysplenia as well as other splenic anomalies are commonly, but not universally, found in patients with an ambiguous or isomeric atrial situs.[15,26,42,44,45,49,55,62,63,82–99] Thus, the four types of atrial situs are: 1) solitus or normal; 2) inversus; 3) bilaterally right; and 4) bilaterally left.

The Clinical Identification of Atrial Situs

The initial task in any segmental and sequential approach to the definition of congenital heart disease is definition of the atrial situs. Without resorting to anatomic inspection, cardiac angiography, or cross-sectional echocardiography, both the electrocardiogram and the abdominal-chest radiograph provide some clues as to the determination of atrial situs. Normally, lateralized atria, and thus assuming a normally positioned sinoatrial node, is suggested by a positive P-wave in leads I, II, III, aVL, and aVF, but negative in aVR in the standard surface electrocardiogram. Conversely, when the P-wave deflection is positive in leads I, II, III, aVR, and aVF, but negative in aVL, this suggests inverted normal atria, and would be consistent with inversus of the atria. A leftward and superior P-wave axis has been found in a substantial number of patients with left atrial isomerism,[100–102] suggesting abnormal morphogenesis of the sinoatrial node.[103] The hepatic and gastric shadows on the plain frontal chest

x-ray may also provide evidence as to atrial localization. The presumption here is that there is viscero-venous-right atrial concordance.[1,3,4,9,13–15,25,30,32,42,44–46,48,50,62,63,72,76,78,81,104] A hepatic shadow lateralized to the right upper quadrant of the abdomen and a gastric air shadow or nasogastric tube in the left upper quadrant are consistent with solitus normal viscera, and by inference a right-sided inferior caval vein and right-sided morphologically right atrium. There are of course exceptions to this, including isolated dextrocardia; the reality is that the determination of visceral, and by deduction, atrial situs from the chest and abdominal x-ray is inaccurate, and that hepatoatrial dissociation will lead to an erroneous conclusion about situs.[79,80,105–110] Isolated atrial inversion in either situs solitus or inversus is a rare congenital cardiac anomaly.[79a,79b] The discordance between atria and ventricles with ventriculoarterial concordance produces transposition physiology (see Chapter 41). In a normal population with atrial situs solitus and levocardia, the left hemidiaphragm is at a lower position than the right hemidiaphragm. There is the widespread view that the liver is responsible for the higher position of the right diaphragm, not the left-sided cardiac apex. This has been challenged by Reddy and colleagues[110a] who concluded that the cardiac mass determines the caudal displacement and lower position of the related hemidiaphragm.

A midline horizontal liver in a patient with congenital heart disease is consistent with incompletely lateralized viscera, and by inference atria as well (see Chapter 41). A midline horizontal liver in a cyanotic infant is considered ominous, raising the specter of complex cardiac disease associated with right atrial isomerism and asplenia (see Chapter 32).[54,55,57,105,106,111,112] Yet a substantial number of patients with necropsy proven asplenia and complex congenital heart disease will appear to have lateralized viscera on a chest radiograph.[105,106] Levocardia with apparent situs inversus of the abdominal viscera in a cyanotic neonate should also provoke concern about the gravity of congenital heart disease.[24]

Indirect determination of atrial situs can be inferred from the disposition of the tracheobronchial tree imaged from either the plain chest radiograph or high kilovoltage filtered films.[26,42,44,45,47,49–51,113,114] The normal short right-sided epiarterial bronchus and the long left-sided hyparterial bronchus are consistent with solitus atria (Fig. 3-16). The appearance of bilateral epiarterial bronchi is consistent with right atrial isomerism, whereas bilaterally long and left-appearing bronchi are consistent with left atrial isomerism.[4,26,47,49–51,55,58,81,84–86,93,113–116] Unequivocally, bronchial anatomy is more consistently predictive of atrial situs than the radiographic appearance of visceral situs, although even bronchial anatomy may not

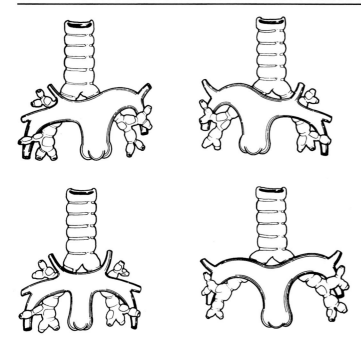

Fig. 3-16: Drawings of lateralized bronchi and pulmonary arteries.
Top, left: Lateralized bronchi in atrial situs solitus with a right-sided epiarterial bronchus and left-sided hyparterial bronchus. **Top, right:** Bronchial situs inversus with atrial situs inversus. **Bottom, left:** Bilateral right-sided or epiarterial bronchi with right atrial isomerism. **Bottom, right:** Bilateral left or hyparterial bronchi with left atrial isomerism.

correlate with atrial anatomy.[47,65,66,68,69,117] The lateral chest radiograph is also helpful in defining the status of the bronchial branching pattern. In situs solitus, the end-on shadow of the right upper lobar bronchus is projected above that of the left upper lobar bronchus. The right pulmonary artery casts a shadow in front of the ipsilateral bronchus, whereas the left pulmonary artery casts a shadow above and behind the ipsilateral bronchus. This hilar anatomy is also seen in situs inversus, as the superior-inferior spatial relationship of the hilar structures is preserved, although the right-left orientation is reversed. In right isomerism, both side upper lobar bronchi are seen at almost the same horizontal level. But in contrast to right isomerism, the pulmonary arteries cast a shadow behind the bronchial shadows in left isomerism.

The cross-sectional echocardiogram is certainly diagnostic of the venous connections to the atria, and even the character of the atrial appendages can be imaged, thus defining with some degree of accuracy the atrial situs.[48,118–120] The recognition of azygous drainage of the inferior caval vein with connection of all the hepatic veins directly to the atrium is highly suggestive of left atrial isomerism (see Chapter 12). Similarly, the cross-sectional recognition of the unusual topography of the aorta and inferior caval vein with both on the same side of the vertebral column is highly suggestive of right atrial isomerism.[121]

The Ventricles

Whereas there is unanimity of opinion as to what constitutes an atrium and a great artery, there is less unanimity as to what constitutes a ventricle. The ventricular mass extends from the atrioventricular junction to the ventriculoarterial junction, and in the normal heart, there are two distinct ventricles, the morphologically right and the morphologically left. About this, there is agreement. Continuing disagreement exists regarding what constitutes a ventricle. Is the morphologically right ventricle a bipartite structure composed of confluent sinus or body portion and an infundibular portion, or is it tripartite, with confluent inlet, apical trabecular, and outlet components? Van Praagh[3–5,7,9,10,122,123] advocates a bipartite perspective, whereas Anderson and others advocate the position of Goor, which views the ventricle as a tripartite structure.[16,17,32,33,35,38,39,41,42,124–126] What confers "rightness" or "leftness" to a ventricle is the character of the mural trabecular component because there are so many variations of the ventricular inlets and outlets that mute their utility in ventricular designation (Figs. 3-3 through 3-6 and Figs. 3-10 through 3-12).[127] It is the coarse trabecular component that confers rightness to the ventricle, and the smooth mural myocardium that confers leftness. Among some hearts with a univentricular atrioventricular connection, the mural trabecular myocardium of some ventricles confers neither rightness nor leftness, and such ventricles, fortunately uncommon, are considered of indeterminate morphology (see Chapter 40).[122]

The Concept of the Ventricular Loop

In their deductive approach to a segmental analysis of congenital heart disease, Van Praagh and colleagues introduced the concept of ventricular loops.[1,3–5,9,10,13–15] A ventricular d-loop indicated that the morphologically right ventricle is to the right of the morphologically left ventricle. Furthermore, in the presence of solitus atria, one would deduce from a d-ventricular loop that the atrioventricular connections are concordant. And in the vast majority of congenitally malformed hearts, this deduction would be correct. But hearts have been described when the apparent type of ventricular loop and type of atrioventricular connection are discordant (see also Chapter 44).[128–132a] These unusual hearts support the position that both the type of internal organization of the ventricle and the type of atrioventricular connection are important elements in any systematized nomenclature. In this regard, Seo and colleagues[131,133] have described several hearts in detail in which the type of atrioventricular connection and internal organization of the ventricle were disharmonious, ie, atrial situs solitus, concordant atrioventricular connection, but with a ventricular loop exhibiting left-hand topography in one case, and in the other a discordant atrioventricular connection, but with right-hand ventricular internal organization (see also Chapter 26, Fig. 26-27 and Chapter 44). In their editorial comment to the first of the two papers,[131] Anderson and Yen Ho point out that those hearts whose ventricular topology are incongruent for the type of atrioventricular connection frequently have juxtaposition of the atrial appendages.[36]

Ventricular Organization

A normal or noninverted ventricular relationship (solitus or d-loop ventricles of Van Praagh) indicates that the morphologically right ventricle(its inlet and trabecular components) are to the right of the morphologically left ventricle. To further characterize the morphologically right ventricle, it is necessary to define the internal organization of the right ventricle; that is, the inlet-outlet axis of the ventricle. Van Praagh uses the concept of a right-hand pattern of internal organization and a left-hand pattern of internal organization (Fig. 3-17).[1,3,4,7–10,13–15,122,123,132] In a normal heart, the thumb of the right hand represents the right ventricular inlet, the palmar surface of the right hand faces the right ventricular septal surface; the back of the right hand faces the free wall of the right ventricle; and the fingers of the right hand represent the right ventricular outlet or infundibulum. In the same normal heart, but now focusing on the left ventricle, the left thumb marks the left ventricular inlet; the palm of the left hand, the left ventricular septal surface; and the fingers of the left hand, the left ventricular outlet. An inverted ventricular relationship has a left-hand pattern for the organization of the morphologically right ventricle.

The Great Arteries

The great arteries are rarely so malformed as to make identification difficult. The normal aorta is that arterial trunk giving origin to the coronary and systemic arteries. The pulmonary trunk supports the right and left pulmonary arteries. Among some malformed hearts, a single, common arterial trunk gives origin to coronary, pulmonary, and systemic arteries (see Chapter 7). Rarely, three great arteries have been identified originating from the base of the heart (see Chapter 19).[133a]

Types of Atrioventricular Connection

Anderson differentiates the type of atrioventricular connection from the mode of connection.[25,30,33,37,38,42] The type of atrioventricular connection indicates only how the atria are connected to the ventricles (ie, concordant, discordant, ambiguous) (Figs. 3-18 and 3-19). The mode refers more specifically to the morphology of the valves at the atrioventricular junction.

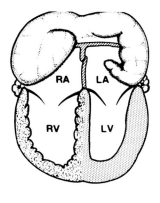
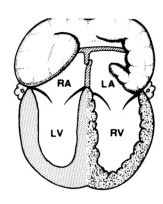
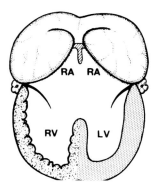
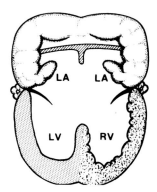

Fig. 3-18: Types of atrioventricular connection in a biventricular heart.
Top, left: A concordant atrioventricular connection with solitus atria. **Top, right:** A discordant atrioventricular connection with solitus atria. **Bottom, left:** Ambiguous atrioventricular connection with right atrial isomerism; the ventricular organization conforms to a d-loop. **Bottom, right:** Ambiguous atrioventricular connection with left atrial isomerism. The ventricular organization conforms to an l-loop.

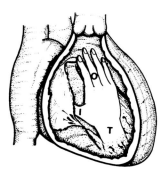
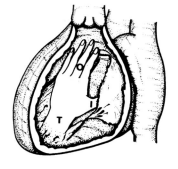

Fig. 3-17: Role of the right or left hand in the determination of the pattern of ventricular organization.
A right-hand pattern or so-called d-ventricular loop is characterized by a right ventricular inlet-outlet axis defined by a right hand placed on the right ventricular septal surface so that the thumb (or wrist) defines the inlet of the right ventricle; the palm defines the septal surface of the morphologically right ventricle; and the fingertips define the outlet of the right ventricle. A left-hand pattern of internal organization for the morphologically right ventricle is defined when the left thumb defines the right ventriclar inlet; the palm of the left-hand placed on the septal surface, and the fingers of the left hand designate the right ventricular outlet.

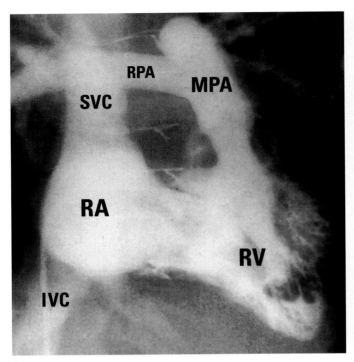

A

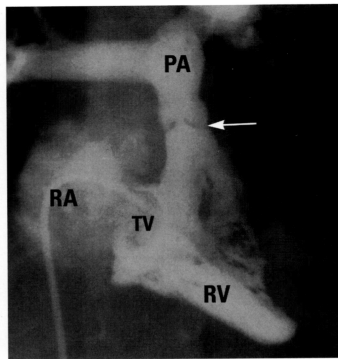

B

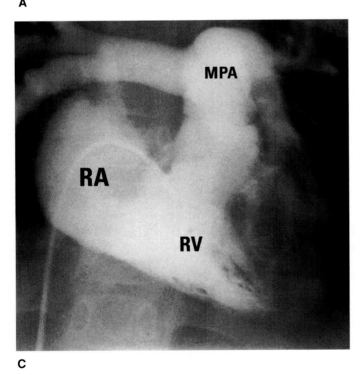

C

Fig. 3-19: Atrioventricular and ventriculoarterial concordant connection between morp hologically right atrium and morphologically right ventricle and right ventricle and pulmonary artery with atrial situs solitus.
A: The right atrium receiving the superior and inferior caval veins connects through a tricuspid valve with the morphologically right ventricle and this ventricle supports the normally connected pulmonary artery. **B:** Another patient showing normal connections with an open tricuspid valve and closed pulmonary valve. **C:** A third patient with atrioventricular and ventriculoarterial concordant connection.

Atrioventricular Connections in a Biventricular Heart

Three types of atrioventricular connection can be defined when the heart is biventricular: 1) concordant atrioventricular connection; 2) discordant atrioventric- ular connection (see also Chapters 36 and 42); 3) am- biguous atrioventricular connection (see Chapter 41) (Fig. 3-18). A concordant atrioventricular connection indicates that the morphogically right atrium connects to a morphologically right ventricle, and left atrium to morphologically left ventricle (Figs. 3-10 and 3-11).

The atrioventricular connection is discordant when the morphologically right atrium connects to a morphologically left ventricle via a mitral valve, and the left atrium to a morphologically right ventricle through a tricuspid valve (see Chapter 36). In those hearts where the atria are not lateralized, the atrioventricular connection is by definition ambiguous (see Chapter 41). In most of the hearts with biventricular atrioventricular connection regardless of the type of connection, the bloodstreams from the atria to the ventricles through the atrioventricular valves are parallel. There are, however, some hearts characterized by their twisted nature of the atrioventricular connection with an unexpected spatial relationship of the cardiac chambers and great arteries for the given segmental connections. The twisted atrioventricular connection is the hallmark of the so-called superoinferior ventricles and criss-cross hearts (see Chapter 44).

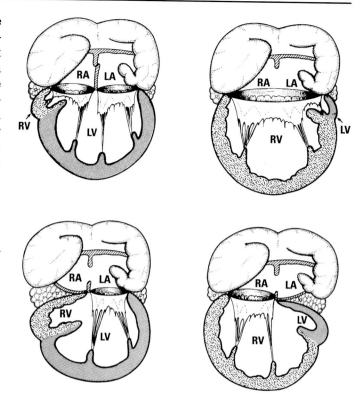

Fig. 3-20: Atrioventricular connections when the heart is not biventricular.
Upper left panel: Double-inlet left ventricle. **Upper right panel**: Double-inlet right ventricle. **Lower left panel**: Absent right atrioventricular connection to a ventricle of left ventricular type. **Lower right panel**: Absent left connection to a ventricle of right ventricular type.

Atrioventricular Connections When the Heart is Not Biventricular

One of the areas where Van Praagh and Anderson and their respective colleagues continue to differ is in the nomenclature applied to those hearts considered by Van Praagh as single ventricle.[1,3–5,9,10,13,15–17,37,38,122–123a] Anderson has used the designation univentricular atrioventricular connection when one atrioventricular connection is absent, or when both atria are connected to one ventricle, he advocates the designation double inlet ventricle. Hearts with a univentricular atrioventricular connection may have a double-inlet connection (see Chapter 40); an absent right (see Chapter 39) or an absent left atrioventricular connection (see Chapter 26) (Fig. 3-19). The ventricular morphology receiving the atrioventricular connection may be that of a dominant left ventricle, a morphologically right ventricle, or a solitary ventricle, usually of indeterminate morphology.

Mode of Atrioventricular Connection

Abnormalities of the mode of atrioventricular connection include perforate vs. imperforate atrioventricular valves; a common atrioventricular orifice; an unguarded atrioventricular orifice; and straddling and/or overriding atrioventricular valve (Figs. 3-20 and 3-21). A straddling atrioventricular valve designates one whose tension apparatus is attached to both sides of the interventricular septum (see Chapter 15, Fig. 15-4 and Chapter 25). The extent of straddling can vary from mild to very severe, and the recognition of the presence and severity of straddling will impact on the choice of

a biventricular repair vs. atriopulmonary connection with atrial separation (Fontan's operation).

Ventricular Topography

The precise spatial relation between the morphologically right and left ventricles can vary considerably. There is the normal or solitus oblique relation, and this varies considerably from the spatial relation observed in those patients with discordant atrioventricular connections (see Chapters 36 and 42). In this condition, the ventricles are aligned about a vertically disposed ventricular septum. In hearts with a superoinferior ventricular relation, the ventricular septum has a horizontal orientation, and the ventricular masses are aligned in the horizontal plane, almost invariably with the often smaller right ventricle on top of the morphologically left ventricle (see Chapter 44).[7,34,134–139] Whether the ventricles have a superoinferior ventricular topography, the so-called topsy-turvy orientation, or the appearance of crossed atrioventricular connections, the characterization of the type of atrioventricular connection is fundamental to the internal organization of the particular heart.

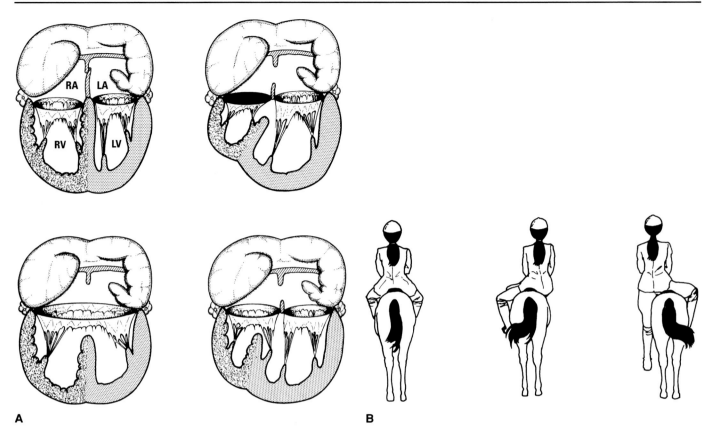

A   **B**

Fig. 3-21: Schematic diagram showing some modes of atrioventricular connection.
A, upper left: Concordant atrioventricular connection. **Lower left**: common atrioventricular orifice. **Upper right**: imperforate tricuspid valve. **Lower right**: Straddling and overriding tricuspid valve. **B:** The difference between straddling and overriding an atrioventricular valve. Straddling indicates that tension apparatus from one valve inserts into the other ventricle. Overriding indicates that the annulus of one atrioventricular valve overrides the ventricular septum. Thus, an atrioventricular valve can straddle, override, or both straddle and override.

Ventriculoarterial Connections

The patterns of ventriculoarterial connections are depicted in Figs. 3-22 and 3-23. Using the same conventions as defining the type and mode of atrioventricular connection, one can characterize the type and mode of ventriculoarterial connection. The four types of ventriculoarterial connection include 1) concordant or normal ventriculoarterial connection; 2) discordant ventriculoarterial connection; 3) double-outlet ventriculoarterial connection; and 4) single-outlet ventriculoarterial connection. When the ventriculoarterial connection is concordant, the morphologically right ventricle supports the pulmonary trunk, and the morphologically left ventricle supports the aorta. A discordant ventriculoarterial connection defines that connection in which the aorta is supported by the morphologically right ventricle, and the pulmonary trunk by the morphologically left ventricle. The more common designation for this type of ventriculoarterial connection is transposition of the great arteries. Double-outlet ventricle indicates that more than half of each great artery has its origin from one ventricle, whether it is right or left, dominant or rudimentary, or indeterminate. Examples of single-outlet connection include hearts with truncus arteriosus, single pulmonary trunk with aortic atresia, and single aortic trunk with pulmonary atresia. In the nomenclature of single outlet of the heart, it is important to state the ventricular origin of the solitary trunk: left or right ventricle, indeterminate ventricle, or a biventricular origin. Among those hearts with an abnormal ventriculoarterial connection, a ventricular septal defect is often present, and thus one or both great arteries may originate above or in juxtaposition to the ventricular septal defect, thus making it difficult to assign with precision or certainty the ventriculoarterial connection (see Chapters 37 and 38).[140–142] Furthermore, because of the malalignment between the outlet and trabecular portions of the ventricular septum that is found in many forms of complex congenital heart disease, this further complicates the assignment of ventriculoarterial connection.[143,144]

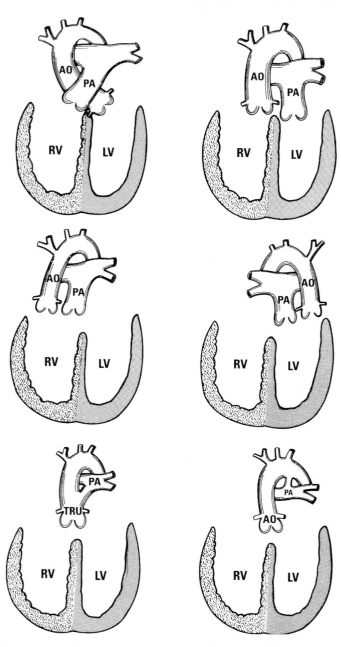

Fig. 3-22: Schematic diagram showing types of ventriculo-arterial connection.
Upper left panel: Concordant ventriculoarterial connection.
Upper right panel: Discordant ventriculoarterial connection.
Middle left panel: Double-outlet right ventricle. **Middle right panel:** Double-outlet left ventricle. **Lower left panel:** truncus arteriosus or common arterial trunk. **Lower right panel:** single-outlet aorta with pulmonary atresia.

Infundibular Anatomy

Of the many fundamental issues that seemingly polarized those followers of Van Praagh from the nucleus of the United Kingdom and Robert Anderson was the former's emphasis on differential conal

growth and infundibular anatomy in the morphogenesis of nontransposed and transposed great arteries.[1–4,6–8,10,11,15,20,25,30,32,37,38] In the system of nomenclature used by Anderson, the infundibulum was and is considered the outlet component of the ventricular mass. It is not that the United Kingdom group did not appreciate the contributions of infundibular development to the morphogenetic disturbances responsible for abnormal ventriculoarterial connections and to obstruction of the arterial outlets, it was that this was not their emphasis.

Van Praagh and colleagues have described a wide range of congenitally malformed hearts, and have catalogued their infundibular anatomy and the anatomy of the normal heart as well. Four types of infundibular anatomy have been described: 1) subpulmonary infundibulum; 2) subaortic infundibulum; 3) bilaterally

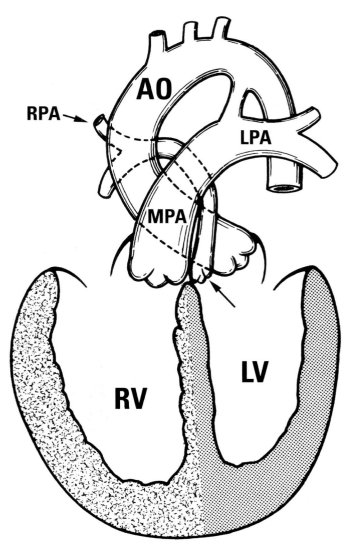

Fig. 3-23: Drawing of triarterial heart. Based on Reference 133A.

present infundibulum; and 4) bilaterally deficient infundibulum. The solitus normal heart has a well-defined subpulmonary infundibulum, whereas the subaortic infundibulum is severely attenuated. This attenuation of the left-sided infundibulum brings the aortic valve into fibrous continuity with the mitral valve. The neonate with complete transposition in isolation has a well-defined subaortic infundibulum that connects the transposed aorta to the morphologically right ventricle (see Chapter 35). Some patients with complex forms of transposition have bilaterally well-expanded infundibulum, and in such hearts semilunar valves and atrioventricular valves are not in fibrous continuity. Rarely, some hearts with transposition of the great arteries will have bilaterally deficient infundibulum in which there is the potential for fibrous continuity between both semilunar and both atrioventricular valves.[145,146] These morphological observations illustrate the reality of differential conal growth and absorption, and the spectrum of normal aortic-mitral fibrous continuity.[147–150]

The infundibulum of the heart is in part responsible for the anterior-posterior disposition of the great arteries relative to one another, and infundibular development or lack thereof is responsible for discontinuity or continuity between semilunar valves and atrioventricular valves. Anderson and colleagues[40] reserve the term crista supraventricularis for normal hearts or those hearts with a normally connected and structured right ventricular outflow tract. For those hearts with complex anatomy, it is useful to view the supraventricular crest in terms of its morphological components: 1) the ventriculo-infundibular fold; 2) infundibular septum; and 3) the septomarginal trabecula. The ventriculoinfundibular fold is derived from the inner curvature of the heart tube and this structure thus separates a semilunar valve from an atrioventricular valve (see also Chapter 29).[151–153] The infundibular septum is a muscular structure separating the arterial outlets. It is this structure whose anterosuperior deviation is the essence of Fallot's tetralogy (see Chapter 20); whose posterior malalignment or displacement produces in the patient with atrioventricular and ventriculoarterial concordance a particular type of muscular subaortic stenosis with the ventricular septal defect inferior to the malaligned infundibular septum (see Chapters 29, 32, and 33); and in the patient with atrioventricular concordance but discordant ventriculoarterial connections, posterior displacement of the infundibular septum produces subpulmonary stenosis, whereas anterior displacement results in subaortic stenosis (see Chapter 35). The infundibular septum is usually a septal structure, but not invariably (see Chapter 37). Finally, the septomarginal trabecula is an intrinsic component of the right ventricular septal surface, and this structure does not dissociate from the morphologically right ventricle.

Arterial Relations

The spatial relations between the aorta and pulmonary artery show a continuum of right-left and anteroposterior coordinates. The exact position of the aortic valve relative to the pulmonary valve does not predict the type of ventriculoarterial connection, although once the spatial relation between the great arteries was considered just this. An extensive literature demonstrates that spatial relations between the great arteries, while important, do not predict the intracardiac anatomy. Thus the great arteries may be l-related (aortic valve to the left of the pulmonary valve) in hearts with concordant atrioventricular, and either concordant or discordant ventriculoarterial connections (so-called loop-rule exceptions).[154–157] And similarly, in patients with discordant atrioventricular and ventriculoarterial connections, where one might anticipate l-related great arteries, the aortic valve may be to the right of the pulmonary valve.[1–4,6–8,12,21,44,45,134–139,154–157] Indeed these so-called loop-rule exceptions became so frequent that the new nomenclature and practitioners thereof 'begged' for a precise connections approach to a segmental analysis, rather than the deductive approach. In the early and halcyon days of the application of a segmental and deductive approach to a patient with solitus atria and an aortic valve unequivocally anterior and to the left of the pulmonary valve, one would think the patient must have a ventricular l-loop and congenitally corrected transposition of the great arteries. A wide array of complex heart malformations with atrial situs solitus, concordant atrioventricular and ventriculoarterial connection, but a levorelated aorta have been catalogued (see Chapters 35, 37, 38, and 42–44).

Heart Positions

Levocardia indicates a heart predominately in the left chest with the apex to the left (see Chapter 44). Dextrocardia indicates a right-sided heart with the cardiac apex pointing to the right.[1,3,4,13,14] A midline heart is designated mesocardia.[23] A very rare type of cardiac malposition is ectopia cordis (see Chapter 48). Rarely, despite a heart predominately in the left chest, the apex of the ventricle will point to the right (Fig. 3-24).[23] The base-axis of a heart may be rotated + 180 degrees so that the great arteries seemingly originate from the apex of the heart. In some patients the cardiac mass will be seemingly lateralized to the left chest, but the cardiac apex is rightward and inferior.[158]

Cardiac Malpositions

The cardiac malpositions include dextrocardia, isolated levocardia, mesocardia, conjoined thorapagi, and ectopia cordis (see Chapter 48 for conjoined thorapagi and ectopia cordis).

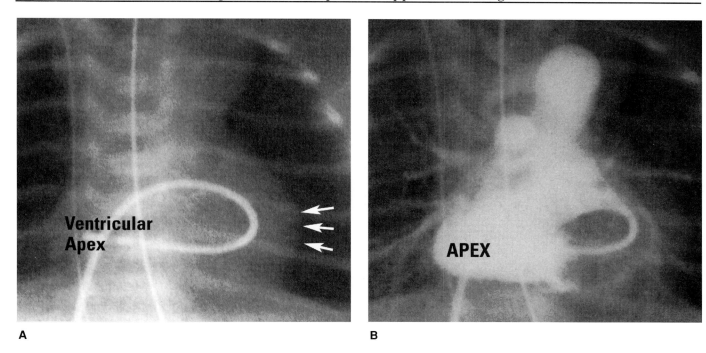

A   B

Fig. 3-24: Discordancy between cardiac apex from chest x-ray and ventricular apex from angiography.
A: Frontal frame showing cardiac apex (arrows) and presumed ventricular apex from catheter position. **B:** The ventriculogram shows a heart predominately in the left chest with a right-sided cardiac apex.

Dextrocardia

Dextro-, meaning right, and cardia, meaning heart, indicate a right-sided heart. This in itself tells us nothing about the atrioventricular or the ventriculoarterial connection. The heart may be in the right chest because of agenesis or hypoplasia of the right lung or because of a left-sided tension pneumothorax. Dextrocardia may occur with normally lateralized atria and viscera (situs solitus), an inversus pattern, or with ambiguous lateralization, hearts with similar atrial appendages (either both right-appearing, or both left-appearing) and incompletely lateralized viscera, often with splenic abnormalities, asplenia or polysplenia (see Chapter 41).

Can one predict the pattern of ventricular organization in the patient with dextrocardia? Does the presence of dextrocardia imply d- or l-ventricular looping? In the comprehensive analysis of dextrocardia published in 1989 by Van Praagh and colleagues,[15] l-loop ventricles were twice as common as ventricular d-loops. This should not be surprising if one considers an l-loop of the ventricles appropriate for the heart in the right chest. The data from this group were interesting in terms of the disposition of ventricular d- and l-loops in the patient with dextrocardia and atrial situs solitus: the frequency of d- and l-loops were almost equal. In those patients with dextrocardia and situs inversus of atria and viscera, an l-ventricular loop was considerably more common than the ventricular d-loop. This predominance of ventricular l-loop was also appreciated in that cohort of patients with dextrocardia and in-

completely lateralized viscera. The ventriculoarterial connection or alignment has been analyzed by Van Praagh and colleagues[15] in 136 cases of dextrocardia. Transposition of the great arteries (complete and corrected) was the most common type of connection, followed by normally connected great arteries, and then by the ventriculoarterial connection of double-outlet right ventricle. Yet, for any given patient with dextrocardia, the atrioventricular and ventriculoarterial connection must be specifically defined.

Mesocardia

In the patient with mesocardia, the cardiac silhouette has a midline position, and it is difficult to determine the cardiac apex from the chest radiograph. This is not a particularly common diagnosis, and as one might anticipate, atrial situs solitus, inversus, or isomeric atrial arrangements have been described in hearts with mesocardia.[23] A wide variety of malformed hearts have been defined in hearts with a midline thoracic position.

Cephalic Orientation of the Cardiac Apex with a Thoracic Heart

We have identified three patients in whom the heart has a thoracic location, but in whom the base-apex axis is most bizarre, a type of heart that we designated topsy-turvy. The three patients had aortopulmonary septal defects, and the apex of the heart was directed cephalad, with the ascending aorta actually descending (see Chapter 44, Fig. 44-4). The final step in the application of a segmental and sequential approach is to catalogue the major and minor cardiac anomalies.

Congenital Pericardial Defect

A congenital defect of the pericardium represents defective formation of the pleuopericardial membrane and may involve the entire pericardium, the left-sided aspect of the pericardium, or the right pericardium (Fig. 3-25).[159-179] Defects of the left pericardium are most commonly involved, but complete and small right-sided defects are well-described.[167,174] Incomplete formation of the septum transversum is thought to be responsible for a diaphragmatic defect. Partial absence of the left pericardium may be suspected clinically in the child and adult because of chest pain and an unusual cardiac silhouette observed on the plain chest radiograph. In patients with partial absence of the left pericardium, either the cardiac ventricles or the left atrial appendage may protrude or herniate through the pleuropericardial defect, leading in some patients to chest pain or syncope, while in others, strangulation of the ventricles or left atrial appendage may lead to death.[161,163,164,167,171,172,174,176,179] Herniation or protrusion of the right lung into the pericardial cavity may obstruct the right superior caval vein.[167] Herniation of the omentum into the pericardial cavity occurs when there is a diaphragmatic pericardial defect and a defect in the diaphragm.[165]

All of these defects are very uncommon, and we are aware of only a few instances of symptomatic right- or left-sided pericardial defect being recognized in the neonate.[180] The chest radiograph in the older child may provide a clue as to the presence of a left-sided defect, and diagnosis may be confirmed by cross-sectional echocardiography and contrast enhanced computed tomography or magnetic resonance imaging. In those symptomatic patients, surgical attention including treatment by thoracoscopic pericardiectomy is required to close, or widely open the pleuropericardial defect.[181]

Dextrocardia, Situs Inversus, and the Syndrome of Kartagener

Kartagener syndrome is the syndrome of dextrocardia with situs inversus totalis, sinusitis, and

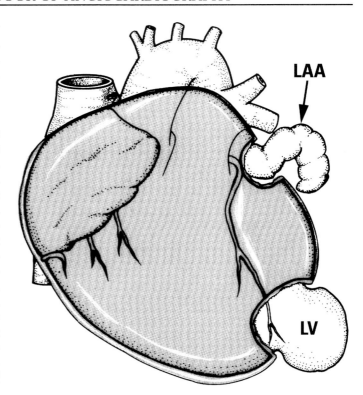

Fig. 3-25: Drawing depicting relatively small congenital pericardial defects causing left atrial and ventricular herniation.

bronchiectasis.[182-195] The respiratory difficulties, including recurrent middle ear infections in this syndrome result from hypomotility or immotility of the tracheobronchial cilia. The basic defect is lack of ciliary dynein.[187,188,194] Males with this disorder are usually infertile, and absence of dynein in the sperm tails accounts for spermatic immotility.[187,188,194] While uncommon to establish this diagnosis in the neonate, in at least one neonate the diagnosis of primary ciliary dyskinesia was confirmed by both ultrastructural and functional investigations.[193] The immotile cilia syndrome was suspected in this patient because of respiratory distress, situs inversus, abnormal nasal discharge, and hyperinflated chest x-ray. Others have also made this diagnosis in the neonate and young infant.[192] In the older patient with Kartagener's syndrome, end-stage bronchiectasis has been treated by heart-lung or double-lung transplantation.[196-198]

References

1. Van Praagh R. The segmental approach to diagnosis in congenital heart disease. *Birth Defects (Original Article Series)* 1972;8:4–23.
2. Van Praagh R. The story of anatomically corrected malposition of the great arteries. *Chest* 1976;69:2–4.
3. Van Praagh R. Terminology of congenital heart disease. Glossary and commentary. *Circulation* 1977;56:139–143.
4. Van Praagh R. Diagnosis of complex congenital heart disease: Morphologic-anatomic method and terminology. *Cardiovasc Intervent Radiol* 1984;7:115–120.
5. Van Praagh R, David I, Van Praagh S. What is a ventri-

cle? The single ventricle trap. *Pediatr Cardiol* 1982;2:79–84.

6. Van Praagh R, Durnin R, Jockin H, Wagner HR, Korns M, Garabedian H, Ando M, Calder AL. Anatomically corrected malposition of the great arteries (S,D,L). *Circulation* 1975;51:20–31.

7. Van Praagh S, LaCorte M, Fellows KE, Bossina K, Busch HJ, Keck EW, Weinberg PM, Van Praagh R. Supero-inferior ventricles: Anatomic and angiocardiographic findings in ten postmortem cases. In: Van Praagh R, Takao A, eds. *Etiology and Morphogenesis of Congenital Heart Disease.* Mount Kisco, NY: Futura Publishing Company, INC; 1980, pp. 317–378.

8. Van Praagh R, Layton WM, Van Praagh S. The morphogenesis of normal and abnormal relationships between the great arteries and ventricles: Pathologic and experimental data. In: Van Praagh R, Takao A, eds. *Etiology and Morphogenesis of Congenital Heart Disease.* Mount Kisco, NY: Futura Publishing Company, Inc.; 1980, pp. 271–316.

9. Van Praagh R, Ongley PA, Swan HJC. Anatomic types of single or common ventricle in man. Morphologic and geometric aspects of sixty autopsied cases. *Am J Cardiol* 1964; 13: 367–386.

10. Van Praagh R, Wise JR Jr, Dahl BA, Van Praagh S. Single left ventricle with infundibular outlet chamber and tricuspid valve opening only into outlet chamber in 44-year-old man with thoracoabdominal ectopia cordis without diaphragmatic or pericardial defect: Importance of myocardial morphologic method of chamber identification in congenital heart disease. In: Van Praagh, Takao A, eds: *Etiology and Morphogenesis of Congenital Heart Disease.* Mount Kisco, NY: Futura Publishing Company, Inc; 1980, pp. 379–420.

11. Van Praagh R, Van Praagh S. Isolated ventricular inversion. A consideration of the morphogenesis, definition and diagnosis of nontransposed and transposed great arteries. *Am J Cardiol* 1966;17:395–406.

12. Van Praagh R, Van Praagh S. Anatomically corrected transposition of the great arteries. *Br Heart J* 1967;29:112–119.

13. Van Praagh R, Van Praagh S, Vlad P, Keith JD. Anatomic types of congenital dextrocardia. Diagnostic and embryologic implications. *Am J Cardiol* 1964;13:510–531.

14. Van Praagh R, Van Praagh S, Vlad P, Keith JD. Diagnosis of the anatomic types of congenital dextrocardia. *Am J Cardiol* 1965;15:234–247.

15. Van Praagh R, Weinberg PM, Smith SD, Foran RB, Van Praagh S. Malpositions of the Heart. In: Adams FH, Emmanouilides GC Riemenschneider, eds. *Moss' Heart Disease in Infants, Children, and Adolescents.* Baltimore: Williams and Wilkins; 1989, pp. 530–580.

15a.Anderson RH, Yen Ho S. Sequential segmental analysis-description and categorization for the millenium. *Cardiol Young* 1997; 7:98–116.

16. Anderson RH, Macartney FJ, Tynan M, Becker AE, Freedom RM, Godman MJ, Hunter S, Quero-Jimenez M, Rigby ML, Shinebourne EA, Sutherland G, Smallhorn JF, Soto B, Thiene G, Wilkinson JL, Wilcox BR, Zuberbuhler JR. Univentricular atrioventricular connection: The single ventricle trap unsprung. *Pediatr Cardiol* 1983;4:273–280.

17. Anderson RH, Becker AE, Freedom RM, Quero-Jimenez M, Macartney FJ, Shinebourne EA, Wilkinson JL, Tynan M. Problems in the nomenclature of the univentricular heart. *Herz* 1979;4:97–106.

18. de la Cruz MV, Anselmi G, Munoz-Castellanos L, Nadal-Ginard B, Munoz-Armas S. Systematization and embryological and anatomical study of mirror-image dextro-

cardias, dextroversions, and laevoversions. *Br Heart J* 1971;33:841–853.

19. de la Cruz MV, Nadal-Ginard B. Rules for the diagnosis of visceral situs, truncoconal morphologies, and ventricular inversions. *Am Heart J* 1972; 84: 19–32.

20. Foran RB, Belcourt C, Nanton MA, Murphy DA, Weinberg AG, Liebman J, Castaneda AR, Van Praagh R. Isolated infundibuloarterial inversion (S,D,I): A newly recognized form of congenital heart disease. *Am Heart J* 1988;116:1337–1350.

21. Freedom RM. The "anthropology" of the segmental approach to the diagnosis of complex congenital heart disease. *Cardiovasc Interventional Radiol* 1984;7:121–123.

22. Lev M. Pathologic diagnosis of positional variations in cardiac chambers in congenital heart disease. *Lab Invest* 1954;3:71–82.

23. Lev M, Liberthson RR, Golden JG, Eckner FAO, Arcilla RA. The pathologic anatomy of mesocardia. *Am J Cardiol* 1971;28:428–435.

24. Liberthson RR, Hastreiter AR, Sinha SN, Bharati S, Novak GM, Lev M. Levocardia with visceral heterotaxy-isolated levocardia: Pathologic anatomy and its clinical implications. *Am Heart J* 1973;85:40–54.

25. Macartney FJ, Shinebourne EA, Anderson RH. Connexions, relations, discordance, and distorsions. *Br Heart J* 1976;38:323–326.

26. Macartney FJ, Zuberbuhler JR, Anderson RH. Morphologic con-siderations pertaining to recognition of atrial isomerism. Consequences for sequential chamber localisation. *Br Heart J* 1980;44:657–667.

27. Shah CV. Recent Trends in malposition terminology. A way out of semantic confusion. *Indian Heart J* 1976;28:201–207.

28. Edwards WD. Classification and terminology of cardiovasculr anomalies. In: Emmanouilides GC, Allen HD, Riemenschneider TA, Gutgesell HP, (eds.) *Moss and Adams Heart Disease in Infants, Children, and Adolescents Including the Fetus and Young Adult.* Baltimore: Williams and Wilkins; 1995, pp. 106–131.

29. Weinber PM. Systematic approach to diagnosis and coding of pediatric cardiac disease. *Pediatr Cardiol* 1986;7:35–48.

30. Shinebourne EA, Macartney FJ, Anderson RH. Sequential chamber localisation—Logical approach to diagnosis in congenital heart disease. *Br Heart J* 1976;38:327–340.

31. Stanger P, Rudolph AM, Edwards JE. Cardiac Malpositions. An overview based on study of sixty-five necropsy specimens. *Circulation* 1977;56:159–172.

32. Tynan MJ, Becker AE, Macartney FJ, Quero Jiminez M, Shinebourne EA, Anderson RH. Nomenclature and classification of congenital heart disease. *Br Heart J* 1979;41:544–553.

33. Wilkinson JL, Acerete F. Terminological pitfalls in congenital heart disease. Reappraisal of some confusing terms, with an account of a simplified system of basic nomenclature. *Br Heart J* 1973;35:1166–1177.

34. Anderson RH. Criss-cross hearts revisited. *Pediatr Cardiol* 1982;3:305–313.

35. Anderson RH. Weasal words in paediatric cardiology. *Int J Cardiol* 1983;2:425–429.

36. Anderson RH, Yen Ho S. Editorial note: Segmental interconnexions versus topological congruency in complex congenital malformations. *Int J Cardiol* 1989;25:229–233.

37. Anderson RH, Becker AE, Freedom RM, Macartney FJ, Quero-Jiminez M, Shinebourne EA, Wilkinson JL, Tynan M. Sequential segmental analysis of congenital heart disease. *Pediatr Cardiol* 1984;5:281–288.

38. Anderson RH, Becker AE, Tynan M, Wilkinson JL. Definitions and terminology—The significance of sequential segmental analysis. In: Anderson RH, Crupi G, Parenzan L, eds: *Double Inlet Ventricle.* New York: Elsevier; 1987, pp, 3–28.

39. Anderson RH, Becker AE, Tynan M, Macartney FJ, Rigby ML, Wilkinson JL. The univentricular atrioventricular connection: Getting to the root of a thorny problem. *Am J Cardiol* 1982;54:822–828.

40. Anderson RH, Becker AE, Van Mierop LHS. What should we call the 'crista'? *Br Heart J* 1977;39:856–859.

41. Anderson RH, Becker AE, Wilkinson JL, Gerlis LM. Morphogenesis of univentricular hearts. *Br Heart J* 1976;37:558–572.

42. Anderson RH, Macartney FJ, Shinebourne EA, Tynan M. *Paediatric Cardiology.* Volume 1. Edinburgh: Churchill Livingstone; 1987, pp. 65–82.

43. Anderson RH, Macartney FJ, Tynan M, Becker AE, Freedom RM, Godman MJ, Hunter S, Quero-Jimenez M, Rigby ML, Shinebourne EA, Sutherland G, Smallhorn JF, Soto B, Thiene G, Wilkinson JL, Wilcox BR, Zuberbuhler JR. Univentricular atrioventricular connection: The single ventricle trap unsprung. *Pediatr Cardiol* 1983;4:273–280.

44. Freedom RM, Culham JAG, Moes CAF. *Angiocardiography of Congenital Heart Disease.* New York: Macmillan Publishing C; 1984, pp. 17–45.

45. Freedom RM, Smallhorn JF. The segmental approach to congenital heart disease. In: Freedom RM, Benson LN, Smallhorn JF, eds: *Neonatal Heart Disease.* London: Springer-Verlag; 1992. Pp. 119–133.

46. Arciniegas JG, Soto B, Coghan HC, Bargeron LMJ. Congenital heart malformations: Sequential angiographic analysis. *AJR* 1981;137:673–681.

47. Caruso G, Becker AE. How to determine atrial situs? Consideration initiated by 3 cases of absent spleen with discordant anatomy between bronchi and atria. *Br Heart J* 1979;41:559–567.

48. Huhta JC, Smallhorn JF, Macartney FJ. Two dimensional echocardiographic diagnosis of situs. *Br Heart J* 1982;48:97–108.

49. Becker AE, Anderson RH. *Pathology of Congenital Heart Disease.* London: Butterworths; 1981, pp. 211–224.

50. Partridge J. The radiological evaluation of atrial situs. *Clin Radiol* 1979;30:95–103.

51. Soto B, Pacifico AD, Souza AS Jr, Bargeron LM Jr, Ermocilla R, Tonkin IL. Identification of thoracic isomerism from the plain chest radiograph. *AJR* 1978;131:995–1002.

52. Bharati S, Lev M. Positional variations of the heart and its component chambers. Circulation 1979;59:886–891.

52a. Victor S, Nayak VM. Sinoatrial malfusion presenting with caudal position of right atrial appendage. *Tex Heart Inst J* 1995;22:192–196

53. Fitzer PM. An approach to cardiac malposition and the heterotaxy syndrome using tc sulfur colloid imaging. *AJR* 1976;127:1021–1025.

54. Forde WJ, Finby N. Roentgenographic features of congenital asplenia: A teratologic syndrome of visceral symmetry. *AJR* 1961;86:523–526.

55. Lucas RV Jr, Neufeld HN, Lester RG, Edwards JE. The symmetrical liver as a roentgen sign of asplenia. *Circulation* 1962;25:973–975.

56. Roberts WC, Anderson RC, Edwards JE. The signifi-

cance of asplenia in the recognition of inoperable congenital heart disease. *Circulation* 1961;26:851–857.

57. Ruttenberg HD, Neufeld HN, Lucas RVJ, Carey LS, Adams PJ, Anderson RC, Edwards JE. Syndrome of congenital cardiac disease with asplenia. Distinction from other forms of congenital cyanotic cardiac disease. *Am J Cardiol* 1964;13:387–406.

58. Van Mierop LHS, Eisen S, Schiebler GL. The radiographic appearance of the tracheobronchial tree as an indicator of visceral situs. *Am J Cardiol* 1970;26:432–435.

59. Van Mierop LHS, Gessner IH, Schiebler GL. Asplenia and polysplenia syndromes. *Birth Defects (Original Article Series)* 1972;8:36–44.

60. Van Mierop LHs, Patterson PR, Reynold RW. Two cases of congenital asplenia with isomerism of the cardiac atria and the sinoatrial nodes. *Am J Cardiol* 1964;13:407–412.

61. Van Mierop LHS, Wiglesworth FW. Isomerism of the cardiac atria in the asplenia syndrome. *Am J Cardiol* 1962;11:1303–1307.

62. Freedom RM, Smallhorn JF. Syndromes of right or left atrial isomerism. In: Freedom RM, Benson LN, Smallhorn JF, eds: *Neonatal Heart Disease.* London: Springer-Verlag; 1992, pp. 543–560.

63. Freedom RM, Culham JAG, Moes CAF. *Angiocardiography of Congenital Heart Disease.* New York: Macmillan Publishing Co; 1984, pp. 643–654.

64. Pelosi G, Guanella S. Isomerism of the left atrial appendages associated with absence of the spleen. *Int J Cardiol* 1990;27:380–382.

65. Pipitone S, Calcaterra G, Grillo R, Thiene G, Sperandeo V. Broncho-atrial discordance: A clinically diagnosed case. *Int J Cardiol* 1985;9:374–378.

66. Stewart PA, Becker AE, Wladimiroff JW, Essed CE. Left atrial isomerism associated with asplenia: Prenatal echocardiographic detection of complex congenital cardiac malformations. *J Am Coll Cardiol* 1984;4: 1015–1020.

67. Zimarino M, Gerboni S, Picchio FM. Left isomerism with absence of the spleen and obstructed pulmonary venous drainage-an uncommon association. *Cardiol Young* 1994;4:160–163.

68. Devine WA, Debich DE, Taylor SR. Symmetrical bronchial pattern with normal atrial morphology. *Int J Cardiol* 1988;20:395–398.

69. Rylaarsdam M, Attie F, Buendia A, Munoz L, Calderon J, Zabal C. Discordancia entre la anatomia bronquial y el situs atrial. *Arch Inst Cardiol Mex* 1990;60:393–399.

70. Van Praagh S, Kreutzer J, Alday L, Van Praagh R. Systemic and pulmonary venous connections in visceral heterotaxy, with emphasis on the diagnosis of the atrial situs: A study of 109 postmortem cases. In: Clark EB, Takao A, eds: *Developmental Cardiology. Morphogenesis and Function.* Mt. Kisco, NY: Futura Publishing Company, Inc; 1990, pp. 671–727.

71. Becker AE, Anderson RH. Isomerism of the atrial appendages-goodbye to asplenia and all that. In: Clark EB, Takao A, eds: *Developmental Cardiology. Morphogenesis and Function.* Mt. Kisco, NY: Futura Publishing Company, Inc; 1990, pp. 659–670.

72. Van Praagh R, Van Praagh S. Atrial isomerism in the heterotaxy syndromes with asplenia, or polysplenia, or normally formed spleen: An erroneous concept. *Am J Cardiol* 1990;66:1504–1506.

73. Geva T, Vick GW III, Wendt RE, Rokey P. Role of spin

echo and cinemagnetic resonance imaging in presurgical planning of heterotaxy syndrome: Comparison with echocardiography and catheterization. *Circulation* 1995;90:348–356.

74. Anderson RH, Devine WA, Uemura H. Diagnosis of heterotaxy syndrome (letter). Circulation 1995;91:906–907.

75. Geva T, Vick GW III, Wendt RE, Rokey P. [Reply to Reference 74]. *Circulation* 1995;91:907–908.

76. Brandt PWT, Calder AL. Cardiac connections: The segmental approach to radiologic diagnosis in congenital heart disease. *Curr Prob Diagn Radiol* 1977;7(3):3–35.

77. Calcaterra G, Anderson RH, Lau KC, Shinebourne EA. Dextrocardia-value of segmental analysis in its categorisation. *Br Heart J* 1979;42:497–507.

78. Ceballos R, Soto B, Bargeron LM Jr. Angiographic anatomy of the normal heart through axial angiography. *Circulation* 1981;64:351–358.

79. Clarkson PM, Brandt PWT, Barratt-Boyes BG, Neutze JM. "Isolated atrial inversion". Visceral situs solitus, visceroatrial discordance, discordant ventricular d loop without transposition, dextrocardia: Diagnosis and surgical correction. *Am J Cardiol* 1972;29:877–882.

79a. Santoro G, Masiello P, Farina R, Baldi C, Di Leo L, Di Benedetto G. Isolated atrial inversion in situs inversus: A rare anatomic arrangement. *Ann Thorac Surg* 1995;59:1019–1021.

80. Akita H, Matsuoka S, Kuroda Y. A rare case of isolated atrial discordance with primary atrial situs inversus. *Tokushima J Exp Med* 1993;40:113–117.

81. Edwards WE. Classification and terminology of cardiovascular anomalies. In: Emmanouilides GC, Allen HD, Riemenschneider TA, Gutgesell HP, eds: *Moss and Adams' Heart Disease in Infants, Children, and Adolescents, Including the Fetus and Young Adult.* Baltimore: Williams and Wilkins; 1995, pp. 106–131.

82. Ivemark BI. Implications of agenesis of the spleen on the pathogenesis of conotruncus anomalies in childhood. *Acta Paediatrica Scand* 1955;44:7–110.

83. Anderson RH, Sharma S, Yen Ho S, Zuberbuhler JR, Macartney FJ. Splenic syndromes, "situs ambiguus: and atrial isomerism (in Spanish). *Rev Latina de Card Inf* 1986;2:97–110.

84. Brandt HM and Liebow AA. Right pulmonary isomerism associated with venous, splenic, and other anomalies. *Lab Invest* 1958;7:469–503.

85. Landing B. Five syndromes (malformation complexes) of pulmonary symmetry, congenital heart disease, and multiple spleens. *Pediatr Pathol* 1984;2:125–151.

86. Landing BH, Lawrence T-YK, Payne VC Jr, Wells TR. Bronchial anatomy in syndromes with abnormal visceral situs, abnormal spleen and congenital heart disease. *Am J Cardiol* 1971;28:456–462.

87. Moller JH, Nakid A, Anderson RC, Edwards JE. Congenital cardiac disease associated with polysplenia: A developmental complex of bilateral "left-sidedness." *Circulation* 1967;36:789–799.

88. Layman TE, Levine MA, Amplatz K, Edwards JE. "Asplenic syndrome" in association with rudimentary spleen. *Am J Cardiol* 1967;20:136–139.

89. Peoples WM, Moller JH, Edwards JE. Polysplenia: A review of 146 cases. *Pediatr Cardiol* 1983;4:129–137.

90. Putschar WGJ, Manion WC. Congenital absence of the spleen and associated Anomalies. *Am J Clin Pathol* 1956;26:429–469.

91. Randall PA, Moller JH, Amplatz K. The spleen and congenital heart disease. *AJR* 1973;119:551–559.

92. Rose V, Izukawa T, Moes CAF. Syndromes of asplenia and polysplenia: A review of cardiac and non-cardiac malformations in 60 cases with special reference to diagnosis and prognosis. *Br Heart J* 1975;37:840–852.

93. Van Mierop LHS, Gessner IH, Schiebler GL. Asplenia and polysplenia syndromes. *Birth Defects (Original Article Series)* 1972;8:36–44.

94. Moller JH. Malposition of the Heart. In: Moller JH, Neal WA, eds: *Fetal, Neonatal, and Infant Cardiac Disease.* Norwalk, CT: Appleton and Lange; 1989, pp. 755–774.

95. Greenberg SD. Multilobulated spleen in association with congenital heart disease. Report of a case. *Arch Pathol* 1957; 63:333–335.

96. Anderson C, Devine WA, Anderson RH, Debich DE, Zuberbuhler JR. Abnomalities of the spleen in relation to congenital malformation of the heart: A survey of necropsy findings in children. *Br Heart J* 1990;63: 122–128.

97. Muir CS. Splenic agenesis and multilobulate spleen. *Arch Dis Child* 1959;34:431–433.

98. Wang J-K, Li Y-W, Chiu I-S, Wu M-H, Chang Y-C, Hung C-R, Lue H-C. Usefulness of magnetic resonance imaging in the assessment of venoatrial connections, atrial morphology, bronchial situs, and other anomalies in right atrial isomerism. *Am J Cardiol* 1994;74:701–704.

99. O'Leary PW, Seward JB, Hagler DJ, Tajik AJ. Echocardiographic documentation of splenic anatomy in complex congenital heart disease. *Am J Cardiol* 1991;68:1536–1538.

100. Freedom RM, Ellison RC. Coronary sinus rhythm in the poly-splenia syndrome. *Chest* 1973;63:952–958.

101. Momma K, Linde L. Abnormal P wave axis in congenital heart disease associated with asplenia and polysplenia. *J Electrocardiol* 1969;2:395–402.

102. Van Der Horst RL, Gotsman MS. Abnormalities of atrial depolarization in infradiaphragmatic interruption of inferior vena cava. *Br Heart J* 1972;34:295–300.

103. Dickinson DF, Wilkinson JL, Anderson KR, Smith A, Ho SY, Anderson RH. The cardiac conduction system in situs ambiguus. *Circulation* 1979;59:879–885.

104. Elliott LP. An angiocardiographic and plain film approach to complex congenital heart disease: Classification and simplified nomenclature. *Curr Prob Cardiol* 1978;3(3):5–64.

105. Freedom RM, Fellows KE. Radiographic visceral patterns in the asplenia syndrome. *Radiology* 1973;107:387–391.

106. Freedom RM, Treves S. Splenic scintigraphy and radionuclide venography in the heterotaxy syndrome. *Radiology* 1973;107:381–386.

107. Hastreiter AR, Rodriguez-Coronel A. Discordant situs of thoracic and abdominal viscera. *Am J Cardiol* 1968;22:111–118.

108. Leachman RD, Angelini P, Cokkinos DV. Hepato-atrial dissociation. Report of two cases and clinical implications. *Chest* 1973;63:926–932.

109. Teplick JG, Wallner RJ, Levine AH, Haskin ME, Teplick SK. Isolated dextrogastria: Report of two cases. *Am J Radiol* 1979;132:124–126.

110. Yen Ho S, Trotter SE, Redington AN. Ectopic accessory liver masquerading as spleen in a case with isomerism of the right atrial appendages. *Cardiol Young* 1993;3:43–46.

110a.Reddy V, Sharma S, Cobanoglu A. What dictates the position of the diaphragm—The heart or the liver? A review of sixty-five cases. *J Thorac Cardiovasc Surg* 1994;108:687–691.

111. Roberts WC, Anderson RC, Edwards JE. The significance of asplenia in the recognition of inoperable congenital heart disease. *Circulation* 1961;26:851–857.

112. Rowe RD, Freedom RM, Mehrizi A. *The Neonate With Congenital Heart Disease.* Philadelphia: WB Saunders Co; 1981, pp. 480–502.

113. Deanfield JE, Leanage R, Stroobant J, Chrispin AR, Taylor JFN, Macartney FJ. Use of high kilovoltage filtered beam radiographs for detection of bronchial situs in infants and young children. *Br Heart J* 1980;44:577–583.

114. Partridge JB, Scott O, Deverall PB, Macartney FJ. Visualization and measurement of the main bronchi by tomography as an objective indicator of thoracic situs in congenital heart disease. *Circulation* 1975;51:188–196.

115. Devine WA, Debich DE, Anderson RH. Dissection of congenitally malformed hearts with comments on the value of sequential segmental analysis. *Pediatr Pathol* 1991;11:235–259.

116. Tonkin ILD, Tonkin AK. Visceroatrial situs abnormalities: Sonographic and computed tomographic appearance. *AJR* 1982;138:509–515.

117. Radhakrishnan S, Singh M, Bajaj R. Discordance between abdominal and atrial arrangement in a case of complex congenital heart disease, *Int J Cardiol* 1992;36:361–363.

118. Huhta JC, Smallhorn JF, Macartney FJ. Cross-sectional echocardiographic Diagnosis of azygos continuation of the inferior vena cava. *Cathet Cardiovasc Diagn* 1984;10:221–232.

119. Huhta JC, Smallhorn JF, Macartney FJ, Anderson RH, De Leval M. Cross-sectional echocardiographic diagnosis of systemic venous return. *Br Heart J* 1982;48:388–403.

120. Stumper OF, Sreeram N, Elzenga NJ, Sutherland GR. Diagnosis of atrial situs by transesophageal echocardiography. *J Am Coll Cardiol* 1990;16:442–446.

121. Elliott LP, Cramer GG, Amplatz K. The anomalous relationship of the inferior vena cava and abdominal aorta as a specific angiocardiographic sign in asplenia. *Radiology* 1966;87:859–863.

122. Van Praah R, Plett JA, Van Praagh S. Single ventricle. pathology, embryology, terminology and classification. *Herz* 1979;4:113–150.

123. Van Praagh R, David I, Gordon D, Wright GB, Van Praagh S. Ventricular diagnosis and designation. In: Godman MJ, ed: *Paediatric Cardiology.* Volume 4. Edinburgh: Churchill Livingstone; 1981, pp. 153–168.

123a.Barlow A, Pawade A, Wilkinson JL, Anderson RH. Cardiac anatomy in patients undergoing the Fontan procedure. *Ann Thorac Surg* 1995;60:1324–1330.

124. Goor DA, Lillehei CW. *Congenital Malformations of the Heart.* New York: Grune and Stratton; 1975, pp. 11–15.

125. Zuberbuhler JR. Double-inlet ventricle. In: Moller JR, Neal WA, eds: *Fetal, Neonatal, and Infant Cardiac Disease.* Norwalk, CT: Appleton and Lange; 1989, pp. 603–619.

126. Freedom RM, Harder J, Culham JAG, Trusler GA, Rowe RD. Ventricular hypoplasia: Angiocardiographic features with surgical implications. In: Godman MJ, ed: *Paediatric Cardiology.* Volume 4, Edinburgh: Churchill Livingstone; 1981, pp. 117–139.

127. Wenink ACG, Gittenberger de Groot AC. Left and right ventricular trabecular patterns. Consequence of ventricular septation and valve development. *Br Heart J* 1982;48:462–468.

128. Weinberg PM, Van Praagh R, Wagner HR, Cuaso CC. New form of criss-cross atrioventricular relation: An expanded view of the meaning of D and l-loops (abstract). World Congress of Pediatric Cardiology. London, 1980, Abstract 319.

129. Anderson RH, Smith A, Wilkinson JL. Disharmony between atrioventricular connections and segmental combinations: Unusual variants of "crisscross" hearts. *J Am Coll Cardiol* 1987;10:1274–1277.

130. Geva T, Sanders SP, Ayres NA, O'Laughlin MP, Parness IA. Two-dimensional echocardiographic anatomy of atrioventricular alignment discordance with situs concordance. *Am Heart J* 1993;125:459–464.

131. Seo JW, Choe GY, Chi JG. An unusual ventricular loop associated with right juxtaposition of the atrial appendages. *Int J Cardiol* 1989;25:219–225.

132. Van Praagh R. When concordant or discordant atrioventricular alignments predict the ventricular situs wrongly. I. Solitus atria, concordant alignments, and l-loop ventricles. II. Solitus atria, discordant alignments, and D-loop ventricles. *J Am Coll Cardiol* 1987;10: 1278–1279.

132a.Sklansky MS, Lucas VW, Kashani IA, Rothman A. Atrioventricular situs concordance with atrioventricular alignment discordance: Fetal and neonatal echocardiographic findings. *Am J Cardiol* 1995;76:202–204.

133. Seo J-W, Yoo S-J, Yen Ho, S, Lee HJ, Anderson RH. Further morphological observations on hearts with with twisted atrioventricular connections (criss-cross hearts). *Cardiovasc Pathol* 1992;1:211–217.

133a.Diaz-Gongora G, Quero-Jimenez M, Espino-Vela J, Arteaga M, Bargeron L. A heart with three arterial trunks (tritruncal heart). *Pediatr Cardiol* 1982;3: 293–299.

134. Freedom RM. Supero-inferior ventricle and criss-cross atrio-ventricular connections: An analysis of the myth and mystery. In: Belloli GP, Squarcia U, eds: *Pediatric Cardiology and Cardiosurgery. Modern Problems in Paediatrics.* Basel: Karger; 1983, pp. 48–62.

135. Freedom RM, Culham G, Rowe RD. The criss-cross and supero-inferior ventricular heart: An angiocardiographic study. *Am J Cardiol* 1978;42:620–628.

136. Freedom RM, Culham JAG, Moes CAF. *Angiocardiography of Congenital Heart Disease.* New York: Macmillan Publishing Co; 1984, pp. 629–642.

137. Freedom RM. Superoinferior ventricles, criss-cross atrioventricular connections, and the straddling atrioventricular valve. In: Freedom RM, Benson LN, Smallhorn JF, eds: *Neonatal Heart Disease.* London: Springer-Verlag; 1992, pp. 667–678.

138. Geva T, Van Praagh S, Sanders SP, Mayer JE Jr., Van Praagh R. Straddling mitral valve with hypoplastic right ventricle, crisscross atrioventricular connections, double-outlet right ventricle and dextrocardia: Morphologic, diagnostic, and surgical considerations. *J Am Coll Cardiol* 1991;17:1603–1612.

139. Anderson RH, Shinebourne EA, Gerlis LM. Criss-cross atrioventricular relationships producing paradoxical atrioventricular concordance or discordance. Their significance to nomenclature of congenital heart disease. *Circulation* 1974;50:176–180.

140. Lecompte Y; Batisse A; Di Carlo D. Double-outlet right ventricle: A surgical synthesis. *Adv Card Surg* 1993;4:109–136.

141. Rubay J, Lecompte Y, Batisse A, Durandy Y, Dibie A, Lemoine G, Vouhe P. Anatomic repair of anomalies of ventriculo-arterial connection (REV). Results of a new technique in cases associated with pulmonary outflow tract obstruction. *Eur J Cardiothorac Surg* 1988;2: 305–311.

142. Sakata R, Lecompte Y, Batisse A, Borromee L, Durandy Y. Anatomic repair of anomalies of ventriculoarterial connection associated with ventricular septal defect. I. Criteria of surgical decision. *J Thorac Cardiovasc Surg* 1988;95:90–95.

143. Zielinsky P, Rossi M, Haertel JC, Vitola D, Lucchese FA, Rodrigues R. Subaortic fibrous ridge and ventricular septal defect: Role of septal malalignment. *Circulation* 1987;75:1124–1129.

144. Roberson DA, Silverman NH. Malaligned outlet septum with subpulmonary ventricular septal defect and abnormal ventriculoarterial connection: A morphologic spectrum defined echocardiographically. *J Am Coll Cardiol* 1990;16:459–468.

145. Garcia Arenal F, Munoz Castellanos L, Kuri Nivon M, Salinas CH. Infundibulos bilaterales en cardiopatias congenitas. *Arch Inst Cardiol Mex* 1992;62:203–214.

146. Freedom RM. Double-outlet left ventricle; Isolated atrioventricular discordance: Anatomically corrected malposition of the great arteries, and syndrome of juxtaposition of the atrial appendages. In: Freedom RM, Benson LN, Smallhorn JF, eds. *Neonatal Heart Disease.* London: Springer-Verlag; 1992, pp. 561–569.

147. Goor DA, Dische R, Lillehei CW. The conotruncus. 1. Its normal inversion and conus absorption. *Circulation* 1972;46:375–384.

148. Goor DA, Edwards JE. The spectrum of transposition of the great arteries with specific reference to developmental anatomy of the conus. *Circulation* 1973;48:406–415.

149. Rosenquist GC, Clark EB, Sweeney LJ, McAllister HA. The normal spectrum of mitral and aortic valve discontinuity. *Circulation* 1976;54:298–301.

150. Rosenquist GC, Clark EB, McAllister HA, Bharati S, Edwards JE. Increased mitral-aortic separation in discrete subaortic stenosis. *Circulation* 1979;60:70–74.

151. Bersch W. On the importance of the bulboauricular flange for the formal genesis of congenital heart defects with special regard to the ventricular septum defects. *Arch Abt A Path Anat* 1971;354:252–267.

152. Meredith MA, Hutchins GM, Moore GW. Role of the left inter-ventricular sulcus in formation of the interventricular septum and crista supraventricularis in normal human cardiogenesis. *Anat Rec* 1979;194:417–428.

153. Anderson RH, Wilkinson JL, Becker AE. The bulbus cordis—A misunderstood region of the developing human heart: Its significance to the classification of congenital cardiac malformations. In: Rosenquist GC, Bergsma D, eds: Morphogenesis and malformation of the cardiovascular system. *Birth Defects (Original Article Series)* 1978;14:1–28.

154. Carr I, Tynan MJ, Aberdeen E, Bonham Carter RE, Graham G, Waterston DG. Predictive accuracy of the loop rule in 109 children with classical complete transposition of the great arteries (abstract). *Circulation* 1968;38(suppl 5):52.

155. Freedom RM, Harrington DP, White RI Jr. The differential diagnosis of levo-transposed or malposed aorta. An angiocardiographic study. *Circulation* 1974;50:1040–1046.

156. Otero Coto E, Jiminez MQ, Cabrera A, Deverall PB, Caffarena JM. Aortic levopositions without ventricular inversion. *Eur J Cardiol* 1978;8:523–541.

157. Freedom RM, Benson LN. Congenitally corrected transposition of the great arteries. In: Freedom RM, Benson LN, Smallhorn JF, eds: *Neonatal Heart Disease.* London: Springer-Verlag; 1992, pp. 523–542.

158. Wood AE, Freedom RM, Williams WG, Trusler GA. The Mustard procedure in transposition of the great arteries associated with juxtaposition of the atrial appendages with and without dextrocardia. *J Thorac Cardiovasc Surg* 1983;85:451–456.

159. Baker WP, Schland HA, Ballenger FP. Congenital partial absence of the pericardium. *Am J Cardiol* 1965;16: 133–137.

160. Bruning EGH. Congenital defect of the pericardium. *J Clin Pathol* 1962;15:133–138

161. Burrows PE, Smallhorn JS, Trusler GA, Daneman A, Moes CAF, Rowe RD. Partial absence of the left parietal pericardium with herniation of the left atrial appendage: Diagnosis by cross-sectional echocardiography and contrast-enhanced computed tomography. *Pediatr Cardiol* 1987;8:205–208.

162. Boxall R. Incomplete pericardial sac: Escape of heart into left pleural cavity. *Trans Obstet Soc Lond* 1887;28:209–212.

163. Carty JE, Deverell PB, Losowsky MS. Pericardial defect presenting as acute pericarditis. *Br Heart J* 1975;37: 98–100.

164. Gehlmann HR, van Ingen GJ. Symptomatic congenital complete absence of the left pericardium. Case report and review of the literature. *Eur Heart J* 1989;10: 670–675.

165. Haider R, Thomas DGT, Ziady G, Cleland WP, Goodwin JF. Congenital pericardioperitoneal communications with herniation of omentum into the pericardium: A rare cause of cardiomegaly. *Br Heart J* 1973;35:981–983.

166. Matsuhisa M, Shimomura K, Beppu S, Nakajima K. Jugular phlebogram in congenital absence of the pericardium. *Am Heart J* 1986;112:1004–1010.

167. Minocha GK, Falicov RE, Nijensohn E. Partial right-sided congenital pericardial defect with herniation of right atrium and right ventricle. Chest 1979;76:484–486 168. Sunderland S, Wright-Smith RJ. Congenital pericardial defects. *Br Heart J* 1944;6:167–169.

169. Talesnick BS, Sutton FJ, Lee Y-C, McLaughlin JS. Pericardial defect mimicking a left atrial mass. *Am J Cardiol* 1985;56:699–701.

170. Victor S, Rajesh PB, Daniel ID, Rajaram S, Lakshmikanthan C. Congenital pericardial defect with accessory lobules in lung and patent ductus anteriosus: A case report. *Indian Heart J* 1979;31:61–64.

171. Bernal JM, Lapiedra JO, Gonzalez I, Saez A, Pastor E, Miralles PJ. Angiocardiographic demonstration of a partial defect of the pericardium with herniation of the left atrium and ventricle. *J Cardiovasc Surg (Torino)* 1986;27:344–346.

172. Finet G, Bozio A, Frieh JP, Cordier JF, Celard P. Herniation of the left atrial appendage through a congenital partial pericardial defect. *Eur Heart J* 1991;12:1148–1149.

173. Salem DN, Hymanson AS, Isner JM, Bankoff MS, Konstam MA. Congenital pericardial defect diagnosed by computed tomography. *Cathet Cardiovasc Diagn* 1985; 11:75–79.

174. Van Son JA, Danielson GK, Schaff HV, Mullany CJ, Julsrud PR, Breen JF. Congenital partial and complete ab-

sence of the pericardium. *Mayo Clin Proc* 1993; 68:743–747.

175. Connolly HM, Click RL, Schattenberg TT, Seward JB, Tajik AJ. Congenital absence of the pericardium: Echocardiography as a diagnostic tool. *J Am Soc Echocardiogr* 1995;8:87–92.

176. Hoorntje JC, Mooyaart EL, Meuzelaar KJ. Left atrial herniation through a partial pericardial defect: A rare cause of syncope. *PACE* 1989;12:1841–1845.

177. Jacob JL, Souza AS Jr, Parro A Jr. Absence of the left pericardium diagnosed by computed tomography. *Int J Cardiol* 1995;47:293–296.

178. Lonsky V, Stetina M, Habal P, Markova D. Congenital absence of the left pericardium in combination with left pulmonary artery hypoplasia, right aortic arch, and secundum atrial septal defect. *Thorac Cardiovasc Surg* 1992;40:155–157.

179. Gassner I, Judmaier W, Fink C, Lener M, Waldenberger F, Scharfetter H, Hammerer I. Diagnosis of congenital pericardial defects, including a pathognomic sign for dangerous apical ventricular herniation, on magnetic resonance imaging. *Br Heart J* 1995;74:60–66.

180. Perez Lorente F, Rodriguez Lambert JL, Burgos R, Juffe A, Moris C, Cortina A. Defecto congenito parcial de pericardio izquierdo con herniacion de orejuela izquierda y porcion basal del ventriculo izquierdo. Asociacion a atresia traqueoesofagica. *Rev Esp Cardiol* 1986;39:234–238.

181. Rees AP, Risher W, McFadden PM, Ramee SR, White CJ. Partial congenital defect of the left pericardium: Angiographic diagnosis and treatment by thoracoscopic pericardiectomy. Case report. *Cathet Cardiovasc Diagn* 1993;28:231–234.

182. Kartagener M. Zur Pathogenese der Bronchiektasian: Bronchiek-tasian bei situs viscerum inversus. *Beitr Klin Tuberk* 1933;83:489–495.

183. Kartagener M, Strucki P. Bronchiectasis with situs inversus. *Arch Pediatr* 1962;79:193–196.

184. Katsuhara K, Kawamoto S, Wakabayashi T, Belsky JL. Situs inversus totalis and Kartagener's syndrome in a Japanese population. *Chest* 1972;61:56–58.

185. Rossman CM, Forrest JB, Lee RMKW, Newhouse AF, Newhouse MT. The dyskinetic cilia syndrome, abnormal ciliary motility in association with abnormal ciliary ultrastructure. *Chest* 1981;80:860–863.

186. Sturgess JM, Chao J, Wong J, Aspin N, Turner JA. Cilia with defective radial spokes: A cause of human respiratory disease. *N Engl J Med* 1979;300:53–56.

187. Afzelius BA, Eliasson R, Johnsen O, Lindholmer C. Lack of dynein arms in immotile human spermatozoa. *J Cell Biol* 1975;66:225–230.

188. Eliasson R, Mossberg B, Cammer P, Afzelius B. The immotile-cilia syndrome, a congenital ciliary abnormality as an etiologic factor in chronic airway infections and male sterility. *N Engl J Med* 1977;297:1–4.

189. Fischer TJ, McAdams JA, Entis GN, Cotton R, Ghory JE, Ausdenmoore RW. Middle ear ciliary defect in Kartagener's syndrome. *Pediatrics* 1978;62:443–445.

190. Armengot M, Escribano A, Carda C, Basterra J. Clinical and ultrastructural correlations in nasal mucociliary function observed in children with recurrent airways infections. *Int J Pediatr Otorhinolaryngol* 1995;32: 143–151.

191. de Iongh RU, Rutland J. Ciliary defects in healthy subjects, bronchiectasis, and primary ciliary dyskinesia. *Am J Respir Crit Care Med* 1995;151:1559–1567.

192. Bhutta ZA Primary ciliary dyskinesia: A cause of neonatal respiratory distress. *J Pak Med Assoc* 1995;45:70–73.

193. Losa M, Ghelfi D, Hof E, Felix H, Fanconi S. Kartagener syndrome: An uncommon cause of neonatal respiratory distress? *Eur J Pediatr* 1995;154:236–238.

194. Aitken J. Reproductive biology. A clue to Kartagener's [news]. *Nature (London)* 1991;353(6342):306.

195. Armengot M, Juan G, Carda C, Basterra J, Cano B. Prevalencia del sindrome de discinesia ciliar primaria en pacientes con sinusitis y bronquiectasias. *An Otorrinolaringol Ibero Am* 1995;22:85–92

196. Miralles A, Muneretto C, Gandjbakhch I, Lecompte Y, Pavie A, Rabago G, Bracamonte L, Desruennes M, Cabrol A, Cabrol C. Heart-lung transplantation in situs inversus. A case report in a patient with Kartagener's syndrome. *J Thorac Cardiovasc Surg* 1992;103:307–313.

197. Macchiarini P, Chapelier A, Vouhe P, Cerrina J, Ladurie FL, Parquin F, Brenot F, Simonneau G, Dartevelle P. Double lung transplantation in situs inversus with Kartagener's syndrome. Paris-Sud University Lung Transplant Group. *J Thorac Cardiovasc Surg* 1994;108: 86–91.

198. Graeter T, Schafers HJ, Wahlers T, Borst HG. Lung transplantation in Kartagener's syndrome. *J Heart Lung Transplant* 1994;13:724–726.

Section II

Specific Conditions

Chapter 4

Atrial Septal Defect

The first description of a communication between atrial chambers is attributed to the Renaissance master Leonardo da Vinci. "I have found from a, left auricle, to b, right auricle, the perforating channel from a to b".[1] The pathological anatomy and its embryological origins was described late in the 19th century by Karl von Rokitansky[2] who distinguished the septum primum from septum secundum defects. The radiological characteristics were described by Assman[3] early in this century. The clinical features of the patient presenting with an isolated lesion were elaborated by Bedford, Papp, and Parkinson[4]; the detailed anatomy was characterized by Hudson[5] and expanded by Sweeney and Rosenquist.[6]

Definition

An atrial septal defect denotes an abnormality in the formation of the atrial septum. The defect may or may not be associated with maldevelopment of the endocardial cushions (detailed descriptions of such atrioventricular septal defects are found in Chapter 5). As an isolated lesion, the location of the defect within the interatrial septum may be used for classification. A centrally (or relatively so) deficiency is referred to as an *ostium secundum* or *fossa ovalis type*; a high and posteriorally positioned defect is referred to as a *sinus venosus type* (often associated with anomalous pulmonary venous return from the right lung); and a posterioinferior defect is referred to as an *inferior caval type.*

An anomaly of the endocardial cushion tissue results in a defect of variable extent involving atrioventricular valves, the ventricular septum (inflow and outflow components), and interatrial septum. The detailed anatomy and angiographic appearance is found in Chapter 5. In this chapter, only isolated defects of the interatrial septum are described.

Embryology and Anatomy

The primitive atrium is divided into two halves as a consequence of the formation of two septa.[7] The first of these two structures, the septum primum, forms from the dorsocephalic atrial wall, to the left of the sinus venosus, and grows causally toward the developing atrioventricular endocardial cushions (Fig. 4-1A). The space (opening) between the inferior margin of this wall and the endocardial cushions is the ostium primum. Just prior to fusion of the septum primum to the centrally forming endocardial tissue, the septum primum fenestrates creating a second communication between the atrial walls, the ostium secundum (Fig. 4-1B). At the same time that the foramen secundum develops, a second septal structure develops with a crescentic lower margin from the ventrocephalic wall of the atrium between the septum primum and sinus venosus— the septum secundum (Figs. 4-1B and 4-1C). This new septum grows caudally to overlap the ostium secundum though stops its caudal migration when it overlaps the ostium secundum. The anterior portion of the septum secundum fuses with the endocardial cushion tissue toward the right of the septum primum. That portion of the ostium primum not covered by the septum secundum becomes the floor of the fossa ovalis (Fig. 4-1D). The opening bounded by the margins of the septum secundum forms the foramen ovale.

At the same time that these septal structures are developing, fenestrating, and involuting, the septum of the atrioventricular canal is evolving. A dorsal and ventral septal cushions grow from their respective walls and gradually fuse, first on the right and then with extension towards the left. Shortly after the appearance of the dorsal and ventral cushions, two additional cushions, one rightward, one leftward, develop and grow into the canal to complete the boundaries of the primitive tricuspid and mitral valves.

From: Freedom RM, Mawson JB, Yoo SJ, Benson LN: *Congenital Heart Disease: Textbook of Angiocardiography.* Armonk NY, Futura Publishing Co., Inc. ©1997.

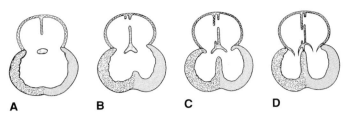

Fig. 4-1: Diagrammatic representation of the formation of the atrial septum.
Although the depiction implies a sequential evolution of structures, coincident formation of septa and foramen is the rule. Modified from Reference 7.

The normal atrial septum, as viewed from the right side, is a spade-like structure with a superior-anterior border guarded by the curvature of the ascending aortic wall, the inferior margin bordered by the mitral annulus, and a posterior margin that is convex.[6] On the left side of the atrial septum, a network of trabeculations are found, formed by the remnants of the septum primum. The fossa ovalis, which is bordered by a limbus and guarded by a valve, represents about 30% of the total septal area. This fetal interatrial communication is normally closed by fusion of the foramen ovale valve with the limbus, as left atrial pressure exceeds that of the right atrium after birth. As such, persistent (or probe) patency of the foramen ovale declines with age from about 33% in the first three decades to 25% through the eighth decade.[8] Functional incompetence, resulting in a potential interatrial communication is distinct from a structural deficiency of the atrial septum; an atrial septal defect. A redundancy of the valve of the foramen ovale can result in an aneurysm of the atrial septum (Fig. 4-2) (see also Chapter 13).[9–13] In children, such atrial wall malformations may disappear with age.[14,15]

Anomalies in the development of the septa forming the atrial septum and atrioventricular canal result in various types of atrial septal defects. The most common type of atrial septal defect is in the ostium secundum location. Either excessive resorption of the septum primum, defective development of the valve of the foramen ovale, or deficiency in the growth of the septum secundum (Figs. 4-1 and 4-3) results in the structural abnormality. The defect, while situated in the region of the fossa ovalis, may vary in size. The mitral and tricuspid valves generally are normal, although rarely an isolated cleft (as distinct from the so-called cleft of the atrioventricular septal defect) may occur in the mitral valve.[16]

In older patients, thickening and structural alterations in the mitral, tricuspid, and pulmonary valves can be seen. Calcification of the tricuspid valve has been noted.[17] An increased incidence of superior displacement (prolapse) of the mitral valve also occurs,[18] the valve thick with fibrotic leaflets and chords is, however, unlike the attenuation and ballooning seen

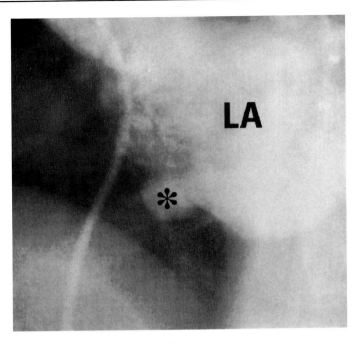

Fig. 4-2: Aneurysms of atrial septum.
Right upper pulmonary vein injection, four-chamber projection. A localized bulge (✱) is seen along the inferolateral left atrial margin, representing an aneurysm of the atrial septum.

with mitral valve prolapse.[19–21] Such lesions increase with age and are related to the abnormal cusp involvement that results from the deformity of the left ventricle (displacement of the interventricular septum from right ventricular volume overload)[18,20] and may in part contribute to the increased mitral regurgitation with age noted in ostium secundum defect.[19,20,22–24] Approximately 10% to 15% of such defects will have partial anomalous pulmonary venous connection.[25]

The next most common defects are in the lower part of the septum, the ostium primum defect. Although these defects may be isolated and behave hemodynamically as ostium secundum defects, they are inevitably components of more profound derangements of the atrioventricular region (see Chapter 5).

Deficiencies in the atrial septum located close to the superior vena cava, and above the fossa ovalis are known as *sinus venosus* defects, and constitute about 2% to 3% of interatrial communications.[26] The superior margin of such defects are absent and there is frequently (80% to 90%) associated anomalous pulmonary venous return from the right lung, usually of the right upper or middle lobe pulmonary veins to either the superior vena cava or right atrium (Fig. 4-3).[25,27–29] The left pulmonary vein(s) can connect anomalously in as few as 10%,[30] usually to the innominate vein or persistent left superior vena cava. They may vary from small (and clinically unrecognizable) to nonrestrictive. The superior caval vein tends to over-

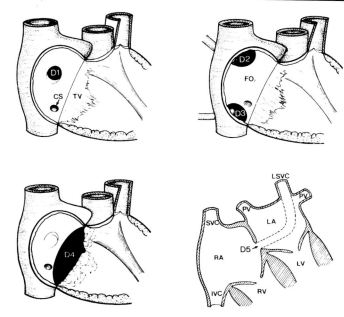

Fig. 4-3: Diagrammatic representation of ASD locations.
Locations of ostium secundum (D1), ostium primum (D4), coronary sinus (D5), and sinus venosus (D2 superior and D3 inferior type) atrial defects. Note the ostium secundum defect, upper left panel, although primarily central, may excavate toward the anterior or posteroinferior septum.

ure of or faulty resorption of the sinus venosus results in an interatrial communication. Additionally, persistence of a large eustachian valve (a rudiment of the right valve of the sinus venosus) that directs fetal inferior caval blood toward the left atrium can, postnatally, participate in the development of right-to-left shunting through an inferior sinus venosus defect (Fig. 4-3).[36,37]

The least common variety of defect is that involving the coronary sinus, which is located at the site normally occupied by the right ostium of the coronary sinus.[11,38–43] The communication allows a shunt from the left atrium through the coronary sinus and into the right atrium, the opening being in the distal portion of the coronary sinus.[11,38] Absence of a portion of wall between left atrial cavity and coronary sinus is termed an "unroofed" coronary sinus (see Chapter 12, Fig. 12-40)[12] with appreciable enlargement of the sinus.[38,39] A left superior caval vein can frequently be found to communicate directly to the left upper corner of the left atrium.[11,38,42] Uncommonly, there may be absence of the coronary sinus, rather than unroofing, and a defect in the atrial septum in the location of the coronary sinus ostium.[43] Whereas the majority of such atrial defects are found in only one location, occasionally there are coexisting defects,[44] particularly in the ostium primum and secundum locations.

Angiography

Echocardiography has largely supplemented the diagnostic utility of angiocardiography in confirming a clinically suspected defect or identifying its presence in the constellation of a more complex malformation.[45–47] Angiography however, can be performed if doubt exists about the diagnosis or during investigation of a more complex malformation.

The lesion may be defined by either a right ventricular or pulmonary artery injection or left atrial angiogram. The levophase of the right-sided study, in the anteroposterior projection will show shunting of a varying amount of contrast from left to right atrium with the inferior margin of the left atrium (the plane of the interatrial septum) becoming indistinct or obliterated (Fig. 4-4). This is in contrast to the appearance when the atrial septum is intact. In this case, the inferior margin of the left atrium is sharply defined as the opacified left atrium abuts on the unopacified right atrium (Fig. 4-5).

A localized bulge in the inferolateral left atrial margin may be visible on occasion and represents an aneurysm of the atrial septum (Fig. 4-2). These aneurysms may involve primum septum and can be quite mobile during the cardiac cycle.

Angiographic definition of the atrial defect is best shown by left atrial angiography, in either a conventional left anterior oblique projection or left anterior

ride the defect, allowing for a biatrial superior caval connection.[31] Various theories have been postulated for the development of this lesion.[5,32–34] Hartley[32] suggested that there was a failure of migration of the sinoatrial orifice from its midline position toward the right. This results in the superior caval vein entering the right atrium closer to the primum septum than normal and restricts development of the secundum septum, so creating a high defect in the atrial septum. Others[5,33] have implicated defective absorption of the right horn of the sinus venosus into the right atrium, or the development of a "fistulous" communication between the right upper pulmonary veins and the superior vena cava. More recently, an echocardiographic study from the Children's Hospital in Boston has demonstrated that sinus venosus defects result from a deficiency in the wall that normally separates the right pulmonary veins from the superior vena cava and the right atrium. This deficiency unroofs the right pulmonary veins, permitting them to drain into the superior vena cava or into the right atrium. An interatrial communication is almost always present and is posterior or posterosuperior to the fossa ovalis. This interatrial communication is the orifice of the unroofed right pulmonary veins rather than a defect in the atrial septum.[34a]

Sinus venous defects of the inferior caval type are located inferior to the fossa ovalis and merge with the floor of the inferior caval vein (Fig. 4-3) (see Chapter 12).[35,36] As in the more superiorly located defect, fail-

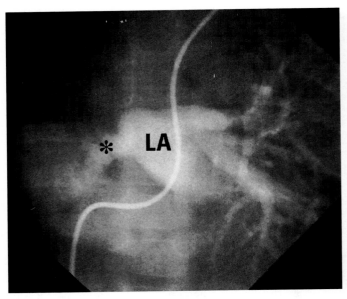

Fig. 4-4: Secundum ASD.
Levophase of LPA injection, frontal projection, demonstrating opacification of the left atrium with shunting of contrast material into the right atrium (∗). See also Chapter 2, Fig. 2-22.

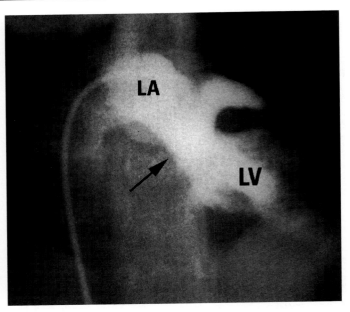

Fig. 4-5: Intact atrial septum.
Left atrial injection, frontal projection. The inferior portion of the atrial septum is intact (arrow), and no contrast is seen in RA.

oblique projection with craniocandal tilt (the so-called four-chambered view (Fig. 4-6).[48] The site of injection is important, and should be performed at the level of or in the right upper pulmonary vein to ensure that the septal wall of the atrium is aligned (Fig 4-6). If contrast is injected into the midposition of the atrium or atrial appendage, unopacified blood will wash out the contrast from the septal aspect of the left atrium and obliterate the margins.

In a secundum defect, contrast can be identified passing through the midposition of the septum into the right atrium (Fig. 4-6). A sinus venosus defect may also be characterized via a left atrial angiogram performed in the left anterior oblique cranially angulated projection. Unlike the ostium secundum defect, the direction of flow is oriented superiorally and to the right, toward the superior vena cava. The defect may also be defined from a superior caval injection (Fig. 4-7), with contrast filling the right atrium, but also crossing the defect into the left atrium.

Demonstration of anomalous pulmonary venous return to the superior vena cava or right atrium in association with a sinus venosus defect may be seen after contrast injection into the right ventricle or main pulmonary artery, but is best detailed from a selective right pulmonary artery injection in the anteroposterior projection. A superior vena caval angiogram may also define a vein filling retrogradely (Fig. 4-7). The presence of an anomalous venous connection is, however, best demonstrated by selective catheterization and opacification of the offending vein(s) (see Chapter 12).

A primum defect in the atrial septum is best outlined in a 45° left anterior oblique projection with 30° craniocardial angulation (four-chambered view[48]). The defect is positioned in the cardial aspect of the septum, bordered inferiorly by the atrioventricular valve(s). If a remnant of tissue is identified between the defect and atrioventricular valve, it is considered a secundum type defect.[49] As noted above, these defects are part of a more comprehensive morphological abnormality.

Defects of the coronary sinus are best demonstrated with a direct injection of contrast into the coronary sinus (see Chapter 12, Fig. 12-40). In the majority of such injections, contrast will be diluted by nonopacified blood originating in the left atrium that originated in the right atrium, or contrast may enter into a left superior caval frequently connected to the roof of the left atrium in this anomaly. The levophase of a pulmonary angiogram will opacify the left atrium and then the coronary sinus, presumptive evidence of a communication between the left atrium and coronary sinus (see Chapter 12, Fig. 12-40).

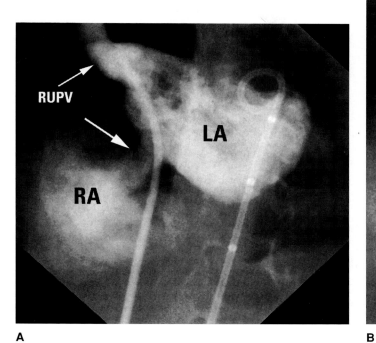

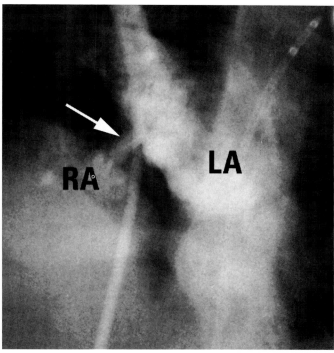

A   **B**

Fig. 4-6: Secundum ASD.
Two different patients. Right upper pulmonary vein injections, four-chamber projections. **A** and **B** both demonstrate the shunt (arrow).

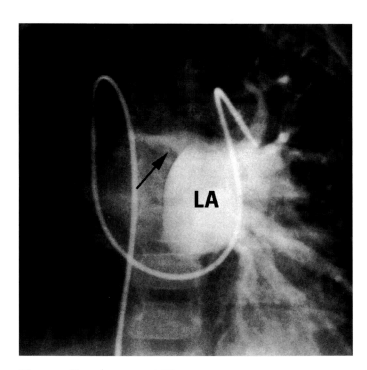

Fig. 4-7: Sinus venosus ASD.
RPA injection (catheter via IVC with azygous continuation), frontal projection. The levophase fills the left atrium with contrast which passes superiorly through a sinus venosus atrial septal defect into the right atrium (arrow).

Transcatheter Therapy: Atrial Septal Defect

The concept of a transcatheter approach for closure of a secundum atrial septal defect has had and continues to have a varied history. Mills and King[50] reported an experimental device for transcatheter therapy and its clinical application more than 20 years ago,[51] but due to its size, it was not suitable for percutaneous application, particularly in children. It wasn't until 1987, that a multcenter clinical trial was begun with a single, self-expanding umbrella device with six stainless steel arms covered by polyurethane foam.[52] However, this device was found to be bulky and difficult to control during implantation. Because of the success of the hookless Bard PDA™ (Bard, Billerica, MA) umbrella in nonduct locations[53,54] the double umbrella concept was used in a redesign in which elbowed stainless steel arms with a Dacron mesh covering was investigated.[55] The clinical experience with this device and its modifications has formed the foundation for an understanding of the impact of atrial septal defect morphology on this and any other catheter-based closure technique.[56] Several other device designs have been conceptualized 0and are undergoing clinical trial.[57,58] All have the same limitations imposed by morphological considerations.

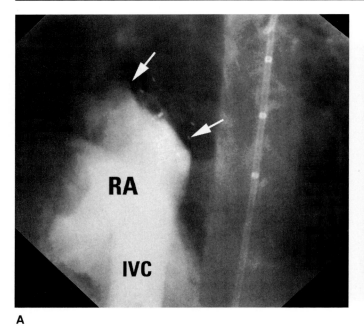

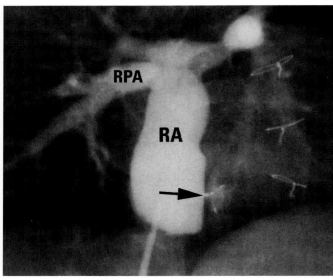

A

B

Fig. 4-8: Device closure of atrial defects.
Two different patients after placement of umbrella occluders. A: Inferior caval vein injection, shallow LAO projection. The device (arrows) is positioned across a secundum atrial defect. Note the left atrial arms flat against the atrial septum. **B:** An injection into the baffle after device occlusion of a fenestrated lateral tunnel atriopulmonary connection shows a residual leak. See also Chapter 2, Fig. 2-22.

Several morphological studies have addressed the feasibility of transcatheter occlusion in the setting of an ostium secundum atrial septal defect.[59,60] Considerable variation in the morphological details has been found including: defects situated in the superior or inferior aspect of the fossa ovalis, those with an attenuated posterior limbus of the atrial septum, subtotal absence of the septum, or complete or partial fenestration of the defect, in addition to the most commonly observed, the central muscular type defect. With such noted variability in form, from 50% to 68% of such ostium secundum defects will be judged suitable for closure. Thus, while angiographic definition is important during the procedure, to delineate the region of the atrial septum (Fig. 4-8), it is inadequate to detail the size of the defect and extent of the muscular rim. The former can be esti-

mated by balloon sizing during fluoroscopy (or echocardiography). During this procedure, an easily deformable balloon is withdrawn through the defect, creating a "waist" that can be measured to define a "stretched" defect diameter. The details of the morphology regarding the position of the defect within the septum and adequacy of the septal rim can only be determined from echocardiography, with the most sensitive being transesophageal approaches.[61,62]

In addition to the secundum atrial septal defect, several additional atrial lesions have been approached with transcatheter techniques for closure. These defects include the baffle fenestration after a modified Fontan operation[63] and the patent foramen ovale after presumed paradoxical embolism.[64]

References

1. Rashkind W. *Congenital Heart Disease*. Stroudsburg, PA: Hutchinson Ross Publishing Company; 1982, pp. 102.
2. Rokitansky K. *Die Defecte der Scheidewande des Herzens*. Vienne, 1875.
3. Assmann H. *Die Klinische Roentgendiagnostik der Innern Erkrankungen*. Leipzig, 1921.
4. Bedford DE, Papp C, Parkinson J. Atrial septal defect. *Br Heart J* 1941;3:37–68
5. Hudson R. Normal and abnormal interatrial septum. *Br Heart J* 1955;17:489–495.
6. Seeney LJ, Rosenquist GC. The normal anatomy of the

atrial septum in the human heart. *Am Heart J* 1979;98:194–200.
7. Langman J. Cardiovascular system. In: *Medical Embryology*. Second edition. Baltimore: Williams and Wilkins Company; 1969, pp. 183–204.
8. Hagen PT, Scholz DG, Edwards WD. Incidence and size of patent foramen ovale during the first 10 decades of life. *Mayo Clin Proc* 1984;59:17–20.
9. Belkin RN, Kisslo J. Atrial septal aneurysm: Recognition and clinical relevance. *Am Heart J* 1990;120:948–957.
10. Hanley PC, Tajik AJ, Hynes JK, Edwards WD, Reeder GS, Haggler DJ, Seward JB. Diagnosis and classification of atrial septal aneurysm by two-dimensional echocardiog-

raphy: Report of 80 consecutive cases. *J Am Coll Cardiol* 1985;6:1370–1382.

11. Mantini E, Grondin CM, Lillehei CW, Edwards JE. Congenital anomalies involving the coronary sinus. *Circulation* 1966;33:317–327.

12. Rice MJ, McDonald RW, Reller MD. Fetal atrial septal aneurysm. A cause of fetal atrial arrhythmias. *J Am Coll Cardiol* 1988;12:1292–1247.

13. Silver MD, Dorsey JS. Aneurysms of the septum primum in adults. *Arch Pathol Lab Med* 1978;102:62–65.

14. Shiraishi I, Hamaoka K, Hayashi S, Koh E, Onouchi Z, Sawada T. Atrial septal aneurysm in infancy. *Pediatr Cardiol* 1990;11:82–85.

15. Brand A, Keren A, Branski D, Abrahamov A, Stern S. Natural course of atrial septal aneurysm in children and the potential for spontaneous closure of associated atrial septal defect. *Am J Cardiol* 1989;64:996–1001.

16. Solomon J, Aygen M, Levy MH. Secundum type of atrial defect with cleft mitral valve. *Chest* 1970;58:540–542.

17. Cooksey J, Parker BM, Weldon CS. Atrial septal defect and calcification of the tricuspid valve. *Br Heart J* 1970;32:409–411.

18. Schreiber TL, Feigenbaum H, Weyman AE. Effect of atrial septal defect repair on left ventricular geometry and degree of mitral valve prolapse. *Circulation* 1980;61:888–896.

19. Boucher CA, Liberthson RR, Buckley MJ. Secundum atrial septal defect and significant mitral regurgitation. Incidence, managment and morphology basis. *Chest* 1979;75:697–702.

20. D'Cruz IA, Arcilla RA. Anomalous venous drainage of the left lung into the inferior vena cava. *Am Heart J* 1964;67:539–544.

21. Nagata S, Nimura Y, Sakakibara H, Beppu S, Park Y, Kawazoe K, Fujita T. Mitral valve lesion associated with secundum atrial septal defect. Br Heart J 1983;49:51–58.

22. Furuta S, Wanibuchi Y, Ino T, Akoi K. Etiology of mitral regurgitation in secundum atrial septal defect. *Jpn Circ J* 1982;46:346–351.

23. Hynes KM, Frye RL, Brandenburg RO, McGoon DC, Titus JL, Giuliani ER. Atrial septal defect (secundum) associated with mitral regurgitation. *Am J Cardiol* 1974;34:333–338.

24. Welch CC, Gibson DC, Fox LM. Atrial septum secundum defects and mitral regurgitation. *Am J Med Sci* 1966;252:45–52.

25. Gotsman MS, Astley R, Parsons CG. Partial anomalous pulmonary venous drainage in association with atrial septal defect. *Br Heart J* 1965;27:566–571.

26. Davia JE, Cheitlin MD, Bedynek JL. Sinus venosus atrial septal defect. *Am Heart J* 1973;85:177–185.

27. Mascarenhas E, Javier RP, Samet P. Partial anomalous pulmonary venous connection and drainage. *Am J Cardiol* 1973;31:512–518.

28. Snellen HA, van Ingen HC, Hoefsmit EC. Patterns of anomalous pulmonary venous drainage. *Circulation* 1968;38:45–63.

29. Stewart JR, Schaff HV, Fortuin NJ, Brawley RK. Partial anomalous pulmonary venous return with intact atrial septum. *Thorax* 1983;38:859–862.

30. Van Meter C, LeBlanc JG, Culpepper WS, Ochsner JL. Partial anomalous pulmonary venous return. *Circulation* 1990;82(suppl IV):IV-195-IV-198.

31. Ettedgui JA, Siewers RD, Anderson RH, Park SC, Pathl E, Zuberbuhler JR. Diagnostic echocardiographic features of the sinus venosus defect. *Br Heart J* 1990;64:329–331.

32. Hartley HRS. The sinus venosus type of atrial interatrial septal defect. *Thorax* 1958;13:12–27.

33. Ross DN. The sinus venosus type of atrial septal defect. *Guy's Hosp Rep* 1952;105:376–380.

34. Shaner RF. The "high" defect in the atrial septum. *Can Med Assoc J* 1958;78:688–690.

35. Bedford DE. The anatomical types of atrial septal defect. Their incidence and clinical diagnosis. *Am J Cardiol* 1960;6:568–574.

36. Gallagher ME, Sperling DR, Gwinn JL, Meyer BW, Flyer DC. Functional drainage of the inferior vena cava into the left atrium. *Am J Cardiol* 1963;12:561–566.

37. Thomas JD, Tabakin BS, Ittleman FP. Atrial septal defect with right-to-left shunt despite normal pulmonary artery pressure. *J Am Coll Cardiol* 1987;9:221–224.

38. Bourdillon PD, Foale RA, Somerville J. Persistent left superior vena cava with coronary sinus and left atrial connections. *Eur J Cardiol* 1980;11:227–234.

39. Lee ME, Sade RM. Coronary sinus septal defect. *J Thorac Cardiovasc Surg* 1979;78:563–569.

40. Maillis MS, Cheng TO, Meyer JF, Crawley IS, Lindsay J. Cyanosis in patients with atrial septal defect due to systemic venous drainage into the left atrium. *Am J Cardiol* 1974;33:674–678.

41. Nath PH, Delaney DJ, Zollikofer C, Ben-Sacher G, Castaneda-Zuniga W, Formanek A, Amplatz K. Coronary sinus-left atrial window. *Radiology* 1980;135:319–322.

42. Quaegebeur J, Kirklin JW, Pacifico AD, Bargeron LM. Surgical experience with unroofed coronary sinus. *Ann Thorac Surg* 1979;27:418–425.

43. Raghib G, Ruttenberg HD, Anderson RC, Amplatz K, Adams P Jr, Edwards JE. Termination of left superior vena cava in left atrium, atrial septal defect, and absence of coronary sinus. A developmental complex. *Circulation* 1965;31:906–918.

44. Sutherland HD. A case with three atrial septal defects. *Br Heart J* 1963;25:267–269.

45. Bierman FZ, Williams RG. Subxyphoid two-dimensional imaging of the interatrial septum in infants and neonates with congenital heart disease. *Circulation* 1979;60:80–90.

46. Lieppe W, Scallion R, Behar VS, Kisslo JA. Two-dimensional echocardiographic findings in atrial septal defects. *Circulation* 1977;56:447–456.

47. Morimoto K, Matsuzaki M, Tohma Y, Ono S, Tanaka N, Michishige H, Murato K, Anno Y, Kusukawa R. Diagnosis and quantitative evaluation of secundum-type atrial septal defect by transesophageal Doppler echocardiography. *Am J Cardiol* 1990;66:85–91.

48. Bargeron LM Jr, Elliott LP, Soto B, Bream PR, Currry GC. Axial angiography in congenital heart disease. *Circulation* 1977;56:1075–1083.

49. Soto B, Bargeron LM Jr, Pacifico AD, Vanini V, Kirklin JW. Angiography of atrioventricular canal defects. *Am J Cardiol* 1981;48:492–499.

50. King TD, Mills NL. Nonoperative closure of atrial septal defects. *Surgery* 1974;75:383–388.

51. Mills NL, King TD. Nonoperative closure of left-to-right shunts. *J Thorac Cardiovasc Surg* 1976;72:371–378.

52. Latson LA. Transcatether closure of atrial septal defects. In: Ras PS, ed: *Transcatehter Therapy in Pediatric Cardiology*. New York: Wiley-Liss; 1993, pp. 335–348.

53. Lock JE, Cockerham JT, Keane JF, et al. Transcatheter umbrella closure of congenital heart defects. *Circulation* 1987;75:593–599.

54. Redington AN, Rigby ML. Novel uses of the Rashkind

ductal umbrella in adults and children with congenital heart disease. *Br Heart J* 1993;69:47–51.

55. Lock JE, Rome JJ, David R, Van Praagh S, Perry SB, Van Praagh R, Keane JF. Transcatheter closure of atrial septal defects: experimental studies. *Circulation* 1989;79:1091–1099.

56. Rome JJ, Keane JF, Perry SB, Spivak PJ, Lock JE. Double umbrella closure of atrial defects: initial clinical applications. *Circulation* 1990;82:751–758.

57. Das GS, Voss G, Jarvis G, Wyche K, Gunther R, Wilson RF. Experimental atrial septal defect closure with a new, transcatheter, self-centering device. *Circulation* 1993;88(1):1754–1764.

58. Sideris EB, Sideris SE, Fowlkes JP, Ehly RL, Smith JE, Gulde RE. Transvenous atrial septal occlusion in piglets using a "buttoned" double-disc device. *Circulation* 1990;81:312–318.

59. Chan KC, Godman MJ. Morphological variations of fossa ovalis atrial septal defects (secundum): Feasibility for transcutaneous closure with the clam-shell device. *Br Heart J* 1993;69:52–55.

60. Ferreira SMAG, Ho Sy, Anderson RH. Morphological study of defects of the atrial septum within the oval fossa: Implications for transcatheter closure of left-to-right shunts. *Br Heart J* 1992;67:316–320.

61. Boutin C, Musewe NN, Smallhorn JF, Dyck JD, Kobayashi T, Benson LN. Echocardiographic follow-up of atrial septal defect after catheter closure by double-umbrella device. *Circulation* 1993;88:621–627.

62. Rosenfeld HM, van der Velde ME, Sanders SP, Colan SD, Parness IA, Lock JE, Spevak PJ. Echocardiographic predictors of candidacy for successful transcatheter atrial septal defect closure. *Cathet Cardiovasc Diagn* 1995;34:29–34.

63. Bridges ND, Mayer JE Jr, Lock JE, Jonas RA, Hanley FL Keane JF, Perry SB, Castenada AR. Effect of baffle fenestration on outcome of the modified Fontan operation. *Circulation* 1992;86:1762–1769.

64. Bridges ND, Hellenbrand W, Latson L, Filiano J, Newburger JW, Lock JE. Transcatheter closure of patent foramen ovale after presumed paradoxical embolism. *Circulation* 1992;86:1902–1908.

Chapter 5

Atrioventricular Septal Defect

Some years ago, in a provocative editorial, Becker and Anderson[1] asked: "What's in a name?" when they suggested that the term atrioventricular septal defect is an appropriate designation for those hearts whose diverse morphology is unified by a deficiency of the atrioventricular muscular and membranous septa (Fig. 5-1). The following designations have been and continue to be used in describing these hearts: endocardial cushion defects; atrioventricular canal defects; atrioventricular communis defects; atrioventricular defects; ostium primum atrial septal defect, etc. Well, there must be something in the name because there is still not unanimity in the nomenclature of these conditions because there are some hearts with pathognomonic features of deficient atrioventricular septation, but with intact septal structures and others only with a hole at the site of atrioventricular membranous septum.[2] Despite the issues of nosology, much has been accomplished in the treatment of patients with atrioventricular septal defect, reflecting our increased knowledge of anatomy, clinical predisposition to early pulmonary vascular damage, the character of the specialized conduction tissue, and appreciation of those particular anatomic risk factors in patients with these heterogeneous malformations. How we have improved on the natural history of this disorder,[3–5] considering that only 54% of patients with the complete form of atrioventricular septal defect were predicted to survive to 6 months of age and 15% were predicted to survive to 2 years without medical and surgical intervention.[6]

Prevalence

Data from the New England Regional Infant Cardiac Program provides a frequency of endocardial cushion defect of 0.118 per 1000 livebirths,[7] while the data from the Baltimore-Washington Infant study defined a prevalence of 0.362 per 1000 livebirths.[8] The New England Regional Infant Cardiac Program did not utilize echocardiography in the diagnosis of this malformation, and this might account for some of the difference in prevalence. Using invasive methodologies, the Alberta Heritage Study defined the prevalence of atrioventricular septal defect as 0.203 per 1000 livebirths; noninvasive methodologies defined the prevalence as 0.242 per 1000 livebirths.[9]

Morphology of the Atrioventricular Septal Defect

A number of studies have addressed the morphological spectrum of patients with atrioventricular septal defect.[10–41A] The pathognomonic feature of this group of malformations is a defect of the atrioventricular septum (Fig. 5-1). Absence or deficiency of the atrioventricular membranous and muscular septum has a significant influence on the morphology of the atrioventricular junction and the contiguous atria and ventricular septa.[1,12–14, 24–27, 32, 36, 42] The atrioventricular septum separates the left ventricle from the right atrium in the normal heart, and has two components: the membranous and the muscular. As emphasized by McGoon,[42] whether one is examining a heart with an ostium primum atrial septal defect (and so-called cleft in the mitral valve) or a heart exhibiting a complete defect, the unifying feature resulting from absence of the atrioventricular septum is a central deficiency between the atrial and ventricular septa. The absence of the atrioventricular septum results in an ostium primum atrial septal defect immediately above the atrioventricular valves and a deficiency or scooped out area in the inlet portion of the ventricular septum immediately below

From: Freedom RM, Mawson JB, Yoo SJ, Benson LN: *Congenital Heart Disease: Textbook of Angiocardiography.* Armonk NY, Futura Publishing Co., Inc. ©1997.

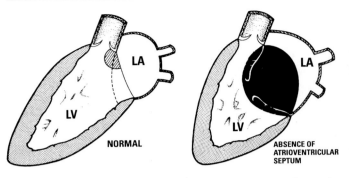

Fig. 5-1: Deficiency of the membranous and muscular atrioventricular septum is the hallmark of the atrioventricular septal defect.
Schematic diagram depicts the normal atrioventricular membranous and muscular septum (left side) and its absence (right side).

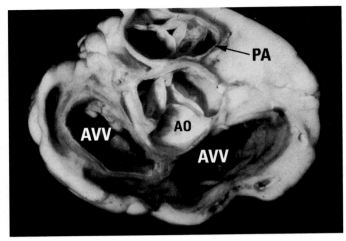

Fig. 5-3: View of the base of the heart with an intact membranous and muscular atrioventricular septum. Note the aorta is wedged between the two atrioventricular valves.

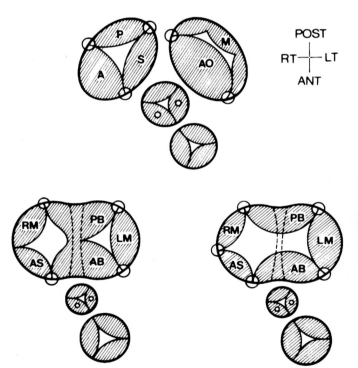

Fig. 5-2: Schematic diagram depicts effect of absence of the membranous and muscular atrioventricular septum on the disposition of the aortic root.
Schematic drawing shows the normal wedged position of the aorta (top diagram) vs. the unwedged aorta in a patient with an atrioventricular septal defect. This unwedging in atrioventricular septal defect reflects absence of the membranous and muscular atrioventricular septum and does not depend on whether the atrioventricular valve is common or partitioned. These diagrams also show the difference in the position of the papillary muscles in the normal heart vs. the heart of a patient with an atrioventricular septal defect. In the latter, they are closer together.

the atrioventricular valves.[1,13,14,21,24–26,43] Thus, the absence of the atrioventricular septum results in lack of continuity between atrial and ventricular septal structures, produces an ovoid common junction, and the aortic outflow tract is no longer wedged between the tricuspid and mitral valves as in the normal heart, but rather the aortic valve is anterosuperior to the common ovoid junction (Figs. 5-2 through 5-4).[13] This anterosuperior elevation and deviation of the aortic valve re-

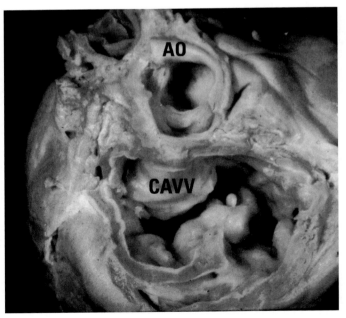

Fig. 5-4: View of the base of the heart with absence of the membranous and muscular atrioventricular septum. Note the aorta is no longer wedged between the common atrioventricular valve. Indeed it is sprung from its usual wedged position.

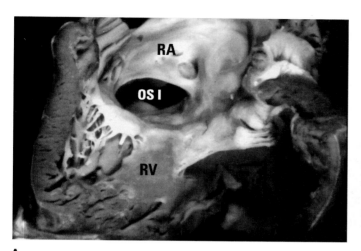

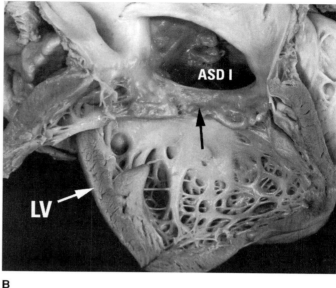

A

B

Fig. 5-5: Large ostium primum atrial septal defect.
A: Large ostium primum atrial septal defect (OS I) viewed from the right atrium and right ventricle. **B:** Internal view of left atrium and left ventricle of a patient with a large primum atrial septal defect and partitioned atrioventricular valves. Note the tongue of tissue (arrow) connecting the partitioned atrioventricular valves.

sults in aortic-mitral fibrous continuity that departs from normal aortic-mitral fibrous continuity.[44,45] The continuity in atrioventricular septal defect was to the base of the noncoronary cusp in about one-fourth of patients and to both the right and noncoronary cusp in about one-third. Absence of the atrioventricular septum also produces a dramatic impact on the form of the valve guarding the atrioventricular junction.[1,10,13,14,19,24–26,35,36,40,43] This deficiency of the atrioventricular septum results in a valve with five leaflets. This is true whether the valve orifice is partitioned or common. The major difference observed in those hearts with partitioned orifices from those with a common atrioventricular orifice is a connecting tongue or bridge of valve tissue linking the superior and inferior bridging leaflets (Fig. 5-5). One of the other most consistent features in atrioventricular septal defect is that the left ventricular inflow tract is shortened in relation to the length of outflow tract, as well as the length of diaphragmatic wall of the left ventricle is shortened when compared with normal. The left ventricular outflow tract is thus elongated and narrow, and thus gives the appearance of a gooseneck deformity (Figs. 5-6 through 5-8).[1,12,13,18,24–26,40, 43,46–49] The left ventricular outflow tract in the atrioventricular septal defect thus departs considerably from the normal (See Chapter 3, Figs. 3-11 and 3-12).

A fundamental difference is noted in the disposition of the papillary muscles in the heart with an atrioventricular septal defect compared with a normal heart. Rather than the paired papillary muscles being located in anterolateral and posteromedial positions as in the normal heart, the papillary muscles are located one in front of the other (Fig. 5-9).[50–55] Another interesting alteration in the cardiac anatomy resulting from an absent atrioventricular septum is obvious disproportion between the inlet and outlet dimensions, a feature recognized for years by left ventricular angiocar-

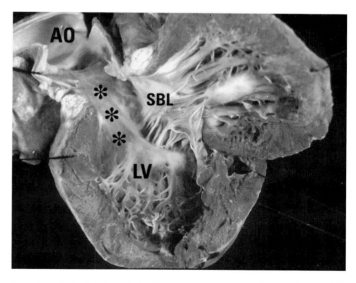

Fig. 5-6: The left ventricular outflow tract of a patient with clinically an ostium primum atrial septal defect. Note the elongated and narrowed left ventricular outflow tract (✳) characteristic of the atrioventricular septal defect and the inlet-outlet disproportion. The superior bridging leaflet (SBL) is firmly attached, preventing an interventricular communication.

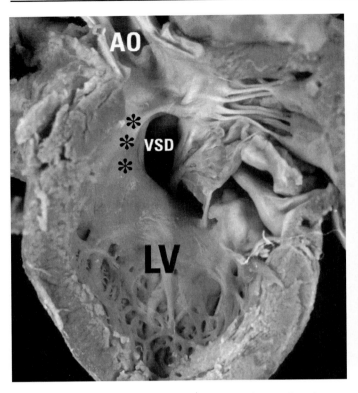

Fig. 5-7: This specimen of a transitional form of atrioventricular septal defect viewed from the left ventricle and outflow tract shows a moderate-sized ventricular septal defect. There is attachment of the atrioventricular valve to the septum. The basic features of the narrowed and elongated left ventricular outflow tract (*) are still present.

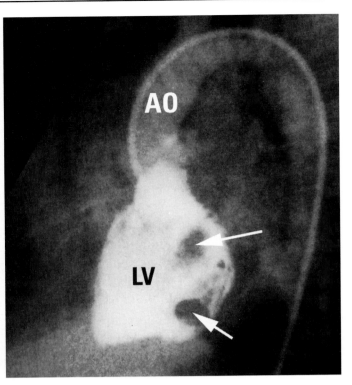

Fig. 5-9: The disposition of the papillary muscles is fundamentally different in the atrioventricular septal defect. Lateral left ventricular angiogram shows the more closely opposed papillary muscles (arrows) in the atrioventricular septal defect (See also Fig. 5-1).

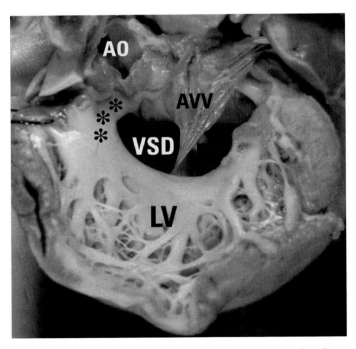

Fig. 5-8: A very large ventricular septal defect and a free-floating common atrioventricular valve do not obscure the characteristic inlet-outlet disproportion and the narrowed and elongated left ventricular outflow tract (*).

diography, with the outlet dimension substantially greater than the inlet (Figs. 5-6 through 5-8 and 5-10 through 5-12).[1,12,13,18,24–26,40,43,46–49] The disposition of the atrioventricular valve leaflets is such in atrioventricular septal defect that the left valve does not represent in any way a normal mitral valve, and because of this Anderson and colleagues eschew the mitral designation for the left component, partitioned or common, of the atrioventricular orifice. The atrioventricular junction in atrioventricular septal defect is guarded by a valve with five leaflets that are so disposed as to divide the common orifice into separate right and left atrioventricular components.[13] It has been difficult to overcome the mitral convention, and thus the designation of the left-sided atrioventricular valve as mitral is still widely applied and endorsed.

One can further categorize or subclassify hearts with atrioventricular septal defects by the presence of a partitioned or common valve orifice, whether a ventricular septal defect is present and its size, the presence and size of the ostium primum atrial septal defect; and whether the defect is balanced or unbalanced, ie, dominant right or left ventricular forms (Fig. 5-13).[43] Currently, there is relatively less emphasis on Rastelli's classification.[28,29] The atrioventricular septal defect in-

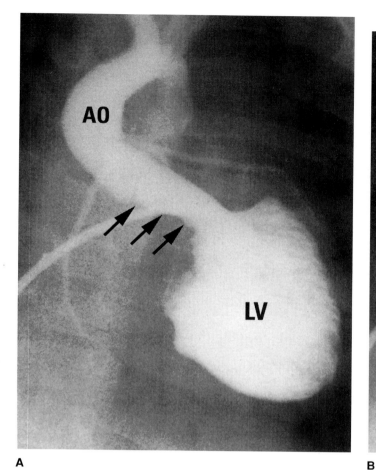

A

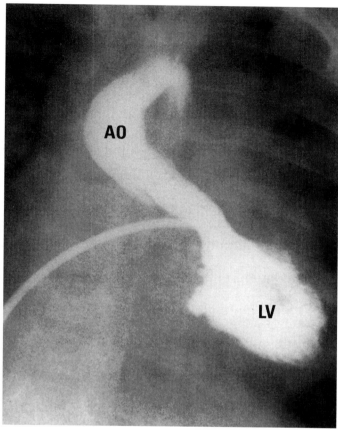

B

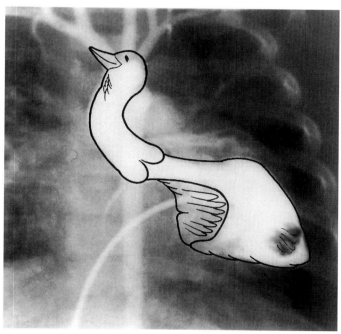

C

Fig. 5-10: The typical elongated left ventricular outflow tract in a patient with an atrioventricular septal defect. The systolic and diastolic frames of the frontal left ventricular angiogram show so clearly those features of the gooseneck or swan's neck deformity, with the inlet-outlet disproportion. The elongated left ventricular outflow tract is seen between the free wall superiorly and the atrioventricular valve leaflet (arrows) in Fig. 5-10A.

A: Diastole. **B:** Systole. **C:** "Korean dove" or gooseneck deformity of left ventricular outflow tract.

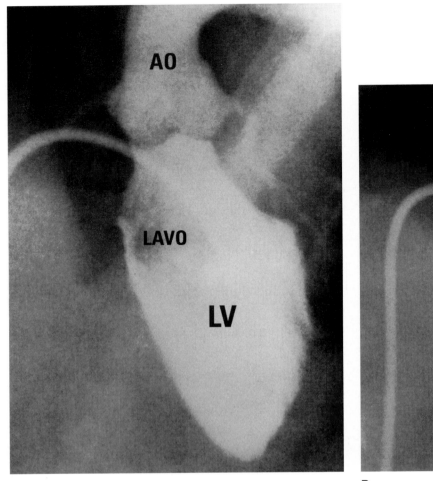

A

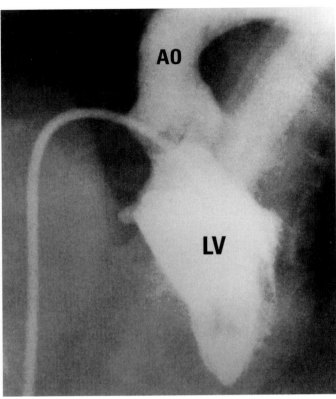

B

Fig. 5-11: Hepatoclavicular left ventriculograms show the medial disposition of the left atrioventricular valve and the inlet-outlet disproportion is readily appreciated. The catheter has been advanced through the left atrioventricular valve.
A: Diastole. **B:** Systole.

cludes a spectrum of abnormalities, ranging from the patient with intact or nearly intact atrial and ventricular septa to the patient with large and usually confluent atrial and ventricular septal defects.[13,30,43,56] This spectrum thus ranges from the patient with ostium primum atrial septal defect with cleft mitral valve to the patient with large confluent atrial and ventricular septal defects and a common atrioventricular orifice. The internal organization of the morphological right ventricle conforms to a right-hand pattern when the atrial relationships are normal or solitus. In the presence of atrial isomerism, about half had a left-hand pattern of internal organization.[57]

The ostium primum atrial septal defect may be very small and in rare instances the atrial septum is intact.[13,30,43,56] In some patients there is gross deficiency of both the primum and secundum portions of the atrial septum resulting in a common atrium (Fig. 5-5). The

usual form of ostium primum atrial septal defect is bounded below by the inferiorly displaced atrioventricular valve leaflets and above by a crescentic ridge of atrial septum that fuses with the atrioventricular valve ring at its extremities.[27] A true defect of the fossa ovalis may be present or a patent foramen ovale will be evident. In the so-called partial or transitional forms of atrioventricular septal defect, a deficiency of the inlet portion of the ventricular septum immediately beneath the atrioventricular valves of variable extent should be evident.[43] The partial form is characterized by the complete attachment of the superior and inferior bridging leaflets that are connected by a tongue of valvar tissue, to the scooped out ventricular septal crest that obliterates the interventricular component, but leaves the ostium primum atrial septal defect. The transitional form, a variant of the partial form, is characterized by the chordal attachments of the bridging leaflets to the ven-

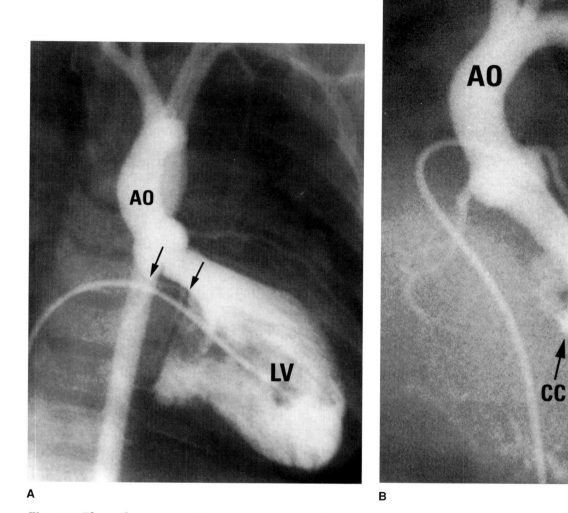

A   **B**

Fig. 5-12: The pathognomonic feature in a patient with an ostium primum atrial septal defect whose left ventricle is studied in the frontal and long axial projections.
A: The left ventricular outflow tract is narrowed and elongated (arrows) as a result of the absence of the atrioventricular septum as seen in this frontal left ventriculogram. **B:** In this axial projection, both the basic nature of the left ventricular outflow tract as well as the inlet-outlet disproportion are seen. Note the wide distance between the aortic valve and the crux cordis and short inlet dimension between the crux cordis and the apex.

tricular septal crest, leaving small interventricular channels between the chords as well as a large ostium primum atrial septal defect. Thus, when the superior and inferior bridging leaflets of the atrioventricular valve are firmly connected and are completely attached to the downwardly and scooped crest of the ventricular septum throughout its length, a ventricular septal defect should not be present (Fig. 5-6). There may be, however, several small ventricular septal defects beneath the attachment of the bridging leaflets to the ventricular septum (Fig. 5-7). The ventricular septal defect may be large and nonrestrictive and in combination with a sub-

stantial primum atrial septal defect, a complete form of atrioventricular septal defect is present (Fig. 5-8). A common atrioventricular orifice is usually present, and thus a tongue of connecting tissue is not present (Fig. 5-8), which produces a bare area on the crest of the ventricular septum. The variable attachment or bridging of the left superior leaflet formed the basis of Rastelli's classification of the atrioventricular septal defect.[28,29]

Those hearts with a deficiency of the atrioventricular septum may have a ventricular septal defect. In the majority of patients, the ventricular septal defect excavates apically and includes the upper portion of the in-

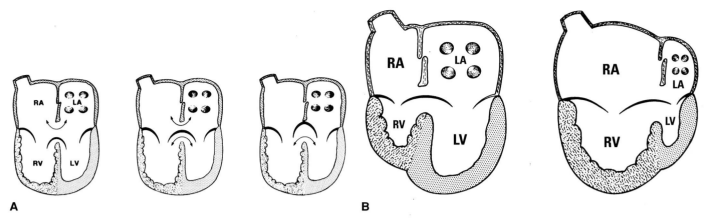

Fig. 5-13: Diagrams shows some variations of the atrioventricular septal defect.
A, left panel: A large primum atrial septal defect; **Middle panel:** Confluent atrial and ventricular septal defects; **Right panel:** A large ventricular septal defect with an intact atrial septum. Not shown is that rare form of atrioventricular septal defect with basically intact atrial and ventricular septum. **B:** Dominant left (left panel) and right ventricular forms (right panel) of atrioventricular septal defect.

let septum; this is responsible for the scooped appearance.[12,13,18,24–26,43,46,47–49] The deficiency of the septum is more conspicuous at the crux of the heart rather than in the antero-superior part. Because of the deficiency at the ventricular inlet, the bridging leaflets are not at the level of the normal septal leaflet, but are rather attached more apically, thus creating a deformity of the ventricular inlets. This explains the inlet-outlet disproportion of the left ventricle, a well-known feature in these hearts. Thus, in hearts with deficiency/absence of the atrioventricular septum, the outlet tract of the left ventricle is always lengthened in relation to the inlet (Figs. 5-2, 5-6, 5-7, 5-8, and 5-10 through 5-12). Almost all hearts with an atrioventricular septal defect and ventricular septal defect show some degree of scooping of the ventricular septum. This scooping is seemingly not related to the morphology of the superior bridging leaflet, nor with the severity of the valvar regurgitation.[47a] Suzuki and colleagues[47a] have found that the scooping to correlate with the morphology of the inferior bridging leaflet.

Anatomic Risk Factors in Atrioventricular Septal Defect

A number of morphological factors may complicate the usual form of atrioventricular septal defect. These include: 1) ventricular hypoplasia[58–75]; 2) left ventricular outflow tract obstruction[13,19,25,26,43,48, 49,76–100]; 3) double-orifice left atrioventricular valve[10, 13,14,19, 101–109]; 4) parachute deformity of left atrioventricular valve[4,13,19,22,24,26,43,50–55,110]; 5) double-outlet atrium, right or left[111–120a]; and 6) association with other forms of congenital cardiac anomalies (tetralogy of Fallot, double-outlet right ventricle, hearts with right or left atrial isomerism, Ebstein's anomaly; etc.[13,15,17,37,38,69,98,121–137]

Ventricular Underdevelopment

Significant underdevelopment of either the right or left ventricle is known to complicate the complete form of atrioventricular septal defect, occurring in about 7% of patients with the complete form of atrioventricular septal defect.[58–75] Usually that component of the atrioventricular orifice ipsilateral to the hypoplastic ventricle is correspondingly underdeveloped.

An extensive literature is devoted to the so-called dominant right form of atrioventricular septal defect in which the morphologically left ventricle is hypoplastic (Figs. 5-14 through 5-21).[58–75] The prevalence of this association is approximately 10%. The conundrum is always how small is too small for a biventricular repair. It is more than ventricular cavity size that impacts on this decision. The left ventricle may be deceivingly large, filling from the ventricular septal defect, not from the left-sided component of the atrioventricular valve that is displaced rightward. The left-sided component of the common atrioventricular orifice is often hypoplastic and obstructive, and the left ventricular outflow tract is frequently diffusely small. While the ventricular septal defect in these patients can be large, it is our experience that the ventricular septal defect tends to be small, and this of course alters the surgical options for palliation. Obstructive anomalies of the aortic arch including coarctation of the aorta and interruption of the aorta are not uncommon in patients with a dominant right form of atrioventricular septal defect (Figs. 5-16, 5-20, and 5-21).[62,67,69] The hemodynamics

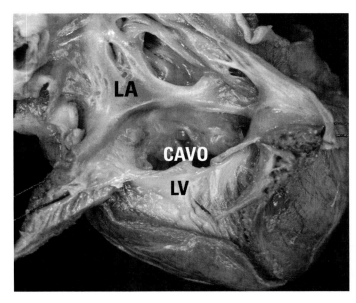

Fig. 5-14: Dominant right form of atrioventricular septal defect.
Internal view of hypoplastic left ventricle with the common atrioventricular orifice (CAVO) committed primarily to the right ventricle.

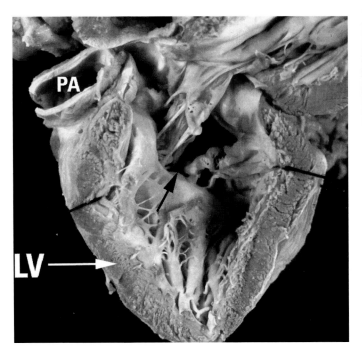

Fig. 5-15: Another specimen with a dominant right form of atrioventricular septal defect.
The left ventricle is better developed than that in Fig. 5-14, nonetheless, the commitment of the common atrioventricular orifice is primarily to the right ventricle.

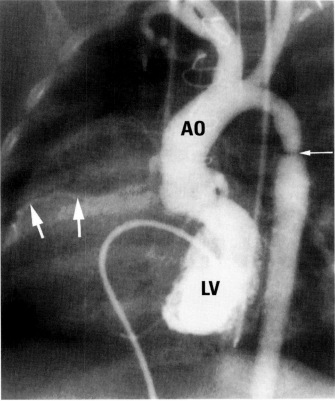

Fig. 5-16: An infant with an ostium primum atrial septal defect and coarctation of the aorta. This infant remained in severe congestive heart failure after repair of the coarctation.
Long axial left ventriculogram confirms an intact ventricular septum and the coarctation of the aorta (small white arrow). Note the epicardial course of the right coronary artery (two white arrows) indicating a very large right ventricle.

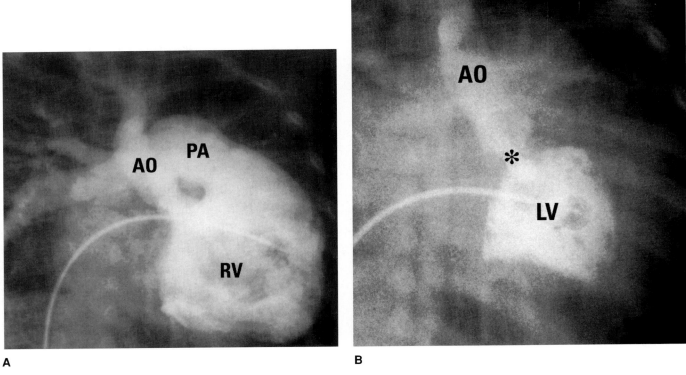

A

B

Fig. 5-17: A dominant right form of atrioventricular septal defect with subaortic stenosis.
A: Frontal right ventriculogram shows a very large right ventricle with right-to-left shunting through the ventricular septal defect explaining the opacification of the aorta. **B:** Frontal left ventriculogram defines a hypoplastic left ventricle with subaortic narrowing (✱).

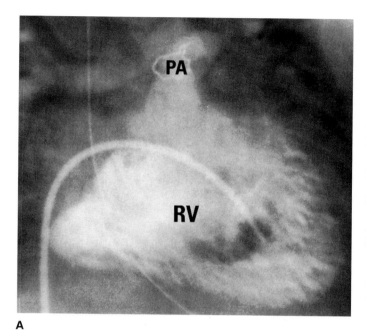

A

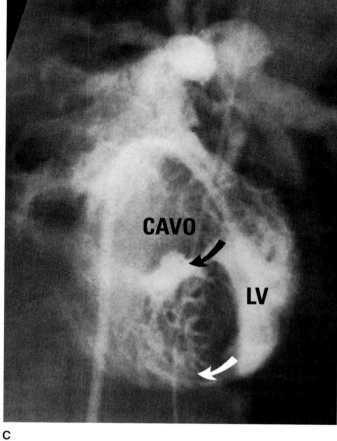

C

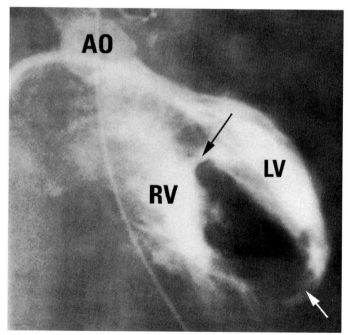

B

Fig. 5-18: A patient with a dominant right form of atrioventricular septal defect palliated with pulmonary artery banding.
A: Frontal right ventriculogram shows the very large ventricle supporting the banded pulmonary artery. **B and C:** Left anterior oblique left ventriculograms define the small left ventricle and the common atrioventricular orifice committed primarily to the right ventricle.

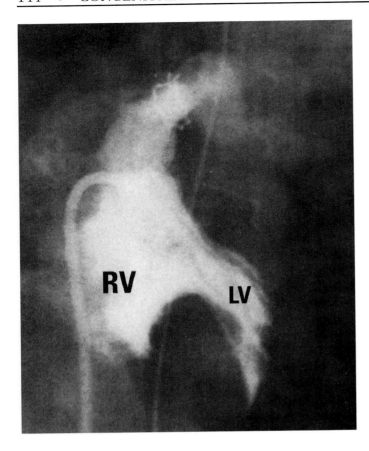

Fig. 5-19: An infant with a hypoplastic left ventricle in the setting of a dominant right form of atrioventricular septal defect palliated with pulmonary artery banding. Note the small, slit-like left ventricle.

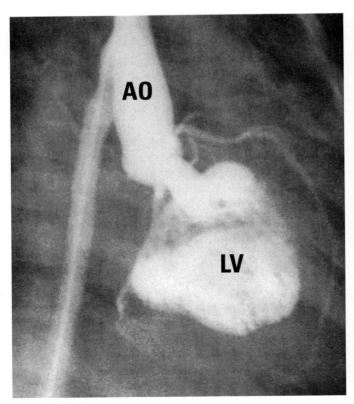

A

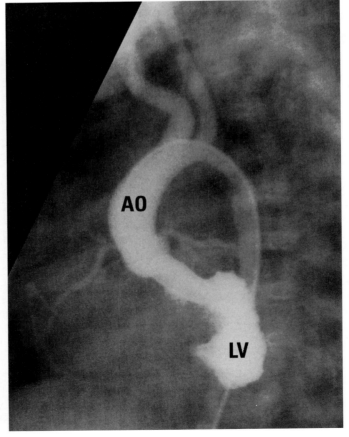

B

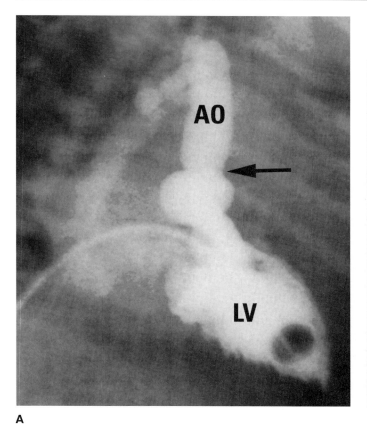

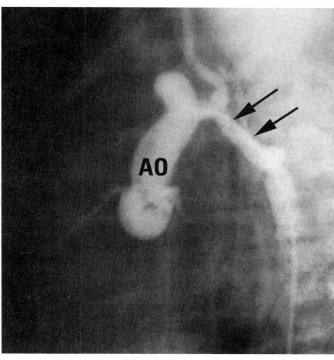

A

B

Fig. 5-21: Another infant with an ostium primum atrial septal defect, a small left ventricle, supra-aortic narrowing, and tubular hypoplasia of the transverse aortic arch.
A: Right anterior oblique left ventriculogram demonstrates the left atrioventricular valve regurgitation and supra-aortic narrowing (arrow). **B:** The aortogram defines the tubular hypoplasia (arrows) of the transverse aortic arch.

do not differentiate between those patients with a large and nonrestrictive ventricular septal defect and those with a restrictive ventricular septal defect. In both situations a large left-to-right shunt is present, and pulmonary artery pressures are at systemic levels. The arbiter of the various surgical algorithms is the size of the ventricular septal defect and the severity of atrioventricular valve regurgitation. Many of these patients are best placed on a Fontan algorithm. The initial form of palliation will depend on the size of the interventricular connection. When the ventricular septal defect is large and in the absence of severe left ventricular outflow tract obstruction despite a very small left ventricle, one could consider pulmonary artery banding followed by construction of bidirectional cavopulmonary anastomosis ± a Damus-Kaye-Stansel connection. A small ventricular septal defect and/or severe left ven-

tricular outflow tract obstruction would necessitate as palliation the Norwood approach (see Chapter 26).

The morphologically right ventricle can also be underdeveloped (Figs. 5-22 through 5-25). Such hypoplasia involves the inlet and trabecular components of the right ventricle. The ventricular septal defect tends to be large, although right ventricular hypoplasia with an intact ventricular septum has been recognized. In those patients with right ventricular hypoplasia and a large ventricular septal defect, the pulmonary outflow tract may or may not be obstructive. There is increasing experience with a biventricular repair of hypoplastic right ventricle assisted by a pulsatile bidirectional cavopulmonary anastomosis in patients with a hypoplastic right ventricle and an atrioventricular septal defect.[74,75] Alvarado and colleagues[74] reported the role of the cavopulmonary connection in the

Fig. 5-20: An infant with an ostium primum atrial septal defect after repair of a coarctation of the aorta. This infant was in refractory congestive heart failure. The left ventricular end-diastolic volume was only 45% of predicted.
A and B: Right anterior and left axial oblique left ventriculogram. The visual image from the right anterior oblique tends to overestimate the cavity size.

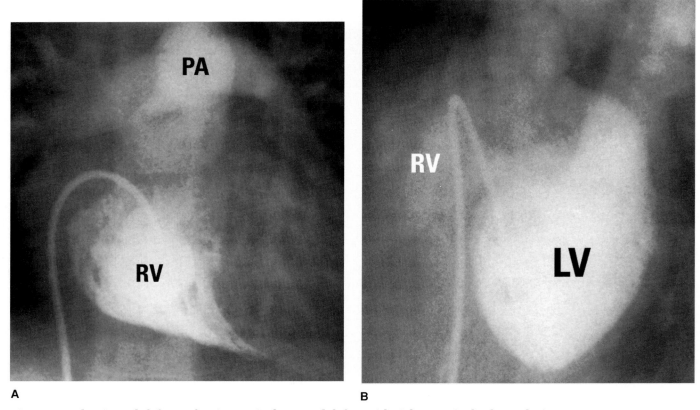

A **B**

Fig. 5-22: A dominant left form of atrioventricular septal defect with right ventricular hypoplasia.
A: The frontal right ventriculogram defines a modestly hypoplastic chamber with attenuation of the apical trabecular zone;
B: The much larger morphologically left ventricle in the hepatoclavicular left ventriculogram.

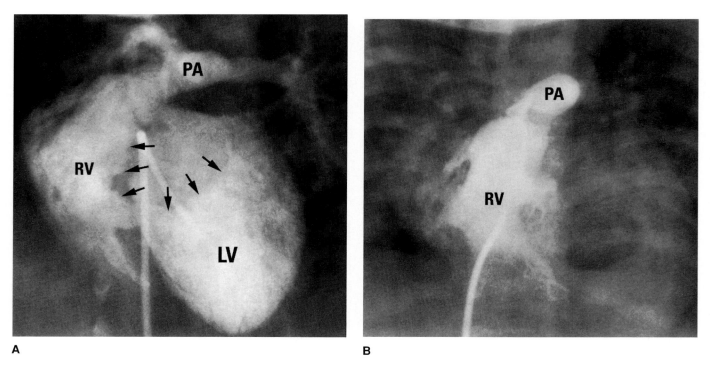

A **B**

Fig. 5-23: Another patient with a dominant left form of atrioventricular septal defect with right ventricular hypoplasia.
A: Left ventricular angiogram in shallow hepatoclavicular projection defines a small right ventricle that does not extend to the apex; note the common atrioventricular orifice (arrows) is committed predominately to the left ventricle. **B:** Selective right ventricular angiocardiogram confirms this chamber's hypoplasia.

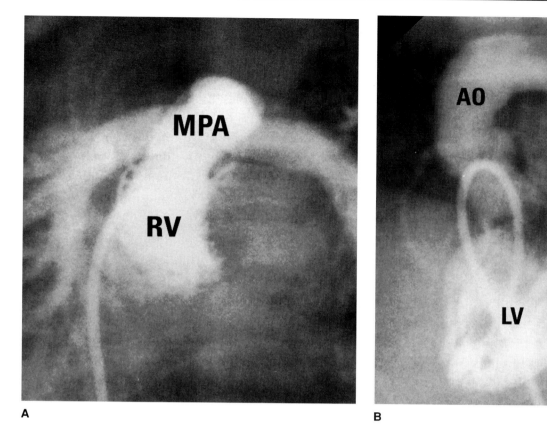

A   **B**

Fig. 5-24: This patient was persistently cyanotic from the newborn period with a dominant left form of atrioventricular septal defect.
A: Right ventricular angiogram. **B:** Left ventricle is much larger than the morphologically right ventricle.

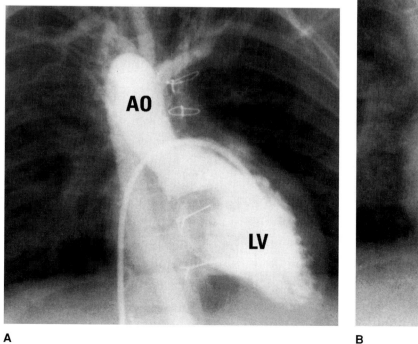
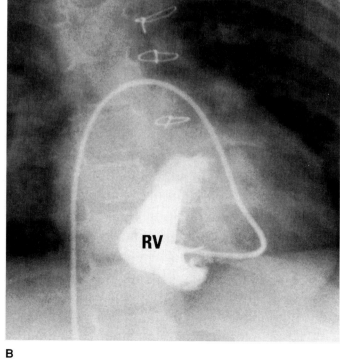

A   **B**

Fig. 5-25: Tricuspid atresia, a dominant left form of atrioventricular septal defect.
A: Left ventriculogram in frontal projection shows the large left ventricle with its elongated outflow tract. **B:** The right ventricle is very small. *(continued on next page)*

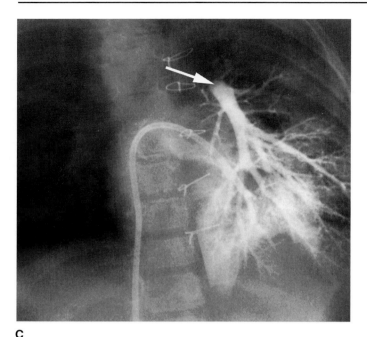

C

Fig. 5-25. *(continued)*
C: Pulmonary vein wedge angiogram demonstrates the left pulmonary artery (arrow).

repair of atrioventricular septal defect and small right ventricle. The majority of these patients had some form of right ventricular outflow tract obstruction, either pulmonary stenosis, double-chambered right ventricle, or tetralogy of Fallot. This should not be surprising because Bharati and colleagues[17] found that 11% of specimens with a complete form of atrioventricular septal defect and tetralogy of Fallot had a hypoplastic right ventricle.

Left Ventricular Outflow Tract Obstruction

Because of the unwedged and anterior position of the aorta in atrioventricular septal defect, the potential for subaortic stenosis in this already elongated left ventricular outflow tract is always present.[76–100] The frequency of subaortic stenosis in the various forms of atrioventricular septal defect ranges from 10% to 30%.[16,53] It is interesting that whereas the left ventricular outflow tract in atrioventricular septal defect is a structure of considerable surgical importance, paradoxically, as pointed out by Ebels, the real anatomy and extent of the left ventricular outflow tract is rarely seen by the surgeon in the usual surgical approach.[48,49] The normal left ventricular outflow tract is very short. We are reminded by Ebels that the posterior border of the normal left ventricular outflow tract is the area of fibrous continuity between the aortic and mitral valves, and this area is of variable length, occasionally being muscularized as shown by Rosenquist.[44,45] The other

anatomic boundaries are the infundibular septum and the left ventricular free wall. This is in distinct contrast to the extensive left ventricular outflow tract in the patient with atrioventricular septal defect, an outflow tract that reflects the unwedged position of the aorta, and the elongated outflow tract (Figs. 5-26 through 5-39). Draulans-Noe and Wenink[138] have observed that the anterolateral muscle bundle of the left ventricle was present between the superior bridging leaflet and left coronary cusp in 128 patients with the complete or partial form of atrioventricular septal defect, and while it was noted to be bulging into the left ventricular outflow tract, it was not prominent enough to result in subaortic obstruction.

The mechanisms responsible for subaortic stenosis in atrioventricular septal defect are diverse, and their specific identification is, of course, surgically relevant (Figs. 5-13, 5-14, and 5-19 through 5-37).[3,19,25,26,43,48,49,76–100,138] The anatomic mechanisms responsible for subaortic stenosis include: 1) abnormal malattachment of the superior bridging leaflet to the ventricular septum; 2) fibromuscular obstruction; 3) displaced papillary muscles; 4) other muscular abnormalities of the left ventricular outflow tract; and 5) tissue tags derived from atrioventricular valve tissue or membranous septum. DeLeon and colleagues[81] reported on 12 patients, 3 with Down syndrome, with subaortic stenosis associated with endocardial cushion defects. In only 2 patients in this series, both with discrete fibromuscular tissue, was the subaortic stenosis recognized preoperatively and dealt with at the initial operation. In the remaining 10 patients the subaortic stenosis was diagnosed at a mean of 6.3 ± 5 years after the primary repair. The mechanism of obstruction was considered to be fibromuscular in 5, mitral valve abnormalities in 3, and tunnel in 2. Reeder and colleagues[92] reported the Doppler echocardiographic findings in 21 patients with fixed subaortic stenosis in atrioventricular septal defect. Ten of 15 patients with the partial form of atrioventricular septal defect and 4 of the 6 with the complete form were recognized as having developed subaortic stenosis after the repair (Figs. 5-32 through 5-39). A discrete fibromuscular membrane was responsible in the majority for the left ventricular outflow tract obstruction. Similar findings have been published by Van Arsdell and colleagues from Toronto.[92a]

In the neonate with severe left ventricular outflow tract obstruction and an atrioventricular septal defect, the left ventricle is often disadvantaged, hypoplastic, and has a very deranged inlet as well.[82,85,94,98–100a] Subaortic atresia has been described in a few of these patients, with the mechanism being a malattached superior bridging leaflet (see Chapter 26, Fig. 26-10).[82,85,94,98–100a] Data from De Biase and colleagues[80] from the Ospedale Bambino Gesu in Rome suggests that patients without Down syndrome, but with atrioventricular

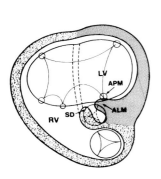
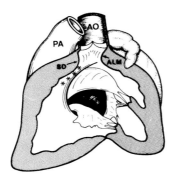
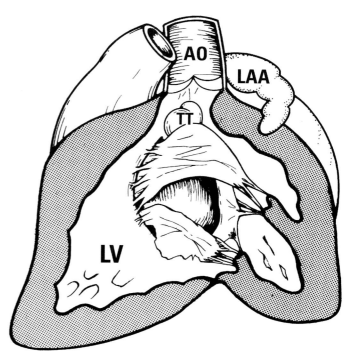

A

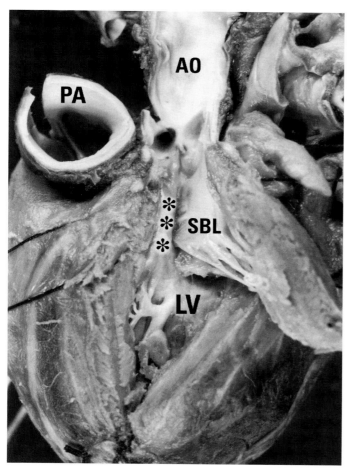

B

Fig. 5-26: Diagrams showing varying bases for left ventricular outflow tract obstruction in atrioventricular septal defect.
A: The left panel shows the spatial relationship between the septal deviation, the anterolateral muscle bundle, and the atrioventricular and aortic valves; middle panel: the outflow tract is intrinsically elongated and narrowed. It may be further compromised by septal deviation and prominence of the anterolateral muscle bundle of Moulaert (the left-sided ventriculoinfundibular fold); the right-hand panel shows accessory tissue tags adjacent to the left atrioventricular valve further compromising the left ventricular outflow tract.
B: Severely narrowed left ventricular outflow tract in an infant with an ostium primum atrial septal defect. Internal view of left ventricle and its outflow tract shows the severely narrowed and elongated subaortic area (✱). The superior bridging leaflet is malattached. *(continued on following page)*

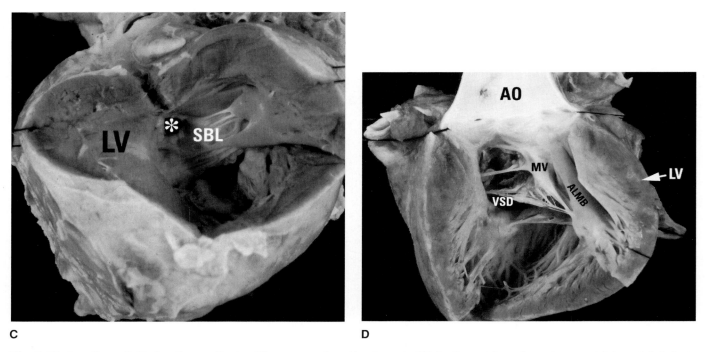

C **D**

Fig. 5-26: *(continued)* **C:** Another patient with severe subaortic stenosis (✱) in the setting of a primum atrial septal defect. **D:** The left ventricular outflow tract of a patient with an atrioventricular septal defect and a nonobstructive anterolateral muscle bundle of Moulaert (ALMB).

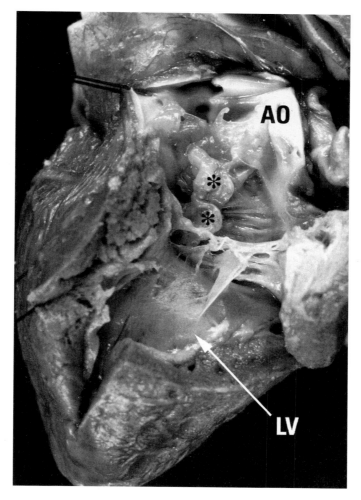

Fig. 5-27: The mechanisms primarily responsible for compromising the left ventricular outflow tract in this infant are multiple tissue tags (*).

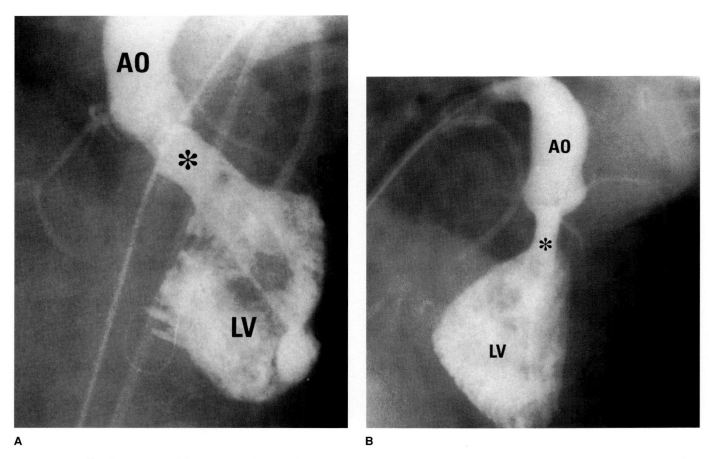

A

B

Fig. 5-28: Diffusely narrowed left ventricular outflow tract in an infant with an ostium primum form of atrioventricular septal defect, and an azygous continuation of the inferior vena cava.
A and B: Left and right anterior oblique left ventriculograms show the diffusely narrowed and elongated outflow tract (*).

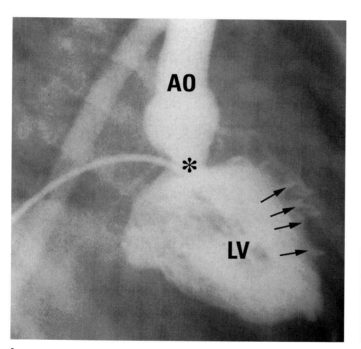

A

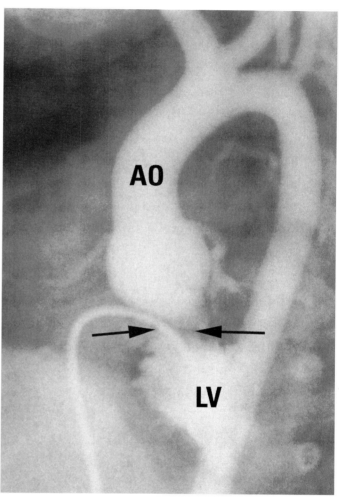

B

Fig. 5-29: Ostium primum atrial septal defect, multiple ventricular septal defects, and left ventricular outflow tract obstruction (✻).
A: Right anterior oblique left ventriculogram defines the multiple anterior wall muscular ventricular septal defects (arrows).
B: The long axial oblique left ventriculogram shows the severe (arrow) subaortic narrowing.

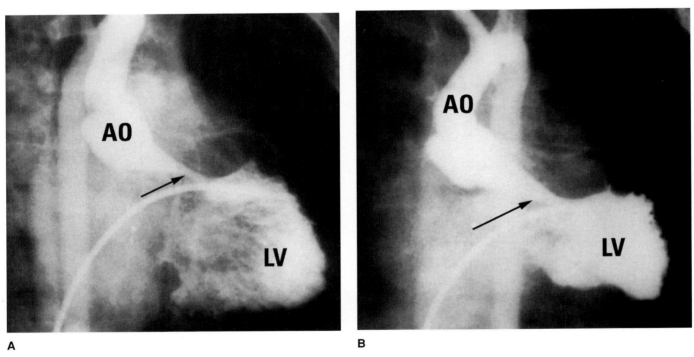

A

B

Fig. 5-30: Severe left ventricular outflow tract obstruction (arrow) in an infant with an ostium primum form of atrio-ventricular septal defect. Little variation in the aortic outflow tract is seen with the cardiac cycle.
A: Diastole. B: Systole.

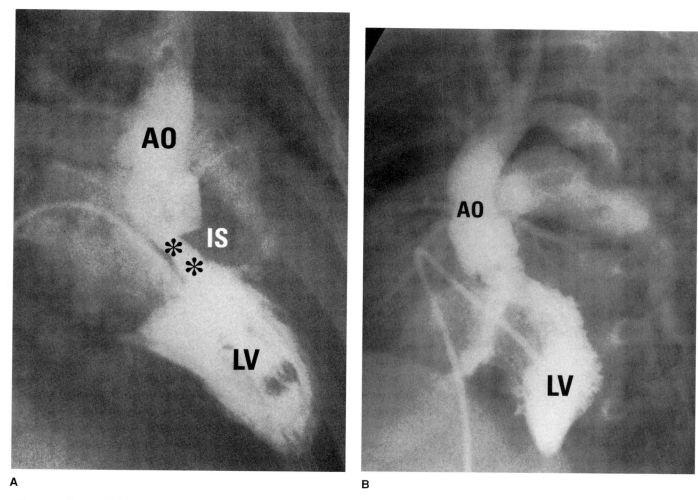

A   **B**

Fig. 5-31: Severe left ventricular outflow tract obstruction in a patient with a complete form of atrioventricular septal defect. **A:** Right anterior oblique left ventriculogram shows the tunnel-form subaortic narrowing (✱). **B:** The ventricular septal defect is evident in this long axial oblique left ventriculogram.

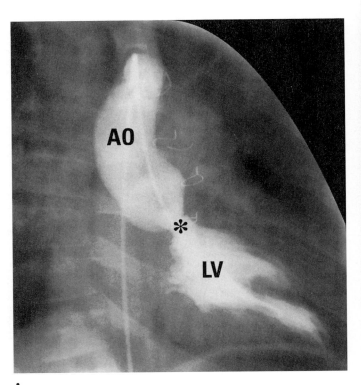

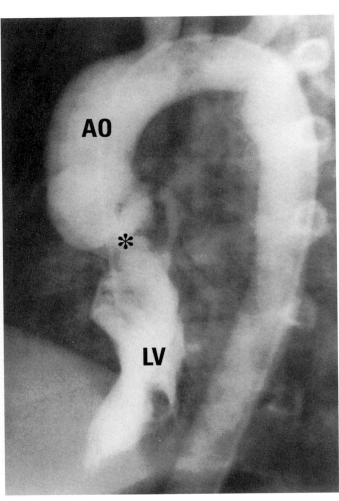

A

B

Fig. 5-32: Subaortic stenosis after repair of a complete form of atrioventricular septal defect.
A and B: Right and left axial oblique left ventriculograms show the discrete form of subaortic stenosis (✻). With cross-sectional echocardiography, one could appreciate that the superior bridging leaflet contributed to the subaortic narrowing.

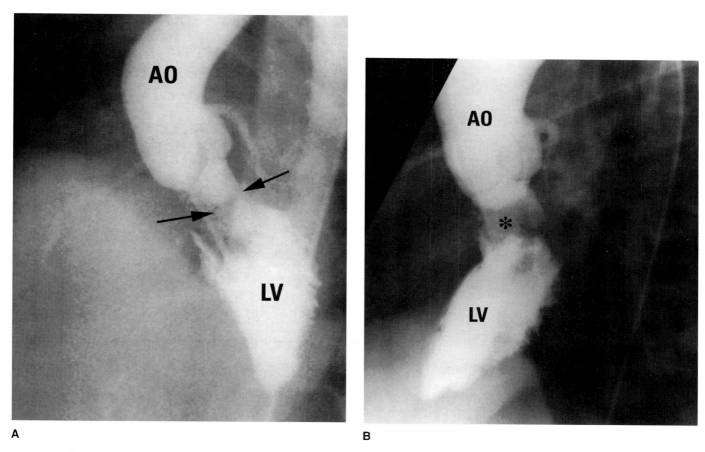

A　　　　　　　　　　　　　　　**B**

Fig. 5-33: Subaortic stenosis after repair of a partial form of atrioventricular septal defect.
Note the subaortic obstruction due to a traversing ridge (arrows in Fig. 5-33A), and a bulbous tissue tag (✻) in Fig. 5-33B.

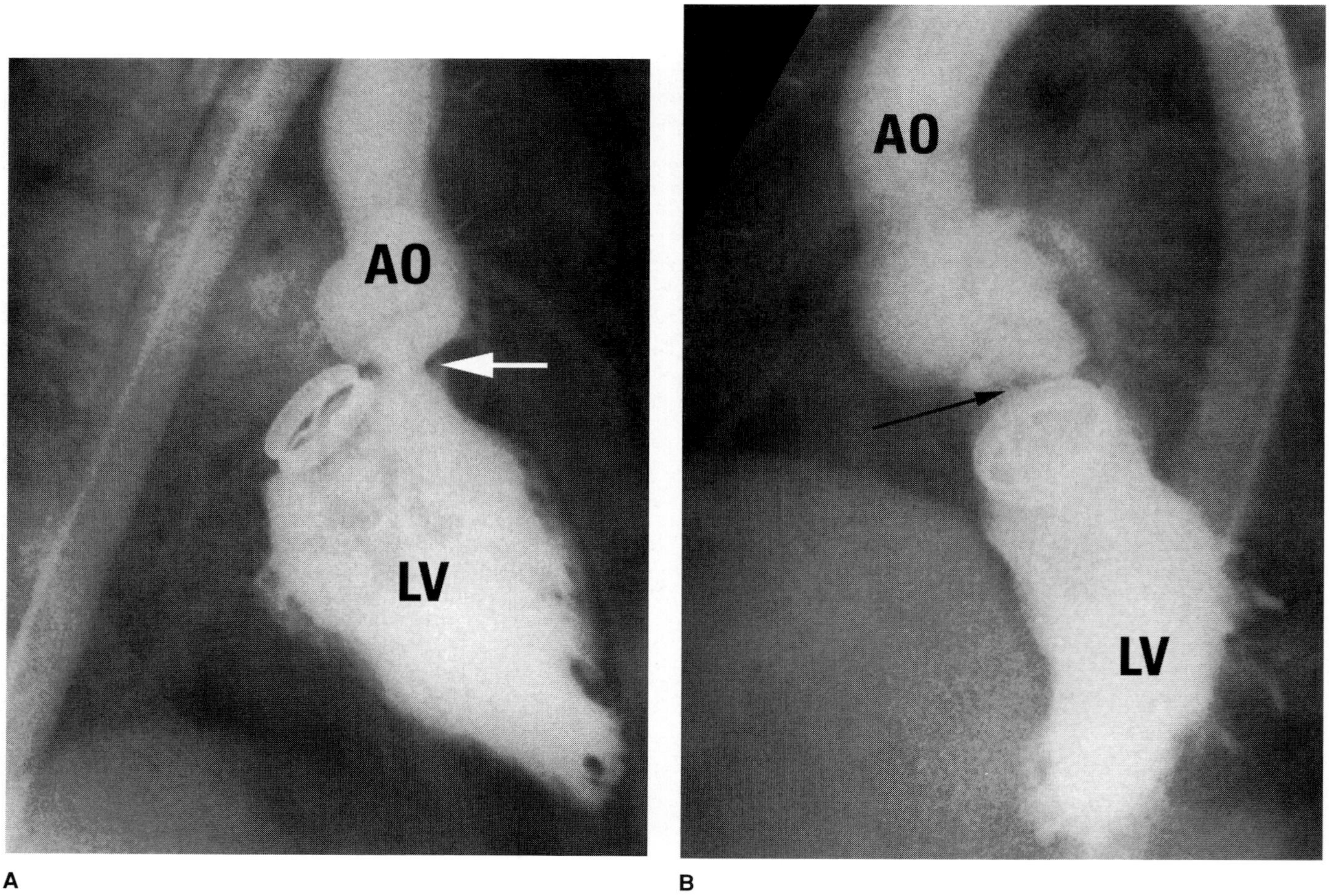

A

B

Fig. 5-34: Subaortic obstruction after mitral valve replacement in a complete form of atrioventricular septal defect.
A and B: Right and left anterior oblique left ventriculograms show the discrete type of subaortic narrowing (arrow).

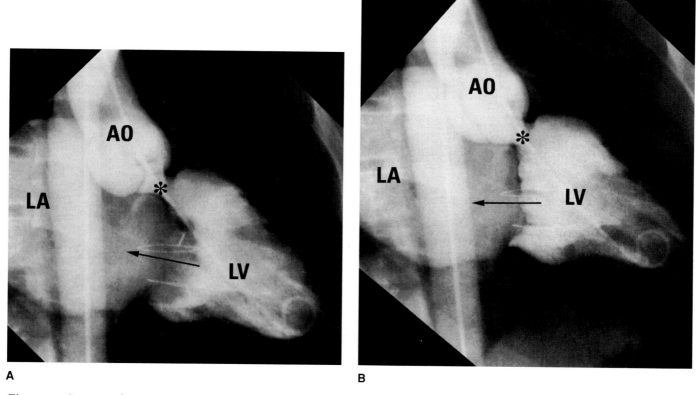

A   **B**

Fig. 5-35: Severe subaortic stenosis and left atrioventricular valve regurgitation after repair of a partial form of atrioventricular septal defect.
A and B: Two frames from right anterior oblique left ventriculograms demonstrate both the fixed subaortic narrowing (✻) and the severe left atrioventricular valve regurgitation (arrow) into a much enlarged left atrium.

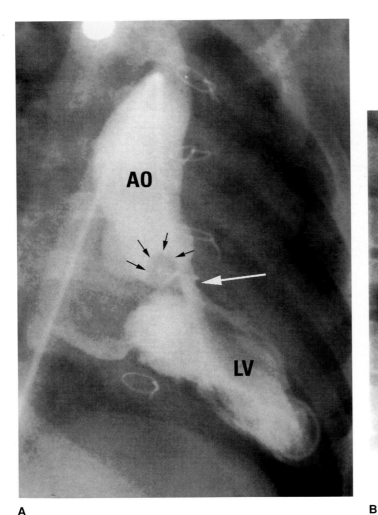

A

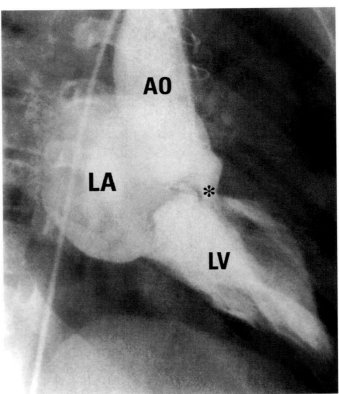

B

Fig. 5-36: Severe subaortic stenosis and left atrioventricular valve regurgitation after repair of a partial form of atrioventricular septal defect.
A: This right anterior oblique left ventriculogram shows the severe subaortic stenosis (white arrow) and tissue (black arrows) probably derived from the left atrioventricular valve herniating into the left ventricular outflow tract. **B:** A later frame shows both the subaortic stenosis (✱) and left atrioventricular valve regurgitation.

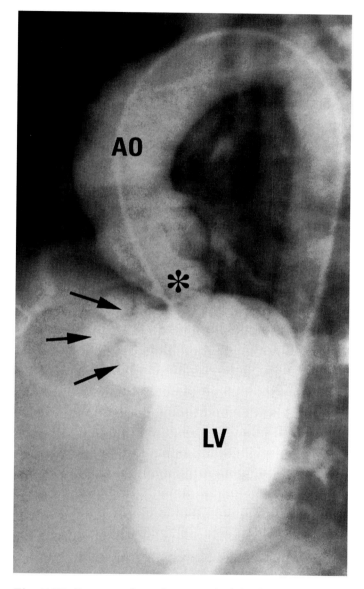

Fig. 5-37: Severe subaortic stenosis (*) after repair of a complete form of atrioventricular septal defect with a residual pouch (arrows) of atrioventricular valve tissue projecting into the right ventricle.

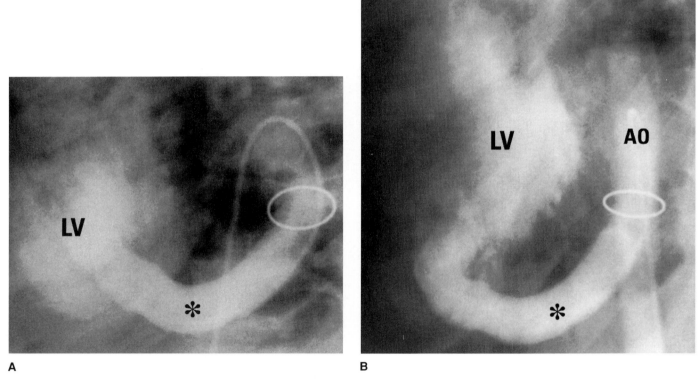

A

B

Fig. 5-38: An apical left ventricular-to-descending aortic conduit was used many years ago to palliate a patient with diffuse left ventricular outflow tract obstruction after repair of a complete form of atrioventricular septal defect.
A and B: These two frames show the functionality of the apical left ventricular-to-descending aortic conduit (✱).

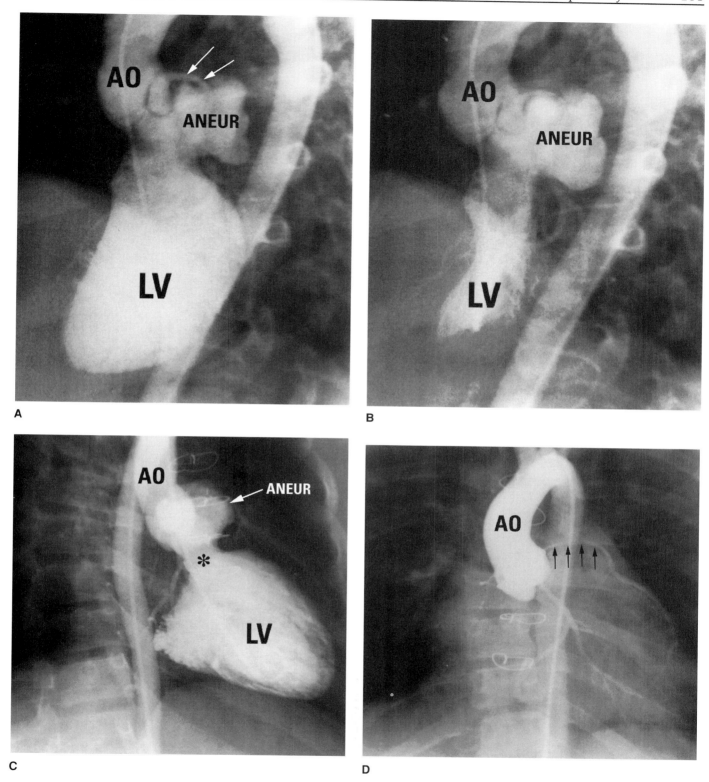

Fig. 5-39: A massive aneurysm in the region of the left-sided ventriculoinfundibular fold (the anterolateral muscle bundle of Moulaert) developed following surgery to relieve post-repair subaortic stenosis.
A and B: Long axial oblique and **C** right anterior oblique left ventriculograms show the very large aneurysm originating from the left-sided ventriculoinfundibular fold. Note the course and proximity of the circumflex coronary artery (arrows) to the aneurysm. The left ventricular outflow tract (✻) in Fig. 5-39C shows only mild narrowing (✻). **D:** This aneurysm displaces and distorts the circumflex coronary artery (arrows).

septal defect have a predilection toward right ventricular dominance and left-sided obstructive lesions. Of 90 consecutive patients seen in their institution with atrioventricular septal defect, 47 had Down syndrome and only one had a left-sided obstructive lesion. Thirteen (30%) of the 43 patients without Down syndrome had left-sided obstructive lesions, many with right ventricular dominance. Subaortic stenosis was particularly common in those infants presenting with congestive heart failure and requiring surgery in the first year of life.[138a] Gallo and colleagues[138b] have provided a pathological and morphometric evaluation of left ventricular outflow tract obstruction in atrioventricular septal defect. These authors pointed out that atrioventricular septal defect is characterized by inflow tract shortening and outflow tract lengthening, and that this latter feature along with the unwedged position of the aorta transforms the left ventricular outflow tract into a long, forward displaced fibromuscular channel, promoting the substrate for subaortic stenosis.

Parachute Deformity of the Left Atrioventricular Valve

The disposition of the papillary muscles in atrioventricular septal defect differs from that in the normal heart (Fig. 5-9; see also Chapter 25, Figs. 25-8 and 25-11).[4,13,19,22,24,26,43,50–55,110] In atrioventricular septal defect, the paired papillary muscles are not in an anterolateral and posteromedial position. Rather they are located one in front of the other, and are more closely disposed than in the normal heart. When all the tension apparatus of the left atrioventricular valve converge onto a solitary papillary muscle or onto abnormally closely opposed papillary muscles, this arrangement results in the so-called potentially parachute deformity (Fig. 5-40) (see also Chapter 25). The prevalence of a so-called parachute mitral valve in atrioventricular septal defect is about 14% based on the analysis of David and colleagues,[51] and 4% of the 155 surgical cases reported by Ilbawi and colleagues.[22] David and colleagues[51] inform us that in patients with an atrioventricular septal defect, there are four types of parachute deformity. These forms of potentially parachute deformity include: 1) one papillary muscle group and one mitral orifice; 2) one papillary muscle group with a double-orifice; 3) two abnormally opposed papillary muscles and one mitral orifice with almost no interpapillary muscle space; and 4) two papillary muscle groups and a double orifice. More than half of the postmortem specimens in the study by David et al[51] had two papillary muscle groups. The consideration of potentially parachute deformity reflects that the functional significance of this valvular abnormality is unmasked by surgical closure of the so-called cleft. In a discussion of the study by David and colleagues,[51] Schaff of the Mayo Clinic indicated that in a series of patients with an atrioventricular septal defect, 8% had either a parachute deformity or potentially parachute deformity of the mitral valve. However, as pointed out by Tandon and his colleagues,[54,55] a solitary left ventricular papillary muscle does not result in a classic parachute deformity because the so-called cleft in the superior bridging leaflet results in an opening on the medial side of the valve. The clinical importance nonetheless is that the surgical reconstruction of the so-called cleft between the superior and inferior bridging leaflets is limited. Closure of the cleft in a parachute deformity may result in stenosis of the valve. Tandon and colleagues[55] addressed the associated anomalies in 52 postmortem cases of parachute mitral valve. These 52 cases stratified into five subgroups: 1) normal great arteries (35 patients); 2) double-outlet right ventricle (8 patients); 3) complete transposition of the great arteries (4 patients); 4) corrected transposition of the great arteries (2 patients); and 5) miscellaneous (3 patients). The most common associated malformation was the ventricular septal defect, identified in 37 cases. A complete form of atrioventricular septal defect was identified in 5 patients.

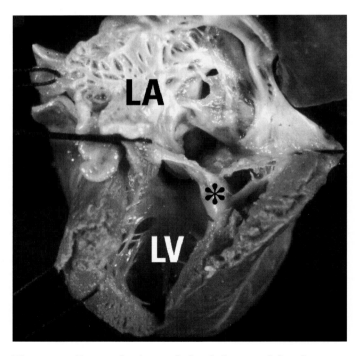

Fig. 5-40: Internal view of the left ventricle shows a parachute configuration (∗) of left atrioventricular valve in atrioventricular septal defect.

Double-Orifice Left Atrioventricular Valve

Double-orifice left atrioventricular valve applies to a group of malformations of the mitral valve that produces or seems to produce two openings in the atrioventricular valve.[10,13,14,19,43,101–109a] In patients with atrioventricular septal defect, the accessory orifice is usually at the posteromedial commissure. A ring of chordae supports and surrounds the accessory orifice and a small papillary muscle is often located beneath the orifice. Kirklin and Barratt-Boyes[43] suggest that the accessory orifice may be conceptualized as an incomplete commissure, and the fibrous tissue bridge between the accessory orifice and the true orifice consists of valvar tissue and chordae. Surgical data from the extensive Mayo Clinic experience indicates it is hazardous to divide that bar or bridge of tissue separating the major from the accessory orifice,[106] and that this would produce severe left atrioventricular valve regurgitation. Accessory orifices predispose patients to inlet obstruction after repair. The valve with the double orifice may be functionally normal, regurgitant, or stenotic.

Double-Outlet Atrium (Right or Left)

While a double-outlet from the atrium may reflect a straddling or overriding atrioventricular valve, in the presence of an atrioventricular septal defect the two most common mechanisms producing a double-outlet atrium are either a double-orifice or malalignment of the atrial septum.[111–120a] Deviation of the atrial septum to the left will result in double-outlet right atrium and produce a variable degree of arterial desaturation. This may confound the assessment of the hemodynamics in the patient with atrioventricular septal defect, pulmonary artery hypertension, and the cause concern about pulmonary vascular obstruction and whether surgery is possible. Indeed a lung biopsy may be the only way of defining the status of the pulmonary vascular bed. Profound leftward deviation of the atrial septum with malattachment can effectively isolate the pulmonary veins from the left atrioventricular valve (see also Chapter 21), producing pulmonary venous obstruction,[112] which simulates cor triatriatum.[120] Starc and colleagues[117] reported three infants with atrioventricular septal defect and pulmonary venous obstruction. Two of the patients had a subdivided left atrium of the classic cor triatriatum type (see Chapter 24), and one patient had leftward deviation and malattachment of the atrial septum to the lateral wall of the left atrium.

Suzuki and colleagues[120a] reported an 18-month-old patient with double-outlet right atrium and complete atrioventricular septal defect. The leftward malaligned atrial septum produced severe obstruction to left atrial egress. Histologic finding at lung biopsy was consistent with pulmonary vascular obstruction. Others have documented double-outlet right atrium with a restrictive ostium primum atrial septal defect and an incomplete supravalvular ring presenting as congenital mitral valve stenosis (see also Chapter 25).[117a] Deviation of the atrial septum to the right will result in an obligatory left-to-right shunt (from left atrium to right ventricle). Double-outlet right atrium is usually associated with an ostium primum atrial septal defect, but has been observed in the patient with a common atrioventricular orifice, an overriding atrioventricular valve, or three atrioventricular valves (see Chapter 15, Fig. 15-5 and Chapter 25, Fig. 25-3). Malalignment of the atrial septum is best recognized by echocardiography.

Associated Lesions

An atrioventricular septal defect can be complicated by other lesions, including Ebstein's anomaly, complete or corrected transposition of the great arteries, cor triatriatum, tetralogy of Fallot, double-outlet right ventricle, single ventricle malformation, and syndromes of right and left atrial isomerism (Figs. 5-41 through 5-43; see also Chapter 20, Fig. 20-22 and Chapter 37, Fig. 37-26).[13,15,17,37,38,69,98,121–137,139] A wide range of systemic and pulmonary venous anomalies have been described in patients with atrioventricular septal defect. Such anomalies are, of course, more frequent when the atria are not normally lateralized (see Chapters 12 and 41). Gow,[83] from the Toronto Hospital for Sick Children, has specifically addressed the association between the complete form of atrioventricular septal defect and coarctation of the aorta. In this association, one should anticipate right ventricular dominance, as well as inlet and outlet obstruction. However, an obstructive anomaly of the aortic arch may be seen in the patient with a balanced form of the defect without any specific risk factors. Additional muscular ventricular septal defects are also known to complicate the atrioventricular septal defect. Such additional muscular defects may occur in any portion of the ventricular septum, but in our experience, additional muscular outlet or juxta-arterial defects are uncommon. Soto and Pacifico[140] have demonstrated the angiography of atrioventricular septal defect in patients with complete and corrected transposition of the great arteries.

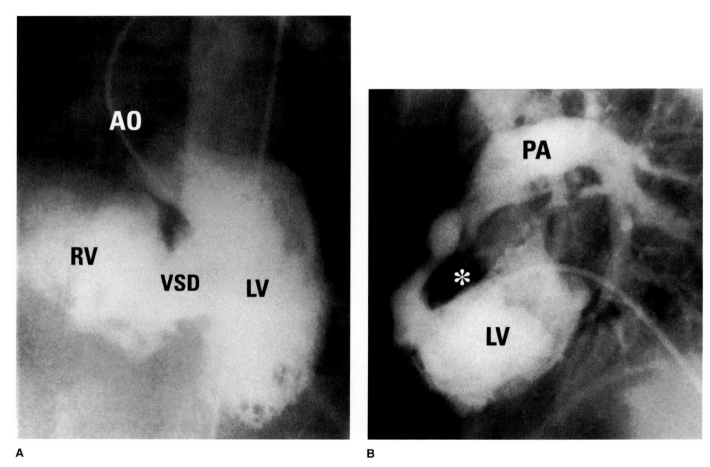

A

B

Fig. 5-41: A patient with tetralogy of Fallot and the complete form of atrioventricular septal defect.
A: Hepatoclavicular left ventriculogram shows the very large ventricular septal defect. **B:** Anterior deviation of the infundibular septum (✱) is conspicuous in this lateral left ventriculogram.

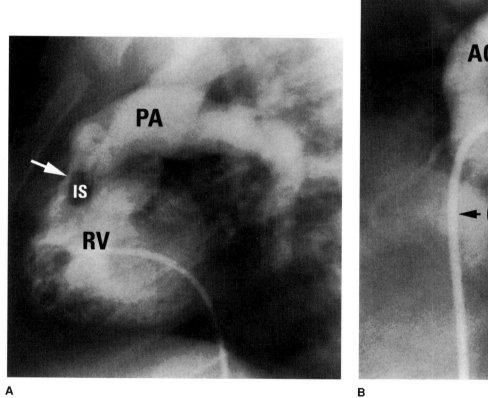

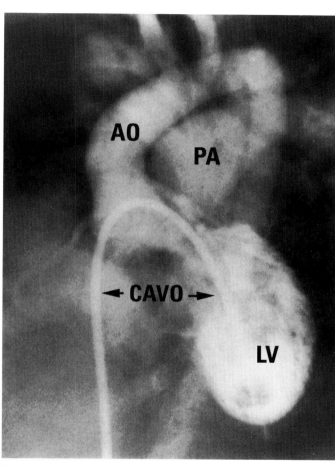

A

B

Fig. 5-42: Severe infundibular obstruction of the tetralogy-type and the complete form of atrioventricular septal defect.
A: Lateral right ventriculogram shows the anteriorly-deviated infundibular septum and the severely narrowed right ventricular outflow tract (arrow). **B:** The overriding aorta in the setting of an atrioventricular septal defect are seen in this long axial left ventriculogram.

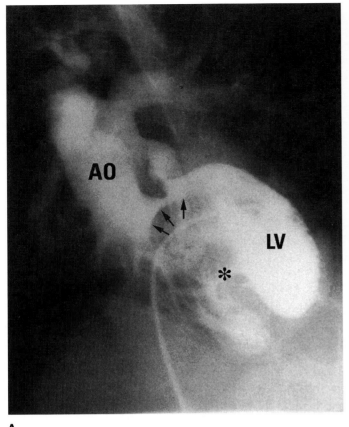

A

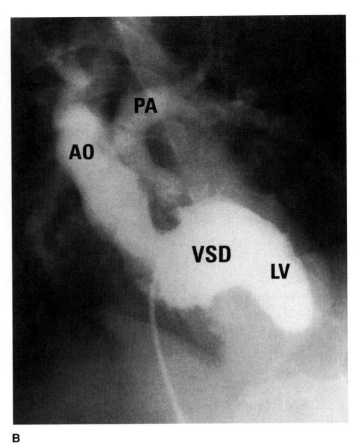

B

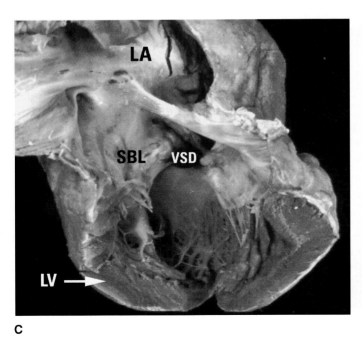

C

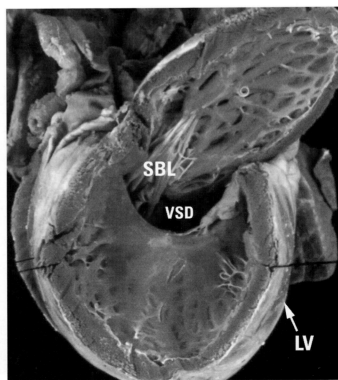

D

Atrioventricular Septal Defect and Tetralogy of Fallot

Kirklin[43] indicated that typical tetralogy of Fallot is present in about 10% of cases with the complete form of atrioventricular septal defects, and approximately 1% of patients with the complete form of atrioventricular septal defect have associated tetralogy of Fallot (Figs. 5-41 and 5-42; see also Chapter 20, Fig. 20-22). The common atrioventricular orifice is not partitioned; the ventricular septal defect is large and juxta-aortic, and the left superior bridging leaflet has extensive bridging and is not attached to the ventricular septal crest (see also Chapter 20).[13,17,37,43,63,131,134,136,137,140]

Atrioventricular Septal Defect and Double-Outlet Right Ventricle

The association of double-outlet right ventricle and atrioventricular septal defect is well established, occurring in about 2% of patients with atrioventricular septal defect (Fig. 5-43; see also Chapter 37, Fig. 37-26). Usually the ventricular septal defect is large and confluent with a juxta-aortic defect. The common atrioventricular orifice is usually not partitioned, and typically there are not chordal attachments to the crest of the ventricular septum.[13,17,37,43,63,129,130,140] We have identified one patient, however, with double-outlet right ventricle, a complete form of atrioventricular septal defect, and a restrictive ventricular septal defect. The mechanism of the restriction was related both to marked attachments of chordal tissue to the septum and an unusually small ventricular septal defect. Pulmonary outflow tract obstruction may or may not be present. It is uncommon to define extension of the ventricular septal defect of the atrioventricular type to the subpulmonary region, ie, the Taussig-Bing form of double-outlet right ventricle. The combination of double-outlet right ventricle and atrioventricular septal defect is rather common in patients with right atrial isomerism (see Chapter 41).

Relation to Down Syndrome

Beyond these issues of nomenclature, however, lies the reality of the management of those patients with cardiac lesions whose unifying feature is absence of the atrioventricular septum, and who are often further compromised by Down syndrome.[141–153] Down syndrome was present in 114 (80%) of 142 infants less than 1 year of age with the complete form of atrioventricular septal defect undergoing surgery in this institution.[151] Similar associations have been recorded elsewhere. When viewed from the opposite perspective, between 35% and 40% of patients with Down syndrome have an atrioventricular septal defect, and in most of these it is with a common, rather than a partitioned atrioventricular orifice. Rosenquist and colleagues[143] have suggested that an enlarged membranous ventricular septum may be an internal stigma of Down syndrome. De Biase and colleagues[80] suggest that there is an increased prevalence of left-sided obstructive lesions in patients with atrioventricular septal defect without Down syndrome (see p. ???, this chapter).[80] Marino and colleagues[147–148] assessed the prevalence of associated cardiac malformations in a large cohort of patients with atrioventricular septal defect compared with patients without Down syndrome. Among 220 patients with atrioventricular septal defect, 130 had a complete form of atrioventricular septal defect; 80 (61.5%) of these had Down syndrome and 50 (38.5%) did not have Down syndrome (38.5%). Of the 90 patients with a partial form of atrioventricular septal defect, 25 (28%) had Down syndrome and 65 (72%) did not have Down syndrome. Thus, Down syndrome was most commonly associated with a complete form of atrioventricular septal defect ($P < 0.01$); patients without Down syndrome tended to have the partial form of the defect. Addressing the entire spectrum of associated cardiac malformations in these 220 patients, 112 had a total of 137 associated malformations. The associated cardiac malformations were significantly more frequent ($P < 0.0001$) in patients without Down syndrome. Among those patients with Down syndrome and the complete form of atrioventricular septal defect, tetralogy of Fallot was more prevalent. In patients without Down syndrome, the hypoplastic left ventricle and coarctation were more common. Marino[147a] has also found that patients without Down syndrome and atrioventricular septal defect have a higher risk of left-sided obstructive lesions. Interestingly, Marino and colleagues[147b] documented the rarity of additional ventricular septal defects in the apical muscular septum of patients with atrioventricular septal defect and Down syndrome.

Fig. 5-43: Double-outlet right ventricle and the complete form of atrioventricular septal defect.
A and B: Two frames from the long axial oblique left ventriculogram demonstrate the ventriculoarterial connection of double-outlet right ventricle, the large ventricular septal defect, and the common atrioventricular orifice. **C and D:** Specimen from a different patient with complete form of atrioventricular septal defect and double-outlet right ventricle. **C:** Internal view of left atrium and left ventricle showing the free-floating superior bridging leaflet, and the large interventricular component of the defect. **D:** This internal view of the left ventricle shows the common atrioventricular valve is not attached to the ventricular septum, and that the only egress of blood from the left ventricle is through the ventricular septal defect. Note that the only outlet of this left ventricle is the ventricular septal defect.

Surgical results for atrioventricular septal defect have been stratified against patients with and without Down syndrome.[146,147,154–156] Again, there is not unanimity of opinion that Down syndrome impacts negatively on surgical outcome. Data provided by Morris[154] suggested a trend toward higher mortality and poorer postoperative hemodynamics in children with Down syndrome, although this was not the conclusion of Vet and Ottenkamp.[156] Data from Castaneda and Clapp, however, indicate an improvement in hemodynamic status after surgical repair.[157–159] Similarly data from Rizzoli[155] did not support the position that surgical outcome was poorer in the patient with Down syndrome.

Bull and colleagues[160] suggested some time ago that patients with Down syndrome and atrioventricular septal defect might do better without surgery because of the inherent risks of surgery. This suggestion provoked considerable discussion.[161,162] In many centers today, repair of the complete form of atrioventricular septal defect can be accomplished with a risk of less than 5%, which is considerably lower than the data provided by Bull.[6,43,63,155,157,158,159,163–165] Shinebourne and Carvalho[160a] have recently provided an overview of atrioventricular septal defect and Down syndrome.

Pulmonary Vascular Disease

The conclusion that patients with Down syndrome and the complete form of atrioventricular septal defect are at increased risk for the development of pulmonary vascular obstructive disease when compared with otherwise normal children with the same heart defect remains debatable.[166–176] Hemodynamic data provided by Chi and Krovetz[166] in 1975 suggested that patients with congenital heart disease and Down syndrome have an unusually high pulmonary vascular resistance and a propensity for early development of severe damage to the pulmonary vascular bed. Also in 1975, Soudon and colleagues[173] came to the same conclusion based on hemodynamic results of pulmonary vascular resistance calculations. More recently and with more follow-up data, Clapp and colleagues[159] concluded that Down syndrome patients with complete atrioventricular septal defect have a greater degree of elevation of pulmonary vascular resistance in the first year of life, and more rapid progression to fixed pulmonary vascular obstruction than patients without Down syndrome,[159] but this was not the case the review by Studer and colleagues.[63] A number of investigators have addressed the morphology of the pulmonary vascular bed in patients with congenital heart disease statified (yes/no) against Down syndrome. Plett and colleagues[175] did not find histological evidence that patients with Down syndrome were at a disadvantage.[175] However, Frescura and colleagues[168] correlated pulmonary vascular resistance determined from catheter-derived hemodynamic

data against pulmonary vascular disease at histology (from autopsy and biopsy material) and concluded that the most severe pulmonary vascular disease was observed in patients with Down syndrome. On the basis of their data, they recommend that surgical correction of the complete form of atrioventricular septal defect be carried out by 6 months of age.

Haworth[169,170] has extensively studied the pulmonary vascular bed in children with complete atrioventricular septal defect, and correlated structural and hemodynamic abnormalities. Her data was not clearly stratified against (yes/no) Down syndrome. The striking finding in this study was the inverse relation between pulmonary artery muscularity, pulmonary artery pressure and resistance, and age. Intimal damage increased with age and cases with the least amount of muscle frequently demonstrated the most severe intimal proliferation and obstruction.[170] Yamaki and colleagues[174] analyzed pulmonary vascular disease morphometrically in 67 patients with the complete form of atrioventricular septal defect, and their data was stratified against Down syndrome. These investigators found the same inverse relation between pulmonary artery muscularity and intimal proliferation and obstruction, defining that the media was thinner in those patients with Down syndrome and that such thinning was of the media of the small pulmonary arteries was generally observed at about 6 months of age. Yamaki and colleagues therefore recommend that intracardiac repair is desirable by 6 months of age, before maximal medial thinning, for patients with the complete form of atrioventricular septal defect and Down syndrome. Whether there is an intrinsic molecular basis for accelerated pulmonary vascular disease in those patients with Down syndrome is uncertain. Chronic upper airway obstruction with macroglossia and an inherently small hypopharynx, hypotonia, the predisposition to chronic infection, an abnormal capillary bed morphology, and the suggestion of pulmonary hypoplasia can all impact on the pulmonary vascular bed.[167,177,178]

Echocardiography

The basic diagnosis of an atrioventricular septal defect is relatively straightforward, requiring recognition of several constant echocardiographic features.[30,41,49,50,57,60,71,92,105,179–188] Inlet-outlet disproportion is appreciated in either the precordial or subcostal long-axis view. Absence of the muscular atrioventricular septum is best imaged from the precordial four-chamber view, with the atrioventricular valves appearing at the same level. The abnormal papillary muscle disposition can be seen in either the precordial or subcostal short-axis view.[50] Finally, the atrioventricular valve morphology, with its bridging leaflets and cleft are clearly imaged in the subcostal or precordial short-axis position with the so-called cleft pointing to the right ventricle, not to the left ventricular outflow tract.[185–188] The so-called cleft of the left atrioventricular valve is easily distinguished from the isolated cleft of the anterior mitral leaflet.[185,189]

We have discussed elsewhere in this chapter the risk factors associated with this disorder. Some are of more significance than others, in particular, hypoplasia of either ventricle and left ventricular outflow tract obstruction. The echocardiogram is ideally suited to define the nature and perhaps the severity of left ventricular outflow tract obstruction, and in the long-axis view, the left ventricular outflow tract is ideally imaged. The recognition of severe ventricular hypoplasia is certainly an echocardiographic prerogative. In those patients with borderline hypoplasia, cardiac angiography with volumetric determination is essential. The disposition of the papillary muscles and the recognition of (or exclusion) of a single papillary muscle is very important in the surgical management of the left atrioventricular valve. The short-axis view usually nicely demonstrates the support structures for the left atrioventricular valve.

Hemodynamics and Angiocardiography

It is our institutional policy and that of some other centers to send most young infants 6 to 8 months of age or younger with a balanced form of atrioventricular septal defect to surgery for complete repair without cardiac catheterization, assuming one is confident in excluding multiple ventricular septal defects, etc.[190,190a] In the neonate and young infant less than 3 months of age, pulmonary hypertension will be present reflecting the large and nonrestrictive ventricular septal defect, but pulmonary vascular obstructive disease is uncommon. Certainly a full hemodynamic and angiographic investigation is warranted at any age if there are concerns about the pulmonary vascular bed, or anatomic considerations not defined by echocardiography and Doppler, and in some patients lung biopsy may be the final arbiter of surgical candidacy. In this regard, one would want to exclude chronic airway difficulties as a confounding variable. When one considers those anatomic risk factors in atrioventricular septal defect including parachute deformity, double-orifice left atrioventricular valve, left ventricular outflow tract obstruction, and double-outlet atrium, echocardiographic imaging provides more information about these particular issues than does angiography. The determination of severity of atrioventricular valve regurgitation is also well suited to echocardiographic assessment, but certainly there is considerable information about the role of left ventricular angiocardiography in this area as well. The echocardiogram may raise the specter of ventricular hypoplasia, but unless the ventricular hypoplasia is pro-

found, we would recommend ventricular angiography with volumetric analysis to aid in the determination of a biventricular repair vs. a univentricular one.

Angiocardiography

The cardinal angiographic features of hearts with atrioventricular septal defect have been beautifully portrayed in many articles and book chapters.[140,190–199] As one reviews these publications in a historical sequence, what becomes obvious is improved understanding of the basic nature of the malformation as well as recognition of the component parts. While angiography may be used to define the presence and size of the ostium primum atrial septal defect, this is rarely necessary because cross-sectional echocardiography is so helpful in this area. The absence of the atrioventricular septum is shown in the left ventriculogram using the elongated right axial oblique projection.[140] The normal smooth line or contour of the posterior aspect of the left ventricular outflow tract is absent, replaced by an irregular border created by the leaflets of the atrioventricular valves in patients with an atrioventricular septal defect (Figs. 5-10 through 5-12, 5-16, 5-18, 5-20, 5-22, 5-23, 5-29, 5-30, 5-41, 5-42, and 5-44 through 5-50). The disproportion between the left ventricular inlet and outlet is evident in this projection as well (Figs. 5-10 through 5-12, 5-16, 5-18, 5-20, 5-22, 5-23, 5-29, 5-30, 5-41, 5-42, and 5-44 through 5-50). When compared with the normal left ventricular outflow tract, the outflow tract of the left ventricle of the patient with an atrioventricular defect appears elongated, narrowed, and at times s-shaped.

The character of the ventricular septum in atrioventricular septal defect is best demonstrated in the hepatoclavicular or four-chamber projection (Figs. 5-11, 5-23, 5-41, 5-44 through 5-47 and 5-49). The normal smoothly contoured septal surface beneath the noncoronary leaflet of the aortic valve is replaced in atrioventricular septal defect by the irregular, scalloped border of the atrioventricular valve leaflets. This appearance is evident whether or not the common atrioventricular orifice is partitioned or not. The characteristic deformity of the left ventricular outflow tract is evident in both ventricular systole and diastole.

The disposition of the common atrioventricular orifice to the ventricular septum is well demonstrated by a left ventriculogram filmed in the four-chamber projection (Figs. 5-11, 5-22, 5-24, 5-25, 5-41, and 5-43 through 5-49). The ring of the atrioventricular valve is seen when contrast material accumulates under the recess formed by the attachment of the leaflets. Much of the information about the disposition of the atrioventricular valve (balanced, dominant right or left forms) should have been provided by the cross-sectional echocardiographic study. This assessment is usually

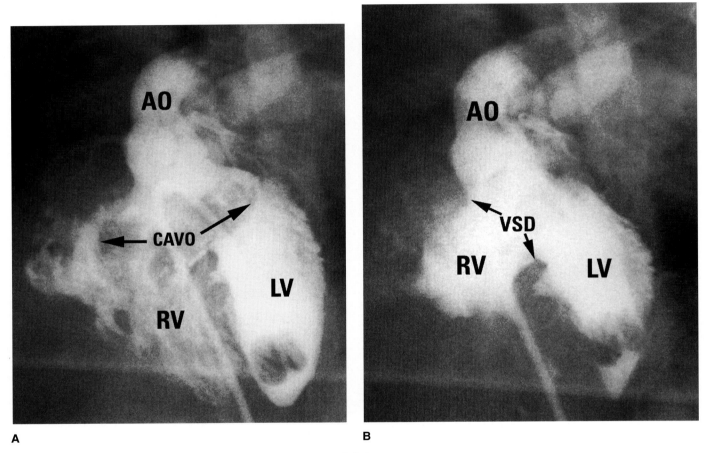

A

B

Fig. 5-44: Complete balanced form of atrioventricular septal defect.
A and B: Two frames from the hepatoclavicular left ventriculogram show the disposition of the common atrioventricular orifice and the large interventricular component of the defect. *(continued on next page)*

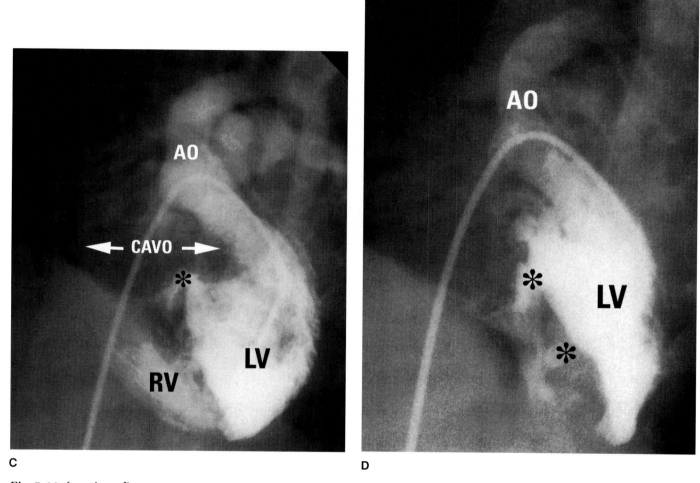

C

D

Fig. 5-44: *(continued)*
C and D: In a different patient, minimal shunting under the inferior bridging leaflet (✳) is seen in this hepatoclavicular left ventriculogram as is the disposition of the common atrioventricular orifice, In D, the most inferior (✳) denotes a separate additional small ventricular septal defect.

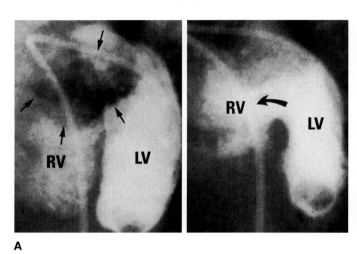

A

Fig. 5-45: Complete balanced form of atrioventricular septal defect.
A: Two frames from a hepatoclavicular left ventriculogram show the common atrioventricular orifice (arrows) has a balanced disposition, and the large ventricular component (curved arrow) is seen. **B:** A different patient with a large ventricular septal defect component shown by a hepatoclavicular left ventriculogram.

B

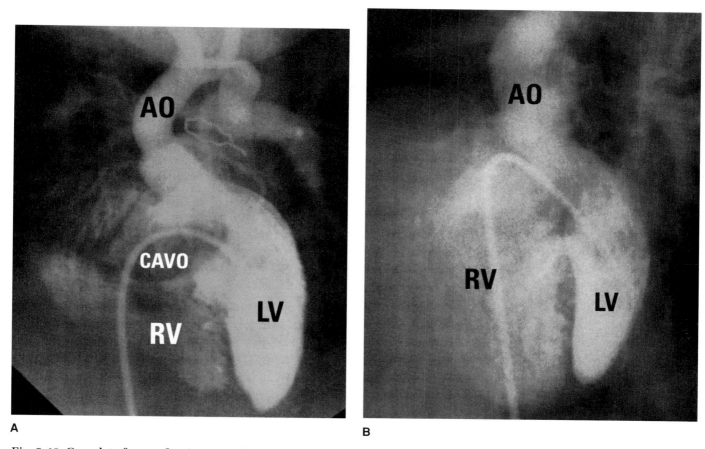

A

B

Fig. 5-46: Complete forms of atrioventricular septal defect in two different patients with a slightly small ventricle.
A: This hepatoclavicular left ventriculogram shows a slightly small right ventricle that doesn't extend to the apex. **B:** In the other patient, a slightly small left ventricle in diastole that doesn't extend to the cardiac apex.

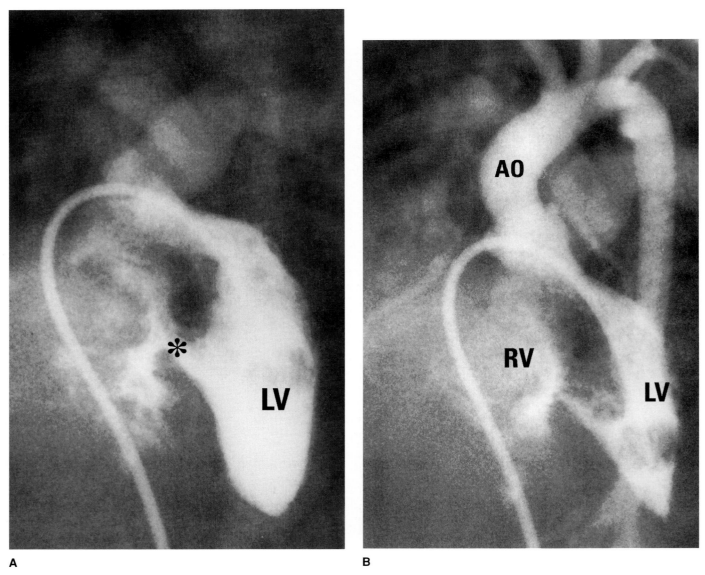

Fig. 5-47: An intermediate form of atrioventricular septal defect studied in the hepatoclavicular projection.
A and B: These two frames show the disposition of the partitioned atrioventricular orifices and the shunting (✱) beneath the inferior bridging leaflet. **C:** Another patient with opacification of the large ventricular septal defect beneath the inferior bridging leaflet.

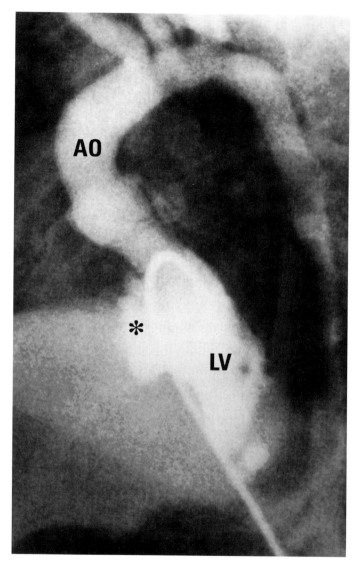

A

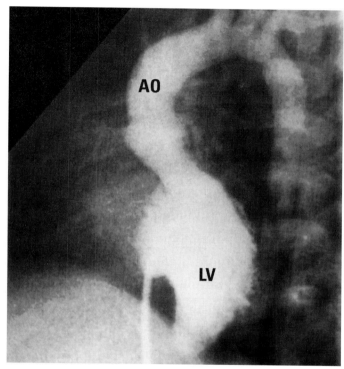

B

Fig. 5-48: So-called tricuspid pouch in atrioventricular septal defect.
These two frames of a long axial left ventriculogram in systole and diastole show the so-called tricuspid pouch (✳) that is produced by the eccentric attachment of the bridging leaflets to the right side of the deficient ventricular septum.

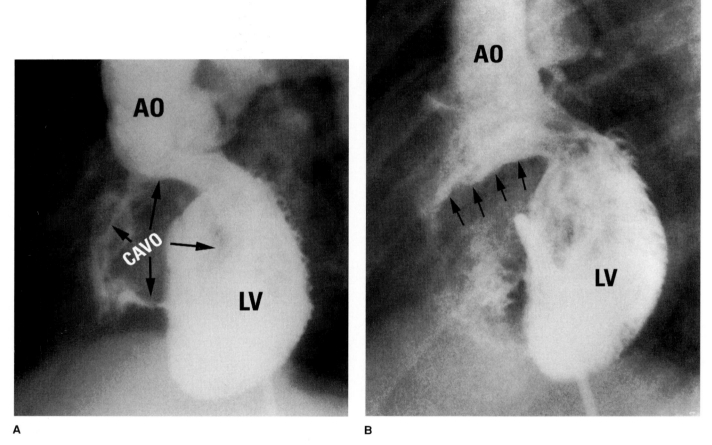

A　　　　　　　　　　　　　　　　　　　　**B**

Fig. 5-49: The appearance of the left ventricle and the common atrioventricular orifice in two patients with tetralogy of Fallot.
A: The disposition of the common atrioventricular orifice is seen in this hepatoclavicular left ventriculogram. B: The superior bridging leaflet (arrows) is seen in this different patient with tetralogy of Fallot and a complete form of atrioventricular septal defect. Note the overriding of the aorta in both frames. See also Figs. 5-41 and 5–42.

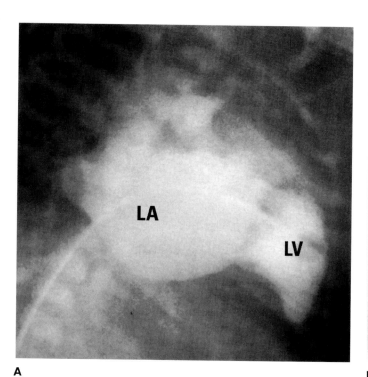

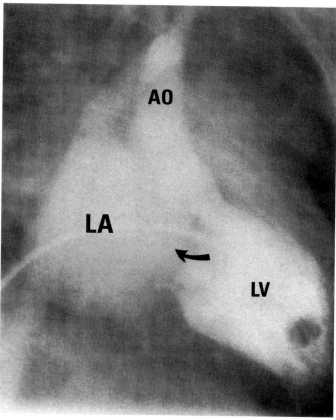

A

B

Fig. 5-50: Left atrioventricular valve regurgitation in two patients with the partial form of atrioventricular septal defect.
A: Severe left atrioventricular valve regurgitation in a 3-week old infant with opacification of a very large left atrium. **B:** Moderately severe left atrioventricular valve regurgitation (arrow). In both patients it is conceivable that the regurgitation is exaggerated by the catheter crossing the atrioventricular valve.

easier in the absence of left atrioventricular regurgitation. Similarly, demonstration of the superior bridging leaflet is best demonstrated by accumulation of contrast material under this leaflet from a left ventriculogram filmed in the four-chamber projection (Figs. 5-43 through 5-45, 5-47, and 5-49). This also serves to demonstrate whether or not the atrioventricular orifice is partitioned, but again, this information is readily and perhaps more easily determined from cardiac ultrasound examination. The attachment of the inferior bridging leaflet is recognizable from the same methodology. The right anterosuperior leaflet and left lateral leaflets are also identified in this projection.

Demonstration of interventricular shunting can be assessed from either the left long axial oblique projection or from the hepatoclavicular four-chamber projection (Figs. 5-29, 5-41, and 5-42 through 5-49). It is important to remember that the jet from left atrioventricular valve regurgitation usually first opacifies the right atrium, and that the use of two projections can separate left ventricle-to-right atrium shunting from left-to-right ventricular shunting. In the assessment and

establishment of the presence and severity of atrioventricular valve regurgitation, the role of cross-sectional echocardiography is of fundamental importance. With the catheter across the left atrioventricular valve, the presence and severity of atrioventricular valve may be influenced by a number of factors including distortion of the valve by the crossing catheter, and the presence of ventricular ectopy may also confound the issues (Fig. 5-50). Thus, ideally, the assessment of the severity of atrioventricular valve regurgitation should utilize a retrograde arterial catheter. While the parachute deformity of the left atrioventricular valve may be suspected from left ventricular angiography, the confirmation of such is clearly in the domain of cross-sectional echocardiography. We also agree with Soto and Pacifico that the demonstration by angiocardiography of a double-orifice left atrioventricular valve is almost always unsuccessful.

The demonstration of ventricular underdevelopment requires selective biplane ventriculography (Figs. 5-14 through 5-25). We would advise using biplane angiocardiography in both ventricles to best glean com-

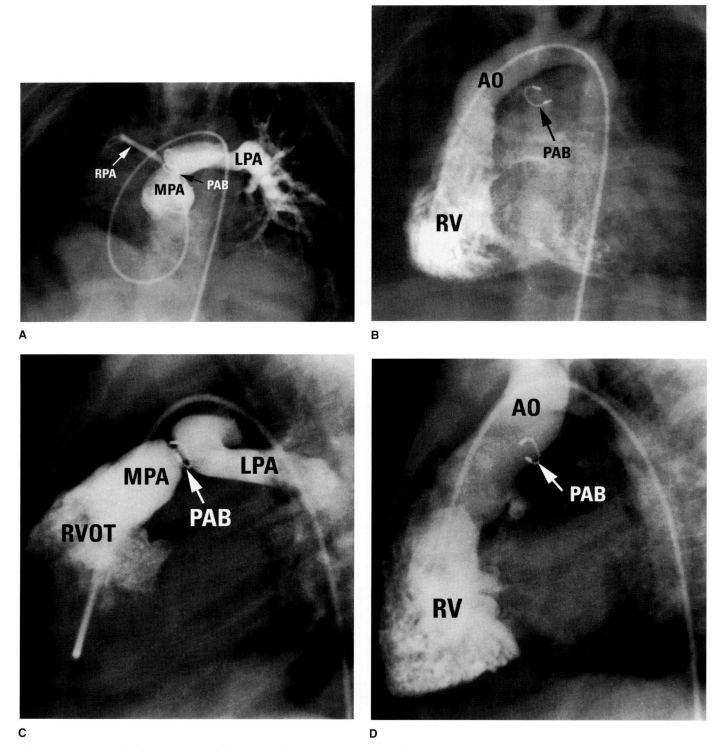

Fig. 5-51: A severely hypertensive left ventricle in the patient with double-outlet right ventricle, a complete form of atrio-ventricular septal defect, a previously banded pulmonary artery performed elsewhere with a dilatable band, and a restrictive ventricular septal defect.
A: Frontal injection into main pulmonary artery performed with a retrograde arterial catheter. Note the severely hypoplastic right pulmonary artery. **B and C:** Frontal and lateral right ventriculogram showing the rightward and anterior aorta. In these figures, the pulmonary artery is not clearly seen because the great arteries are in a direct anteroposterior spatial relationship. **D:** This lateral frame from the pulmonary arteriogram shows reflux into the distal right ventricular infundibulum that supports the pulmonary artery. *(continued on next page)*

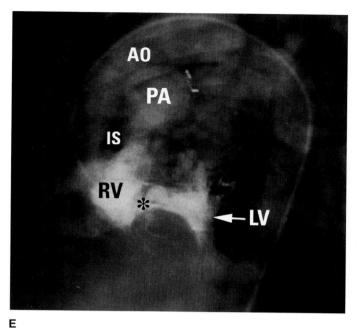

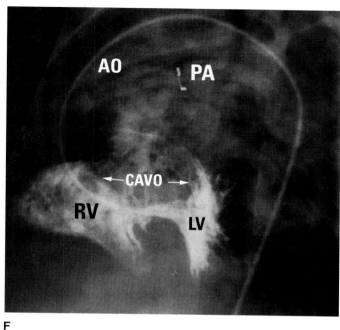

E   F

Fig. 5-51: *(continued)*
E: Retrograde left ventriculogram in long axial oblique shows the disposition of the common atrioventricular orifice. **F:** In this systolic frame, the severely restrictive character of the ventricular septal defect (✱) is seen.

parative information about ventricular dominance and also because one can apply volumetric analysis. Because the left ventricular outflow tract appears elongated and narrowed, there is always the angiographic appearance of subaortic narrowing. Frank and unequivocal subaortic stenosis is rarely recognized preoperatively, especially in the patient with the complete form of the defect where the left ventricle may decompress through the ventricular septal defect into the right ventricle and hemodynamic considerations may thus be misleading (Figs. 5-28 through 5-37). One must view the left ventricular outflow tract with considerable suspicion in those patients with an associated obstructive malformation of the aortic arch, coarctation, or interruption. There is considerable information about the postoperative recognition of left ventricular outflow tract obstruction in these patients, and those diverse mechanisms responsible for it. Left ventricular angiography in the biplane long axial oblique projections are ideal for recognition of this occurrence and for determination of the particular mechanism(s) (Figs. 5-32 through 5-37).

Right ventricular angiocardiography should be performed in any patient where there are concerns about possible right ventricular underdevelopment; ie, in the patient whose electrocardiogram does not show significant R-wave voltage in V_4R or V_1 or echocardiographic evidence of a small right atrioventricular orifice and/or inlet and trabecular hypoplasia, or in the patient with

right ventricular outflow tract obstruction (Figs. 5-22 through 5-25). Right ventricular angiocardiography should be performed in frontal and lateral projection, perhaps with cranial angulation, with calibration grids. When the degree of right ventricular hypoplasia is only mild-to-moderate, biventricular repair can be achieved by unloading the right ventricle with a bidirectionl cavopulmonary connection. Thus it is important to define the nature of the superior caval venous connection(s) (see Chapter 12). Certainly, right ventricular angiography is required for the patient with previous pulmonary artery banding or naturally occurring pulmonary outflow tract obstruction.

Left ventricular angiocardiography using the axial four-chamber projection can almost always diagnose atrioventricular septal defect (Figs. 5-10, 5-11, 5-12, 5-16, 5-18, 5-20, 5-22, 5-23, 5-29, 5-30, 5-41, 5-42, and 5-44 through 5-50).[140,190–200] The characteristic elongation of the left ventricular outflow tract, the disproportion between inlet and outlet septum, and the so-called gooseneck or swan's neck appearance of the left ventricular outflow tract are very specific for this diagnosis. The ventricular septal defect is profiled in relation to the superior and posterior bridging leaflets in the four-chamber projection, its size can be appreciated, and also, one can readily detect the gap or space between the leaflets guarding the left atrioventricular junction, and the presence or absence of atrioventricular valve regurgitation. The aortic arch is best imaged from selective aortography filmed in the biplane long axial oblique projections. While the elongation of the left ventricular outflow tract is best appreciated during diastole, it can also be recognized during the systolic phase of the cardiac cycle. During the cardiac cycle, one can appreciate changes in the appearance and caliber of the left ventricular outflow tract. However, in patients with fixed left ventricular outflow tract obstruction, systolic and diastolic variation is minimal.[83]

We have previously described the appearance of left ventricular outflow tract obstruction occurring after repair of an atrioventricular septal defect. Resection in the area of the left-sided ventriculoinfundibular fold in an attempt to enlarge the intrinsically narrowed and elongated outflow tract reminds us how vulnerable this area is. Because this area is in the muscular fibrosa between aortic and mitral valves, too vigorous a resection could result in a false aneurysm (see Chapters 3 and 29) (Fig. 5-39).

Atrioventricular septal defect can complicate tetralogy of Fallot (see Chapter 20), double-outlet right ventricle (see Chapter 37) (Figs. 5-43 and 5-51); and complex heart malformations with visceral heterotaxy and right or left atrial isomerism (see Chapter 41). Lastly, there is evidence that a fetus with an atrioventricular septal defect may develop a hypoplastic left ventricle (see Chapter 26).[200]

References

1. Becker AE, Anderson RH. Atrioventricular septal defect: What's in a name? *J Thorac Cardiovasc Surg* 1982;83: 461–469.

2. Anderson RH, Ebels T, Yen Ho S. The surgical anatomy of atrio-ventricular septal defect. In: Yacoub M, Pepper J, eds: *Annual of Cardiac Surgery*. Seventh edition. London: Current Science; 1994, pp. 71-79.

3. Collmann RD, Stoller A. A life table for mongols in Victoria, Australia. *J Ment Defic Res* 1963;7:53–59.

4. Freedom RM, Benson LN, Olley PM, Rowe RD. The natural history of the complete atrioventricular canal defect: An analysis of selected genetic, hemodynamic, and morphological variables. In: Gallucci V, Bini RM, Thiene G, eds. *Selected Topics in Cardiac Surgery*. Bologna: Patron Editore Bologna; 1980, pp. 45–72.

5. Fabia J, Drolette M. Life tables up to age 10 for mongols with and without congenital heart defect. *J Ment Defic Res* 1970;14:235–241.

6. Berger TJ, Blackstone EH, Kirklin JW, Bargeron LM Jr, Hazelrig JB, Turner ME Jr. Survival and probability of cure without and with operation in complete atrioventricular canal. *Ann Thorac Surg* 1979;27:104–111.

7. Fyler DC. Report of the New England Regional Infant Cardiac Program. *Pediatrics* 1980;65(Suppl):376–461.

8. Ferencz C, Rubin JD, McCarter RJ, Brenner JI, Neill CA, Perry LW, Hepner SI, Downing JW. Congenital heart disease: Prevalence at livebirth. The Baltimore-Washington Infant Study. *Am J Epidemiol* 1985;121:31–36.

9. Grabitz RG, Joffres MR, Collins-Nakai R. Congenital heart disease: Incidence in the first year of life. The Alberta Heritage Pediatric Cardiology Program. *Am J Epidemiol* 1986;128:381–386.

10. Akiba T, Becker AE, Neirotti R, Tatsuno K. Valve morphology in complete atrioventricular septal defect: Variability relevant to operation. *Ann Thorac Surg* 1993;56: 295–299.

11. Alfieri O and Subramanian S. Successful repair of complete atrio-ventricular canal with undivided anterior common leaflet in a 6-month-old infant. *Ann Thorac Surg* 1975;19:92–97.

12. Allwork SP. Anatomical-embryological correlates in atrioventricular septal defect. *Br Heart J* 1982;47: 419–429.

13. Anderson RH, Macartney FJ, Shinebourne EA, Tynan M. *Paediatric Cardiology*. Edinburgh: Churchill Livingstone; 1987, pp. 571–613.

14. Anderson RH, Zuberbuhler JR, Penkoske PA, Neches WH. Of clefts, commissures and things. *J Thorac Cardiovasc Surg* 1985;90:605–610.

15. Seo J-W, Jung WH, Park YW. Imperforate Ebstein's malformation in atrioventricular septal defect. *Cardiol Young* 1991;1:152–154.

16. Bharati S, Lev M. The spectrum of common atrioventricular orifice (canal). *Am Heart J* 1973;86:553–561.

17. Bharati S, Kirklin JW, McAllister HA Jr, Lev M. The surgical anatomy of common atrioventricular orifice associated with tetralogy of Fallot, double outlet right ventricle and complete regular transposition. *Circulation* 1980;61:1142–1149.

18. Draulans-Noe HAY, Wenink ACG, Quaegebeur JM. Ventricular septal deficiency in atrioventricular(AV) septal defect-a correlation with AV-valve morphology. *Pediatr Cardiol* 1984;5:227–228.

19. Ebels T, Ho SY, Anderson RH, Devine WA, Debich DE, Penkoske PA, Zuberbuhler JR. Anomalies of the left atrioventricular valve and related ventricular septal morphology in atrioventricular septal defects. *J Thorac Cardiovasc Surg* 1990;99:299–307.

20. Ebert PA, Goor DA. Complete atrioventricular canal malformation: Further clarification of the anatomy of the common leaflet and its relationship to the VSD in surgical correction. *Ann Thorac Surg* 1978;25:134–143.

21. Goor D, Lillehei CW, Edwards JE. Further observations on the pathology of the atrioventricular canal malformation. *Arch Surg* 1968;97:954–962.

22. Ilbawi MN, Idriss FS, DeLeon SY, Riggs TW, Muster AJ, Berry TE, Paul MH. Unusual mitral valve abnormalities complicating surgical repair of endocardial cushion defects. *J Thorac Cardiovasc Surg* 1983;85:697–704.

23. Omeri MA, Bishop M, Oakley C, Bentall HH, Cleland WP. The mitral valve in endocardial cushion defects. *Br Heart J* 1965;27:161–176.

24. Penkoske PA, Neches WH, Anderson RH, Zuberbuhler JR. Further observations on the morphology of atrioventricular septal defects. *J Thorac Cardiovasc Surg* 1985; 90:611–622.

25. Piccoli GP, Gerlis LM, Wilkinson JL, Lozsadi K, Macartney FJ, Anderson RH. Morphology and classification of atrioventricular defects. *Br Heart J* 1979;42:621–632.

26. Piccoli GP, Wilkinson JL, Macartney FJ, Gerlis LM, Anderson RH. Morphology and classification of complete atrioventricular defects. *Br Heart J* 1979;42:633–639.

27. Pillai R, Ho SY, Anderson RH, Lincoln C. Ostium pri-

mum atrio-ventricular septal defect: An anatomical and surgical review. *Ann Thorac Surg* 1986;41:458–461.

28. Rastelli GC, Kirklin JW, Titus JL. Anatomic observations of complete form of persistent common atrioventricular canal. With special reference to atrioventricular valves. *Mayo Clin Proc* 1966;41:296–308.

29. Rastelli GC, Ongley PA, McGoon DC. Surgical repair of complete atrioventricular canal with anterior common leaflet undivided and unattached to ventricular septum. *Mayo Clin Proc* 1969;44:335–341.

30. Silverman NH, Ho SY, Anderson RH, Smith A, Wilkinson JL. Atrioventricular septal defect with intact atrial and ventricular septal structures. *Int J Cardiol* 1984; 5:567–573.

31. Thiene G, Mazzucco A, Grisolia EF, Bortolotti U, Stellin G, Chioin R, Pellegrino PA, Gallucci V. Postoperative pathology of complete atrio-ventricular defects. *J Thorac Cardiovasc Surg* 1982;83:891–900.

32. Thiene G, Wenink ACG, Frescura C, Wilkinson JL, Gallucci V, Ho S-Y, Mazzucco A, Anderson RH. Surgical anatomy and pathology of the conduction tissues in atrioventricular defects. *J Thorac Cardiovasc Surg* 1981;82: 928–937.

33. Towbin R, Schwartz D. Endocardial cushion defects: Embryology, anatomy, and angiography. *Am J Radiol* 1981;136:157–162.

34. Ugarte M, Enriquez de Salamanca F, Quero M. Endocardial cushion defects. An anatomical study of 54 specimens. *Br Heart J* 1976;38:674–682.

35. Van Mierop LHS, Alley RD. The management of the cleft mitral valve in endocardial cushion defects. *Ann Thorac Surg* 1966;2:416–421.

36. Van Mierop LHS, Alley RD, Kansel HW, Stranahan A. The anatomy and embryology of endocardial cushion defects. *J Thorac Cardiovasc Surg* 1962;43:71–80.

37. Van Praagh S, Antoniadis S, Otero-Coto E, Leidenfrost RD, Van Praagh R. Common atrioventricular canal with and without conotruncal malformations: An anatomic study of 251 postmortem cases. In: Takao A, Nora JJ, eds. *Congenital Heart Disease: Causes and Processes.* Mount Kisco, NY: Futura Publishing Company, Inc; 1984; pp. 599–639.

38. Van Praagh S, Vangi V, Sul JH, Metras D, Parness I, Castaneda AR, Van Praagh R. Tricuspid atresia or severe stenosis with partial common atrioventricular canal: Anatomic data, clinical profile and surgical considerations. *J Am Coll Cardiol* 1991;17:932–943.

39. Virdi IS, Keeton BR, Shore DF. Atrioventricular septal defect with a well developed primary component of the atrial septum ("septum primum"). *Int J Cardiol* 1985; 9:243–247.

40. Wakai CS, Edwards JE. Pathology study of persistent common atrioventricular canal. *Am Heart J* 1958;56: 779–787.

41. Wenink ACG, Ottenkamp J, Guit GL, Draulans-Noe Y, Doornbos J. Correlation of morphology of the left ventricular outflow tract with two-dimensional Doppler echocardiography and magnetic resonance imaging in atrioventricular septal defect. *Am J Cardiol* 1989;63: 1137–1140.

41a. Anderson RH, Ebels T, Yen Ho S. The surgical anatomy of atrioventricular septal defect. In: Yacuoub M, Pepper J, (eds.) *Annual of Cardiac Surgery.* Seventh Edition. London: Current Science; 1994, pp. 71–79.

42. McGoon DC, McMullan MH, Mair DD, Danielson GK. Correction of complete atrioventricular canal in infants. *Mayo Clin Proc* 1973;48:769–772.

43. Kirklin JW, Barratt-Boyes BG. *Cardiac Surgery.* Second edition. New York: Churchill Livingstone; 1993, pp. 693–747.

44. Rosenquist GC, Clark EB, McAllister HA, Bharati S, Edwards JE. Increased mitral-aortic separation in discrete subaortic stenosis. *Circulation* 1979;60:70–74.

45. Rosenquist GC, Clark EB, Sweeney LJ, McAllister HA. The normal spectrum of mitral and aortic valve discontinuity. *Circulation* 1976;54:298–301.

46. Anderson RH, Neches WH, Zuberbuhler JR, Penkoske PA. Scooping of the ventricular septum in atrioventricular septal defect (letter). *J Thorac Cardiovasc Surg* 1989; 95:146.

47. Blieden LC, Randall PA, Castaneda AR, Lucas RC Jr, Edwards JE. The "goose neck" of the endocardial cusion defect: Anatomic basis. *Chest* 1974;65:13–17.

47a. Suzuki K, Tatsuno K, Mimori S, Murakami Y, Mori K, Takahashi Y, Kikuchi T. Relationship between scooping of the ventricular septum, morphology of the inferior bridging leaflet and electrocardiographic findings in atrioventricular septal defect with common valvar orifice. *Cardiol Young* 1996;6:37–43.

48. Ebels T, Ho SY, Anderson RH, J ME, Eijgelaar A. The surgical anatomy of the left ventricular outflow tract in atrioventricular septal defect. *Ann Thorac Surg* 1986;41: 483–488.

49. Ebels T, Meijboom EJ, Anderson RH, Schasfoort-van Leeuwen MJM, Lenstra D, Eijgelaar A, Bossina KK, Homan-van der Heide JN. Anatomic and functional "obstruction" of the outflow tract in atrioventricular septal defects with separate valve orifices ("ostium primum atrial septal defect"): An echocardiographic study. *Am J Cardiol* 1984;54:843–847.

50. Chin AJ, Bierman FZ, Sanders SP, Williams RG, Norwood WI, Castaneda AR. Subxyphoid 2-dimensional echocardiographic identification of left ventricular papillary muscle anomalies in complete common atrioventricular canal. *Am J Cardiol* 1983;51:1695–1699.

51. David I, Castaneda AR, Van Praagh R. Potentially parachute mitral valve in common atrioventricular canal. *J Thorac Cardiovasc Surg* 1982;84:178–186.

52. Draulans-Noe HAY, Wenink ACG, Quaegebeur J. Single papillary muscle (parachute valve) and double-orifice left atrioventricular valve in atrioventricular septal defect convergence of chordal attachment: Surgical anatomy and results of surgery. *Pediatr Cardiol* 1990;11: 29–35.

53. Piccoli GP, Ho SY, Wilkinson JL, Macartney FJ, Gerlis LM, Anderson RH. Left-sided obstructive lesions in atrioventricular septal defects. An anatomic study. *J Thorac Cardiovasc Surg* 1982;83:453–460.

54. Tandon R, Moller JH, Edwards JE. Single papillary muscle of the left ventricle associated with persistent common atrioventricular canal: Variant of parachute mitral valve. *Pediatr Cardiol* 1986;7:111–114.

55. Tandon R, Moller JH, Edwards JE. Anomalies associated with the parachute mitral valve: A pathologic analysis of 52 cases. *Can J Cardiol* 1986;2:278–281.

56. Ho SY; Russell G; Gerlis LM. Atrioventricular septal defect with intact septal structures in a 74-year-old. *Int J Cardiol* 1990;26:371–373.

57. Carvalho JS, Rigby ML, Shinebourne EA, Anderson RH. Cross sectional echocardiography for recognition of ventricular topology in atrioventricular septal defect. *Br Heart J* 1989;61:285–288.

58. Baum D, Roth GJ, Creighton SA. Right axis deviation. Clockwise QRS loop, and signs of left ventricular underdevelopment in a child with complete type of persistent common atrioventricular canal. *Circulation* 1964; 30:755–758.

59. Quero Jimenez M, Perez Martinez VM, Maitre Azcarate MJ, Merino Batres G, Moreno Granados F. Exaggerated displacement of the atrioventricular canal towards the bulbus cordis. *Br Heart J* 1973;35:453–460.

60. Bloom KR, Freedom RM, Williams CM, Trusler GA, Rowe RD. Echocardiographic recognition of atrioventricular valve stenosis associated with endocardial cushion defect: Pathologic and surgical correlates. *Am J Cardiol* 1979;44:1326–1331.

61. Thanopoulos BD, Fisher EA, DuBrow IW, Hastreiter AR. Right and left ventricular volume characteristics in common atrioventricular canal. *Circulation* 1978;57: 991–995.

62. Rowe RD, Freedom RM, Mehrizi A. *The Neonate with Congenital Heart Disease.* New York: WB Saunders Company; 1981, pp. 373–396.

63. Studer M, Blackstone EH, Kirklin JW, Pacifico AD, Soto B, Chung GKT, Kirklin JK, Bargeron LM Jr. Determinants of early and late results of repair of atrioventricular septal (canal) defects. *J Thorac Cardiovasc Surg* 1982;84: 523–542.

64. Corno A, Marino B, Catena G, Marcelletti C. Atrioventricular septal defects with severe left ventricular hypoplasia. Staged palliation. *J Thorac Cardiovasc Surg* 1988;96:249–252.

65. Espinosa-Caliani JS, Alvarez-Guisado L, Munoz-Castellanos L, Aranega-Jimenez A, Kuri-Nivon M, Sanchez RS, Aranega-Jimenez AE. Atrioventricular septal defect: Quantitative anatomy of the right ventricle. *Pediatr Cardiol* 1991;12:106–13.

66. Fisher EA, Doshi M, DuBrow IW, Silverman N, Levitsky S. Effect of palliative and corrective surgery on ventricular volumes in complete atrioventricular canal. *Pediatr Cardiol* 1984;5:159–166.

67. Freedom RM, Bini M, Rowe RD. Endocardial cushion defect and significant hypoplasia of the left ventricle: A distinct clinical and pathological entity. *Eur J Cardiol* 1978;7:263–281.

68. Freedom RM, Bini R, Dische R, Rowe RD. The straddling mitral valve: Morphological observations and clinical implications. *Eur J Cardiol* 1978;8:27–50.

69. Freedom RM, Perrin DG, Smallhorn JF. A consideration of certain anatomic risk factors in patients with atrioventricular septal defect. In: D'alessandro LC, ed. *Heart Surgery 1985.* Rome: Casa Editrice Scientifica Internazione; 1985, pp. 351–368.

70. Jarmakani JM, George B, Wheller J. Ventricular volume characteristics in infants and children with endocardial cushion defects. *Circulation* 1978;58:153–157.

71. Mehta S, Hirschfeld S, Riggs T, Liebman J. Echocardiographic estimation of ventricular hypoplasia in complete atrioventricular canal. *Circulation* 1979;59: 888–893.

72. Troconis CJ, Di Donato R, Marino B, Vairo U, Marcelletti C. Atrioventricular septal defects with severe left ventricular hypoplasia-clinical findings and surgical options. *Cardiol Young* 1992;2:53–55.

73. Williams HJ Jr, Tandon R, Edwards JE. Persistent ostium primum coexisting with mitral or tricuspid atresia. *Chest* 1974;66:39–43.

74. Alvarado O, Sreeram N, McKay R, Boyd IM. Cavopul-

75. Muster AJ; Zales VR; Ilbawi MN; Backer CL; Duffy CE; Mavroudis C. Biventricular repair of hypoplastic right ventricle assisted by pulsatile bidirectional cavopulmonary anastomosis. *J Thorac Cardiovasc Surg* 1993; 105:112–119.

76. Ben-Shachar G, Moller JH, Castaneda-Zuniga W, Edwards JE. Signs of membranous subaortic stenosis appearing after correction of persistent common atrioventricular canal. *Am J Cardiol* 1981;48:340–344.

77. Bembom MC, Paulista PP, Kiyose AT, Falcao HC, Bembom J da C, Esteves CA, Guerra AL, Fontes VF. Estenose subaortica associada a defeito do septo atrioventricular. Uma condicao pouco referida. *Arq Bras Cardiol (Brazil)* 1993;60:257–260.

78. Chang C-I, Becker AE. Surgical anatomy of left ventricular outflow tract obstruction in complete atrioventricular septal defect. A concept for operative repair. *J Thorac Cardiovasc Surg* 1987;94:897–903.

79. Freedom RM, Culham JAG, Rowe RD. Angiocardiography of subaortic obstruction in infancy. *AJR* 1977;129: 813–824.

80. De Biase L, Di Ciommo V, Ballerini L, Bevilacqua M, Marcelletti C, Marino B. Prevalence of left-sided obstructive lesions in patients with atrioventricular canal without Down's syndrome. *J Thorac Cardiovasc Surg* 1986;91:467–472.

81. De Leon SY, Ilbawi MN, Wilson WR Jr, Arcilla RA, Thilenius OG, Bharati S, Lev M, Idriss FS. Surgical options in subaortic stenosis associated with endocardial cushion defects. *Ann Thorac Surg* 1991;52:1076–1082; discussion 1082–1083

82. Freedom RM, Dische MR, Rowe RD. Pathologic anatomy of subaortic stenosis and atresia in the first year of life. *Am J Cardiol* 1977;39:1035–1044.

83. Gow RM, Freedom RM, Williams WG, Trusler GA, Rowe RD. Coarctation of the aorta or subaortic stenosis with atrioventricular septal defect. *Am J Cardiol* 1984;53: 1421–1428.

84. Heydarian M, Griffith BP, Zuberbuhler JR. Partial atrioventricular canal associated with discrete subaortic stenosis. *Am Heart J* 1985;109:915–918.

85. Jue KL, Edwards JE. Anomalous attachment of mitral valve causing subaortic atresia. Observations in a case with other cardiac anomalies and multiple spleens. *Circulation* 1967;35:928–932.

86. Lappen RS, Muster AJ, Idriss FS, Riggs TW, Ilbawi M, Paul MH, Bharati S, Lev M. Masked subaortic stenosis in ostium primum atrial defect: Recognition and treatment. *Am J Cardiol* 1983;52:336–340.

87. Mace L, Dervanian P, Folliguet T, Grinda JM, Losay J, Neveux JY. Atrioventricular septal defect with native subaortic stenosis: Correction by extended valvular detachment (letter). *J Thorac Cardiovasc Surg* 1994;107: 943–945.

88. Marino B. Left-sided cardiac obstruction in patients with Down syndrome (letter). *J Pediatr* 1989;115: 834–835.

89. Marino B. Anterolateral muscle bundle of the left ventricle in atrioventricular septal defect: Left ventricular outflow tract and subaortic stenosis (letter). *Pediatr Cardiol* 1992;13:192.

90. Molthan ME, Paul MH, Lev M. Common A-V orifice

with pulmonary valvular and hypertrophic subaortic stenosis. *Am J Cardiol* 1962;10:291–297.

91. Neveux JY, Hazan E, Baillot F, Bourdillat N, Chauvaud S. Ostium primum et fente mitrale avec stenose sous-valvulaire aortique. A propos de 2 cas operes. *Arch Mal Coeur* 1977;70:411–414.

92. Reeder GS, Danielson GK, Seward JB, Driscoll DJ, Tajik AJ. Fixed subaortic stenosis in atrioventricular canal defect: A Doppler echocardiographic study. *J Am Coll Cardiol* 1992;20:386–394.

92a. Van Arsdell GS, Williams WG, Boutin C, Trusler GA, Coles JG, Rebeyka IM, Freedom RM. Subaortic stenosis in the spectrum of atrioventricular septal defects: Solutions may be complex and palliative. *J Thorac Cardiovasc Surg* 1995;110:1513–1520.

93. Sellers RD, Lillehei CW, Edwards JE. Subaortic stenosis caused by anomalies of the atrioventricular valves. *J Thorac Cardiovasc Surg* 1964;48:289–301.

94. Silberberg B. Coexistent aortic and mitral atresia associated with persistent common atrioventricular canal. *Am J Cardiol* 1965;16:754–757.

95. Spanos PK, Fiddler CI, Mair DD, McGoon DC. Repair of atrioventricular canal associated with membranous subaortic stenosis. *Mayo Clin Proc* 1977;52:121–124.

96. Starr A and Hovaguimian H. Surgical repair of subaortic stenosis in atrioventricular canal defects. *J Thorac Cardiovasc Surg* 1994;108:373–376.

97. Taylor NC, Somerville J. Fixed subaortic stenosis after repair of ostium primum defects. *Br Heart J* 1981;45:689–697.

98. Freedom RM. Aortic valve and arch anomalies in the congenital asplenia syndrome. Case report, literature review and re-examination of the embryology of the congenital asplenia syndrome. *Johns Hopkins Med J* 1974;135:124–135.

99. Freedom RM & Benson LN: The Hypoplastic left heart syndrome. In: Emmanouilides GC, Allen HD, Riemenschneider TA, Gutgesell HP, (eds.) *Moss and Adams' Heart Disease in Infants, Children, and Adolescents, Including the Fetus and Young Adult.* Baltimore: Williams and Wilkins; 1995, pp. 1133–1153.

100. Freedom RM, Williams WG, Dische MR, Rowe RD. Anatomical variants in aortic atresia. Potential candidates for ventriculoaortic reconstitution. *Br Heart J* 1976;38:821–826.

100a. Houyel L, Zupan V, Roset F. Aortic atresia with normal left ventricle and intact ventricular septum—a major form of subaortic stenosis complicating an atrioventricular septal defect with intact septal structures. *Cardiol Young* 1995;5:282–285.

101. Warnes C, Somerville J. Double mitral valve orifice in atrioventricular defects. *Br Heart J* 1983;49:59–64.

102. Trowitzsch E, Bando-Rodrigo A, Burger BM, Colan SD, Sanders SP. Two-dimensional echocardigraphic findings in double orifice mitral valve. *J Am Coll Cardiol* 1985;6:383–387.

103. Mehrizi A, Hutchins GM, Rowe RD. Double orifice of the mitral valve. *Johns Hopkins Med J* 1965; 117: 8–15.

104. Rowe DW, Desai B, Bezmalinovic Z, Desai JM, Wessel RJ, Grayson LH. Two-dimensional echocardiography in double orifice mitral valve. *J Am Coll Cardiol* 1984; 4:429–433.

105. Cooke RA; Chambers JB; Curry PV. Doppler echocardiography of double orifice of the left atrioventricular valve in atrioventricular septal defect. *Int J Cardiol* 1991;32:254–256.

106. Lee C-N, Danielson GK, Schaff HV, Puga FJ, Mair DD. Double orifice mitral valve in AV canal defect: Surgical experience in 25 patients. *J Thorac Cardiovasc Surg* 1985;90:700–705.

107. Ancalmo N, Ochsner JL, Mills NL, King TD. Double mitral valve. Report of a case and review of the literature. *Angiology* 1977;28:95–100.

108. Bano-Rodrigo A, Van Praagh S, Trowitzsch E, Van Praagh R. Double-orifice mitral valve: A study of 27 postmortem cases with developmental, diagnostic and surgical considerations. *Am J Cardiol* 1988;61:152–160.

109. Yamaguchi M, Tachibana H, Hosokawa Y, Ohoshi H, Oshima Y, Obo H. Ebstein's anomaly and partial atrioventricular canal associated with double orifice mitral valve. *J Cardiovasc Surg* 1989;30:790–792.

109a. Brieger DB, Ward C, Cooper SG, Nunn GR, Cartmill TB, Sholler GF. Double orifice left atrioventricular valve-diagnosis and management of an unexpected lesion. *Cardiol Young* 1995;5:267–271.

110. Szulc M, Poon E, Cooper R, Kaplovitz H, Frenkel M, Tranbaugh R. Single papillary muscle and ostium primum defect. *Pediatr Cardiol* 1990;11:96–97.

111. Horiuchi T, Saji K, Osuka Y, Sato K, Okada Y. Successful correction of double outlet left atrium associated with complete atrioventricular canal and l-loop double outlet right ventricle with stenosis of the pulmonary artery. *J Cardiovasc Surg* 1976;17:157–161.

112. Ahmadi A, Mocellin R. Spillner G. Gildein HP. Atrioventricular septal defect with double-outlet right atrium. *Pediatr Cardiol* 1989;10:170–173.

113. Alivizatos P, Anderson RH, Macartney FJ, Zuberbuhler JR, Stark J. Atrioventricular septal defect with balanced ventricles and malaligned atrial septum: Double-outlet right atrium. *J Thorac Cardiovasc Surg* 1985;89:295–297.

114. Buchler J, Rabelo R, Marino R, David I, Van Praagh R. Double outlet right atrium: Autopsied case of newly recognised entity (abstract). In: *World Congress of Pediatric Cardiology.* London: 1980, p. 223.

115. Corwin RD, Singh AK, Karlson KE. Double-outlet right atrium: A rare endocardial cusion defect. *Am Heart J* 1983;106:1156–1157. 116. Nunez L, Gil Aguado M, Sanz E, Perez Martinez V. Surgical repair of double-outlet right atrium. *Ann Thorac Surg* 1984;37:164–166.

117. Starc TJ, Bierman FZ, Bowman Jr FO, Steeg CN, Wang NK, Krongrad E. Pulmonary venous obstruction and atrioventricular canal anomalies: Role of cor triatriatum and double outlet right atrium. *J Am Coll Cardiol* 1987; 9:830–833.

117a. Radermecker MA, Chauvaud S, Carpentier A. Double-outlet right atrium with restrictive ostium primum and incomplete supravalvular ring presenting as congenital mitral valve stenosis. *J Thorac Cardiovasc Surg* 1995; 109:804–805.

118. Suzuki Y, Hamada Y, Miura M, Haneda K, Horiuchi T, Ogata H. Double-outlet left atrium with intact ventricular septum. *Ann Thorac Surg* 1988;45:332–334.

119. Westerman GR, Norton JB, Van Devanter SH. Double-outlet right atrium associated with tetralogy of Fallot and common atrioventricular valve. *J Thorac Cardiovasc Surg* 1986;91:205–207.

120. Thilenius OG, Vitullo D, Bharati S, Luken J, Lamberti JJ, Tatooles C, Lev M, Carr I, Arcilla RA. Endocardial cushion defect associated with cor triatriatum sinistrum or supravalve mitral ring. *Am J Cardiol* 1979;44:1339–1343.

120a. Suzuki K, Kikuchi T, Mimori S. Double outlet right

atrium and complete atrioventricular septal defect with abnormal findings of the biopsied lung. *Cardiol Young* 1994;4:402–440.

121. Binet J-P, Losay J, Hvass U. Tetralogy of Fallot with type C complete atrioventricular canal. *J Thorac Cardiovasc Surg* 1980;79:761–764.

122. Caruso G, Losekoot TG, Becker AE. Ebstein's anomaly in persistent common atrioventricular canal. *Br Heart J* 1978;40:1275–1279.

122a. Guenthard J, Wyler F. Complete atrioventricular septal defect and Ebstein anomaly. *Pediatr Cardiol* 1996;17: 67–69.

123. Handler JB, Berger TJ, Miller RH, Hagan AD, Peniston RL, Vieweg WVR. Partial atrioventricular canal in association with Ebstein's anomaly. Echocardiographic diagnosis and surgical correction. *Chest* 1981;80:515–517.

124. Hartyanszky IL, Lozsadi K, Kadar K, Huttl T, Kiraly L. Ebstein's anomaly and intermediate-form atrioventricular septal defect with double-orifice mitral valve (letter). *J Thorac Cardiovasc Surg* 1992;104:1496–1497.

125. Fisher RD, Bone DK, Rowe RD, Gott VL. Complete atrioventricular canal associated with tetralogy of Fallot. Clinical experience and operative methods. *J Thorac Cardiovasc Surg* 1975;70:265–271.

126. LeBlanc JG, Williams WG, Freedom RM, Trusler GA. Results of total correction in complete atrioventricular septal defects with congenital or surgically induced right ventricular outflow tract obstruction. *Ann Thorac Surg* 1986;41:387–391.

127. Nath PH, Soto B, Bini RM, Bargeron LM Jr, Pacifico AD. Tetralogy of Fallot with atrioventricular canal. An angiographic study. *J Thorac Cardiovasc Surg* 1984;87: 421–430.

128. Sade RM, Riopel DA, Lorenzo R. Tetralogy of Fallot associated with complete atrioventricular canal. *Ann Thorac Surg* 1980;30:177–180.

129. Sridaromont S, Feldt RH, Ritter DG, Davis GD, McGoon DC, Edwards JE. Double-outlet right ventricle associated with persistent common atrioventricular canal. *Circulation* 1975;52:933–942.

130. Toussaint M, Planche C, Graff WC, Royon M, Ribierre M. Double outlet right ventricle associated with common atrioventricular canal: Report of nine anatomic specimens. *J Am Coll Cardiol* 1986; 8: 396–401.

131. Tandon R, Moller JH, Edwards JE. Tetralogy of Fallot associated with persistent common atrioventricular canal (endocardial cushion defect). *Br Heart J* 1974;36: 197–206.

132. Roach RM, Tandon R, Moller JH, Edwards JE. Ebstein's anomaly of the tricuspid valve in persistent common atrioventricular canal. *Am J Cardiol* 1984;53:640–642.

133. Thomas R, Van Wesep R. Intracardiac epithelial cyst in association with an atrioventricular canal defect. *Am J Cardiovasc Pathol* 1990;3:325–328.

134. Uretzky G, Puga FJ, Danielson GK, Feldt RH, Julsrud PR, Seward JB, Edwards WD, McGoon DC. Complete atrioventricular canal associated with tetralogy of Fallot. Morphologic and surgical considerations. *J Thorac Cardiovasc Surg* 1984;87:756–766.

135. Utley JR, Noonan JA, Walters LR, Frist RA. Anomalous position of atrial septum with anomalous pulmonary and systemic venous drainage. *J Thorac Cardiovasc Surg* 1974;67:730–732.

136. Vargas FJ, Coto EO, Mayer JE Jr, Jonas RA, Castaneda AR. Complete atrioventricular canal and tetralogy of Fallot:
Surgical considerations. *Ann Thorac Surg* 1986;42: 258–263.

137. Vogel M, Sauer U, Buhlmeyer K, Sebening FJ. Atrioventricular septal defect complicated by right ventricular outflow tract obstruction. Analysis of risk factors regarding surgical repair. *J Cardiovasc Surg* 1989;30: 34–39.

138. Draulans-Noe HAY and Wenink ACG. Anterolateral muscle bundle of the left ventricle in atrioventricular septal defect: Left ventricular outflow tract and subaortic stenosis. *Pediatr Cardiol* 1991;12:83–88.

138a. Manning PB, Mayer JE Jr., Sanders SA, Coleman EA, Jonas RA, Keane JF, Van Praagh S, Castaneda AR. Unique features and prognosis of primum ASD presenting in the first year of life. *Circulation* 1994;90(Part 2):II-30-II-35.

138b. Gallo P, Formigari R, Hokayem NJ, D'Offizi F, Allesandro D, Francalanci P, d'Amati G, Colloridi V, Pizzuto F. Left ventricular outflow tract obstruction in atrioventricular septal defects: A pathologic and morphometric evaluation. *Clin Cardiol* 1991;14:513–521.

138c. Giamberti A, Marino B, di Carlo D, Iorio FS, Formigari R, De Zorzi A, Marceletti C. Partial atrioventricular canal with congestive heart failure in the first year of life: Surgical options. *Ann Thorac Surg* 1996; 62:151–154.

139. Cloez JL, Ravault MC, Worms AM, Marcon F, Pernot C. Complete atrioventricular canal defect associated with congenitally corrected transposition of the great arteries: Two-dimensional echocardiographic identification. *J Am Coll Cardiol* 1983;1:1123–1128.

140. Soto B, Pacifico AD. *Angiocardiography in Congenital Heart Malformations*. Mount Kisco, NY: Futura Publishing Company, Inc; 1990, pp. 161–184.

141. Cullum L, Liebman J. The association of congenital heart disease with Down's syndrome (Mongolism). *Am J Cardiol* 1969;24:354–357.

142. Tandon R, Edwards JE. Cardiac malformations associated with Down's syndrome. *Circulation* 1973;47: 1349–1355.

143. Rosenquist GC, Sweeney LJ, Amsel J, McAllister HA. Enlargement of the membranous ventricular septum: An internal stigma of Down's syndrome. *J Pediatr* 1974;85: 490–493.

144. Park SC, Mathews RA, Zuberbuhler JR, Rowe RD, Neches WH, Lenox CC. Down syndrome with congenital heart malformation. *Am J Dis Child* 1977;131:29–33.

145. Laursen HB. Congenital heart disease in Down's syndrome. *Br Heart J* 1976;38:32–38.

146. di Carlo DC; Marino B. Atrioventricular canal with Down syndrome or normal chromosomes: Distinct prognosis with surgical management (letter)? *J Thorac Cardiovasc Surg* 1994;107:1368–1370.

147. Marino B. Complete atrioventricular septal defect in patients with and without Down's syndrome (letter). *Ann Thorac Surg* 1994;57:1687–1688.

147a. Marino B. Atrioventricular septal defect-anatomic characteristics in patients with and without Down's syndrome. *Cardiol Young* 1992;2:308–310.

147b. Marino B, Corno A, Guccione P, Marcelletti C. Ventricular septal defect and Down's syndrome. *Lancet* 1991; 2:245–246.

148. Marino B, Vairo U, Corno A, Nava S, Guccione P, Calabro R, Marcelletti C. Atrioventricular canal in Down syndrome. Prevalence of associated cardiac malformations compared with patients without Down syndrome. *Am J Dis Child* 1990;144:1120–1122.

149. Shah RM, Farina MA, Porter IH, Bishop M. Clinical as-

pects of congenital heart disease in Mongolism. *Am J Cardiol* 1972;29:497–503.

150. Greenwood RD, Nadas AS. The clinical course of cardiac disease in Down's syndrome. *Pediatrics* 1976;58:893–897.

151. Freedom RM, Smallhorn JF, Rebeyka I, Thompson L, Trusler GA, Williams WG, Coles J. Atrioventricular septal defect: Late postoperative functional results after complete repair in infancy. Abstracts of 1st World Congress of Pediatric Cardiac Surgery. Bergamo, Italy; 1988, pp. 39–40.

152. Katlic MR, Clark EB, Neill C, Haller JA Jr. Surgical management of congenital heart disease in Down's syndrome. *J Thorac Cardiovasc Surg* 1977;74:204–209.

153. Cronk CE. Growth of children with Down's syndrome: Birth to age 3 years. *Pediatrics* 1978;61:564–568.

154. Morris CD; Magilke D; Reller M. Down's syndrome affects results of surgical correction of complete atrioventricular canal. *Pediatr Cardiol* 1992;13:80–84.

155. Rizzoli G, Mazzucco A, Maizza F, Daliento L, Rubino M, Tursi V, Scalia D. Does Down syndrome affect prognosis of surgically managed atrioventricular canal defects? *J Thorac Cardiovasc Surg* 1992;104:945–953.

156. Vet TW, Ottenkamp J. Correction of atrioventricular septal defect. Results influenced by Down syndrome? *Am J Dis Child* 1989;143(11):1361–1365. (see comments in Am J Dis Child 1990;144(7):752; *Am J Dis Child* 1990; 144(8):849–850.

157. Castaneda AR, Mayer JE, Jonas RA. Repair of atrioventricular canal in infancy. *World J Surg* 1985;9:590–597.

158. Clapp SK, Perry BL, Farooki AQ, Jackson WL, Karpawich PP, Hakimi M, Arciniegas E, Green EW. Surgical and medical results of complete atrioventricular canal." A ten year review. *Am J Cardiol* 1987;59:454–458.

159. Clapp S, Perry BL, Farooki ZQ, Jackson WL, Karpawich PP, Hakimi M, Arciniegas E, Green EW, Pinsky WW. Down's syndrome, complete atrioventricular canal, and pulmonary vascular obstructive disease. *J Thorac Cardiovasc Surg* 1990;100:115–121.

160. Bull C, Rigby ML, Shinebourne EA. Should management of complete atrioventricular canal defect be influenced by coexistent Down syndrome? *Lancet* 1985; 1:1147–1149.

160a. Shinebourne EA and Carvalho JS. Atrioventricular septal defect and Down's syndrome. In: Yacoub M, Pepper J, (eds.) *Annual of Cardiac Surgery.* Seventh edition. London: Current Science; 1994, pp. 66–70.

161. Wilson NJ, Gavalaki E, Newman CGH. Complete atrioventricular canal defect in the presence of Down syndrome (letter). *Lancet* 1985;1:834.

162. Menahem S, Mee RBB. Complete atrioventricular canal defect in the presence of Down syndrome (letter). *Lancet* 1985;1:834.

163. Kirklin JW, Blackstone EH, Bargeron Jr LM, Pacifico AD, Kirklin JK. The repair of atrioventricular septal defects in infancy. *Int J Cardiol* 1986;13:333–351.

164. Berger TJ, Kirklin JW, Blackstone EH, Pacifico AD, Kouchoukos NT. Primary repair of complete atrioventricular canal in patients less than 2 years old. *Am J Cardiol* 1978;41:906–913.

165. Gallucci V, Mazzucco A, Stellin G, Faggian G, Bortolotti U. Repair of complete atrioventricular canal: 1975–1985. *J Card Surg* 1986;1:261–269.

166. Chi TPL, Krovetz LJ. The pulmonary vascular bed in children with Down syndrome. *J Pediatr* 1975;86:533–538.

167. Cooney TP, Thurlbeck WM. Pulmonary hypoplasia in Down's syndrome. *N Engl J Med* 1982;307:1170–1173.

168. Frescura C, Thiene G, Franceschini E, Talenti E, Mazzucco A. Pulmonary vascular disease in infants with complete atrioventricular septal defect. *Int J Cardiol* 1987;15:91–100.

169. Haworth SG. Understanding pulmonary vascular disease in young children. *Int J Cardiol* 1987;15:101–103.

170. Haworth SG. Pulmonary vascular bed in children with complete atrioventricular septal defect: Relation between structural and hemodynamic abnormalities. *Am J Cardiol* 1986;57:833–839.

171. Newfeld EA, Sher M, Paul MH, Nikaidoh H. Pulmonary vascular disease in complete atrioventricular canal defect. *Am J Cardiol* 1977;39:721–726.

172. Rosengart RM. Pulmonary vascular involvement in Down syndrome. *J Pediatr* 1976;88:161.

173. Soudon P, Stijns M, Tremouroux-Wattiez M, Vliers A. Precocity of pulmonary vascular obstruction in Down's syndrome. *Eur J Cardiol* 1975;2:473–476.

174. Yamaki S, Yasui H, Kado H, Yonenaga K, Nakamura Y, Kikuchi T, Ajiki H, Tsunemoto M, Mohri H, Pulmonary vascular disease and operative indications in complete atrioventricular septal defect in early infancy. *J Thorac Cardiovasc Surg* 1993;106:398–405.

175. Plett JA, Tandon R, Moller JH, Edwards JE. Hypertensive pulmonary vascular disease. *Arch Pathol* 1974;97:187–188.

176. Noonan JA and Walters LR. Hemodynamic studies in Down's syndrome patients with congenital heart disease. *Pediatr Res* 1974;79:353.

177. Kontras SB, Bodenbender JA. Abnormal capillary morphology in congenital heart disease. *Pediatrics* 1966;37:316–322.

178. Ugazio AG, Lanzavecchia A, Jayakar S, Plebani A, Duse M, Burgio GR. Immunodeficiency in Down's syndrome. Titres of natural antibodies in *E. coli* and rabbit erythrocytes at different ages. *Acta Paediatr Scand* 1978;67:705–708.

179. Alboliras ET, Seward JB, Hagler DJ, Danielson GK, Puga FJ, Tajik AJ. Impact of two-dimensional and Doppler echocardiography on care of children aged two years and younger. *Am J Cardiol* 1988;61:166–169.

180. Ebels T. Echocardiography and surgery for atrioventricular septal defect. *Int J Cardiol* 1986;13:353–360.

181. Eshaghpour E, Turnoff HB, Kingsley B, Kawai N, Linhart JW. Echocardiography in endocardial cushion defects: A preoperative and postoperative study. *Chest* 1975;68:172–177.

181a. Cohen MS, Jacobs ML Weinberg PM, Rychik J. Morphometric analysis of unbalanced common atrioventricular orifice using two-dimensional echocardiography. *J Am Coll Cardiol* 1996; 28:1017–1023.

182. Hagler DJ, Tajik AJ, Seward JB, Mair DD, Ritter DG. Real-time wide-angle sector echocardiography: Atrioventricular canal defects. *Circulation* 1979;59:140–150.

183. Mortera C, Rissech M, Payola M, Miro C, Perich R. Cross sectional subcostal echocardiography: Atrioventricular septal defects and short axis cut. *Br Heart J* 1987;58:267–273.

184. Silverman NH, Zuberbuhler JR, Anderson RH. Atrioventricular septal defects: Cross-sectional echocardiographic and morphologic comparisons. *Int J Cardiol*

1986;13:309–331.

185. Smallhorn JF, de Leval M, Stark J, Somerville J, Taylor JFN, Anderson RH, Macartney FJ. Isolated mitral cleft. Two dimensional echocardiographic assessment and differentiation from "clefts" associated with atrioventricular septal defect. *Br Heart J* 1982;48:109–116.

185a.Sigfusson G, Ettedgui JA, Silverman NH, Anderson RH. Is a cleft in the anterior leaflet of an otherwise normal mitral valve an atrioventricular canal malformation? *J Am Coll Cardiol* 1995;26:508–515.

186. Smallhorn JF, Sutherland GR, Anderson RH, Macartney FJ. Cross-sectional echocardiographic assessment of conditions with atrioventricular valve leaflets attached to the atrial septum at the same level. *Br Heart J* 1982;48: 331–341.

187. Smallhorn JF, Tommasini G, Anderson RH, Macartney FJ. Assessment of atrioventricular septal defects by two dimensional echocardiography. *Br Heart J* 1982;47: 109–121.

188. Smallhorn JF, Tommasini G, Macartney FJ. Two-dimensional echocardiographic assessment of common atrioventricular valves in univentricular hearts. *Br Heart J* 1981;46:30–34.

189. Di Segni E and Edwards JE. Cleft anterior leaflet of the mitral valve with intact septa. A study of 20 cases. *Am J Cardiol* 1983;51:919–926.

190. Freedom RM, Smallhorn JF. Atrioventricular septal defect. In: Freedom RM, Benson LN, Smallhorn JF. *Neonatal Heart Disease*. London: Springer-Verlag; 1992, pp. 611–632.

190a.Zellers TM, Zehr R, Weinstein E, Leonard S, Ring WS, Nikaidoh H. Two-dimensional and Doppler echocardiography alone can adequately define preoperative anatomy and hemodynamic status before repair of complete atrioventricular septal defect in infants < 1 year old. *J Am Coll Cardiol* 1994;24:1565–1570.

191. Baron MG, Wolf BS, Steinfeld L, Van Mierop LHS. Endocardial cushion defects. Specific diagnosis by angio-cardiography. *Am J Cardiol* 1964;13:162–175.

192. Somerville J, Jefferson K. Left ventricular angiocardiography in atrioventricular defects. *Br Heart J* 1968;30: 446–457.

193. Brandt PWT, Clarkson PM, Neutze JM, Barratt-Boyes BG. Left ventricular cineangiocardiography in endocardial cushion defect (persistent common atrioventricular canal). *Aust Radiol* 1972;16:367–376.

194. Fellows K, Henschel WG, Keck EW, Lassrish A. Left ventricular angiocardiography in endocardial cushion defects: Emphasis on the lateral projection. *Ann Radiol* 1972;15:223–230.

195. Freedom RM, Culham JAG, Moes CAF. *Angiocardiography of Congenital Heart Disease*. New York: Macmillan Publishing Company; 1984, pp. 141–160.

196. Yoo S-J, Choi Y-H. *Angiocardiograms in Congenital Heart Disease. Teaching File of Sejong Heart Institute*. Oxford: Oxford Medical Publications; 1991, pp. 123–132.

197. Girod D, Raghib G, Wang Y, Adams P Jr, Amplatz K. Angiocardiographic characteristics of persistent common atrioventricular canal. *Radiology* 1965;85:442–447.

198. Macartney FJ, Rees PG, Daly K, Piccoli GP, Taylor JFN, De Leval MR, Stark J, Anderson RH. Angiocardiographic appearances of atrioventricular defects with particular reference to distinction of ostium primum atrial septal defect from common atrioventricular orifice. *Br Heart J* 1979;42:640–656.

199. Lipschultz SE, Sanders SP, Mayer JE, Colan SD, Lock JE. Are routine preoperative cardiac catheterization and angiocardiography necessary before repair of ostium primum atrial septal defect? *J Am Coll Cardiol* 1988;11: 373–378.

200. Yates RWM, Sharland GK, Qureshi SA. The evolution of a hypoplastic left ventricle in an infant with an atrioventricular septal defect detected antenatally. *Cardiol Young* 1995;5:360–362.

Chapter 6

Ventricular Septal Defect

Ventricular septal defects are the most ubiquitous of all significant congenital cardiac malformations. The relative incidence as a proportion of total congenital heart disease ranges from approximately 16% to 50%.[1-7] Although bicuspid aortic valve and mitral valve prolapse are more prevalent, both lesions uncommonly produce symptoms in infants and children, and mitral valve prolapse is not classified as a congenital defect in most series.[6,7] Ventricular septal defect occurs as either an isolated defect or part of a more complex lesion. In this chapter, the discussion is confined to those hearts with concordant atrioventricular and ventriculoarterial connections.

Prevalence

The reported incidence of isolated ventricular septal defect ranges from approximately 0.4 to 3.3 per 1000 livebirths.[1,2] The variations in the reported incidence relate mainly to the case finding methodology and the reporting system, both of which have been ever improving. A recent study reported an overall incidence of 4.68 per 1000 livebirths, which is the highest rate of all.[8] The increased incidence in this study has been attributed to the high-risk population of the study. The fact that ventricular septal defects often close spontaneously either in the fetus or postnatally also accounts for the differences in incidence between the studies, which are almost certainly based on populations consisting of different age groups.[2,8-11] It is noteworthy that ventricular septal defects are more common in premature and low birth weight infants.[1,2,8,12,13] However, the incidence rates are not related significantly to race, sex, maternal age, birth order, and socioeconomic status.

Anatomy of Normal Ventricular Septum and Angiocardiographic Projections

Before discussing the anatomy of the ventricular septum, it is worthwhile to recall the four fundamental features of normal hearts (Figs. 6-1 and 6-2).

1. The pulmonary valve is separated from the tricuspid valve by a prominent muscular crest that is commonly called the crista supraventricularis,[14] and more specifically the ventriculoinfundibular fold (Figs. 6-1A and 6-2B).[15,16] Thus, the right ventricular outlet is a conspicuous structure surrounded by a completely muscular cone (see also Chapter 3). In contrast, the aortic valve is in direct fibrous continuity with the mitral valve (Figs. 6-1B and 6-2B). Thus, the left ventricular outlet is less conspicuous than the right ventricular outlet, and is partly muscular and partly fibrous.

2. The four cardiac valves are arranged in a single plane that is called the base of the ventricles (Fig. 6-2).[14] In this plane, the aortic valve occupies a deeply wedged position between the anterior aspects of the tricuspid and mitral valves. This allows the fibrous continuity between the aortic and mitral valves and aortic and tricuspid valves as well. A dense fibrous core is present at the junction of the aortic, mitral, and tricuspid valves. This is called the central fibrous body.[14,15]

3. On cross section of the ventricles through the short axis of the heart, the crescent right ventricle wraps itself around the circular left ventricle (Fig. 6-2B). Thus, the interventricular septum sustains an arc of approximately 100° to 120°.

4. The left side of the ventricular septum from its apex to the aortic valve has more or less a sigmoid configuration.[14,15a] The sigmoid character of the ventricular septum becomes more pronounced with age.

The ventricular septum consists of the membranous

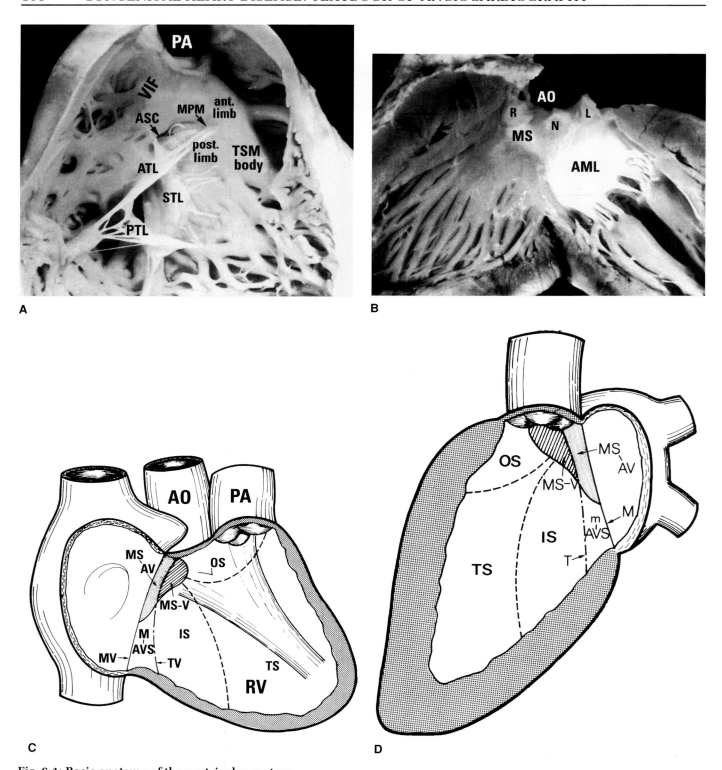

Fig. 6-1: Basic anatomy of the ventricular septum.
A: Opened right ventricle of a normal specimen. The right ventricle is characterized by heavy trabeculations. The trabecula septomarginalis (TSM) is the most stout septal trabeculation and consists of a body and anterior and posterior limbs. The crista supraventricularis is a saddle-shaped muscular crest intervening between the tricuspid valve (TV) and the pulmonary valve (PV). The crista consists of the septal and parietal components, ie, the outlet septum and the ventriculoinfundibular fold (VIF). The medial papillary muscle (MPM) arises from the area of bifurcation of the anterior and posterior limbs of the TSM, and supports the anterior and septal tricuspid leaflets (ATL and STL, respectively). The membranous septum occupies the area around the anteroseptal (ASC) commissure of the tricuspid valve. PTL indicates posterior tricuspid leaflet. **B:** Opened left ventricle of a normal specimen. The left ventricle is characterized by fine trabeculations. The noncoronary cusp (N) of the aortic

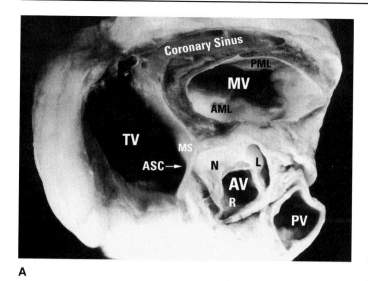
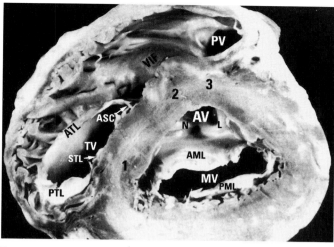

Fig. 6-2: Base of the ventricles.
A: Base of the ventricles photographed from above. The atria and great arteries are removed. Notice that the aortic valve (AV) is wedged between the tricuspid valve (TV) and the mitral valve (MV). The membranous septum (MS) is closely related to the anteroseptal commissure (ASC) of the tricuspid valve. **B:** Base of the ventricles photographed from below. The major part of the ventricular apex is removed. The ventriculoinfundibular fold (VIF) is seen between the tricuspid valve and the pulmonary valve (PV). The ventricular septum has an arc configuration between the round left ventricle and the crescent right ventricle. The inlet component (area 1) of the ventricular septum is best profiled in four-chamber view, whereas the outlet component (area 3) below the semilunar valves is best profiled in lateral or right anterior oblique view. The trabecular part (area 2) is best profiled in long axial oblique view. AML and PML indicate anterior and posterior mitral leaflets; ATL, PTL, and STL, anterior, posterior, and septal tricuspid leaflets respectively; R, L, and N indicate right, left, and noncoronary cusps of the aortic valve, respectively.

and muscular parts (Figs. 6-1 and 6-2). The membranous septum is the septal extension of the of the central fibrous body. Thus, the membranous septum is closely related to the anterior leaflet of the mitral valve and the septal leaflet of the tricuspid valve around its anteroseptal commissure, and is located immediately below the right and noncoronary cusps of the aortic valve. The muscular septum is arbitrarily divided into the inlet, trabecular, and outlet components (Figs. 6-1C and 6-1D). Each component occupies a triangular area with a common apex at the membranous septum. As the left ventricular outlet is less conspicuous than the right ventricular outlet, the extent of the outlet septum when seen from the left ventricle is significantly smaller than that seen from the right ventricle. The right ventricular aspect of the septum is characterized by heavy trabeculations, whereas its left ventricular aspect is characterized by fine trabeculations. There is a constant stout trabeculation, which is called a trabecula septomarginalis, in

the right ventricular septal surface. It consists of a body and two limbs with a shape of the letter Y. Its body runs obliquely toward the ventricular apex and gives rise to the moderator band. The cranial end of the body bifurcates to become the posterior and anterior limbs. The bifurcation of the two limbs is demarcatd by the insertion of the medial or conal papillary muscle (of Lancisi). The posterior limb extends to the membranous septum and the anterior limb supports the pulmonary valve.

As the ventricular septum is between the circular left ventricle and the crescent right ventricle, it is not a flat structure but has an arc configuration (see Chapter 2). Thus, the angiocardiographic projection should be tailored in such a way that the part of the septum to be visualized is placed in tangent to the x-ray beam (Fig. 6-2B).[17–19] The inlet component of the ventricular septum is best profiled in the four-chamber projection (cranially tilted shallow left anterior oblique projection). The trabecular component around the trabecula sep-

valve (AV) is in direct contact with the anterior leaflet of the mitral valve (AML). The membranous septum (MS) is transilluminated from the right atrial and ventricular aspect. It is located immediately below the right (R) and noncoronary cusps (N) of the aortic valve. L indicates left coronary cusp of the aortic valve. **C and D:** Diagrams showing the right and left aspects of the atrial, atrioventricular and ventricular septum. The ventricular septum is divided into the inlet (IS), trabecular (TS), and outlet (OS) components. M-AVS indicates muscular part of atrioventricular septum; MS-AV, atrioventricular membranous septum; MS-V, interventricular membranous septum; MV, septal attachment of mitral valve; TV, septal attachment of tricuspid valve.

tomarginalis is best profiled in the long axial oblique projection (cranially tilted mid left anterior oblique projection). The outlet component below the semilunar valves is best profiled in the right anterior oblique or lateral projection. The membranous septum is profiled predominately in long axial oblique projections; the hepatoclavicular four-chamber projection profile the basal aspect of the membranous septum.

Because the septal leaflet of the tricuspid valve is more apically attached than the anterior leaflet of the mitral valve, the posterior part of the septal surface seen from the left ventricle is not between the two ventricles, but between the left ventricle and the right atrium (Figs. 6-1C and 6-1D).[20] This part of the septum is the atrioventricular septum, which, again, consists of the membranous part anteriorly and the muscular part posteriorly. The membranous atrioventricular septum is the posterior extension of the interventricular membranous septum. The atrioventricular septum is profiled in the four-chamber projection as is the atrial and ventricular inlet septae.

Classification

The classification of ventricular septal defects remains controversial. More than a dozen different systems of classification have been introduced (Table 6-1).[21–32] However, just as mankind can be classified in various ways according to various criteria (such as sex, age, race, nationality, religion, skin color, etc.), it is not unusual for ventricular septal defects to be classified in various ways according to various criteria (such as location, size, shape, relations to certain antomic structure, embryological implication, etc.). Among the numerous criteria, the size of the defect is the most important factor that determines the physiologic status of the patient.[33] The criteria of classification, other than the defect size and shape, is determined by the purpose of classification. Thus, in classifying ventricular septal defects, we should reiterate why we are classifying them. In clinical cardiology, we classify them to elicit better understanding of the clinical presentation, the natural history, and the findings at diagnostic imaging; to decide the surgical approach and technique when surgery is contemplated; and to facilitate communication. However, there will not be any ideal system that fully satisfies these multiple purposes. Neverthless, we should come to an agreement to use a single system even if it is not the ideal one. In this regard, the system proposed by Soto et al[29] and subsequently revised by Anderson and colleagues[34–36] would be most useful in clinical diagnosis, treatment, and communication

(Fig. 6-3) (Table 6-2). The critera for this classification system are:

1. The relation of the defect to the atrioventricular conduction axis, ie, the membranous septum.
2. The relation of the defect to the atrioventricular valves.
3. The relation of the defect to the arterial valves.
4. The position of the defect within the ventricular septum, ie, the inlet, trabecular, or outlet part of the septum.

According to the first three criteria, ventricular septal defects are classified into four types: perimembranous, juxtatricuspid (and non-perimembranous), doubly committed juxta-arterial, and muscular defects. The perimembranous defect involves the interventricular membranous septum and the adjacent muscular septum. The aortic and tricuspid valves are virtually in direct contact through the defect. The mitral valve is usually separated from the defect by the intervening atrioventricular membranous septum. In rare occasions with a perimembranous defect that extends extensively toward the ventricular inlet to the crux cordis, ie, the so-called ventricular septal defect of the persistent common atrioventricular canal type, the mitral and tricuspid valves are in direct contact through the defect.[37] In all cases with a perimembranous defect, the atrioventricular conduction axis is intimately related to the posteroinferior margin of the defect, regardless of its subtype.[38] The juxtatricuspid (and nonperimembranous) defect involves the inlet muscular septum along the tricuspid annulus without direct contact with the membranous septum.[32] In this particular defect, the conduction axis is located at the anterior aspect of the defect along the posteroinferior margin of the intact membranous septum. The doubly committed juxta-arterial defect involves the most cranial part of the outlet septum. The aortic and pulmonary valves are in direct contact above the defect. The muscular defect is surrounded completely by a muscular rim when it is seen from the right ventricle. Defects that are not perimembranous have no direct contact with the atrioventricular conduction axis. Among these four types, perimembranous and muscular defects need further categorization according to the last criterion: the position of the defect within the ventricular septum. When defining the position of the defect within the ventricular septum, it should be done as seen from the right ventricle. This is because the septal boundaries seen from the right ventricle are not necessarily identical to those seen from the left ventricle.[35,36]

Table 6-1

Various Classifications of Isolated Ventricular Septal Defect

Taussig HB, et al. (1947)
 Simple defect: congenital perforation of the ventricular wall
 High defect: failure of the aortic septum to meet the ventricular septum

Selzer A[21] (1949)
 Defect underneath aortic valve
 — Leading to tricuspid region
 — Leading to conus arteriosus
 — Membranous portion of septum (multiple perforations)
 Defect in lower or muscular portion of ventricular septum

Becu LM, et al.[22] (1956)
 Defects related to the ventricular outflow tracts
 — Posterior to the crista supraventricularis
 — Anterior to the crista supraventricularis
 Defects involving the regions not related to the ventricular outflow tracts
 —Related to the atrioventricular valves
 —Involving the apical portion of the ventricular septum
*Multiple defects

Kirklin JW et al.[23] (1957)
 Defects related to ventricular outflow tracts---
 Inferior to crista supraventricularis
 Superior to crista supraventricularis = "High" defects
 Defects related to ventricular inflow tracts
 —Beneath septal leaflet of tricuspid valve
 —Near apex of muscular septum = "Low" defects

Warden HE et al.[24] (1957); after Karl Freherr von Rokintansky (1875)
 Complete absence of ventricular septum (single ventricle)
 Defect in the posterior ventricular septum
 Defect in the anterior ventricular septum
 —Absence of the entire anterior septum
 —Defect in the posterior part of the anterior septum
 —Defect in the anterior part of the anterior septum
 Defect in unusual positions (including muscular defects)
 (Defect in anomalous septum)

Goor DA, et al.[25] (1970)
 Infundibular ventricular septal defect
 —VSD in the inferior (proximal) margin of the crista supraventricularis (infundibular VSD Type 1)
 —Midcristal VSD (infundibular VSD type II)
 —Supracristal VSD (infundibular VSD type III)
 —VSD characterized by complete absence of the crista supraventricularis (infundibular VSD type IV)
 —VSD between the conus septum and the posterior septum (infundibular VSD type V)
 VSD of septum membranaceum interventriculare
 Smooth VSD
 —VSD of posterior smooth septum with coincident involvement of septum membranaceum (smooth VSD type I)
 —Complete absence of the posterior smooth septum (smooth VSD type II)
 —VSD at the junction of the smooth and trabeculated septa (smooth VSD type III)
 —VSD in the body of the posterior smooth septum (smooth VSD type IV)
 —VSD at the junction of the smooth and the anterior septa (smooth VSD type V)
 Trabeculated VSD
 Left ventricular-right atrial communication (atrioventricular septal defect)

Lincoln C, et al.[26] (1977)
 Membranous and membranous/malalignment defects
 Infundibular septal defects
 Posterior defects
 Apical muscular defects

Moulaert AJ[27] (1978)
 Defects of the posterior (inlet) septum
 Defects of the trabecular septum
 —Apical muscular trabecular defect
 —Posterior muscular trabecular defect
 —Anterior muscular trabecular defect
 —Multiple muscular trabecular defect (Swiss cheese-type)
 Defects of the membranous septum
 Defects of the infundibular septum
 —Proximal infundibular septal defect
 —Distal infundibular septal defect
 —Complete infundibular septal defect

Wenink ACG, et al.[28] (1979); classification of muscular defects
 Central muscular defects
 Posterior muscular defects
 Marginal muscular defects

Soto B, et al.[29] (1980)
 Perimembranous defects
 —Defects extending into the inlet septum
 —Defects extending into the trabecular septum
 —Defects extending into the infundibulum
 Muscular defects
 —Defects in inlet area of muscular septum
 —Defects in trabecular area of muscular septum
 —Defects in infundibular area of septum
 Subarterial infundibular defects

Capelli H, et al.[30] (1983)
 Subvalvular VSD
 —Inlet
 —Subtricuspid
 —Subaortic
 —Subpulmonary
 —Doubly committed subarterial
 Muscular VSD
 —Apical
 —Central
 —Outlet
 —Defects in the posterior part of the septum

Smolinksy A, et al.[31] (1988)
 Membranous VSD
 Infundibuloventricular (conoventricular) VSD
 Muscular VSD
 Atrioventricular canal type of VSD
 Infundibular (conal) VSD

Soto B, et al.[32] (1989)
 Conoventricular (infundibuloventricular or junctional) defects
 Defects in the right ventricular outlet
 —Juxta-aortic
 —Juxtapulmonary
 —Juxta-arterial
 —Muscular in the conal septum
 —Muscular in the trabecular septum (anterosuperior position)
 Inlet septal defects
 —Juxtatricuspid and juxtamitral
 —Juxtacrucial
 —Muscular
 Trabecular defects
 —Anterior
 —Midseptal
 —Apical

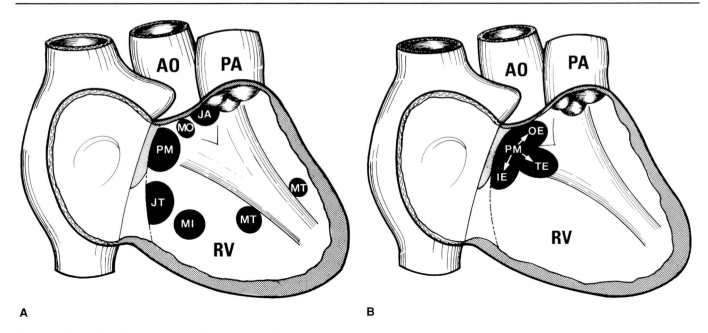

Fig. 6-3: Classification of ventricular septal defects.
A: Ventricular septal defects seen from the right ventricular aspect. **B:** Subdivision of the perimembranous ventricular septal defects. Abbreviations for types of ventricular septal defect are listed in Table 6-2.

Concept of Malalignment Defect

Ventricular septal defects are most commonly a simple punched-out hole (Fig. 6-4A). Less commonly, the defect is associated with the malalignment of a part of the septum (Figs. 3C and 6-4B).[27] Malalignment usually involves the outlet or infundibular septum (see also Chapters 20, 33, and 35). The malalignment of the outlet septum may occur either anteriorly toward the right ventricle or posteriorly toward the left ventricle.

Table 6-2

Modified Soto's Classification of Ventricular Septal Defects

Perimembranous defects (PM)
 –Extending toward the inlet of the right ventricle (PM-IE)
 –Extending toward the trabecular part of the right ventricle (PM-IE)
 –Extending toward the outlet of the right ventricle (PM-OE)
 –Confluent defects

Juxtatricuspid, nonperimembranous defects (JT)

Doubly committed juxta-arterial defects (JA)

Muscular defects
 –In inlet septum (MI)
 –In trabecular septum (MT)
 –In outlet septum (MO)

Malalignment occurs as if there is a door that moves on a hinge.

The anterior malalignment of the outlet septum is the most common type of malalignment. In this situation, the outlet septum that is supported by a hinge along its left anterior aspect is pulled anteriorly toward the right ventricular outflow tract (Fig. 6-4B).[27,39,40] This anterior malalignment results in a large ventricular septal defect and overriding of the aortic valve, which are seen in Eisenmenger type of ventricular septal defect. More typically, the anterior malalignment is severe enough to encroach on the subpulmonary outflow tract, and the morphology of tetralogy of Fallot results (see Chapter 20).

The posterior malalignment is a less common situation in which the outlet septum is pushed backwards into the left ventricular outflow tract, a hinge is present along the aortic valve (Fig. 6-4C).[27,39,41–45] This posterior malalignment results in a ventricular septal defect and muscular subaortic stenosis (see Chapter 33). If the malalignment is severe, the pulmonary valve may override the ventricular septum. The posterior malalignment defect is frequently associated with the obstructive lesion of the aortic arch, and is called the coarctation type of ventricular septal defect.

Rarely, the malalignment occurs between the atrial and the muscular ventricular septal structures. This atrioventricular septal malalignment is associated with overriding and/or straddling of the tricuspid valve,[46] which will be discussed in detail in Chapter 15.

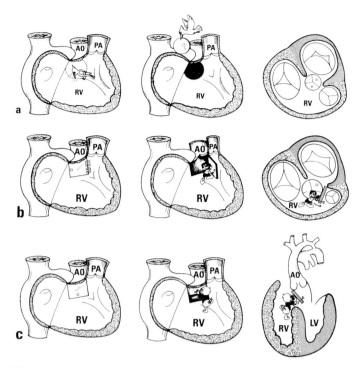

Fig. 6-4: Pathological mechanisms of simple and malaligned ventricular septal defects.
A: Ventricular septal defect as a simple punched-out hole. A piece of ventricular septum is not formed, as if it is simply removed. **B:** Anterior malalignment type of ventricular septal defect in tetralogy of Fallot. The outlet septum is supported by a hinge along its left anterior margin. It is pulled anteriorly into the right ventricular outflow tract, which is encroached on by the deviated outlet septum. **C:** Posterior malalignment type of ventricular septal defect. The outlet septum is supported by a hinge along its junction with the aortic valve. It is pushed backwards into the left ventricular outflow tract. Because of the encroachment of the latter structure, the obstructive lesion of the aortic arch is commonly associated.

Natural History of Ventricular Septal Defects

The natural history of most patients with ventricular septal defect is not static, but may be characterized by changes in its form and function, the changes either being advantageous or disadvantageous (Table 6-3).[11,47]

Table 6-3

Natural History of Ventricular Septal Defects

1. Spontaneous closure.
2. Left ventricle to right atrial shunt.
3. Aortic valve prolapse and regurgitation.
4. Right ventricular outflow tract obstruction.
5. Left ventricular outflow tract obstruction.
6. Pulmonary vascular obstructive disease.

Various factors such as the location of the defect within the septum, the initial size of the defect, the anatomic structure or structures in the vicinity of the defect, and the association of other malformation are responsible for the functional as well as the morphologic changes.

Spontaneous Closure

The most advantageous change is the reduction of defect size ultimately leading to spontaneous closure. The reported rate of closure varies depending on the population studied and method of investigation.[8–11,48,49] The true rate of closure, however, can only be ascertained by following a large number of patients from birth to adulthood. Moe and Guntheroth[8] found a true rate of closure of at least 45%. Four mechanisms have been described as responsible for closure of ventricular septal defects (Fig. 6-5). The first mechanism is the adhesion of the tricuspid valve leaflet to the rim of a perimembranous defect.[50–52] The adhesion is facili-

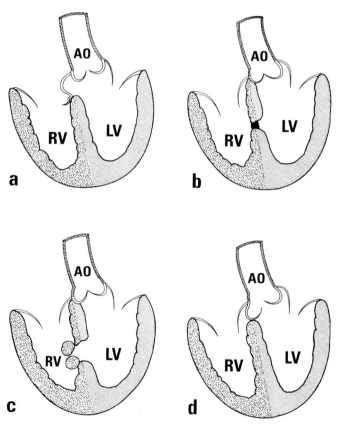

Fig. 6-5: Mechanisms of spontaneous closure of ventricular septal defect.
A: Closure of a perimembranous defect by adhesion of the tricuspid leaflet to the defect rim. **B:** Closure of a small muscular defect by a fibrous tissue plug. **C:** Closure of a muscular trabecular defect by hypertrophy of right ventricular septal trabeculations. **D:** Closure of a subaortic defect by prolapsing aortic valve.

tated by sticky endothelial damage along the rim of the defect and the adjacent tricuspid valve leaflet; the endothelial damage is a result of high-velocity jet through the defect. The involved tricuspid valve leaflet is frequently redundant or duplicated and forms an aneurysm-like pouch at the right ventricular aspect of the defect. The second mechanism is the obliteration of the defect by a fibrous tissue plug occurring in small muscular defects. The fibrous tissue plug is also a product of a high-velocity jet lesion. There is no difference in rate of closure of a single muscular defect with respect to anatomic locations.[49] The first and second mechanisms account for most of the cases with spontaneous closure. The third mechanism is the obliteration of the defect by the hypertrophied septal trabeculations of the right ventricle. Closure by this mechanism occurs when the muscular defect involves the apical trabecular part or is associated with aberrant muscle bundles. The last mechanism is the closure by a prolapsing aortic valve leaflet and/or sinus.[53–55] Once the aortic valve or sinus prolapses, the size of the defect is reduced and the flow velocity through the defect increases. The high-velocity jet produces sticky endocardial damage that facilitates adhesion of the prolapsed aortic valve cusp or cusps to the defect margin. However, this last mechanism of closure is not advantageous, as the aortic valve eventually becomes incompetent.

Left Ventricle to Right Atrial Shunt

The process of spontaneous closure of a perimembranous ventricular septal defect may be complicated by the perforation of the adherent tricuspid valve leaflet (Fig. 6-6).[56–57] In this circumstance, the shunt from the left ventricle is no longer in the right ventricle but in the right atrium, or both, and an obligatory left-to-right shunt ensues. Similar hemodynamic effects may be produced when the adhesion of the tricuspid valve leaflet itself or duplicated leaflet tissue to the rim of perimembranous defect occurs in such a way that the commisure between the anterior and septal leaflets of the tricuspid valve becomes a fixed gap throughout the cardiac cycle. Less frequently, the left ventricle to right atrial shunt is encountered as an initial lesion. This occurs when the perimembranous defect is associated with hypoplasia of the septal leaflet of the tricuspid valve leaving a gaping anteroseptal commissure or when there is a cleft in the septal leaflet of the tricuspid valve. Thus, most of the cases with left ventricle to right atrial shunting are considered as the variants of perimembranous defects. An isolated defect of the atrioventricular membranous septum, a so-called Gerbode defect, is considered extremely rare.[58,59] It should also be differentiated from atrioventricular septal defect (see Chapter 5).

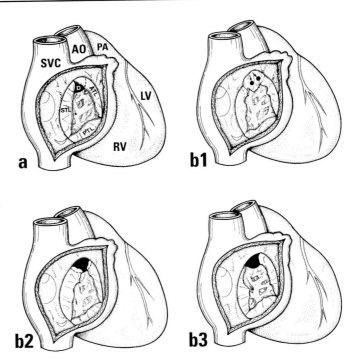

Fig. 6-6: Mechanisms of development of left ventricle to right atrial shunt in perimembranous defects.
a: Diagram of an uncomplicated perimembranous defect seen through an incised opening in the right atrial free wall. Notice that this perimembranous defect (D) is in close proximity with the anterior tricuspid leaflets (ATL) and septal tricuspid leaflets (STL) and the intervening anteroseptal commissure. PTL indicates posterior leaflet of tricuspid valve. **b:** Left ventricle to right atrial shunt: (1) through the perforations (arrows) in the adherent tricuspid valve leaflet; (2) through a wide anteroseptal commissure produced by abnormal adhesion of the anterior and septal tricuspid leaflets to the apical margin of the defect, and (3) through a wide anteroseptal commissure produced by congenital or acquired hypoplasia of the septal tricuspid leaflet. Rarely, a cleft may be present in the septal tricuspid leaflet.

Aortic Valve Prolapse

Aortic valve prolapse is an important complication of ventricular septal defect that is in direct contact with the aortic valve.[11,53–55,60–64] Thus, it is worthwhile to recall that all the perimembranous and doubly committed juxta-arterial defects and most of the muscular outlet defects are virtually in direct contact with the aortic valve. Among these subaortic defects, those defects that have more extensive contact with the aortic valve are the most prone to develop aortic valve prolapse because of the deficiency of the muscle supporting the aortic valve. The prolapse usually involves the right coronary cusp, and less frequently the noncoronary cusp. Prolapse of the noncoronary cusp occurs when the defect is a perimembranous type. Involvement of the left coronary cusp is extremely rare. When the muscular support of the valve sinus as well as the valve leaflets is

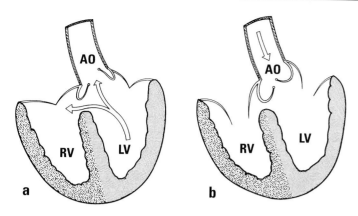

Fig. 6-7: Pathogenetic mechanism of aortic valve prolapse.
a: Systolic prolapse. Any defect in the subaortic location is prone to prolapse due to the Venturi effect by the rapid shunt flow in the systolic phase. **b:** Diastolic prolapse. When the valve cusp is damaged by the systolic prolapse or when the aortic sinus is devoid of muscular support, the prolapse occurs also in the diastolic phase.

compromised as in cases with a doubly committed juxta-arterial defect or in some cases with a muscular outlet defect, the whole or a part of the valve sinus may prolapse. In its early stage, the prolapse occurs only in the systolic phase due to the Venturi effect resulting from the rapid shunt flow through the defect (Fig. 6-7). In its late stage, the prolapse also occurs in diastole, as the valve cusp cannot stand the intra-aortic pressure. Eventually the prolapsing valve becomes incompetent because of the significant damage to the valve cusps and annulus. As the prolapsing aortic valve may completely close the ventricular septal defect, the shunt physiology may disappear with the progressive development of aortic regurgitation. Some or perhaps many of the cases reported as aneurysms of the sinus of Valsalva might in fact be ventricular septal defects complicated by aortic valve prolapse with complete obliteration of the defect (see also Chapter 31). Rarely, the prolapsed valve cusp may perforate with resultant aortic regurgitation into the right ventricle. Occasionally the prolapsing valve may contribute to the right ventricular outflow tract obstruction.

Right Ventricular Outflow Tract Obstruction

Right ventricular outflow tract obstruction can occur as a consequence of developing pulmonary hypertension and right ventricular hypertrophy, especially when the defect is an anterior malalignment type or when the defect is associated with anomalous muscle bundles in the right ventricle (see also Chapter 17).[11,47,65–67] This change reduces the amount of left-to-right shunting and may prevent further development of pulmonary vascular obstructive disease. As previously mentioned, the prolapsing aortic valve may play an ad-

ditional role in the development of the right ventricular outflow tract obstruction. When an aneurysmal pouch of the adherent tricuspid leaflet is prominent, it seems to exert an additional contibution to the obstruction already present, although its hemodynamic significance is not clear. There is evidence published from the Toronto Hospital for Sick Children that the most common mechanism responsible for acquired right ventricular outflow tract obstruction is hypertrophy of anomalous muscle bundles.[67]

Left Ventricular Outflow Tract Obstruction

Various lesions are responsible for left ventricular outflow tract obstruction in association with a ventricular septal defect (Table 6-4) (see Chapters 29 and 33). The obstruction is usually localized above the defect and occasionally below the defect.[68–70] The obstruction may be evident in the immediate postnatal period, may be a progression of the pre-existing lesion that was potentially obstructive, or may be an acquired lesion.[71] The nature of obstruction is either muscular or fibromuscular. Three major structures may be responsible for the muscular subaortic stenosis: the posteriorly malaligned outlet or infundibular septum, the septal deviation or anteroseptal twist, and the anterolateral muscle bundle. The obstruction by the posteriorly malaligned outlet septum is described elsewhere in this chapter. The septal deviation or anteroseptal twist is a muscular protrusion of the left ventricular aspect of the septum along the anterior and superior aspect of the defect.[27,43,44,72,73] It is most commonly associated with a central muscular defect and is often associated with additional trabeculae crossing the outflow tract. The anterolateral muscle bundle is a muscular protrusion found between the left coronary cusp of the aortic valve and the anterior leaflet of the mitral valve, extending into the anterolateral wall of the left ventricle.[44,72,73] It is present in approximately 40% of normal hearts. When it is unusually prominent in association with a

Table 6-4

Various Lesions Responsible for Left Ventricular Outflow Tract Obstruction in Association with Ventricular Septal Defect

1. Muscular lesions
   a. Posteriorly malaligned outlet septum
   b. Septal deviation or anteroseptal twist
   c. Anterolateral muscle bundle
   d. Muscular bundle along the septal insertion of the anterior leaflet of mitral valve
   e. Mitral arcade
3. Fibromuscular shelf
4. Fibrous ridge or tissue tag

ventricular septal defect, it may cause obstruction of both the left ventricular inflow and outflow tracts. The development or aggravation of muscular subaortic stenosis after pulmonary artery banding has been reported. Rarely, the muscular stenosis is below the ventricular septal defect.[69] The responsible muscle extends along the septal insertion of the anterior mitral valve in a gradual fibromuscular transition. In this occurrence, the clinical picture simulates double outlet right ventricle. Very rarely, the abnormal muscular bundle extending from the anterior leaflet of the mitral valve to the septal surface, a kind of the so-called mitral arcade, is responsible for subaortic obstruction.[74] Discrete subaortic stenosis is most commonly due to a fibrous shelf and less commonly due to a fibromuscular shelf or diaphragm.[75] The obstruction may be again either above or below the defect.[68,70] The discrete stenosis due to a fibrous ridge or diaphragm is often associated with spontaneous closure or reduction in size of a perimembranous defect.[70,76,77] It is particularly common when the defect is associated with right ventricular anomalous muscle bundle (see also Chapter 29). Less frequently, the discrete lesion is an abnormal tissue tag derived from either the mitral or tricuspid valve leaflet.[45,76]

Pulmonary Vascular Obstructive Disease

When the amount of left-to-right shunting through a ventricular septal defect is significant and at or near systemic pressures, pulmonary vascular changes develop.[11,47,78–82] These changes include progressive medial hypertrophy of the small pulmonary arteries with increases in arterial wall thickness, obstructive intimal fibrosis, and reduction in number of small pulmonary arteries with formation of thrombi. With the progression of pulmonary vascular changes that increase the pulmonary vascular resistance, the amount of left-to-right shunting decreases and ultimately overt right-to-left shunting develops. As the right ventricular ejection is against the high pulmonary resistance, the right ventricle hypertrophies.

Angiocardiographic Findings

As previously discussed, tailored angiocardiographic projections should be used for the proper demonstration of the ventricular septal defects (Fig. 6-2B)(see also Chapter 2).[17–19] Noninvasive cross-sectional images provide better understanding of the ideal angiocardiographic projections.[30,52,83–85]

The perimembranous ventricular septal defect is best profiled in the long axial oblique left ventriculogram as a septal discontinuity immediately below the right and noncoronary cusps of the aortic valve (Figs.

6-8 through 6-10).[29,86,87] The aortic valve and the tricuspid valve are in direct contact through the defect. It should be remembered that an intact atrioventricular septum intervenes beween the perimembranous defect and the anterior leaflet of the mitral valve, although the septum can be attenuated in defects with inlet extension. The main extension of the defect may be determined by observing which component of the right ventricle the initial shunt flow opacifies and which leaflet of the tricuspid valve the initial shunt flow delineates. When the perimembranous defect extends toward the inlet of the right ventricle, the initial shunt flow opacifies the right ventricular inlet between the septal leaflet of the tricuspid valve and the profiled septum (Fig. 6-8). When the defect extends toward the outlet of the right ventricle, the initial shunt flow opacifies the right ventricular outlet and delineates the anterior leaflet of the tricuspid valve (Fig. 6-9). When the defect extends toward the trabecular part of the right ventricle, the initial shunt flow delineates neither the septal nor the anterior leaflet of the tricuspid valve but tends to cross the tricuspid orifice and opacifies the right ventriclar body (Fig. 6-10). However, a large perimembranous defect may involve more than one of the septal components and the characteristic angiocardiographic features may not be appreciated.

An aneurysmal pouch formed by the adherent tricuspid leaflets typically bulges into the right ventricle, as the left ventricular pressure is greater than the right ventricular pressure (Fig. 6-11).[51] On the rare occasions that the right ventricular pressure exceeds the left ventricular pressure as a result of severe pulmonary vascular obstructive disease or after pulmonary artery banding, the aneurysmal pouch may bulge into the left ventricular outflow tract (Fig. 6-12). The aneurysmal pouch bulging into the low-pressure ventricle is well profiled by the long axial oblique projection. It may be seen as a round filling defect around the junction between the aortic and tricuspid valve in the right anterior oblique right ventriculogram.

Most of the cases with left ventricle to right atrial shunting are considered as the variants of perimembranous ventricular septal defects that are complicated by adhesion of the tricuspid valve leaflets.[56–57] The shunt direction in these circumstances is best defined in the long axial or right anterior oblique left ventriculogram (Fig. 6-13).

The juxtatricuspid ventricular septal defect is very rare.[32] It might be best defined in the four-chamber view. However, it might not be differentiated from a perimembranous defect. As this particular defect may coexists with a straddling or overriding tricuspid valve, special attention should be paid to the tricuspid valve. In this situation, right atriography in four-chamber view may be helpful.

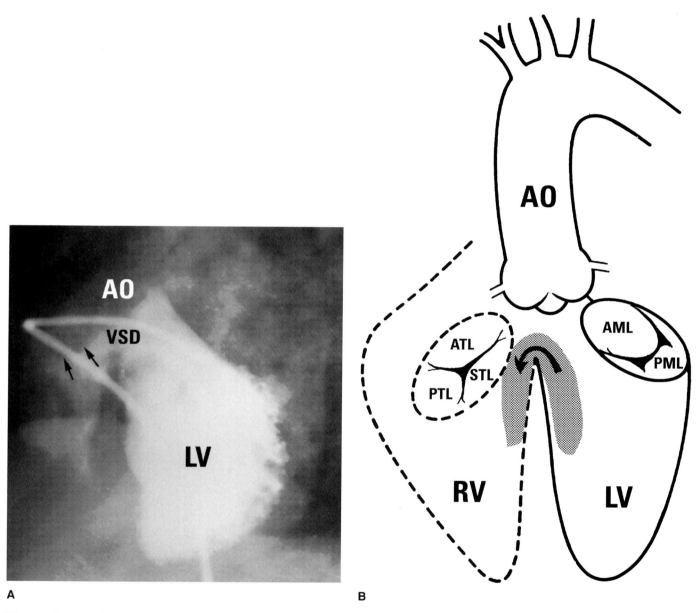

A

B

Fig. 6-8: Perimembranous ventricular septal defect extending toward the right ventricular inlet.
A and B: Left ventriculogram in long axial oblique view and diagrammatic representation. The defect is seen immediately below the aortic valve. The initial shunt flow opacifies the right ventricular inlet along the ventricular septum and delineates the septal leaflet (arrows) of the tricuspid valve.

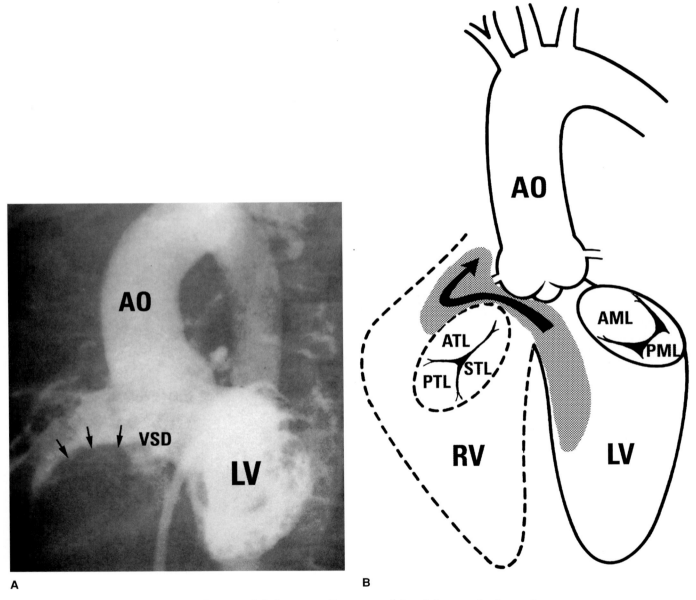

A

B

Fig. 6-9: Perimembranous ventricular septal defect extending toward the right ventricular outlet.
A and B: Left ventriculogram in long axial oblique view and diagrammatic representation. The initial shunt flow through this perimembranous defect opacifies the right ventricular outlet and delineates the anterior leaflet (arrows) of the tricuspid valve.

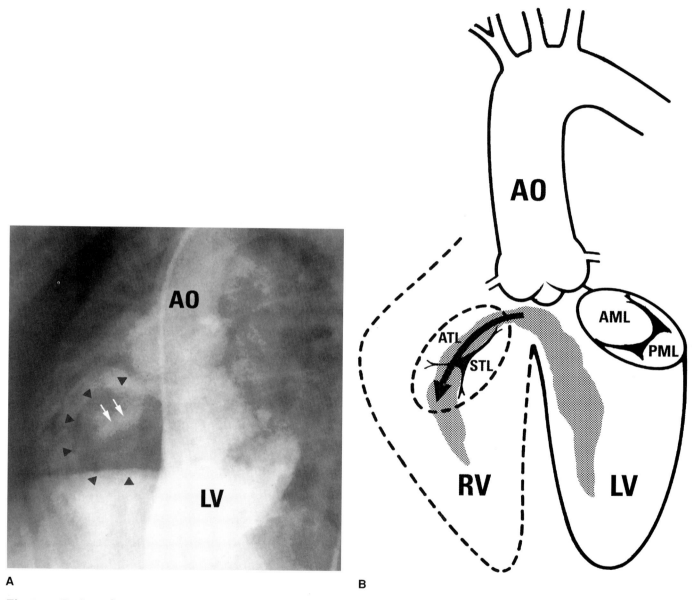

A

B

Fig. 6-10: Perimembranous ventricular septal defect extending toward the trabecular part of the right ventricle.
A and B: Left ventriculogram in long axial oblique view and diagrammatic representation. The shunt flow (arrow) through this perimembranous defect delineates neither the septal nor the anterior leaflet of the tricuspid valve. The shunt flow in early systolic phase crosses the tricuspid orifice (arrowheads).

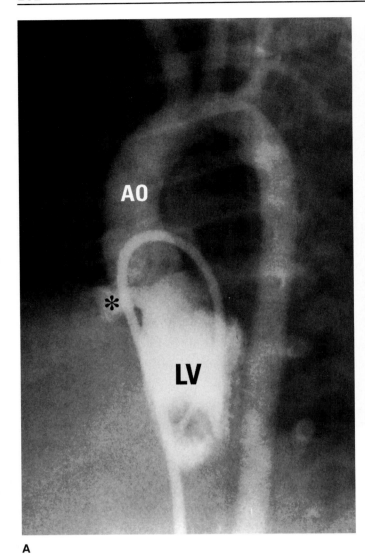

A

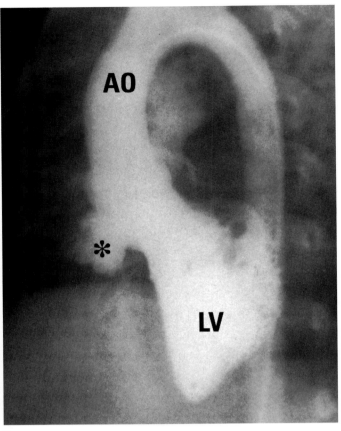

B

Fig. 6-11: Perimembranous ventricular septal defects spontaneously closed by adhesion of the tricuspid valve tissue.
Left ventriculograms in long axial oblique view. An aneurysmal pouch (asterisk) bulges into the right ventricle because of higher pressure in the left ventricle.

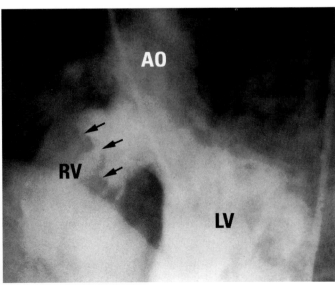

A

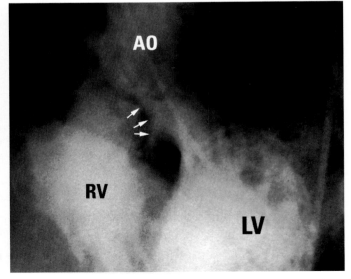

B

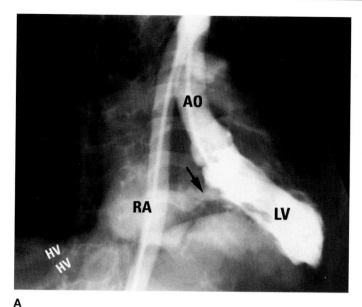

A

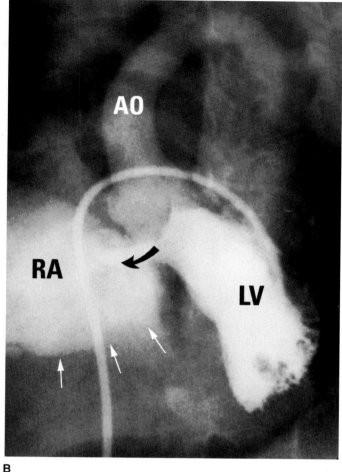

B

Fig. 6-13: Perimembranous ventricular septal defects complicated by left ventricle-to-right atrial shunt.
A: Left ventriculogram in right anterior oblique view. A direct shunt flow (arrow) from the left ventricle opacifies the right atrium. The regurgitant shunt flow also opacifies the hepatic veins (HV). **B:** Left ventriculogram in long axial oblique view from another patient. There is a direct shunt from the left ventricle into the right atrium (curved arrow). Although the direction of the shunt flow in this view is similar to that seen in patients with simple perimembranous defect, the initial opacification is safely considered to be into the right atrium which is demarcated by the tricuspid valve (arrows).

The muscular defect involving the inlet or trabecular septum is best profiled by the four-chamber or long axial oblique pojection and, less frequently, in right anterior oblique view (Fig. 6-14) (see also Chapter 2).[86,88,89] Frequently, the muscular defect, especially when it involves the central trabecular septum, has a conical configuration with a narrower opening at its right ventricular aspect (Fig. 6-14). When the conical defect is small, it may be completely obliterated at the time of full ventricular contraction (Fig. 6-15). Occasionally, the defect is an oblique tunnel that cannot be profiled in a single projection. This is especially true when the defect involves the apical or high anterior aspects of the ventricular septum. Such defects are well demonstrated in the right anterior oblique or long axial oblique projections.[52,89] A single muscular defect may have multiple openings at its right ventricular aspect

because of the traversing right ventricular septal trabeculations (Fig. 6-16). As the muscular defects are often multiple, it is advisable to obtain left ventriculograms in four-chamber, long axial oblique and right anterior oblique views. Multiple defects in the muscular septum have been termed "swiss-cheese defects" (Fig. 6-17). When the defect involves the central trabecular septum, it is often associated with left ventricular outflow tract obstruction. The muscular defect involving the outlet septum is rare in Caucasians, but is relatively common in Asians and South Americans. Most of the muscular outlet defects are seen immediately below the right coronary cusp of the aortic valve. It is best profiled by cranially tilted steep left anterior oblique or lateral projection. A small remnant of the outlet septum is seen to intervene between the defect and the pulmonary valve. Although its lower aspect may sometimes be profiled in

Fig. 6-12: Perimembranous ventricular septal defect partially closed by adherent tricuspid valve tissue.
In this case with severe pulmonary hypertension, an aneurysmal pouch shows phasic displacement. **A:** In some phase during the cardiac cycle, the aneurysmal sac (arrows) bulges into the right ventricle. **B:** In another phase during the ventricular systole when the right ventricular pressure is equal to or greater than the left ventricular pressure, the sac recoils to the margin of the defect.

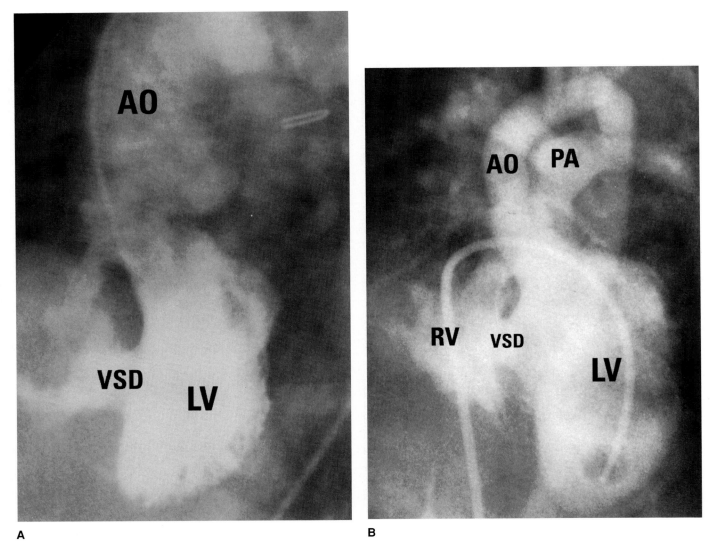

Fig. 6-14: Muscular ventricular septal defects.
A: Left ventriculogram in long axial oblique view shows a punched-out hole in the midtrabecular septum. **B:** Left ventriculogram in long axial oblique view from another patient shows a conical muscular defect. When the defect is conical, its apex usually points the right ventricular aspect. *(continued)*

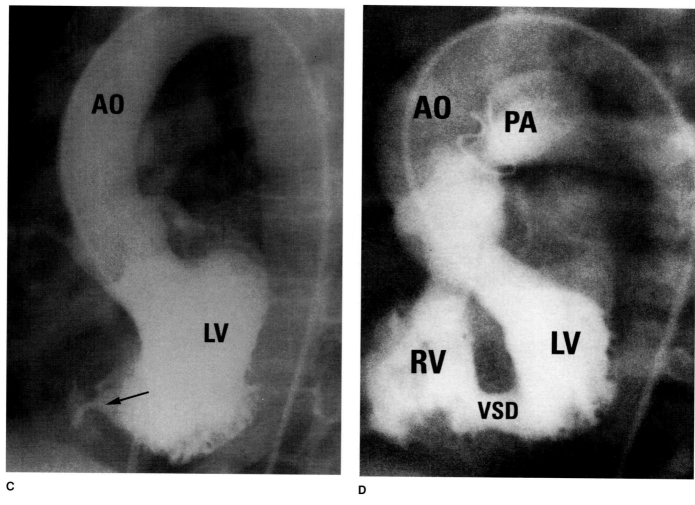

C   **D**

Fig. 6-14: *Continued.* **C:** Left ventriculogram in long axial oblique view from another patient shows a large muscular defect nearly completely obliterated at its right ventricular aspect (arrow). Note the large size of the defect at its left ventricular aspect. **D:** Left ventriculogram in long axial oblique view from another patient shows an apical muscular defect. *(continued)*

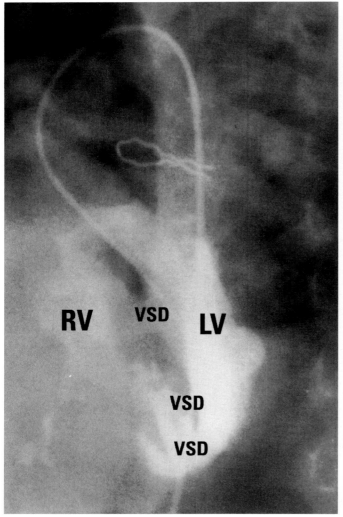

E

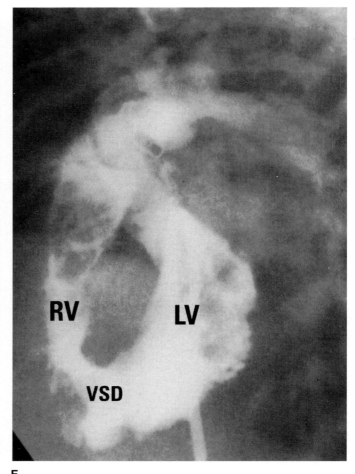

F

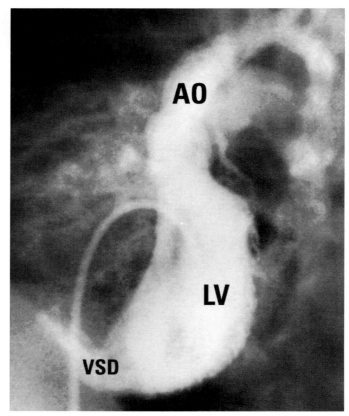

G

Fig. 6-14: *Continued.* **E:** Multiple ventricular septal defects demonstrated by this long axial oblique left ventriculogram. **F and G:** Two other patients with apical and near apical defects.

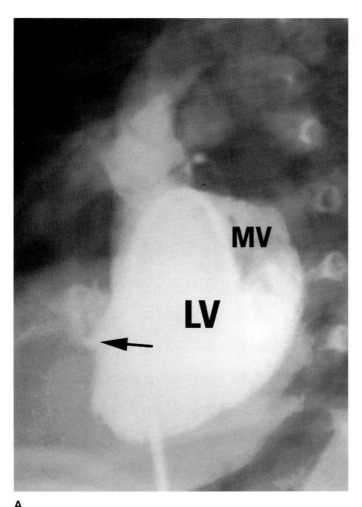

A

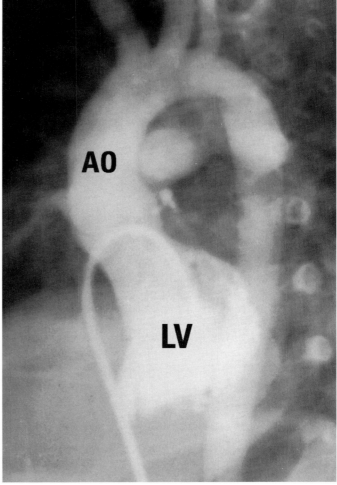

B

Fig. 6-15: **Obliteration of a small muscular ventricular septal defect on full ventricular contraction.**
A: Left ventriculogram obtained in the early systolic phase shows a small defect (arrow) in the trabecular septum. It has an oblique tract and its right ventricular aspect is irregular. **B:** The defect is completely obliterated at the time of full ventricular contraction.

Fig. 6-16: **A single muscular ventricular septal defect with multiple right ventricular openings.**
Left ventriculogram in long axial oblique view shows a large muscular defect. Its right ventricular side is divided into two tracts (arrows) by hypertrophied septal trabeculations (✱).

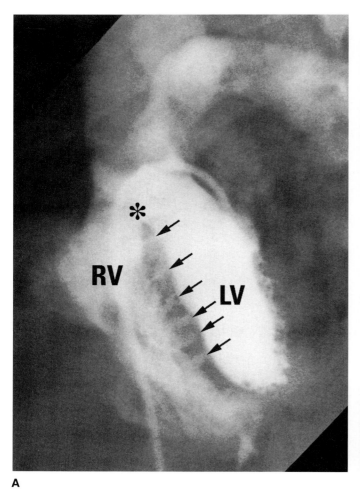

A

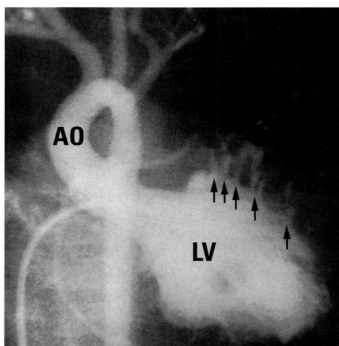

B

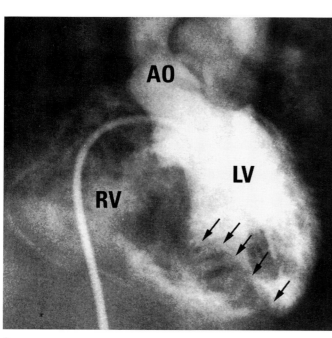

C

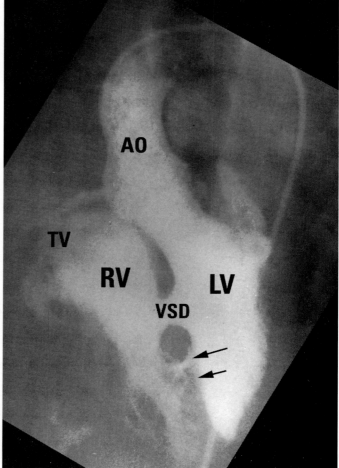

D

the long axial oblique view, the initial shunt flow does not directly delineate the anterior leaflet of the tricuspid valve.

The doubly committed juxta-arterial defect is also common in Asians and South Americans, but is certainly less common in Caucasians.[90] It is best defined in the right anterior oblique or cranially tilted steep left anterior oblique or lateral projection (Fig. 6-18).[19,52,86] The key finding is the direct continuity of the aortic and pulmonary valves above the defect without any intervening muscular structure. The septal contour seen in the long axial oblique view is intact when the defect is small. When the juxta-arterial defect is large, it may extend into the perimembranous septum.

Aortic valve prolapse is characterized angiographically by the downward displacement and lobulated contour of a part or all of the involved cusp and/or sinus that is usually larger than the uninvolved ones (Figs. 6-19 and 6-20).[52,87] Occasionally, the prolapsed part of the aortic cusp or sinus accumulates the contrast medium in the systolic phase of the aortogram, when the contrast medium in the other area of the aorta is washed out by the unopacified blood from the left ventricle (Fig. 6-21A). Similarly, the prolapsed part is not opacified in the systolic phase of the very first part of the left ventriculogram, when the other area of the aorta starts opacified (Fig. 6-21B). The direction of prolapse vary according to the location of the defect. In the doubly committed juxta-arterial defect, the prolapsed part faces more toward the subpulmonary outflow tract and is more clearly demonstrated in the right anterior oblique view (Fig. 6-20). Conversely, when the defect is predominately perimembranous, the prolapsed part faces more toward the tricuspid valve and is more readily demonstrated in the left anterior oblique view (Fig. 6-19). The size of the defect through which a left-to-right shunt occurs becomes smaller as the prolapse progresses. Occasionally, the defect may be completely obliterated by the prolapsing valve. With time, the prolapsing valve is complicated by aortic regurgitation. Thus, it is important to perform a retrograde aortography in patients with suspected aortic valve prolapse. Rarely, the aortic regurgitation is directly into the right ventricle (Fig. 6-22).[87] We have identified several cases in which the regurgitation into the right ventricle was through the perforation(s) of the prolapsed right coronary cusp.

The right ventricular outflow tract obstruction that develops in patients with an isolated ventricular septal defect is most often due to the hypertrophy of the right ventricular anomalous muscle bundles (Fig. 6-23) and less commonly due to the hypertrophy of the anteriorly malaligned outlet septum (Fig. 6-24).[67] Rarely, a prolapsing aortic valve or an aneurysmal pouch of the adherent tricuspid valve leaflets in spontaneously closing perimembranous defect may play an additional role in the development of the right ventricular outflow tract obstruction (Fig. 6-20). These obstructive lesions within the right ventricle are best defined by the right ventriculography obtained in the right anterior oblique and long axial oblique views.

The left ventricular outflow tract obstruction caused by the posteriorly malaligned outlet septum is best defined by the left ventriculography in the long axial oblique view (see Chapter 33, Fig. 33-15).[87] The outlet septum, which normally cannot be profiled by the long axial oblique view, is seen to encroach on the left ventricular outflow tract below the aortic valve in patients with posterior malalignment type of ventricular septal defect. The hypertrophied anterolateral muscle bundle is extremely difficult to demonstrate by angiocardiography. When it is prominent, it may produce a band-like filling defect running along the inferior margin of the left coronary cusp of the aortic valve in the right anterior oblique left ventriculogram. So-called septal deviation or anteroseptal twist is suspected when the septum above the defect has bulbous expansion. The fibrous ridge or membrane is often seen as a thin negative defect traversing the left ventricular outflow tract either above or below the defect in the long axial oblique left ventriculograms (Fig. 6-25) (see also Chapter 29). The so-called fibrous ridge is particularly common when a perimembranous defect is in the process of spontaneous closure or associated with right ventricular anomalous muscle bundles (see also Chapter 29, Figs. 29-28 and 29–29).

The angiographic features of pulmonary vascular obstructive disease include tortuosity of the pulmonary arterial branches, decreased number of and irregular intervals between the side branches of the segmental and subsegmental pulmonary arteries with the apprearance of pruned tree, and delayed opacification of the pulmonary veins on pulmonary artery wedge angiography (Fig. 6-26).[78] As the pulmonary vascular obstructive

Fig. 6-17: Swiss cheese-type of multiple muscular ventricular septal defects.
A: Left ventriculogram in long axial oblique view shows numerous tiny defects (arrows) involving the muscular septum. An additional large defect (✳) involves the perimembranous part of the ventricular septum. **B:** Left ventriculogram in frontal view from another patient shows tiny muscular defects (arrows) projecting superiorly from the left ventricular margin. **C:** A different patient with multiple midapical to apical muscular ventricular septal defects (arrows). **D:** A final patient with multiple ventricular septal defects (arrows) shown by a hepatoclavicular left ventriculogram.

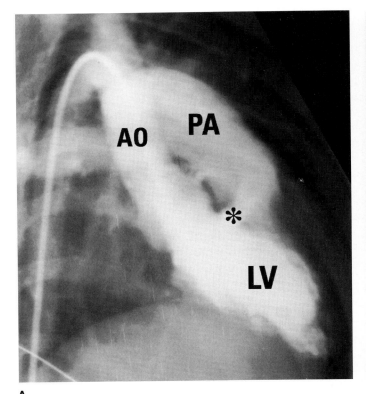

A

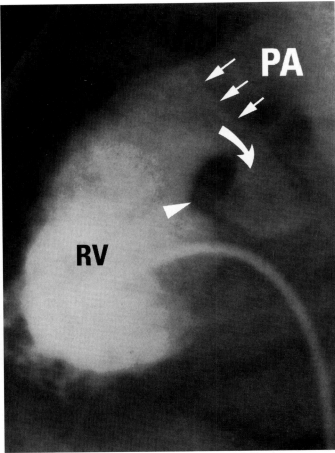

C

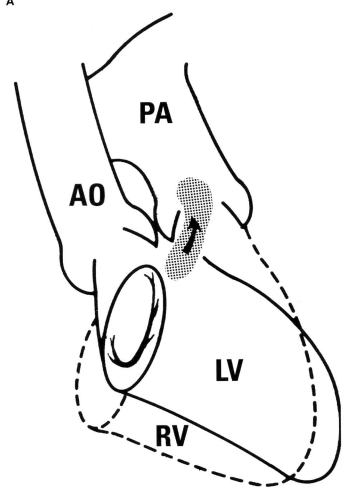

B

Fig. 6-18: Doubly committed juxta-arterial ventricular septal defect.
A and B: Left ventriculogram in right anterior oblique view and diagramatic representation shows a defect (✻) in the outlet or infundibular septum. The pulmonary valve and aortic valve are in direct contact above the defect. The initial shunt flow delineates the pulmonary valve. **C:** Right ventriculogram in lateral view from antother patient with systemic right ventricular pressure. There is a right-to-left shunt through the ventricular septal defect. It is immediately below the pulmonary valve (arrows), but is well above the tricuspid valve.

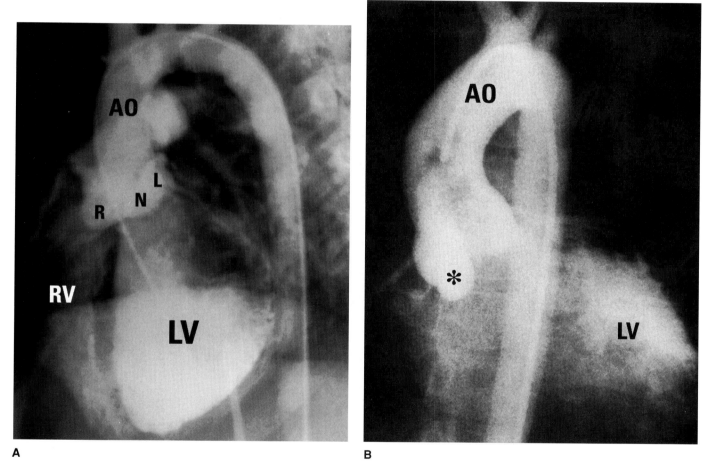

Fig. 6-19: Aortic valve prolapse complicating perimembranous ventricular septal defects.
A: Left ventriculogram in long axial oblique view shows the prolapsed right coronary cusp (R) of the aortic valve. It is larger than the left (L) and noncoronary cusps (N) and shows a lobulated contour. **B:** Aortogram in frontal view from another patient shows the prolapsed noncoronary cusp (✳) of the aortic valve. There is a large amount of aortic regurgitaion.

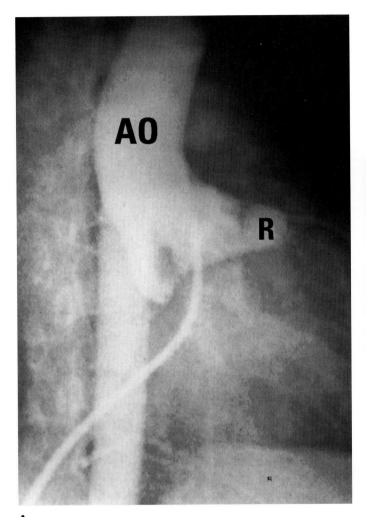

A

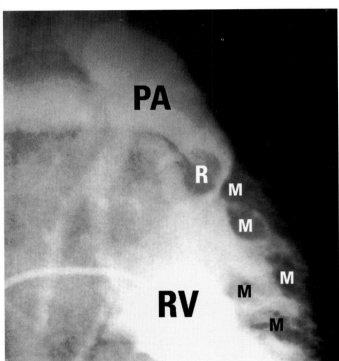

B

Fig. 6-20: Aortic valve prolapse complicating a doubly committed juxta-arterial ventricular septal defect.
A: Aortogram in right anterior oblique view shows the prolapsed right coronary cusp (R). It projects left anteriorly into the right ventricular outflow tract. **B:** Right ventriculogram in the same projection as in A. The prolapsed right coronary cusp is seen as a negative filling defect (R) immediately below the pulmonary valve. The right ventricular outflow tract is significantly encroached on by the prolapsed valve together with the hypertrophied muscle bundles (M).

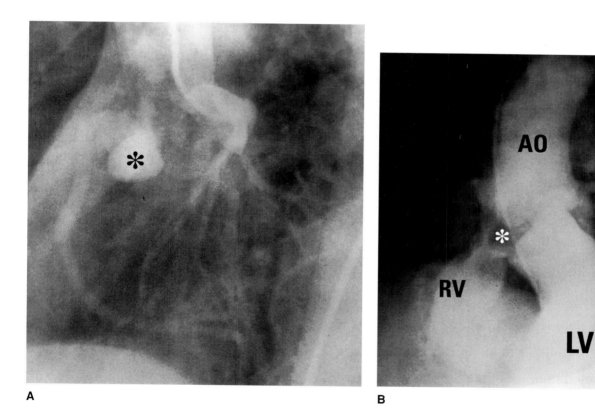

A

B

Fig. 6-21: Ancillary angiographic features of aortic valve prolapse in two different patients.
A: On aortography, most of the contrast medium is washed out by the unopacified blood from the left ventricle. The prolapsed part may be identified when there is an area of abnormal persistence of contrast accumulation (✳). **B:** On left ventriculography, the unopcaified blood in the ascending aorta is replaced by the opacified blood from the left ventricle by the first ventricular systole. The prolapsed part of the aortic valve may be identified, when there is an area of delayed opacification in the aortic sinus (✳).

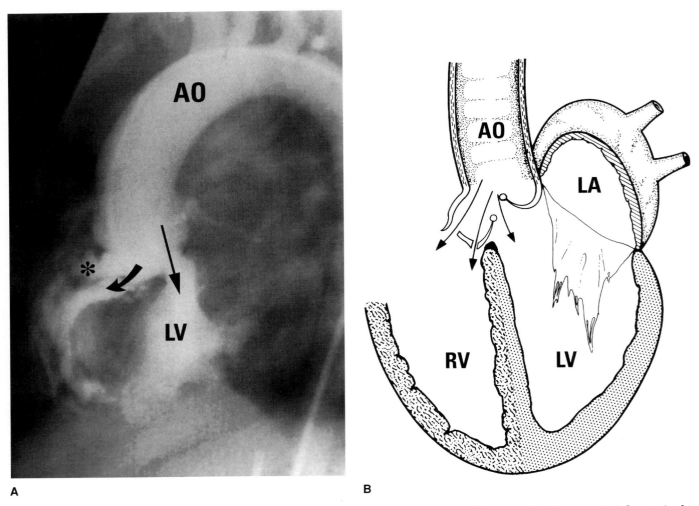

A

B

Fig. 6-22: Aortic regurgitation into the left and right ventricles complicating a doubly committed juxta-arterial ventricular septal defect.
A: Aortogram in left anterior oblique view shows the prolapsed right coronary cusp (✱) of the aortic valve. Both the right and left ventricles are opacified by the regurgitant flow (arrows) from the aorta. **B:** Diagrammatic representation of the case. The aortic regurgitation into the right ventricle is usually through the perforations in the aortic cusp and/or denuded sinus, in contrast to the regurgitation into the left ventricle, which is through the incompletely coaptated valve opening.

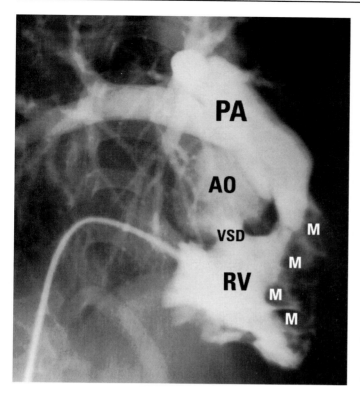

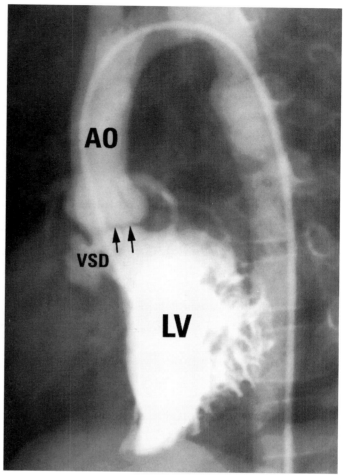

Fig. 6-23: Right ventricular outflow tract obstruction complicating a ventricular septal defect.
Right ventriculogram in right anterior oblique view shows multiple anomalous muscle bundles (M) seen as filling defects along the left anterior margin of the right ventricle. There is right-to-left shunting through a muscular outlet defect, which is spatially committed to the proximal high-pressure chamber.

Fig. 6-25: Fibrous ridge in the left ventricular outflow tract above the perimembranous ventricular septal defect.
Left ventriculogram in long axial oblique view shows a perimembranous defect. It is completely closed by the adherent tricuspid valve. A linear ridge (arrows) traverses the left ventricular outflow tract immediately below the aortic valve.

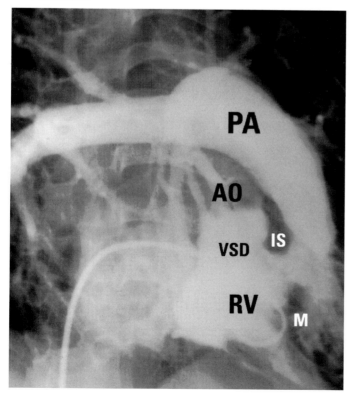

Fig. 6-24: Right ventricular outflow tract obstruction due to hypertrophy of the malaligned outlet septum.
Right ventriculogram in right anterior oblique view shows that the outlet septum (OS) is anteriorly malaligned and hypertrophied. Additional anomalous muscle bundle (M) contributes to the obstruction. There is right-to-left shunting through the perimembranous ventricular septal defect.

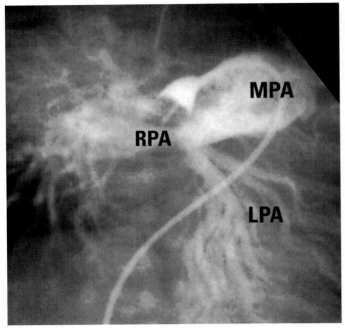

A

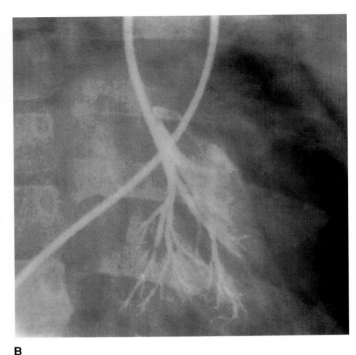

B

Fig. 6-26: Angiographic findings of pulmonary vascular obstructive disease in two different patients.
A: Pulmonary arteriogram shows severe tortuosity of the pulmonary artery branches. **B:** Selective injection into the pulmonary artery branch to a basal segment of the left lower lobe shows the pruned tree appearance with decreased number and irregular interval of origins of peripheral twigs. The capillary staining is nonhomogenous.

disease progresses, the shunt direction through the defect becomes bidirectional or from the right to the left ventricle. As a result of severe right ventricular hypertrophy, the right ventricular cavity may be significantly obliterated and its diastolic dimension is greatly reduced. When the defect is the anterior malalignment type, the right ventricular outflow tract morphology is not unlike that of tetralogy of Fallot except for the dilated pulmonary artery.

References

1. Fyler DC, Buckley LP, Hellenbrand WE, et al. Report of the New England Regional Infant Cardiac Program. *Pediatrics* 1980;65(suppl):376–461.
2. Newman TB. Etiology of ventricular septal defects: An epidemiologic approach. *Pediatrics* 1985;76:741–749.
3. Ferencz C, Rubin JD, McCarter RJ, et al. Congenital heart disease: Prevalence at live birth. The Baltimore-Washington infant study. *Am J Epidemiol* 1985;121:31–36
4. Grabitz RG, Joffres MR, Collins-Nakai RL. Congenital heart disease: Incidence in the first year of life. The Alberta heritage pediatric cardiology program. *Am J Epidemiol* 1988;128:381–388.
5. Hoffman JIE. Incidence of congenital heart disease: I. Postnatal incidence. *Pediatr Cardiol* 1995;16:103–113.
6. Freedom RM, Benson LN. Ventricular septal defect. In: Freedom RM, Benson LN, Smallhorn JF, eds. *Neonatal Heart Disease*. London: Springer-Verlag; 1992, pp. 571–591.
7. Rosenthal A, Bank ER. Ventricular septal defect. In: Moller JH, Neal WA, eds. *Fetal, Neonatal, and Infant Cardiac Disease*. Norwalk, CT: Appleton & Lange; 1990, pp. 371–390.
8. Moe DG, Guntheroth WG. Spontaneous closure of uncomplicated ventricular septal defect. *Am J Cardiol* 1987; 60:674–678
9. Hoffman JIE. Natural history of congenital heart disease. Problems in its assessment with specific reference to ventricular septal defect. *Circulation* 1968;37:97–125.
10. Mitchell SC, Korones SB, Berendes HW. Congenital heart disease in 56,109 births: Incidence and natural history. *Circulation* 1971;43:323–332.
11. Corone P, Doyon F, Gaudeau S, Guerin F, Vernant P, Ducam H, et al. Natural history of ventricular septal defect. *Circulation* 1977;55:908–915.
12. Mitchell SC, Berendes HW, Clark WM. The normal closure of the ventricular septum. *Am Heart J* 1967;73: 334–338.
13. Levy RJ, Rosenthal A, Fyler DC, et al. Birth weight of infants with congenital heart disease. *Am J Dis Child* 1978; 132:249–254.
14. Goor DA, Lillehei CW. The anatomy of the heart. In: *Congenital Malformations of the Heart. Embryology, Anatomy and Operative Considerations*. New York: Grune & Stratton; 1975, pp. 1–37.
15. Anderson RH, Becker AE. The fibrous skeleton of the heart. In: *Cardiac Anatomy. An Integrated Text and Atlas*. Edinburgh: Chuchill Livingstone; 1980, pp. 5.2–5.13.

15a. Goor D, Lillehei CW, Edwards JE. The "sigmoid septum": variation in the contour of the left ventricular outlet. *AJR* 1969;107:366–376.

16. Anderson RH, Becker AE, Van Mierop LHS. What should we call the "crista"? *Br Heart J* 1977;39:856–859.

17. Fellows KE, Keane JE, Freed MD. Angled view in cineangiography of congenital heart disease. *Circulation* 1977; 56:485–490.

18. Bargeron LM, Elliott LP, Soto B, Bream PR, Curry GC. Axial cineangiography in congenital heart disease. Section I: Technical and anatomic considerations. *Circulation* 1977;56:1075–1083.

19. Ceballos R, Soto B, Bargeron LM. Angiographic anatomy of the normal heart through angiography. *Circulation* 1981;64:351–359.

20. Becker AE. Atrioventricular septal defects. What's in a name? *J Thorac Cardiovasc Surg* 1982;83:461–469.

21. Selzer A. Defect of the ventricular septum. *Arch Intern Med* 1949;84:798–823.

22. Becu LM, Fontana RS, DuShane JW, Kirklin JW, Burchell HB, Edwards JE. Anatomic and pathologic studies in ventricular septal defect. *Circulation* 1956;14:349–364.

23. Kirklin JW, Harshbarger HG, Donald DE, Edwards JE. Surgical correction of ventricular septal defect: Anatomic and technical considerations. *J Thorac Surg* 1957;33: 45–59.

24. Warden HE, DeWall RA, Cohen M, Varco RL, Lillehei CW. A surgical-pathologic classification for isolated ventricular septal defects and for those in Fallot's tetralogy based on observations made on 120 patients during repair under direct vision. *J Thorac Surg* 1957;33:21–44.

25. Goor DA, Lillehei CW, Rees R, Edwards JE. Isolated ventricular septal defect. *Chest* 1970;58:468–482.

26. Lincoln C, Jamieson S, Joseph M, Shinebourne E, Anderson RH. Transatrial repair of ventricular septal defects with reference to their anatomic classification. *J Thorac Cardiovasc Surg* 1977;74:183–190.

27. Moulaert AJ. Anatomy of ventricular septal defect. In: Anderson RH, Shinebourne eds. *Pediatric Cardiology 1977*. Edinburgh: Churchill Livingstone; 1978, pp. 113–124.

28. Wenink ACG, Oppenheimer-Dekker A, Moulaert AJ. Muscular ventricular septal defects: A reappraisal of the anatomy. *Am J Cardiol* 1979;43:259–264.

29. Soto B, Becker AE, Moulaert AJ, Lie JT, Anderson RH. Classification of ventricular septal defects. *Br Heart J* 1980;43:332–343.

30. Capelli H, Andrade JL, Somerville J. Classification of the site of ventricular septal defect by 2-dimensional echocardiography. *Am J Cardiol* 1983;51:1474–1480.

31. Smolinsky A, Castaneda AR, Van Praagh R. Infundibular septal resection: Surgical anatomy of the superior approach. *J Thorac Cardiovasc Surg* 1988;95:486–494.

32. Soto B, Ceballos R, Kirklin JW. Ventricular septal defects: A surgical viewpoint. *J Am Coll Cardiol* 1989;14: 1291–1297.

33. Lev M. The pathologic anatomy of ventricular septal defects. *Dis Chest* 1959;35:533–545.

34. Anderson RH, Becker AE, Tynan M. Description of ventricular septal defects or how long is piece of string? *Int J Cardiol* 1986;13:267–278.

35. Becker AE, Anderson RH. Classification of ventricular septal defects—A matter of precision. *Heart Vessels* 1985; 1:120–121.

36. Anderson RH, Wilcox BR. The surgical anatomy of ventricular septal defect. *J Card Surg* 1992;7:17–35.

37. Neufeld HN, Titus JL, Dushane JW, Burchell HB, Edwards JE. Isolated ventricular septal defect of the persistent common atrioventricular canal type. *Circulation* 1961;23:685–696.

38. Milo S, Ho SY, Wilkinson JL, Anderson RH. Surgical anatomy and atrioventricular conduction tissues of hearts with isolated ventricular septal defects. *J Thorac Cardiovasc Surg* 1980;79:244–255.

39. Becu LM, Tauxe WN, DuShane JW, Edwart JE. A complex of congenital anomalies: Ventricular septal defect, biventricular origin of the pulmonary trunk, and subaortic stenosis. *Am Heart J* 1955;50:901–911.

40. Becker AE, Connor M, Anderson RH. Tetralogy of Fallot. A morphometric study. *Am J Cardiol* 1975;35:402–412.

41. Jaffe RB, Scherer JL. Supracristal ventricular septal defects: Spectrum of associated lesions and complications. *AJR* 1977;128:629–637.

42. Anderson RH, Lenox CC, Zuberbuhler JR. Morphology of ventricular septal defect associated with coarctation of aorta. *Br Heart J* 1983;50:176–181.

43. Moulaert AJ, Bruins CC, Oppenheimer-Dekker A. Anomalies of the aortic arch and ventricular septal defects. *Circulation* 1976;53:1011–1015.

44. Moulaert AJ, Oppenheimer-Deekker A. Anterolateral muscle bundle of the left ventricle, bulboventricular flange and subaortic stenosis. *Am J Cardiol* 1976;37: 78–81.

45. Freedom RM, Bain HH, Esplugas E, Dische R, Rowe RD. Ventricular septal defect in interruption of aortic arch. *Am J Cardiol* 1977;39:572–582.

46. Anderson RH, Wilcox BR. The surgical anatomy of ventricular septal defects associated with overriding valvar orifices. *J Card Surg* 1993;8:130–142.

47. Somerville J. Congenital heart disease: Changes in form and function. *Br Heart J* 1979;41:1–22.

48. Nir A, Driscoll DJ, Edwards WD. Intrauterine closure of membranous ventricular septal defects: Mechanism of closure in two autopsy specimens. *Pediatr Cardiol* 1994; 15:33–37.

49. Ramaciotti C, Vetter JM, Bornemeier RA, Chin AJ. Prevalence, relation to spontaneous closure, and association of muscular ventricular septal defect with other cardiac defects. *Am J Cardiol* 1995;75:61–65.

50. Freedom RM, White RD, Pieroni DR, Varghese JP, Krovetz JL, Rowe RD. The natural history of so-called aneurysm of the membranous ventricular septum in childhood. *Circulation* 1974;49:375–384.

51. Anderson RH, Lenox CC, Zuberbuhler JR. Mechanisms of closure of perimembranous ventricular septal defect. *Am J Cardiol* 1983;52:341–345.

52. Freedom RM, Moes CAF, Burrows PE, Perrin DE, Smallhorn JF. The angiocardiographic recognition of types of ventricular septal defects. In: Anderson RH, Neches WH, Park SC, Zuberbuhler JR, eds. *Perspectives in Pediatric Cardiology*. Volume 1. Mt. Kisco, NY: Futura Publishing Company, Inc; 1988, pp. 35–55.

53. Van Praagh R, McNamara JJ. Anatomic types of ventricular septal defect with aortic insufficiency. *Am Heart J* 1968;75:604–619.

54. Ando M, Takao A. Pathological anatomy of ventricular septal defect associated with aortic valve prolapse and regurgitation. *Heart Vessels* 1986;2:117–126.

55. Menahem S, Johns JA, Torso SD, et al. Evaluation of aortic valve prolapse in ventricular septal defect. *Br Heart J* 1986;56:242–249.

56. Burrows PE, Fellows KE, Keane JF. Cineangiography of the perimembranous ventricular septal defect with left ventricular-right atrial shunt. *J Am Coll Cardiol* 1983; 1:1129–1134.

56a. Riemenschneider TA, Moss JR. Left ventricular-right atrial communication. *Am J Cardiol* 1967;19:710–718.

57. Leung MP, Mok CK, Lo RNS, Lau KC. An echocardiographic study of perimembranous ventricular septal defect with left ventricular to right atrial shunting. *Br Heart J* 1986;55:45–52.

58. Gerbode F, Hultgren H, Melrose D, Osborn J. Syndrome of left ventricular-right atrial shunt. Successful surgical repair of defect in five cases, with observation of bradycardia on closure. *Ann Surg* 1958;148:433–446.

59. Mckay R, Battistessa SA, Wilkinson JL, Wright JP. A communication from the left ventricle to the right atrium: A defect in the central fibrous body. *Int J Cardiol* 1989;23:117–123.

60. Nadas A, Thilenius O, LaFarge C, Hauck A. Ventricular septal defect with aortic regurgitation: Medical and pathologic aspects. *Circulation* 1964;29:862–870.

61. Somerville J, Brandao A, Ross D. Aortic regurgitation with ventricular septal defect. *Circulation* 1970;41:317–330.

62. Tatsuno K, Konno S, Sakakibara S. Ventricular septal defect with aortic insufficiency: Angiographic aspects and a new classification. *Am Heart J* 1973;85:13–21.

63. Keane J, Plauth W, Nadas A. Ventricular septal defect with aortic regurgitation. *Circulation* 1977;56(suppl):72–77.

64. Okai Y, Miki S, Kusuhara K, et al. Long-term results of aortic valvuloplasty for aortic regurgitation associated with ventricular septal defect. *J Thorac Cardiovasc Surg* 1988;96:769–774.

65. Gasul BM, Dillon RF, Vrla V, Hait G. Ventricular septal defects. *JAMA* 1957;164:847–853.

66. Grant RP, Downey FM, Macmahon H. The architecture of the right ventricular outflow tract in the normal human heart and in the presence of ventricular septal defects. *Circulation* 1961;24:223–235.

67. Pongiglione G, Freedom RM, Cook D, Rowe RD. Mechanisms of acquired right ventricular outflow tract obstruction in patients with ventricular septal defects, An angiographic study. *Am J Cardiol* 1982;50:776–780.

68. Lauer RM, DuShane JW, Edwards JE. Obstruction of left ventricular outlet in association with ventricular septal defect. *Circulation* 1960;22:110–125.

69. Dirksen T, Moulaert AJ, Buis-Liem TN, Brom AG. Ventricular septal defect associated with left ventricular outflow tract obstruction below the defect. *J Thorac Cardiovasc Surg* 1978;75:688–694.

70. Vogel M, Freedom RM, Brand A, Trusler GA, Williams WG, Rowe RD. Ventricular septal defect and subaortic stenosis: An analysis of 41 patients. *Am J Cardiol* 1983; 52:1258–1263.

71. Freedom RM, Pelech A, Brand A, et al. The progressive nature of subaortic stenosis in congenital heart disease. *Int J Cardiol* 1985;8:137–143.

72. Moene RJ, Oppenheimer-Dekker A, Moulaert AJ, Wenink ACG, Gittenberger-de Groot AC, Roozendaal H. The concurrence of dimensional aortic arch anomalies and abnormal left ventricular muscle bundle. *Pediatr Cardiol* 1982;2:107–114.

73. Oppenheimer-Dekker A. Septal architecture in hearts with ventricular septal defects. In: Wenink ACG, Oppenheimer-Dekker A, Moulaert AJ, eds. *The Ventricular Septum of the Heart*. Hague: Leiden University Press; 1981, pp. 47–56.

74. Morais P. Westaby S, Hallidie-Smith KA. Left ventricular outflow tract obstruction due to anomalous mitral valve: Successful mitral valve replacement in a four month old infant. *Br Heart J* 1986;56:385–387.

75. Neufeld EA, Muster AJ, Paul MH, Idriss FS, Riker WL. Discrete subvalvular aortic stenosis in childhood. *Am J Cardiol* 1976;39:53–61.

76. Nanton MA, Belcourt CL, Gillis DA, Krause VW, Roy DL. Left ventricular outflow tract obstruction owing to accessory endocardial cushion tissue. *J Thorac Cardiovasc Surg* 1979;78:537–541.

77. Chung KJ, Fulton DR, Kreidberg MB, Payne DD, Creveland RJ. Combined discrete subaortic stenosis and ventricular septal defect in infants and children. *Am J Cardiol* 1984;53:1429–1432.

78. Rabinovitch M, Hawarth SG, Vance Z, et al. Early pulmonary vascular changes in congenital heart disease studied in biopsy tissue. *Human Pathol* 1980; 11(suppl):499–509.

79. Rabinovitch M, Keane JF, Fellows KE, Castaneda AR, Reid L. Quantitative analysis of the pulmonary wedge angiogram in congenital heart defects. Correlation with hemodynamic data and morphometric findings in lung biopsy tissue. *Circulation* 1981;63:152–164.

80. Haworth SG. Pulmonary vascular disease in different types of congenital heart disease. Implications for interpretation of lung biopsy findings in early childhood. *Br Heart J* 1984;52:557–571.

81. Haworth SG, Hall SM. Occlusion of intra-acinar pulmonary arteries in pulmonary hypertensive congenital heart disease. *Int J Cardiol* 1986;13:207–217.

82. Bush A, Busst CM, Haworth SG, et al. Correlations of lung morphology, pulmonary vascular resistance, and outcome in children with congenital heart disease. *Br Heart J* 1988;59:480–485.

83. Sutherland GR, Godman MJ, Smallhorn JF, Guiterras P, Anderson RH, Hunter S. Ventricular septal defects: Two dimensional echocardiographic and morphological correlations. *Br Heart J* 1982;47:316–328.

84. Baker EJ, Leung MP, Anderson RH, Fischer DR, Zuberbuhler JR. The cross sectional anatomy of ventricular septal defects: A reappraisal. *Br Heart J* 1988;59:339–351.

85. Yoo S-J, Lim T-H, Park I-S, Hong CY, Song MG, Kim SH. Defects of the interventricular septum of the heart: En face MR imaging in the oblique coronal plane. *AJR* 1991; 157:943–946.

86. Santamaria H, Soto B, Ceballos R, Bargeron LM, Coghlan HC, Kirklin JW. Angiographic differentiation of types of ventricular septal defects. *AJR* 1983;141:273–281.

87. Yoo S-J, Choi Y-H. Ventricular septal defect. In: *Angiocardiograms in Congenital Heart Disease*. Oxford: Oxford University Press; 1991, pp. 29–54.

88. Green CE, Elliott LP, Bargeron LM. Axial cineangiographic evaluation of the posterior ventricular septal defect. *Am J Cardiol* 1981;48:331–335.

89. Fellows KE, Westerman GR, Keane JF. Angiocardiography of multiple ventricular septal defects in infancy. *Circulation* 1982;66:1094–1099.

90. Griffin ML, Sullivan ID, Anderson RH, Macartney FJ. Doubly committed subarterial ventricular septal defect: New morphological criteria with echocardiographic and angiocardiographic correlation. *Br Heart J* 1988;59:474–479.

Chapter 7

Truncus Arteriosus or Common Arterial Trunk

The anomaly of truncus arteriosus, or common arterial trunk, is characterized by a single arterial trunk supported by the ventricular mass from which the coronary arteries, at least one pulmonary artery, and the brachiocephalic arteries originate.[1-11] With rare exception a ventricular septal defect is present.[3,12-15] Indeed, the reality of truncus arteriosus with an intact ventricular septum is one of those morphological considerations that led to the revision of the initial classification of truncus arteriosus provided by Collett and Edwards.[1] Untreated truncus arteriosus has a high mortality rate with many babies dying in the neonatal period or early infancy of congestive heart failure, often with an ischemic myocardium. The causes of myocardial ischemia are complex, reflecting both an unusual physiology as well as an often abnormal coronary arterial anatomy. About 65% of patients treated medically do not survive beyond 6 months of life, and more than 90% die before 1 year of age.[3,9,16-18] Data from Butto et al,[19] Collett and Edwards,[1] and Van Praagh and Van Praagh[9] summarized by Stanger[20] suggests that of 100 babies born with truncus arteriosus who are not treated surgically, 20 will die in the first week and at least 86 will die by 1 year of age. Rarely, a rare patient will survive with pulmonary vascular obstructive disease into the fourth decade of life or beyond.[17] Clinical experience also indicates that some patients with truncus arteriosus will survive past infancy without developing pulmonary vascular obstructive disease, but such patients are not common.[21,22]

Prevalence

Truncus arteriosus is an uncommon cardiac anomaly with a prevalence of 0.030 per 1000 live births.[16]

This defect, also designated as common aorticopulmonary trunk, truncus arteriosus, or common arterial trunk, is not usually genetically transmitted, nor is familial aggregation common.[23-29] However, the association between truncus arteriosus and the DiGeorge syndrome has been thoroughly documented.[28] This disorder has occasionally been recognized in siblings, and the prevalence of truncus arteriosus is thought higher in pregnancies complicated by maternal diabetes.[23,26,27] The Report of the New England Regional Infant Cardiac Program indicated that 33 of the 2251 infants (1.4%) with heart disease had truncus arteriosus.[16] These data also reported the prevalence at livebirth of 0.030 per 1000 for this lesion. The prevalence at livebirth data from the more current Baltimore-Washington Infant study was 0.056 per 1000.[24] Data from the Hospital for Sick Children in Toronto reported an incidence for truncus arteriosus of 0.7% of congenital heart disease.[30]

Classification of Truncus Arteriosus

The classification proposed by Collett and Edwards[1] in 1949 had been widely accepted, but in the past 15 years some important modifications to this original classification system have taken place (Table 7-1).

The original classification of Collett and Edward described four types of truncus arteriosus. Type 1: truncus arteriosus with a main pulmonary trunk; types 2 and 3: different sites of origin of the right and left pulmonary arteries from the ascending truncus arteriosis; and type 4: truncus arteriosis without any pulmonary arteries (Fig. 7-1). However, there current opinion is that type 4 truncus arteriosus is really a type of pulmonary atresia with ventricular septal defect. Calder

From: Freedom RM, Mawson JB, Yoo SJ, Benson LN: *Congenital Heart Disease: Textbook of Angiocardiography.* Armonk NY, Futura Publishing Co., Inc. ©1997.

Table 7-1

Collett and Edwards' Classification of Truncus Arteriosus*

Type 1: A single pulmonary trunk and ascending aorta arise from the truncus arteriosus.

Type 2: The right and left pulmonary arteries arise close together from the dorsal wall of the truncus arteriosus.

Type 3: One or both pulmonary arteries arise independently from either side of the truncus arteriosus.

Type 4: There are no pulmonary arteries and there is apparent congenital absence of the sixth aortic arches.

* From Collett and Edwards, 1949

Table 7-2

Modification of Collett and Edward's Classification of Truncus Arteriosus*

Type A: Ventricular septal defect present.

Type B: Ventricular septum intact.

Subgroup 1: Partially separate main pulmonary trunk.

Subgroup 2: Both pulmonary arteries arise separately from the truncus.

Subgroup 3: Absence of one pulmonary artery from the ascending aorta.

Subgroup 4: Underdevelopment of the aortic arch.

* From Calder et al, 1976

and colleagues with Van Praagh[3] from the Children's Hospital in Boston used material from the Cardiac Registry and surveyed the published records. They developed a classification that focuses on the presence of a ventricular septal defect (type A) or its absence (type B), as well as on the site of origin of the pulmonary arteries (Table 7-2).[3]

Type A1 has a partially separate main pulmonary trunk because of the presence of an incompletely formed aortopulmonary septum (Figs. 7-1 through 7-3). The short main pulmonary trunk usually originates from the left posterolateral aspect of the common arterial trunk, and only rarely, anteriorly. In Type A2, the aortopulmonary septum is absent and the pulmonary arteries originate separately from the truncus. Type A3 is characterized by absence of either the right or left pulmonary artery. The absent pulmonary artery will originate from either a ductus arteriosus or a major aortopulmonary collateral; the more common is a ductal origin.[1,9,31–40] Those patients with truncus arteriosus and either interruption of the aortic arch, atresia of the aortic arch, preductal coarctation of the aortic arch, or severe diffuse hypoplasia of the aortic arch are classified as type A4 (Fig. 7-3). The classification of Collett and Edwards did not mention obstructive anomalies of the aortic arch, a not insignificant population.[3,10,11,41–43] This particular population has a well-documented correlation with DiGeorge syndrome.[28]

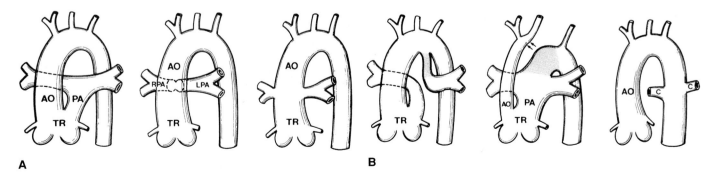

A   **B**

Fig. 7-1: Classification of types of truncus arteriosus or common arterial trunk.
A: Left panel: The two right-sided diagrams have been grouped as one form of truncus arteriosus. **B:** Right panel: That form with so-called pulmonary arteries originating from the descending aorta is more appropriately considered pulmonary atresia and ventricular septal defect.

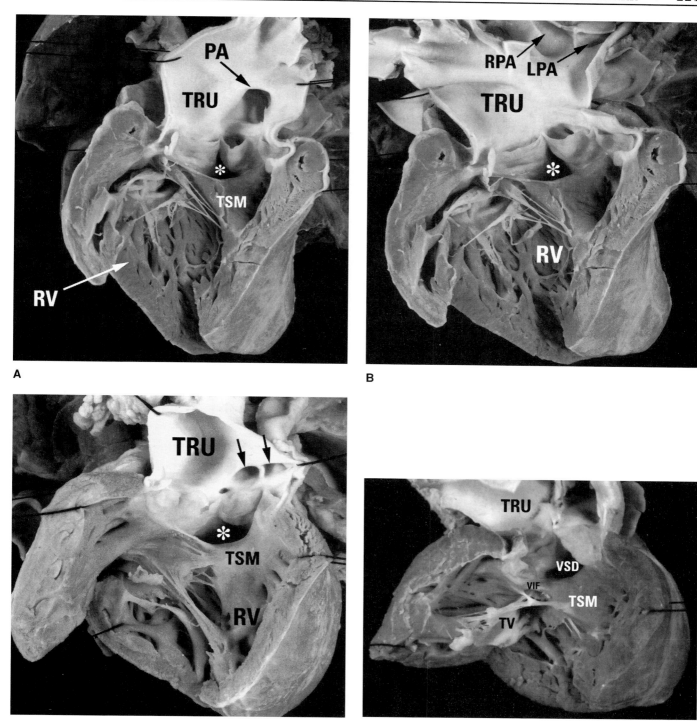

Fig. 7-2: The morphology of truncus arteriosus.
A: Right ventricular view of a patient with a short main pulmonary trunk (arrow); the ventricular septal defect is roofed by the common arterial trunk (✳). **B**: A long main pulmonary trunk bifurcating into right and left pulmonary arteries (arrows). **C**: That form of truncus arteriosus with separate origins of both pulmonary arteries (arrows). **D and E**: The ventricular septal defect in truncus arteriosus viewed from the right and left ventricle. The right-sided ventriculoinfundibular fold is attenuated, and thus the truncal and tricuspid valves are nearly in continuity with the ventricular septal defect cradled in the limbs of the trabecula septo-marginalis. The ventricular septal defect does not extend into the membranous septum (see Chapter 6). From the left ventricle, the truncal valve roofs the ventricular septal defect, and continuity between the mitral and truncal valves is conspicuous.

(continued on next page)

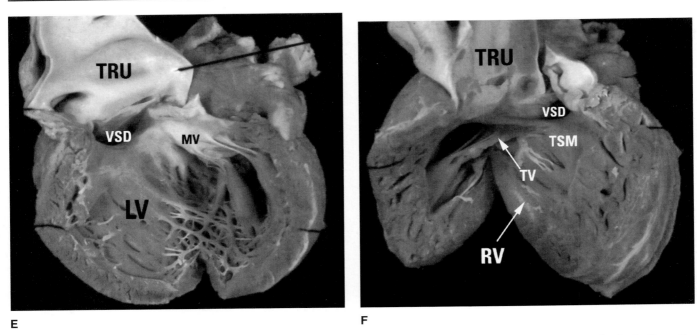

Fig. 7-2: *Continued.* **F:** A relatively small ventricular septal defect in a patient whose truncus originates exclusively from the right ventricle.

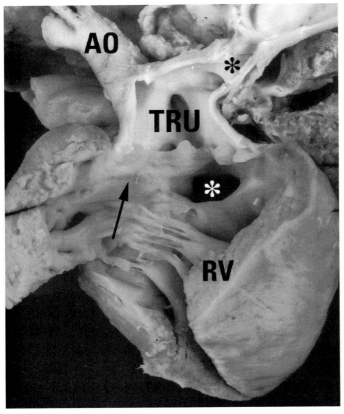

Fig. 7-3: Truncus arteriosus with interruption of the aortic arch.
A: Internal view of truncus with interruption of the aortic arch showing the arterial duct (✱) confluent with the descending aorta and the left subclavian artery originating from the descending aorta; the tricuspid valve is separated from the truncal valve by the attenuated right-sided ventriculoinfundibular fold (black arrow). *(continued)*

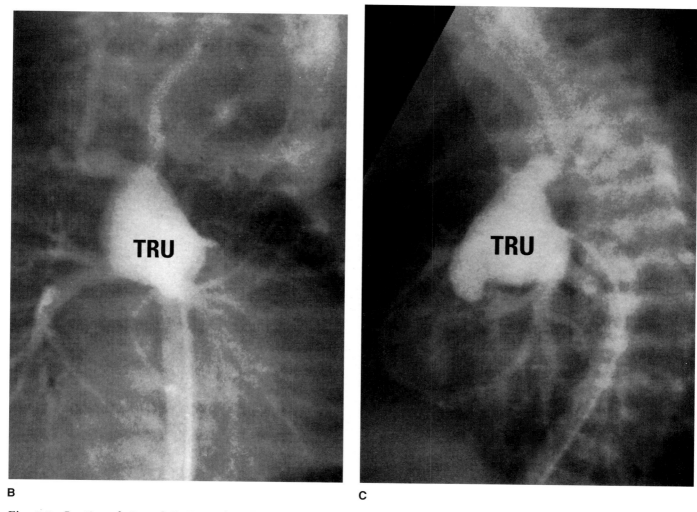

Fig. 7-3: *Continued.* **B and C**: Frontal and lateral truncal root angiograms of a newborn with truncus arteriosus with interruption of the aortic arch.

Morphology and Morphogenesis

Three hypotheses have been used to explain the development of this lesion. 1) This defect represents partial or total absence of the aorticopulmonary septum, complete absence of fusion of the truncal swellings and the conal ridges that normally join to form the arterial valves and the distal infundibulum. 2) Van Praagh and colleagues consider truncus arteriosus to be closely related to tetralogy of Fallot, and thus, truncus arteriosus represents absence or severe attenuation of the distal pulmonary infundibulum, with defects of the aortopulmonary septum, and ventricular septum. 3) This defect represents the absence of a common arterial vessel downstream from the semilunar valve.[3,9,10,41,44]

Segmental Analysis

Hearts with truncus arteriosus are usually left-sided and the atrial situs is solitus.[2–11] With rare exception, the hearts are biventricular, the atrioventricular connections are concordant, and there is often fibrous continuity between mitral valve and the truncal valve. The right-sided ventriculoinfundibular fold may be attenuated, thus permitting continuity or nearly so between truncal valve and tricuspid valve (Figs. 7-2 and 7-3).[2,4,8] Occasionally, the single arterial root originates entirely above the right ventricle.[1,3,5,7,9,10,31,34,35,45] Truncus arteriosus has been observed in the patient with right atrial isomerism and presumed asplenia.[46] Truncus arteriosus has also been observed in the patient with tricuspid atresia, as well as other forms of double-inlet ventricle.[2,6,47-50] A common arterial trunk has also been identified in the patient with hypoplastic left ventricle and intact ventricular septum as well as in the patient with mitral atresia and a hypoplastic left ventricle (see Table 7-2).[14,15,51] Another rare variant is common arterial trunk with a discordant atrioventricular connection.[51a]

The Truncal Valve

The truncal valve can theoretically possess one to six cusps, but the unicommissural, pentacuspid, and hexacuspid valves are uncommon.[2-4,9-11,20-21,52-61] Calder and colleagues from Boston Children's Hospital reported that 61% of their patients had a tricuspid truncal valve; 31% had a quadricuspid valve; and 8% had a bicuspid valve (Fig. 7-4).[3] Among the 54 cases reported from the United Hospital in Minneapolis, 42% had a tricuspid truncal valve, 30% had a bicuspid valve, and 24% had a quadricuspid valve.[19]

The truncal valve may guard the ventriculoarterial junction normally, or the valve may be stenotic or regurgitant, or both. Truncal valve leaflet thickening may

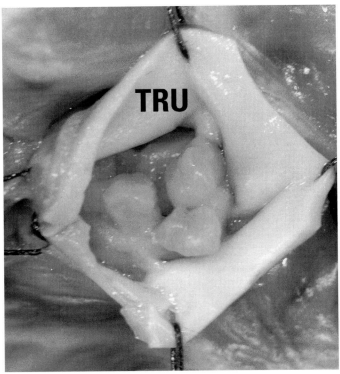

A

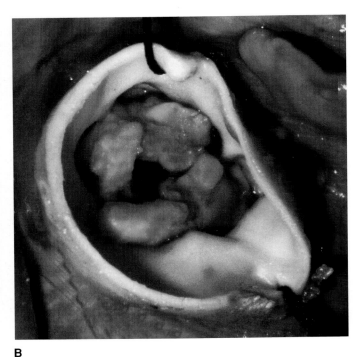

B

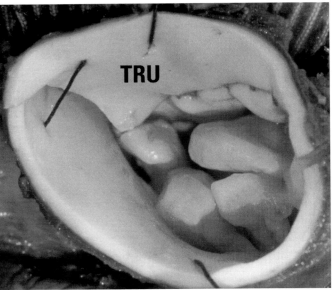

C

Fig. 7-4: Severe truncal valve stenosis in neonates.
A through C: Three different patients with severely abnormal quadricuspid truncal valves. Commissural fusion is relatively mild.

be mild, moderate, or severe (Fig. 7-4). In this last group the truncal valve may be nodular, polypoid, and myxomatous.[52–61] Severe truncal valve regurgitation has been reported as a serious complication[55] and truncal valve replacement has been required in the symptomatic infant.

The Ventricular Septum

With very rare exceptions a ventricular septal defect is present in truncus arteriosus.[10–15] When the ventricular septum is intact, the common arterial trunk may originate either above the right or left ventricle. In the patient with an intact ventricular septum and left ventricular origin of the arterial trunk as reported by Zeevi and colleagues,[15] the right ventricle was small, hypertensive, and there were extensive ventriculocoronary connections. In those patients with exclusive origin of the truncus above the morphological right ventricle and intact ventricular septum, the left ventricle is usually underdeveloped. The ventricular septal defect results from absence of the infundibular septum and is found in the limbs of the trabecula septomarginalis (Figs. 7-2 and 7-3). When viewed from the right ventricle, the ventricular septal defect is beneath the truncal valve, and is cradled in the superior and posterior limbs of the trabecula septomarginalis.[2–4,9–11,19,21,31] Usually the posterior rim of the ventricular septal defect is muscular, reflecting fusion of the posterior limb of the trabecula septomarginalis with the ventriculoinfundibular fold, and the defect is therefore separated from the annulus of the tricuspid valve, and thus from the conduction tissue. Less frequently the ventricular septal defect extends to the tricuspid valve and thus is both perimembranous and subarterial. Ventricular septal defects may be present remote from this area, but are uncommon. Truncus may be found with atrioventricular septal defect. The infundibular ventricular septal defect is usually large, but may be actually or potentially restrictive, especially in those patients where the truncus originates almost entirely above the right ventricle.[62,62a] Multiple ventricular septal defects have been described in patients with truncus arteriosus.[21]

Pulmonary Artery Anomalies or Ostial Stenosis

Most patients with persistent truncus arteriosus have excessive pulmonary blood flow, and if not treated, die of congestive heart failure. The pulmonary blood flow is restrictive in about 10% of patients with truncus arteriosus. The mechanism responsible for limiting the pulmonary blood flow in most of these patients is ostial stenosis resulting from an obstructive truncal leaflet.[3,9,10,19,21,31,35,37] Less commonly the pulmonary arteries will be truly underdeveloped. Significant pulmonary artery anomalies include distal ductal

Table 7-3

Pulmonary Artery Abnormalities in Truncus Arteriosus

Distal ductal or ligamental origin
Origin of one pulmonary artery from direct aortopulmonary collateral
Pulmonary artery stenosis
Pulmonary ostial stenosis
Pulmonary artery hypoplasia
Crossed pulmonary arteries

origin of one pulmonary artery; origin of a pulmonary artery from an aortopulmonary collateral; unilateral absence of one pulmonary artery; or hypoplasia of one pulmonary artery, and pulmonary arterial stenosis (Table 7-3).[31–37a]

In those patients with distal ductal origin of one pulmonary artery and origin of the other pulmonary artery from the ascending aorta, it may be difficult to differentiate this anomaly from a complex form of pulmonary atresia with ventricular septal defect (see Chapter 21). True pulmonary atresia has been observed in truncus arteriosus.[39] In this situation, the atretic main pulmonary trunk originates from the truncus, not the ventricular mass, and an imperforate pulmonary valve should not be present. The pulmonary arteries may be crossed—a most unusual situation—usually in those patients with associated interruption of the aortic arch (see also Chapter 19, Fig. 19-40).[63–65] The pulmonary arteries may be distorted by palliative pulmonary artery banding, and for this reason Litwin and others[66,67] had advocated surgical creation of ostial stenosis, although today this procedure is rarely required because of the widely accepted approach of primary repair in the neonate.[4,21,36,37]

The Coronary Arterial Circulation

The coronary arteries exhibit a variable pattern of origin independent of the number of truncal valve leaflets.[3,4,9–11,68–75] An abnormally high origin of a coronary artery, usually the right, has been observed in this disorder. Frank myocardial ischemia reflects the disordered hemodynamics with a torrential pulmonary blood flow, a volume loaded left ventricle, and a low aortic diastolic or coronary artery driving pressure. Rarely, a coronary ostium will be congenitally stenotic and this will promote an ischemic myocardium. Uncommonly, the coronary ostium will be just superior to the truncal valve commissure, and a bulky, fleshy truncal valve leaflet will obstruct the coronary ostium, resulting in coronary insufficiency.[21,54,71–75] Anderson, McGoon, and Lie[68] described large infundibular branches of the right coronary artery that crossed the upper anterior surface of the right ventricle to supply the anterobasal surface of both ventricles and the upper portion of the ventricular septum, indicating the vulnerability of these arteries to surgical right ventriculotomy. Lenox, Debich, and Zuberbuhler[69,73] and others have examined the role of coronary artery abnormalities in the prognosis of truncus arteriosus. A substantial instance of coronary ostial and arterial abnormalities was found in the study of Lenox and colleagues[73] of 30 pathological specimens of truncus arteriosus including the left coronary ostium in a posterior and high position; proximity of the left coronary ostium to the pulmonary artery segment in trileaflet truncal valves; stenosis of the coronary ostium; acute angle take-off of the cononary artery; single coronary artery, etc.[73] Daskaloupoulos and colleagues[72] described a patient who died of acute myocardial ischemia at the time of pulmonary banding. The pulmonary artery band compromised flow into a circumflex coronary artery originating from the right pulmonary artery. Ventriculocoronary connections have been identified in the patient with truncus arteriosus and an intact ventricular septum.[15] The findings in this patient are similar to those in patients with pulmonary atresia and intact ventricular septum (see Chapter 23); double-outlet left ventricle (see Chapter 38), and aortic atresia with a discordant ventriculoarterial connection (see Chapters 26 and 35).

Laterality of the Aortic Arch

A right-sided aortic arch is present in 20% to 30% of patients with truncus arteriosus.[3,4,9,10] An occasional patient with a common arterial trunk has a double aortic arch.[3a]

Obstructive Anomalies of the Aortic Arch

Coarctation of the aorta, aortic arch atresia, and interruption of the aortic arch, usually type B, can complicate the basic morphologic expression of truncus arteriosus. Ductus arteriosus is also usually present.[2–4,9–11,19,21,31,36,38,41–44] Interruption of a right-sided aortic arch has also been noted.

Uncommon Lesions

Persistent truncus arteriosus has been described in patients with associated complete form of atrioventricular septal defect; tricuspid atresia; single ventricle; hypoplastic left ventricle; double-orifice mitral valve, and total anomalous pulmonary venous return.[3,19,31] Crossed pulmonary arteries have been described in truncus arteriosus, usually but not invariably with associated interruption of the aortic arch (see also Chapter 19).[63–65]

Imaging of Truncus Arteriosus

The majority of babies with uncomplicated truncus arteriosus are referred to surgery at the Toronto Hospital for Sick Children on the basis of the clinical examination and cross-sectional echocardiography with Doppler and color interrogation. The classic echocardiographic features of truncus arteriosus in its many variations have been widely documented, including fetal recognition.[4,21,76–81] Rao and colleagues[82] have reviewed the association between truncus arteriosus and tricuspid atresia, and have documented the echocardiographic features in one such case.[82]

Angiocardiography of Truncus Arteriosus

In our institution, there must be specific indications before a cardiac catheterization with angiography is performed in the patient with truncus arteriosus.[21] A hemodynamic study is indicated to determine surgical candidacy in the older infant or child where pulmonary vascular obstructive disease is being considered or in the older patient with one pulmonary artery.[32,33] The specific anatomic indications relate to the demonstration of ventricular anatomy, pulmonary artery anatomy, or to definition of a specific coronary artery anomaly.

Angiography performed in patients with truncus arteriosus should demonstrate the morphology and functional competency of the truncal valve, the disposition of the coronary arteries and their epicardial distribution, the integrity of the aortic arch, and the topography of the pulmonary arteries (Figs. 7-3, and 7-5 through 7-17).

The truncal origins and length of the main pulmonary trunk are readily defined by selective injection of contrast either into the truncal root, the main pulmonary artery, or selective injection of right or left pulmonary arteries (Figs. 7-5 through 7-8). If only one pulmonary artery is visualized by aortography performed in the ascending portion of the truncus, then aortography performed in the descending thoracic aorta and/or direct aortopulmonary collaterals or pulmonary vein wedge angiography may be necessary to demonstrate the caliber of the non-visualized pulmonary artery (Figs 7-9 through 7-11). For those patients with pulmonary arterial stenosis or hypoplasia, a selective pulmonary artery injection may be necessary (Figs. 7-12 and 7-13).

In those patients with either a type 1 or type 2 truncus arteriosus, but with a normal transverse aortic arch and isthmus, the pulmonary arteries seem to be an appendage of the much larger aortic component of the common arterial trunk (Figs. 7-5 through 7-14). Among those patients with aortic arch interruption, the ascending aortic component often appears to be an appendage of the much larger pulmonary artery compo-

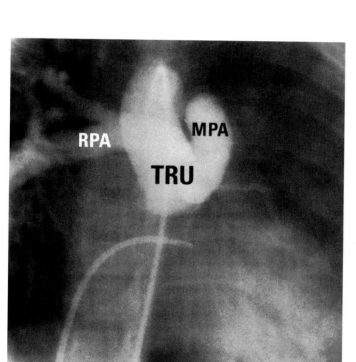

A

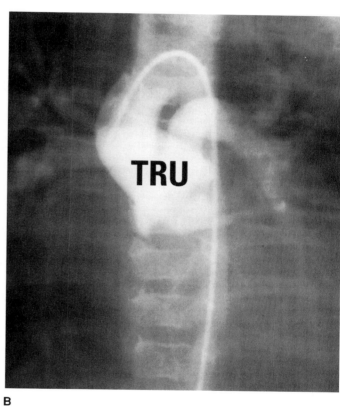

B

Fig. 7-5: Angiographic appearance of truncus arteriosus with well-developed main pulmonary trunk (A), and with short main pulmonary trunk (B).

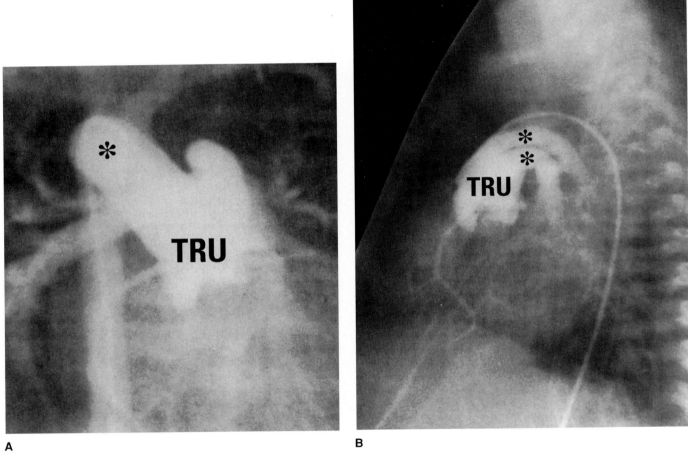

A

B

Fig. 7-6: Angiographic appearance of truncus arteriosus with well-developed main pulmonary trunk and right aortic arch in frontal (A) and lateral projections (B).

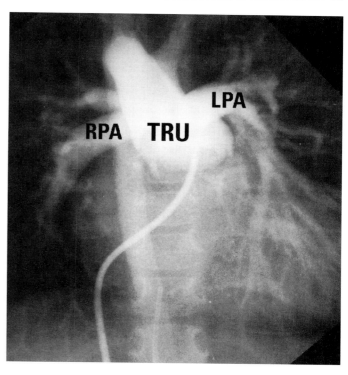

Fig. 7-8: Angiographic appearance of truncus arteriosus with separate origins of right and left pulmonary arteries and right aortic arch in frontal projection.

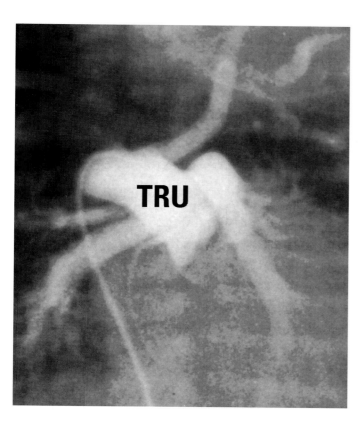

Fig. 7-7: Angiographic appearance of truncus arteriosus with short main pulmonary trunk and right aortic arch in frontal projection.

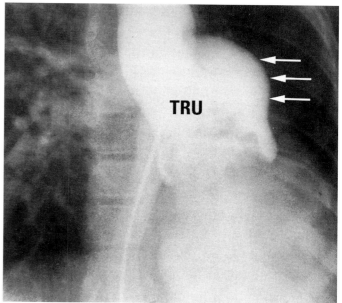

Fig. 7-9: An older child with a type I truncus and so-called absent left pulmonary artery (arrows).

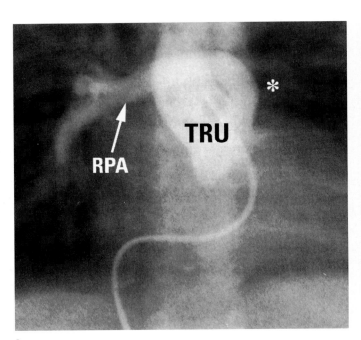 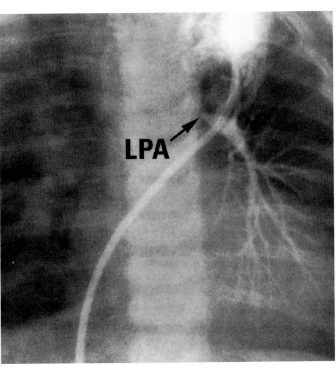

A   **B**

Fig. 7-10: A young infant with a common arterial trunk and so-called absent left pulmonary artery, ie, distal ductal origin.
A: Frontal injection of contrast into the truncal root from the venous approach demonstrates absence of the left pulmonary artery (✱). **B:** A left pulmonary vein wedge angiogram demonstrates the hilar pulmonary artery with its somewhat superior orientation, consistent with a ligamental origin.

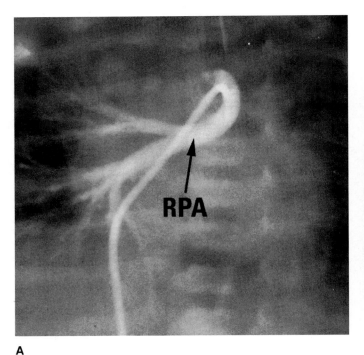 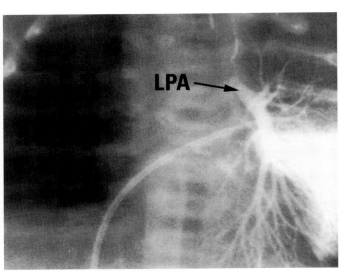

A   **B**

Fig. 7-11: Another young infant with with a common arterial trunk and so-called absent left pulmonary artery, ie, distal ductal origin.
A: Selective injection into the main pulmonary trunk shows an unusual course to the solitary right pulmonary artery. **B:** A left pulmonary vein wedge angiogram demonstrates the hilar pulmonary artery with its somewhat superior orientation, consistent with a ligamental origin.

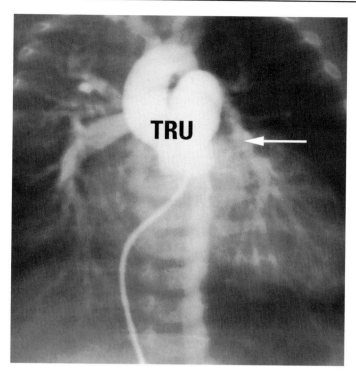

Fig. 7-12: Truncus arteriosus with hypoplasia of the left pulmonary artery (arrow).
(This figure was kindly provided by Dr. G. Cumming, Winnipeg, Manitoba.)

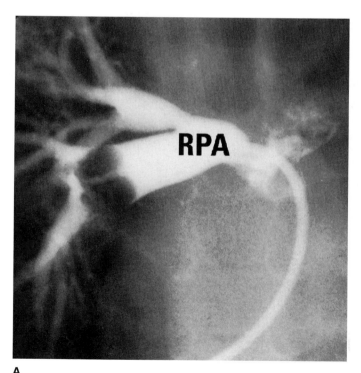

A

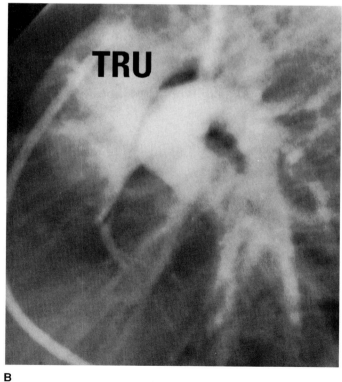

B

Fig. 7-13: Truncus arteriosus with right pulmonary artery stenosis. This 5-year-old child underwent correction because the vascular bed had been protected.

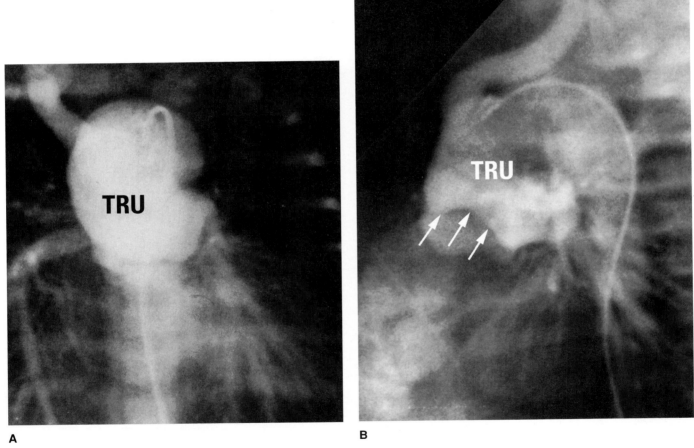

A   **B**

Fig. 7-14: Truncal root angiogram of a patient with severe and fatal truncal valve stenosis.
A: The truncal root is very dilated. **B:** Doming of the truncal valve is evident (arrows).

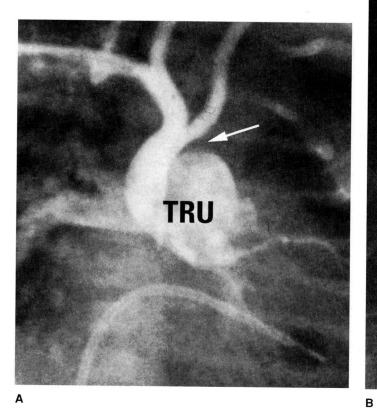

A

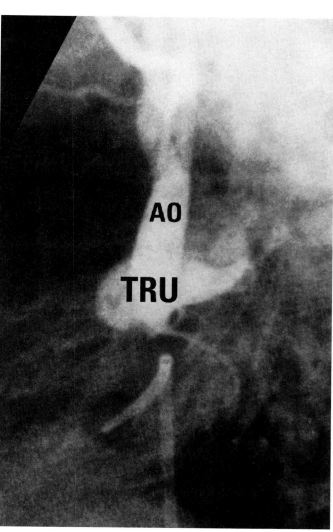

B

Fig. 7-15: Truncus arteriosus with interruption of the aortic arch (arrow).
A and B: Frontal and lateral injections into the truncal root. Note the aortic portion of the truncus seemingly originates from the pulmonary component and the aorta seems relatively small (see also Fig.7–3).

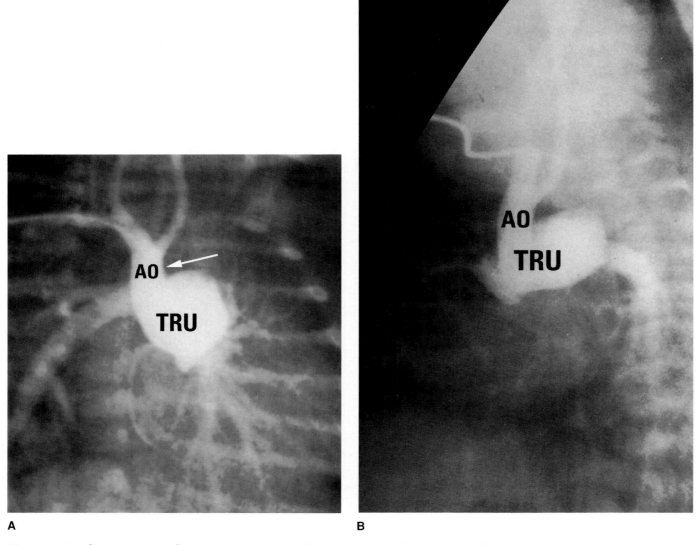

A

B

Fig. 7-16: Another neonate with truncus arteriosus with interruption of the aortic arch (arrow).
A and B: Frontal and lateral injections into the truncal root. As in Figs. 7-3 and 7–15, the aortic portion of the truncus seemingly originates from the pulmonary component and the aorta is small.

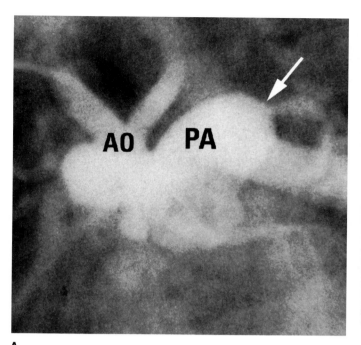

A

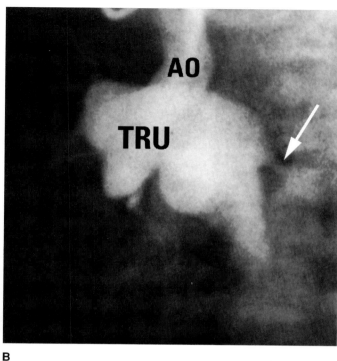

B

Fig. 7-17: A severely constricted arterial duct in a newborn with truncus arteriosus with interruption of the aortic arch (arrow).
A: Left anterior oblique. **B:** Lateral injection into truncal root demonstrates the ductal anatomy (arrow).

nent of the truncus (Figs. 7-3, 7-15 through 7-17).[21,41] Furthermore, in the lateral projection, the course of the retrograde arterial catheter takes a considerably more inferior course into the truncal root when there is interruption, remembering the spatial distribution between the fourth and sixth arches.[21,41]

The ventricular anatomy is remarkably constant in truncus arteriosus. Biplane right and left ventricular angiocardiography should demonstrate the intracardiac anatomy, although as stated earlier, this is rarely required today.[3,20,83–87] The infundibular ventricular septal defect is best profiled by right and left long axial oblique angiography. Whether the ventricular septal defect extends to the tricuspid valve annulus or if it has a just a muscular posteroinferior rim can be determined by observing the continuity or discontinuity of the truncal valve with the tricuspid valve in the elongated right axial oblique view. Occasionally, multiple ventricular

septal defects are present (Fig. 7-18). If echocardiographic examination suggests an inlet muscular ventricular septal defect or an atrioventricular septal defect, then the hepatoclavicular projection should be utilized (see Chapters 2 and 5). An excellent review of the angiographic features of truncus arteriosus was published by Yoshizato and Julsrud.[87] Peculiar origins and course of the pulmonary arteries will be demonstrated by selective injection of contrast into the truncal root or directly into the pulmonary arteries (Fig. 7-19). When truncus arteriosus is associated with airway compression, other imaging modalities may be required to determine the mechanism of bronchial compression.[88] Common arterial trunk has been reported in patients with underdeveloped right or left ventricle (Fig. 7-20). There is only limited experience with percutaneous balloon dilatation of a stenotic truncal valve in a newborn.[89]

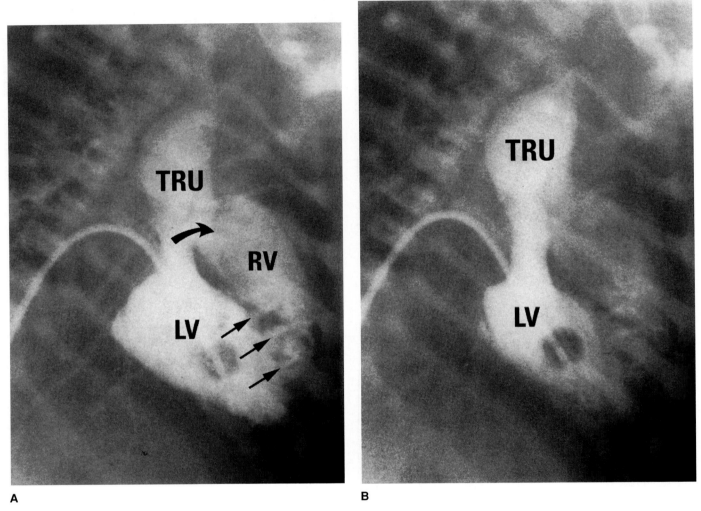

A   **B**

Fig. 7-18: Multiple ventricular septal defects in a neonate with truncus arteriosus.
A and B: Frames from a right axial oblique left ventriculogram show multiple anterior muscular ventricular septal defects (straight arrows) in addition to the usual defect resulting from an absent infundibular septum (curved arrow).

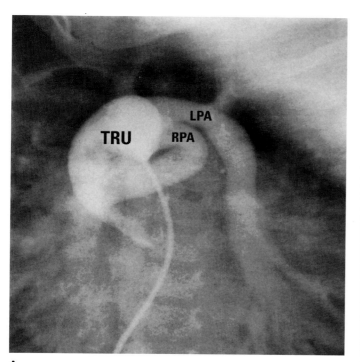

A

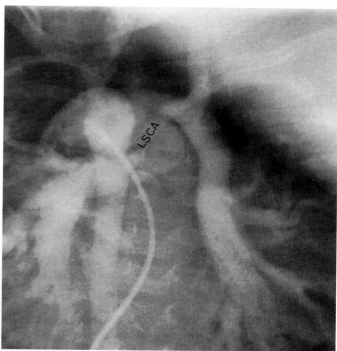

B

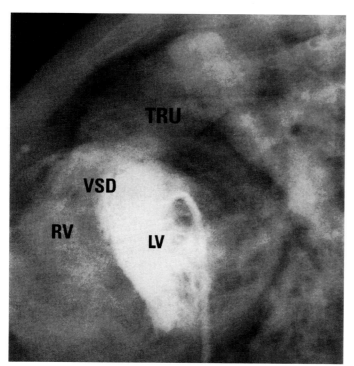

C

Fig. 7-19: Unusual course of pulmonary arteries in a patient with truncus arteriosus.
A and B: The injection of contrast into the truncal root shows the peculiar course of the right and left pulmonary arteries. **C**: Left ventriculogram shows the typical ventricular septal defect.

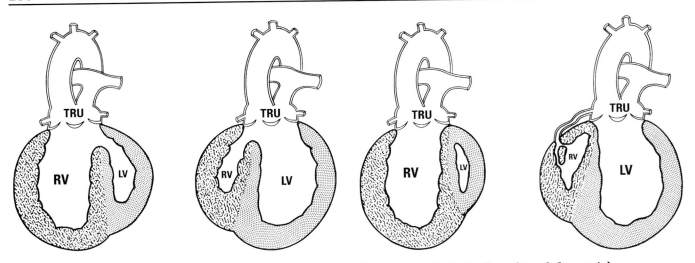

Fig. 7-20: Diagram showing common arterial trunk with hypoplasia of morphologically right or left ventricle.
The right drawing shows a patient with hypoplasia of the morphologically right ventricle, an intact ventricular septum, and ventriculocoronary connections

Differential Diagnoses

Before the application of either cross-sectional echocardiography or angiocardiography, any substantial left-to-right shunt at great artery level should be included in the differential diagnosis of truncus arteriosus. Thus, the clinical differentia diagnoses include patent arterial duct; aortopulmonary window; origin of one pulmonary artery from the ascending aorta; arteriovenous fistula; aortico-left ventricular tunnel, etc. Certain very rare entities must be considered including aortic atresia with aortopulmonary window, aortic atresia with aortico-left venticular tunnel, aortic origin of both right and left pulmonary arteries but with a main pulmonary trunk, and the triarterial heart.[90–93] Finally, there is increasing experience with the echocardiographic identification of thymic tissue, an issue germane to the management of those patients with conotruncal abnormalities associated with DiGeorge syndrome.[94]

References

1. Collett RW, Edwards JE. Persistent truncus arteriosus: A classification according to anatomic types. *Surg Clin North Am* 1949;29:1245–1270.

2. Anderson RH, Thiene G. Categorization and description of hearts with a common arterial trunk. *Eur J Cardiothorac Surg* 1989;3:481–487.

3. Calder L, Van Praagh R, Van Praagh S, Sears WP, Corwin R, Levy A, Keith JD, Paul MH. Truncus arteriosus communis. *Am Heart J* 1976;92:23–38.

3a.Albolaris ET, Lombardo S, Antillon J. Truncus arteriosus ith double aortic arch: Two-dimensional and color flow Doppler echocardiographic diagnosis. *Am Heart J* 1995;129:415–417.

4. Anderson RH, Macartney FJ, Shinebourne EA, Tynan M. *Paediatric Cardiology*. Volume 2. Edinburgh: Churchill Livingstone; 1987, pp. 913–929.

5. Crupi G, Macartney FJ, Anderson RH. Persistent truncus arteriosus. *Am J Cardiol* 1977;40:569–578.

6. Tandon R, Edwards JE. Tricuspid atresia: A re-evaluation and classification. *J Thorac Cardiovasc Surg* 1974;67:530–542.

7. Thiene G, Bortolotti U, Gallucci V, Terribile V, Pellegrino PA. Anatomical study of truncus arteriosus communis with embryological and surgical considerations. *Br Heart J* 1976;38:1109–1123.

8. Thiene G. Truncus arteriosus communis: Eleven years later. *Am Heart J* 1977;93:809.

9. Van Praagh R, Van Praagh S. The anatomy of common aorticpulmonary trunk (truncus arteriosus communis) and its embryologic implications. *Am J Cardiol* 1965;16:406–425.

9a.Berdjis F, Wells WJ, Starnes VA. Truncus arteriosus with total anomalous pulmonary venous return and interrupted arch. *Ann Thorac Surg* 1996;61:220–222.

10. Van Praagh R. Classification of Truncus arteriosus communis. *Am Heart J* 1976;92:129–132.

11. Van Praagh R. Truncus arteriosus: What is it and how should it be classified? *Eur J Cardiothorac Surg* 1987;1:65–70.

12. Carr I, Bharati S, Kusnoor VS, Lev M. Truncus arteriosus communis with intact ventricular septum. *Br Heart J* 1979;42:97–102.

12a.Murdison KA, McLean DA, Carpenter B, Duncan WJ. Truncus arteriosus communis associated with mitral valve and left ventricular hypoplasia without ventricular septal defect: Unique combination. *Pediatr Cardiol* 1996;17:322–326.

13. Swift LFR, Shimomura S, Ryan SF, Van Praagh R. New type of truncus arteriosus communis with two semilunar valves, aortic valvar atresia and no ventricular septal defect. *Circulation* 1969;40(suppl III):199.

14. Alves PM, Ferrari AH. Common arterial trunk arising ex-

clusively from the right ventricle with hypoplastic left ventricle and intact ventricular septum. *Int J Cardiol* 1987;16(1):99–102.

15. Zeevi B, Dembo L, Berant M. Rare variant of truncus arteriosus with intact ventricular septum and hypoplastic right ventricle. *Br Heart J* 1992;68:214–215.

16. Fyler DC. Report of the New England Regional Infant Cardiac Program. *Pediatrics* 1980;65(suppl):376–461.

17. Hicken P, Evans D, Heath D. Persistent truncus arteriosus with survival to the age of 38 years. *Br Heart J* 1966;28:284–286.

18. Marcelletti C, McGoon DC, Mair DD. The natural history of truncus arteriosus. *Circulation* 1976;54:108–111.

19. Butto F, Lucas RV, Edwards JE. Persistent truncus arteriosus: Pathologic anatomy in 54 cases. *Pediatr Cardiol* 1986;7:95–101.

20. Stanger P. Truncus arteriosus. In: Moller JH, Neal WA, eds. *Fetal, Neonatal, and Infant Cardiac Disease.* Norwalk, CT: Appleton and Lange; 1989, pp. 587–602.

21. Freedom RM. Anomalies of aortopulmonary septation: Persistent truncus arteriosus, aortopulmonary septal defect, and hemitruncus arteriosus. In: Freedom RM, Benson LN, Smallhorn JF, eds. *Neonatal Heart Disease.* London: Springer-Verlag; 1992, pp. 428–452.

22. Juaneda E, Haworth SG. Pulmonary vascular disease in children with truncus arteriosus. *Am J Cardiol* 1984;54:1314–1320.

23. Ferencz C, Rubin JD, McCarter R J, Clark EB. Maternal diabetes and cardiovascular malformations: Predominance of double outlet right ventricle and truncus arteriosus. *Teratology* 1990;41:319–326.

24. Ferencz C, Rubin JD, McCarter RJ, Brenner JI, Neill CA, Perry LW, Hepner SI, Downing JW. Congenital heart disease: Prevalence at livebirth. The Baltimore-Washington Infant Study. *Am J Epidemiol* 1985;121:31–36.

25. Grabitz RG, Joffres MR, Collins-Nakai RL. Congenital heart disease: Incidence in the first year of life. The Alberta Heritage Pediatric Cardiology Program. *Am J Epidemiol* 1988;128:381–388.

26. le Marec B, Odent S, Almange C, Journel H, Roussey M. Defawe G. Truncus arteriosus: An autosomal recessive disease? *J Genet Hum* 1989;37:225–230.

27. Pierpont MEM, Gobel JW, Moller JH, Edwards JE. Cardiac malformations in relatives with truncus arteriosus or interruption of the aortic arch. *Am J Cardiol* 1988;61:423–427.

28. Radford DJ, Perkins L, Lachman R, Thong YH. Spectrum of DiGeorge syndrome in patients with truncus arteriosus: Expanded DiGeorge syndrome. *Pediatr Cardiol* 1988;9:95–101.

29. Thomas IT, Jewett T, Raines KH, Gash C, Garber-P. New lethal syndrome of fetal akinesia with characteristic facial appearance, severe microphthalmia, microtia, and truncus arteriosus in two male sibs. *Am J Med Genet* 1993;46:180–181.

30. Keith JD. Prevalence, incidence, and epidemiology. In: Keith JD, Rowe RD, Vlad P, eds. *Heart Disease in Infancy and Children.* Third edition. New York: MacMillan; 1978, pp. 3–13.

31. Bharati S, McAllister HA Jr, Rosenquist GC, Miller RA, Tatooles CJ, Lev M. The surgical anatomy of truncus arteriosus communis. *J Thorac Cardiovasc Surg* 1980;67:501–510.

31a. Di Segni E, Lew S, Shapira H, Kaplinsky E. Double mitral valve orifice. *Pediatr Cardiol* 1986;6:215–217.

32. Fyfe DA, Driscoll DJ, Di Donato RM, Puga FJ, Danielson GK, McGoon DC, Mair DD. Truncus arteriosus with single

pulmonary artery: Influence of pulmonary vascular obstructive disease on early and late operative results. *J Am Coll Cardiol* 1985;5:1168–1172.

33. Mair DD, Ritter DG, Danielson GK, Wallace RB, McGoon DC. Truncus arteriosus with unilateral absence of a pulmonary artery: Criteria for operability and surgical results. *Circulation* 1977;55:641–647.

34. Van Der Horst RL, Gotsman MS. Type 3C truncus arteriosus: Case report with clinical and surgical implications. *Br Heart J* 1974;36:1046–1048.

35. Rossiter SJ, Silverman JF, Shumway NE. Patterns of pulmonary arterial supply in patients with truncus arteriosus. *J Thorac Cardiovasc Surg* 1978;75:73–79.

36. Bove EL, Lupinetti FM, Pridjian AK, Beekman RH III, Callow LB, Snider AR, Rosenthal A. Results of a policy of primary repair of truncus arteriosus in the neonate. *J Thorac Cardiovasc Surg* 1993;105:1057–1066.

37. Gerlis LM, Ho SY, Smith A, Anderson RH. The site of origin of nonconfluent pulmonary arteries from a common arterial trunk or from the ascending aorta: Its morphological significance. *Am J Cardiovasc Pathol* 1990;3:115–120.

37a. Luisi VS, Vanini V, Del Sarto P, Giusti S. Truncus arteriosus con inusuale anatomia delle arterie polmonari: descrizione di un caso trattato chirurgicamente. *G Ital Cardiol* 1993;23:899–903.

38. Hanley FL, Heinemann MK, Jonas RA, Mayer JE Jr, Cook NR, Wessel DL, Castaneda AR. Repair of truncus arteriosus in the neonate. *J Thorac Cardiovasc Surg* 1993;105:1047–1056.

39. Schofield DE, Anderson RH. Common arterial trunk with pulmonary atresia. *Int J Cardiol* 1988;20:290–294.

40. Ziemer G, Luhmer I, Siclari F, Kallfelz HC. Truncus arteriosus type A3: Complex repair with cryopreserved pulmonary homograft. *Eur J Cardiothorac Surg* 1987;1:100–115.

41. Moes CAF, Freedom RM. Aortic arch interruption with truncus arteriosus or aorticopulmonary septal defect. *AJR* 1980;135:1011–1016.

42. Rothko K, Moore GW, Hutchins GM. Truncus arteriosus malformation: A spectrum including fourth and sixth aortic arch interruptions. *Am Heart J* 1980;99:17–24.

43. Thiene G, Cucchini F, Pellegrino PA. Truncus arteriosus communis associated with underdevelopment of the aortic arch. *Br Heart J* 1975;37:1268–1274.

44. Van Mierop LHS, Patterson DF, Schnarr WR. Pathogenesis of persistent truncus arteriosus in light of observations made in a dog embryo with the anomaly. *Am J Cardiol* 1978;41:755–762.

45. Angelini P, Verdugo AL, Illera JP, Leachman RD. Truncus arteriosus communis: Unusual case associated with transposition. *Circulation* 1977;56:1107–1110.

46. Gumbiner CH, McManus BM, Latson LA. Associated occurrence of persistent truncus arteriosus and asplenia. *Pediatr Cardiol* 1991;12:192–195.

47. Areias JC, Lopes JM. Common arterial trunk associated with absence of one atrioventricular connexion. *Int J Cardiol* 1987;17:329–333.

48. Diogenes TCP, Atik E, Aiello VD. Common arterial trunk associated with absence of right atrioventricular connexion. *Int J Cardiol* 1990;27:385–388.

49. Rao PS. Tricuspid atresia with common arterial trunk. *Int J Cardiol* 1991;30:367–368.

50. Sreeram N, O Alvarado O, Peart I. Tricuspid atresia with common arterial truck: Surgical palliation in a neonate. *Int J Cardiol* 1991;32:251–253.

51. Rice MJ, Andrilenas K, Reller MD, McDonald RW. Truncus arteriosus associated with mitral atresia and a hypoplastic left ventricle. *Pediatr Cardiol* 1991;12:128–130.

51a. Marino B, Ballerini L, Soro A. Ventricular inversion with truncus arteriosus. *Chest* 1990;98:239–241.

52. Becker AE, Becker MJ, Edwards JE. Pathology of the semilunar valve in persistent truncus arteriosus. *J Thorac Cardiovasc Surg* 1971;62:16–26.

53. Burnell RH, McEnery G, Miller GAH. Truncal valve stenosis. *Br Heart J* 1971;33:423–424.

54. Chernausek SD, Swan DS, Moller JH, Vlodaver Z, Edwards JE. Clinical pathologic conference. *Am Heart J* 1976;91:249–254.

55. Deely WJ, Hagstom JM, Engle MA. Truncus insufficiency. Common truncus arteriosus with regurgitant truncal valves. Report of 4 cases. *Am Heart J* 1963;65:542–548.

56. Elami A, Laks H, Pearl JM. Truncal valve repair: Initial experience with infants and children. *Ann Thorac Surg* 1994;57:397–402.

57. Fugelstad SJ, Puga FJ, Danielson GK, Edwards WD. Surgical pathology of the truncal valve: A study of 12 cases. *Am J Cardiovasc Pathol* 1988;2:39–47.

58. Gelband H, Van Meter S, Gersony WM. Truncal valve abnormalities in infants with persistent truncus arteriosus. *Circulation* 1972;45:397–403.

59. Ledbetter MK, Tandon R, Titus JL, Edwards JE. Stenotic semilunar valve in persistent truncus arteriosus. *Chest* 1976;69:182–187.

60. Lee MH, Bellon EM, Liebman J, Perrin EV. Truncal valve stenosis. *Am Heart J* 1973;85:397–400.

61. Patel RG, Freedom RM, Bloom KR, Rowe RD. Truncal or aortic valve stenosis in functionally single arterial trunk. *Am J Cardiol* 1978;42:800–809.

62. Rosenquist GC, Bharati S, McAllister HA, Lev M. Truncus arteriosus communis: Truncal valve anomalies associated with small conal or truncal septal defects. *Am J Cardiol* 1976;37:410–412.

62a. Delius RE, Embry RP, Behrendt DM. Late development of functional subvalvar stenosis after repair of truncus arteriosus. *Pediatr Cardiol* 1996;17:393–395.

63. Becker AE, Becker MJ, Edwards JE. Malposition of pulmonary arteries (crossed pulmonary arteries) in persistent truncus arteriosus. *Am J Radiol* 1970;110:509–514.

64. Jue KL, Lockman LA, Edwards JE. Anomalous origins of pulmonary arteries from pulmonary trunk ("crossed pulmonary arteries"). *Am Heart J* 1966;71:807–812.

65. Wolf WJ, Casta A, Nichols M. Anomalous origin and malposition of the pulmonary arteries (crisscross pulmonary arteries) associated with complex congenital heart disease. *Pediatr Cardiol* 1986;6:287–291.

66. Litwin SB, Friedberg DZ. Pulmonary artery plication: A new surgical procedure for small infants with type 1 truncus arteriosus. *Ann Thorac Surg* 1983;35:192–196.

67. Mistrot JJ, Varco RL, Nicoloff DM. Palliation of infants with truncus arteriosus through creation of a pulmonary artery ostial stenosis. *Ann Thorac Surg* 1976;22:495–497.

68. Anderson KR, McGoon DC, Lie JT. Surgical significance of the coronary arterial anatomy in truncus arteriosus communis. *Am J Cardiol* 1978;41:76–81.

69. Bogers AJJC, Bartelings MM, Bokenkamp R, Stijnen T, van Suylen RJ, Poelmann RE, Gittenberger-de Groot A. Common arterial trunk, uncommon coronary arterial anatomy. *J Thorac Cardiovasc Surg* 1993;106:1133–1137.

69a. Oddens JR, Bogers AJ, Witsenburg M, Bartelings MM, Bos E. Anatomy of the proximal coronary arteries as a risk factor in primary repair of common arterial trunk. *J Cardiovasc Surg* 1994;35:295–299.

70. Daskalopoulos DA, Edwards WD, Driscoll DJ, Schaff HV, Danielson GK. Fatal pulmonary artery banding in truncus arteriosus with anomalous origin of circumflex coronary artery from right pulmonary artery. *Am J Cardiol* 1983;52:1363–1364.

71. de la Cruz MV, Cayre R, Angelini P, Noriega Ramos N, Sadowinski S. Coronary arteries in truncus arteriosus. *Am J Cardiol* 1990;66:1482–1486.

72. Deshpande J, Desai M, Kinare S. Persistent truncus arteriosus—an autopsy study of 16 cases. *Int J Cardiol* 1992;37:395–399.

73. Lenox CC, Debich DE, Zuberbuhler JR. The role of coronary arterial abnormalities in the prognosis of truncus arteriosus. *J Thorac Cardiovasc Surg* 1992;104:1728–1742.

74. Shrivastava S, Edwards JE. Coronary arterial origin in persistent truncus arteriosus. *Circulation* 1977;55:551–554.

75. Suzuki A, Ho SY, Anderson RH, Deanfield JE. Coronary arterial and sinusal anatomy in hearts with a common arterial trunk. *Ann Thorac Surg* 1989;48:792–797.

76. de Araujo LML, Schmidt KG, Silverman NH, Finkbeiner WE. Prenatal detection of truncus arteriosus by ultrasound. *Pediatr Cardiol* 1987;8:261–263.

77. Hagler DJ, Tajik AJ, Seward JB, Mair DD, Ritter DG. Wide-angle two-dimensional echocardiographic profiles of conotruncal abnormalities. *Mayo Clin Proc* 1980;55:73–82.

78. Rice MJ, Seward JB, Hagler DJ, Mair DD, Tajik AJ. Definitive diagnosis of truncus arteriosus by two-dimensional echocardiography. *Mayo Clin Proc* 1982;57:476–481.

79. Riggs TW, Paul MH. Two-dimensional echocardiographic prospective diagnosis of common truncus arteriosus in infants. *Am J Cardiol* 1982;50:1380–1384.

80. Silverman N. *Pediatric Echocardiography.* Baltimore: Williams and Wilkins; 1993, pp. 229–243.

81. Smallhorn JF, Anderson RH, Macartney FJ. Two dimensional echocardiographic assessment of communications between ascending aorta and pulmonary trunk or individual pulmonary arteries. *Br Heart J* 1982;47:563–572.

82. Rao PS, Levy JM, Nikicicz E, Gilbert-Barness EF. Tricuspid atresia: Association with persistent truncus arteriosus. *Am Heart J* 1991;122:829–835.

83. Ceballos R, Soto B, Kirklin JW, Bargeron Jr LM. Truncus arteriosus: An anatomical-angiographic study. *Br Heart J* 1983;49:589–599.

84. Freedom RM, Culham JAG, Moes CAF. *Angiocardiography of Congenital Heart Disease.* New York: MacMillan Publishing Company; 1984, pp. 437–452.

85. Soto B, Pacifico A. *Angiocardiography in Congenital Heart Malformations.* Mt. Kisco, NY: Futura Publishing Company, Inc; 1990.

86. Hallermann FJ, Kincaid OW, Tsakiris AG, Ritter DG, Titus JL. Persistent truncus arteriosus: A radiographic and angiocardiographic study. *Anat Pathol* 1968;107:827–834.

87. Yoshizato T, Julsrud PR. Truncus arteriosus revisited: An angiographic demonstration. *Pediatr Cardiol* 1990;11:36–40.

88. Habbema L, Losekoot TG, Becker AE. Respiratory distress due to bronchial compression in persistent truncus arteriosus. *Chest* 1980;77:230–232.

89. Ballerini L, Cifarelli A, Di Carlo D. Percutaneous balloon dilatation of stenotic truncal valve in a newborn. *Int J Cardiol* 1989;23:270–272.

90. Bricker DL, King SM, Edwards JE. Anomalous aortic origin of the right and left pulmonary arteries in a normally septated truncus arteriosus. *Chest* 1975;68:591–594.

91. Beitzke A and Shinebourne EA. Single origin of right and left pulmonary arteries from ascending aorta, with main pulmonary artery from right ventricle. *Br Heart J* 1980;43:363–365.

92. Aotsuka H, Nagai Y, Saito M, Matsumoto H, Nakamura T. Anomalous origin of both pulmonary arteries from the ascending aorta with a nonbranching main pulmonary artery arising from the right ventricle. *Pediatr Cardiol* 1990;11:156–158.

93. Diaz-Gongora G, Quero-Jimenez M, Espino-Vela J, Arteaga M, Bargeron L. A heart with three arterial trunks (tritruncal heart). *Pediatr Cardiol* 1982;3:293–299.

94. Yeager SB, Sanders SP. Echocardiographic identification of thymic tissue in neonates with congenital heart disease. *Am Heart J* 1995;129:837–838.

Chapter 8

Aortopulmonary Window

The aortopulmonary window (septal defect or fenestration)[1] is an uncommon cardiac anomaly characterized by a communication, often large, between the ascending aorta and pulmonary trunk.[2–8] While considered clinically related to truncus arteriosus and located in the same area of the heart, evidence provided by Kutsche and Van Mierop[4] suggests that these two anomalies are probably pathogenetically unrelated. The shape and size of the aortopulmonary window are variable, but it is always related to the aortic wall above the aortic sinuses containing the coronary arteries. The aortopulmonary window can occur in isolation, but it has been found with a wide variety of other cardiac anomalies. Yen Ho and colleagues[9] remind us that the designation of this defect as an aortopulmonary septal defect is inappropriate because there is no or little septum between the arterial trunks.

Prevalence

The New England Regional Infant Cardiac Program identified only 7 of 2251 infants with an aortopulmonary window.[10] Two of these occurred in isolation; 3 were in patients with associated interruption of the aortic arch, and 1 each with coarctation of the aorta and tetralogy of Fallot. Kutsche and Van Mierop[4] defined an incidence of this anomaly of 0.2% (13 of 6522 children with congenital heart disease). The incidence for this lesion from the Hospital for Sick Children in Toronto is 0.171 per 1000.[11] Of 4390 patients surveyed by the Baltimore-Washington Infant Study, an aortopulmonary window was identified in only 8.[12]

Morphology and Morphogenesis

Kutsche and Van Mierop[4] define three types of aortopulmonary window: 1) a defect with a more or less circular border, located between the arterial valves and the bifurcation of the main pulmonary artery; 2) a similarly located fenestration in which the border represents a helix, and 3) a large defect with no posterior or distal border. These authors suggest a different pathogenesis for each of the three types. The first type may reflect nonfusion of the embryonic aorticopulmonary and truncal septa. The second type suggests malalignment of the embryonic aorticopulmonary and truncal septi, while the third type results from total absence of the embryonic aorticopulmonary septum.

Yen Ho[9] and colleagues have examined 25 specimens with aortopulmonary window. The window was in a proximal position in 3 specimens, intermediate in 3 specimens, distal in 16 specimens, and confluent in 3 specimens (Fig. 8-1). Of the 16 specimens with the distal type of aortopulmonary window, the right pulmonary artery arose from the aorta in 7. This is a well-known association.[4]

Associated Malformations

Data compiled by Kutsche and Van Mierop[4] in a review of 249 patients with aorticopulmonary window (including 13 of their own) showed that in about 48% of the patients where information was available, no other cardiac lesions were identified, whereas associated cardiac malformations were present in 52%. Perhaps the most common associated lesion was either type A interruption of the aortic arch or severe preductile coarctation of the aorta (see Chapter 33).[3,4,9,13–18] Other lesions included anomalous origin of one or both coronary arteries from the pulmonary trunk, right pulmonary artery from the ascending aorta, especially in those with a distal type of aortopulmonary window (see Chapter 9), tetralogy of Fallot, bicuspid aortic valve, ventricular septal defect, pulmonary atresia and ven-

From: Freedom RM, Mawson JB, Yoo SJ, Benson LN: *Congenital Heart Disease: Textbook of Angiocardiography.* Armonk NY, Futura Publishing Co., Inc. ©1997.

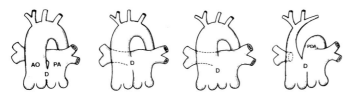

Fig. 8-1: Schematic diagram showing types of aortopulmonary window.

tricular septal defect, or cor triatriatum.[4,9,19–36A] Aortic atresia has been found in patients with an aortopulmonary septal defect and interruption of the aortic arch (see Chapter 26).[37–39] Delayed recognition of anomalous origin of the circumflex coronary artery originating from the pulmonary artery many years after repair of aortopulmonary window has been reported.[35a] Transposition of the great arteries has been complicated by a large aortopulmonary communication.[28,28a]

Gerlis and colleagues[33] have reviewed the literature on the presence or absence of the arterial duct in the patient with an aortopulmonary window. Obviously an arterial duct is present in those patients with an aortopulmonary septal defect and interruption of the aortic arch. Gerlis reminds us that Coleman and colleagues[40] consider the association between aortopulmonary window and patent arterial duct to be rare. However, data compiled by Neufeld and colleagues[7] indicated that among 66 cases of aortopulmonary window, a patent arterial duct was found in 8 cases, similar to that reported by Deverall and colleagues[41] who reported that 2 of 8 had an arterial duct. A fifth aortic arch with a systemic-to-systemic connection was identified in a patient with an aortopulmonary septal defect, discordant ventriculoarterial connections, pulmonary atresia, a right aortic arch, and an aortic coarctation.[33,42,43]

The timing of clinical presentation of patients with aortopulmonary window may be determined by the associated lesions.[2,3,7,44] Those with associated interruption of the aortic arch or severe preductile coarctation of the aorta will present in the neonatal period. The defect is small in about 10% of all patients with aortopulmonary septal defect, and thus, these fortunate few would present considerably later, much like the child with a small- to moderate-sized patent arterial duct in isolation. Remembering that in most patients with this anomaly of aortopulmonary septation, the defect is large, one is not surprised when symptoms related to a large pulmonary blood flow and pulmonary hypertension, tachypnea, dyspnea, poor feeding, and diphoresis are observed late in the first month of life coincident with maturation of the fetal pulmonary vascular bed.

Nonassociation with DiGeorge Syndrome

There is a well-known association between abnormalities of the third and fourth phayngeal pouch and interruption of the aortic arch (see Chapter 33), truncus arteriosus (see Chapter 7), and other conotruncal abnormalities. This association has **not** been documented with aortopulmonary septal defect.[4,44]

Echocardiography

In the newborn period while the pulmonary arterial pressure is high, this the aortopulmonary window type of lesion can be missed if the echocardiographer relies solely on Doppler echocardiography. It is therefore imperative that a thorough examination of the aortopulmonary septum is performed. It is also important to understand which lesions occur in association with aortopulmonary window (see above, p.***). The diagnosis of aortopulmonary window is readily made by echocardiography when a combination of subcostal, precordial, and suprasternal views are used.[44–53a] The aortopulmonary window with interruption of the aortic arch and aortic origin of the right pulmonary artery has also been diagnosed by magnetic resonance imaging.[54]

Hemodynamics and Angiocardiography

Before the routine application of echocardiography, the first suggestion of the existence of the possibility of the existence of an aortopulmonary window was often an unusual catheter course.[2,3,6,7,20,26,36,38] The venous catheter would advance into the main pulmonary trunk, and then, to the operator's surprise, to the ascending aorta through the defect (Fig. 8-2). The hemodynamics reflect the presence of the associated lesions, but in the patient with an isolated large fenestration, arterial oxygen saturation is normal or nearly so. Substantial left-to-right shunting at atrial level is not uncommon, reflecting a large pulmonary blood flow and shunting through a stretched patent foramen ovale.

Pulmonary artery and right ventricular pressures are at systemic levels. A higher pressure in the main pulmonary trunk than in the descending thoracic aorta is consistent with an obstructive anomaly of the aortic arch and a narrowed or closing arterial duct.

The role of cardiac angiography is to demonstrate the presence of the aortopulmonary window and to demonstrate or exclude the presence of important associated anomalies (Figs. 8-3 through 8-5).[38,44,55] Biplane right ventricular angiography with some craniocaudal angulation will demonstrate the origin of the main pul-

Fig. 8-3: Large aortopulmonary window demonstrated by lateral aortogram.
A: Early and **(B)** later frames showing very large aortopulmonary window (✱) in a patient who developed pulmonary vascular obstruction after surgical closure.

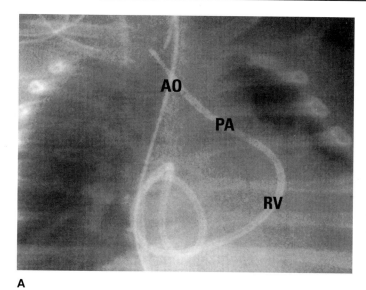

A

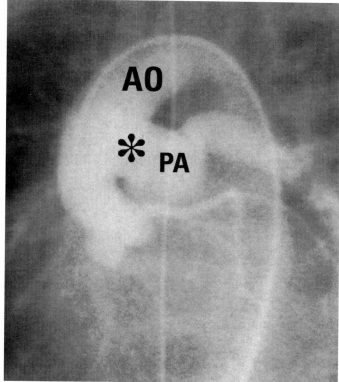

B

Fig. 8-2: **Course of venous catheter in a patient with aortopulmonary window.**
A: The venous catheter has been advanced from the right ventricle to the pulmonary artery and through the aortopulmonary window to the ascending aorta. **B:** The retrograde lateral aortogram shows the aortopulmonary window (✻) in this patient.

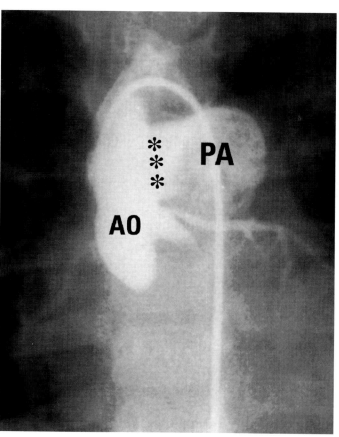

A

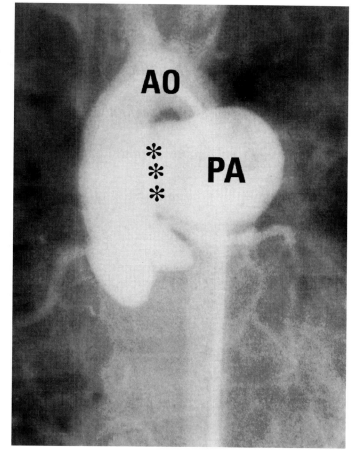

B

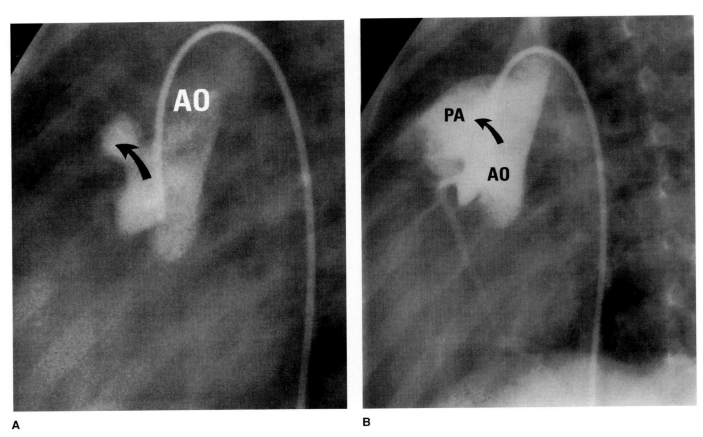

A

B

Fig. 8-4: A different patient with a large aortopulmonary window.
A and B: The aortopulmonary window is shown (arrow) by an aortogram filmed in the lateral and (**C**) right anterior oblique (✱) projections.

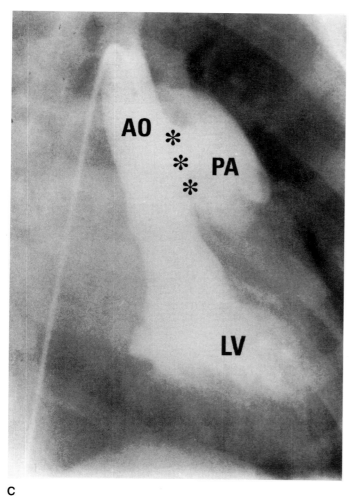

C

Fig. 8-4: *Continued.*

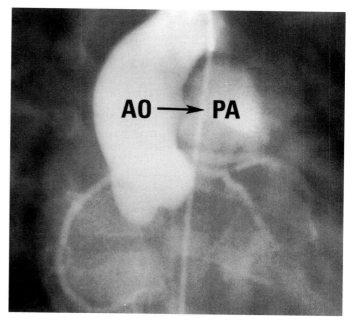

Fig. 8-5: A small aortopulmonary window (arrow) successfully closed in the cardiac catheterization laboratory

monary trunk from the right ventricular infundibulum, and in the lateral projection, the main pulmonary trunk can be seen crossing in front of the aorta. Selective injection of contrast into the ascending aorta demonstrates the size and extent of the aortopulmonary window, and with varying obliquity, one should be able to exclude aortic origin of a pulmonary artery (see Chapter 9). Aortography should as well demonstrate the integrity of the aortic arch and the aortic origin of the coronary arteries. Balloon occlusion aortography may be useful in enhancing contrast delivery to the coronary arteries. An aortopulmonary fistulous tract in distinction from an aortopulmonary window has been identified in the patient with aortic atresia and interruption of the aortic arch.[37–39,56] It is likely that this fistulous connection represents a fifth aortic arch with a systemic-to-pulmonary artery connection.[57,58] Finally, in the patient with interruption of the aortic arch and an apparently intact ventricular septum, this situation is so uncommon that it is likely that an aortopulmonary septal defect has gone unrecognized (see also Chapter 33). The small aortopulmonary window has been closed in the catheter laboratory (Fig. 8-5).[59] We have shown elsewhere the angiographic features of the most peculiar topsy-turvy hearts with superoinferior ventricles and large aortopulmonary windows (see Chapter 44, Fig. 44-2). The aortopulmonary window may be the sole source of pulmonary blood flow in the patient with pulmonary atresia (see Chapter 21, Fig. 21-16), or the sole source of ascending aortic blood flow in the patient with aortic atresia and interruption of the aortic arch (see Chapter 26, Fig. 26-12).

References

1. Belcourt CL, Aterman K, Gillis DA, Roy DL. Aortopulmonary window or aortopulmonary fenestration. *Chest* 1979;75:397–399.
2. Baronofsky ID, Gordon AJ, Grishman A, Steinfeld L, Kreel I. Aorticopulmonary septal defect: Diagnosis and report of case successfully treated. *Am J Cardiol* 1960;5:273–276.
3. Blieden LC, Moller JH. Aorticopulmonary septal defect. An experience with 17 patients. *Br Heart J* 1974;36:630–635.
4. Kutsche LM, Van Mierop LHS. Anatomy and pathogenesis of aorticopulmonary septal defect. *Am J Cardiol* 1987;59:443–447.

5. Lau KC, Calcaterra G, Miller GAH, Lennox SC, Panneth M, Anderson RH, Shinebourne EA, Lincoln C. Aortopulmonary window. *J Cardiovasc Surg* 1982;23:21–27.

6. Mori K, Ando M, Takao A, Ishikawa S, Imai Y. Distal type of aortopulmonary window. Report of 4 cases. *Br Heart J* 1978;40:681–689.

7. Neufeld HN, Lester RG, Adams PJ, Anderson RC, Lillehei CW, Edwards JE. Aorticopulmonary septal defect. *Am J Cardiol* 1962;9:12–25.

8. Richardson JV, Doty DB, Rossi NP, Ehrenhaft JL. The spectrum of anomalies of aortopulmonary septation. *J Thorac Cardiovasc Surg* 1979;78:21–27.

9. Yen Ho S, Gerlis LM, Anderson C, Devine WA, Smith A. The morphology of aortopulmonary windows with regard to their classification and morphogenesis. *Cardiol Young* 1994;4:146–155.

10. Fyler DC. Report of the New England Regional Infant Cardiac Program. *Pediatrics* 1980;65:377–461.

11. Keith JD. Prevalence, incidence, and epidemiology. In: Keith JD, Rowe RD, Vlad P. *Heart Disease in Infancy and Childhood.* Third Edition. New York: MacMillan Publishing Co; 1978, pp. 3–13.

12. Perry LW, Neill CA, Ferencz C, Rubin JD, Loffredo CA. Infants with congenital heart disease: The cases. In: Ferencz C, Rubin JD, Loffredo CA, Magee CA, eds. *Perspectives in Pediatric Cardiology. Volume 4: Epidemiology of Congenital Heart Disease. The Baltimore-Washington Infant Study 1981–1989.* Mt. Kisco, NY: Futura Publishing Company, Inc; 1993, pp. 33–62.

13. Berry TE, Bharati S, Muster AJ, Santucci B, Lev M, Paul MH. Distal aortopulmonary septal defect, aortic origin of the right pulmonary artery, intact ventricular septum, patent ductus arteriosus and hypoplasia of the aortic isthmus: A newly recognized syndrome. *Am J Cardiol* 1982;49:108–116.

14. Boonstra PW, Talsma M, Ebels T. Interruption of the aortic arch, distal aortopulmonary window, arterial duct and aortic origin of the right pulmonary artery in a neonate: Report of case successfully repaired in a one-stage operation. *Int J Cardiol* 1992;34:108–110.

15. Braunlin E, Peoples WM, Freedom RM, Fyler DC, Goldblatt A, Edwards JE. Interruption of the aortic arch with aorticopulmonary septal defect. An anatomic review. *Pediatr Cardiol* 1982;3:329–335.

16. Jacobsen JG, Trusler GA, Izukawa TI. Repair of interrupted aortic arch and aortopulmonary window in an infant. *Ann Thorac Surg* 1979;28:290–294.

17. Fisher EA, Dubrow IW, Eckner FAO, Hastreiter AR. Aorticopulmonary septal defect and interrupted aortic arch. A diagnostic challenge. *Am J Cardiol* 1974;34:356–359.

18. Tabak C, Moskowitz W, Wagner H, Weinberg P, Edmunds LHJ. Aortopulmonary window and aortic isthmus hypoplasia. Operative management in newborn infants. *J Thorac Cardiovasc Surg* 1983;86:273–279.

19. Burroughs JT, Schmutzer KJ, Linder F, Neuhaus G. Anomalous origin of the right coronary artery with aortico-pulmonary window and ventricular septal defect. Report of a case with complete operative connection. *J Cardiovasc Surg* 1962;3:142–148.

19a. D'Souza VJ, Chen MY. Anomalous origin of coronary artery in association with aorticopulmonary window. *Pediatr Cardiol* 1996;17:316–318.

20. Hurwitz RA, Ruttenberg HD, Fonkalsrud E. Aortopulmonary window, ventricular septal defect and mesoversion. Surgical correction in an infant. *Am J Cardiol* 1967;20:566–570.

21. Luisi SV, Ashraf MH, Gula G, Radley-Smith R, Yacoub M. Anomalous origin of the right coronary artery with aortopulmonary window: Functional and surgical considerations. *Thorax* 1980;35:446–448.

22. Perez-Martinez VM, Burgueros M, Quero M, Perez Leon J, Hafer G. Aorticopulmonary window associated with tetralogy of Fallot. Report of one case and review of the literature. *Angiology* 1976; 27:526–534.

23. Kutsche LM, Van Mierop LH. Anomalous origin of a pulmonary artery from the ascending aorta: Associated anomalies and pathogenesis. *Am J Cardiol* 1988;61:850–856.

24. Shore DF, Yen Ho S, Anderson RH, de Leval M, Lincoln C. Aortopulmonary septal defect coexisting with ventricular septal defect and pulmonary atresia. *Ann Thorac Surg* 1983;35:132–137.

25. Sreeram N and Walsh K. Aortopulmonary window with aortic origin of the right pulmonary artery. *Int J Cardiol* 1991; 31:249–251.

26. Tandon R, da Silva CL, Moller JH, Edwards JE. Aorticopulmonary septal defect coexisting with ventricular septal defect. *Circulation* 1974;50:188–191.

27. Lloyd TR, Marvin WJ Jr, Lee J. Total anomalous origin of the coronary arteries from the pulmonary artery in an infant with aortopulmonary septal defect. *Pediatr Cardiol* 1987;8:153–154.

28. Krishnan P, Airan B, Sambamurthy S, Shrivastava S, Rajani M, Rao IM. Complete transposition of the great arteries with aortopulmonary window: Surgical treatment and embryologic significance. *J Thorac Cardiovasc Surg* 1991; 101:749–751.

28a. Amato JJ. Complete transposition of the great arteries with aorto-pulmonary window (letter; comment). *J Thorac Cardiovasc Surg* 1992;104:1490–1491.

29. Clarke CP, Richardson JP. The management of aortopulmonary window. Advantages of transaortic closure with a Dacron patch. *J Thorac Cardiovasc Surg* 1976;72:48–51.

30. Putnam TC, Gross RE. Surgical management of aortopulmonary fenestration. *Surgery* 1966;59:727–735.

31. van Son JAM, Puga FJ, Danielson GK, Mair DD, Schaff HV, Ilstrup DM. Aortopulmonary window: Factors associated with early and late success after surgical treatment. *Mayo Clin Proc* 1993;68:128–133.

32. Castaneda AR, Kirklin JW. Tetralogy of Fallot with aorticopulmonary window. *J Thorac Cardiovasc Surg* 1977; 74:467–468.

33. Gerlis LM, MacGregor CC d'A, Yen Ho S. An anatomical study of 110 cases with deficiency of the aorticopulmonary septum with emphasis on the role of the arterial duct. *Cardiol Young* 1992;2:342–352.

34. Geva T, Ott DA, Ludomirsky A, Argyle SJ, O'Laughlin MP. Tricuspid atresia associated with aortopulmonary window: Controlling pulmonary blood flow with a fenestrated patch. *Am Heart J* 1992;123:260–262.

35. Corno A, Pierli C, Lisi G, Biagioli B, Grossi A. Anomalous origin of the left coronary artery from an aortopulmonary window (letter). *J Thorac Cardiovasc Surg* 1988;96:669–671.

35a. Chopra PS, Reed WH, Wilson AD, Rao PS. Delayed presentation of anomalous circumflex coronary artery arising from pulmonary artery following repair of aortopulmonary window in infancy. *Chest* 1994;106:1920–1922.

36. Doty DB, Richardson JV, Falkovsky GE, Gordonova MI, Burakovsky VI. Aortopulmonary septal defect: Hemodynamics, angiography, and operation. *Ann Thorac Surg* 1981;32:244–250.

36a. Bhagwat AR, Pinto RJ, Sharma S. Tetralogy of Fallot with pulmonary atresia associated with aortopulmonary window and major aortopulmonary collaterals. *Cardiol Young* 1995;5:289–290.

37. Rosenquist GC, Taylor JFN, Stark J. Aortopulmonary fenestration and aortic atresia: Report of an infant with ventricular septal defect, persistent ductus arteriosus, and interrupted aortic arch. *Br Heart J* 1974;36:1146–1148.

38. Freedom RM, Culham JAG, Moes CAF. *Angiocardiography of Congenital Heart Disease.* New York: MacMillan Publishing Company; 1984, pp. 431–436.

39. Redington AN, Rigby ML, Ho SY, Gunthard J, Anderson RH. Aortic atresia with aortopulmonary window and interruption of the aortic arch. *Pediatr Cardiol* 1991; 12: 49–51.

39a. Bertolini A, Dalmonte P, Bava GL, Moretti R, Cervo G, Marasini M. Aortopulmonary septal defects. A review of the literature and report of ten cases. *J Cardiovasc Surg* 1994;35:207–213.

40. Coleman EN, Barclay RS, Reid JM, Stevenson JG. Congenital aorto-pulmonary fistula combined with persistent ductus arteriosus. *Br Heart J* 1967;29:571–576.

41. Deverall PB, Aberdeen E, Bonham-Carter RE, Waterston DJ. Aortic pulmonary window. *J Thorac Cardiovasc Surg* 1960;57:479–486.

42. Gerlis LM, Dickinson DF, Wilson N, Gibbs JL. Persistent fifth aortic arch. A report of two new cases and review of the literature. *Int J Cardiol* 1987;16:185–192.

43. Gerlis LM, Ho S-Y, Anderson RH, Da Costa P. Persistent fifth aortic arch-a great pretender: Three new covert cases. *Int J Cardiol* 1989;16:185–192.

44. Freedom RM. Anomalies of aortopulmonary septation: Persistent truncus arteriosus, aortopulmonary window, and hemitruncus arteriosus. In: Freedom RM, Benson LN, Smallhorn JF, eds. *Neonatal Heart Disease.* London: Springer-Verlag; 1992, pp. 429–452.

45. Aboliras ET, Chin AJ, Barber G, Gregg Helton J, Pigott JD. Detection of aortopulmonary window by pulsed and color Doppler echocardiography. *Am Heart J* 1988;115: 900–902.

46. Carminati M, Borghi A, Valsecchi O, Quattrociocchi M, Balduzzi A, Rusconi P, Russo MG, Festa P, Preda L, Tiraboschi R. Aortopulmonary window coexisting with tetralogy of Fallot: Echocardiographic diagnosis. *Pediatr Cardiol* 1990;11:41–43.

47. King DH, Huhta J, Gutgesell HP, Ott DA. Two-dimensional echocardiographic diagnosis of anomalous origin of pulmonary artery from the aorta: Differentiation from aortopulmonary window. *J Am Coll Cardiol* 1984; 4:351–355.

48. Rice MJ, Seward JB, Hagler DJ, Mair DD, Tajik AJ. Visualization of aortopulmonary window by two-dimensional echocardiography. *Mayo Clin Proc* 1982;57:482–487.

49. Smallhorn JF, Anderson RH, Macartney FJ. Two-dimensional echocardiographic assessment of communications between ascending aorta and pulmonary trunk or individual pulmonary arteries. *Br Heart J* 1982;47:563–572.

50. Rein AJJT, Gotsman MS, Simcha A. Echocardiographic diagnosis of interrupted aortic arch with an aortopulmonary communication. *Int J Cardiol* 1989;24:238–241.

51. Balaji S, Burch M, Sullivan ID. Accuracy of cross-sectional echocardiography in diagnosis of aortopulmonary window. *Am J Cardiol* 1991;67:650–653.

52. Satomi G, Nakamura K, Imai Y, Takao A. Two-dimensional echocardiographic diagnosis of aortopulmonary window. *Br Heart J* 1980;43:351–356.

53. Mendoza DA, Ueda T, Nishioka K, Yokota Y, Mikawa H, Nomoto S, Yamazato A, Fukumasu H, Ban T. Aortopulmonary window, aortic origin of the right pulmonary artery, and interrupted aortic arch: Detection by two-dimensional and color Doppler echocardiography in an infant. *Pediatr Cardiol* 1986;7:49–52.

53a. Alva-Espinoza C, Jimenez-Arteaga S, Diaz-Diaz E, Martinez-Sanchez A, Jimenez-Zepeda D, Mojarro-Rios J, Melendez-Lopez C. Diagnosis of Berry syndrome in an infant by two-dimensional and color Doppler echocardiography. *Pediatr Cardiol* 1995;16:42–44.

54. Yoo S-J, Choi HY, Park I-S, Hong CY, Song MG, Kim SH. Distal aortopulmonary window with aortic origin of the right pulmonary artery and interruption of the aortic arch (Berry syndrome): Diagnosis by MR imaging. *AJR* 1991; 157:835–836.

55. Moes CAF and Freedom RM. Aortic arch interruption with truncus arteriosus or aorticopulmonary septal defect. *AJR* 1980;135:1011–1016.

56. Donofrio MT, Ramaciotti C, Weinberg PM, Murphy JD. Aortic atresia with interruption of the aortic arch and an aortopulmonary fistulous tract: Case report. *Pediatr Cardiol* 1995;16:147–149.

57. Freedom RM, Silver M, Miyamura H. Tricuspid and pulmonary atresia with coarctation of the aorta: A rare combination possibly explained by persistence of the fifth aortic arch with a systemic-to-pulmonary arterial connection. *Int J Cardiol* 1989;24:241–245.

58. Yoo SJ, Moes CA, Burrows PE, Molossi S, Freedom RM. Pulmonary blood supply by a branch from the distal ascending aorta in pulmonary atresia with ventricular septal defect: Differential diagnosis of fifth aortic arch. *Pediatr Cardiol* 1993;14:30–33.

59. Stamato T, Benson LN, Smallhorn JF, Freedom RM. Transcatheter closure of an aortopulmonary window with a modified double umbrella occluder system. *Cathet Cardiovasc Diagn* 1995;35:165–167.

Chapter 9

Origin of One Pulmonary Artery from the Ascending Aorta

In patients with normal truncal septation, consideration of abnormal arteries originating from the ascending aorta proximal to the origin of the first brachiocephalic artery includes one or both pulmonary arteries, or rarely, the fifth aortic arch. This chapter considers the origin of either the right or left pulmonary artery from the ascending aorta (Table 9-1) (Fig. 9-1). Specific comments about the fifth aortic arch can be found in Chapters 7, 8, 21, 33, 34, and 39. Discussions of normal truncal septation with ascending aortic origin of both right and left pulmonary arteries can be found in Chapters 7, 19, and 21.

Anomalous origin of one pulmonary artery from the ascending aorta in isolation is uncommon. Anomalous origin of one pulmonary artery from the ascending aorta has been identified in patients with aortopulmonary window and/or aortic arch hypoplasia, tetralogy of Fallot and tetralogy with absent pulmonary valve, and in pulmonary atresia and ventricular septal defect. The pathological anatomic features and associated cardiovascular anomalies of patients with anomalous origin of one pulmonary artery from the ascending aorta have been thoroughly reviewed by Kutsche and Van Mierop and others.[1–19] From the 99 cases in the literature and 9 from their own institution, Kutsche and Van Mierop conclude that anomalous origin of the right pulmonary artery from the ascending aorta was far more common (89 cases) than origin of the left (19 cases).[1] The anomalous right pulmonary artery usually originated from the posterior aspect of the ascending aorta close to the aortic valve. Occasionally, it arose from the lateral ascending aorta just proximal to the innominate artery. Aorticopulmonary septal defect and patent arterial duct are commonly associated with anomalous origin of the right pulmonary artery, whereas other cardiovascular anomalies are rare.[1–19] Among patients with anomalous origin of the left pulmonary artery from the ascending aorta, right aortic arch and tetralogy of Fallot are common (Table 9-2) (see Chapters 20 and 21).[6,8–10]

It has been suggested that the origin of the right or left pulmonary artery from the ascending aorta results from origin of these arteries from the aortic sac instead of the confluent sixth arches.[1–3,7,18,20,21] These conditions must be distinguished from distal ductal origin of the pulmonary artery or origin of a so-called pulmonary artery from a segmental artery originating from the descending thoracic aorta (see Chapters 19 and 21).[9,10,18] Distal ductal origin of a pulmonary artery is discussed and illustrated in considerable detail in Chapter 19, Figs. 19-10 through 19-15. This condition may of course be seen in patients with tetralogy of Fallot and complex forms of pulmonary atresia (see Chapters 20 through 22, and 41).

When one pulmonary artery originates from the ascending aorta in isolation, that pulmonary artery is usually hypertensive, with a driving pressure equal to that in the aorta, unless there is a proximal obstruction or stenosis in the abnormally connected pulmonary artery.[8–10,13,15–18,22–25] The contralateral pulmonary is also usually hypertensive.[8–10,13,15–18,22–25] The reasons for the hypertension in the lung not connected to the aorta is unclear. Reflex vasoconstriction or some circulating vasoconstrictor agents have been suggested as causal, but these have not been substantiated. Somewhat surprisingly, lung biopsies have not consistently demonstrated significant differences between the two lungs in the young baby or infant, but in the older child,

Table 9-1

Conditions with Origin of One Pulmonary Artery from the Ascending Aorta

Tetralogy of Fallot
Pulmonary atresia with ventricular septal defect
Truncus arteriosus
Aortopulmonary window
Isolated origin of one pulmonary artery from the ascending aorta

Table 9-2

Common Associated Cardiac Anomalies in Patients with Origin of a Single Pulmonary Artery from the Ascending Aorta

Origin of Right Pulmonary Artery from Ascending Aorta

Usually occurs in isolation

Less common associations: tetralogy of Fallot; interruption of aortic arch; aorticopulmonary septal defect

Origin of Left Pulmonary Artery from Ascending

¾ of patients have tetralogy of Fallot

Aorticopulmonary septal defect and/or interruption of the aortic arch are very rare

both lungs may exhibit severe pulmonary vascular damage. Occasionally the protected lung (ie, that with right ventricular origin) will demonstrate the more advanced histopathological changes. In a review of their own experience and the literature, Fontana and colleagues[25a] reported 65 patients with the right pulmonary artery originating from the ascending aorta. This review showed a 1-year survival without surgery of 30%, and a 1-year survival with surgery of 84%. Fontana and colleagues have provided an excellent review of this disorder through 1986.

Imaging Modalities

The diagnosis of origin of one pulmonary artery from the ascending aorta has been made by echocardiography and by magnetic resonance imaging.[8,10,26–34c] Long and associates[35] have published pertinent radionuclide findings in a patient with origin of one pulmonary artery from the ascending aorta. Cardiac catheterization with angiography has been advocated for two reasons: to define the hemodynamic status of the pulmonary circulation and to exclude other cardiac malformations.[8–10,13,15–18,22–25]

Angiocardiography

The angiographic diagnosis of origin of either the right or left pulmonary artery arising from the ascending aorta can be established either by aortography performed in the ascending aorta or by left ventriculography (Figs. 9-2 and 9-3). The aortogram will be guided by the echocardiographic determination and this will aid in the axial projection. When the right pulmonary artery originates anomalously from the ascending aorta, a left ventriculogram filmed in the right axial oblique will demonstrate this artery and its point of origin to ad-

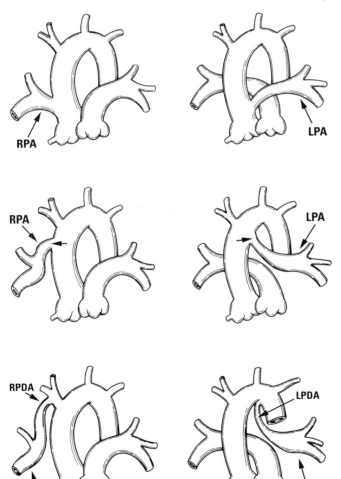

Fig. 9-1: Diagram showing types of aortic origin of pulmonary artery from aorta. This particular drawing shows only a left aortic aortic arch.
Top left: Origin of right pulmonary artery from ascending aorta. **Top right:** Origin of left pulmonary artery from ascending aorta. **Center left:** Origin of right pulmonary artery from ascending aorta with mild proximal narrowing (arrow). **Center right:** Origin of left pulmonary artery from ascending aorta with mild proximal narrowing (arrow). **Bottom left:** Distal right ductal origin (RPDA) of right pulmonary artery. Note the right ductus originates from the base of the innominate artery. **Bottom right:** Distal left ductal origin of the left pulmonary artery.

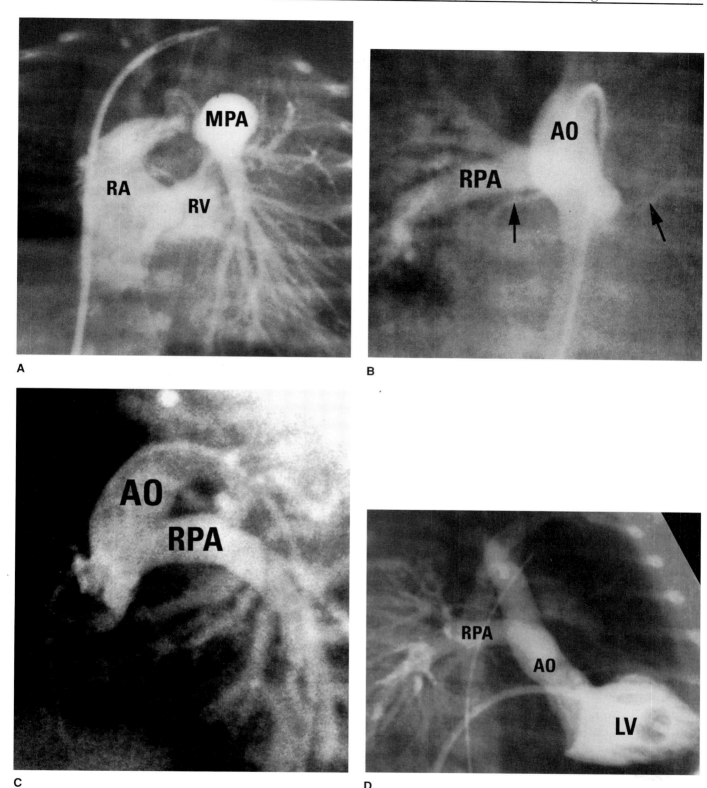

Fig. 9-2: Origin of right pulmonary artery from ascending aorta.
A: Venogram showing sequential opacification of right atrium, right ventricle, and main and left pulmonary artery. Note from the venogram the right pulmonary artery is not seen. **B and C:** Frontal and lateral aortogram demonstrates ascending aortic origin of right pulmonary artery. **D:** Right anterior oblique left ventriculogram demonstrates ascending aortic origin of right pulmonary artery from a different infant.

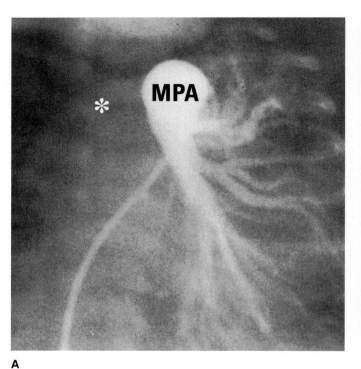

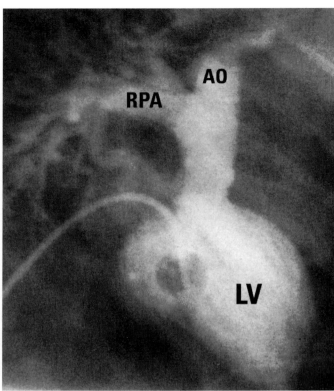

A   **B**

Fig. 9-3: Origin of right pulmonary artery from ascending aorta.
A: Selective injection in main pulmonary artery trunk shows only opacification of left pulmonary artery; the absence of the right pulmonary artery is noted (*). **B:** Left ventriculogram in shallow right anterior oblique clearly demonstrates aortic origin of right pulmonary artery

vantage (Fig. 9-3). Selective right ventriculography or angiography performed in the main pulmonary artery will demonstrate the solitary pulmonary artery (Fig. 9-3). Dodo and colleagues[35a] have provided beautiful angiography of anomalous origin of the main left pulmonary artery from the ascending aorta in two infants, both with DiGeorge syndrome. Tagliente and colleagues [35b] have summarized the literature pertinent to isolated anomalous origin of the left pulmonary artery from the ascending aorta, and demonstrated both the echocardiographic and angiographic findings in their patient. Origin of the left pulmonary artery from the ascending aorta in the patient with tetralogy of Fallot and absent pulmonary valve is shown in Chapter 22, Fig. 22-9.

Differential Diagnoses

It is apparent that the foremost consideration is to differentiate origin of one pulmonary artery from the ascending aorta from a common arterial trunk with nonconfluent pulmonary arteries. Other considerations must be given to those very uncommon situations of truncal septation, but with aortic origin of the branch

pulmonary arteries, and right ventricular origin of the main pulmonary trunk.[36–38] The fifth aortic arch originates from the ascending aorta, and while it usually has a systemic-to-systemic connection, it may rarely have a systemic-to-pulmonary artery connection.[39–41]

In those patients where the origin of the right pulmonary artery is from the ascending aorta, one must exclude the more common associated conditions that may confuse or confound the diagnosis, including aorticopulmonary septal defect. Tetralogy of Fallot is identified in about 75% of those patients in whom the left pulmonary artery originates from the ascending aorta.[1,6] Some of these patients will have the so-called absent pulmonary valve variant.

Anomalous origin of the right pulmonary artery from the ascending aorta may promote profound respiratory distress. Ben-Shachar and colleagues[42] described a 2-month-old girl with a so-called hemitruncal sling who presented with congestive heart failure and respiratory distress. The right pulmonary artery in this patient with complex pulmonary atresia and ventricular septal defect originated from the left lateral aspect of the aorta, wrapped around the trachea passing lateral to the trachea in a dorsocranial fashion, then coursed to the right and passed dorsal to the trachea and ventral to the esophagus. Transnasal bronchoscopy demonstrated a large ventrolateral pulsating extrinsic compression of the trachea above the carina severely reducing the intratracheal luminal diameter.[42]

After repair of anomalous origin of the right pulmonary artery from the ascending aorta, there has been potential for stenosis at the site of reanastomosis. van Son and Hanley[43] have used autogenous main pulmonary artery flaps for repair of anomalous origin of the right pulmonary artery from the ascending aorta to avoid this complication.

References

1. Kutsche LM, Van Mierop LHS. Anomalous origin of a pulmonary artery from the ascending aorta: Associated anomalies and pathogenesis. *Am J Cardiol* 1988;61: 850–856.

2. Anderson RC, Char F, Adams PJ. Proximal interruption of a pulmonary artery 1 (Absence of one pulmonary artery): Case report and a new embryologic interpretation. *Dis Chest* 1958;34:73–86.

3. Anderson RH, Macartney FJ, Shinebourne EA, Tynan M. *Paediatric Cardiology.* Volume 2. Edinburgh: Churchill Livingstone; 1987, pp. 818–825.

4. Berry TE, Bharati S, Muster AJ, Idriss FS, Lev M, Paul MH. Distal aortopulmonary septal defect, aortic origin of the right pulmonary artery, intact ventricular septum, patent ductus arteriosus and hypoplasia of the aortic isthmus: A newly recognized syndrome. *Am J Cardiol* 1982; 49:108–116.

5. Bjork VO, Rudhe U, Zetterquist P. Aortic origin of the right pulmonary artery and wide patent ductus arteriosus. *Scand J Thorac Cardiovasc Surg* 1970;4:87–95.

6. Calder AL, Brandt PWT, Barratt-Boyes BG, Neutze JM. Variants of tetralogy of Fallot with absent pulmonary valve leaflet and origin of one pulmonary artery from the ascending aorta. *Am J Cardiol* 1980;46:106–116.

7. Cucci CE, Doyle EF, Lewis EW. Absence of a primary division of the pulmonary trunk. An ontogenic theory. *Circulation* 1964;29:124–131.

8. Fong LV, Anderson RH, Siewers RD, Trento A, Park SC. Anomalous origin of one pulmonary artery from the ascending aorta: A review of echocardiographic, catheter, and morphological features. *Br Heart J* 1989;62:389–395.

9. Freedom RM, Culham JAG, Moes CAF. *Angiocardiography of Congenital Heart Disease.* New York: MacMillan Publishing Company; 1984, pp. 453–456.

10. Freedom RM. Anomalies of aortopulmonary septation: Persistent truncus arteriosus, aortopulmonary septal defect, and hemitruncus arteriosus. In: Freedom RM, Benson LN, Smallhorn JF, eds. *Neonatal Heart Disease.* London: Springer-Verlag; 1992, pp. 429–452.

11. Gula G, Chew C, Radley-Smith R, Yacoub M. Anomalous origin of the right pulmonary artery from the ascending aorta with aortopulmonary window. *Thorax* 1978;33: 459–461.

12. Jew EW Jr, Gross P. Aortic origin of the right pulmonary artery and absence of the transverse aortic arch. *AMA Arch Pathol* 1952;53:191–194.

13. Keane JF, Maltz D, Bernhard WF, Corwin RD, Nadas AS. Anomalous origin of one pulmonary artery from the ascending aorta. Diagnostic, physiological and surgical considerations. *Circulation* 1974;50:588–594.

14. McKim JS, Wiglesworth FW. Absence of the left pulmonary artery. A report of six cases with autopsy findings in three. *Am Heart J* 1954;47:845–849.

15. Mee RBB. Surgical repair of hemitruncus: Principles and techniques. *J Cardiovasc Surg* 1987;2:247–256.

16. Nakamura Y, Yasui H, Kado H, Yoneaga K, Shiokawa Y, Tokunaga S. Anomalous origin of the right pulmonary artery from the ascending aorta. *Ann Thorac Surg* 1991; 52:1285–1291.

17. Nashef SAM, Jamieson MPG, Pollock JCS. Aortic origin of right pulmonary artery: Successful surgical correction in three consecutive patients. *Ann Thorac Surg* 1987;44: 536–538.

18. Penkoske PA, Castaneda AR, Fyler DC, Van Praagh R. Origin of pulmonary artery branch from ascending aorta. Primary surgical repair in infancy. *J Thorac Cardiovasc Surg* 1983;85:537–545.

19. Rowe RD, Freedom RM, Mehrizi A. *The Neonate with Congenital Heart Disease.* Philadelphia: WB Saunders Company; 1981, pp. 646–649.

20. Congdon ED. Transformation of the aortic-arch system during development of the human embryo. *Contributions in Embryology, Carnegie Institute of Washington.* 1922; pp. 47–111.

21. Schneiderman LJ. Isolated congenital absence of the right pulmonary artery: A caution as to its diagnosis and a proposal for its embryogenesis—report of a case with review. *Am Heart J* 1958;55:772–780.

22. Agarwala B, Waldman JD, Sand M, Loe WA Jr, Ruschaupt DG. Aortic origin of the RPA: Immediate resolution of severe pulmonary artery hypertension by surgical repair. *Pediatr Cardiol* 1994;15:41–44.

23. Fucci C, Di Carlo D, Di Donato R, Marino B, Calcaterra, Marcelletti C. Anomalous origin of the right pulmonary artery from the ascending aorta: Repair without cardiopulmonary bypass. *Int J Cardiol* 1989;23:309–313.

24. Pool PE, Vogel JHK, Blount SG Jr. Congenital unilateral absence of a pulmonary artery. The importance of Flow in Pulmonary Hypertension. *Am J Cardiol* 1962;10:706–732.

25. Yamaki S, Suzuki Y, Ishizawa E, Kagawa Y, Horiuchi T, Sato T. Isolated aortic origin of the right pulmonary artery. Report of a case with special reference to pulmonary vascular disease in the left and right lungs. *Chest* 1983;83:575–578.

25a. Fontana G, Spach MS, Effmann EL, Sabiston DC Jr. Origin of the right pulmonary artery from the ascending aorta. *Ann Surg* 1987;206:102–113.

26. Duncan WJ, Freedom RM, Olley PM, Rowe RD. Two-dimensional echocardiographic identification of hemitruncus: Anomalous origin of one pulmonary artery from ascending aorta with the other pulmonary artery arising normally from the right ventricle. *Am Heart J* 1981;102: 892–896.

27. Juredini S, Nouri S, Goel DP. Similarity of anomalous origin of right pulmonary artery from the ascending aorta to d-transposition of the great arteries: 2D echocardiographic and Doppler study. *Am Heart J* 1986;112: 175–176.

28. King DH, Huhta JC, Gutgesell HP, Ott DA. Two-dimensional echocardiographic diagnosis of anomalous origin of the right pulmonary artery from the aorta: Differentiation from aortopulmonary window. *J Am Coll Cardiol* 1984;4:351–355.

29. Lo RNS, Mok CK, Leung MP, Lau KC, Cheung DLC. Cross-sectional and pulsed Doppler features of anomalous origin of right pulmonary artery from the ascending aorta. *Am J Cardiol* 1987;60:921–924.

30. Mendoza DA, Ueda T, Nishioka K, Yokata Y, Mikawa H, Nomoto S, Yamazato A, Fukumasu H, Ban T. Aortopulmonary window, aortic origin of the right pulmonary artery, and interrupted aortic arch: Detection by two-dimensional and color Doppler echocardiography in an infant. *Pediatr Cardiol* 1986;7:49–52.

31. Rice MJ, Seward JB, Hagler DJ, Mair DD, Tajik AJ. Visualization of aorticopulmonary window by two-dimensional echocardiography. *Mayo Clin Proc* 1982;57:482–487.

32. Satomi G, Nakamura K, Imai Y, Takao A. Two-dimensional echocardiographic diagnosis of aorticopulmonary window. *Br Heart J* 1980;43:351–356.

33. Saxena A, Fong LV, Keeton BR. Identification of anomalous origin of one pulmonary artery from ascending aorta by two-dimensional and colour Doppler echocardiography. *Eur Heart J* 1991;12:835–837.

34. Smallhorn JF, Anderson RH, and Macartney FJ. Two dimensional echocardiographic assessment of communications between ascending aorta and pulmonary trunk or individual pulmonary arteries. *Br Heart J* 1982;47:563–572.

34a. Volker H, Kohler E. Hemitruncus arteriosus bei einem asymptomatischen jungen Mann—Diagnostischer Wert der transosophagealen Echokardiographie. *Z Kardiol* 1994;83:610–614.

34b. Kim TK, Choe YH, Kim HS, Ko JK, Lee YT, Lee HJ, Park JH. Anomalous origin of the right pulmonary artery from the ascending aorta: Diagnosis by magnetic resonance imaging. *Cardiovasc Intervent Radiol* 1995;18:118–121.

34c. Lin M-H, Shen C-T, ang N-K, Ling Y-M, Jeng C-M. Magnetic resonance imaging of anomalous origin of the right pulmonary artery from the ascending aorta in association with ventricular septal defect. *Am Heart J* 1996;132:1073–1078.

35. Long WA, Perry JR, Henry GW. Radionuclide diagnosis of anomalous origin of right pulmonary artery from the as-cending aorta (so-called hemitruncus). *Int J Cardiol* 1985;8:492–496.

35a. Dodo H, Alejos JC, Perloff JK, Laks H, Drinkwater DC, Williams RG. Anomalous origin of the left main pulmonary artery from the ascending aorta associated with the DiGeorge syndrome. *Am J Cardiol* 1995;75:1294–1297.

35b. Tagliente MR, Troise D, Millella L, Vairo U. Isolated anomalous origin of left pulmonary artery from the ascending aorta. *Am Heart J* 1996;132:1289–1292.

36. Bricker DL, King SM, Edwards JE. Anomalous Aortic origin of the right and left pulmonary arteries in a normally septated truncus arteriosus. *Chest* 1975;68:591–594.

37. Beitzke A, Shinebourne EA. Single origin of right and left pulmonary arteries from ascending aorta, with main pulmonary artery from right ventricle. *Br Heart J* 1980;43:363–365.

38. Aotsuka H, Nagai Y, Saito M, Matsumoto H, Nakamura T. Anomalous origin of both pulmonary arteries from the ascending aorta with a nonbranching main pulmonary artery arising from the right ventricle. *Pediatr Cardiol* 1990;11:156–158.

39. Freedom RM, Silver M, Miyamura H. Tricuspid and pulmonary atresia with coarctation of the aorta: A rare combination possibly explained by persistence of the fifth aortic arch with a systemic-to-pulmonary arterial connection. *Int J Cardiol* 1989;24:241–245.

40. Yoo S-J, Moes CAF, Burrows PE, Molossi S, Freedom RM. Pulmonary blood supply by a branch of the distal ascending aorta in pulmonary atresia and ventricular septal defect: Differential diagnosis of fifth aortic arch. *Pediatr Cardiol* 1993;14:230–233.

41. Schulze-Neick I, Hausdorf G, Lange PE. Maldevelopment of conotruncal and aorto-pulmonary septum with absent left central pulmonary artery: Anatomical and clinical implications. *Br Heart J* 1994;71:89–91.

42. Ben-Schachar G, Beder SD, Liebman J, Van Heecheren D. Hemitruncal sling: A newly recognized anomaly and its surgical correction. *J Thorac Cardiovasc Surg* 1985;90:146–148.

43. van Son JAM, Hanley FL. Use of autogenous aortic and main pulmonary artery flaps for repair of anomalous origin of the right pulmonary artery from the ascending aorta. *J Thorac Cardiovasc Surg* 1996;111:675–676.

Chapter 10

The Patent Arterial Duct

Through a series of misinterpretations and careless translations, the name of Leo Bottali has become, quite unjustifiably, attached to the term ductus arteriosus.[1] Indeed, a recent re-examination of Galen's original Greek text[2] indicates that Galen realized that in the fetus, some blood entered the right ventricle and pulmonary artery and was shunted into the aorta through a special fetal channel. Although he did not appreciate that blood circulated, Galen did understand that dramatic readjustments occurred in the circulation at the time of birth. It was not until the appearance of Rokitansky's handbook in 1844 and monograph in 1852 that it has become well recognized that patent ductus arteriosus should be considered an isolated congenital malformation.[3]

It has been argued that the terms "patent" or "persistent" are redundancies, and should be avoided, but this is an oversimplification; both terms remain useful. Persistent implies the arterial duct is present beyond the time of expected closure, and is therefore, a pathological state. The term patent remains useful, particularly in the perinatal period, where it may signify a ductus that is functionally open as opposed to one that is functionally closed, but retains the potential to re-open.

Incidence

The estimated incidence of an isolated persistent arterial duct is subject to potential error, especially due to the inclusion of cases of prematurity or maternal rubella. Anderson[4] estimated the incidence between 1 in 2500 and 1 in 5000 births, and accounted for 12% of all congenital malformations. In a more extensive, relatively homogeneous population, Carlgren[5] found the overall incidence of all cardiac malformations to be 6.4 per 1,000 births, with persistent arterial duct the third most common lesion seen representing about 0.04% of livebirths. More recently, Mitchell[6] reported the incidence at 0.06%, but may have included cases of prematurity or the influence of maternal rubella as well. The incidence in the general population may indeed be found to be higher, however, as more sensitive imaging techniques are applied.[7]

Embryological Considerations

During fetal life, six arterial arches link the paired ventral aorta with the paired dorsal aorta, although all six arches are never present simultaneously (see Chapter 34).[8] The normal arterial duct develops from the dorsal portion of the left sixth arch. The sixth arch develops bilaterally from the vascular connection between the aortic sac and dorsal aorta. When the common arterial trunk partitions to form the aorta and pulmonary trunk, the sixth arch remains continuous with the pulmonary trunk. On the right side, the ventral portion ultimately becomes the proximal portion of the right pulmonary artery, while the dorsal segment regresses. On the left side, the ventral portion is absorbed into the pulmonary trunk, and the dorsal segment becomes the ductus arteriosus. When the aortic arch is left sided, the dorsal portion of the right sixth arch usually disappears, whereas the dorsal part of the left sixth arch persists to form the ductus arteriosus. If the aortic arch is right sided, the ductus may be on the right and connect the right pulmonary artery to the right arch, although it is more common for the arterial duct to persist on the left and connect to the left pulmonary artery and proximal left subclavian artery.

From: Freedom RM, Mawson JB, Yoo SJ, Benson LN: *Congenital Heart Disease: Textbook of Angiocardiography.* Armonk NY, Futura Publishing Co., Inc. ©1997.

Developmental Anomalies

Anomalies of the aortic arch may be associated with an abnormally situated arterial duct, either a patent structure or one represented by a ligament. In such cases the ductus may form part of a vascular ring (see Chapter 34).[9] A right aortic arch with mirror-image arterial branching, exemplified by tetralogy of Fallot (25% to 30% of cases have a right aortic arch), is associated with intracardiac anomalies in up to 98% of cases. In this case, the arterial duct (or ligament) is left sided. The arterial duct may connect the left pulmonary artery to either the subclavian portion of the brachiocephalic (innominate) artery or to the upper descending aorta, or aberrant left subclavian artery by a remnant of the left dorsal aortic root. In the latter two cases, a vascular ring can occur.[10] A right-sided arterial duct, with a right ascending and descending arch has also been described.[11] A right-sided duct (or ligament) occurs less frequently with a right arch and mirror image branching, but is also associated with the presence of intracardiac anomalies (Fig. 10-1).

A right aortic arch with an aberrant left subclavian artery and a left arterial duct is the most common form of a complete vascular ring and is probably an independent developmental error. It is, however, commonly associated with intracardiac lesions.[9] A rare ductal anomaly, also associated with a vascular ring, is the so-called ductal sling[12] in which the ductus connects a left descending aorta to the right pulmonary artery, passing between the trachea and esophagus (see Chapter 19). A right aortic arch with an aberrant left subclavian artery and a right sided duct is exceedingly rare, but does occur.[13,14] This combination also forms a ring and is discussed more fully in Chapter 34.

In a double aortic arch, with both arches patent (in the usual situation, the right arch is larger than the left), the upper descending aorta is also usually to the left, and a left-sided patent arterial duct (or ligament) may also connect on the left to the left pulmonary artery. Double aortic arches in which both limbs are patent with either a right ductus or bilateral ductus have not been reported. Atresia of one of the arch branches may also occur[15] between the left ductus and descending aorta, the left subclavian artery and ductus, or the left common carotid and subclavian arteries. If the atresia is between the left subclavian artery and ductus or between the left common carotid and subclavian artery, the ductus passes between the left pulmonary artery and the caudal end of the left dorsal aortic root (descending aortic diverticulum). An atretic right arch is exceedingly rare,[16,17] and in two cases, the atresia involved segments of the subclavian artery and right ductus.

A right arterial duct with a normal left aortic arch (with normal branching) has also been observed, as has the combination of a left aortic arch, right descending aorta (the so-called circumflex aorta; see Chapter 34), and left ductus.[18,19] A vascular ring does not occur when the arterial duct connects the right pulmonary artery to the base of the brachiocephalic artery. However, if the connection is to the descending aorta by means of a persistent dorsal aortic root, a complete vascular ring results (see Chapter 34).

Bilateral arterial ducts can rarely occur in isolation. However, these unique anomalies are more often reported[20,21] in association with pulmonary atresia and nonconfluent pulmonary arteries (Fig. 10-2), although there is a wide spectrum of congenital malformations in which they can occur (see also Chapter 21). There is a continuum of bilateral arterial ducts in which they: 1) are required to provide blood flow for the entire systemic circulation (as in patients with aortic arch atresia; type C interruption of the aortic arch) (see Chapters 26 and 33) and 2) are required for the entire supply of the pulmonary circulation (see Chapter 21). In addition, there are other conditions for which bilateral ducts can be found (without pulmonary atresia) with complex intracardiac malformations and include: ectopic origin of one pulmonary artery (see Chapter 9); interruption of

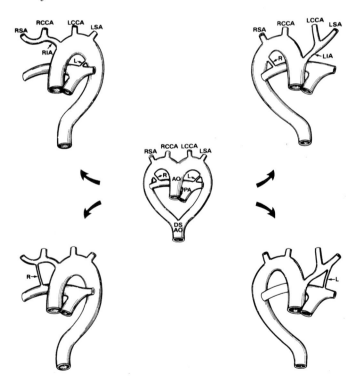

Fig. 10-1: Diagrams of typical arterial ducts with a usual branching pattern of arch vessels.
The interrelationship between the systemic and pulmonary circulations is demonstrated for a right and left arterial duct, in a left aortic arch (left upper and lower panels) or a right aortic arch (right upper and lower panels). Note that the duct from the underside of the arch is a posterior structure whereas while that from the innominate artery is anterior. In neither does a vascular ring exist.

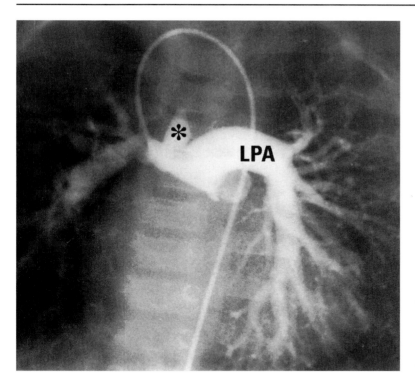

Fig: 10-2: Right-sided ductus. Frontal projections, with tetralogy-type pulmonary atresia and left-sided aortic arch.
Retrograde pulmonary artery injection via a right-sided Blalock-Taussig shunt. The right ductus is indicated by the ductal diverticulum (✳) connected to the superior aspect of the right pulmonary artery.

the left or right aortic arch with isolation of a subclavian artery; and isolation of a subclavian artery (usually but not inevitably the left).[21-28] As discussed in Chapter 20, bilateral ductus may be both patent, both occluded, or one patent and one occluded. This latter rare situation has been described in a patient with dextrocardia, pulmonary atresia with ventricular septal defect, and a patent right arterial duct and left ligamentum.[24] Bilateral arterial ducts with a right aortic arch and right descending aorta or isolated left subclavian artery has also been reported,[28,29] as has the combination of the additional anomaly of absence of the proximal left pulmonary artery.[30]

Persistent right, left, or bilateral ductus may replace the proximal pulmonary artery, whereas the origin of one pulmonary artery from a ipsilateral ductus arteriosus is not uncommon[31] (see also Chapter 19), particularly in pulmonary atresia and ventricular septal defect.[32,33] Bilateral ductal origins of the pulmonary arteries are uncommon (see Chapters 21 and 41).[21,34-36] Absence of the arterial duct was first described in 1671[37] in an infant with apparent tetralogy of Fallot. Emmanouilides et al[38] reported its occurrence in tetralogy of Fallot with absent pulmonary valve, and postulated the absence of the duct a component in the etiology of the massive pulmonary artery dilatation seen in this condition (see Chapter 22),[38-40] although there are examples of this situation in the presence of a patent ar-

terial duct (see Chapter 22, Fig. 22-8).[41] The arterial duct may also be absent in about 70% of patients with a common arterial trunk (truncus arteriosus) or rarely as an isolated lesion.[42] In more complex examples of a single arterial trunk, the pulmonary arteries may originate from ipsilateral patent arterial ducts, and in those patients with an associated arch interruption or arch atresia, the presence of the arterial duct is essential for systemic perfusion (see Chapter 33).[31,32] Rarely, a fifth aortic arch with a systemic-to-pulmonary artery connection may simulate an arterial duct.[42a]

Anatomy

In the fetus, the arterial duct is a short wide vessel of variable length. It is usually a posterior structure connecting the pulmonary artery to the lesser curve of the aortic arch at the point of transition from the arch to the descending aorta (just beyond and opposite the origin of the left subclavian artery). The duct appears very much as a direct continuation of the pulmonary artery, while the left and right pulmonary arteries are seen as smaller branches of the main trunk. The duct is related posteriorly to the left main bronchus, while anteriorly it is crossed by the vagus nerve. In fetal life, with the ventricles working in parallel, the fetal ductus carries most of the right ventricular output (about two-thirds). The relative sizes of the great arteries and ductus are dependent on the magnitude of this flow and impact significantly on the form of many cardiovascular malformations.[43]

The arterial duct to the contralateral side of the aortic arch is situated anteriorly if arising from the brachiocephalic or subclavian artery, or posteriorly if arising from an aberrant vessel in association with a diverticulum of Kommerell, which is the remnant of the dorsal aortic root. At the aortic end, a posterior contralateral arterial duct can also communicate directly with the aorta via the remnant of the dorsal aortic root.

In the normally developing heart, the arterial duct meets the aorta at the proximal acute angle (<45°) and the distal angle is obtuse (110° to 120°)[44] in contrast to the situation of many cardiac malformations. For example, in patients with pulmonary atresia, when pulmonary arterial flow is ductal-dependent from the aorta, the proximal angle is usually obtuse and the distal angle acute[45] and often longer, more tortuous and narrow. When this is not the case, the development of pulmonary atresia is thought to have occurred late in fetal life.[46,47] However, even with normal intracardiac anatomy, the ductus may be long, narrow, short or wide, or even aneurysmal with all gradations in between.[48–50] The persistently patent arterial duct is characteristically larger at its aortic insertion and tends to have the shape of a truncated cone (Fig. 10-3). This is because ductal closure begins at the pulmonary artery end[51,52] except when there is associated right ventricular outflow obstruction, when a prominent pulmonary diverticulum can be seen (Fig. 10-4).[53] Ductal closure may be associated with stenosis of the vessel at either end. At the pulmonary artery end, stenosis may involve the proximal left pulmonary artery (see also Chapter 21).[46,54–56] Isolation of a pulmonary artery may occur when nonconfluent pulmonary arteries are perfused *in utero* by an arterial duct and become separated from the central circulation by ductal closure (so-called "absent" pulmonary artery) (see also Chapter 19, Figs. 19-10 through 19–15). At the aortic end, ductal closure has been associated with coarctation. When the arterial duct originates from a subclavian or brachiocephalic artery, the only indication of its presence may be the course of the subclavian artery, where it is tethered down by the ligamentum rather than having a straight course (Fig. 10-5). The aortic insertion of the arterial duct occasionally remains widely patent after the pulmonary artery end is sealed, with aneurysm formation within the remaining ampulla.[48,49,57–61,61a] Patency confined to the pulmonary artery end is rare.[52] True aneurysms of the arterial duct are rare, and manifest in two distinct forms. Present at or shortly after birth,[57,61,62] a "spontaneous" infantile aneurysm has been described (Fig. 10-6), that has also been noted as an incidental finding at autopsy. The aneurysm involves the length of the ductus, usually occluded at its pulmonary end. It is a true aneurysm, often containing thrombus. It is thought to be due to delayed closure of the aortic end, exposing the wall to systemic pres-

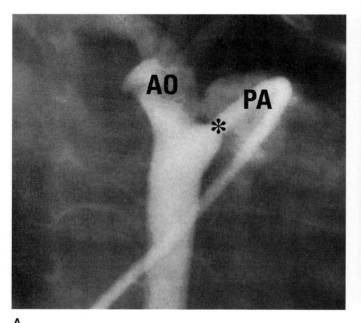

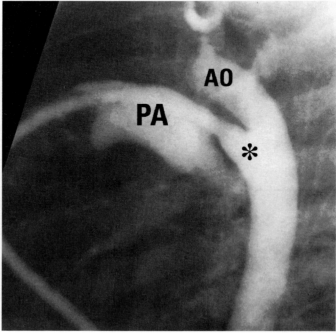

A

B

Fig. 10-3: Left posterior arterial duct.
Aortogram obtained by cannulating the patent arterial duct from the right heart. **A:** Frontal projection. Note the duct (✳) oriented leftward and superiorly. **B:** Lateral projection. The cone-shaped configuration, widest at the arterial end is seen (✳).

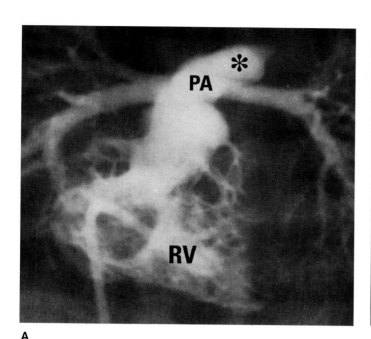

A

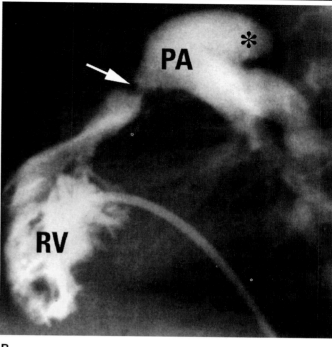

B

Fig. 10-4: Pulmonary ductal diverticulum. Right ventriculogram in a patient with pulmonary valve stenosis.
A: Frontal projection. The pulmonary valve stenosis is obscured due to the projection but the hypertrophied heavily trabeculated right ventricle is outlined and the diverticulum prominent (✳). **B:** Lateral projection. The valvar pulmonary stenosis is evident (arrow) as is the diverticulum of the ductus (✳). The arterial end of the ductus in this patient was closed.

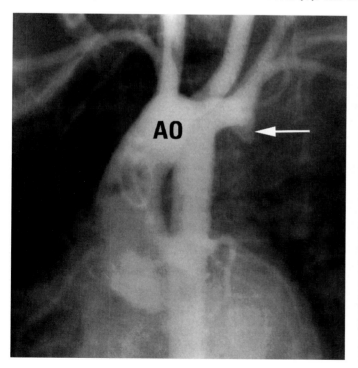

Fig. 10-5: Diverticulum associated with a left anterior ductus.
A retrograde aortogram in shallow anterior oblique projection. The left subclavian artery is pulled down and the aortic ampula of the obliterated arterial duct is identified by the residual diverticulum. Note how the left subclavian artery changes direction acutely (arrow) at the point where it is tethered by the ductal diverticulum and ligamentum.

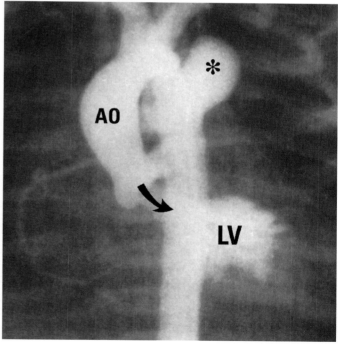

Fig. 10-6: Ductal aneurysm.
A retrograde aortogram in the frontal projection. The ductal aneurysm projects leftward and superiorly. Note the associated aortic insufficiency and prominent ascending aorta reflecting associated aortic valve disease.

sures—a wall weakened by the changes occurring within the structure during normal involution,[57] although additional structural abnormalities or sepsis may play a role. Aneurysms in later childhood and adulthood are also very rare and unrelated to the infantile form. The ductus may be patent at both ends, but usually closed at the pulmonary end.[63,64] These may represent arrested closure with persistence of an aortic diverticulum, infective endarteritis, or external trauma.[65] As in the infantile forms, complications of rupture, thromboembolism, infection, and nerve palsy can occur[57,59] and in addition, there may be erosion into the lung, esophagus, or vertebral body, and/or calcification and compression of the left bronchus.[48,57,63,66]

Angiographic Features

Diagnostic catheterization with angiography is rarely performed in the patient with typical clinical and echocardiographic findings of a persistently patent arterial duct. Such procedures are indicated only in atypical cases where the pulmonary vascular resistance is to be determined or associated anomalies to be characterized. For the most part, cardiac catheterization is now limited to transcatheter therapies for occlusion or techniques to maintain patency.

Ductal patency can be demonstrated by the passage of a catheter, either antegrade from the pulmonary artery or retrograde from the aorta. Occasionally, by torquing the catheter from the main pulmonary artery, the ascending aorta can be entered.[67] The antegrade catheter tip should be advanced well into the aorta, below the diaphragm, to confirm that the catheter is in the descending aorta rather than the left lower pulmonary artery branch. Ductal anatomy can be defined by aortography (Fig. 10-7). The size and the length of the ductus can be defined by retrograde aortography or left ventriculography. In the isolated form, the best projection is the steep left anterior oblique projection or the lateral, with the catheter either in the aortic end of the ductus or its tip just into the descending aorta. At times, a left anterior oblique projection with cranial angulation may be required. Should the arterial duct be difficult to visualize on these views, especially if superimposed on the aortic arch, caudal angulation is helpful. In the presence of a large ventricular septal defect, ventriculography may not outline the coexistent duct, and its presence can only be confirmed if the catheter traverses the structure.[68,69] Ductal patency may also be demonstrated by negative washout of contrast in the descending aorta or pulmonary artery by unopacified blood (see Chapter 2, Fig. 2-5). As noted above, normal ductal closure begins at the pulmonary artery end and with its closure one sees a conical "bump" or ampulla arising from the aortic connection (Fig. 10-8).[70] The arterial duct may provide an access route to the descending aorta for balloon occlusion aortography to delineate an arch anomaly or aortopulmonary collaterals[71] in tetralogy-type or more complex forms of pulmonary atresia (see Chapter 21).

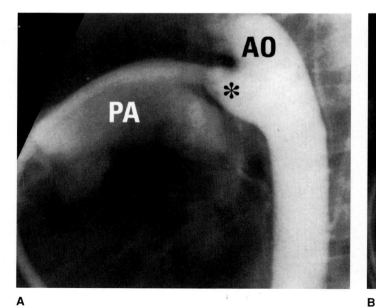

A

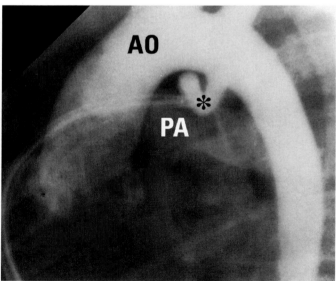

B

Fig. 10-7: Ductal morphology.
Five different patients. **A:** Antegrade aortogram, lateral projection shows a truncated cone-shaped aortic ductal ampula (✱). **B:** Retrograde aortogram, lateral projection, shows a tortuous duct (✱) originating from the under surface of the transverse arch; note the venous catheter for delivery of an umbrella occluder.

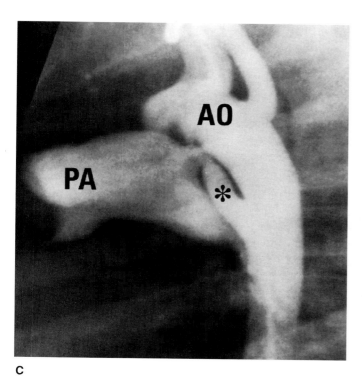

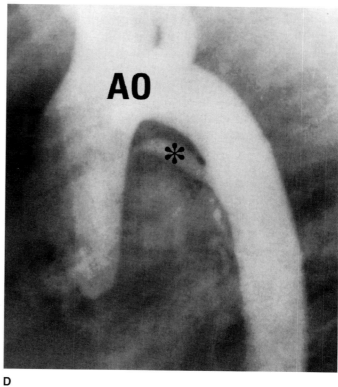

C

D

E

Fig. 10-7: *(continued)*
C: Retrograde aortogram, lateral projection. Bizarre appearing long thin ductus (✱) with an acute angle communication (✱) to the main pulmonary artery. **D:** Retrograde aortogram, lateral projection. Small ductal communication with a relatively flat aortic ampula. **E:** Retrograde ventriculogram, mid-LAO projection. A large unrestrictive arterial duct is shown (✱).

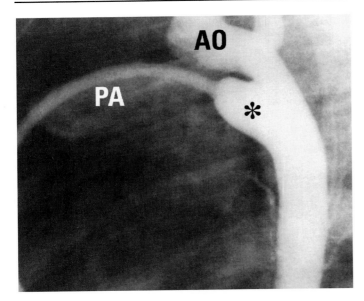

Fig. 10-8: Patent arterial duct prior to transcatheter occlusion.
Lateral projection of a descending aortic injection, the catheter passed through the right heart and patent arterial duct. The pulmonary end is restrictive, the catheter nearly completely occludes the orifice. There is a typical conical "bump" or ampula, arising from the aortic end (*).

Transcatheter Therapies

Catheter Closure

Porstmann[72–75] first advocated a percutaneous technique for permanent closure of the arterial duct that could be achieved via the femoral artery. Closure was accomplished with an Ivalon (polyvinyl alcohol) plug introduced by catheterization from the femoral artery. A prerequisite for this approach is that the lumen of the duct must be conical in shape and smaller than the lumen of the femoral artery. A technically complicated procedure, it requires a large-gauge sheath to be placed into the femoral artery and the formation of a femoral artery-ductal-femoral vein wire loop; it has not been found suitable for infants and small children.[76] Other devices, such as polyvinyl alcohol umbrellas with steel wires, umbrella-sponge plugs or shape-memory polymers, and detachable silicone double-balloons have been used to close artificial patent ductus arteriosus in dogs from either the arterial or venous circulations.[77–80] Magal and colleagues[81] described a device that consisted of a small nylon sack that could be filled with segments of guidewire and fixed with a distal flexible crossbar. Rao[82] described a successful modification of a single-disk device originally designed for atrial defect closure. An early approach proposed by Rashkind and Cuaso[83] used a device that consisted of a stainless steel grappling hook filled with a cone of foam. The prosthesis was intro-

duced in a collapsed state and expanded when released from the tip of the catheter. Since that initial clinical application and improved equipment design, experience from a multicenter clinical trial[84] has defined when successful catheter occlusion could take place and has led to its use as an effective alternative to surgery. Most recently, spring coils, whose initial application was in peripheral vascular embolization, have been used with great success as well in transcatheter arterial duct closure.[85]

The Rashkind Ductal Occluder

Ductal closure can be accomplished with the catheter delivery system from either the venous or arterial entry,[84] although the use of a long sheath placed across the ductus from a transvenous route[86] has become the technique of choice. Catheter closure is applicable in infants and young children, but is restricted to an arterial duct no larger than 8 or 9 mm in diameter, and not applicable in the premature infant. The occluder consists of two open-pore medical grade polyurethane foam disks (USCI Angiographic Systems, Billerica, MA) mounted on two opposing three-arm spring assemblies, resembling two opposing umbrellas. When released, the arms spring perpendicular to the catheter shaft and self-seal (Fig. 10-9). Two prostheses are available in 12- and 17-mm diameters, the latter made with four wire arms per disk, but with the same spring and attachment mechanism.

As with surgical management, the clinical diagnosis should be confirmed noninvasively prior to catheterization by color Doppler echocardiography with particular emphasis placed on the presence of associated lesions that could complicate the procedure (eg, azygous continuation of the inferior cava), require an additional interventional procedure (such as balloon pulmonary valvotomy), or preclude catheter closure (eg, an additional lesion that requires surgical intervention or the presence of pulmonary vascular disease) (Fig. 10-10). Special attention should also be directed to the transverse arch and isthmal region, where an unsuspected coarctation may be present (Fig. 10-11). The procedure is ideally suited for patients weighing 10 kg or more, and should not be performed in smaller infants because compromise of the left pulmonary artery can occur, with the potential for late arterial stenosis.[87,88]

There is considerable variation in procedural details as practiced among centers (for example, the use of coincident arterial cannulation and the number and type of angiograms) however, the majority of procedures can be performed in an outpatient setting with discharge the afternoon of study.[89,90]

A number of clinical series have been published involving hundreds of patients.[84,89,90–102] Successful implantation can be accomplished in the majority of cases (>98%), with the elimination of clinical signs of left-to-

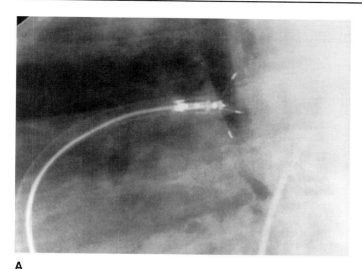

A

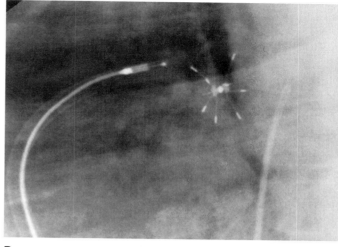

B

Fig. 10-9: Placement of umbrella occluder.
A: Lateral projection of a retrograde descending aortogram just prior to release of the proximal arms of a double umbrella occluder in the aortic ampulla. The proximal arms of the umbrella remain folded within the delivery sheath by the locking mechanism and delivery sheath. **B:** After device release, with proximal and distal arms expanded.

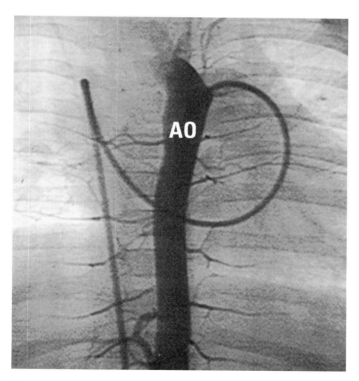

Fig. 10-10: Unusual approach to transcatheter ductal closure.
Frontal projection of an antegrade descending aortogram obtained through a patent arterial duct in a child with azygous continuation of the inferior vena cava. Transvenous ductal occlusion was achieved.

right shunting (Fig. 10-12). Within the first 48 hours, a few patients retain ductal murmurs despite correct placement, although a number may have residual shunts without murmurs. Doppler evidence of residual shunting is often over the superior aspect of the device.[87,92]

Complications are few. Acute bacterial endarteritis has occurred after implantation when appropriate procedural coverage was not applied.[92,93] Embolization to both systemic and pulmonary circulations has been encountered, with several patients requiring surgical referral. Catheter retrieval has been accomplished in both situations, using snares, baskets, or grasping forceps.[84,93]

Using pulsed and color-flow Doppler techniques, occlusion rates have been evaluated.[87,91,98,103,104] In a study by Hosking,[103] 38% had Doppler evidence of shunting detected 1 year after the procedure, falling to 18% at 2 years and 8% at 40 months. Similar observations from several studies have been reported.[91,104] A number of patients have undergone additional procedures with successful placement of a second device.[103,104] The potential for long-term complications associated with a residual shunt, which is clinically silent but detected by color-flow Doppler mapping in the presence of a foreign body remains unknown. A few patients have increased Doppler velocity shifts at the origin of the left pulmonary artery postimplantation due to turbulence or encroachment into the ostium of the left pulmonary artery, with an increased incidence when placement was performed in children under 10 kg in weight (Fig. 10-13).[105] Finally, and rarely, few patients have experienced hemolysis after device placement, with coexistent residual shunting.[106–108]

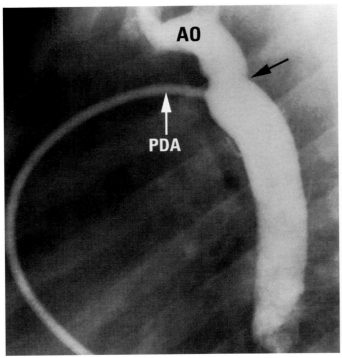

A

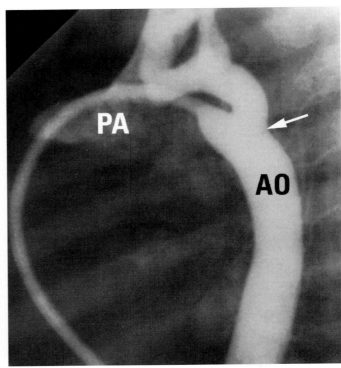

B

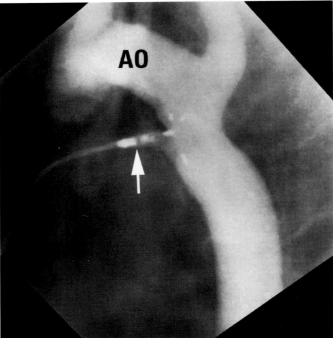

C

Fig. 10-11: Transcatheter closure of patent arterial ducts in three different patients with variant arch anatomy.
A and B: Antegrade aortograms, lateral projection. Note the mild isthmal hypoplasia and posterior shelf (arrow). There was no hemodynamic obstruction to flow and transcatheter occlusion in both patients was achieved without complication. **C:** Retrograde aortogram, lateral projection. Note the dilatation of the left subclavian artery and posterior shelf without arch or isthmal hypoplasia. The distal arms are positioned in the aortic ampulla prior to opening the proximal limbs (arrow) and release of the device.

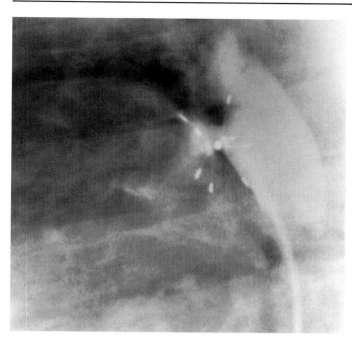

Fig. 10-12: Occlusion of arterial duct by umbrella device. Aortogram in the lateral projection with residual shunt following device occlusion. Residual flow is over the superior aspect of the device.

Transfemoral Plug Closure

In the Porstmann method, a catheter is inserted from the femoral artery across the ductus into the right side of the heart. Either the catheter itself or an exchange length guidewire is snared from the contralateral vein and exteriorized forming a femoral artery-ductal-femoral artery loop. The polyvinyl alcohol plug is introduced through a tubular applicator and threaded over the track wire. The lower age limit for transfemoral plug closure is between 3 and 4 years.[74,76,109,110] The success of the technique depends on the ratio of the lumen of the femoral artery to that of the ductus, allowing an appropriately sized plug to be placed retrograde.[111]

Several hundred cases of persistently patent ductus arteriosus have undergone occlusion with this method. In 109 cases commented upon by Porstmann,[74] no mortality and only minor morbidity were noted. In eight cases the method was unsuccessful. In five cases the ductus was too large and the plug slipped into the pulmonary artery. Because the plug was still attached to the guidewire, it could be maneuvered into the femoral vein and removed by venectomy. In the remaining three cases, because of the rigidity or small size

of the ductus, the plug could not be fixed and was allowed to embolize to the aortic bifurcation and was removed by arteriotomy.

Disadvantages of the Porstmann technique include arterial entry with arterial exposure under certain circumstances and possible arterial damage, the requirement for a transductal arterial-venous loop (venectomy for device retrieval), and the limitation on age for closure. Advantages, however, include a secured delivery system that avoids free embolization with placement and little or no residual or recurrent shunting.[76,110,112] Despite the early clinical trials and success of this approach, it remains technically complex, and except for a few centers world-wide, has not achieved a large clinical application.

The Spring Coil

Using embolization spring coils (Gianturco, Cook Inc, Bloomington, IN), Cambier[113] reported successful occlusion of small ductal communications (<2.5 mm) using a retrograde approach in 3 of 4 children. Lloyd[85] and Moore[114] expanded the early experience with this technique, noting the approach to be effective and simple, and that this technique can be performed in an outpatient setting (Fig. 10-14).

Catheter Techniques to Maintain Ductal Patency

Percutaneous balloon dilation has also been proposed as a method to maintain ductal patency.[115–119] Temporary patency can be achieved, but abrupt closure, thrombosis, or rupture can occur, making this a less reliable means to assure patency. Except for special instances, this technique has not been pursued clinically except in the Toronto Hospital for Sick Children.

To provide a mechanical scaffold for the ductal wall resistant to the constrictive forces of ductal closure, Coe and Olley[120] proposed the implantation of endovascular stents. This approach (either self- or balloon expandable stents) has had limited clinical application. The implantation in anatomically uncomplicated ductus arteriosus, such as in pulmonary atresia/critical pulmonary stenosis or the hypoplastic left heart syndrome (Fig. 10-15), has been encouraging.[121–123] The application in more complex ductal topologies as occurs in pulmonary atresia with ventricular septal defect, however, can be technically difficult,[122] and its role in the management of these infants has yet to be defined.

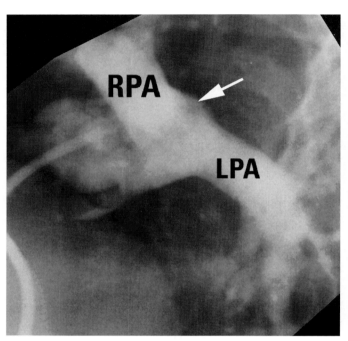

A

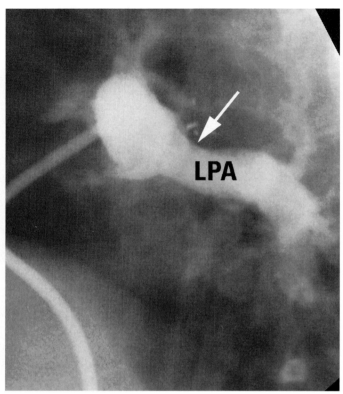

B

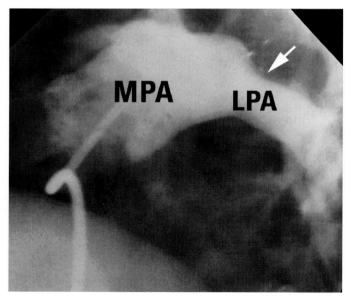

C

Fig. 10-13: Effect of umbrella occluder on the left pulmonary artery.
Two different patients. **A:** Pulmonary artery injection, cranially-tilted steep LAO projection. The proximal left pulmonary artery is normal prior to implantation. **B:** Antegrade pulmonary artery injection, steep LAO projection, following device placement. There is mild superior scalloping of the proximal left pulmonary artery due to the proximal arms of the implant (arrow). **C:** Another patient after ductal umbrella implantation, no deformity of the proximal left pulmonary artery is seen (arrow).

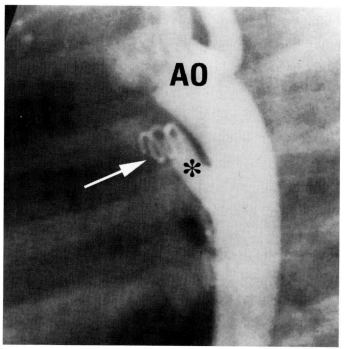

A

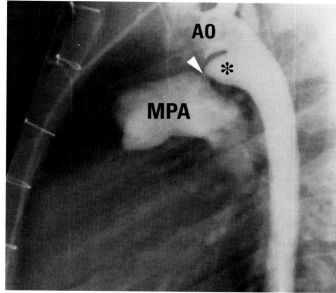

B

C

Fig. 10-14: Coil placement within an arterial duct.
A: A lateral projection descending aortogram after spring coil implantation (arrow). One coil loop is near the posterior wall of the main pulmonary artery at the ductal ostium (✳), while the remainder of the coil loops are implanted within the ampulla of the arterial duct (arrow). In **B**, (projection similar to **A**), a small patent arterial duct (arrowhead) with a prominent ampulla (✳) is occluded with a single coil (**C**). A tiny leak persists acutely (arrowheads).

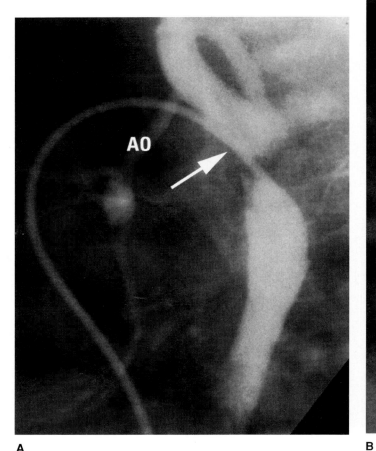

A

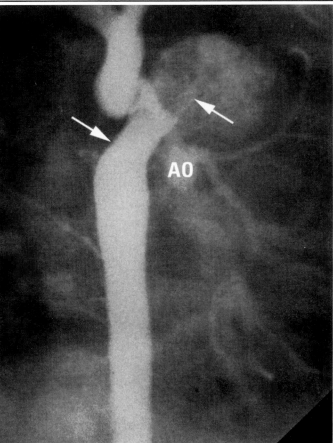

B

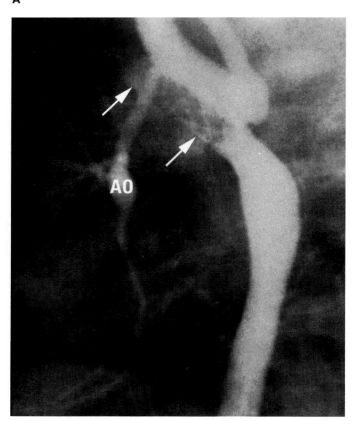

C

Fig. 10-15: Stenting of arterial duct.
Patient with the hypoplastic left heart syndrome. **A:** Lateral projection of antegrade descending aortogram with the catheter via a venous approach through the patent duct (arrow). **B:** Retrograde aortogram in near frontal and (**C**)lateral projections following stent placement (arrow). Note the hypoplastic aortic root.

References

1. Franklin K J. Ductus venosus (Arantii) and ductus arteriosus (Botalli). *Bull History Med* 1941;9:580–584.
2. Siegal RE. Galen's experiments and observations on pulmonary blood flow and respiration. *Am J Cardiol* 1962; 10:738–745.
3. Marquis RM. The continuous murmur of persistence of the ductus arteriosus—An historical review. *Eur Heart J* 1980;91:465–478.
4. Anderson RC. Causative factors underlying congenital heart malformations. I: patent ductus arteriosus. *Pediatrics* 1954;14:143–151.
5. Carlgren LE. The incidence of congenital heart disease in children born in Gothenburg 1941–1950. *Br Heart J* 1959;21:40–50.
6. Mitchell SC, Korones SB, Berendes HW. Congenital heart disease in 56 109 births. Incidence and natural history. *Circulation* 1971;43:323–332.
7. Houston AB, Gnanapragasam JP, Lim MK, Doig WB, Coleman EN. Doppler ultrasound and the silent ductus arteriosus. *Br Heart J* 1991;65:97–99
8. Congdon ED. Transformation of the aortic-arch system during the development of the human embryo. *Contrib Embryol* 1922;14:47–110.
9. Stewart JR, Kincaid OW, Edwards JE. *An Atlas of Vascular Rings and Related Malformations of the Aortic Arch System.* Sprinfield: Thomas; 1964
10. Edwards JE. Malformations of the aortic arch system manefested as "vascular rings". *Lab Invest* 1953;2:56–75.
11. Akiyama K, Hasegawa T, Kitamura S, Shindo S, Orime Y, Harada Y, Kurihara K, Nakazawa S, Sezai Y, Okada T. Right-sided patent ductus arteriosus with a right aortic arch and right descending aorta (in Japanese). *Jpn J Thorac Surg* 1992;45:442–445.
12. Binet JP, Conso JF, Losay J. Ductus arteriosus sling: Report of a newly recognized anomaly and its surgical correction. *Thorax* 1978;33:72–75.
13. Gross RE, Neuhauser ED. Compression of the trachea or esophagus by vascular anomalies: Surgical therapy in 40 cases. *Pediatrics* 1951;7:69–88.
14. Sones FM Jr, Effler DB. Diagnosis and treatment of aortic rings. *Cleve Clin Quart* 1951–1952;18–19:310–320.
15. Shulford WH, Sybers RG, Weens HS. The angiographic features of double aortic arch. *AJR* 1972;116:125–140.
16. Burrows PE, Moes CAF, Freedom RM. Double aortic arch with atretic right dorsal segment. *Pediatr Cardiol* 1986;6:331–334.
17. Ergin MA, Jayaram N, LaCorte M. Left aortic arch and right descending aorta: Diagnostic and therapeutic implications of a rare type of vascular ring. *Ann Thorac Surg* 1981;31:82–85.
18. Airan B, Bhan A, Rao IM. The combination of a left aortic arch, a right-sided descending thoracic aorta with a left-sided arterial duct. *Int J Cardiol* 1989;24:107–109.
19. Sanchez Torres G, Roldan Conesa D. Left aortic arch without a circumflex segment and a right descending aorta: A hypothetical case a real example (in Spanish). *Archivos Del Institution De Cardiologia De Mexico* 1989; 59:125–131.
20. Formigari R, Vairo U, de Zorzi A, Santoro G, Marino B. Prevalence of bilateral patent ductus arteriosus in patients with pulmonic valve atresia and asplenia syndrome. *Am J Cardiol* 1992;70:1219–1220.
21. Freedom RM, Moes CAF, Pelech A. Bilateral ductus arteriosus (or remnant): An analysis of 27 patients. *Am J Cardiol* 1984;53:884–889.
22. Penkoske PA, Castenada AR, Fyler DC Van Praagh R. Origin pulmonary artery branch from ascendong aorta. Primary surgical repair in infancy. *J Thorac Cardiovasc Surg* 1983;85:537–545.
23. Pierpont ME, Zollikofer CL, Moller JH, Edwards JE. Interruption of the aortic arch with right descending aorta. A rare condition and a cause of bronchial compression. *Pediatr Cardiol* 1982;2:153–159.
24. Kelsey JR Jr, Gilmore CE, Edwards JE. Bilateral ductus arteriosus representing persistence of each sixth aortic arch. *AMA Arch Pathol* 1953;55:154–161.
25. Keagy KS, Schall SA, Herrington RT. Selective cyanosis of the right arm. Isolation of right subclavian artery from aorta with bilateral ductus arteriosus and pulmonary hypertension. *Pediatr Cardiol* 1982;3:301–303.
26. Neye-Bock S Fellows KE. Aortic arch interruption in infancy: Radio- and angiographic features. *AJR* 1980;135: 1005–1010.
27. Rodriquez L, Izukawa T, Moes CAF, Trusler GA, Williams W. Surgical implications of right aortic arch with isolation of left subclavian artery. *Br Heart J* 1975; 37:931–936.
28. Barger JD, Bregman EH, Edwards JE. Bilateral ductus arteriosus with right aortic arch and right-sided descending aorta. *Am J Roentgen Rad Ther Nucl Med* 1956;76: 758–761.
29. Nair SK, Subramanyam R, Venkitachalam CG, Valiathan MS. Right aortic arch with isolation of the left subclavian artery and bilateral patent ductus arteriosus. A case report. *J Cardiovasc Surg* 1992;33:242–244.
30. Steinberg I, Miscall L, Goldberg HP. Congenital absence of left pulmonary artery with patent ductus arteriosi. *JAMA* 1964;190:394–396.
31. Freedom RM, Smallhorn JF, Burrows PE. Pulmonary atresia and ventricular septal defect. In: Freedom RM, Benson LN, Smallhorn JF, eds. *Neonatal Heart Disease.* London: Springer-Verlag; 1992, pp. 229–256.
32. Frescura C, Talenti E, Pellegrino PA, Mazzucco A, Faggian G, Thiene G. Coexistence of ductal and systemic pulmonary arterial supply in pulmonary atresia with ventricular septal defect. *Am J Cardiol* 1984;53:884–889.
33. Thiene G, Frescura C, Bortolotti U, Del Maschio A, Valente M. The systemic pulmonary circulation in pulmonary atresia with ventricular septal defect: Concept of reciprocal development of the fourth and sixth aortic arches. *Am Heart J* 1981;101:339–344.
34. Murray CA, Korns ME, Amplatz K, Edwards JE. Bilateral origin of the pulmonary artery from the homolateral ductus arteriosus. *Chest* 1970;57:310–317.
35. Berry BE, McGoon DC, Ritter DG, Davis GD. Absence of anatomic origin from heart of pulmonary arterial supply: Clinical application of classification. *J Thorac Cardiovasc Surg* 1974;68:119–125.
36. Todd EP, Lindsay WG, Edwards JE. Bilateral ductus origin of the pulmonary arteries. Systemic pulmonary arterial anastomosis as first stage in planned total correction. *Circulation* 1976;54:834–836.
37. Steno N. Reprinted with historical note: An unusually early description of the so-called tetralogy of Fallot. *Proc Staff Meetings Mayo Clin* 1948;23:316–320.
38. Emmanouilides G C, Thanopoulos B, Siassi B, Fishbein M. 'Agenesis' of ductus arteriosus associated with the syndrome of tetralogy of Fallot and absent pulmonary valve. *Am J Cardiol* 1976;37:403–409.

39. Fischer DR, Neches WH, Beerman LB. Tetralogy of Fallot with absent pulmonary valve: Analysis of 17 patients. *Am J Cardiol* 1984;53:1433–1437.

40. Ettedgui JA, Sharland GK, Chita SK, Cook A, Fagg N, Allan L D. Absent pulmonary valve syndrome with ventricular septal defect: Role of the arterial duct. *Am J Cardiol* 1990;15:233–234.

41. Mainwaring RD, Lamberti JJ, Spicer RL. Management of absent pulmonary valve syndrome with patent ductus arteriosus. *J Card Surg* 1993;8:148–155.

42. Lacina SJ, Hamilton WT, Thilenius OG, Bharati S, Lev M, Arcilla RA. Angiographic evidence of absent ductus arteriosus in severe right ventricular outflow obstruction. *Pediatr Cardiol* 1983;4:5–11.

42a.Wu JR, Chiu CC, Lin YT, Huang TY. Isolated persistent fifth aortic arch with right-sided aortic arch. *Jpn Heart J* 1995;36:813–817.

43. Heymann MA, Rudolph AM. Ductus arteriosus dilatation by prostaglandin E_1 in infants with pulmonary atresia. *Pediatrics* 1973;59:325–329.

44. Cassels De. *The Ductus Arteriosus.* Springfield: Thomas; 1973.

45. Calder AL, Kirker JA, Netuze JM, Starling MB. Pathology of the ductus arteriosus treated with prostaglandis: Comparisons with untreated cases. *Pediatr Cardiol* 1984; 5:85.

46. Elzenga NJ. *The Ductus Arteriosus and Stenoses of the Adjacent Great Vessels.* The Netherlands: University of Leiden; 1986. Thesis.

47. Santos MA, Moll JN, Drummond C, Aranjo WB, Romano N, Reiss NB. Development of the ductus arteriosus in right ventricular outflow tract obstruction. *Circulation* 1988;62:818–822.

48. Cruickshank B, Marquis RM. Spontaneous aneurysm of the ductus arteriosus. *Am J Med* 1958;25:140–149.

49. Holman E, Gerbode F, Purdy A. The patent ductus. A review of seventy-five cases with surgical treatment including an aneurysm of the ductus and one of the pulmonary artery. *J Thorac Surg* 1953;25:111–142.

50. Oldham HN Jr, Collinns NP, Pierce GE, Sabiston DC Jr, Blalock A. Giant patent ductus arteriosus. *J Thorac Cardiovasc Surg* 1964;47:331–336.

51. Gittenberger-de Groot AC, Strengers JL, Mentink M. Histologic studies on normal and persistent ductus arteriosus in the dog. *J Am Coll Cardiol* 1985;6:394–404.

52. Jager BV, Wollenman 0J. An anatomical study of the closure of the ductus arteriosus. *Am J Pathol* 1942;18: 595–613.

53. Quiroga C. Partial persistence of the ductus arteriosus. *Acta Radiol* 1961;55:103–108.

54. Gittenberger-de Groot AC. Structual variations of the ductus arteriosus in congenital heart disease and in persistent fetal circulation. In: Godman MJ, ed. *Pediatric Cardiology.* Volume 4. Edinburgh: Churchill Livingstone; 1981, pp. 53–63.

55. Presbitero P, Bull C, Haworth SG, et al. Absent or occult pulmonary artery. *Br Heart J* 1984;52:178–185.

56. Elzenga NJ, Gittenberger-de Groot AC. The ductus arteriosus and stenoses of the pulmonary arteries in pulmonary atresia. *Int J Cardiol* 1986;11:195–208.

57. Falcone MW, Perloff JK, Roberts WC. Aneurysm of the non-patent ductus arteriosus. *Am J Cardiol* 1972;29: 422–426.

58. Lund JT, Hansen D, Brocks V, Jensen MB, Jacobson JR. Aneurysm of the ductus arteriosus in the neonate: Three case reports with a review of the literature. *Pediatr Cardiol* 1992;13:222–226.

59. Lund JT, Jensen MB, Hjelms E. Aneurysm of the ductus arteriosus: A review of the literature and the surgical implications. *Eur J Cardiothorac Surg* 1991;5:566–570.

60. Ohtsuka S, Kahihana M, Ishikawa T, et al. Aneurysm of patent ductus arteriosus in an adult case: Findings of cardiac catheterization, angiography, and pathology. *Clin Cardiol* 1987;10:537–540.

61. Heikkinen ES, Simila S, Laitinen J, et al. Infantile aneurysm of the ductus arteriosus. *Acta Paediatr Scand* 1974;63:241–248.

61a.Sattar P, Ehrensperger J, Ducommun JC. Thrombosed aneurysmal nonpatent arteriosus: A case report. *Pediatr Radiol* 1996;26:207–209.

62. Das JB, Chesterman JT. Aneurysms of the ductus arteriosus. *Thorax* 1956;11:295–302.

63. Tutassaura H, Goldman B, Moes CAF, et al. Spontaneous aneurysm of the ductus arteriosus. *J Thorac Cardiovasc Surg* 1969;57:180–184.

64. Ueno Y, Shinozaki T, Shimamoto M, Ohkubo K, Ueda M, Akiyama F. Aneurysm of the diverticulum of the ductus arteriosus in the adult (in Japanese). *J Jpn Assoc Thorac Surg* 1990;83:1356–1361.

65. Rangel-Abundis A, Badui E, Verdin R, Escobar CV, Enciso R, Valdespino A. Spontaneous aneurysm of the patent ductus arteriosus with endarteritis. A case report (in Spanish). *Archives Del Instituto De Cardiologia De Mexico* 1991;61:59–64.

66. Taskar VS, John PJ, Mahashur AA. Ductal aneurysm presenting as acute lung callopse. *J Assoc Physicians India* 1992;40:475–476.

67. Mardini MK, Rao PS. Aortic arch angiography in patients with patent ductus arteriosus: A new technique. *Pediatr Cardiol* 1983;4:53–54.

68. Anand NK, Soloria M, Braudo JL, et al. Nonvisualization by aortography of patent ductus arteriosus associated with a large proximal left-to-right shunt. *Chest* 1971;60: 156–160.

69. Rao PS, Thapar MK, Strong WB. Nonopacification of patent ductus arteriosus by aortography in patients with large ventricular septal defects. *Angiology* 1978;29: 888–897.

70. Goodman PC, Jeffrey RB, Minagi H et al. Angiographic evaluation of the ductus diverticulum. *Cardiovasc Intervent Radiol* 1982;5:1–4.

71. Keane JF, McFaul R, Fellows K, et al. Balloon occlusion angiography in infancy: Methods, uses and limitations. *Am J Cardiol* 1985;56:495–497.

72. Porstmann W, Wierny L, Warnke H. Der Verschluss des Ductus arteriosus persistens ohne Thorakotomie (vor l a ufige Mitterlung). *Thoraxchicurgie* 1967;15:199–203.

73. Porstmann W, Wierny L, Warnke H. Der Vershlussdes Ductus arteriosus persistens ohne Thorakotomie (zweite Mitterlung). *Fortschr Rontgenstr* 1968;109:133–148.

74. Porstmann W, Wierny L, Warnke H. Gerstberger G, Romaniuk PA: Catheter closure of patent ductus arteriosus. *Radiol Clin North Am* 1971;9:203–218.

75. Porstmann W, Hieronymi K, Wierny L, Warnke H. Nonsurgical closure of oversized patent ductus arteriosus with pulmonary hypertension. Report of a case. *Circulation* 1974;50:346–381

76. Schrader R, Kneissl GD, Sievert H, Bussmann W-D, Kaltenbach M. Nonoperative closure of the patent ductus arteriosus: The Frankfurt experience. *J Intervent Cardiol* 1992;5:89–98.

77. Leslie J, Lindsay W, Amplatz K. Nonsurgical closure of patent ductus arteriosus: An experimental study. *Invest Radiol* 1977;12:142–145.

78. Mills ML, King TD. Nonoperative closure of left-to-right shunts. *J Thorac Cardiovasc Surg* 1976;72:371–378.

79. Echigo S, Matsuda T, Kamiya T, Tsuda E, Suda K, Kuroe K, Ono Y, Yazawa K. Development of a new transvenous patent ductus arteriosus occluder technique using a shape memory polmer. *ASAIO Trans* 1990;36:M195-M198.

80. Warnecke I, Frank J, Hohle R, Lemm W, Bucherl ES. Transvenous double-balloon occlusion of the persistent ductus arteriosus: An experimental study. *Pediatr Cardiol* 1984;5:79–84.

81. Magal C, Wright KC, Dupart G Jr, Wallace S, Gianturco C. A new device for transcatheter closure of the patent ductus arteriosus: A feasibility study in dogs. *Invest Radiol* 1989;24:272–276.

82. Rao PS, Wilson AD, Sideris ED, Chopra PS. Transcatheter closure of patent ductus arteriosus with 'buttoned' device: First successful clinical application in a child. *Am Heart J* 1991;121:1799–1802.

83. Rashkind WJ, Cuaso CC. Transcatheter closure of patent ductus arteriosus: Successful use in a 3.5 kilogram infant. *Pediatr Cardiol* 1979;1:3–7.

84. Rashkind WJ, Mullins CE, Hellenbrand WE, Tait MA. Nonsurgical closure of the patent ductus arteriosus: Clinical application of the Rashkind PDA Occluder System. *Circulation* 1987;75:583–592.

85. Lloyd TR, Fedderly R, Mendelson AM, Sandhu S, Beekman RH. Transcatheter occlusion of patent ductus with Gianturco coils. *Circulation* 1993;88:1412–1420.

86. Bash GE, Mullins CE. Insertion of patent ductus occluder by transvenous approach: A new technique. *Circulation* 1984;70(suppl II):II-285.

87. Musewe NN, Benson LN, Smallhorn JF, Freedom RM. Two-dimensional echocardiographic and color flow Doppler evaluation of ductal occlusion with the Rashkind prosthesis. *Circulation* 1989;80:1706–1710.

88. Ottenkamp J, Hess J, Talsma MD, Buis-Liem TN. Protrusion of the device: A complication of catheter occlusion of patent ductus arteriosus. *Br Heart J* 1992;68:301–303.

89. Wessel DL, Keane JF, Parness I, Lock JE. Outpatient closure of the patent ductus arteriosus. *Circulation* 1988;77:1068–1071.

90. Benson LN, Dyck J, Hecht B. Technique for closure of the small patent ductus arteriosus using the Rashkind occluder. *Cathet Cardiovasc Diagn* 1988;14:82–84.

91. Anonymous. Transcatheter occluasion of persistent arterial duct. Report of the European Registry. *Lancet* 1992;340:1062–1066.

92. Dyck JD, Benson LN, Smallhorn JF, McLaughlin P, Freedom PM, Rowe RD. Catheter occlusion of the persistently patent ductus arteriosus: Initial experience and early follow up. *Am J Cardiol* 1988;62:1089–1092.

93. Latson LA, Hofschire PJ, Kugler JD, Cheatham JP, Gumbiner CH, Danford DA. Transcatheter closure of patent ductus arteriosus in pediatric patients. *J Pediatr* 1989;115:549–553

94. Rohmer J, Hess J, Talsma MD. Closure of the persistent ductus arteriosus (Botalli) using a catheter procedure: The initial 50 patients treated in The Netherlands. *Nederlands Tijdschrift Voor Geneeskunde* 1990;134:2347–2351.

95. Ballerini L, Mullins CE, Cifarelli A, Pasquini L, Vairo U, Bermudez Canete R, Picchio FM, Boncivini M, Marzocchi A, Piovaccari G. Non-surgical closure of patent ductus arteriosus in children with the Rashkind double disk occluder. *Gionale Italian Di Cardiologia* 1990;20:805–809.

96. Rey C, Piechaud, JF, Bourlon F. Endoluminal closure of ductus arteriosus. A cooperative study. *Archives Des Maladies Du Coeur Et Des Vaisseaux* 1990;83:615–619.

97. Hosking MCK, Benson LN, Musewe N, Dyck JD, Freedom RM. Transcatheter occlusion of the persistent patent ductus arteriosus: Forty month follow-up and prevalence of residual shunting. *Circulation* 1991;84:2312–2317.

98. Ali Khan MA, Al Yousef S, Mullins CE, Sawyer W. Experience with 205 procedures of transcatheter closure of the ductus areteriosus with special reference to residual shunts and long term follow up. *J Thorac Cardiovasc Surg* 1992;104:1721–1727.

99. Ng MP, Wong KY, Tan A, Ong KK. Non-surgical closure of patent ductus arteriosus with the Rashkind PDA occluder system. *J Singapore Paediatric Soc* 1992;34:185–190.

100. Moore JW, Cambier PA. Transcatheter occlusion of patent ductus arteriosus: *J Intervent Cardiol* 1995;8:517–531.

101. Verin V, Friedli B, Oberhansli I, Urban P, Meier B. Closure of patent ductus arteriosus using interventional catheterization. *Schweizerische Medizinische Wochenschrift—Journal Suisse De Medecine* 1993;123:530–532.

102. Wilson NJ, Neutze JM, Mawson JB, Calder AL. Transcatheter closure of patent ductus arteriosus in children and adults. *New Zealand Med J* 1993;26:299–301.

103. Hosking MCK, Benson LN, Musewe N, Freedom RM. Reocclusion for persistent shunting after catheter placement of the Rashkind patent ductus arteriosus occluder. *Can J Cardiol* 1989;5:340–342.

104. Huggon IC, Tabatabaei AH, Qureshi SA, Bakker EJ, Tynan M. Use of a second Rashkind arterial duct occluder for persistent flow after implantation of the first device. *Br Heart J* 1993;69:544–550.

105. Fadley F, Al Halees Z, Galal O, Kumar N, Wilson N. Left pulmonary artery stenosis after transcatheter occlusion of the persistent arterial duct. *Lancet* 1993;341:559–560.

106. Ladusans EJ, Murduch I, Franciosi J. Severe haemolysis after percutaneous closure of a ductus arteriosus (arterial duct). *Br Heart J* 1989;61:548–550.

107. Hayes AM, Redington AN, Rigby ML. Severe haemolysis after transcatheter duct occlusion: A non-surgical remedy. *Br Heart J* 1992;67:321–322.

108. Grifka RG, O'Laughlin MP, Mullins CE. Late transcatheter removal of a Rashkind PDA occlusion device for persistent hemolysis using a modified transseptal sheath. *Cathet Cardiovasc Diagn* 1992;25:140–143.

109. Sato K, Fujino M, Kozuka T, Naito Y, Kitamura S, Makano S, Ohyama C, Kawashima Y. Transfemoral plug closure of patent ductus arteriosus. *Circulation* 1975;51:337–341.

110. Kitamura S, Sato K, Naito Y, Shimizu, Y, Fujino M, Oyama C, Nakano S, Kawashima Y. Plug closure of patent ductus arteriosus by transfemoral catheter method. *Chest* 1976;70:631–635.

111. Qian J. Catheter closure of patent ductus arteriosus without thoracotomy. *Chung-Hua Hsin Hsueh Kuan Ping Tsa Chih* 1992;20:167–168.

112. Wang Y. Transfemoral plug closure in 45 cases of patent ductus arteriosus. *Chung-Hua Hsin Hsueh Kuan Ping Tsa Chih* 1991;19:18–20.

113. Cambier PA, Kirby WC, Wortham DC, Moore JW. Percutaneous closure of the small (less than 2.5 mm) patent ductus arteriosus using coil embolization. *Am J Cardiol* 1992;69:815–816.

114. Moore JW, George L, Kirkpatrick SE, Mathewson JW, Spicer RL, Uzark K, Rothman A, Slack MC, Kirby WC. Percutaneous closure of small patent ductus arteriosus using occluding spring coils. *J Am Coll Cardiol* 1993;23: 759–765.

115. Lund G, Rysavy J, Cragg A. Long-term patency of the ductus arteriosus after balloon dilatation: An experimental study. *Circulation* 1989;69:772–774.

116. Corwin RD, Singh AK, Karlson KE. Balloon dilation of ductus arteriosus in a newborn with interrupted aortic arch and ventricular septal defect. *Am Heart J* 1981;102: 446–447.

117. DeLezo JS, Lopez-Rubio F, Guzman J. Percutaneous transluminal angioplasty of stenotic ductus arteriosus. *Cathet Cardiovasc Diagn* 1985;11:493–500.

118. Walsh KP, Abrams SE, Arnold R. Arterial duct angioplasty as an adjunct to dilatation of the valve for critical pulmonary stenosis. *Br Heart J* 1993;69:260–263.

119. Walsh KP, Sreeram N. Franks R, Arnold R. Balloon dilatation of the arterial duct in congenital heart disease. *Lancet* 1992;339:331–332.

120. Coe JY, Olley PM. A novel method to maintain ductus arteriosus patency. *J Am Coll Cardiol* 1991;18:837–841.

121. Ruiz CE, Zhang HP, Larsen RL. The role of interventional cardiology in pediatric heart transplantation. *J Heart Lung Transplant* 1993;12:S164-S167.

122. Gibbs JL, Rothman MT, Rees MR, Parsons JM, Blackburn ME, Ruiz CE. Stenting the arterial duct: A new approach to palliation for pulmonary atresia. *Br Heart J* 1992;67: 240–245.

123. Gibbs JL, Wren C, Watterson KG, Hunter S, Hamilton JR Leslie. Stenting of the arterial duct combined with banding of the pulmonary arteries and atrial septectomy or septostomy: A new approach to palliation for the hypoplastic left heart syndrome. *Br Heart J* 1993:69; 551–555.

Chapter 11

Arteriovenous Fistula

With Cathy MacDonald, MD, FRCPC

Introduction

Congenital extracardiac arteriovenous malformations are relatively rare lesions. Since the majority do not present until adult life, progressive enlargement occurs throughout childhood. In the infant or child, large malformations may present with intractable congestive heart failure, cyanosis, dyspnea, abnormal bounding, or diminished peripheral pulses. The diagnosis of these malformations may be elusive because the clinical picture in the newborn often mimics a variety of congenital cardiac diseases. The delay in diagnosis has often been implicated as a major reason for the high mortality of these lesions. Although favorable long-term outcome particularly of the cerebral fistula remains guarded, sophisticated interventional radiological techniques have increased survival rates.[1,2]

Definition

The term vascular lesion covers a wide range of anomalies that can be subclassified as capillary or cavernous hemangiomas and arteriovenous malformations.[3–5] Hemangiomas are tumor-like masses characterized by endothelial proliferation and spontaneous involution. Arteriovenous malformations are congenital vascular anomalies that are characterized by abnormal communications between arterial and venous systems with lack of normal capillary development; they have no potential for cellular proliferation or involution. Hemangiomas may be stimulated to involute by the administration of systemic or intralesional corticosteroids, laser therapy, and embolization. Vascular malformations show no response to steroids; they are often

difficult to resect completely and are often treated by combined embolization and surgery.[4]

In early fetal life, extensive anastomoses exist between the arterial and venous systems.[6] The underlying causative factor in the development of arteriovenous fistulas is disordered embryogenesis resulting in persistence of these primitive connections.

Incidence

The vascular malformations that present with congestive heart failure in infancy most commonly involve the brain, liver, or lungs.[7,8] The intracranial arteriovenous malformations associated with an aneurysm of the great vein of Galen are the most frequent malformations encountered. Other rarer types of high-flow cerebrovascular fistula include intrahemispheric, dural, vertebrovertebral, external carotid, and giant capillary hemangiomas of the head and neck.[9–11]

Less often, arteriovenous malformations are multiple and may have multisystem involvement. Hereditary hemorrhagic telangiectasia, also known as Osler-Weber-Rendu disease, is a condition with autosomal dominant inheritance that occurs with an estimated frequency of 1–2:100,000. It is characterized by telangiectasias, arteriovenous fistulas, and aneurysms. The skin and mucosa, as well as blood vessels of the liver, lungs, and central nervous system may be involved. Hepatic arteriovenous fistulas occur in approximately 30% of patients with the disease; pulmonary malformations 15% to 20%, and central nervous system in less than 10% of patients. There is a strong association between pulmonary arteriovenous malformations and hereditary hemorrhagic telangiectasia, approximately

From: Freedom RM, Mawson JB, Yoo SJ, Benson LN: *Congenital Heart Disease: Textbook of Angiocardiography.* Armonk NY, Futura Publishing Co., Inc. ©1997.

40% to 70% of patients with pulmonary arteriovenous malformations have hereditary hemorrhagic telangiectasia.[12–14]

Congenital Arteriovenous Malformations

An extracardiac arteriovenous fistula is a rare cause of congestive heart failure and should be kept in mind in cases of unexplained heart failure in infancy. The clinical manifestation depends on the pathophysiology and hemodynamic influence of the arteriovenous malformation, which depends on the size, number, and nature of vessels within the lesion.[15–17]

Cerebral Arteriovenous Fistula

Although a rare lesion, the vein of Galen aneurysm is the most common cerebrocranial vascular lesion presenting with cardiac manifestations. The vein of Galen is a midline structure that drains the internal cerebral venous system and basal veins of Rosenthal, emptying into the straight sinus. During development of the cerebral circulation, arteries and veins cross in close proximity allowing for abnormal fistulous connections to occur.[18] The size and number of arteriovenous connections determine the degree of aneurysmal enlargement of the vein of Galen. The massive dilatation of the great

vein of Galen may be a result of true aneurysmal enlargement due to primary connections from arteries feeding directly into the vein or secondary dilatation in which a nearby angiomatous malformation drains through the Galenic system.[19] The distinction is important as they require different surgical treatments: the secondary dilatation is directed to excision of the angioma, whereas the primary aneurysm is directed to occlusion of the feeding arteries. The arteriovenous fistula may be supplied from the carotid artery through terminal branches of the anterior cerebral circulation however, the main blood supply is usually from the vertebrobasilar circulation.[20] The malformation may contain a convolution of thin-walled vessels without a capillary network representing a true arteriovenous malformation or it may consist of a direct arteriovenous fistula.[21] The cerebral arteries involved are enlarged with multiple feeding arteries into the vein of Galen. The vein of Galen drains into large straight and lateral sinuses (Fig. 11-1). Often there is associated obstructive anomalies of the dural venous sinuses or jugular vein. The end result is a complex vascular mass surrounded by ischemic and edematous brain tissue.[8,22]

Intracranial arteriovenous malformation of the epidural vessels are exceedingly rare.[23] Dural arteriovenous malformations are characterized by increased abnormal blood vessels within the dura mater, represent-

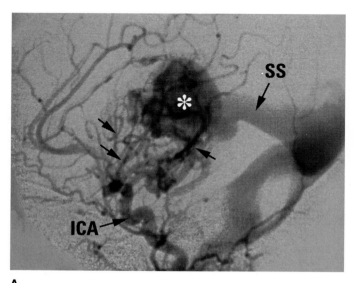

A

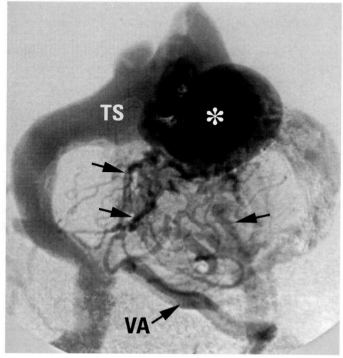

B

Fig. 11-1: Cerebral arteriovenous malformation of the vein of Galen type.
Internal carotid arteriogram lateral view (**A**) and vertebral arteriogram frontal view (**B**) demonstrate multiple arterial feeders (arrows) supplying a markedly enlarged vein of Galen (✻) that rapidly drains into the dural sinuses.

ing approximately 10% of intracranial arteriovenous malformations. These malformations are supplied by branches of internal and external carotid and vertebral arteries and drain into the dural sinuses (Figs. 11-2 and 11-3).[24] High-flow dural and mixed dural-pial arteriovenous malformations most commonly present in adulthood with symptoms ranging from cranial nerve palsy to impaired cortical function.[25] Cases of massive dural fistula presenting in the neonatal period with cardiac failure pose an extremely difficult problem. Attempts at embolization, resection, and a combination of staged procedures have been used to control cardiac failure.[11,25] The lesions involve multiple arterial feeders and most frequently involve the posterior dura. These lesions are high risk and have generally been fatal.[8,11]

The clinical presentation of a cerebral arteriovenous fistula depends on its hemodynamic impact, which in turn is associated with the patient's age and the severity of the lesion. The neonatal presentation of a cerebrovascular malformation is often fatal due to severe refractory cardiac failure associated with subendocardial ischemia or transmural infarction.[18,26] High-output congestive heart failure in the neonatal period, a reflection of a large left-to-right shunt, is the most common presentation of a cerebral arteriovenous fistula.[8,27-29] Cardiac failure is usually absent in utero; this may relate to low-resistance cerebral and placental circulations that are in competition for blood flow, resulting in lower volumes flowing through the fistula. After birth, with removal of the low-resistance placental circulation, flow is directed toward the cerebral fistula.[27] The cerebral circulation may have flows of 80% or more of the cardiac output, resulting in large vol-

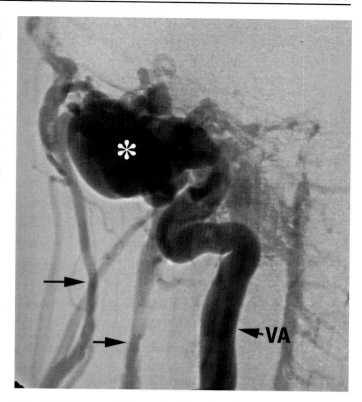

Fig. 11-3: Congenital vertebral-jugular fistula.
Frontal right vertebral angiogram demonstrates an ectatic vertebral artery supplying a large fistulous pouch at the skull base (✳) that rapidly shunts into multiple draining veins (arrows).

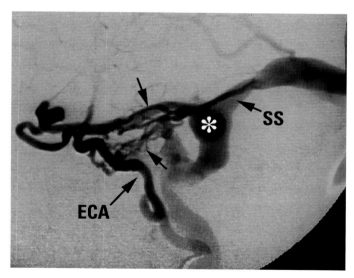

Fig. 11-2: Dural arteriovenous fistula.
Selective right external carotid angiogram demonstrates the major arterial feeders (arrows) supplying the arteriovenous malformation (✳).

umes of oxygenated blood under high pressure returning to the right side of the heart and pulmonary circulation.[8] In addition, it is hypothesized that in utero the left ventricle supplies the fistula and the right ventricle supplies the placenta, which results in parallel circulations; after birth there are complex adjustments with each ventricle having to sustain the entire circulation, contributing to cardiac failure.[30,31] The high flow through the fistula may compromise blood flow to the coronary circulation and also the myocardium during diastole. The increased ventricular pressures reducing subendocardial perfusion and reduced coronary flow causing myocardial ischemia are important factors contributing to persistent congestive heart failure.[16,21,26] In addition to the intractable heart failure, the tremendous shunt through the fistula deprives the cerebrum of blood resulting in ischemic parenchymal brain damage.[32]

Cyanosis may be present because of persistent fetal circulation.[27,33] An arteriovenous fistula lowers the mean systemic arterial blood pressure and results in increased pulmonary arterial and right atrial mean pressures. The markedly increased systemic venous return to the right atrium elevates right atrial pressure above left atrial pressure, causing right-to-left shunting through a patent foramen ovale.[17] The low systemic resistance also causes unoxygenated blood to stream from the high-pressure pulmonary artery through the ductus arteriosus into the low-pressure descending aorta. The combination of left-to-right shunt hemodynamics and central cyanosis should raise a flag for the diagnosis of an arteriovenous malformation.

The large fistula proximal to the ductus results in lowered pressure within the aorta beyond the origin of the subclavian artery. This leads to reduced stimulus for the aortic isthmus to enlarge and hence to isthmus hypoplasia or discrete coarctation.[34]

When the presentation appears later in infancy, obstructive hydrocephalus, seizures, subarachnoid hemorrhage, or venous congestion of the scalp and facial veins may be observed. Older children are more likely to present with mild heart failure, hydrocephalus, headache, or focal neurological signs. The pathogenesis of the hydrocephalus may be due to compression of the aqueduct of Sylvius by the venous aneurysm, elevated sinus pressure that impedes absorption of cerebrospinal fluid, recurrent subclinical episodes of subarachnoid hemorrhage, or a combination of factors.[8,25] Neurological deterioration is primarily due to "cerebral steal phenomenon," which implies a state of insufficient perfusion of brain tissue. The arteriovenous fistula consists of afferent feeding arteries that also emit arteries to adjacent brain tissue. The shunt flow through an arteriovenous malformation is pressure-dependent in contrast to flow through normal vasculature, which is autoregulated. The characteristic flow-pressure relationship results in passive dilatation of the involved vascular channels. The intravascular pressure throughout the feeding arterial system is low; it is the low intravascular pressure within nutrifying arteries that results in an intracerebral steal phenomena.[35] The nutrifying arterioles in an attempt to maintain adequate blood flow in the face of low pressure are in a state of maximal dilatation. It is this theory that is the basis for the postoperative complication of "normal perfusion pressure breakthrough." After conversion of shunt flow to perfusion flow, the maximally dilated arterioles may have an impaired vasomotor regulation that leads to overperfusion or a circulatory breakthrough.[35,36] Results of other studies that demonstrate decreasing flow velocities, rising peripheral resistance, and vasomotor response in the arterioles arising from feeding arteries question the assumption of the breakthrough phenomenon.[35] Arterial and/or venous thrombosis may lead to postoperative ischemia, swelling, and hemorrhage. The mass effect of the venous aneurysm directly compressing brain parenchyma may contribute to focal neurological deficits.[18,32,37] Fibrous thickening, calcification, thrombus and gliosis in adjacent neural tissue is more common in the older child.[23,38]

On examination cranial bruits are heard in one-third of patients.[8] The peripheral pulses are generally decreased in amplitude except in arteries near the fistula, which are of large volume. In the presence of a cerebral arteriovenous fistula, most of the cardiac output is diverted to the arteries supplying the fistula, resulting in decreased lower limb pressure, features mimicking an aortic coarctation.[39] As previously described, if descending aortic flow is significantly reduced, then anatomic coarctation of the aorta or hypoplasia of the aortic isthmus may occur.[40]

The electrocardiogram may show signs of ventricular hypertrophy, myocardial ischemia or infarction.[26] Chest radiography demonstrates a constellation of features due to the volume overload in patients with an intracranial arteriovenous fistula. There is cardiomegaly with specific signs of right-chamber dilatation and increased pulmonary vascularity. A more specific feature is widening of the superior mediastinum with both retrosternal fullness and retropharyngeal soft tissue thickening due to dilatation of the ascending aorta and brachiocephalic vessels.[8,27,41]

Noninvasive imaging techniques including ultrasound, computed tomography, and magnetic resonance imaging (MRI) have facilitated diagnosis in these patients. The cross-sectional echocardiogram is valuable in confirming a structurally normal heart.[16] Routine echocardiography has demonstrated an unsuspected sinus venosus atrial septal defect in an infant with a vein of Galen malformation.[42] In patients with large intracerebral shunts, echocardiographic features include dilated hyperdynamic cardiac chambers with increased runoff to the upper half of the body and abnormal dilatation of the superior vena cava, ascending aorta, aortic arch, and brachiocephalic vessels.[8,39,43] Focal narrowing of the aortic isthmus may be observed. Doppler assessment demonstrates retrograde diastolic steal in the descending aorta with continuous forward flow in the aortic arch and brachiocephalic vessels due to the low resistance to flow through the fistula.[8,39,44,45] Contrast (bubble) echocardiography increases diagnostic sensitivity and shows early recirculation of microbubbles from the left side of the heart to the superior vena cava after passing through the cerebral malformation.[17,18,43] Right-to-left shunting across a patent foramen ovale or patent ductus arteriosus may also be observed.

Cardiac catheterization and angiography play little role in the evaluation of extracardiac arteriovenous fistula and are often poorly tolerated by the critically ill neonate. Cardiac catheterization unfortunately may be performed with the view of evaluating congenital heart disease. Catheterization reveals increased oxygen saturation in the superior vena cava without signs of intracardiac shunting and pulmonary artery hypertension.[28]

Two-dimensional cranial ultrasound with color-flow Doppler provides a rapid and accurate demonstration of the cerebral arteriovenous malformation and plays a role in screening neonates with congestive heart failure of undetermined etiology. Color-flow Doppler demonstrates flow in feeding arteries and their convergence into the large confluent vein. Pulsed-wave Doppler shows continuous flow in the feeding arteries and nonpulsating, low-velocity continuous flow in the venous aneurysm.[46] The results have been used to assess blood flow within the malformation pre- and post-staged endovascular embolization procedures and to plan further interventions.[21]

Cross-sectional imaging with computed tomography and MRI provides valuable information regarding the nature and location of the intracerebral malformation including the morphology of the dural sinuses, as well as identifying associated ventriculomegaly or the presence of ischemic infarction. Serial magnetic resonance scans have demonstrated progressive thrombosis in vein of Galen malformations after embolotherapy.[21]

Selective neuroarteriography continues to be required to complete the diagnostic evaluation and provide precise information regarding the angioarchetecture necessary for planning the most effective surgical or embolization therapy.[47] A diagnostic angiogram, however, is not warranted in early infancy because cross-sectional imaging provides all the necessary diagnostic information. In evaluating a high-flow arteriovenous fistula, the arterial digital subtraction technique offers several advantages that include rapid film rates and less contrast per injection, which enables selective studies of multiple vessels with reduced risk of exacerbating the cardiac failure.[25]

Despite prompt recognition and aggressive treatment of symptomatic newborns with arteriovenous malformations, the natural history of the disease has high morbidity and mortality rates. Early therapy is important to avoid or minimize systemic complications, as well as nervous system complications. Treatment is directed toward correcting both cardiac failure and cerebral ischemia. The vein of Galen aneurysm represents a therapeutic challenge, due in part to its difficult surgical access as well as to severe clinical symptomatology.[48] The cerebrovascular malformations can be treated by surgery, embolization, or a combination of methods. Occasionally, spontaneous thrombosis of the arteriovenous malformations may occur. Comprehensive reviews report a mortality of over 90% in patients presenting with cardiac failure in the newborn period from a vein of Galen aneurysm.[16,23,48] In the past, surgical treatment consisted of clipping identifiable feeding vessels and leaving the venous portion intact, as it represents a normal channel for venous drainage. Although there are reports of staged surgical successes, mortality approached 100%. There are encouraging results with advances in endovascular embolization techniques. Embolization offers a primary therapeutic approach that can successively occlude arterial vessels feeding the fistula.[23,49] This allows for stabilization of cardiac function, as well as favors thrombosis of the arteriovenous nidus. Proper analysis of the angioarchitecture is imperative for planning appropriate treatment. There are a variety of different materials that may be used for embolization that include administration of thrombogenic materials such as acrylic glue and solid particles proximal to or directly into the lesion, detachable coils, detachable silicone balloons, silk suture, or silicone beads.[8,49,50] Initial embolotherapy is directed toward the arterial side of the malformation; if this is contraindicated or unsuccessful, a transtorcular or transfemoral venous approach may be performed. The transtorcular approach requires a craniotomy for access to the straight or falcine sinus. Complications of this procedure include perforation of the vein of Galen and perforation of the torcula Herophili or sinus resulting in subarachnoid hemorrhage. Advantages include the ability to use larger coils.[6,8,23,51–54]

Treatment strategies favor a staged approach that improves the cardiovascular status and also slowly redistributes intracranial blood flow to normal brain tissue.[18,22] Congestive heart failure has been successfully treated and normal neurological development has been reported. It is felt that at least 30% of the lesion must be controlled in one procedure.[9] Rapid ligation of arterial feeders may potentially lead to fatal hemodynamic changes. An acute increase in systemic vascular resistance worsens the cardiac failure, this is further aggravated by aggressive vasodilation which compromises coronary perfusion. In addition rapid ligation of afferent vessels may redirect cerebral blood flow too abruptly leading to massive cerebral edema and/or venous infarction.[6,18] After staged embolization, cardiac symptoms resolved or improved in over 90% of cases in one series. Mortality in the embolized group was 9%.[9] The major risks of the embolotherapy includes intraventricular bleed, inadvertent embolization of an uninvolved vessel, and intra- or postoperative cardiac ischemia.[6] Although embolization may be effective in controlling the shunt and the congestive heart failure, it may not always completely obliterate the lesion. After embolization, surgical excision may then be performed in an older, more stable patient.[4,8,23] Endovascular therapy may not be appropriate in all cases and may be rejected in cases of preexisting severe brain damage or arterial feeders inaccessible for safe embolization.[9] Permanent parenchymal damage that occurred in utero cannot be reversed. Close follow-up with computed tomography or MRI is important in guiding the success of treatment.[21,23] When there is persistent cardiac failure, the arteriovenous fistula must be reevaluated carefully for any residual shunt as additional sources of blood supply to the fistula may be unmasked following occlusion of large feeding vessels, if there are no signs of a persistent fistula than an associated cardiac defect should be considered. Uncommon associated lesions have been described including a sinus venosus atrial septal defect.[42] Late neurological sequelae remains unknown, influenced by the prenatal cerebral status and effect of revascularization and development of the cerebral circulation to the normal brain tissue.[37]

Embolization of dural arteriovenous fistulas has a lower morbidity and mortality than surgical treatment. Dural arteriovenous malformations in children are difficult lesions to treat, there is a high incidence of secondary complications that include hydrocephalus due to venous hypertension, cerebral ischemia and atrophy, hemorrhage, and progressive cardiac failure. The treatment goal is to obliterate the malformation before secondary complications occur.[4] The best chance of cure is through combined embolization of the arterial tributaries with subsequent resection of the malformation and preservation of the venous drainage.[21]

To obtain the optimal outcome, it is important that the presence of an intracranial arteriovenous fistula be recognized early so that prompt diagnostic evaluation and appropriate therapy can be performed.

Hepatic Arteriovenous Fistula

There are a variety of vascular lesions that arise within the liver parenchyma. Vascular tumors of the liver are rare in childhood. Hepatic hemangiomas or hemangio-endotheliomas are benign vascular tumors that may be part of a clinical syndrome described as multinodular hemangiomatosis of the liver (Fig. 11-4). The syndrome consists of hepatomegaly, congestive heart failure, and cutaneous hemangioma. Associated disorders include a consumptive coagulopathy, thrombocytopenia, and liver dysfunction.[55–57] An uncommon complication is portal hypertension, which may relate to increased flow within the portal system.[58] The great variability in the severity and extent of the lesions, associated complications, and the occurrence of spontaneous regression often pose problems in both diagnosis and management. Hemodynamically, more than 50% of the total cardiac output may be shunted through the liver causing high-output congestive heart failure.[8] It is the congestive heart failure that is often the dominant clinical and prognostic feature in patients with hepatic hemangioendotheliomas. The hemodynamic changes are simply the response of the cardiovascular system to a large left-to-right shunt. Commonly, the presentation is an abdominal mass or a pulsatile liver.[8] Less common presenting features are transient obstructive jaundice, intestinal obstruction, or intestinal bleeding.[59] Clinical audible bruits over the right upper quadrant are uncommon. Peripheral pulses are usually normal.

The arteriovenous malformations within the liver may be single, multiple, or diffuse ranging in diameter from a few millimeters to several centimeters. The group of hepatic malformations that present with congestive heart failure contain direct arteriovenous fistulas. The arterial feeders arise from the hepatic artery with drainage into the hepatic veins both of which become massively enlarged. There are many cases of hepatic hemangiomas that involute; however, those presenting early with congestive heart failure have a poor prognosis.[8]

A chest radiograph demonstrates features of high-output cardiac failure, with cardiomegaly and pulmonary congestion. In contrast to the widened superior mediastinum seen in intracranial malformations, hepatic fistulas may lead to dilatation of the descending thoracic aorta.[8,16]

Sonography demonstrates an abnormally dilated hepatic artery and intrahepatic arteries, with abnormal echogenicity of the liver.[60] The aorta above the celiac trunk is dilated, tapering to a small diameter inferiorly. Visualization of the arteriovenous fistulas depends on their size. Conglomerate arterial masses are difficult to differentiate from arteriovenous fistulas. Doppler tracing or spectral analysis of feeding arteries and draining veins are helpful in making a distinction. The spectral analysis of large feeding arteries reveals arterial signal, while flow through the arteriovenous fistulas exhibits spectral broadening as well as mixed arterial and venous signal.[14]

The diagnosis of a hemangioendothelioma of the liver is confirmed by hepatic scanning, angiography, and/or biopsy. Computerized tomography and MRI are useful in diagnosing and defining the site and extent of hepatic fistula. MRI of hepatic hemangiomas depicts the hepatic vascular anatomy modifying the role of angiography.[61] The findings at angiography include dilated hepatic arteries, abnormal pooling of contrast material throughout the liver, and early opacification of hepatic and/or portal veins. Angiography is necessary if surgical intervention or arterial embolotherapy are considerations.[57,62]

The prognosis for children with hemangioendotheliomas of the liver is poor. The rarity of the disorder and absence of standard treatment contribute to the low survival rate.[62] If complications are absent, careful observation is appropriate as spontaneous resolution is known to occur even in large tumors.[59] If congestive cardiac failure develops, anticongestive medical therapy should be first line treatment. If cardiac failure is refractory to medical management, then hepatic artery ligation or embolization is recommended in infants less than 6 weeks of age due to the high associated mortality.[8] Although there are hepatic hemangiomas successfully treated with embolization particle techniques, the results are less uniform in infantile lesions presenting with massive arteriovenous shunting. Strict guidelines must be adhered to in developing appropriate particle

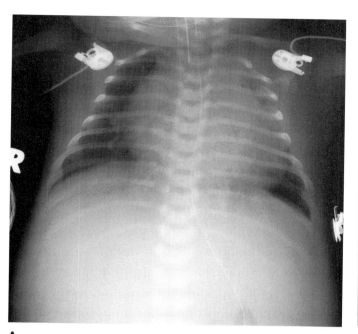

A

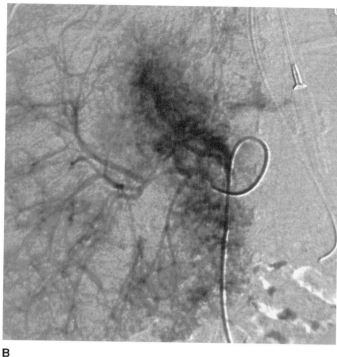

B

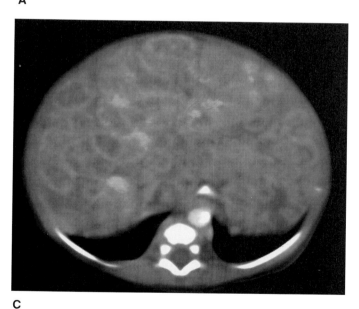

C

Fig. 11-4: Infantile hepatic hemangiomatosis with congestive cardiac failure.
A: Frontal chest and abdominal radiograph which demonstrate moderate cardiomegaly with pulmonary overcirculation and pulmonary edema. The large abdominal mass is due to marked hepatomegaly. **B**: Late arterial phase of a selective hepatic arteriogram demonstrates widespread intrahepatic arteriovenous malformations. **C**: Transverse enhanced CT image depicts the diffuse intrahepatic hemangiomas as multiple ring enhancing nodules.

suspensions for embolization therapy.[63–66] Radiolabeled polyvinyl alcohol particles have been used to embolize an hepatic arteriovenous malformation. Scintigraphic imaging after the procedure allowed determination of particle position, establishing documentation of placement within the liver and the absence of embolic particles to the lungs.[67]

In infants more than 6 weeks old, prednisone in combination with anticongestive therapy has been shown to be an effective method of treatment.[57] The mechanisms by which corticosteroids cause involution of hepatic hemangiomas is unclear, however, one proposal is that the systemic steroids have a vasoconstrictive effect on the rapidly proliferating endothelial cells lining the vascular spaces. Complete surgical resection is reserved for localized tumors.[68]

Pulmonary Arteriovenous Fistula

Pulmonary arteriovenous malformation is a vascular anomaly of the pulmonary circulation that conveys pulmonary arterial blood into the pulmonary veins resulting in a right-to-left shunt (see also Chapters 19, 24, and 41). Typically, a pulmonary arteriovenous malformation comprises a conglomerate of dilated vessels in the peripheral lung parenchyma associated with a variable number of afferent and efferent connections, the malformation however may range from a large arteriovenous fistula to a myriad of microscopic shunts (Figs. 11-5 and 11-6). The pulmonary vascular abnormalities include four major types of lesions: primary pulmonary telangiectasia, hereditary hemorrhagic telangiectasia, discrete arteriovenous fistula, and hepatogenic pul-

monary angiodysplasia. The afferent vessels generally arise from the pulmonary artery with rare additional connections from bronchial or intercostal arteries.[8,69] Large malformations may result from a single large feeding pulmonary artery and a single draining vein connected by a nonseptated vascular space. Alternatively the malformation may be more complex consisting of multiple feeding arteries and draining veins connected by a septated communication.[12,70] In classic discrete pulmonary arteriovenous fistulas and hereditary hemorrhagic telangiectasia, the malformations are

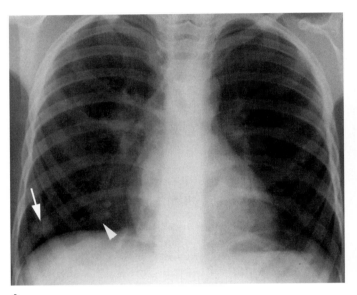

A

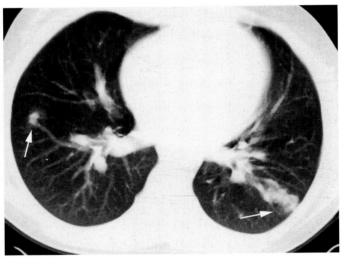

B

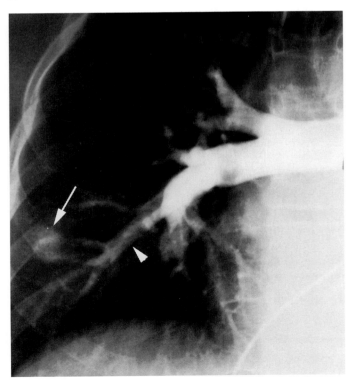

C

Fig. 11-5: Simple multiple pulmonary arteriovenous malformations.
A: Frontal chest radiograph demonstrating the pulmonary artery malformation within the right lower lobe (arrow) and adjacent dilated vessel (arrowhead). **B:** Transverse unenhanced CT image depicting the multiple simple pulmonary arteriovenous malformations (arrows). **C:** Right pulmonary arteriogram frontal view which demonstrates supply to the simple pulmonary arteriovenous malformation within the right lower lobe (arrow) from the pulmonary artery (arrowhead).

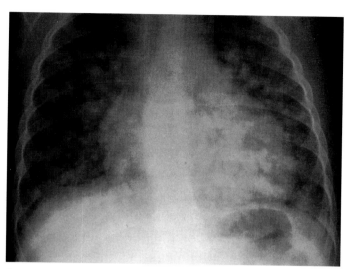

A

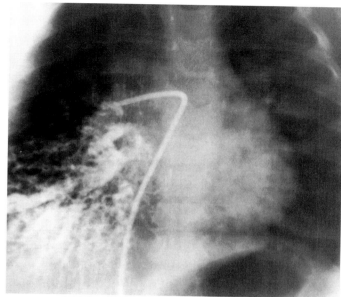

B

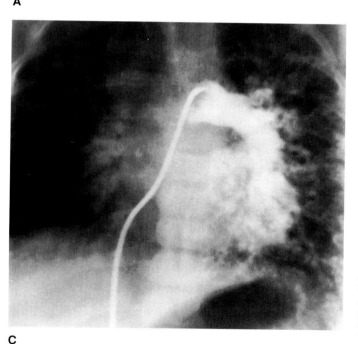

C

Fig. 11-6: Diffuse pulmonary arteriovenous malformations.
A: Frontal chest radiograph demonstrating a myriad of pulmonary arteriovenous malformations and moderate cardiomegaly. **B**: Selective right lower and left main (**C**) pulmonary arteriograms confirm the widespread bilateral pulmonary arteriovenous malformations.

generally localized rather than diffuse, although they may be multiple. The lesions typically seen in primary pulmonary telangiectasia and hepatogenic pulmonary angiodysplasia are evenly disseminated throughout both lungs.

Cyanosis is reported as the presenting sign of a pulmonary fistula in approximately 25% of cases, most often later in infancy.[12,71,72] Only very large fistula or those involving the proximal pulmonary arteries present with cyanosis in the neonatal period.[73] There is a rare situation where a direct communication between a central pulmonary artery and a common pulmonary vein or left atrium occurs, leading to a physiologic pul-

monary steal. Neonates with this unusual anomaly present with cyanosis within hours or days after birth. An important factor in determining survival and correction of this anomaly is the degree of hypoplasia of the peripheral pulmonary arteries, which occurs as the result of a physiologic pulmonary arterial steal in utero.[74,75] In the symptomatic group, other presenting problems include exertional dyspnea, fatigue, recurrent lower respiratory tract infections, and congestive heart failure.[8] Severe complications may occur later that include brain abscess, embolism, hemoptysis, and hemothorax.[12] The neurological complications arise due to the absence of an intrapulmonary filter.[16,76] The latter two complications result from thin-walled malformations rupturing into a bronchus or pleural space.[76] Secondary polycythemia may lead to headache and dizziness, as well as increasing the risk of stroke.[8] A significant number of patients are asymptomatic and are only identified with an abnormal chest radiograph. On examination, cyanosis and finger clubbing are often found. A pulmonary bruit may be heard with large malformations, with the bruit typically increasing in intensity during inspiration. The peripheral pulses are usually normal. The right heart pressures and pulmonary arterial pressures are typically normal, due to the low-resistance channels of the malformation. Characteristically there is marked arterial hypoxemia at rest, which increases in the upright position due to the prevalence of malformations in the lower lobes. A normal chest radiograph and normal arterial saturation excludes a significant pulmonary shunt. A clinical presentation of congestive failure with deep cyanosis is suggestive of pulmonary arteriovenous malformations.

There are a number of reports of congestive heart failure due to pulmonary sequestration or to an isolated anomalous systemic-pulmonic arterial connection (see Chapter 19). The hemodynamics are similar to a left-to-right shunt across a patent ductus arteriosus. The blood from the systemic artery supplying the lung returns through the pulmonary veins to the left atrium causing volume overload and congestive heart failure. This differs from a systemic arteriovenous fistula where the increased blood volume returns to the right heart, as well this is in contrast to a pulmonary arteriovenous fistula where desaturated blood enters the systemic arterial circulation. A pulmonary sequestration should be considered in an infant with congestive heart failure in which there is a persistent focal confluent opacity on the chest radiograph. The treatment should be individualized, in some cases surgical ligation or embolotherapy of the abnormal artery is sufficient, others may require surgical resection of the sequestered or involved lung segment.[77,78]

A unique subgroup of pulmonary arteriovenous shunting is seen in patients with severe liver disease. The term "hepatogenic pulmonary angiodysplasia" has been proposed to describe the syndrome of hepatic failure with cyanosis, clubbing, and arterial desaturation caused by intrapulmonary right-to-left shunting.[79,80] The changes in the pulmonary vessels are mainly at the precapillary level affecting arterial branches less than 500 μm in diameter.[79] The etiology of hypoxemia and hepatogenic angiodysplasia in patients with liver failure is unclear. A chest radiograph may demonstrate spidery pulmonary vessels distributed evenly throughout both lungs. The diagnosis is confirmed with pulmonary angiography, the central and middle sized arteries are dilated and untapered, filling a myriad of spidery small branches. There is patchy staining of the parenchyma

during the capillary phase, with rapid filling of pulmonary veins. The arteriovenous fistulas are minute and widely disseminated throughout the lungs, with discrete pulmonary arteriovenous fistula rarely identified.

In contrast to systemic arteriovenous fistulas the cardiac silhouette in patients with pulmonary arteriovenous malformations is normal. The pulmonary vascularity is often decreased. An intrapulmonary mass-like opacity may be seen with large pulmonary arteriovenous fistula or alternatively a myriad of spider-like vessels may be seen with diffuse small fistulas. The characteristic plain film findings of tortuous vessels leading to a lobulated mass seen in older children and adults is rarely seen in infants.

Contrast (bubble) echocardiography may show signs suggestive of right-to-left shunting through pulmonary arteriovenous fistula. Dense echoes appear in the left atrium later than in intracardiac shunts, but earlier than normal.[12,81]

In pulmonary arteriovenous malformations right-to-left shunting can be demonstrated with radionuclide imaging using radiolabeled albumin microspheres or macroaggregates. Quantification of the shunt is calculated by comparing uptake in the pulmonary and systemic circulations.[8]

Computed tomography of the chest is a noninvasive method of screening for pulmonary arteriovenous malformation in patients with unexplained neurological symptoms resulting from paradoxical emboli. Computed tomography is also a useful screening tool in detecting pulmonary fistula in family members with a positive history of hereditary hemorrhagic telangiectasia. Computed tomography is very accurate in identifying pulmonary arteriovenous malformations and providing accurate segmental location.[82–84] MRI of pulmonary arteriovenous fistula has been reported; specifically, MRI was useful in separating nonvascular from vascular lesions in the lung. MRI, however, is unreliable in demonstrating small pulmonary arteriovenous malformations or lesions with high blood flow due to absence of signal.[85] Definitive evaluation of pulmonary arteriovenous fistulas with bilateral pulmonary angiography is mandatory. The pulmonary angiogram is necessary to delineate the exact number and location of all malformations and define the caliber and morphology of the feeding vessels prior to embolization or surgical resection.[8,12,86]

The favored therapy in pulmonary arteriovenous malformations with arteries exceeding 3 mm in diameter is occlusion with embolotherapy. Embolization therapy is particularly useful in patients with multiple or bilateral pulmonary arteriovenous malformations obviating extensive pulmonary resection. Embolization for treatment of pulmonary arteriovenous malformations has been described in a patient with hepatogenic pulmonary angiodysplasia, where a selected number of the arteriovenous fistulas were coil occluded.[80] Embolization therapy may be advised in essentially asymptomatic pulmonary arteriovenous malformations to avoid paradoxical embolization and to correct symptomatic hypoxemia.[12,13,87] Embolization of anomalous systemic-pulmonic arterial vessels has improved cardiac failure.[8] Most reports favor embolization of pulmonary arteriovenous malformations with detachable balloons because of the ability to exactly place the balloon before detachment. Additionally, compared with coils, the more distal placement of the balloon prevents occlusion of normal branches which may result in pulmonary infarction. Coil embolization, however, may be technically easier and appropriate for occluding multiple small vessel arteriovenous malformations. The combination of the coil method with the detachable balloon technique has also been used successfully.[76]

The morbidity and mortality of pulmonary arteriovenous malformations is high if the lesion is unrecognized or untreated. The most significant complications are cerebrovascular events, which primarily are a result of paradoxical emboli. Polycythemia causing hyperviscosity may also contribute to cerebral ischemia.

Miscellaneous Arteriovenous Fistula

There are a variety of rare congenital systemic arteriovenous fistula that have presented with congestive heart failure during infancy. In the developing embryo there are multiple communications between arteries and veins. It is the persistence of these channels that may be the basis for congenital arteriovenous fistulas that can occur virtually anywhere in the body.[88] The vascular abnormality is determined by the site of maldevelopment. If the abnormality is on the venous side, a venous angioma results. If on the other hand the abnormal differentiation involves the capillary system, capillary or cavernous hemangioma occur. It is the presence of vascular channels bypassing the usual capillary connection, that leads to micro or macro arteriovenous fistula.

The clinical presentation of the more peripheral arteriovenous malformations varies. Increased blood flow through the fistula may result in local growth disturbance, pain is a common complaint and cosmetic disfigurement is often seen in cases of macrofistulas. The lesions may result in a local teratogenic effect resulting in abnormalities of the adjacent mesenchyma and neuroectodermal tissues, as seen in Klippel-Trenaunay-Parkes-Weber syndrome. It is a low proportion of intrathoracic, extremity and extrahepatic intra-abdominal fistulas which are associated with cardiac failure. An arteriovenous fistula however, anywhere in the body represents a path of low resistance and potentially can result in hemodynamic changes leading to high-output cardiac failure in infancy.

Cutaneous hemangiomas are common pediatric lesions most of which occur in the head and neck region, however to have a hemangioma functioning as an arteriovenous fistula is extremely rare. There are reports of chest wall arteriovenous fistulas involving the intercostal, internal mammary and subclavian vessels causing cardiac failure.[8,89–93] In addition, significant heart failure has been reported in large shunts across pelvic and extremity malformations.[92–95]

Arteriography should be performed to delineate the extent of the arteriovenous malformation and to facilitate an appropriate treatment plan. Surgical cure is achieved by complete excision of the lesion, this is often not possible due to the size and location of the malformation. Partial excision and ligation of arterial feeders without obliteration of the vascular nidus has been ineffective due to regrowth of new collateral vessels.[87] Attempts at therapy for the control or cure of peripheral arteriovenous malformations with transcatheter embolization alone or in combination with limited surgery has been successful and has provided relief of congestive failure. Multiple embolic agents have been used, recommended is both proximal and distal occlusion of the arteriovenous malformation with permanent embolic agents.[87]

Finally, one should remember that uncommon and indeed curious association between multiple cutaneous hemangiomas and coarctation of the aorta with right aortic arch. We have seen this association in a patient with multiple cutaneous hemangiomas and coarctation of the right fourth arch in a patient with a double aortic arch and an atretic left arch (see Chapters 32 and 34).[96–98]

References

1. Nielsen G. Arteriovenous malformations as a cause of congestive heart failure in the newborn and infant. *Eur J Pediatr* 1984;142:298–300.
2. Knudson RP, Alden ER. Symptomatic arteriovenous malformation in infants less than 6 months of age. *Pediatrics* 1979;64(2):238–241.
3. Liu P, Daneman A, Stringer DA, Smith CR. Computed tomography of hemangiomas and related soft tissue lesions in children. *J Can Assoc Radiol* 1986;37:248–255.
4. Burrows PE, Lasjaunias PL, TerBrugge KG, Flodmark O. Urgent and emergent embolization of lesions of the head and neck in children: Indications and results. *Pediatrics* 1987;80(3)386–394.
5. Mulliken JB, Glowacki J. Hemangiomas and vascular malformations in infants and children: A classification based on endothelial characteristics. *Plast Reconstr Surg* 1982;69:412–420.

6. King WA, Wackym PA, Vinuela F, Peacock WJ. Management of vein of Galen aneurysms—Combined surgical and endovascular approach. *Childs Nerv Syst* 1989; 5:208–211.

7. O'Donnabhain D, Duff DF. Aneurysms of the vein of Galen. *Arch Dis Child* 1989;64:1612–1617.

8. Musewe NN, Burrows PE, Culham JAG, Freedom RM. Arteriovenous fistulae: A consideration of extracardiac causes of congestive heart failure. In: Freedom RM, Benson L, Smallhorn J, eds. *Neonatal Heart Disease.* London: Springer Verlag; 1992, pp. 759–775.

9. Garcia-Monaco R, De Victor D, Mann C, Hannedouche A, TerBrugge K, Lasjaunias P. Congestive cardiac manifestations from cerebrocranial arteriovenous shunts. *Childs Nerv Syst* 1991;7:48–52.

10. Pearse LA, Sondeheimer HM, Washington RL, Robertson D, Clarke DR. Congenital vertebral-jugular fistula in an infant. *Pediatr Cardiol* 1989;10:229–231.

11. Chan ST, Weeks R. Dural arteriovenous malformations presenting as cardiac failure in a neonate. *Acta Neurochir* 1988;91:134–138.

12. Schlemmer M, Tulzer G, Wimmer M. Pitfalls in the diagnosis of pulmonary arteriovenous malformations. *Cardiol Young* 1994;4:408–410.

13. Dines DE, Sweard JB, Bernatz PE. Pulmonary arteriovenous fistulas. *Mayo Clin Proc* 1983;58(3):176–181.

14. Ralls PW, Johnson MB, Radin DR, Lee KP, Boswell WD. Hereditary hemorrhagic telangiectasia: Findings in the liver with color Doppler sonography. *AJR* 1992;159: 59–61.

15. Nielsen G. Arteriovenous malformations as a cause of congestive heart failure in the newborn and infant. Three cases with different hemodynamic mechanisms. *Eur J Pediatr* 1984;142(4):298–300.

16. Melville C, Walsh K, Sreeram N. Cerebral arteriovenous malformations in the neonate: Clinical presentation, diagnosis and outcome. *Int J Cardiol* 1991;31:175–180.

17. Stanbridge RDL, Westaby S, Smallhorn J, Taylor JFN. Intracranial arteriovenous malformation with aneurysm of the vein of Galen as cause of heart failure in infancy—Echocardiographic diagnosis and results of treatment. *Br Heart J* 1983;49:157–162.

18. Matjasko J, Robinson W, Eudaily D. Successful surgical and anesthetic management of vein of Galen aneurysm in a neonate in congestive heart failure. *Neurosurgery* 1988; 22(5):908–910.

19. Amacher AL, Shillito J. The syndromes and surgical treatment of aneurysms of the great vein of Galen. *J Neurosurg* 1973;39:89–98.

20. Wiggins CW, Loisel D, Budock AM. Intracranial arteriovenous malformation in a neonate: Aneurysm of the great vein of Galen. *Neonatal Network* 1991;9(8):7–17.

21. Ciricillo SF, Edwards MSB, Schmidt KG, et al. Interventional neuroradiological management of vein of Galen malformations in the neonate. *Neurosurgery* 1990; 27(1):22–28.

22. Lasjaunias P, TerBrugge K, Ibor LL, et al. The role of dural anomalies in vein of Galen aneurysms: Report of six cases and review of the literature. *AJNR* 1987;8:185–192.

23. McConnell ME, Aronin P, Vitek JJ. Congestive heart failure in neonates due to intracranial arteriovenous malformation: Endovascular treatment. *Pediatr Cardiol* 1993;14: 102–106.

24. Albright AL, Latchaw RE, Price RA. Posterior dural arteriovenous malformations in infancy. *Neurosurgery* 1983; 13(2):129–135.

25. Godersky JC, Menezes AH. Intracranial arteriovenous anomalies of infancy: Modern concepts. *Pediatr Neurosci* 1987;13:242–250.

26. Jedeikin R, Rowe RD, Freedom RM, Olley PM, Gillan JE. Cerebral arteriovenous malformation in neonates—The role of myocardial ischemia. *Pediatr Cardiol* 1983; 4:29–35.

27. Pellegrino PA, Milanesi O, Saia OS, Carollo C. Congestive heart failure secondary to cerebral arteriovenous fistula. *Childs Nerv Syst* 1987;3:141–144.

28. Holden AM, Fyler DC, Shillito J, Nadas AS. Congestive heart failure from intracranial arteriovenous fistula in infancy. *Pediatrics* 1972;49(1):30–39.

29. Johnston IH, Whittle IR, Besser M, Morgan MK. Vein of Galen malformation: Diagnosis and management. *Neurosurgery* 1987;20(5):747–758.

30. Milstein JM, Juris AL. Aortic diastolic pressure decay in congenital arteriovenous malformations. *Pediatr Cardiol* 1993; 14:204–207.

31. Cumming GR. Circulation in neonates with intracranial arteriovenous fistula and cardiac failure. *Am J Cardiol* 1980;45:1019–1024.

32. Hoffman HJ, Chuang S, Hendrick B, Humphreys RP. Aneurysms of the vein of Galen—Experience at the hospital for sick children, Toronto. *J Neurosurg* 1982;57: 316–322.

33. Long WA, Schall SA, Henry GW. Cerebral arteriovenous malformation presenting as persistent fetal circulation: Diagnosis by cross-sectional echo. *Am J Perinatol* 1984; 1(3):236–241.

34. Walker WJ, Mullins C. Cyanosis, cardiomegaly and weak pules: A manifestation of massive congenital systemic arteriovenous fistula. *Circulation* 1964;29:777–781.

35. Hassler W, Steinmetz H. Cerebral hemodynamics in angioma patients: An intraoperative study. *J Neurosurg* 1987;67:822–831.

36. Nornes H, Grip A. Hemodynamic aspects of cerebral arteriovenous malformations. *J Neurosurg* 1980;53:456–464.

37. Eiras J, Carcavilla LI, Gomez J, Goni A, Salazar J, Marco A. Surgical treatment of an aneurysm of the vein of Galen in a newborn with heart failure. *Childs Nerv Syst* 1985; 1:126–129.

38. Takashima S, Becker LE. Neuropathology of cerebral arteriovenous malformations in children. *J Neurol Neurosurg Psychiatry* 1980;43(5):380–585.

39. Sapire DW, Casta A, Donner RM, Markowitz RI, Capitanio MA. Dilatation of the descending aorta: A radiologic and echocardiographic diagnostic sign in arteriovenous malformations in neonates and young infants. *Am J Cardiol* 1979;44:493–497.

40. Deverall PB, Taylor JFN, Sturrock GS, Aberdeen E. Coarctation-like physiology with cerebral arteriovenous fistula. *Pediatrics* 1960;44:1024–1028.

41. Swischuk LE, Crowe JE, Mewborne EB Jr. Large vein of Galen aneurysms in the neonate: A constellation of diagnostic chest and neck radiologic findings. *Pediatr Radiol* 1977;6:4–9.

42. Friedman DM, Rutkowski M, Madrid M, Berenstein A. Sinus venosus atrial septal defect associated with vein of Galen malformations: Report of two cases. Pediatr Cardiol 1994;15:50–52.

43. Vaksmann G, Decoulx E, Mauran P, Jardin M, Rey C, Dupuis C. Evaluation of vein of Galen arteriovenous malformation in newborns by two dimensional ultrasound, pulsed and colour Doppler method. *Eur J Pediatr* 1989; 148:510–512.

44. Starc TJ, Krongrad E, Bierman FZ. Two-dimensional echocardiography and doppler findings in cerebral arteriovenous malformation. *Am J Cardiol* 1989;64:252–254.

45. Snider AR, Soifer SJ, Silverman NH. Detection of intracranial arteriovenous fistula by two-dimensional ultrasonography. *Circulation* 1981;63(5):1179–1185.

46. Hegesh J, Kuint J, Frand M, et al. Cerebral arteriovenous malformation diagnosis by two-dimensional color-coded doppler ultrasonography of the head. *Pediatr Cardiol* 1991;12:107–109.

47. Godersky JC, Menezes AH. Intracranial arteriovenous anomalies of infancy: Modern concepts. *Pediatr Neurosci* 1987;13:242–250.

48. Lasjaunias P, Rodesch G, Pruvost P, Laroche FG, Landrieu P. Treatment of vein of Galen aneursymal malfomation. *J Neurosurg* 1989;70:746–750.

49. Luessenhop AJ, Roas L. Cerebral arteriovenous malformations: Indications for and results of surgery, and the role of intravascular techniques. *J Neurosurg* 1984;60:14–22.

50. Widlus DM, Murray RR, White RI, et al. Congenital arteriovenous malformations: Tailored embolotherapy. *Radiology* 1988;169:511–516.

51. Kaufman SL, Kumar AA, Roland JM, et al. Transcatheter embolization in the management of congenital arteriovenous malformations. *Radiology* 1980;137:21–29.

52. Burrows PE, Lasjaunias P, Terbrugge KG. A 4-F coaxial catheter system for pediatric vascular occlusion with detachable balloons. *Radiology* 1989;170:1091–1094.

53. Dowd CF, Halbach VV, Barnwell SL, Higashida RT, Edwards MSB, Hieshmia GB. Transfemoral venous embolizations of vein of Galen malformations. *AJNR* 1990;11:643–648.

54. Mickle JP, Quisling RG. The transtorcular embolization of vein of Galen aneurysms. *J Neurosurg* 1986;64:731–735.

55. Lofland GK, Filston H. Giant cutaneous hemangioma associated with axillary arteriovenous fistula causing congestive heart failure in the newborn infant. *J Pediatr Surg* 1987;22(5):458–460.

56. McLean RH, Moller JH, Warwich WJ, Satran L, Lucas RV. Multinodular hemangiomatosis of the liver in infancy. *Pediatrics* 1972;49(4)563–573.

56a. Boon LM, Burrows PE, Paltiel HJ, Lund DP, Ezekowitz RA, Folkmann J, Mulliken JB. Hepatic vascular anomalies in infancy: A twenty-seven year experience. *Pediatrics* 1996;129:346–354.

57. Rocchini AP, Rosenthal A, Issenberg HJ, Nadas AS. Hepatic hemangioendothelioma: Hemodynamic observations and treatment. *Pediatrics* 1976;57(1):131–135.

58. Shulman RJ, Holmes R, Ferry GD, Finegold M. Splanchinc bed malformations and the development of portal hypertension. *J Pediatr Surg* 1986;21(4):355–357.

59. Larcher VF, Howard ER, Mowat AP. Hepatic haemangiomata: Diagnosis and management. *Arch Dis Child* 1981;56:7–14.

60. Cloogman HM, DiCapo RD. Hereditary hemorrhagic telangiectasia: sonographic findings in the liver. *Radiology* 1984;150:521–522.

61. Varma DG, Schoenberger SG, Kumra A, Agrawal N, Robinson AE. Osler-Weber-Rendu disease: MR findings in the liver. *J Comput Assist Tomogr* 1989;13(1):134–135.

62. Adler J, Goodgold M, Mitty H, Gordon D, Kinkhabwala M. Arteriovenous shunts involving the liver. *Radiology* 1978;129:315–322.

63. Derauf BJ, Hunter DW, Sirr SA, Cardella JF, Castaneda-Zuniga W, Amplatz K. Peripheral embolization of diffuse hepatic arteriovenous malformations in a patient with hereditary hemorrhagic telangiectasia. *Cardiovasc Intervent Radiol* 1987;10(2):80–83.

64. Stanley P, Grinnell VS, Stanton RE, Williams KO, Shore NA. Therapeutic embolization of infantile hepatic hemangioma with polyvinyl alcohol. *AJR* 1983;141: 1047–1051.

65. Repa I, Moradian GP, Dehner LP, Tadvarthy SM, et al. Mortalities associated with use of a commercial suspension of polyvinyl alcohol. *Radiology* 1989;170:395–399.

66. Burrows PE, Rosenberg HC, Chuang HS. Diffuse hepatic hemangiomas: Percutaneous transcatheter embolization with detachable silicone balloons. *Radiology* 1985;156: 85–88.

67. Whiting JH, Morton KA, Datz FL, Patch GG, Miller FJ Jr. Embolization of hepatic arteriovenous malformations using radiolabeled and nonradiolabeled polyvinyl alcohol sponge in a patient with hereditary hemorrhagic telangiectasia: Case report. *J Nucl Med* 1992;33(2):260–262.

68. Matolo NM, Johnson DG. Surgical treatment of hepatic hemangioma in the newborn. *Arch Surg* 1973;106: 725–727.

69. Chilvers ER. Clinical and physiological aspects of pulmonary arteriovenous malformations. *Br J Hosp Med* 1988;39:188–192.

70. Audenaert SM, Wood BP. Radiological case of the month. *Am J Dis Child* 1990;144:575–576.

71. Taylor GA. Pulmonary arteriovenous malformation: An uncommon cause for cyanosis in the newborn. *Pediatr Radiol* 1983;13:339–341.

72. Allen SW, Whitfield JM, Clarke DR, Sujansky E, Wiggins JW. Pulmonary arteriovenous malformation in the newborn: A familial case. *Pediatr Cardiol* 1993;14:58–61.

73. Clarke CP, Goh TH, Blackwood A, Venables AW. Massive pulmonary arteriovenous fistula in the new born. *Br Heart J* 1976;38:1092–1095.

74. Jimenez M, Fournier A, Choussat A. Pulmonary artery to the left atrium fistula as an unusual cause of cyanosis in the newborn. *Pediatr Cardiol* 1989;10:216–220.

75. Fried R, Amberson JB, O'Loughlin JE, Cruz SB, Sniderman DW, Firpo AB, Engle MA. Congenital pulmonary arteriovenous fistula producing pulmonary arterial steal syndrome. *Pediatr Cardiol* 1982;2:313–318.

76. White RI, Lynch-Nyhan A, Terry P, et al. Pulmonary arteriovenous malformations: Techniques and long-term outcome of embolotherapy. *Radiology* 1988;169:663–669.

77. Levine MM, Nudel DB, Gootman N, Wolpowitz A, Wisoff W. Pulmonary sequestration causing congestive heart failure in infancy: A report of two cases and review of the literature. *Ann Thorac Surg* 1982;34(5):581–585.

78. Burrows PE, Freedom RM, Rabinovitch M, Moes CAF. The investigation of abnormal pulmonary arteries in congenital heart disease. *Radiol Clin North Am* 1985; 23(4):689–717.

79. Sang Oh K, Bender TM, Bowen A, Ledesma-Medina J. Plain radiographic, nuclear medicine and angiographic observations of hepatogenic pulmonary angiodysplasia. *Pediatr Radiol* 1983;13:111–115.

80. Felt RW, Kozak BE, Bosch J, et al. Hepatogenic pulmonary angiodysplasia treated with coil-spring embolization. *Chest* 1987;91(6):920–922.

81. Teragaki M, Akioka K, Yasuda M, Ikuno Y, Oku H, Takeuchi K, Takeda T. Hereditary hemorrhagic telangiectasia with growing pulmonary arteriovenous fistulas followed for 24 years. *Am J Med Sci* 1988;295(6):545–547.

82. Love BB, Biller J, Landas SK, Hoover WW. Diagnosis of pulmonary arteriovenous malformation by ultrafast chest

computed tomography Rendu-Osler-Weber syndrome with cerebral ischemias—A case report. *Angiology* 1992; 43(6):522–528.

83. Remy J, Remy-Jardin M, Wattinne L, Deffontaines C. Pulmonary arteriovenous malformations: Evaluation with CT of the chest before and after treatment. *Radiology* 1992;182(3):809–816.

84. Remy J. Angioarchitecture of pulmonary venous malformations: Clinical utility of three-dimensional helical CT. *Radiology* 1994;191:657–664.

85. Gutierrez FR, Glazer HS, Levitt RG, Moran JF. NMR imaging of pulmonary arteriovenous fistulae. *J Comput Assist Tomogr* 1984;8(4):750–752.

86. Higgins CB, Wexler L. Clinical and angiographic features of pulmonary arteriovenous fistulas in children. *Radiology* 1976;119:171–175.

87. Gomes AS, Mali WP, Oppenheim WL. Embolization therapy in the management of congenital arteriovenous malformations. *Radiology* 1982;144:41–49.

88. Bopp P, Faidutti B, Fournet PC, Tollenaere P. Congenital arteriovenous fistula of the internal mammary vessels. *J Cardiovas Surg* 1977;18:79–82.

89. Atwood GF, King TD, Graham TP, et al. Thoracic arteriovenous fistula: Venous connection to the right iliac vein. *Am J Dis Child* 1975;129:233–236.

90. Glass IH, Rowe RD, Duckworth JWA. Congenital arteriovenous fistula between the left internal mammary artery and the ductus venosus: Unusual cause of congestive heart failure in the newborn infant. *Pediatrics* 1960;26:604–610.

91. Sapire DW, Lobe TE, Swischuk LE. Subclavian-artery-to-innominate-veing fistula presenting with congestive failure in a newborn infant. *Pediatr Cardiol* 1983; 4:155–157.

92. Woolley MM, Stanley P, Wesley JR. Peripherally located congenital arteriovenous fistulae in infancy and childhood. *J Pediatr Surg* 1977;12(2):165–176.

93. Romero M, Pán M, Suarez de Lezo J, Gomez S, Concha M, Romanos A. Fistula congenita entre la arteria subclavia izquierda y la vena innominada. Una rara causa de insuficiencia intratable en el recien nacido. *Rev Esp Cardiol* 1988;41:630–632.

94. Gutierrez FR, Monaco MP, Hartmann AF Jr, McKnight RC. Congenital arteriovenous malformations between brachiocephalic arteries and systemic veins. *Chest* 1987; 92:897–899.

95. Israel PG, Armstrong BE, Effman EL, Newman GE, Anderson PA. Retroperitoneal arteriovenous malformation, a rare cause of heart failure in infancy: Consideration of therapeutic approaches. *Pediatr Cardiol* 1993;14:49–52.

96. Vaillant L, Lorette G, Chantepie A, Marchand M, Alison D, Vaillant M-C, Laughier J. Multiple cutaneous hemangiomas and coarctation of the aorta with right aortic arch. *Pediatrics* 1988;81:707–709.

97. Schneeweiss A, Blieden LC, Shem-Tov A, Motro M, Feigl A, Neufeld HN. Coarctation of the aorta with congenital hemangioma of the face and neck and aneurysm or dilatation of a subclavian or innominate artery. A new syndrome? *Chest* 1982;82:186–187.

98. Honey M, Lincoln JCR, Osborne MP, de Bono DP. Coarctation of the aorta with right aortic arch. Report of surgical correction in 2 cases; one with associated anomalous origin of left circumflex coronary artery from the right pulmonary artery. *Br Heart J* 1975;37:937–945.

Part 2

Malformations of the Right Side of the Heart

Chapter 12

Anomalies of Systemic Venous Connections, Coronary Sinus, and Divided Right Atrium (Cor Triatriatum Dexter)

Anomalies of the superior and inferior caval veins, hepatic veins, and coronary sinus can complicate almost any form of congenital heart disease. Their recognition and incorporation into surgical management has become perhaps even more important since the benchmark contribution of Fontan and Baudet[1] in 1971 in their successful application of atrial separation and atriopulmonary connection (see Chapters 39 and 40). Before the Fontan principle or any one of its modifications was applied to many forms of complex heart malformations, hepatic venous connection to the coronary sinus or left atrium or an unroofed coronary sinus assumed just another line in the diagnosis of these patients. However, it is evident that some of these abnormalities complicated the surgical management and postoperative follow-up of the more common congenital heart malformations. Now, if unrecognized preoperatively, these uncommon malformations may contribute to an obligatory right-to-left shunt and varying degrees of arterial hypoxemia after Fontan's operation or any of its many modifications. Similarly, there is increasing recognition of abnormal systemic venous connections and collaterals that develop and enlarge after either a bidirectional cavopulmonary anastomosis or Fontan's operation. Some of these unusual systemic venous collaterals may connect to the pulmonary venous circulation resulting in progressive hypoxemia. Recognition of a wide range of abnormalities of the coronary sinus has been made possible by radiofrequency catheter ablation therapy for cardiac rhythm disturbances and from the very large worldwide experience in coronary arteriography.

Anomalies of the Right Superior Vena Cava

Anomalies of the right superior vena cava (assuming lateralized atria and atrial situs solitus) are uncommon (Figs. 12-1 through 12-9). Some of the recorded anomalies include absence of the right superior vena cava;[2-8] saccular dilatation of the right superior vena cava with or without distal obstruction;[9-15] anomalous termination of the right superior vena cava into the left atrium,[2,12,14,16-28] and anomalous low insertion of the right superior vena cava.[29,30] A diverticulum of the right superior caval vein is a rare vascular abnormality.[30a,30b] Aneurysmal transformation of the superior caval vein and brachiocephalic vein have also been recorded.[31] Hidvegi and colleagues reviewed the literature relevant to this unusual entity (Figs. 12-4 and 12-8).[31a] The course and contour of the right superior caval vein may be altered by a right aortic arch (Fig. 12-3). Significant enlargement of the right superior caval vein may reflect abnormal connection of all the pulmonary veins to a vertical vein and the substantial blood flow from this (see also Chapter 24). We have also seen tremendous dilatation of the right superior caval vein many years after creation of an axillary artery-vein fistula to augment flow through a classical Glenn opera-

From: Freedom RM, Mawson JB, Yoo SJ, Benson LN: *Congenital Heart Disease: Textbook of Angiocardiography*. Armonk NY, Futura Publishing Co., Inc. ©1997.

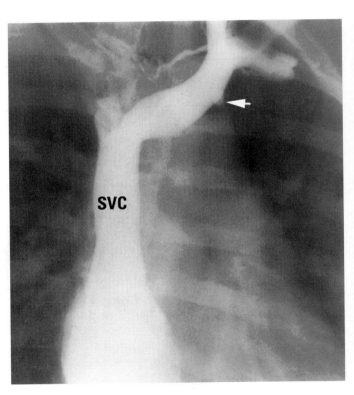

Fig. 12-1: Disposition of the normal right superior vena cava in the patient with solitus atria. The arrow notes a diminutive superior intercostal vein.

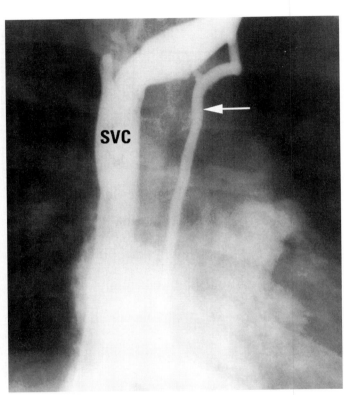

Fig. 12-2: A normal superior vena cava, but with a dilated left-sided hemiazygous vein (arrow). The lateral (not shown) indicated that this vein did not connect with the coronary sinus.

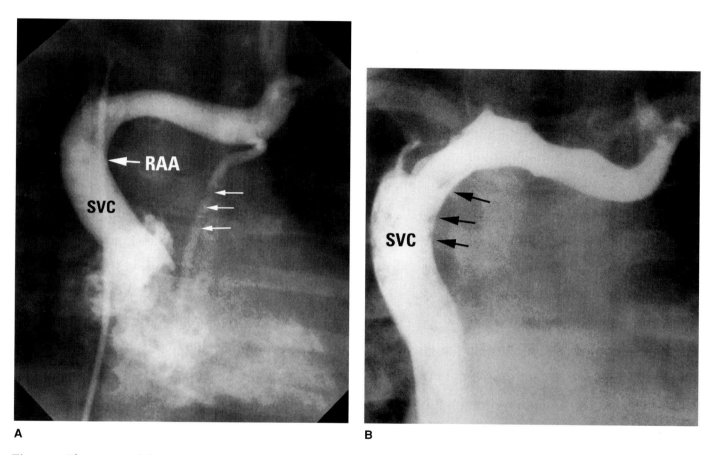

Fig. 12-3: The course of the right superior vena cava may be altered by a right-sided aortic arch, especially one dilated as in tetralogy of Fallot, or complex pulmonary atresia; note the small hemiazygous vein (arrows) in Fig. 12-3A.
A and B: Frontal injections into the superior caval veins of two different patients.

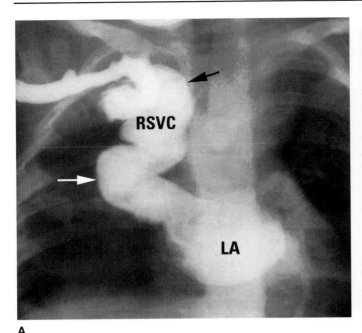

A

Fig. 12-4: Aneurysmal transformation of the right superior vena cava with termination in the left atrium.
A and B: Frontal and lateral injection into the right superior vena cava. Note the very dilated and tortuous superior caval vein.

B

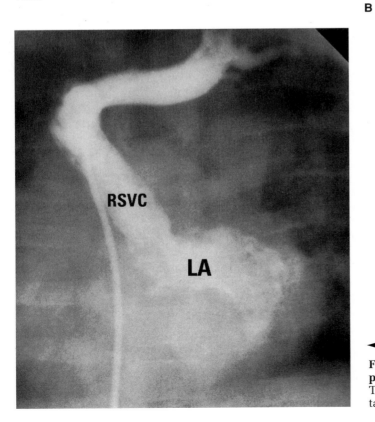

Fig. 12-5: A different patient with termination of the right superior vena cava into the left atrium.
This figure provided by Dr. M. Frommelt, Children's Hospital, Milwaukee, Wisconsin.

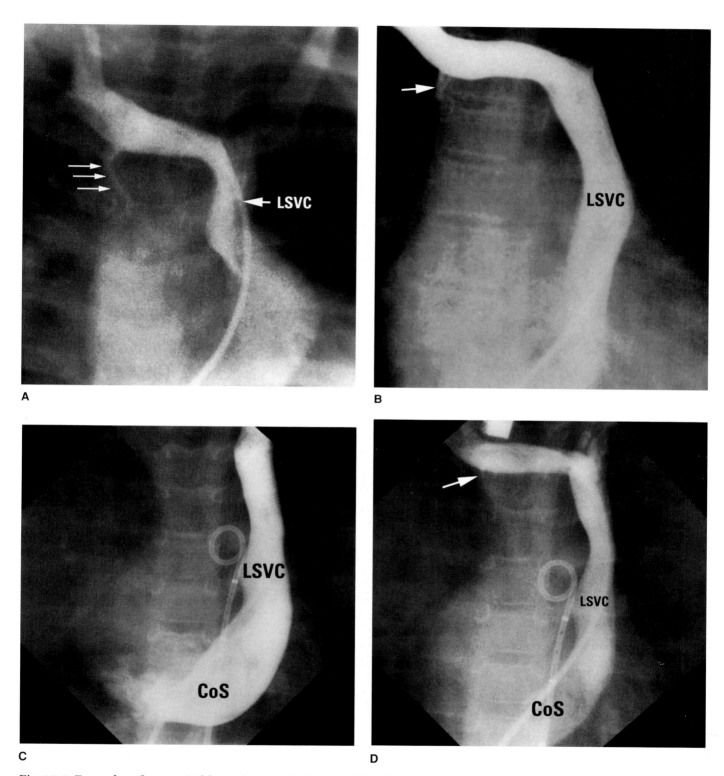

Fig. 12-6: Examples of congenital hypoplasia and absence of the right superior vena cava in patients with atrial situs solitus.
A: A miniscule remnant of the right superior caval vein (arrows). **B:** Another patient with an atretic remnant (arrow). **C and D:** Another patient with a remnant of the right superior caval vein, with termination of the left superior vena cava in the coronary sinus.

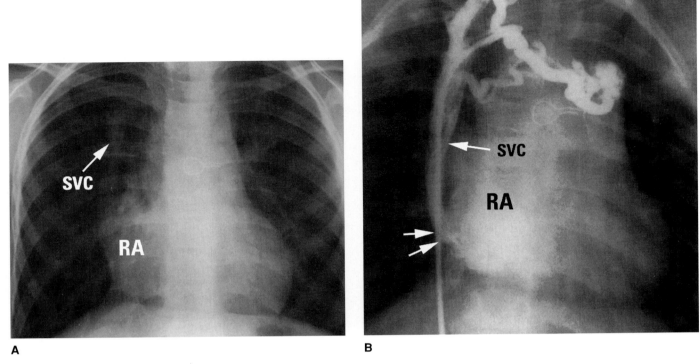

Fig. 12-7: So-called anomalous low insertion of the right superior vena cava.
A: Frontal chest radiograph shows an unusual band of opacity along the right mediastinum, which is confirmed as the superior vena cava. **B:** The venogram shows the low insertion (arrows) of the superior vena cava and tortuous mediastinal veins.

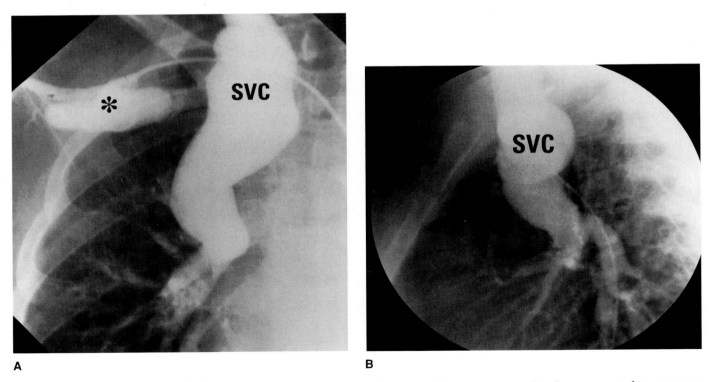

Fig. 12-8: Aneurysmally dilated superior vena cava many years after an axillary artery-vein fistula was created to augment pulmonary blood flow through a classical Glenn anastomosis.
A: Peripheral arteriogram in frontal projection shows a very dilated right subclavian vein (∗) and superior vena cava. **B:** Lateral view shows very dilated superior vena cava.

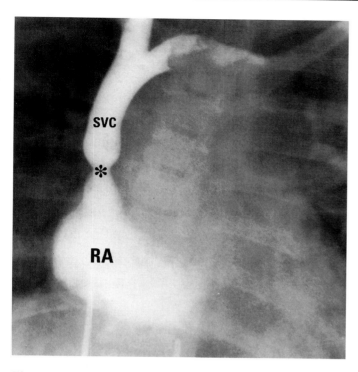

Fig. 12-9: Congenital mild stenosis of right superior vena cava-right atrial junction (✳).

tion (see Chapter 19) (Fig. 12-8). Peculiar communications between systemic venous collaterals and pulmonary venous channels have been observed after superior caval obstruction.[31b]

When the right superior vena cava is hypoplastic or represented by a fibrous cord, systemic venous flow from the head and neck necessitates the presence of a left-sided superior caval vein, a bridging innominate or brachiocephalic vein, and termination or connection of this caval vein in the coronary sinus, or rarely the left atrium directly (Fig 12-6).[3–7,32–34a] Thus, this unusual anomaly will usually result in a dilated coronary sinus.[35] While the usual course of the left superior vena cava with absent right superior caval vein is termination in the right atrium via the coronary sinus, the coronary sinus may be unroofed in some of these patients, thus promoting an obligatory right-to-left atrial shunt. Another implication of a hypoplastic right superior vena cava or fibrous cord with a left-sided superior caval vein, a bridging innominate or brachiocephalic vein, and termination in the coronary sinus: the sinoatrial node may be hypoplastic or abnormally formed.[5,6,32–34] Thus, rhythm disturbances reflecting sinus node dysfunction should be anticipated in these patients.[5,6,32–34]

Anomalous low insertion of the superior vena cava is a most uncommon congenital anomaly probably reflecting developmental failure of the right sinoatrial fold and incomplete absorption of the right anterior cardinal vein into the right limb of the sinus venosus (Fig. 12-7).[29,30] In this condition, the right superior caval vein connects with the right atrium just proximal to the inferior caval-right atrial junction. The patient being described from this institution had electrocardiographic evidence of an ectopic atrial pacemaker consistent with an abnormality of the sinoatrial node.

Saccular dilatation of the right superior caval vein or brachiocephalic vein is uncommon and is rarely observed in the neonate. Braudo and colleagues[12] reported striking dilatation of the right superior caval vein in a patient in whom this vein terminated in the left atrium, both very unusual findings (Fig. 12-4). Yokomise and colleagues[31] have also observed aneurysmal changes in both the right superior caval vein and left brachiocephalic vein.

Termination of the right superior caval vein exclusively in the left atrium in patients with unequivocally lateralized atria or with biatrial connections is also uncommon (Figs. 12-4 and 12-5).[2,12,14,16–20,22–28,36] The majority of the reported patients with this condition have been adults who presented clinically with cyanosis of unknown etiology, with a quiet heart, no heart murmur, and a normal electrocardiogram. This condition has been diagnosed by selective venography or radionuclide angiography. We are not aware of a neonate with this condition *in isolation* who was symptomatic, although this anomaly has been identified and treated in the infant and child. Bharati and Lev[14] described a baby dying 3 hours after birth who had direct entry of the right superior vena cava into the left atrium with aneurysmal dilatation and stenosis at its entry into the right atrium. This patient was also found to have stenosis of the individual pulmonary veins as well (see also Chapter 24). As emphasized by Bharati and Lev, in most patients with termination of the right superior caval vein exclusively in the left atrium, the right upper pulmonary veins connect to the right superior vena cava as well. Biatrial drainage of the right superior caval vein with anomalous connection of the right pulmonary veins has been reported.[35a] We have identified one patient with mild congenital stenosis of the superior vena cava just proximal to the cavoatrial junction (Fig. 12-9).

Anomalous Location or Course of the Brachiocephalic Vein Below the Aortic Arch

The spatial relationship between the brachiocephalic vein and the aorta has been explored and de-

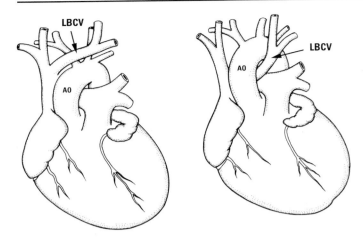

Fig. 12-10: Diagram showing position of the left brachiocephalic vein in relation to the aortic arch

tailed (Fig. 12-10).[37–40] The left brachiocephalic vein usually runs above and in front of the aortic arch and the innominate, left common carotid and left subclavian arteries. Less commonly, the left brachiocephalic vein is found below the aortic arch. While this anomalous position of the left brachiocephalic vein was rec-

ognized more than 100 years ago, the echocardiographic findings were first described by Smallhorn and colleagues in 1985.[37] Choi and colleagues[40] found this subaortic course of the brachiocephalic vein in 24 of 2457 patients with congenital heart disease (0.98%); this anatomic finding was more common in patients with tetralogy of Fallot or pulmonary atresia and ventricular septal defect, both with a right-sided aortic arch. Other abnormalities of the brachiocephalic vein are perhaps better imaged with angiography (Figs. 12-10 through 12-13).

Very rarely the innominate vein is compressed by the arteries originating from the aortic arch, producing a superior vena cava syndrome (Fig. 12-11).[41,41a] The patient reported by Moes from this institution had left innominate vein compression by a leftward origin of a brachiocephalic artery with an aberrant right subclavian artery.[41a] Duplication of the left brachiocephalic vein has also been observed (Fig. 12-12).[41b] In a number of patients small mediastinal veins have been observed in the absence of a brachiocephalic vein connecting the right to the left superior vena cava (Fig. 12-12). These mediastinal veins probably serve as one mechanism permitting ligation of a left superior vena cava in the absence of a well-formed left brachiocephalic vein. We

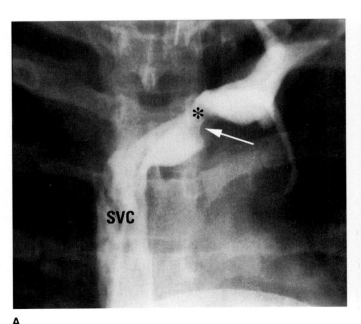

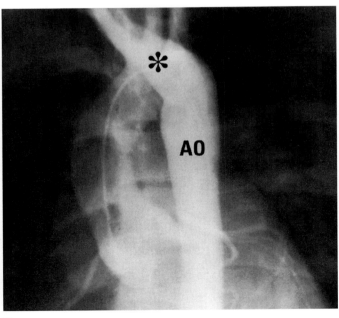

A   **B**

Fig. 12-11: Compression of the brachiocephalic (innominate) vein by the brachiocephalic artery.
A: Venogram shows site of compression (arrow) and narrowed (✱) brachiocephalic (innominate) vein. **B:** The aortogram shows the brachiocephalic arterial trunk (✱) arising aberrantly from the descending aorta.

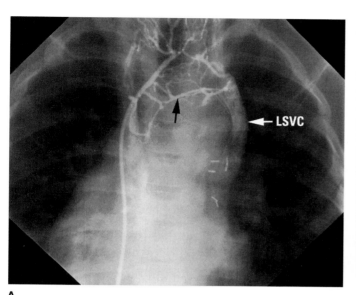

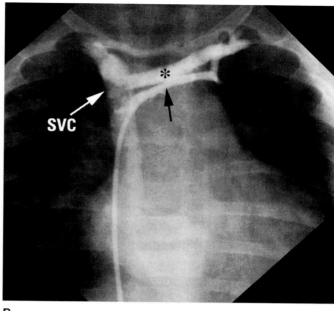

A   **B**

Fig. 12-12: A: A network of small venous collaterals (arrow) connect the right superior vena cava to the left superior vena cava. B: Duplication of the brachiocephalic (innominate) vein as noted by the (✻) and arrow.

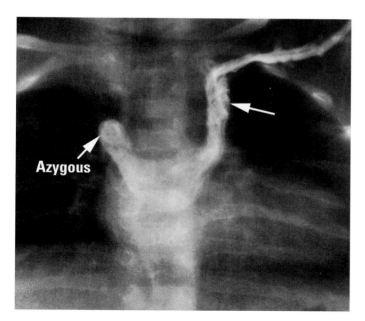

Fig. 12-13: A most peculiar connection of the left subclavian vein and left superior vena cava to the right-sided azygous vein. The pulmonary venous connections were normal.

have also seen one patient in whom the left subclavian vein and brachiocephalic vein communicated with the right-sided azygous vein (Fig. 12-13).

Persistence of the Left Superior Vena Cava and Related Anomalies

Abnormalities of the left superior caval vein are relatively common (Figs. 12-14 through 12-20). These abnormalities include connection with the coronary sinus (Figs. 12-14 through 12-18); termination in the left atrium with a normal coronary sinus; and termination in the left atrium with an unroofed coronary sinus (Fig. 12-19). Less commonly the left superior caval vein is aneurysmal, sometimes reflecting anomalous connection of pulmonary veins (see also Chapter 24) (Fig. 12-20).

Persistence of the left superior caval vein with termination in the coronary sinus occurs in about 4.0% of patients with congenital heart disease, and in approximately 0.3% of the general population.[42–49] With lateralized atria and solitus relations, the left superior caval vein can terminate in the left atrium directly, or rarely, through a systemic-pulmonary venous malformation.[2,17,19,20,24,46,48,50–59] Termination of the left superior caval vein into the roof of the left atrium is usually

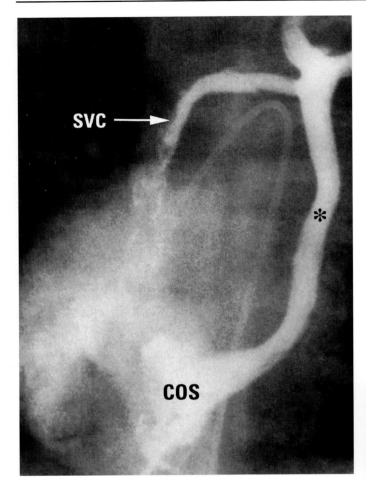

Fig. 12-14: Left superior vena cava (✳) connecting to coronary sinus in a patient with dextrocardia and atrial situs solitus. A small right superior vena cava is also seen.

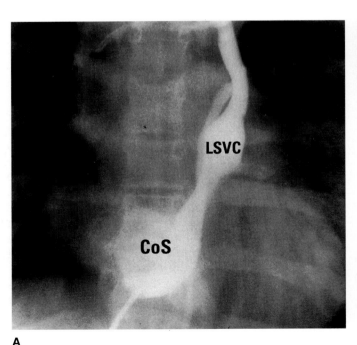

A

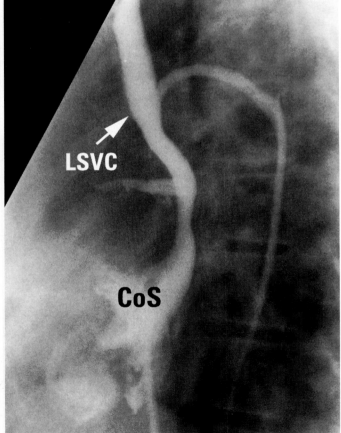

B

Fig. 12-15: Left superior vena cava connecting to coronary sinus with a conspicuous hemiazygous vein.
A and B: Frontal and lateral injection into left superior caval vein.

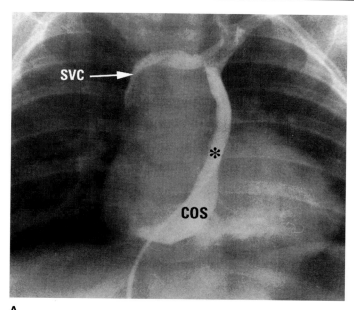

A

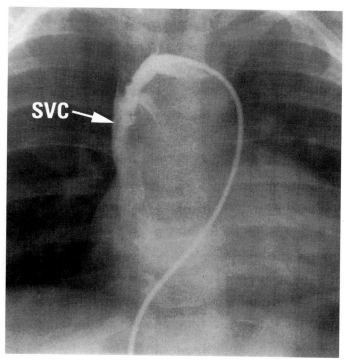

B

Fig. 12-16: A and B: Access to the left brachiocephalic vein and right superior vena cava via the coronary sinus and left superior vena cava (✳).

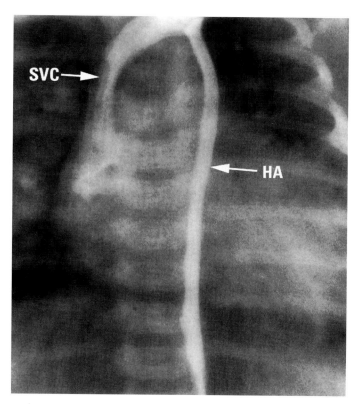

Fig. 12-17: Access to the left brachiocephalic vein and right superior vena cava via the left-sided hemiazygous vein.

accompanied by an unroofed coronary sinus. This is not invariably so, and there is considerable documentation of a left superior caval vein terminating in the left atrium with a normal coronary sinus (Fig. 12-19).[60]

When the left superior vena cava connects in isolation to the left atrium, the patient may be clinically cyanosed, demonstrating nail-bed clubbing, and may be hypoxemic, without obvious cause. Patients with connection of a left superior vena cava to the left atrium are predisposed to paradoxical emboli and brain abscess. The presence of this abnormal communication may be masked by those congenital cardiac anomalies which normally produce hypoxemia (ie, tetralogy of Fallot) or in those conditions where there is a large pulmonary blood flow, ie, atrial septal defect or ventricular septal defect.

Gerlis and colleagues[50] have described anomalous connection of the left atrial appendage with a persistent left superior vena cava that terminated in the coronary sinus (see Chapter 41, Fig. 41-20). In this patient, the left atrial appendage was demarcated from the rest of the atrial chamber. Treatment of the abnormal connection of the left superior caval vein to the left atrium can

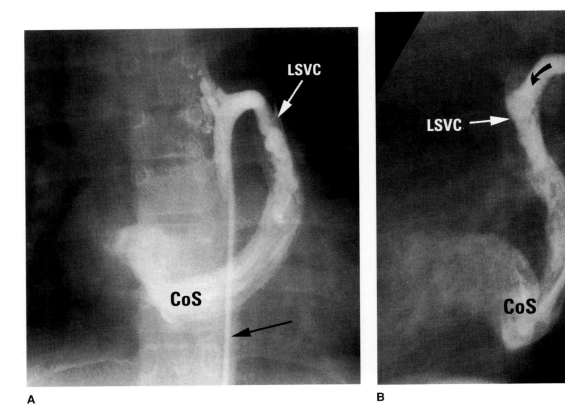

Fig. 12-18: A left hemiazygous vein (arrow) connects to the left superior vena cava and then the coronary sinus.
A and B: Frontal and lateral views with injection in the left-sided hemiazygous continuation demonstrating connection to the coronary sinus.

take one of several forms: surgical ligation if there is an adequate bridging innominate vein; or diversion of the left superior vena cava to the right atrium with an intra-atrial baffle; construction of a left-sided cavopulmonary connection (assuming appropriate hemodynamics) or catheter occlusion of the venous channel. Sibley and colleagues[61] reported the surgical correction of an isolated persistent left superior vena cava draining into the left atrium in a neonate. This infant, who had a hypoplastic right superior caval vein, presented at 28 hours of age with cyanosis. The repair consisted of ligation of the left superior vena cava and surgical anastomosis of the innominate vein to the right atrial appendage. Ascuitto and colleagues[62] have reported the unusual finding of a left superior vena cava that promoted a subdivided left atrium. In their patient, the left superior caval vein impinged on the left atrium posteriorly, producing a subdivided left atrium. Total anomalous systemic venous return to the left atrium has been reported by de Leval and colleagues.[2] This condition is very un-

common, and both of the patients reported by de Leval and colleagues[2] had hypoplasia of the right ventricle, as one might anticipate as a result from underfilling of this chamber. A significant degree of right ventricular hypoplasia was also observed in the patient reported by Freedom and colleagues.[9]

Recognition of the presence of a left superior caval vein is important before the consideration of either a classic right superior cavopulmonary connection or a bidirectional cavopulmonary connection. Failure to recognize the presence of left superior caval vein prior to the construction of a cavopulmonary connection will certainly compromise the efficacy of this type of shunt. Clearly this venous connection to the left atrium, even if very small, has to be recognized and dealt with, in the consideration of Fontan's operation. Even a small left superior vena cava connecting with the coronary sinus may enlarge dramatically after Fontan's operation especially when the coronary sinus is left on the systemic venous side of the Fontan circulation.

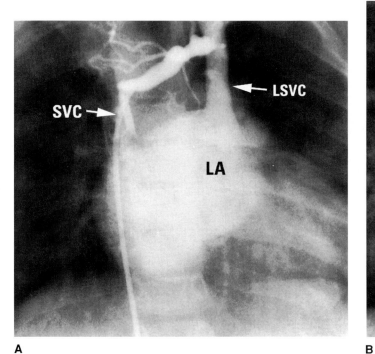

A

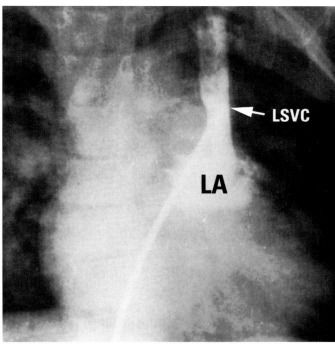

B

C

Fig. 12-19: Examples of termination of the left superior vena cava in the left atrium.
A: A patient with lateralized atria and an unroofed coronary sinus, the classic Raghib complex. **B:** Left superior vena cava to left atrium in a patient with tetralogy of Fallot. **C:** A patient with left atrial isomerism whose left superior vena cava terminates in the left atrium. Note in this patient the left-sided inferior vena cava.

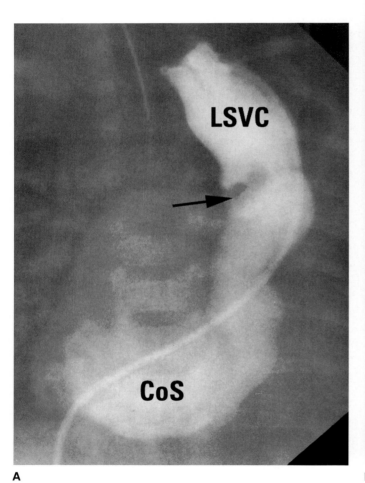

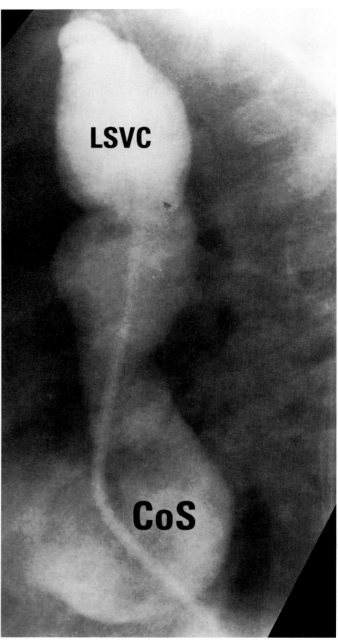

A

B

Fig. 12-20: Aneurysmally dilated left superior vena cava to coronary sinus in a patient with anomalous pulmonary venous connection to this vein.
A and B: Frontal and lateral cavograms. Note in Fig. 12-20A, the unopacified blood (arrow) from the anomalously connected pulmonary veins washing into the left superior vena cava (see also Chapter 24, Figs. 24-4 and 24–5).

The Levoatrial Cardinal Vein

The so-called levoatrial cardinal vein is very uncommon, and its presence is pathologic (see also Chapter 26).[19,26,63–67] This vein, probably derived from persistence of anastomotic channels connecting the capillary plexus of the embryonic foregut to the cardinal veins, is a pulmonary-systemic connection that provides an egress for pulmonary venous blood in left-sided obstructive lesions (see Chapter 26, Fig. 26-9).[66a] This unusual vein connects the left atrium or pulmonary vein to the left brachiocephalic vein in the setting of mitral atresia and a restrictive interatrial communication. It is considered an alternative pathway for pulmonary venous drainage in the presence of a severe left-sided obstructive lesion. This vein differs from a left superior vena cava terminating in the left atrium because the levoatrial cardinal vein ascends dorsal to the left pulmonary artery and more importantly the pulmonary veins connect with the left atrium.[63] This vein shares many similarities to that vein connecting a left upper pulmonary vein to the innominate vein.[64,65] Pinto and colleagues[66] recently described three patients with a levoatrial cardinal vein or pulmonary-to-systemic collateral vein. In two of these patients this unusual vein occurred in hypoplastic left heart syndrome, and in the third patient, in septation or division of the left atrium. In one patient with mitral atresia, this vein simulated a vertical vein in obstructive total anomalous pulmonary venous connection to the right superior caval vein.[64a]

Anomalies of the Inferior Vena Cava

The inferior caval vein has a large number of anatomical variations (Figs. 12-21 through 12-34).[68–71] Those anomalies most commonly associated with congenital heart disease include azygous continuation of the inferior vena cava; stenosis at the junction of the right atrium and inferior caval vein; termination of the inferior vena cava in the left atrium, and anomalous high insertion of the inferior caval vein. We have identified a number of patients in whom the inferior caval vein ascends on one side of the spine, only to cross the midline to enter the atrium (Figs. 12-21 and 12-22; see also Chapter 41, Fig. 41-12). The inferior caval vein is left-sided in those patients with situs inversus of atria and may be left-sided as well in patients with either dextrocardia or levocardia, but not clearly lateralized atria (Fig. 12-24). A network of vessels have been identified in some patients connecting the inferior caval vein with a hemiazygous vein or to a paravertebral plexus (Figs. 12-25 and 12-26).

Azygous Continuation of the Inferior Vena Cava: Absence of the Hepatic Segment of the Inferior Vena Cava

The most common anomaly of the inferior vena cava in patients with congenital heart disease is absence of the infrahepatic segment of the inferior vena cava with azygous continuation to the superior vena cava (Figs. 12-27 through 12-34; see also Chapter 41, Figs. 41-6 through 41-8, 41-10, 41-11, 41-17, 41-20, and 41-22,).[9,10,18,19,67,72–78] In this condition, the dilated azygous vein serves as the major venous conduit for

systemic venous return from the lower half of the body, and the hepatic veins usually connect directly to the atrium (see Chapter 41, Figs. 41-7 through 41-11, 41-17, 41-18, and 41-20). Azygous continuation of the inferior vena cava has been identified in 0.6% of patients with congenital heart disease, but occurs in more than 80% of patients with left atrial isomerism, often with polysplenia or multiple spleens (see Chapter 41). Azygous continuation of the inferior vena cava is only rarely identified in patients with right atrial isomerism and asplenia. The sinoatrial node is often abnormally formed in patients with left atrial isomerism and azygous continuation of the inferior vena cava.[79] This is reflected in the electrocardiogram by so-called coronary sinus rhythm with negative P-waves in leads II, III, and aVF.[80,81] Complete atrioventricular block is a major complicating factor in some patients with left atrial isomerism, a finding noted by Garcia and colleagues[82] (see also Chapter 41). The characteristics and natural history of abnormal or ectopic atrial rhythms in a large cohort of patients with left atrial isomerism have been detailed by Momma and colleagues.[83] The azygous continuation may be right-sided or left-sided, or less commonly bilateral.[84] A rare patient with azygous continuation of the inferior vena cava will still have direct continuity with the right atrium (Fig. 12-27).[76] Anomalous high insertion of the inferior caval vein has been described,[85] perhaps analogous to the situation of anomalous low insertion or connection of the superior caval vein), both reflecting some immaturity in the incorporation of the sinus venosus (Fig. 12-23). Azygous continuation of the inferior caval vein has been noted infrequently in the patient with juxtaposition of the right-sided atrial appendage (Fig. 12-28) (see also Chapter 13).

Azygous continuation of the inferior vena cava may be suspected in any neonate with complex congenital heart disease and coronary sinus rhythm. Absence of the inferior vena caval shadow on the lateral of the plain chest radiograph has not been particularly sensitive nor specific for this diagnosis in the neonate.[77,78,86] Cross-sectional echocardiographic imaging is diagnostic of this condition,[57,87–90] as is angiocardiography.[9,10,63,71,74,75,78]

Connection of the Inferior Caval Vein with the Left Atrium

An obligatory right-to-left shunt at atrial level may reflect connection of the inferior vena cava with the left atrium. This is a rare anomaly that may occur with or without an atrial septal defect.[91–94a] Fischer and Zuberbuhler[21] correctly pointed out that this condition must be differentiated from that in which the inferior caval

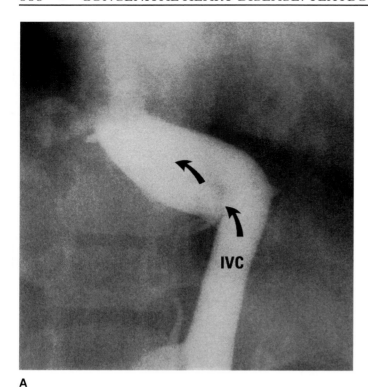

A

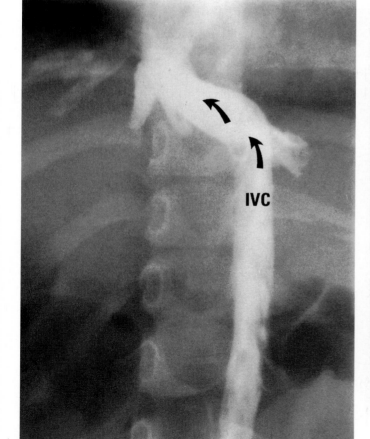

B

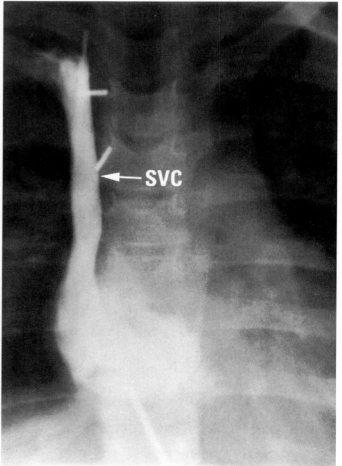

C

Fig. 12-21: The 'crossing' inferior vena cava (from left to right).
A: A patient with an uncomplicated secundum atrial septal defect. The left-sided inferior vena cava crosses the midline (arrows). **B and C:** A different patient with complex congenital heart disease, a 'crossing' inferior vena cava, and a right superior vena cava without a bridging innominate vein.

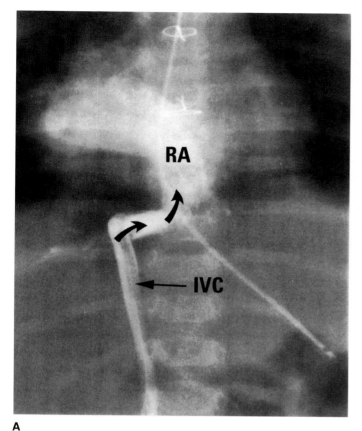

A

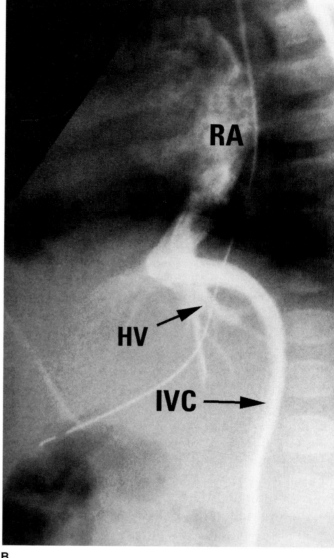

B

Fig. 12-22: The 'crossing' inferior vena cava (from right to left).
A patient with dextrocardia and an inferior vena cava 'crossing' from right to left. **A and B:** Frontal and lateral inferior vena cavograms show that the hepatic veins connect to the inferior caval vein, not the right atrium.

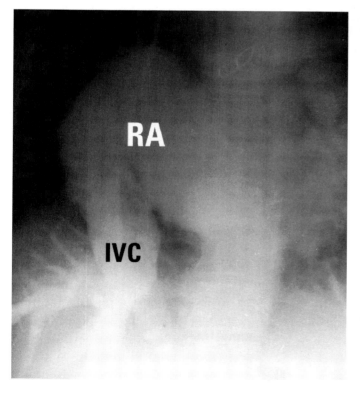

Fig. 12-23: Anomalous high insertion of the inferior caval vein (perhaps analogous to low insertion of the superior caval vein). This figure provided by Dr. M. Ando, Tokyo Women's Hospital, Tokyo, Japan.

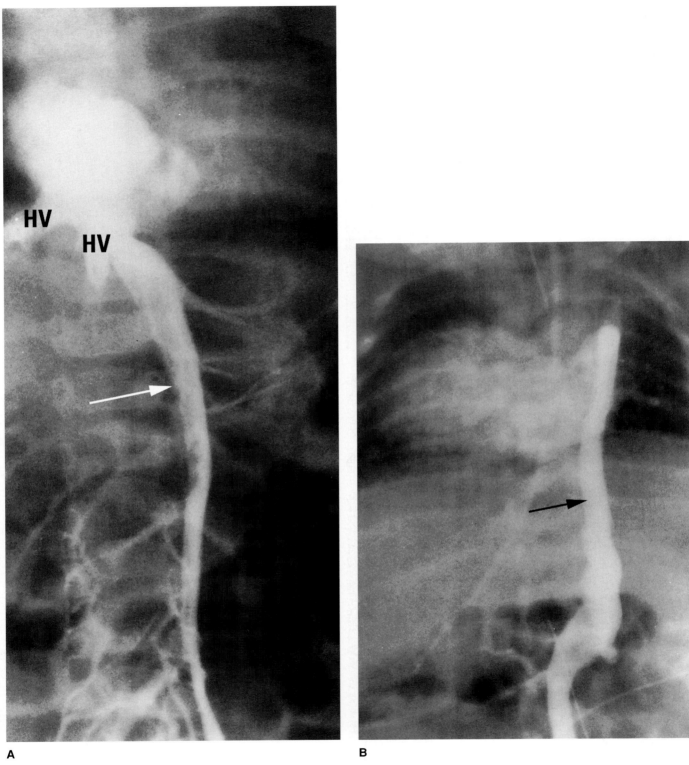

A   **B**

Fig. 12-24: A: Patient with right atrial isomerism and left-sided inferior caval vein (arrow). Note that the hepatic veins have multiple openings in the diaphragmatic wall of the atrium in this patient with isomerism. B: Hemiazygous continuation of left-sided inferior caval vein (arrow) to left superior caval vein in this patient with dextrocardia and presumed left atrial isomerism.

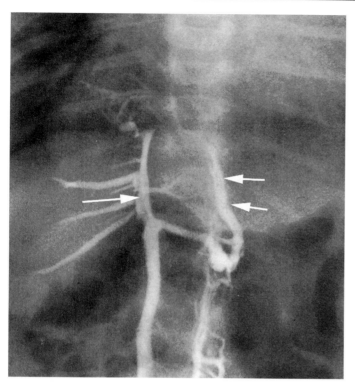

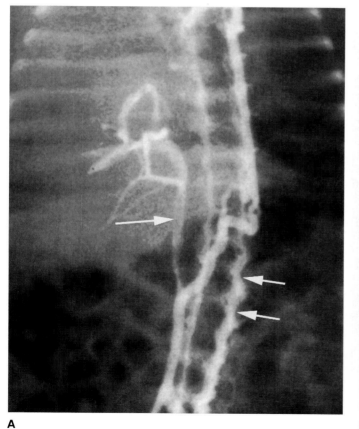

Fig. 12-25: Connection of right-sided inferior caval vein with left-sided hemiazygous vein (arrows).

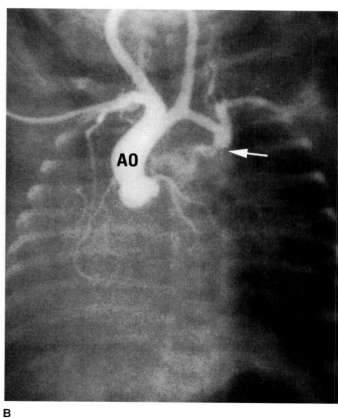

A

B

Fig. 12-26: Peculiar inferior caval vein (single arrow) with connections to paravertebral venous plexus in a patient with dextrocardia and aortic arch atresia.
A: Inferior vena cavogram shows the unusual caval configuration with connections to paravertebral venous plexus (arrows).
B: Aortogram performed from right axillary artery demonstrates aortic arch atresia (arrow) or severe coarctation.

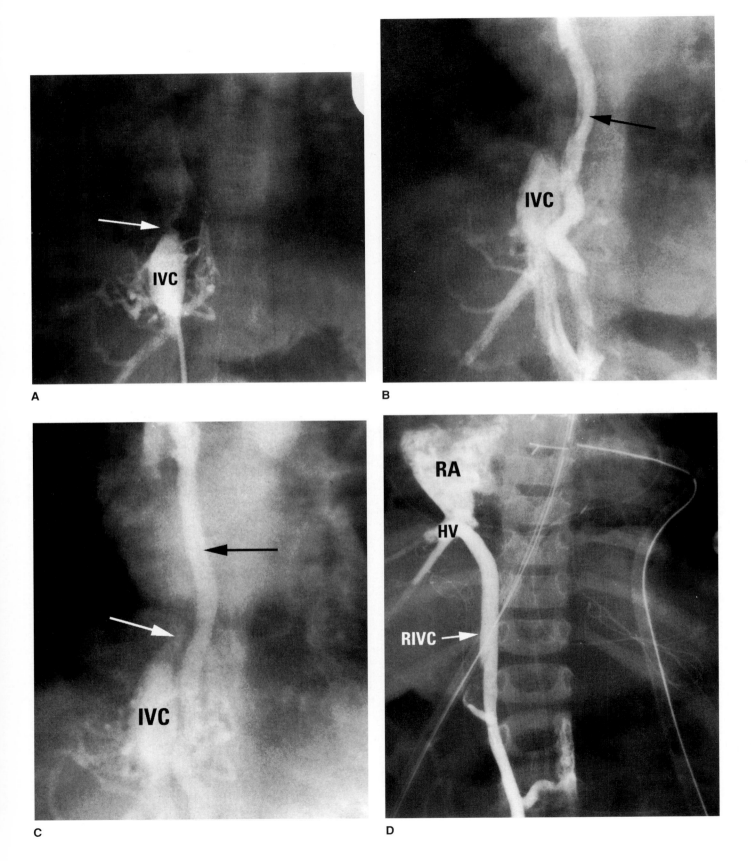

A

B

C

D

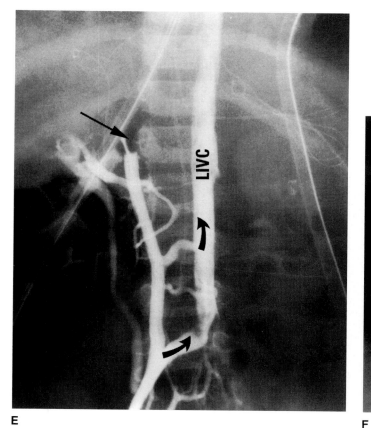

E

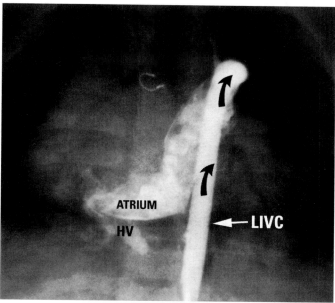

F

Fig. 12-27: Two different patients with an inferior vena cava connecting to atrium and an azygous continuation of the inferior caval vein.

A through C: A patient with the scimitar syndrome and an inferior vena cava connecting directly to the right-sided atrium and an azygous vein connecting to the superior vena cava. A: Inferior vena cavogram shows a focal stenosis (arrow) of the inferior caval vein. B and C: Later frames showing azygous vein (black arrow). **D through F:** Another patient with a left-sided hemiazygous continuation to the left superior vena cava and a right-sided inferior vena cava connecting to the right-sided atrium with the hepatic veins. D: Injection into the right-sided inferior vena cava (RIVC) demonstrates its connection to the right-sided atrium with the hepatic veins. E: A balloon occlusion (straight arrow) venogram shows the connection (lower curved arrow) with the left-sided inferior vena cava (LIVC). **F:** The left-sided inferior vena cava connects to the left superior caval vein via the hemiazygous vein. Note the reflux from the atrium into the hepatic veins.

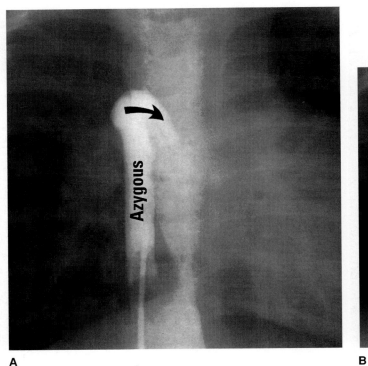

A

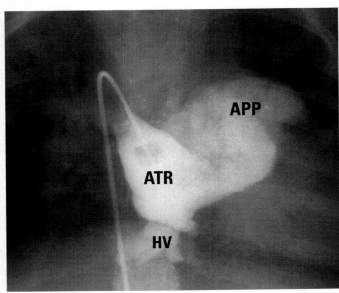

B

Fig. 12-28: Azygous continuation of the right-sided inferior caval vein with juxtaposition of the right-sided atrial appendage. **A:** Injection into the right-sided azygous continuation. **B:** The frontal injection of the right-sided atrium shows the juxtaposed atrial appendage and direct connection of the hepatic veins to the atrium.

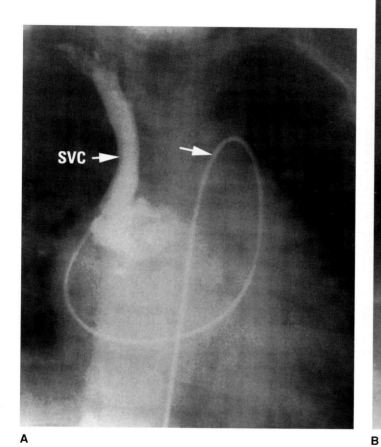

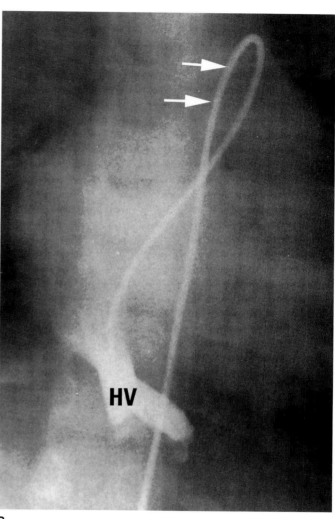

A

B

Fig. 12-29: Left-sided hemiazygous continuation to a left superior vena cava with a right-sided superior vena cava connecting to the right-sided atrium and direct connection of the hepatic veins to the atrium.
A: The catheter course confirms a left-sided hemiazygous continuation (arrow) with the catheter then advanced from the left-sided atrium into a right-sided superior vena cava. **B:** Direct connection of the hepatic veins to the atrium is demonstrated by selective injection. These findings are consistent with presumed left atrial isomerism.

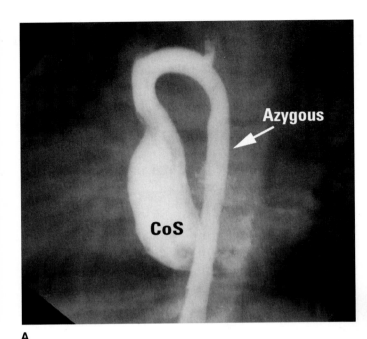

A

Fig. 12-30: **A patient with dextrocardia, left atrial isomerism and interruption of the inferior vena cava. The azygous vein that receives the inferior vena cava is connected to the right-sided superior vena cava and then to the coronary sinus.**
A and B: Frontal and lateral views show the azygous continuation of the inferior caval vein to the right-sided superior vena cava and the coronary sinus. **C:** Direct connection of the hepatic veins to the atrium is demonstrated.

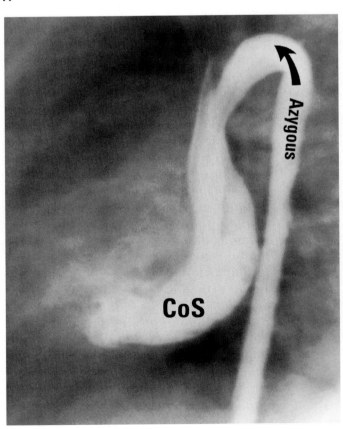

B

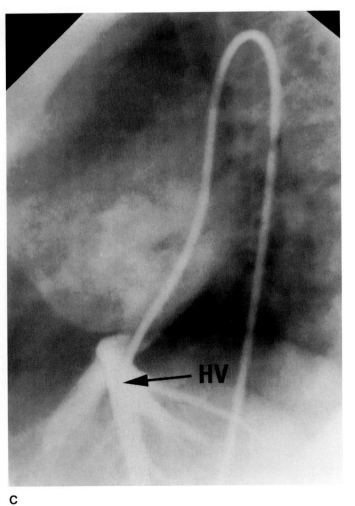

C

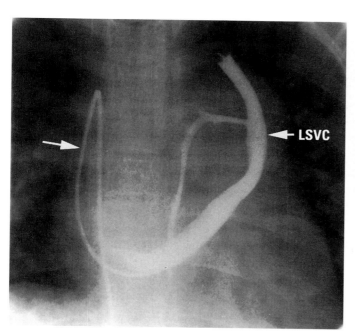

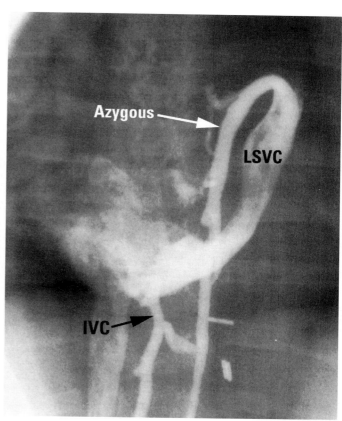

Fig. 12-31: A patient with levocardia, left atrial isomerism, interruption of the inferior vena cava with azygous continuation (arrow). The catheter was advanced into the right-sided superior vena cava, to the coronary sinus and then into the left-sided superior vena cava. A small left-sided hemiazygous vein is opacified.

Fig. 12-32: A patient with presumed left atrial isomerism, connection of a small left-sided hemiazygous continuation to a left superior vena cava, and also direct inferior caval connection to the atrium.

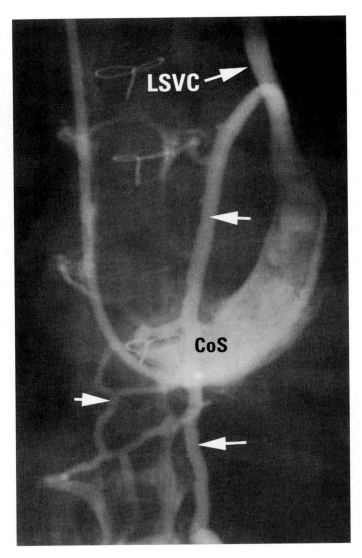

Fig. 12-33: A patient with presumed left atrial isomerism, interruption of the inferior vena cava, and left-sided hemiazygous continuation. The left superior vena cava is connected to the coronary sinus and a number of small venous connections are seen (small arrows) to the right-sided paravertebral plexus.

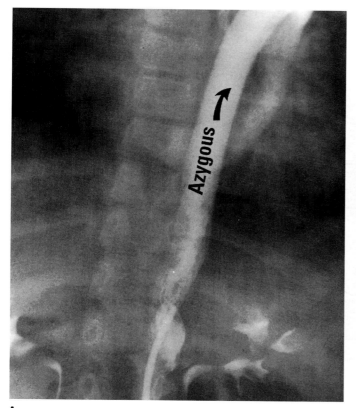

A

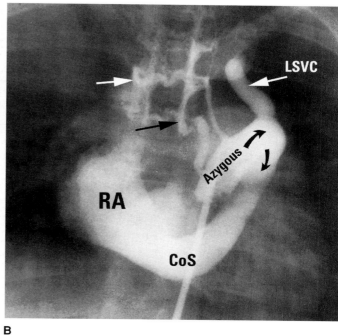

B

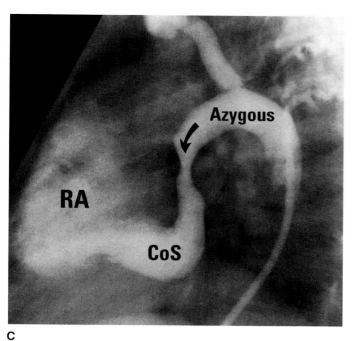

C

Fig. 12-34: Left-sided hemiazygous continuation of the interrupted inferior caval vein draining into the left-sided superior vena cava that connects to coronary sinus. A myriad of small mediastinal veins (black arrow) connect to the right-sided superior caval vein (white arrow).
A: Injection in the abdominal inferior cava at the level of the renal veins showing the left-sided hemiazygous continuation. B: A frontal injection just proximal to the connection with the left superior vena cava. C: Lateral to Fig. 12-34B.

vein is adjacent to a low lying atrial septal defect that functionally directs venous return to the left atrium.

Connection of Inferior Caval Vein with the Coronary Sinus

Connection of the inferior caval vein with the coronary sinus is very unusual, but this has been reported in a patient with visceroatrial heterotaxy in whom the inferior caval vein drained into the coronary sinus, while the majority of the hepatic veins drained into the right-sided atrium.[95] We have also identified connection of the entirety of the systemic venous return to the coronary sinus in an infant with an absent right superior caval vein.[95a] In those rare situations of inferior vena caval connection to the coronary sinus, the coronary sinus is usually unroofed.[95b]

We and others have observed congenital stenosis of the inferior caval vein at its junction with the right atrium in a patient with the scimitar syndrome.[95c] This patient, shown in Fig. 12-27, has seemingly massively dilated hepatic veins (Fig. 12-35). As pointed out by Jolly and colleagues[96] referring to the developmental observations of

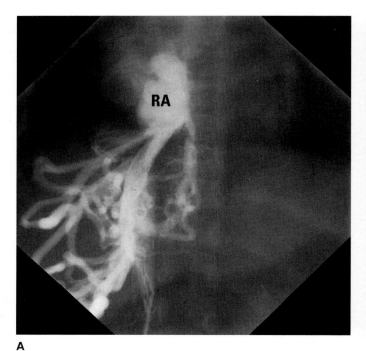

A

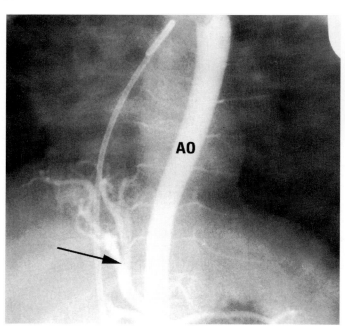

C

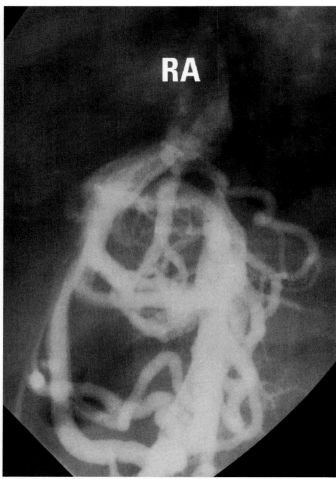

B

Fig. 12-35: This child with the scimitar complex has a peculiar plexus of hepatic veins, as well as both direct continuity of a stenotic inferior caval vein with the atrium and an azygous continuation. Same patient as shown in Fig. 12-27.
A and B: The peculiar developmental plexus of hepatic veins (see also Chapter 40, Fig. 40-45). **C:** The anomalous systemic artery supplies a basal segment of the right lower lobe.

Huntington and McClure,[97] a plexus of hepatic veins is likely a precursor in hepatic vein development, and this plexus probably contributes to the hepatic segment of the inferior cava vein.

Membranous stenosis of the inferior caval vein has been described in a young child with Budd-Chiari syndrome.[98] Massive hemoptysis has been attributed to congenital absence of a segment of the inferior vena cava.[99]

Abnormalities of Hemiazygous Vein

The hemiazygous vein may be enlarged either naturally or because of femoral-iliac-inferior caval venous occlusion (Figs. 12-2, 12-15, 12-17, 12-18, 12-25, 12-29, 12-31 through 12-34). The most common cause for such venous occlusion is a previous cardiac catheterization or venous cannulation at the time of cardiac surgery, etc. The hemiazygous vein may also dilate in response to superior caval vein narrowing after Mustard's repair for transposition of the great arteries (Fig. 12-36). The hemiazygous vein may ascend to connect with a left-sided superior caval vein, or it may cross the midline to enter a right-sided superior caval vein.[99a] We have most commonly observed the crossing hemiazygous vein in patients with left atrial isomerism. Progressive dilatation of the hemiazygous vein has been observed after Fontan's operation or construction of a bidirectional cavopulmonary connection. We have also observed rather spectacular enlargement of the superior or supreme intercostal vein and a tiny left superior caval vein after Fontan's operation or con-

struction of a bidirectional cavopulmonary connection (Fig. 12-37).

Other abnormalities of the inferior vena cava in the occasional patient with lateralized atria include bilateral inferior caval veins and a left-sided inferior caval vein that crosses to the right of the spine to enter the morphologically right atrium.[100,100a] Day and colleagues[100b] have described a persistent subcardinal anastomosis as a source of right-to-left shunting promoting arterial hypoxemia after Fontan's operation.

Anomalies of the Hepatic Veins

The most common anomaly of the hepatic veins is direct connection of these veins to the atrium when the atria are not completely lateralized; ie, left atrial isomerism (see Chapter 41). Other abnormalities include connection of the hepatic veins with the coronary sinus or with the left atrium.[101-104]

Hepatic Venous Connection to the Coronary Sinus

Connection of the left hepatic vein to the coronary sinus has been observed in a child with other systemic venous anomalies.[102-104] In isolation this should not compromise the patient. Conversely, should the pulmonary veins also terminate in the coronary sinus, the

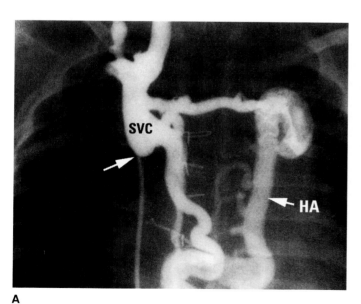

A

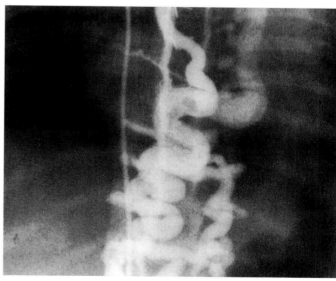

B

Fig. 12-36: Significant venous collateralization after nearly complete surgical occlusion of the right-sided superior vena cava with decompression by way of a right-sided azygous and left-sided hemiazygous veins.
A: Injection into the right-sided superior vena cava; the catheter completely occludes flow into the right atrium (arrow). **B:** The paravertebral venous plexus has extensively dilated.

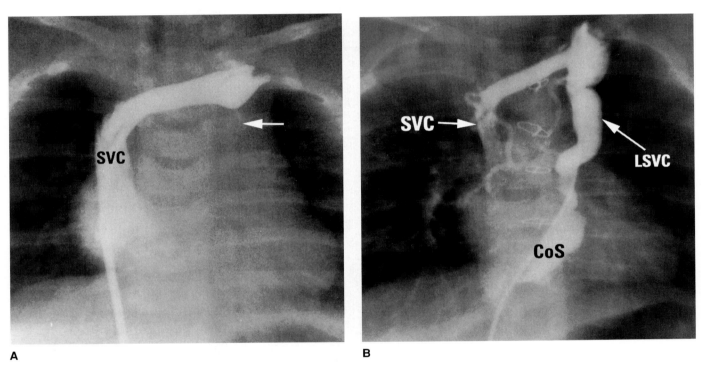

A   **B**

Fig. 12-37: Spectacular dilatation of a very tiny left superior vena cava found a few weeks after construction of a bidirectional cavopulmonary connection.
A: Before construction of a bidirectional cavopulmonary connection, a tiny left superior vena cava was seen (arrow). **B and C:** Frontal and lateral injection into the left superior vena cava entered via the coronary sinus. The left-sided superior vena cava is markedly dilated postoperatively.

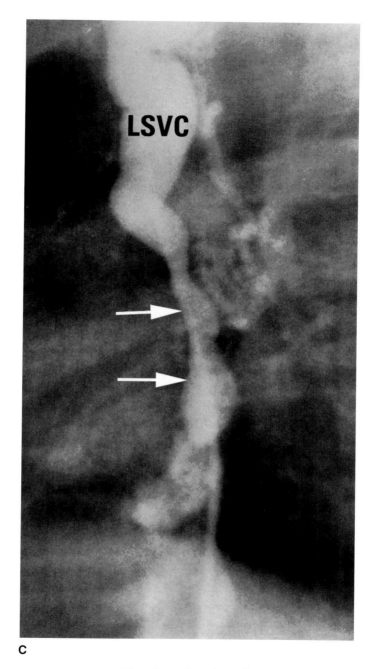

C

Fig. 12-37 *(continued)*

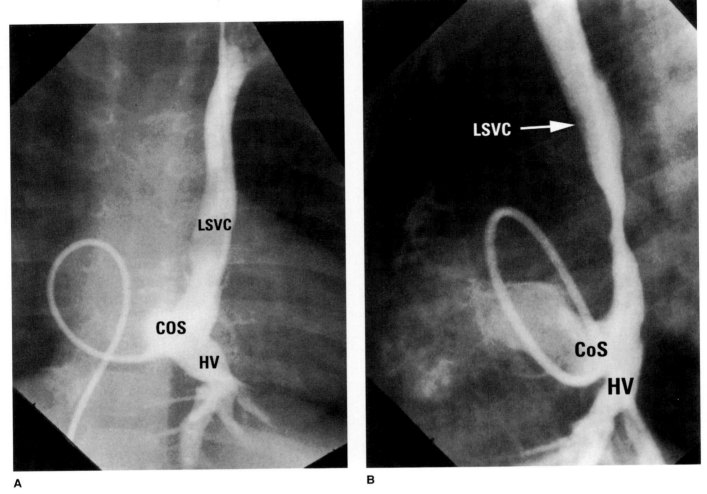

Fig. 12-38: Connection of left-sided hepatic veins into coronary sinus also receiving a left-sided superior vena cava.
A and B: Frontal and lateral views with an injection into the coronary sinus show the connection of the left-sided hepatic veins with the coronary sinus.

presence of a hepatic vein-coronary sinus connection could compromise surgical repair. Furthermore, if hepatic vein-coronary sinus connections were not diagnosed prior to a Fontan-type operation, the decision to leave the coronary sinus draining into the left atrium would promote arterial hypoxemia (Fig. 12-38).

Hepatic Venous Connection to the Left Atrium

In 1968, Yee[101] described the postmortem finding of anomalous termination of a hepatic vein in the left atrium.[101a] This patient also had tetralogy of Fallot with total anomalous pulmonary venous connections to the right atrium. Clearly the effect of this anomalously connected hepatic vein was masked in this particular pa-

tient by the Fallot malformation and the anomalously connected pulmonary veins.

Persistence of the Hepatic Venous Plexus as the Terminal Part of the Inferior Caval Vein

Jolly and colleagues[96] have reported a 10-year-old boy with a patent arterial duct in whom the prerenal segment of the inferior vena cava was replaced by an intrahepatic plexus of vessels draining into the right atrium.[96] We have studied two patients with similar hepatic venous findings. In one patient with the scimitar syndrome the connection between the right atrium and inferior vena caval vein was hypoplastic (Fig. 12-27) (see Chapter 19). Slavik and colleagues[96a] have described a patient with an azygous continuation of the

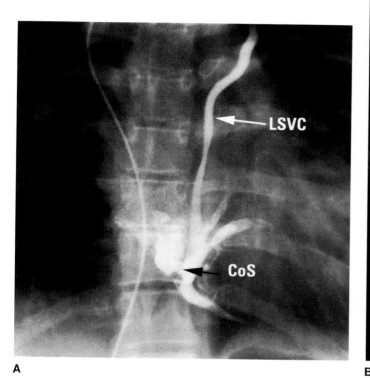

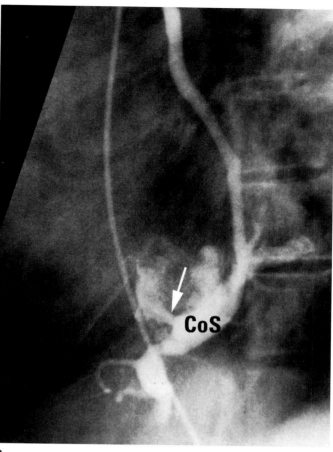

A

B

Fig. 12-39: Stenosis of the coronary sinus ostium in a patient with an unbalanced form of atrioventricular septal defect. A and B: Frontal and lateral views with injection into a left-sided superior caval vein show the stenotic ostium (arrow) of the coronary sinus.

inferior vena cava who became severely and persistently cyanotic after a bidirectional superior cavopulmonary anastomosis. They attributed this to an intrahepatic venovenous malformation. Clinical improvement followed transcatheter deployment of two Rashkind double umbrella devices into the malformation. The venous angiography in this patient is certainly reminiscent of the findings reported by Jolly and colleagues[96] and that shown in Fig. 12-35 and Chapter 40, Fig. 40-45. Similar angiographic findings have just been reported by Reed and colleagues.[96b] Again, these findings have been attributed to a sequelae of the Fontan or Kawashima modification of bidirectional cavopulmonary anastomosis procedure, but in the case of Jolly and colleagues[96] and in one of our cases, this finding was of a congenital nature, not associated with either a Fontan nor a Kawashima modification of the bidirectional cavopulmonary anastomosis procedure.

Anomalies of the Coronary Sinus

The coronary sinus exhibits a wide range of congenital and acquired abnormalities some of which are minor, but others have important clinical implications (Figs. 12-39 through 12-41).[105–124] The ostium of the coronary sinus may be enlarged,[35] absent, displaced from its usual position,[105] stenotic or atretic,[56,57,106–112] aneurysmal,[122–124] or doubled.[108a] Enlargement of the coronary sinus can reflect right atrial volume or pressure overload, but more commonly reflects abnormal communication between the coronary sinus and systemic or pulmonary veins (see Chapter 24, Fig. 24-9).[35] It has been suggested that a dilated coronary sinus can produce left ventricular inflow obstruction.[112a] The basis for the obstruction was a coronary sinus dilated by connection of a left superior caval vein to the coronary sinus. Cochrane and colleagues[112a] have reported four

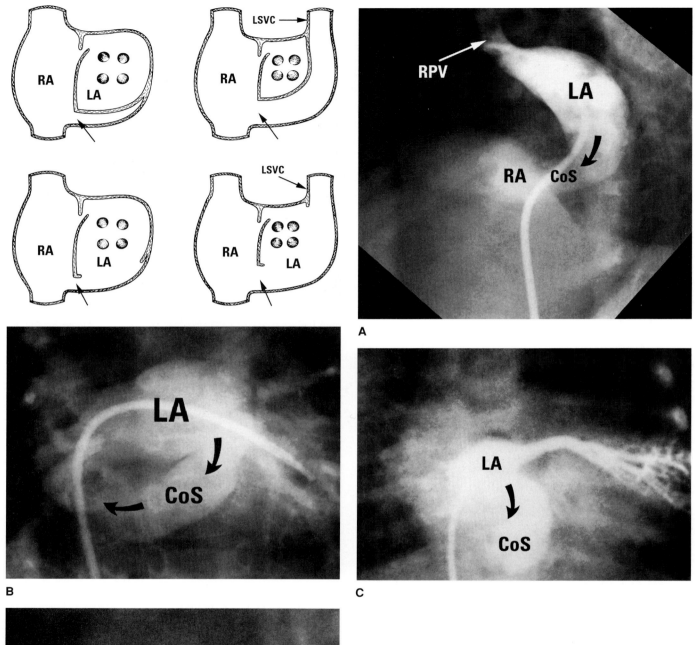

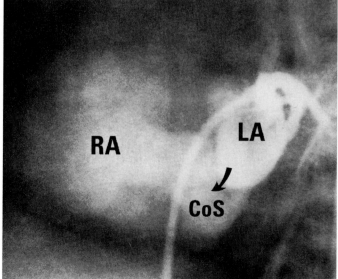

Fig. 12-40: Unroofed coronary sinus in the absence of a left superior vena cava connecting to the left atrium.

Diagram of coronary sinus and its unroofing. **Left upper panel:** Normal coronary sinus draining to right atrium. **Upper right panel:** Left superior caval vein connecting to coronary sinus which drains to the right atrium. **Lower left panel:** Left atrial-coronary sinus communication without a persistent left superior caval vein. **Lower right panel:** Unroofed coronary sinus with left superior caval vein connecting to left atrium. **A and B:** A patient with a left atrium-coronary sinus communication. A: Left atrial injection shows the communication with the coronary sinus (arrow). B: Another view demonstrates this unusual communication. **C and D:** A different patient with an unroofed coronary sinus. Frontal and lateral projections with an injection into the left atrium shows direct flow into the coronary sinus. *(continued)*

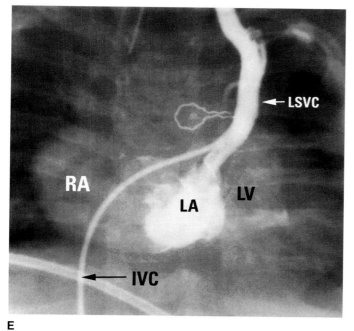

E

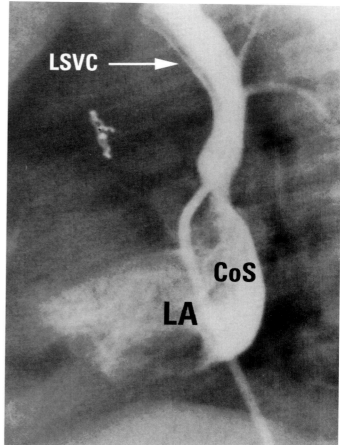

F

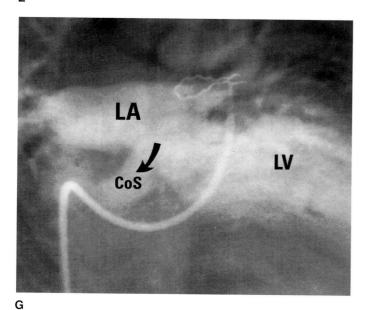

G

Fig. 12-40 *(continued):* **E through G:** Yet another patient with multiple ventricular septal defects, pulmonary artery banding, and an unroofed coronary sinus with the left superior vena cava connecting to the left atrium. **E and F:** The venous catheter is advanced from the right atrium to the left atrium and the left superior vena cava. Contrast injected into the left superior vena cava in frontal and lateral projections opacifies the left atrium and the left ventricle. **G:** The levophase of the main pulmonary arteriogram shows the left atrium with opacification of the coronary sinus. **H:** Specimen showing a coronary sinus-left atrial communication. This internal view of the left atrium shows the unroofed coronary sinus communicating with the left atrium.

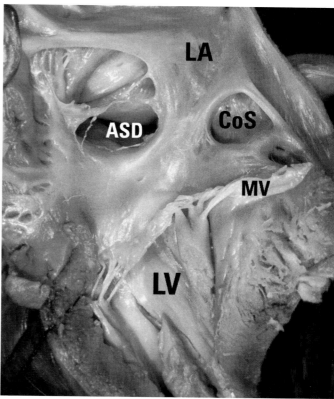

H

patients where they suggested that a markedly dilated coronary sinus produced left ventricular inflow obstruction. This has been seen by others as well.[112b] We have seen a massively dilated coronary sinus in a patient who underwent a Fontan operation. The coronary sinus was left on the systemic venous side of the atriopulmonary connection, and a left superior caval vein connecting to the coronary sinus was inadvertently not addressed at the time of the Fontan (personal communication. John P. Finley, MD, Division of Cardiology, The Izaak Walton Killam Children's Hospital, Halifax, Nova Scotia). Stenosis of the coronary sinus ostium has been identified in isolation,[111,112] but has also been documented in a patient with pulmonary atresia, intact ventricular septum, and left superior vena cava to the coronary sinus with an unroofed coronary sinus (Fig. 12-39, see also Chapter 23, Fig. 23-12).[56] Chiang and colleagues[113] reported stenosis and angulation of the coronary sinus in adult patients undergoing radiofrequency ablation of supraventricular tachycardia. Conventional teaching has suggested that if pulmonary venous obstruction is present in the patient with total anomalous pulmonary venous return to the coronary sinus, the obstruction must occur at the level of the interatrial septum. However, the coronary sinus may also be stenotic in the patient with total anomalous pulmonary venous connection to the coronary sinus (see also Chapter 24).[114,115] This uncommon cause for pulmonary venous obstruction in this setting has been documented both by Arciniegas and colleagues[114] as well as Jonas and colleagues.[115] The coronary sinus may be absent, and in this condition, the cardiac veins drain directly into the atrium via thebesian veins. Atresia of the coronary sinus ostium may be associated with a persistent left superior caval vein.[116–117b] When this vein provides the major source of egress for coronary venous blood, ligation of the left superior caval vein may prove fatal as it did in the case reported by Yokota.[112] Donor coronary sinus atresia has been noted at the time of cardiac transplantation.[118] Rarely the coronary sinus may have a congenital fistulous connection with the left ventricle,[119–121] remembering that such a connection may be acquired after mitral valve replacement.[121a,121b] The coronary sinus may be aneurysmal,[122] and diverticulum of the coronary sinus may be present; in both conditions, these abnormalities may be associated with the Wolff-Parkinson-White syndrome (see also Chapter 50, Fig. 50-1).[122–124] Others have suggested that coronary sinus morphology is different in patients with atrioventricular junctional reentry tachycardia and other supraventricular tachyarrhythmias when compared with normal patients.[123a] Doig and coauthors[123a] found that the ostium of the coronary sinus was larger and its appearance like a windsock in atrioventricular junctional reentry tachycardia. Petit and colleagues[124a] have recognized a congenital diverticulum of the right atrium situated on the floor of the coronary sinus in a baby with hypoplastic left heart syndrome. In one patient with absent right superior caval vein, a double coronary sinus was recognized at postmortem.[124b] The coronary sinus is usually absent in patients with isomerism of the morphologically right atrial appendage, but is more likely to be normal in patients with morphologically left atrial appendage (see Chapter 41).

The coronary sinus may be wholly or partially unroofed, communicating with the floor of the left atrium.[9,10,21,26,56,59,67,72,109,125–133] The complex of the so-called unroofed coronary sinus is usually but not invariably associated with a left superior caval vein connecting to the left atrium (See Left Superior Caval Vein) (Figs. 12-40 and 12-41).

Peculiar communications between the coronary sinus and left atrium have developed after Fontan's operation, and in one patient in whom the coronary sinus was left on the right atrial side, these communications promoted a right-to-left shunt (Fig. 12-41).[134] Hayes and colleagues[134] documented these communications and then interrupted them with transcatheter techniques. These vessels probably reflect coronary venous channels dilated by high right atrial pressures. We have stated before that in patients with complex congenital heart disease, both de novo and after heart surgery there is increasing appreciation of unusual communications between the systemic and pulmonary venous circulations and the development of systemic venous collaterals after construction of a bidirectional cavopulmonary connection, a classic Glenn, or Fontan (Figs. 12-41 through 12-43).[135–136a] In addition, right-to-left shunting from systemic venous to pulmonary venous system has been observed developing after superior caval obstruction.[136b]

Some of the anomalies of the coronary sinus can be demonstrated by cross-sectional echocardiography, whereas angiocardiography is required for recognition of others. Selective coronary arteriography, left atrial angiography, and/or selective injection of contrast into the left superior caval vein have helped to define those abnormalities of the coronary sinus.[9,19,21,56,111,130] An excellent study of retrograde coronary venography in patients with posteroseptal and left-sided accessory atrioventricular pathways has been published by Schumacher and colleagues.[130a]

The Divided Right Atrium: So-called Cor Triatriatum Dexter

Septation of the right atrium that produces a divided right atrium has received considerable attention in the past two decades, perhaps more since the intro-

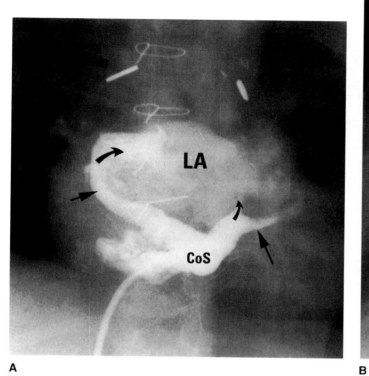

A

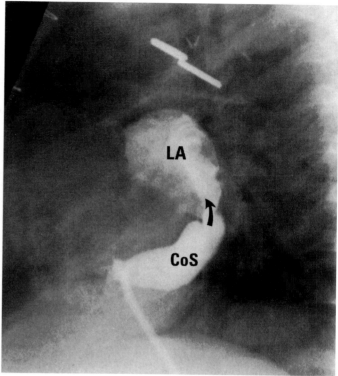

B

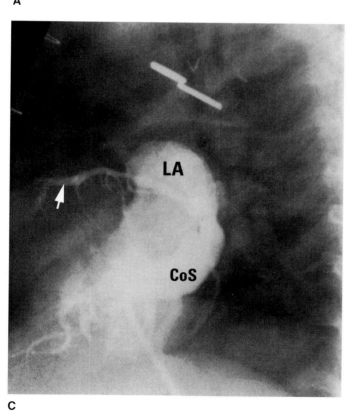

C

Fig. 12-41: A small fenestration between the coronary sinus and left atrium was unmasked after Fontan's operation. This patient also developed coronary venous connections promoting a right-to-left shunt after Fontan's operation.
A and B: Frontal and lateral angiograms with an injection into coronary sinus show the fenestration (curved arrow) of its party wall with the left atrium; superiorly coronary veins connect with the left atrium. **C:** A slightly later frame than Fig. 12-41B.

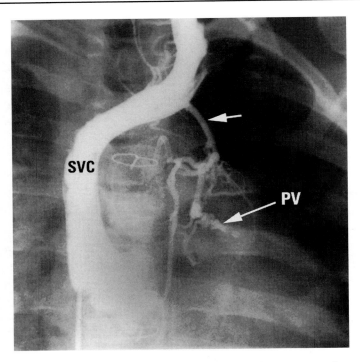

Fig. 12-42: Some years after Fontan's operation, progressive arterial hypoxemia could be explained by development of an enlarged supreme intercostal vein (arrow) connecting to the pulmonary vein.

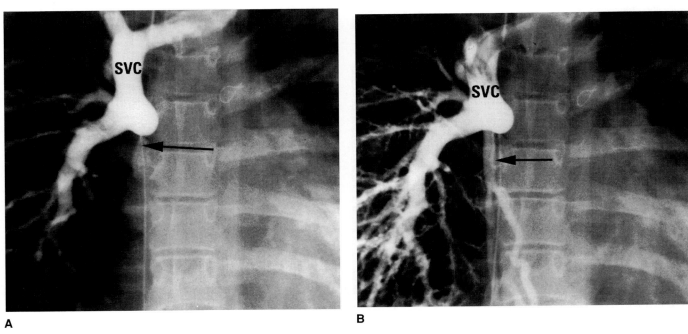

A   **B**

Fig. 12-43: Reasons for late deterioration of a cavopulmonary connection (see also Chapter 19).
A: Residual recannulation of the ligated superior vena cava-right atrial connection (arrow). **B:** Development of systemic venous collaterals bypassing the right pulmonary artery (arrow). **C and D:** Another patient who developed extensive systemic venous collaterals (arrows) bypassing the right pulmonary artery some years after construction of a classic Glenn operation (same patient as in Fig. 12-39). **E:** Another patient some years after construction of a classic Glenn operation developed systemic venous collateralization to the left pulmonary veins.

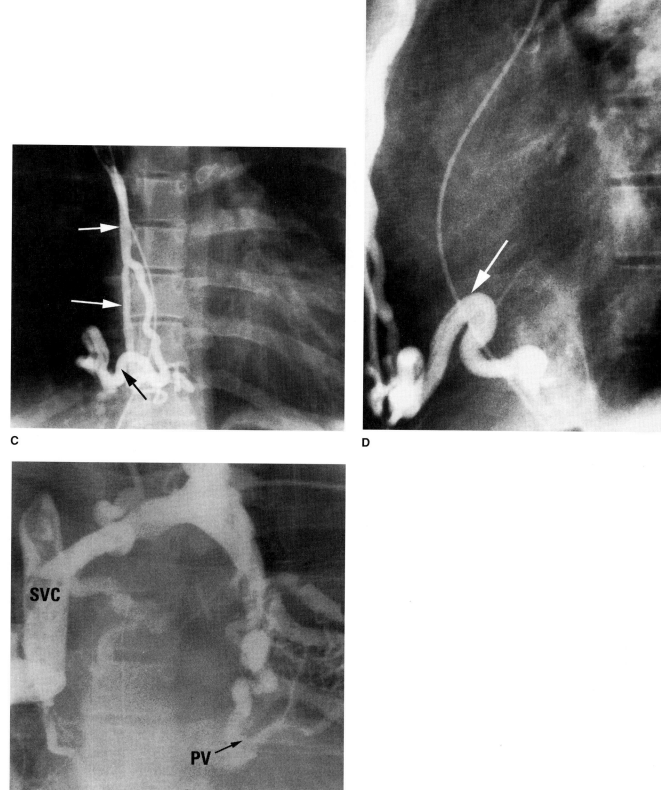

Fig. 12-43 *(continued)*

duction of cross-sectional echocardiography in routine imaging armamentarium.[137–159] The septation is produced by a fibrous membrane derived embryologically from the right venous valve (Fig. 12-44).[9,10,137,138] This right atrial diaphragm partitions the morphologically right atrium into two chambers: the trabeculated portion of the right atrium and the tricuspid valve orifice, which is more or less separated from the sinus venarum portion of the atrium receiving the great veins. Trento and colleagues[160] have reviewed 14 hearts from the cardiac museum of the Children's Hospital of Pittsburgh.[160] They suggested three subgroups: 1) valves prominent in the formation of Chiari network and probably of no functional significance; 2) valves of considerable prominence dividing the right atrium, and these valves themselves posed the impediment to flow through the right side of the heart, and 3) persistent venous valves in hearts with either atresia or stenosis of the right-sided pathways. Kauffman and Anderson, a quarter-of-a-century earlier, had noted the presence of persistent venous valves in patients with maldevelopment of the right heart, and coronary artery-ventricular communications.[161] They speculated that the persistence and prominence of these venous valves might be causal to inflow and outflow right heart obstruction. Others have imaged the prominent Eustachian valve in the patient with right heart obstruction.[162,163]

Absent Ductus Venosus

The ductus venosus, a fetal structure, connects the umbilical vein and the portal vein to the inferior caval vein.[164–166] In the normal growing infant, the ductus venosus obliterates and is transformed into the ligamentum venosum. However, an absent ductus venosus or one that obliterates in the fetus implies that the oxygenated blood from the umbilical vein has to circulate through the liver, severely jeopardizing the fetus. Jorgensen and Andolf[166] summarized the literature of this rare condition, adding four cases of their own. Three of the patients provided by Jorgensen and Andolf had extreme hydrops, especially hydrothorax. Thrombosis of the umbilical cord vessels is a rare but life-threatening event, usually leading to the death of the fetus. Hasaart and colleagues[167] report a case of an intra-partum fetal death due to thrombosis of the ductus venosus, an entity previously not described in the literature. Chandar and Wolfe[168] report the displacement of a thrombus originating in either the ductus venosus or hepatic vein by umbilical vein catheterization to perform a balloon septostomy. Finally, the ductus venosus may persist as well.[169]

The surgical anatomy of coronary venous return in hearts with isomeric atrial appendages has been examined in detail (see also Chapter 41) (Fig. 12-45).[170]

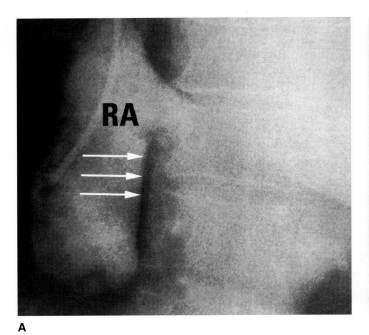

A

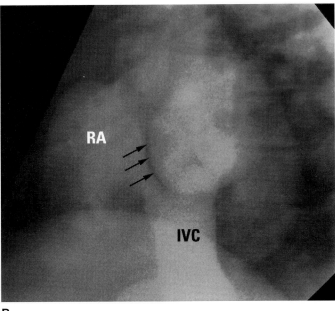

B

Fig. 12-44: Divided right atrium from a persistent right venous valve.
A: Frontal right atriogram shows the well-developed right venous valve (arrows). **B:** Lateral angiogram with an injection into the inferior vena cava from another patient shows a membrane (arrows) dividing the right atrium.

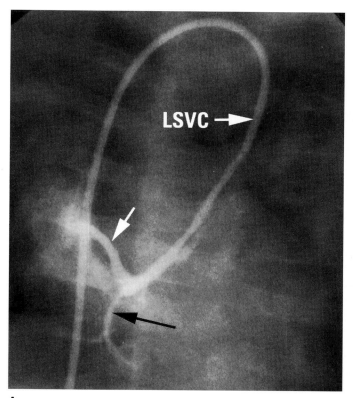

A

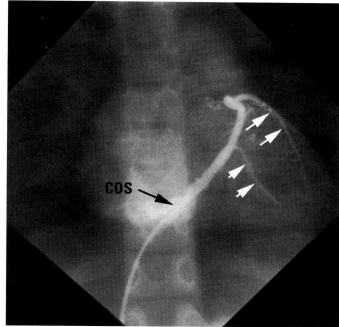

B

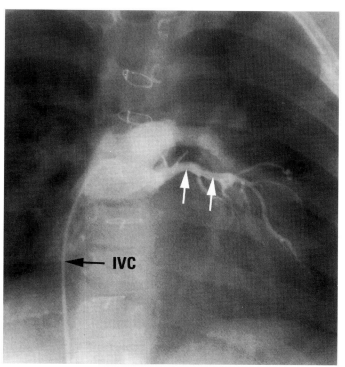

C

Fig. 12-45: Appearance of coronary veins after surgery to palliate complex cardiac malformations.
A: Catheter advanced to a small left superior vena cava to coronary sinus where coronary sinus venogram shows coronary veins (arrows). **B:** Coronary sinus venogram from another patient shows opacification of some coronary veins after a bidirectional cavopulmonary shunt. **C:** Either a coronary vein or right atrial vein developed after an atriopulmonary connection and atrial separation.

References

1. Fontan F, Baudet E. Surgical repair of tricuspid atresia. *Thorax* 1971;26:240–248.

2. de Leval MR, Ritter DG, McGoon DC, Danielson GK. Anomalous systemic venous connection; surgical considerations. *Mayo Clin Proc* 1975;50:599–610.

3. Fleming JS, Gibson RV. Absent right superior vena cava as an isolated anomaly. *Br J Radiol* 1964;37:696.

4. Karnegis JN, Wang Y, Winchell P, Edwards JE. Persistent left superior vena cava, fibrous remnant of the right superior vena cava and ventricular septal defect. Am J Cardiol 1964;14:573–578.

4a. Alhan HC, Kayacioglu I, Tayyareci G, Cakalagaoglu C, Idiz M, Tarcan S, Yigiter B. Absent right suprior vena cava with hypoplastic proximal inferior vena cava. *Ann Thorac Surg* 1996;62:566–568.

5. Lenox CC, Hashida Y, Anderson RH, Hubbard JD. Conduction tissue anomalies in absence of the right superior caval vein. *Int J Cardiol* 1985;8:251–260.

6. Lenox CC, Zuberbuhler JR, Park SC, Neches WH, Mathews RA, Fricker FJ, Bahnson HT, Siewers RD. Absent right superior vena cava with persistent left superior vena cava: Implications and management. *Am J Cardiol* 1980;45:117–122.

7. Marin-Garcia J, Sanmarti J, Moller JH. Congenital absence of the right superior vena cava: Report of two cases. *Eur J Cardiol* 1978;7:293–297.

8. Tuma S, Samanek M, Voriskova M, Benesova D, Prazsky F, Hucin B. Anomalies of systemic venous return. *Pediatr Radiol* 1977;5:193–197.

9. Freedom RM, Benson LN. Anomalies of systemic venous connections, persistence of the right venous valve and silent cardiovascular causes of cyanosis. In: Freedom RM, Benson LN, Smallhorn JF. *Neonatal Heart Disease*. London: Springer-Verlag; London, 1992, pp. 484–495.

10. Freedom RM, Culham JAG, Moes CAF. *Angiocardiography of Con-genital Heart Disease*. New York: MacMillan Publishing Co; 1984, pp. 46–66.

11. Bell MJ, Gutierrez JR, DuBois JJ. Aneurysm of the superior vena cava. *Radiology* 1970;95:317–318.

12. Braudo M, Beanlands DS, Trusler GA. Anomalous drainage of the right superior vena cava into the left atrium. *Can Med Assoc J* 1968;99:715–719.

13. Polansky S, Gooding CA, Potter B. Idiopathic dilatation of the superior vena cava. *Pediatr Radiol* 1974; 2:167–174.

14. Bharati S, Lev M. Direct entry of the right superior vena cava into the left atrium with aneurysmal dilatation and stenosis at its entry into the right atrium with stenosis of the pulmonary veins: A rare case. *Pediatr Cardiol* 1984; 5:123–126.

15. Modry DL, Hidvegi RS, LaFleche LR. Congenital saccular aneurysm of the superior vena cava. *Ann Thorac Surg* 1980;29:258–262.

16. Alpert B, Rao PS, Moore HV, Covitz W. Surgical correction of anomalous right superior vena cava to the left atrium. *J Thorac Cardiovasc Surg* 1981;82:301–305.

16a. Alday LE, Maisuls H, De Rossi R. Right superior caval vein draining into the left atrium—Diagnosis by color flow mapping. *Cardiol Young* 1995;5:345–349.

17. Blank E, Zuberbuhler JR. Left to right shunt through a left atrial left superior vena cava. *AJR* 1968;103: 87–92.

18. Edwards JE. Malformations of the thoracic veins. *Pathol-*

19. Edwards JE, Dushane JW. Thoracic venous anomalies. *Arch Pathol* 1950;49:517–537.

20. Ezekowitz MD, Alderson PO, Bulkley BH. Isolated drainage of the superior vena cava into the left atrium in a 52-year-old man. *Circulation* 1978;58:751–756.

21. Fischer DR, Zuberbuhler JR. Anomalous systemic venous return. In: Anderson RH, Macartney FJ, Shinebourne EA, Tynan M, eds. *Paediatric Cardiology*. Edinburgh: Churchill Livingstone; 1987, pp. 867–888.

22. Park HM, Smith ET, Silberstein EB. Isolated right superior vena cava draining into left atrium diagnosed by radionuclide angiography. *J Nucl Med* 1973;14:240–242.

23. Park HM, Summerer MH, Preuss K, Armstrong WF, Mahomed Y, Hamilton DJ. Anomalous drainage of the right superior cava into the left atrium. *J Am Coll Cardiol* 1983;2:358–362.

24. LePere RH, Kohler CM, Klinger P, Lowry JK. Intrathoracic Venous Anomalies. *J Thorac Cardiovasc Surg* 1965;49:599–614.

25. Shapiro EP, Al-Sadir J, Campbell NPS, Thilenius OG, Anagnostopoulos CE, Hays P. Drainage of right superior vena cava into both atria. Review of the literature and description of a case presenting with polycythemia and paradoxical embolization. *Circulation* 1981;63: 712–717.

26. Taybi H, Kurlander GJ, Lurie PR, Campbell JA. Anomalous systemic venous connection to the left atrium or to a pulmonary vein. *AJR* 1965;94:62–77.

27. Vargas FJ, Mayer JE Jr, Jonas RA, Castaneda AR. Anomalous systemic and pulmonary venous connection in conjunction with atriopulmonary anastomosis (Fontan-Kreutger). *J Thorac Cardiovasc Surg* 1987;93:523–527.

28. Vazquez-Perez J, Frontera-Izquierdo P. Anomalous drainage of the right superior vena cava into the left atrium as an isolated anomaly. *Am Heart J* 1979;97: 89–93.

29. Dupuis C, Risbourg B, Demougeot C. "Absence d'amarrage" de la veine superieure au mediastin. A propos de 2 observations. *Arch Mal Coeur* 1977;70:415–417.

30. Freedom RM, Schaffer MS, Rowe RD. Anomalous low insertion of the right superior vena cava. *Br Heart J* 1982; 48:601–603.

30a. Sai S, Yoshida I, Itoh Y, Niibori K, Ninomiya M, Tabayashi K, Mohri H. Diverticulum of the superior vena cava. *Ann Thorac Surg* 1994;58:889–890.

30b. Hidvegi RS. Diverticulum of the superior vena cava (letter). *AJR* 1995;164:1553.

31. Yokomise H, Nakayama S, Aota M, Daitoh N, Katsura H. Systemic venous aneurysms. *Ann Thorac Surg* 1990;50: 460–462.

31a. Hidvegi RS, Modry DL, LaFleche L. Congenital saccular aneurysm of the superior vena cava: Radiographic features. *AJR* 1979;133:924–927.

31b. Stockberger SM, West KW, Cohen MD. Right-to-left shunt from systemic venous to pulmonary venous system developing after SVC obstruction. *J Comput Assist Tomogr* 1995;19:312–315.

32. Bernardis C, Chatzis A, Treasure T. Absence of the right superior caval vein associated with disease of the sinus node. *Int J Cardiol* 1992;16:115–117.

33. Camm AJ, Dymond D, Spurrell RA. Sinus node dysfunction associated with absence of right superior vena cava. *Br Heart J* 1979;41:504–507.

34. Choi JY, Anderson RH, Macartney FJ. Absent right supe-

rior caval vein with normal atrial arrangement. *Br Heart J* 1987;57:474–478.

34a. Kaemmerer H, Prokop M, Schirg E, Emter M, Hesel C, Daniel W, Kallfelz HC. Unilaterale linke Vena cava superior bei fehlender rechter Vena cava superior. Moderne bildgebende Diagnostik und klinische Relevanz. *Z Kardiol* 1994;83:386–391.

35. Fellows KE, Sigmann J, Stern AM, Bookstein JJ. Coronary sinus enlargement in infants. A diagnostic note. *Radiology* 1970;94:347–349.

35a. Khanna SN, Pandey RB, Khandeparkar JM, Agarwal NB, Magotra RA. Biatrial drainage of right superior vena cava with anomalous right pulmonary venous connection. *Thorac Cardiovasc Surg* 1994;42:247–249.

36. Akalin H, Uysalel A, Ozyurda U, Corapcioglu T, Eren NT, Emiroguliari N, Erol C, Sonel A. The triad of persistent left superior vena cava connected to coronary sinus, right superior vena cava draining into the left atrium, and atrial septal defect: Report of a successful operation for a rare anomaly. *J Thorac Cardiovasc Surg* 1987;94:151–153.

37. Smallhorn JF, Zielinsky P, Freedom, RM, Rowe RD. Anomalous subaortic position of the brachiocephalic vein. *Am J Cardiol* 1985;55:234–236.

38. Gerlis LM, Ho SY. Anomalous subaortic position of the brachiocephalic (innominate) vein: A review of published cases and report of three new cases. *Br Heart J* 1989;61:540–545.

39. Mill MR, Wilcox BR, Detterbeck FC, Anderson RH. Anomalous course of left brachiocephalic vein. *Ann Thorac Surg* 1993;55:600–602.

40. Choi JY, Jung MJ, Kim YH, Noh CI, Yun YS. Anomalous subaortic position of the brachiocephalic vein (innominate vein): An echocardiographic study. *Br Heart J* 1990;64:385–387.

41. Wurtz A, Quandalle P, Lemaitre L, Robert Y. Innominate vein compression. *Br J Surg* 1989;76:575–576.

41a. Moes CAF, MacDonald C, Mawson JB. Left innominate vein compression by a brachiocephalic artery anomaly. *Pediatr Radiol* 1995;16:291–293.

41b. Subirana MT, de Leval M, Somerville J. Double left innominate vein: An unusual cross-sectional ehocardiographic finding. *Int J Cardiol* 1986;12:263–265.

42. Basu BN. Persistent "left superior vena cava," "left duct of Cuvier," and "left horn of the sinus venosus." *J Anat* 1932;66:268–274.

43. Campbell M, Deuchar DC. The left-sided superior vena cava. *Br Heart J* 1954;16:423.

44. Cha EM, Khoury GH. Persistent left superior vena cava. *Radiology* 1972;103:375–381.

45. Davis D, Pritchett ELC, Klein GJ, Benson DW, Gallagher JJ. Persistent left superior vena cava in patients with congenital atrioventricular pre-excitation conduction abnormalities. *Am Heart J* 1981;101:677–679.

46. Fraser RS, Dvorkin J, Rossall RE, Eidem R. Left superior vena cava: A review of associated congenital heart lesions, catheterization data and roentgenologic findings. *Am J Med* 1961;31:711–716.

47. McCotter R. Three cases of the persistence of the left superior vena cava. *Anat Rec* 1916;10:371–383.

48. Stevens JS and Mishkin FS. Persistent left superior vena cava demonstrated by radionuclide angiography: Case report. *J Nucl Med* 1975;16:469–471.

49. Winter FS. Persistent left superior vena cava: Survey of world literature and report of thirty additional cases. *Angiology* 1954;5:90–97.

50. Gerlis LM, Partridge JB, Fiddler GI. Anomalous connection of left atrial appendage with persistent left superior vena cava. *Br Heart J* 1982;48:73–74.

51. Konstam MA, Levine BW, Strauss HW, McKurick KA. Left superior vena cava to left atrial communication diagnosed with radionuclide angiography and with differential right to left shunting. *Am J Cardiol* 1979;43:149–153.

52. Looyenga DS, Lacina SJ, Gebuhr CJ, Stockinger GS. Persistent left superior vena cava communicating with the left atrium through a systemic-pulmonary venous malformation. *J Am Coll Cardiol* 1986;8:621–626.

53. Meadows WR, Sharp JT. Persistent left superior vena cava draining into the left atrium without arterial oxygen unsaturation. *Am J Cardiol* 1965;16:273.

54. Meadows WR. Isolated anomalous connection of a great vein to the left atrium. *Circulation* 1961;24:669–676.

55. Sherafat M, Friedman S, Waldhausen JA. Persistent left superior vena cava draining into the left atrium with absent right superior vena cava. *Ann Thorac Surg* 1971;11:160–164.

56. Freedom RM, Culham JAG, Rowe RD. Left atrial to coronary sinus fenestration. (Partially unroofed coronary sinus). Morphological and angiocardiographic observations. *Br Heart J* 1981;46:63–68.

57. Snider AR, Ports TA, Silverman NH. Venous anomalies of the coronary sinus: Detection by M-mode, two-dimensional, and contrast echocardiography. *Circulation* 1979;60:721–725.

58. Tuchman H, Brown JF, Huston JH, Weinstein AB, Rowe GG, Crumpton CW. Superior vena cava draining into left atrium: Another cause for left ventricular hypertrophy with cyanotic congenital heart disease. *Am J Med* 1956;21:481–484.

59. Raghib G, Ruttenberg HD, Anderson RC, Amplatz K, Adams P Jr, Edwards JE. Termination of left superior vena cava in left atrium, atrial septal defect, and absence of coronary sinus. *Circulation* 1965;31:906–911.

60. Wiles HB. Two cases of left superior vena cava draining directly to a left atrium with a normal coronary sinus. *Br Heart J* 1991;65:158–160.

61. Sibley YD, Roberts KD, Silove ED. Surgical correction of isolated persistent left superior vena cava draining to left atrium in a neonate. *Br Heart J* 1986;55:605–606.

62. Ascuitto RJ, Ross-Ascuitto NT, Kopf GS, Fahey J, Kleinman CS, Hellenbrand WE, Talner NS. Persistent left superior vena cava causing subdivided left atrium: Diagnosis, embryologic implications, and surgical management. *Ann Thorac Surg* 1987;44:546–549.

63. Lucas RV Jr, Lester RG, Lillehei CW, Edwards JE. Mitral atresia with levoatriocardinal vein. A form of congenital pulmonary venous obstruction. *Am J Cardiol* 1962;9:607–613.

63a. Blieden LC, Schneeweiss A, Deutsch V, Neufeld HN. Anomalous venous connection from the left atrium or to a pulmonary vein. *AJR* 1977;129:937–938.

63b. McIntosh CA. Cor biatriatum triloculare. *Am Heart J* 1926;1:735–744.

64. Hunt CE, Rao S, Moller JH, Edwards JE. Anomalous pulmonary vein serving as collateral channel in aortic stenosis with hypoplastic left ventricle and endocardial fibroelastosis. *Chest* 1970;57:185–189.

64a. Lee ML, Wang JK, Lue HC. Levoatriocardinal vein in mitral atresia mimicking obstructive total anomalous pulmonary venous connection. *Int J Cardiol* 1994;47:1–4.

65. Beitzke A, Machler H, Stein JI. Mitral atresia with premature closure of the oval foramen, right-sided levoatri-

ocardinal vein and thrombus formation in the left atrium. *Int J Cardiol* 1987;14:221–224.

66. Pinto CAM, Yen Ho S, Redington A, Shinebourne EA, Anderson RH. Morphological features of a levoatrialcardinal(or pulmonary-to-systemic collateral) vein. *Pediatr Pathol* 1993;13:751–761.

66a. Bernstein HS, Moore P, Stanger P, Silverman NH. The levoatrialcardinal vein: Morphology and echocardiographic identification of the pulmonary-systemic connection. *J Am Coll Cardiol* 1995;26:995–1001.

67. Lucas RV Jr, Krabill KA. Anomalous Venous Connections, Pulmonary and Systemic. In: Adams FH, Emmanoulides GC, Riemenschneider TA, eds. *Moss' Heart Disease in Infants, Children, and Adolescents.* Baltimore: Williams and Wilkins; 1989, pp. 580–617.

68. McClure CFW and Butler EG. The Development of the Vena Cava Inferior in Man. *Am J Anat* 1925;35:331–383.

69. McClure CFW, Huntington GS. The mammalian vena cava posterior. *Am Anat Memoirs* 1929;15:2–148.

70. Milloy FJ, Anson BJ, Cauldwell EW. Variations in the inferior vena caval veins and in their renal and lumbar communications. *Surg Gynecol Obstet* 1962;115:131–141.

71. Mayo J, Gray R, St. Louis E, Grosman H, McLoughlin M, Wise D. Anomalies of the inferior vena cava. *AJR* 1983; 140:339–345.

72. Mazzucco A, Bortolotti U, Stellin G, Gallucci V. Anomalies of the systemic venous return: A review. *J Card Surg* 1990;5:122–133.

73. Anderson RH, Adams PJ, Burke B. Anomalous inferior vena cava with azygos continuation (infrahepatic interruption of the inferior vena cava). Report of 15 new cases. *J Pediatr* 1961;59:370–383.

74. Dupuis C, Nuyts JP, Christiaens L. "Continuation azygos" de la veine cave inferieure. *Arch Mal Coeur* 1964; 57:28–33.

75. Floyd GD and Nelson WP. Developmental interruption of the inferior vena cava with azygos and hemiazygos substitution. *Radiology* 1976;119:55–57.

76. Schneeweiss A, Bleiden LC, Deutsch V, Shem-Tov A, Neufeld HN. Uninterrupted inferior vena cava with azygos continuation. *Chest* 1981;80:114–115.

77. Heller RM, Dorst JP, James AE, Rowe RD. A useful sign in the recognition of azygos continuation of the inferior vena cava. *Radiology* 1971;101:519–522.

78. Merrill WH, Pieroni DP, Freedom RM, Ho CS. Diagnosis of infrahepatic interruption of the inferior vena cava. *Johns Hopkins Med J* 1973;133:329–338.

79. Dickinson DF, Wilkinson JL, Anderson KR, Smith A, Ho SY, Anderson RH. The cardiac conduction system in situs ambigus. *Circulation* 1979;59:879–885.

80. Van der Horst RL, Gotsman MS. Abnormalities of atrial depolarization in infradiaphragmatic interruption of the inferior vena cava. *Br Heart J* 1972;34:295–300.

81. Freedom RM, Ellison RC. Coronary sinus rhythm in the polysplenia syndrome. *Chest* 1973;63:952–958.

82. Garcia OL, Mehta AV, Pichoft A. Left isomerism and complete atrioventricular block: A report of six cases. *Am J Cardiol* 1981;48:1103–1107.

83. Momma K, Takao A, Shibata T. Characteristics and natural history of abnormal atrial rhythms in left isomerism. *Am J Cardiol* 1990;65:231–236.

84. Roguin N, Milo S, Vidne B. Unusual drainage of the inferior caval vein in left atrial isomerism. *Int J Cardiol* 1989;24:35–39.

85. Takanashi Y, Anzai N, Okada T, Sano A, Ando M,

Konno S. Common atrium associated with anomalous high insertion of the inferior vena cava. *J Thorac Cardiovasc Surg* 1975;69:912–918.

86. O'Reilly RJ and Grollman JH Jr. The lateral chest film as an unreliable indicator of azygos continuation of the inferior vena cava. *Circulation* 1976;53:891–895.

87. Foale R, Bourdillon PD, Somerville J. Anomalous systemic venous return: Recognition by two-dimensional echocardiography. *Eur Heart J* 1983;4:186–190.

88. Huhta JC, Smallhorn JF, Macartney FJ. Cross-sectional echocardiographic diagnosis of systemic venous return. *Br Heart J* 1982;48:388–395.

89. Sanders SP. Echocardiography and related techniques in the diagnosis of congenital heart defects. Part I. Veins, atria, and interatrial septum. *Echocardiography* 1984; 1:185–196.

90. Huhta JC, Smallhorn JF, Macartney FJ. Cross sectional echo-cardiographic diagnosis of azygous continuation of the inferior vena cava. *Cathet Cardiovasc Diagn* 1984;10: 221–226.

91. Gardner DL and Cole L. Longterm survival with inferior vena cava draining into the left atrium. *Br Heart J* 1955; 17:93–97.

92. Kim YS, Serratto M, Long DM, Hastreiter AR. Left atrial inferior vena cava with atrial septal defect. *Ann Thorac Surg* 1971;11:165–170.

93. Sanches HE, Human DG. Drainage of the inferior vena cava to the left atrium. *Pediatr Cardiol* 1986;6:207–209.

94. Chantapie A, Marchand M, la Tour R, Verney RN, Faidutti B, Ashori K, Fauchier JP. Inferior vena cava return to the left atrium with intact interauricular septum. Apropos of 2 cases surgically treated with success. *Arch Mal Coeur Vaiss* 1986;79:684–691.

94a. Cabrera A, Arriola J, Llorente A. Anomalous connection of inferior vena cava to the left atrium. *Int J Cardiol* 1994; 46:79–81.

95. Van Praagh S, Kreutzer J, Alday L, Van Praagh R. Systemic and pulmonary venous connections in visceral heterotaxy, with emphasis on the diagnosis of the atrial situs: A study of 109 postmortem cases. In: Clark EB, Takao A, eds. *Developmental Cardiology. Morphogenesis and Function.* Mount Kisco, NY: Futura Publishing Company, Inc; 1990, pp. 671–727.

95a. Kadletz M, Black MD, Smallhorn J, Freedom RM, Van Praagh R. Systemic venous anoamlies and hypoplastic left heart disease: More than just a mere coincidence. *Ann Thorac Surg* (In press).

95b. Rubino M, Van Praagh S, Kadoba K, Pessoto R, Van Praagh R. Systemic and pulmonary venous connections in visceral heterotaxy with asplenia. *J Thorac Cardiovasc Surg* 1995;110:641–650.

95c. Jimenez M, Hery E, van Doesberg NH, Guerin R, Spier S. Inferior vena cava stenosis in Scimitar sydrome: A case report. *J Am Soc Echo* 1988;1:152–154.

96. Jolly N, Kumar P, Arora R. Persistence of hepatic venous plexus as the terminal part of inferior caval vein. *Int J Cardiol* 1991;31:110–111.

96a. Slavik Z, Lamb RK, Webber SA, Delaney DJ, Salmon AP. A rare cause of profound cyanosis after Kawashima modification of bidirectional cavopulmonary anastomosis. *Ann Thorac Surg* 1995;60:435–437.

96b. Reed MK, Leonard SR, Zellers TM, Nikaidoh H. Major intrahepatic venovenous fistulas after a modified Fontan operation. *Ann Thorac Surg* 1996;61:713–715.

97. Huntington GS and McClure CFW. The development of the veins in the domestic cat. *Anat Rec* 1920;20: 1–20.

98. Amodeo A, Di Donato R, Dessanti A, Caccia G, Zaltron D, Alberti D, Callea F, Marcelletti C. Relief of membranous obstruction of the inferior vena cava in a 5-year-old child. *J Thorac Cardiovasc Surg* 1986;92:1101–1103.

99. Ashour MH, Jain SK, Kattan KM, el-Bakry AK, Khoshim M, Mesahel FM. Massive hemoptysis caused by congenital absence of a segment of inferior vena cava. *Thorax* 1993;48:1044–1045.

99a. Kim HJ, Ahn IO, Park ED. Hemiazygos continuation of a left inferior vena cava draining into the right atrium via persistent left superior vena cava: Demonstration by helical computed tomography. *Cardiovasc Intervent Radiol* 1995;18:65–67.

100. Van Tellingen C, Verzijlbergen F, Plokker HWM. A patient with bilateral superior and inferior caval veins. *Int J Cardiol* 1984;5:366–373.

100a. Mantri RR, Bajaj R, Shrivastava S. Multiple anomalies of the caval veins in a patient with pulmonic stenosis. *Int J Cardiol* 1994;46:172–174.

100b. Day RW, Harake B, Laks H. Cyanosis following a modified Fontan procedure secondary to anomalous inferior systemic venous return. *Cardiol Young* 1991;1:149–151.

101. Yee KF. Anomalous termination of a hepatic vein in the left atrium. *Arch Path* 1968;85:219–223.

101a. Fernandez-Martorell P, Sklansky MS, Lucas VW, Kashani IA, Cocalis MW, Jamieson SW, Rothman A. Accessory hepatic vein to pulmonary venous atrium as a cause of cyanosis after the Fontan operation. *Am J Cardiol* 1996;77:1386–1387.

102. Heinemann MK, Oldhafer KJ, Ziemer G. Partial "anomalous" hepatic venous drainage associated with secundum atrial septal defect. *Thorac Cardiovasc Surg* 1992;40:105–107.

103. Sanders SP. Anomalous hepatic venous connection to the coronary sinus diagnosed by two-dimensional echocardiography. *Am J Cardiol* 1984;54:458–459.

104. Van der Horst RL, Winship WS, Gotsman MS. Drainage of left hepatic vein into coronary sinus associated with other systemic venous anomalies. *Br Heart J* 1971;33:164–166.

105. Yokoyama M, Ando M, Takao A, Sakakibara S. The location of the coronary sinus orifice in endocardial cushion defects. *Am Heart J* 1973;85:302–307.

106. Foale RA, Baron DW, Rickards AF. Isolated congenital absence of the coronary sinus. *Br Heart J* 1979;42:355–358.

107. Harris WG. A case of bilateral superior venae cavae with a closed coronary sinus. *Thorax* 1960;15:172–173.

108. Falcone MW, Roberts WC. Atresia of the right atrial ostium of the coronary sinus unassociated with persistence of the left superior vena cava: A clinicopathologic study of 4 adult patients. *Am Heart J* 1972;83:604–611.

108a. Sahinoglu K, Cassell MD, Miyauchi R, Bergman RA. Human persistent left superior vena cava with doubled coronary sinus. *Anat Anz* 1994;176:451–454.

109. Mantini E, Grondin CM, Lillehei CW, Edwards JE. Congenital anomalies involving the coronary sinus. *Circulation* 1966;33:317.

110. Watson GH. Atresia of the Coronary sinus orifice. *Pediatr Cardiol* 1985;6:99–102.

111. Yeager SB, Balian AA, Gustafson RA, Neal WA. Angiocardiographic diagnosis of coronary sinus ostium atresia. *Am J Cardiol* 1986;56:996.

112. Yokota M, Kyoku I, Kitano M, Shimada I, Mizuhara H, Sakamoyo K, Nakano H, Hamazaki M. Atresia of the coronary sinus orifice. Fatal outcome after intraoperative division of the drainage left superior vena cava. *J Thorac Cardiovasc Surg* 1989;98:30–32.

112a. Cochrane AD, Marath A, Mee RBB. Can a dilated coronary sinus produce left ventricular inflow obstruction? An unrecognised entity. *Ann Thorac Surg* 1994;58:1114–1116.

112b. Comas JV, Pawade A, Karl TR. Obstruction from persistent superior vena cava (letter). *Ann Thorac Surg* 1995;59:793.

113. Chiang C-E, Chen S-A, Yang C-R, Cheng C-C, Wu T-R, Tsai D-S, Chiou C-W, Chen C-Y, Wang S-P, Chiang BN, Chang M-S. Major coronary sinus abnormalities: Identification of occurrence and significance in radiofrequency ablation of supraventricular tachycardia. *Am Heart J* 1994;127:1279–1289.

114. Arciniegas E, Henry JG, Green EW. Stenosis of the coronary sinus ostium. An unusual site of obstruction in total anomalous pulmonary venous drainage. *J Thorac Cardiovasc Surg* 1980;79:303–305.

115. Jonas RA, Smolinsky A, Mayer JE, Castaneda AR. Obstructed pulmonary venous drainage with total anomalous pulmonary venous connection to the coronary sinus. *Am J Cardiol* 1987;59:431–435.

116. Gerlis LM, Gibbs JL, Williams GJ, Thomas GDH. Coronary sinus orifice atresia and persistent left superior vena cava. A report of two cases, one associated with atypical coronary thrombosis. *Br Heart J* 1984;52:648–653.

117. Sunaga Y, Okuba N, Hayashi K, Taniichi Y, Sugiura T, Iwasaka T, Inada M. Transesophageal echocardiographic diagnosis of coronary sinus orifice atresia. *Am Heart J* 1992;124:794–796.

117a. Adatia I, Gittenberger-de Groot AC. Unroofed coronary sinus and coronary sinus orifice atresia. Implications for management of complex congenital heart disease. *J Am Coll Cardiol* 1995;25:948–953.

117b. Santoscoy R, Walters HL III, Ross RD, Lyons JM, Hakimi M. Coronary sinus ostial atresia with persistent left superior vena cava. *Ann Thorac Surg* 1996;61:879–882.

118. Buckels NJ, Vosloo, Rose AG, Odell JA. Donor heart coronary sinus ostium atresia in a successful cardiac transplant. *Ann Thorac Surg* 1992;53:1096–1097.

119. McGarry KMJ, Stark J, Macartney FJ. Congenital fistula between left ventricle and coronary sinus. *Br Heart J* 1981;45:101–104.

120. Gnanapragasam JP, Houston AB, Lilley S. Congenital fistula between the left ventricle and coronary sinus: Elucidation by colour flow mapping. *Br Heart J* 1989;62:406–408.

121. Fetter JE, Backer CL, Muster AJ, Weigel TJ, Mavroudis C. Successful repair of congenital left ventricle-to-coronary sinus fistulas. *Ann Thorac Surg* 1994;57:757–758.

121a. Wright DH, Nipper M, Baisden CE. Left ventricular-coronary sinus fistula after mitral valve replacement: Case report and ultrafast CT findings. *J Thorac Imaging* 1994;9:85–87.

121b. Tokunaga S, Yoshitoshi M, Mayumi H, Nakano E, Toshima Y, Kawachi Y, Yasui H. Left ventricular-coronary sinus shunt through a septal aneurysm after mitral valve re-replacement. *Ann Thorac Surg* 1995;59:224–227.

122. Ho SY, Gupta I, Anderson RH, Lendon M, Kerr I. Aneurysm of the coronary sinus. *Thorax* 1983;38:686–689.

123. McGiffen DC, Masterson ML, Stafford WJ. Wolff-Parkinson-White syndrome associated with a coronary sinus diverticulum. *PACE* 1990;13:966–969.

123a.Doig JC, Saito J, Harris L, Downar E. Coronary sinus morphology in patients with atrioventricular junctional reentry tachycardia and other supraventricular tachyarrhythmias. *Circulation* 1995;92:436–441.

124. Guiraudon GM, Klein GJ, Sharma AD, Yee R. The coronary sinus diverticulum, a pathologic entity associated with the Wolff-Parkinson-White syndrome. *Am J Cardiol* 1988;62:733–735.

124a.Petit A, Eicher JC, Louis P. Congenital diverticulum of the right atrium situated on the floor of the coronary sinus. *Br Heart J* 1988;59:721–723.

124b.Sahinoglu K, Cassell MD, Miyauchi R, Bergman RA. Human persistent left superior vena cava with doubled coronary sinus. *Anat Anz* 1994;176:451–454.

125. Allmendinger P, Dear WE, Cooley DA. Atrial septal defect with communication through the coronary sinus. *Ann Thorac Surg* 1974;17:193–196.

126. Beckman CB, Moller JH, Edwards JE. Alternate pathways to pulmonary venous flow in left-sided obstructive lesions. *Circulation* 1975;52:509–516.

127. Franz C, Mennicken U, Dalichau H, Hirsh H. Abnormal communication between the left atrium and coronary sinus. Presentation of two cases and review of the literature. *Thorac Cardiovasc Surg* 1985;33:113–117.

128. MacMahon HE. Communication of the coronary sinus with the left atrium. *Circulation* 1963;28:947.

129. Matsuwaka R, Tomukuni T, Ishikawa S, Watanabe F, Matsushita T, Matsuda H. Partially unroofed coronary sinus associated with tricuspid atresia. An important associated lesion in the Fontan operation. *Eur J Cardiothorac Surg* 1987;1:180–182.

130. Nath PH, Delaney DJ, Zollikofer C, Ben-Sachar B, Castaneda-Zuniga W, Formanek A, Amplatz K. Coronary sinus-left atrial window. *Radiology* 1980;135:319–322.

130a.Schumacher B, Tebbenjohanns, Pfieffer D, Omran H, Jung W, Luderitz B. Prospective study of retrograde coronary venography in patients with posteroseptal and left-sided accessory atrioventricular pathways. *Am Heart J* 1995;130:1031–1039.

131. Rose AG, Beckman CB, Edwards JE. Communication between coronary sinus and left atrium. *Br Heart J* 1974;36:182–185.

132. Rumisek JD, Pigott JD, Weinberg PM, Norwood WI. Coronary sinus septal defect associated with tricuspid atresia. *J Thorac Cardiovasc Surg* 1986;92:142–145.

133. Schmidt KG, Silverman NH. Cross-sectional and contrast echocardiography in the diagnosis of interatrial communications through the coronary sinus. *Int J Cardiol* 1987;16:193–199.

134. Hayes AM, Burrows PE, Benson LN. An unusual cause of cyanosis after the modified Fontan procedure—closure of venous communications between the coronary sinus and left atrium by transcatheter techniques. *Cardiol Young* 1994;3:172–174.

135. Holmes G, Wagman AJ, Epstein ML. Anomalous systemic venous to left atrial connection in tricuspid atresia with severely restrictive interatrial communication. *Pediatr Cardiol* 1991;12:241–242.

136. Weber HS, Markowitz RI, Hellenbrand WE, Kleinman CS, Kopf G. Pulmonary venous collaterals secondary to superior cava stenosis: A rare cause of right-to-left shunting following repair of a sinus venosus atrial septal defect. *Pediatr Cardiol* 1989;10:49–51.

136a.Gatzoulis MA, Shinebourne EA, Redington AN, Rigby ML, Ho SY, Shore DF. Increasing cyanosis after cavopul-

monary connection caused by abnormal systemic venous channels. *Br Heart J* 1995;73:182–186.

136b.Stockberger SM, West KW, Cohen MD. Right-to-left shunt from systemic venous to pulmonary venous system developing after SVC obstruction. *J Comput Assist Tomogr* 1995;19:312–315.

137. Yater WM. Variations and anomalies of the venous valves of the right atrium of the human heart. *Arch Pathol* 1929;7:418–441.

138. Odgers PNB. The formation of the venous valves, the foramen secundum and the septum secundum in the human heart. *J Anat* 1935;69:412–422.

139. Folger GMJ. Supravalvular tricuspid stenosis. Association with developmental abnormalities of the right heart and derivatives of the sixth aortic arch. *Am J Cardiol* 1968;21:81–87.

140. Doucette J and Knoblich R. Persistent right valve of the sinus venosus. So-called cor triatriatum dextrum: Review of the literature and report of a case. *AMA Arch Pathol* 1963;75:105–112.

141. Anderson RH. Understanding the nature of congenital division of the atrial chambers (editorial). *Br Heart J* 1992;68:1–3.

142. Gerlis LM, Anderson RH. Cor triatriatum dexter with imperforate Ebstein's anomaly. *Br Heart J* 1976;38:108–111.

143. Freedom RM, Patel RG, Bloom KR, Duckworth JWA, Silver MM, Dische R, Rowe RD. Congenital absence of the pulmonary valve associated with imperforate membrane type of tricuspid atresia, right ventricular tensor apparatus and intact ventricular septum: A curious developmental complex. *Eur J Cardiol* 1979;10:171–196.

144. Hansing CE, Young WP, Rowe GG. Cor triatriatum dexter. Persistent Right Sinus Venosus Valve. *Am J Cardiol* 1972;30:559–564.

145. Jones RN, Niles NR. Spinnaker formation of sinus venosus valve. Case report of a fatal anomaly in a ten-year-old boy. *Circulation* 1968;38:468–473.

146. Imachi T, Arimitsu K, Minami M, Hayakawa M, Kawaguchi A. Cor triatriatum dexter with anomalous pulmonary venous drainage and sinus venosus atrial septal defect. *J Thorac Cardiovasc Surg* 1988;95:734–737.

147. Mazzucco A, Bortolotti U, Gallucci V, Del Torso S, Pellegrino P. Successful repair of symptomatic cor triatriatum dexter in infancy. *J Thorac Cardiovasc Surg* 1983;85:140–145.

148. Morishita Y, Yamashita M, Yamada K, Arikawa K, Taira A. Cyanosis in atrial septal defect due to persistent eustachian valve. *Ann Thorac Surg* 1985;40:614–616.

149. Ott DA, Cooley DA, Angelini P, Leachman RD. Successful surgical repair of symptomatic cor triatriatum dexter. *J Thorac Cardiovasc Surg* 1979;78:573–575.

150. Raffa H, Al-Ibrahim K, Kayali MT, Sorefan AA, Rustom M. Central cyanosis due to prominence of the eustachian and thebesian valves. *Ann Thorac Surg* 1992;54:159–160.

151. Roguin N, Milo S, Isserles S. Atrial septal defect associated with a remnant of the valve of the sinus venosus producing unusual drainage of the inferior caval vein. *Int J Cardiol* 1986;13:369–372.

152. Smith NM, Byard RW, Vigneswaran R, Bourne AJ, Knight B. Parachute-like sinus venosus remnant: Echocardiographic and pathological appearance. *Pediatr Cardiol* 1993;14:82–85.

153. Sutherland RD, Stanger P, Climie ARW, Quinn MHF,

Edwards JE. Large anomalous fibrous sac in the right side of the heart. *Circulation* 1969;39:837–840.

154. Trakhtenbroit A, Majid P, Rokey R. Cor triatriatum dexter: antemortem diagnosis in an adult by cross sectional echocardiography. *Br Heart J* 1990;314–316.

155. Burton DA, Chin A, Weinberg PM, Pigott PD. Identification of cor triatriatum dexter by two-dimensional echocardiography. *Am J Cardiol* 1987;60:409–410.

156. Battle-Diaz J, Stanley P, Kratz C, Fouron J-C, Guerin R, Davignon A. Echocardiographic manifestations of persistence of the right sinus venosus valve. *Am J Cardiol* 1979;43:850–853.

157. Bashour T, Kabbani S, Saalouke M, Cheng TO. Persistent eustachian valve causing severe cyanosis in atrial septal defect with normal right heart pressures. *Angiology* 1983;34:79–83.

158. Alboliras ET, Edwards WD, Driscoll DJ, Seward JB. Cor triatriatum dexter: Two-dimensional echocardiographic diagnosis. *J Am Coll Cardiol* 1987;9:334–337.

159. Verel D, Pilcher J, Hynes DM. Cor triatriatum dexter. *Br Heart J* 1970;32:714–716.

160. Trento A, Zuberbuhler JR, Anderson RH, Park SC, Siewers RD. Divided right atrium (prominence of the eustachian and thebesian valves). *J Thorac Cardiovasc Surg* 1988;96:457–463.

161. Kauffman SL, Anderson DH. Persistent venous valves, maldevelopment of the right heart, and coronary artery-ventricular communications. *Am Heart J* 1963;66:664–669.

162. Brook MM and Silverman NH. Echocardiography of the prominent Eustachian valve-association and complications with cyanosis and right heart obstruction. *Cardiol Young* 1993;3:417–421.

163. Muhler EG, Franke A, Messmer BJ. Divided right atrium ('cor triatriatum dexter') with azygous drainage of the superior caval vein. *Cardiol Young* 1996;6:80–83.

164. MacMahon HE. The congenital absence of the ductus venosus. *Lab Invest* 1960;9:1227–1231.

165. Leonidas JC, Fellows RA. Congenital absence of the ductus venosus with direct connection between the umbilical vein and the distal inferior vena cava. *AJR* 1976;126:892–895.

166. Jorgensen C and Andolf E. Four cases of absent ductus venosus: Three in combination with severe hydrops fetalis. *Fetal Diagn Ther* 1994;9:395–397.

167. Hasaart TH, Delarue MW, de Bruine AP. Intra-partum fetal death due to thrombosis of the ductus venosus: A clinicopathological case report. *Eur J Obstet Gynecol Reprod Biol* 1994;56:201–203.

168. Chandar JS, Wolfe SB. Displacement of preexisting thrombus by umbilical vein catheterization. *Pediatr Cardiol* 1994;15:311–312.

169. Mitchell IM, Pollock JC, Gibson AA. Patent ductus venosus. *Pediatr Cardiol* 1991;12:181–183.

170. Uemura H, Yen Ho S, Anderson RH, Devine WA, Smith A, Shinohara T, Yagihara T, Kawashima Y. The surgical anatomy of coronary venous return in hearts with isomeric atrial appendages. *J Thorac Cardiovasc Surg* 1995; 110:436–444.

Chapter 13

Juxtaposition of Atrial Appendages and Abnormalities of the Right Atrial Wall

Juxtaposition of the atrial appendages is an uncommon anomaly characterized by abnormal laterality of the atrial appendages. This peculiar arrangement of the atrial appendages is almost always associated with abnormal segmental connections.[1-15] As we discussed in Chapter 3, the normal arrangement of the atrial appendages is that each atrial appendage normally stands as a phalanx at the side of the great arteries, the morphologically right atrial appendage to the right side and the morphologically left atrial appendage to the left in the individual with solitus atria. In juxtaposition of the atrial appendages, yet with atrial situs solitus, both atrial appendages are usually to the left of the great arteries, with right juxtaposition of the left atrial appendage considerably less common (Fig. 13-1). Right juxtaposition of the left atrial appendage has been observed in the absence of a conotruncal anomaly.[15a]

Juxtaposition of the atrial appendages can occur with relatively modest congenital heart disease, but as pointed out more than 25 years ago by Melhuish and Van Praagh,[1] juxtaposition of the atrial appendages is usually associated with severe congenital heart malformations. These malformations include tricuspid atresia or stenosis, discordant ventriculoarterial connections, anatomically corrected malposition of the great arteries, and patients with superoinferior ventricles (see Chapter 44) and crossed atrioventricular connections.[16-19] Juxtaposition of the atrial appendages usually occurs with solitus atria, less commonly with inversus atria, and only a few instances of juxtaposed atrial appendages have been observed in patients with left or right atrial

isomerism (see also Chapters 12 and 41). Juxtaposition of the right-sided atrial appendage with a right-sided azygous continuation of the inferior vena cava is shown in Chapter 12, Fig. 12-28.

In two recently completed studies of atrial appendage juxtaposition, Van Praagh and colleagues[19a,19b] suggest that it is more appropriate to define the condition as juxtaposition of the morphologically right or left atria appendage. In these studies, juxtaposition of the morphologically right atrial appendage was always left sided in patients with solitus atria and was found in patients with tricuspid valve anomalies, hypoplasia of the right ventricle and an abnormal infundibulum (subaortic or bilateral). Juxtaposition of the morphologically left appendage was typically right sided (in situs solitus) and identified in patients with left atrial outlet obstruction, left ventricular hypoplasia, left ventricular hypoplasia, and a normal subpulmonary infundibulum.

Clinical Recognition of Juxtaposition of the Atrial Appendages

One may suspect the presence of left juxtaposition of the right atrial appendage from the frontal chest x-ray (Fig. 13-2).[20,21] An unusual contour to the left heart border, together with a relatively flat or even concave right lower heart border may suggest left juxtaposition of the right atrial appendage. Not infrequently, the right upper heart border shows an outward bulge due to the lateral

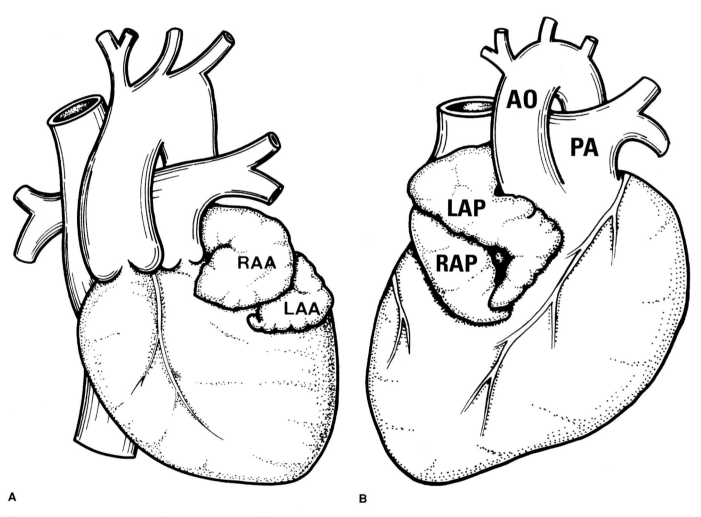

A

B

Fig. 13-1: Juxtaposition of the atrial appendages.
A: Schematic diagram of left juxtaposition of the right atrial appendage. **B:** Schematic diagram of right juxtaposition of left atrial appendage. **C:** Left juxtaposition of the right atrial appendage is seen with the right atrial appendage somewhat superior to the smaller left atrial appendage, and both atrial appendages are lateralized to the left of the aorta. **D:** Right juxtaposition of the left atrial appendage.

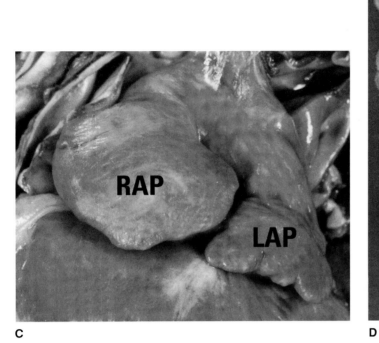

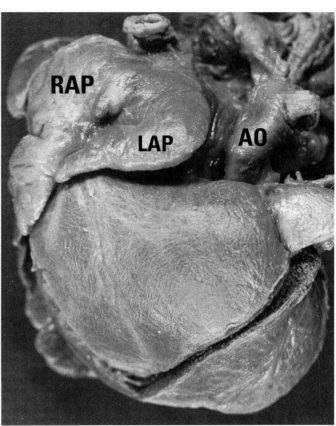

C

D

Fig. 13-1 *(continued)*

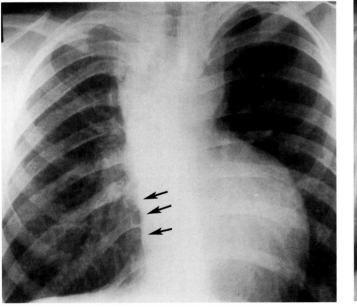

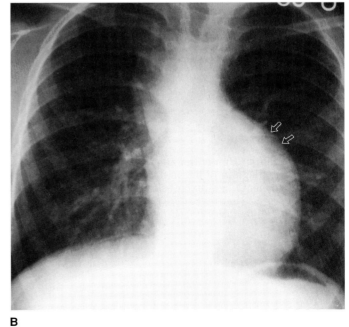

A

B

Fig. 13-2: Chest radiographs of patients with left juxtaposition of the right atrial appendage.
A: This chest radiograph shows a flat right heart border (arrows) in a patient with left juxtaposition of the right atrial appendage. **B:** Note the unusual left heart contour (arrows).

displacement of the superior vena cava. A systematic approach to atrial echocardiography may also demonstrate left juxtaposition of the right atrial appendage, especially in the young infant where the echocardiographic window may still be opened to the examiner's advantage.[22–24] Magnetic resonance imaging has also defined juxtaposed atrial appendages, although this methodology is used less commonly in everyday practice.

The diagnosis of left juxtaposition of the right atrial appendage can be suggested by the abnormal catheter course and catheter tip position. The definitive diagnosis of juxtaposition is made by selective injection into the right atrium, the juxtaposed right atrial appendage, or superior or inferior caval vein (Figs. 13-3 through 13-6). On the frontal angiogram, the atrial septum shows a characteristic oblique orientation from the inferior vena caval orifice right inferiorly to the right

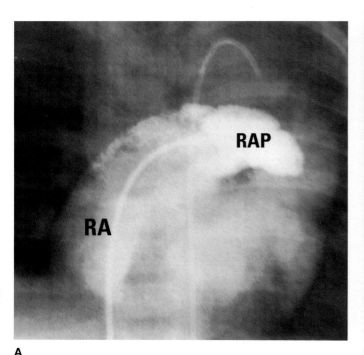

A

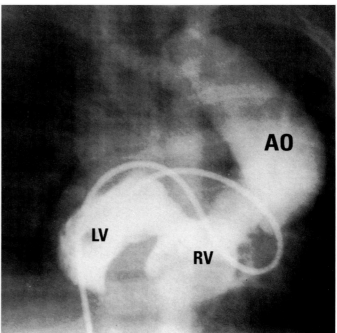

B

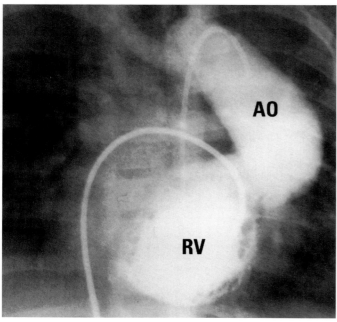

C

Fig. 13-3: **Left juxtaposition of the right atrial appendage in a patient with atrioventricular discordance and single-outlet aorta and pulmonary atresia.**
A: Injection of contrast into the right atrial appendage demonstrates to advantage its juxtaposition. **B and C:** Selective left and right ventriculography characterize the intracardiac malformations.

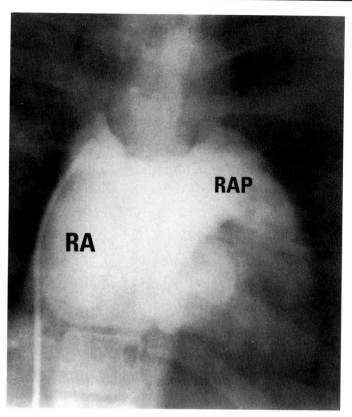

Fig. 13-4: Another patient with left juxtaposition of the right atrial appendage demonstrated by right atriography.

atrial appendage left superiorly. The right atrial appendage is always seen above and more or less medial to the left atrial appendage. As the displacement of the right atrial appendage occurs through the transverse sinus of the pericardial space behind the great arterial trunks, the roof or superior wall of the right atrium between the superior caval orifice and the juxtaposed atrial appendage demonstrates a round concavity due to an indentation from the great arteries. This round indentation is a signal finding of the juxtaposition. When the right atrial appendage has its unusual anteromedial location in front of the great arterial trunks as in cases with severe rightward rotation of the heart, this may simulate left juxtaposition. In this situation, the round indentation of the superior wall is not seen.[25–27] The volume of the right atrium will seem absolutely small, and the left juxtaposed atrial appendage will occupy the left heart border, superior in position to the morphologically left atrial appendage. Whenever the atrial appendages are juxtaposed, the character of the atrioventricular and ventriculoarterial connections as well as the size of each cardiac chamber should be defined.[1–5,19]

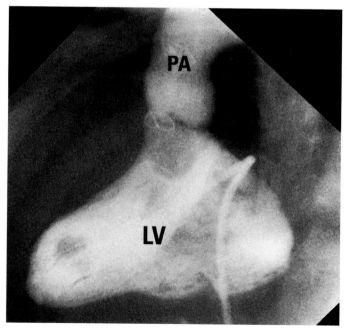

B

Fig. 13-5: Juxtaposition of the right atrial appendage in a patient with dextrocardia after Mustard's operation for transposition of the great arteries.
A: Injection of contrast into the inferior limb of baffle shows the inferior caval vein and the systemic venous atrium (SVA) which constitutes in part the juxtaposed right atrial appendage; **B:** Left ventriculogram demonstrates the discordantly connected pulmonary artery.

A

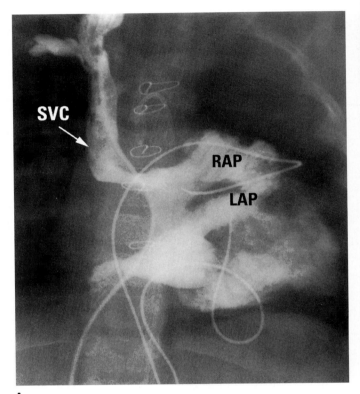

A

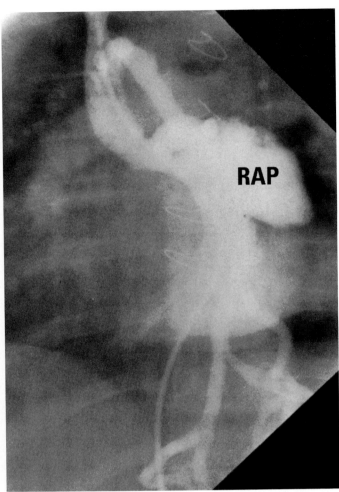

B

Fig. 13-6: Two different patients after Mustards operation for transposition of the great arteries.
A: Both atrial appendages are shown by this injection into the systemic venous atrium. **B:** The enlarged juxtaposed right atrial appendage is evident in this patient with some narrowing of the superior baffle limb and retrograde flow down the azygous venous system (see also Chapter 35).

Clinical Relevance of Juxtaposition of the Atrial Appendages

The clinical relevance of juxtaposition of the atrial appendages is its importance to balloon atrial septostomy and to surgical considerations. Tyrell and Moes[28] have reported the difficulty in performing balloon atrial septostomy in the presence of left juxtaposition of the right atrial appendage. Some of the difficulties can of course be obviated if two-dimensional echocardiography guides or directs the course of the catheter to the left atrium, not to the relatively posteriorly positioned juxtaposed right atrial appendage. This of course requires the perception that one is dealing with left juxtaposition of the right atrial appendage.

Among hearts with left juxtaposition of the right atrial appendage, the morphologically right atrium is smaller than normal, an observation made some years ago by Rosenquist and colleagues.[29] This observation has certainly been confirmed by any cardiovascular surgeon performing atrial surgery for transposition of the great arteries. The Mustard or Senning operation has to be modified in those patients with a small right atrium (Figs. 13-5 and 13-6).[30–31a] Finally, the topography of the juxtaposed right atrial appendage lends itself to an atriopulmonary connection as part of the Fontan operation.[5,32,33]

Atrial Aneurysms or Diverticulum

Atrial diverticulum or multiple aneurysms are very uncommon (see also Chapter 50).[34–38] They have been identified in patients with atrial tachycardia. The aneurysms were multiple in the signal case reported by

Varghese and his colleagues, but may originate in the coronary sinus (see Chapter 12 and 50). In the adult, successful treatment of incessant atrial tachycardia has been accomplished by excision of a giant right atrial aneurysm.[39] Kim and colleagues[39a] have reported the echocardiographic and surgical findings of a solitary large right atrial aneurysm in a child with paroxysmal supraventricular tachycardia. A substantial mural thrombus was found at surgical exploration in this aneurysm. Finally, the right atrial appendage may be bifid.

The so-called aneurysm of the atrial septum is con-sidered fully in Chapter 4. In the patient with tricuspid atresia or pulmonary atresia and intact ventricular sep-tum, profound restriction at the level of the ovale fora-men may lead to aneurysmal herniation of septum pri-mum from right to left, promoting mitral inflow obstruction in some patients (see also Chapters 23 and 39).[40–45] The atrial septal aneurysm has been observed in the absence of more complex heart lesions in the fe-tus, child and adult, and the association between atrial rhythm disturbances, untoward cerebrovascular events, and the atrial septal aneurysm have been ex-plored.[46–64]

References

1. Melhuish BPP, Van Praagh R. Juxtaposition of the atrial appendages. A sign of severe cyanotic congenital heart disease. *Br Heart J* 1968;30:269–284.
2. Mendelsohn G, Hutchins GM. Juxtaposition of atrial ap-pendages. *Arch Pathol Lab Med* 1977;101:490–492.
3. Allwork SP, Urban AE, Anderson RH. Left juxtaposition of the auricles with l-position of the aorta. Report of 6 cases. *Br Heart J* 1977;39:299–303.
4. Anderson RH, Smith A, Wilkinson JL. Right juxtaposition of the auricular appendages. *Eur J Cardiol* 1976; 4:495–503.
5. Anjos RT, Yen Ho, S, Anderson RH. Surgical Implications of juxtaposition of the atrial appendages. A review of forty-nine autopsied hearts. *J Thorac Cardiovasc Surg* 1990;99:897–904.
6. Baehrel B, Eisenmann B, Kieny R. Juxtaposition driote des auricules. *Arch Mal Coeur* 1977;4:399–404.
7. Becker AE, Becker MJ. Juxtaposition of atrial appendages associated with normally oriented ventricles and great ar-teries. *Circulation* 1970;41:685–688.
8. Charuzi Y, Spanos PK, Amplatz K, Edwards JE. Juxtapo-sition of the Atrial Appendages. *Circulation* 1973;47: 620–626.
9. Coto EO, Wilkinson JL, Rufilanchas JJ, Marquez J. Gross distortion of atrioventricular and ventriculo-arterial rela-tions associated with left juxtaposition of atrial ap-pendages. Bizarre form of atrioventricular criss-cross. *Br Heart J* 1979;41:486–492.
10. Ellis K and Jameson AG. Congenital levoposition of the right atrial appendage. *Am J Cardiol* 1963;89:984–988.
11. Embree J, Aterman K, Belcourt C. Right-sided juxtaposi-tion of the atrial appendages in an anencephalic. *J Pathol* 1979;129:157–160.
12. Freedom RM, Harrington DP. Anatomically corrected malposition of the great arteries: Report of 2 cases, one with congenital asplenia, frequent association with juxta-position of atrial appendages. *Br Heart J* 1974;36: 207–212.
13. Ho SY, Monro JL, Anderson RH. Disposition of the sinus node in left-sided juxtaposition of the atrial appendages. *Br Heart J* 1979;41:129–132.
14. Mathew R, Replogle R, Thilenius OG, Arcilla RA. Right juxtaposition of the atrial appendages. *Chest* 1975;67: 483–486.
15. Stewart AM and Wynn-Williams A. Combined tricuspid and pulmonary atresia with juxtaposition of the auricles. *Br J Radiol* 1956;29:326–330.
15a. Konishi M, Nobuoka W, Asazuma S, Iwamoto T, Hama-jima T, Otabe E, Nakanoin H. [A case of right juxtaposi-tion of the atrial appendages, without conotruncal anom-aly]. *Kyobu Geka* 1985;38:307–311.
16. Anderson RH, Smith A, Wilkinson JL. Disharmony be-tween atrioventricular connections and segmental combi-nations: Unusual variants of "crisscross" hearts. *J Am Coll Cardiol* 1987;10:1274–1277.
17. Seo JW, Choe GY, Chi JG. An unusual ventricular loop as-sociated with right juxtaposition of the atrial appendages. *Int J Cardiol* 1989;25:219–228.
18. Anderson RH and Yen Ho S. Editorial Note: Segmental in-ter-connexions versus topological congruency in com-plex congenital malformations. *Int J Cardiol* 1989;25: 229–233.
19. Wagner HR, Alday LE, Vlad P. Juxtaposition of the atrial appendages. A report of 6 necropsied cases. *Circulation* 1970;42:157–162.
19a. Van Praagh R, O'Sullivan J, Brili S, Van Praagh R. Juxta-position of the morphologically right atrial appendage in solitus and inversus atria: A study of 35 postmortem cases. *Am Heart J* 1996;132:382–390.
19b. Van Praagh R, O'Sullivan J, Brili S, Van Praagh R. Juxta-position of the morphologically left atrial appendage in solitus and inversus: A study of 18 postmortem cases. *Am Heart J* 1996;132:391–402.
20. Lind TA, Pitt MJ, Groves BM, White JE, Quinn E. The ab-normal left hilum. *Circulation* 1975;51:183–187.
21. Bream PR, Elliott LP, Bargeron LM Jr. Plain film findings of anatomically corrected malposition: Its association with juxtaposition of the atrial appendages and right aor-tic arch. *Radiology* 1978;126:589.
22. Chin AJ, Bierman FZ, Williams RG, Sanders SP, Lang P. Two-dimensional echocardiographic appearance of com-plete left-sided juxtaposition of the atrial appendages. *Am J Cardiol* 1983;52:346–348.
22a. Lee M-L, Wu M-H, Wang J-K, Chiu I-S, Lue H-C. Echocar-diographic features of juxtaposed atrial appendages asso-ciated with dextro-transposition of the great arteries. *Pe-diatr Cardiol* 1995;17:63–66.
23. Rice MJ, Seward JB, Hagler DJ, Edwards WD, Julsrud PR, Tajik AJ. Left juxtaposed atrial appendages: Diagnostic two-dimensional echocardiographic features. *J Am Coll Cardiol* 1983;1:1330–1336.
24. Stumper O, Rijlaarsdam M, Vargas-Barron J, Romero A, Hess J, Sutherland GR. The assessment of juxtaposed atrial appendages by transesophageal echocardiography. *Int J Cardiol* 1990;29:365–371.

25. Deutsch V, Shem-Tov A, Yahini JH, Neufeld HN. Juxtaposition of atrial appendages: Angiocardiographic observations. *Am J Cardiol* 1974;34:240–244.

26. Freedom RM, Culham JAG, Moes CAF. *Angiocardiography of Congenital Heart Disease*. New York: Macmillan Publishing Company; 1984, pp. 72–76.

27. Hunter AS, Henderson CB, Urquhart W, Farmer MB. Left-sided juxtaposition of the atrial appendages: Report of 4 cases diagnosed by cardiac catheterization and angiocardiography. *Br Heart J* 1973;35:1184–1189.

28. Tyrrell MJ, Moes CAF. Congenital levoposition of the right atrial appendage. *Am J Dis Child* 1971;121:508–510.

29. Rosenquist GC, Stark J, Taylor JFN. Anatomical relationships in transposition of the great arteries. *Ann Thorac Surg* 1974;18:456–461.

30. Urban AE, Stark J, Waterston DJ. Mustard's operation for transposition of the great arteries complicated by juxtaposition of the atrial appendages. *Ann Thorac Surg* 1976; 21:304–310.

31. Wood AE, Freedom RM, Williams WG, Trusler GA. The Mustard procedure in transposition of the great arteries associated with juxtaposition of the atrial appendages with and without dextrocardia. *J Thorac Cardiovasc Surg* 1983;85:451–456.

31a. Dihmis WC, Eldridge J, Jordan SC, Wisheart JD. Modification of the Senning repair in a case of transposition of the great arteries with juxtaposition of the atrial appendages. *Eur J Cardiothorac Surg* 1995;9:50–51.

32. Leu MR, Chiu IS, Hung CR, Wu MH. Surgical implications of juxtaposed atrial appendages and the associated anomalies. *Ann Thorac Surg* 1992;54:134–136.

33. Thoele DG, Ursell PC, Ho SY, Smith A, Bowman FO, Gersony WM, Anderson RH. Atrial morphologic features in tricuspid atresia. *J Thorac Cardiovasc Surg* 1991;102:606–610.

34. Varghese PJ, Simon AL, Rosenquist GC, Berger M, Rowe RD, Bender HW. Multiple saccular congenital aneurysms of the atria causing persistent atrial tachyarrhythmia in an infant. Report of a case successfully treated by surgery. *Pediatrics* 1969;42:157–159.

35. Okita Y, Miki S, Tamura T, Kusuhara K, Ueda Y, Tahata T, Yamanaka K, Sasakabe H. Multiple congenital aneurysms of the atria. *Ann Thorac Surg* 1990;49:672–763.

36. Gayet C, Pillot M, Revel D, Finet G, Buisson P, Milon H. Diverticule de l'oreillette droite: Description d'un cas et revue de la litterature. *Arch Mal Coeur Vaiss (France)* 1992;85:1479–1482.

37. Morishita Y, Kawashima S, Shimokawa S, Taira A, Kawagoe H, Nakamura K. Multiple diverticula of the right atrium. *Am Heart J* 1990;120:1225–1227.

38. Petit A, Eicher JC, Louis P. Congenital diverticulum of the right atrium situated on the floor of the coronary sinus. *Br Heart J* 1988;59:721–723.

39. Scalia GM, Stafford WJ, Burstow DJ, Carruthers T, Tesar PJ. Successful treatment of incessant atrial flutter with excision of congenital giant right atrial aneurysm diagnosed by transesophageal echocardiography. *Am Heart J* 1995; 129:834–835.

39a. Kim YJ, Kim H, Choi JY. Right atrial aneurysm. *Cardiol Young* 1995;5:354–356.

40. Freedom RM, Rowe RD. Aneurysm of the atrial septum in tricuspid atresia. *Am J Cardiol* 1976;38:265–267.

41. Rowe RD, Freedom RM, Mehrizi A. *The Neonate with*
Congenital Heart Disease. New York: WB Saunders Company; 1981, pp. 193–203.

42. Lev M. *Autopsy Diagnosis of Congenitally Malformed Hearts*. Charles C. Thomas: Springfield, IL; 1953, p. 22.

43. Sahn DJ, Allen HD, Anderson R, Goldberg SJ. Echocardiographic diagnosis of atrial septal aneurysm in an infant with hypoplastic right heart syndrome. *Chest* 1978; 73:227–229.

44. Casta A. Atrial septal aneurysm herniation across the mitral valve orifice in pulmonary atresia. *Am Heart J* 1988; 115:1136–1138.

45. Freedom RM. General morphologic considerations. In: Freedom RM. *Pulmonary Atresia with Intact Ventricular Septum*. Mt. Kisco, NY: Futura Publishing Company, Inc; 1989, pp. 17–36.

46. Silver MD, Dorsey JS. Aneurysms of the septum primum in adults. *Arch Pathol Lab Med* 1978;102:62–65.

47. Topaz O, Feigl A, Edwards JE. Aneurysm of the fossa ovalis in infants: A pathologic study. *Pediatr Cardiol* 1985;6:65–68.

48. Shiraishi I, Hamaoka K, Hayashi S, Koh E, Onouchi Z, Sawada T. Atrial septal aneurysm in infancy. *Pediatr Cardiol* 1990;11:82–85.

49. Wolf WJ, Casta A, Sapire DW. Atrial septal aneurysms in infants and children. *Am Heart J* 1987;113:1149–1153.

50. Rice MJ, McDonald RW, Reller MD. Fetal atrial septal aneurysm: A cause of fetal atrial arrhythmias. *J Am Coll Cardiol* 1988;12:1292–1297.

51. Hanley PC, Tajik AJ, Hynes JK, Edwards WD, Reeder GS, Hagler DJ, Seward JB. Diagnosis and classification of atrial septal aneurysm by two-dimensional echocardiography: Report of 80 consecutive cases. *J Am Coll Cardiol* 1985;6:1370–1382.

52. Toro L, Weintraub RG, Shiota T, Sahn DJ, Sahn C, McDonald RW, Rice MJ, Hagen-Ansert S. Relation between persistent atrial arrhythmias and redundant septum primum flap (atrial septal aneurysm) in fetuses. *Am J Cardiol* 1994; 73:711–713

53. Brand A, Keren A, Branski D, Abrahamov A, Stern S. Natural course of atrial septal aneurysm in children and the potential for spontaneous closure of associated septal defect. *Am J Cardiol* 1989;64:996–1001.

54. Belohlavek M, Foley DA, Gerber TC, Greenleaf JF, Seward JB. Three-dimensional ultrasound imaging of the atrial septum: Normal and pathologic anatomy. *J Am Coll Cardiol* 1993;22:1673–1678.

55. Abinader EG, Rokey R, Goldhammer E, Kuo LC, Said E. Prevalence of atrial septal aneurysm in patients with mitral valve prolapse. *Am J Cardiol* 1988;62:1139–1140.

56. Cabanes L, Mas JL, Cohen A, Amarenco P, Cabanes PA, Oubary P, Chedru F, Guerin F, Bousser MG, de Recondo J. Atrial septal aneurysm and patent foramen ovale as risk factors for cryptogenic stroke in patients less than 55 years of age. A study using transesophageal echocardiography. *Stroke* 1993;24:1865–1873.

57. Mas JL. Patent foramen ovale, atrial septal aneurysm and ischaemic stroke in young adults (editorial). *Eur Heart J* 1994;15:446–449.

58. Belkin RN; Kisslo J. Atrial septal aneurysm: Recognition and clinical relevance. *Am Heart J* 1990;120:948–957.

59. Yeoh JK, Appelbe AF, Martin RP. Atrial septal aneurysm mimicking a right atrial mass on transesophageal echocardiography. *Am J Cardiol* 1991;68:827–828.

60. Pearson AC, Nagelhout D, Castello R, Gomez CR, Labovitz

AJ. Atrial septal aneurysm and stroke: A transesophageal echocardiographic study. *J Am Coll Cardiol* 1991;18: 1223–1229.

61. Angelini P, Wilansky S, Gaos C, Montazavi A, Boncompagni E, Cooley DA. Prolapsing large aneurysm of the atrial septum simulating a right atrial mass. *Cathet Cardiovasc Diagn* 1992;26:122–126.

62. Zabalgoitia M, Norris LP, Garcia M. Atrial septal aneurysm as a potential source of neurological ischemic events. *Am J Card Imaging* 1994;8:39–44.

63. Schneider B, Hofmann T, Meinertz T, Hanrath P. Diagnostic value of transesophageal echocardiography in atrial septal aneurysm. *Int J Card Imaging* 1992;8:143–152

64. Mugge A, Daniel WG, Angermann C, Spes C, Khanderia BK, Kronzon I, Freedberg RS, Keren A, Dennig K, Engberding R, et al. Atrial septal aneurysm in adult patients. A multicenter study using transthoracic and transesophageal echocardiography. *Circulation* 1995;91: 2785–2792.

Chapter 14

Ebstein's Malformation of the Tricuspid Valve

Dr. Wilhelm Ebstein, then in his 30th year, published the case report of a 19-year-old laborer named Joseph Prescher who had pronounced cyanosis. The focus of this report was Prescher's congenitally malformed heart.[1] Ebstein described the very peculiar tricuspid valve that now bears his name, and his contribution has subsequently been translated into English.[2–5] In the 130 years since this publication, the definition of the tricuspid valve demonstrating features of the Ebstein malformation conveys the physiology of a regurgitant valve of varying severity.[6–8] This is partly true, but there is now ample morphological as well as clinical data indicating that an imperforate valve, a stenotic valve, as well as a regurgitant valve are encompassed by the designation of Ebstein's malformation of the tricuspid valve.[9–24] Thus, this morphological heterogeneity translates into a diverse clinical experience. In an editorial comment to the article by Celermajer and colleagues,[25] Mair states: "Perhaps no other congenital heart lesion encompasses as broad a spectrum of clinical significance as does Ebstein's malformation."[26]

The Anatomy of the Tricuspid Valve

The essence of Ebstein's malformation of the tricuspid valve is displacement of part of the origin of its leaflets from the atrioventricular junction into the cavity of the right ventricle; this displacement is accompanied by varying degrees of valvular dysplasia and abnormal attachments of the valvular distal margins (Figs 14-1 to 14-3).[7–14,16,24,27] An extensive literature is devoted to the Ebstein's anomaly of the tricuspid valve.[7–16,18–20,24–28a] While the hallmark of Ebstein's

anomaly is displacement from its annulus part of the tricuspid valve into the cavity of the right ventricle, the degree of displacement varies from just minimal displacement to extremely severe. As Becker and colleagues[29] and others[7–14,16,25–28] have pointed out, other confounding features include dysplasia of the tricuspid valve, and more recently, attention has focused on the abnormal distal attachments of the tricuspid valve as well. Indeed, Zuberbuhler and Anderson[14] indicated that displacement, dysplasia, and abnormalities of distal attachment are all integral aspects of Ebstein's anomaly and the severity is reflected in the morphological and clinical expression of this disorder.

The normal tricuspid valve has three leaflets: the posterior or mural leaflet, the septal leaflet, and the anterosuperior leaflet (Figs. 14-1 and 14-2). There are numerous observations that it is the posterior or mural and septal leaflets of the tricuspid valve that are usually displaced, whereas the anterosuperior leaflet retains its normal annular attachment. The observations of Zuberbuhler and Anderson[14] about displacement of the tricuspid valve indicate that in some hearts the mural leaflet is not displaced, but that displacement is confined to the septal leaflet. The septal leaflet displays considerable variability from displacement, to virtual absence, to resembling a supernumerary hammock-like structure that fuses with the leaflet. Becker and colleagues[29] and the more recent observations of Anderson point out that some degree of dysplasia of the tricuspid valve is virtually always present in the neonatal expression of this disorder.[10,12–14,24] In some hearts the displaced mural and septal leaflets are plastered to the wall of the right ventricle, whereas in others the valve tissue is recognizable as excrescences marking the level

From: Freedom RM, Mawson JB, Yoo SJ, Benson LN: *Congenital Heart Disease: Textbook of Angiocardiography.* Armonk NY, Futura Publishing Co., Inc. ©1997.

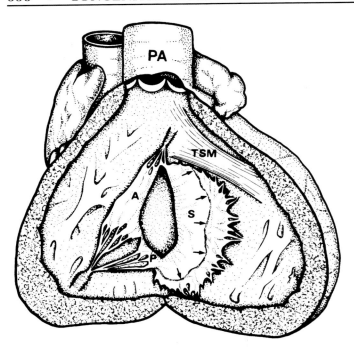

Fig. 14-1: Schematic diagram showing internal view of right ventricle and tricuspid valve in Ebstein's anomaly.

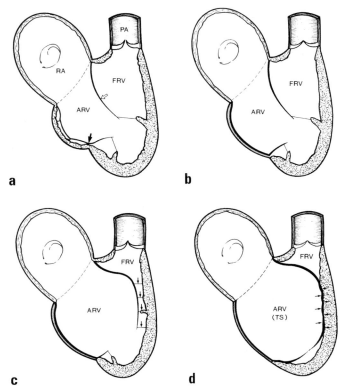

Fig. 14-3: This drawing depicts the various forms of Ebstein's anomaly of the tricuspid valve.
A: Moderate displacement of the attachment of the septal and posterior leaflets with a mobile anterior leaflet. The wall of the atrialized ventricle is not devoid of the myocardium. **B:** Marked displacement of the attachment of the septal and posterior leaflets with a mobile myocardium. The wall of the atrialized ventricle is devoid of myocardium and is not contractile. **C:** Marked displacement of the attachment of the septal and posterior leaflets with a nonmobile anterior leaflet. Multiple chords are seen to tether the anterior leaflet to the ventricular wall. The atrialized ventricle is not contractile. **D:** Severely stenotic or imperforate Ebstein's anomaly with a large tricuspid sac.

of the displaced orifice (Figs. 14-4 through 14-7). The nondisplaced anterosuperior leaflet is usually large, redundant, and sail-like (Fig. 14-7). Finally, the distal attachment of the anterosuperior and/or mural leaflets to the junction between the inlet and trabecular components of the right ventricle may exhibit what Zuberbuhler and Anderson[14] characterized as linear attach-

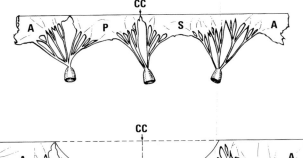

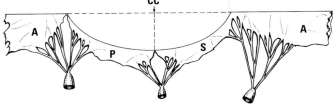

Fig. 14-2: The top drawing depicts the normal tricuspid valve and the bottom drawing the tricuspid valve of Ebstein's anomaly. Note that the septal and posterior leaflets have displaced attachement and that the maximal displacement is at the crux cordis (CC). Note also that the anterior leaflet is grossly enlarged, although it shows no displaced attachment.

ments. When such linear attachments are extensive, functional tricuspid stenosis may result, as well as posing a degree of functional obstruction to pulmonary blood flow.[12,13,15,16,24] The most florid manifestation of these linear attachments is the so-called imperforate type of Ebstein's malformation that in effect produces functional tricuspid atresia.[12,13,18–20,30,31] For the majority of affected patients, however, the displacement of the tricuspid valve, the characteristic dysplasia, and abnormal distal attachments produces a valve that is regurgitant. The most conspicuous alteration resulting from displacement is atrialization of a portion of the right ventricle, a process that reduces the size of the functional right ventricle.

The impact of this disorder in the severely affected neonate can be profound. The atrialized portion of the

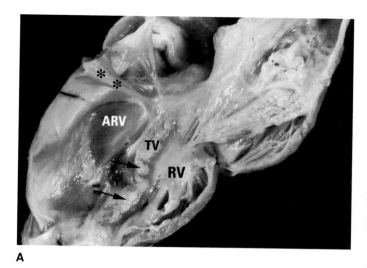

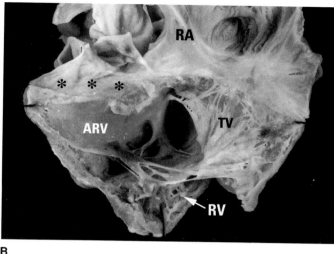

Fig. 14-4: Ebstein's anomaly of the tricuspid valve in the neonate.
A: The mural leaflet is displaced (arrows) producing a large atrialized component of the right ventricle. **B:** The tricuspid valve is not only displaced but also thickened and dysplastic. The right atrium is capacious. The atrioventricular annulus is marked by ✱ in both pictures.

right ventricle may be very thinned, virtually devoid of myocardium, and consistent with Uhl's malformation of the right ventricle (Fig. 14-5).[7–14,16,25,27,31,32–40] Whether such striking attenuation of the inferior parietal wall indicates a congenital malformation or a secondary one is uncertain. Abnormalities of left ventricular form and function are also present, although perhaps less frequently recognized in the neonate. These include angiocardiographic evidence of an abnormal contour and wall motion, as well as mitral valve

prolapse and other mitral valve anomalies including orificial, leaflet, chordal, and papillary muscle anomalies.[41–44] More recently, Celermajer and colleagues[44] have found increased left ventricular fibrosis in neonates who died of Ebstein's anomaly when compared with a similarly-aged normal infant.

The severely affected neonatal heart is tremendously enlarged, with the right atrium assuming gigantic proportions, and completely filling the right hemithorax. At the necropsy table, the atrialized portion of the right ventricle is conspicuous, being much thinner than the infundibular muscle. The pulmonary arteries are small, reflecting the underdeveloped lungs, a consequence of intrauterine compression by the very much enlarged right heart chambers.[7,10,11,14,16,45–50]

Prevalence

Ebstein's anomaly is an uncommon disorder, and we have estimated its prevalence among patients with congenital heart disease at the Hospital for Sick Children in Toronto to be about 0.5%.[51] The New England Regional Infant Cardiac Program identified 18 patients with Ebstein's disease of 2251 infants with congenital heart disease, but 5 of these 18 had associated pulmonary atresia.[52] The Baltimore-Washington Infant Study enrolled 4390 infants with congenital heart disease from 1981–1989; 43 (1%) had Ebstein's malformation.[53,53a] The Baltimore-Washington study indicates the prevalence of Ebstein's anomaly was 5.2 per 100,000 livebirths.[53a]

Fig. 14-5: The morphologically right ventricle is usually very thin in the neonate with florid Ebstein's anomaly.
This transilluminated right ventricle from a newborn with Ebstein's anomaly shows how very thinned and disadvantaged the myocardium is.

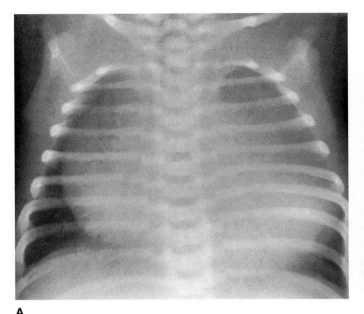

A

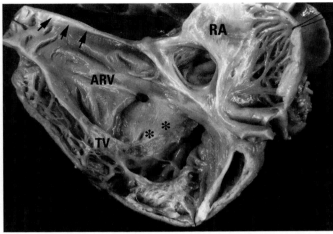

B

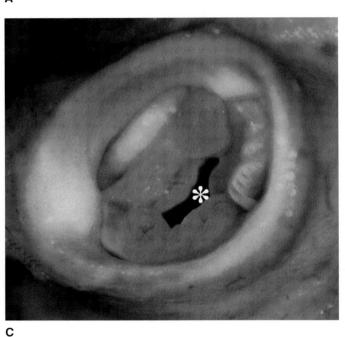

C

Fig. 14-6: Ebstein's anomaly of the tricuspid valve and congenital pulmonary valve insufficiency in the newborn.
A: Massive cardiomegaly on the chest radiograph. **B:** The internal view of the right ventricle shows the severe displacement and dysplasia of the tricuspid valve. **C:** The pulmonary valve leaflets are somewhat thickened and do not coapt (✻).

Etiology and Morphogenesis

There are reports of an unexpectedly high frequency of Ebstein's anomaly of the tricuspid valve among infants born to mothers who ingested lithium during pregnancy.[54–57] However, a review of infants born with this disorder and examined at our institution has not supported these observations.[58]

Associated Anomalies

Ebstein's malformation of the tricuspid valve can be found with a wide variety of congenital cardiac mal-

formations. These include an ovale foramen; a secundum atrial septal defect; aneurysm of the atrial septum; pulmonary stenosis or atresia; coarctation of the aorta; congenital pulmonary valvular regurgitation; divided right ventricle; mitral stenosis; single or multiple ventricular septal defect; tetralogy of Fallot (see Chapter 20), and complete (see Chapter 35) or corrected transposition (see Chapter 36) of the great arteries.[7–14,16,18,23,24,27,28,30,31,43–44,59–71] Ebstein's malformation of the tricuspid valve has also been seen in the patient with an atrioventricular septal defect, occasionally with a double-orifice left atrioventricular valve or an overriding and straddling tricuspid valve.[65,66,69,72–76]

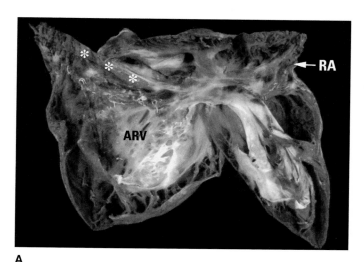
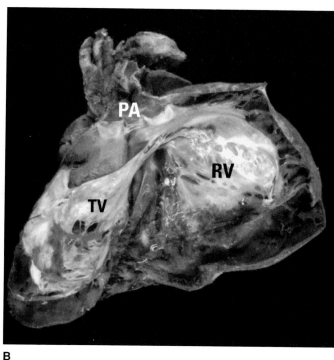

A **B**

Fig. 14-7: Ebstein's anomaly in the adult.
A: Internal view of the right atrium and ventricle shows that the tricuspid annulus (✱) is partly unguarded with the anterior leaflet displaced. **B:** The right ventricle seen from below shows that the anterior leaflet is sail-like. These figures provided by M. D. Silver, MD, Department of Pathology, the Toronto Hospital, Toronto, Canada.

Duplication of the tricuspid valve with Ebstein's malformation has been reported in the Japanese literature.[77] Bashour and colleagues[78] have described a patient with an apical left ventricular diverticulum and Ebstein's malformation of the tricuspid valve. The relationship between Ebstein's abnormality of the tricuspid valve and an unguarded tricuspid orifice has been explored elsewhere (see Chapter 23). There are obvious similarities between these two conditions, and in those severely affected neonates it may be difficult to differentiate these conditions even with echocardiography.[79–82]

Prognosis

A number of articles have addressed the natural history of patients with Ebstein's anomaly of the tricuspid valve and those morphological features influencing outcome.[14,16,17,22–26,44,47,57,83,84] To determine which morphological features are associated with early death, the complete echocardiograms and medical records of 16 consecutive patients with Ebstein's anomaly and concordant atrioventricular connections who presented in the fetal (n = 5) or neonatal (n = 11) period were reviewed by Roberson and Silverman.[47] The cohort was classified into two groups on the basis of survival at 3 months. Group 1 consisted of 7 patients who

died at or less than 3 months of age, and group 2 consisted of the 9 surviving patients. Comparing Groups 1 and 2, the respective incidence rates of morphological features that correlated with early death ($P<0.05$) included tethered distal attachments of the anterosuperior tricuspid leaflet (86% vs. 11%), right ventricular dysplasia (86% vs. 0%), left ventricular compression by right heart dilation (71% vs. 11%), and the area of the combined right atrium and atrialized right ventricle being greater than the combined area of the functional right ventricle, left atrium, and left ventricle (57% vs. 0%) measured in the apical four-chamber view. Right ventricular dysplasia was present in all patients with marked right atrial and atrialized right ventricular enlargement, in 86% of patients with tethered anterior leaflets, and in 83% of those with left ventricular compression; 86% of patients with right ventricular dysplasia had tethered distal attachments. These authors suggest that echocardiography defines those specific morphological features in the fetus and neonate that are highly predictive of death by 3 months of age. One must always urge some caution in these retrospective studies. Russo and colleagues[84] have addressed those factors affecting mortality of babies with Ebstein's anomaly diagnosed in infancy. Analysis of survival of 42 patients symptomatic at a mean age of 6 days demonstrated 69% survival at 14 days; 52% at 1 year, and only

37% at 5 years. Their data showed that early death was most influenced by morphological features including absence or hypoplasia of the trabecular portion of the right ventricle, a small and tethered anterior tricuspid leaflet, and associated anomalies. Others have suggested that early cyanosis with associated lesions conveys a poorer prognosis.[84a]

Imaging

Cross-sectional echocardiographic imaging has become the contemporary imaging modality of choice for the diagnosis of Ebstein's anomaly of the tricuspid valve.[11,45a,47,83,85–100] This technique permits the differentiation of functional from organic or anatomic pulmonary atresia that so often accompanies the neonatal expression of severe Ebstein's anomaly.[88–93,96,98–100] Furthermore, this technique allows the assessment of the mobility of the anterosuperior leaflet of the tricuspid valve. Increasing experience with the application of magnetic resonance imaging in the recognition of this disorder has also been recorded.[101]

Angiocardiography

Despite the contributions of echocardiography to the recognition of Ebstein's malformation of the tricuspid valve, angiocardiography retains a vital role in the imaging algorithm for Ebstein's malformation, especially and perhaps more for the evaluation of those complex forms of Ebstein's malformation.[10,11,16,24,31,89,90,102–108] These include the assessment of those patients with Ebstein's complicated by ventricular septal defect; tetralogy of Fallot; atrioventricular septal defect; etc. Also angiography may be helpful in assessing those distal linear attachments promoting an obstructive valve limiting pulmonary blood flow.[11,16,24,109–111]

Right ventriculography in frontal and lateral projections should permit recognition of Ebstein's anomaly of the tricuspid valve in all but the most mild (ie, offsetting of the tricuspid valve) expressions of this disorder (Figs. 14-8 through 14-19).[102–108] With injection of contrast material into the right atrium, tricuspid valve regurgitation of varying severity will opacify the en-

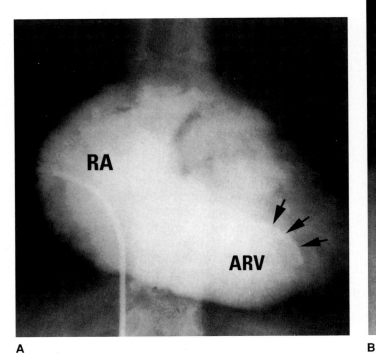

A

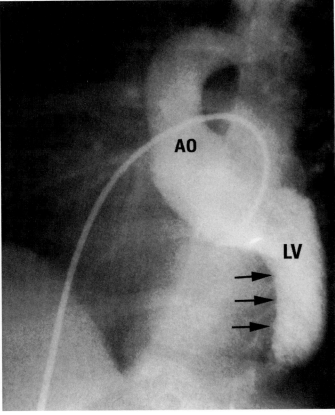

B

Fig. 14-8: Ebstein's anomaly of the tricuspid valve with a sail-like anterior leaflet.
A: Frontal right atriogram shows the level of the displaced tricuspid valve (arrows) producing an atrialized portion of the right ventricle and the huge right atrium. **B:** Left anterior oblique left ventriculogram shows that the left ventricle is distorted (arrows) by the very much enlarged right ventricle.

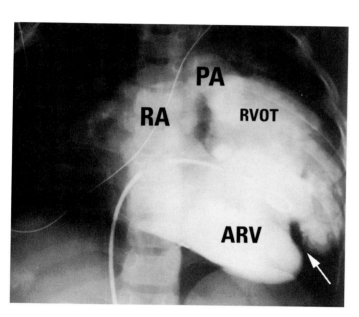

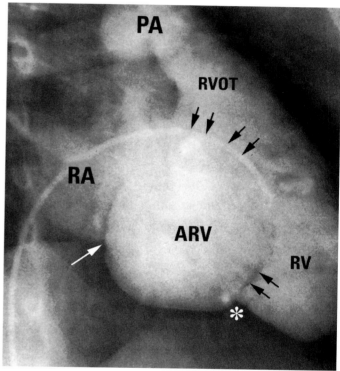

Fig. 14-9: Ebstein's anomaly of the tricuspid valve with profound notching of the right ventricle.
This frontal right ventriculogram shows the level of the displaced tricuspid valve producing the notch (white arrow) on the diaphragmatic surface of the right ventricle. The atrialized portion of the right ventricle is quite large and the right atrium opacifies from regurgitation. The displaced leaflet is thickened. The right ventricular outflow tract is widely patent with unimpeded flow into the pulmonary arteries.

Fig. 14-10: Ebstein's anomaly of the tricuspid valve with a sail-like anterior leaflet.
Right anterior oblique right ventriculogram shows significant displacement (✱) of the tricuspid valve from the annulus (white arrow). The sail-like anterior leaflet and the displaced leaflets together with the annulus form a complete ring (black arrows).

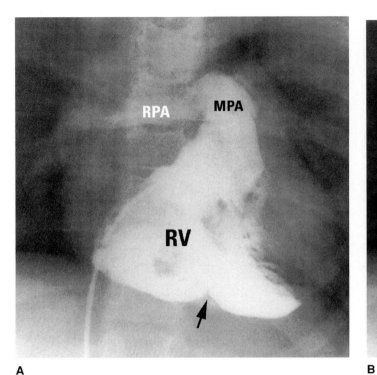

A

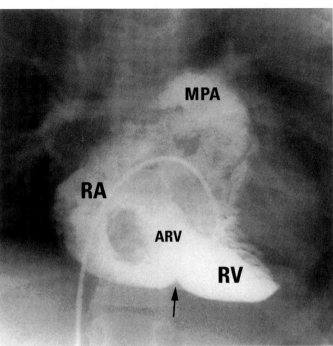

B

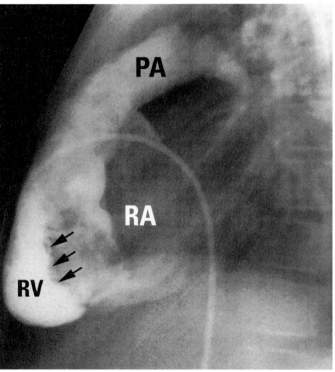

C

Fig. 14-11: Ebstein's anomaly of the tricuspid valve.
A and B: Right ventriculograms in frontal projection show a notch between the functional and atrialized parts of the right ventricle. **C:** The lateral view shows the displaced (arrows) tricuspid valve.

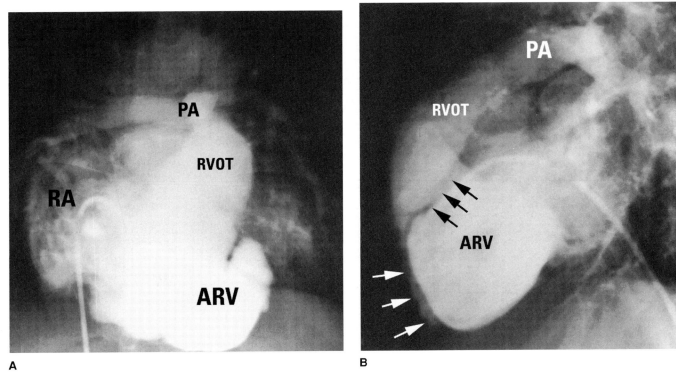

Fig. 14-12: Stenotic Ebstein's anomaly of the tricuspid valve.
A: Frontal right ventriculogram shows an unusual-shaped ventricle. The atrialized part of the right ventricle is a confined space of tricuspid sac. **B:** The lateral view shows the level of the displaced tricuspid valve (white arrows) and the anterosuperior infundibular attachments (black arrows).

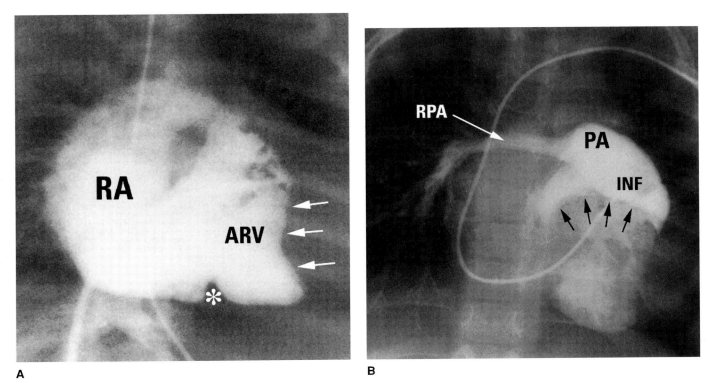

Fig. 14-13: Stenotic Ebstein's anomaly of the tricuspid valve with significant distal attachments.
A: Right ventriculogram shows the typical notch on the right ventricular diaphragmatic surface (✱) and the level of the atrialized right ventricle (white arrows). **B:** From a later study, the level of the distal attachments of the tricuspid valve are well seen (arrows), separating the infundibulum from the remainder of the ventricle.

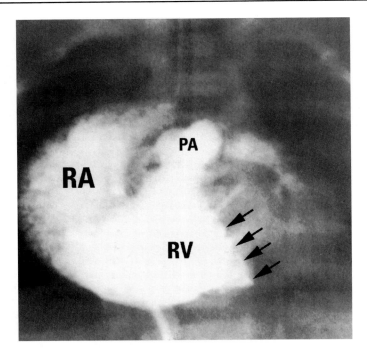

Fig. 14-14: Stenotic Ebstein's anomaly of the tricuspid valve with significant distal attachments.
This frontal right ventriculogram shows the distal attachments (arrows) of the tricuspid valve, with flow into the pulmonary artery. No trabecular component of the right ventricle is seen.

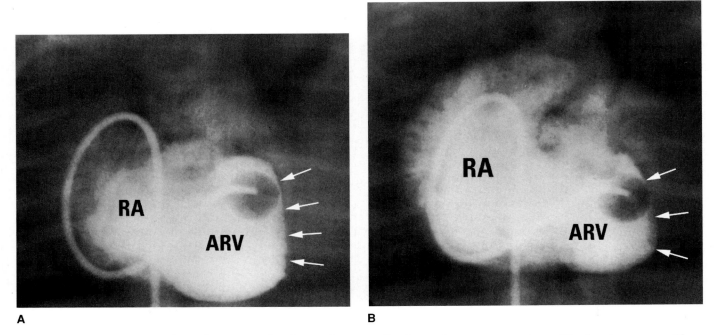

A   B

Fig. 14-15: Ebstein's anomaly of the tricuspid valve with severe distal attachments promoting critical pulmonary outflow tract obstruction.
A and B: Two frames from injection of contrast into atrialized portion of the right ventricle with almost no contrast in the pulmonary arteries.

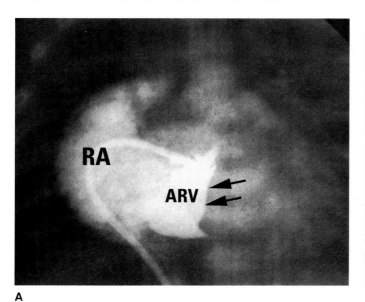

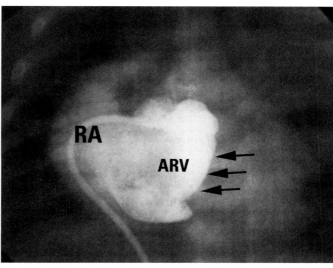

A

B

Fig. 14-16: Imperforate form of Ebstein's anomaly of the tricuspid valve.
A and B: Two frames with injection of contrast into atrialized portion of the right ventricle in frontal view. The distal linear attachments of the tricuspid valve completely separate and isolate the trabecular and infundibular components of the right ventricle from the atrialized portion.

larged right atrium (Figs. 14-8 and 14-13). The right atrium is usually enlarged in patients with this disorder, usually markedly so especially in those with the neonatal expression of this disorder. In the lateral projection, right-to-left shunting is evident at the atrial level, although this information is obtained from blood gas analysis as well as from color Doppler interrogation of the interatrial septum. With injection of contrast material into the trabecular portion of the right ventricle, regurgitation will opacify the smooth atrialized portion of the right ventricle, as well as the much enlarged right atrium (Figs. 14-8, 14-9, 14-14, and 14-15). Characteris-

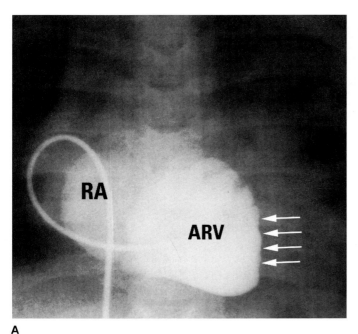

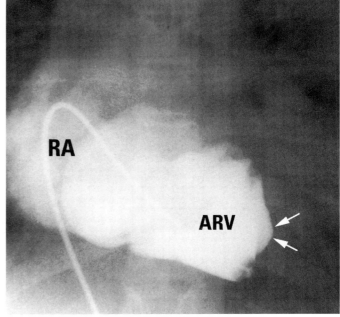

A

B

Fig. 14-17: Imperforate form of Ebstein's anomaly of the tricuspid valve.
A and B: Two frames with injection of contrast into atrialized portion of the right ventricle in frontal view. Note the motion of the imperforate tricuspid valve (arrows). No opacification of the right ventricular trabecular or infundibular components is seen.

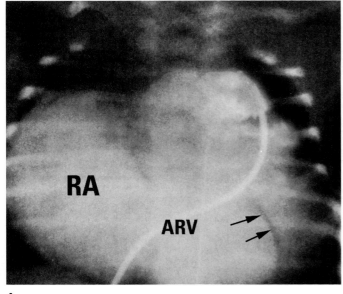

A

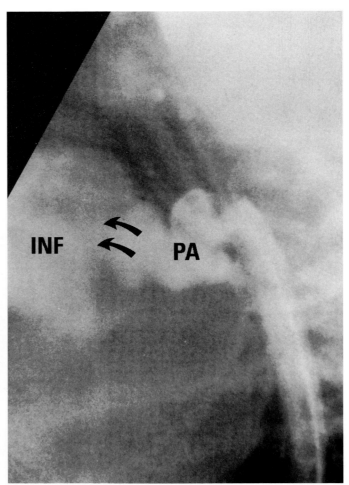

B

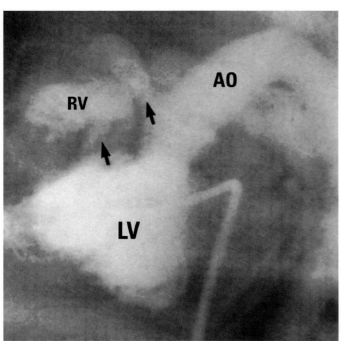

C

Fig. 14-18: Ebstein's anomaly of the tricuspid valve and multiple ventricular septal defects.
A: The frontal right ventriculogram shows the displaced tricuspid valve (arrows) with regurgitation into the enlarged right atrium, with no forward flow into the pulmonary arteries. **B:** The prostaglandin-enhanced aortogram demonstrates regurgitation of contrast (curved arrows) from the pulmonary artery into the infundibulum of the right ventricle. **C:** The left ventriculogram shows several ventricular septal defects (arrows).

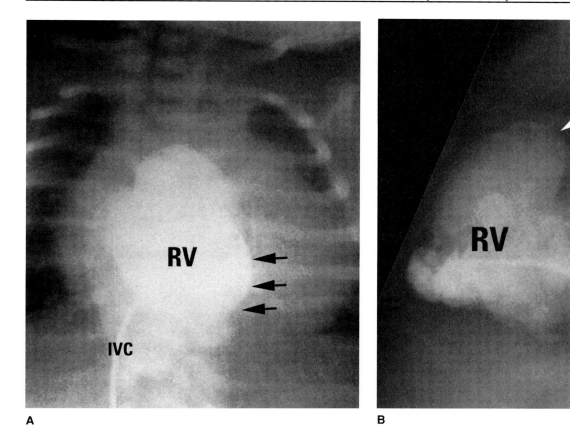

A

B

Fig. 14-19: Uhl's anomaly of the right ventricle with functional pulmonary atresia.
A and B: Frontal and lateral right ventriculograms show no flow from the right ventricle into the pulmonary arteries; the right ventricle is virtually devoid of trabeculations and on magnetic resonance imaging was very thinned. Arrows in frontal view indicate absence of trabeculation in the apical zone. There is virtually no forward flow through the pulmonary valve (arrow in lateral view).

tically there is a notch on the inferior or diaphragmatic surface of the right ventricle (Figs. 14-9 through 14-11, and 14-13).[102-107] This notch represents the distal attachment of the displaced tricuspid valve. That smooth area between the notched diaphragmatic surface of the right ventricle and the right atrioventricular groove (identified from the course of the right coronary artery) is the atrialized portion of the right ventricle. Because the atrialized portion of the right ventricle is invested with ventricular myocardium, it contracts synchronously with the functional right ventricle. That portion distal to the notch representing the apical trabecular portion of the right ventricle and the infundibular or outlet portion comprise the functional right ventricle. Elliott and Hartmann[104] have focused attention on the right ventricular infundibulum in patients with Ebstein's anomaly of the tricuspid valve. Their angiocardiographic evaluation showed that the right ventricular infundibulum demonstrated an extreme degree of volume variation to the point that the infundibulum rose above the pulmonary trunk during ventricular diastole and below the pulmonary trunk in systole. This finding is not specific solely for Ebstein's malformation as it has

been seen in patients with profound volume overload of the right ventricle (ie, congenitally absent pulmonary valve). They also pointed out that the right atrial appendage and the infundibulum exhibit reciprocal expansion, the so-called "teeter-totter" phenomenon.

Dilatation of the main pulmonary trunk is infrequent patients with uncomplicated Ebstein's anomaly of the tricuspid valve. If such dilatation is present, one should be suspicious of co-existing pulmonary valve stenosis or pulmonary hypertension reflecting a large arterial duct or ventricular septal defect. The angiographic studies of Deutsch and colleagues[103] indicated that the pulmonary vessels tended to be normal in size, or in those with significant right-to-left atrial shunting, the vessels were small. Another reason for small pulmonary arteries is hypoplastic lungs, reflecting fetal compression of the lungs by a very much enlarged heart. The transit time through the lungs is usually very prolonged because of the ineffective right ventricle.

In the obstructive forms of Ebstein's malformation, the distal attachments of the atrioventricular valve promote a pinhole anatomy between the inlet of the right ventricle and the infundibulum (Figs. 14-12 through

14-17; see also Chapter 23, Fig. 23-14).[11,16,24,110,111] This pinhole effectively limits pulmonary blood flow from the right ventricle into the pulmonary arteries, and thus the caliber of the pulmonary arteries should reflect the severity of the obstruction. This obstructive form of Ebstein's malformation can be recognized from injection of contrast material into the atrialized portion of the right ventricle. The forward margin of contrast is 'trapped' against the distally tethered tricuspid valve, and this veil of tissue effectively partitions the inlet of the right ventricle from its apical trabecular component. This provides an excellent example of the divided right ventricle where the division is valvular in origin, not muscular (see Chapter 17). The Ebstein form of imperforate tricuspid valve is diagnosed from selective injection into the atrialized portion of the right ventricle. Unless there is an associated ventricular septal defect as in the patient reported by Rao and colleagues[18] in 1973, the patient with an imperforate, Ebstein tricuspid valve will also have pulmonary atresia (as in the patient reported by Gerlis and Anderson[19]). There is complete separation of the right ventricular inlet from its apical trabecular component in the patient with Ebstein form of imperforate tricuspid valve, and from the injection of contrast material into the atrialized portion of the right ventricle, there is no opacification of the trabecular component (nor of the right ventricular infundibulum).[31]

Leung and colleagues[24] have catalogued patients with Ebstein's anomaly of the tricuspid valve according to their cineangiographic appearance. It was possible to classify patients into three groups with focal, hyphenated, and linear attachments reflecting the type and extent of distal attachments of the tricuspid valve. In those with so-called normal or focal attachments, there was free communication between the inlet (atrialized) and the remainder of the right ventricle between the focal attachments. These authors felt that they could recognize linear as opposed to focal attachment of the anterosuperior and mural leaflets by the linear trapping of contrast material within the functional right ventricle. One is not surprised that those patients with linear distal attachments had lower oxygen levels at rest, or cyanosis at rest, and reduced exercise tolerance. These are the patients with the smallest functional right ventricle as well as 'keyhole' communications between the inlet and outlet of the right ventricle.

The differentiation of functional from organic or anatomic pulmonary atresia can usually be addressed and resolved by cross sectional echocardiography with Doppler/color Doppler interrogation of the pulmonary outflow tract (see also Chapter 23).[96,98–100] The role of prostaglandin-enhanced retrograde aortography is certainly less today than 15 years ago when we first advocated this technique to make this differentiation (Fig. 14-18).[89,90]

Left ventricular angiocardiography is rarely required to demonstrate wall-motion abnormalities or mitral valve prolapse, both of which are so prevalent in any cohort of patients with Ebstein's malformation that these features can be imaged by echocardiography.[41–43,112] The other leaflet anomalies, papillary muscle anomalies, and cord anomalies are perhaps best addressed by cross-sectional echocardiography.[43] The right ventricle devoid of its normal trabecular pattern and suggestive of Uhl's anomaly is best demonstrated by selective right ventricular angiography (Fig. 14-19).

Differential Diagnosis

Today the almost immediate application of cross-sectional echocardiography makes definition of a differential diagnosis an almost academic relic of the educational algorithm (how sad!). Any abnormality of the tricuspid valve promoting congenital tricuspid regurgitation must be considered in this differential including tricuspid valve dysplasia; an unguarded tricuspid orifice; isolated tricuspid cleft; etc.[113–116] Those very unusual conditions including isolated dilatation or enlargement of the right atrium or Uhl's anomaly of the right ventricle must be considered as well.[32–41] Finally, displacement and dysplasia of the mitral valve can occur, promoting congenital mitral valve regurgitation (see Chapter 25).[117–123]

References

1. Ebstein W. Ueber einen sehr seltenen Fall von insuffizienz der Valvula tricuspidalis, bedingt durch eine angeborene hochgradige Missbildung derselben. *Arch Anat Physiol* 1866;238–254.
2. Schiebler GL, Gravenstein JS, Van Mierop LHS. Ebstein's anomaly of the tricuspid valve, translation of original description with comments. *Am J Cardiol* 1968; 22:867–873.
3. Mann RJ and Lie JT. The life story of Wilhelm Ebstein (1836–1912) and his almost overlooked description of a congenital disease. *Mayo Clin Proc* 1979;54:197–204.
4. Shampo MA. Wilhelm Ebstein. Internist, pathologist, and medical historian. *Prog Pediatr Cardiol* 1993;2:1.
5. Feldt RH. Ebstein's anomaly. A historical overview. *Prog Pediatr Cardiol* 1993;2:2–4.
6. Schiebler GL, Adams PAJ, Anderson RC, Amplatz K, Lester RG. Clinical study of twenty-three cases of Ebstein's anomaly of the tricuspid valve. *Circulation* 1959; 19:165–187.
7. Lev M, Liberthson RR, Joseph RH, Seten CE, Kunske RD, Eckner FAO, Miller RA. The pathologic anatomy of Ebstein's disease. *Arch Pathol* 1970;90:334–343.
7a. Becker AE. Ebstein's malformation-What's in a name? *Cardiovasc Pathol* 1995;4:25–28.

7b. Anderson RH. Ebstein's malformation (letter to the editor). *Cardiovasc Pathol* 1995;4:225–226.

8. Anderson KR, Lie JT. Pathologic anatomy of Ebstein's anomaly of the heart revisited. *Am J Cardiol* 1978;41:739–745.

9. Anderson KR, Zuberbuhler JR, Anderson RH, Becker AE, Lie JT. Morphologic spectrum of Ebstein's anomaly of the heart. A review. *Mayo Clin Proc* 1979;54:174–180.

10. Anderson RH, Macartney FJ, Shinebourne EA, Tynan M. *Paediatric Cardiology.* Edinburgh: Churchill Livingstone; 1987, pp. 721–736.

11. Freedom RM, Smallhorn JF. Ebstein's malformation of the morphologically tricuspid valve: A consideration of regurgitant and obstructive forms in patients with concordant and discordant atrioventricular connections. In: Anderson RH, Neches WH, Park SC, Zuberbuhler JR, eds. *Perspectives in Pediatric Cardiology.* Volume 1. Mt. Kisco, NY: Futura Publishing Company, Inc; 1988, pp. 127–146.

12. Zuberbuhler JR, Allwork SP, Anderson RH. The spectrum of Ebstein's anomaly of the tricuspid valve. *J Thorac Cardiovasc Surg* 1979;77:202–211.

13. Zuberbuhler JR, Becker AE, Anderson RH, Lenox CC. Ebstein's malformation and the embryological development of the tricuspid valve. With a note on the nature of "clefts" in the atrioventricular valves. *Pediatr Cardiol* 1984;5:289–296.

14. Zuberbuhler JR, Anderson RH. Ebstein's malformation of the tricuspid valve: Morphology and natural history. In: Anderson RH, Neches WH, Park SC, Zuberbuhler JR, eds. *Perspectives in Pediatric Cardiology.* Volume 1. Mt. Kisco, NY: Futura Publishing Company, Inc; 1988, pp. 99–112.

15. Takayasu S, Obunai Y, Konno S. Clinical classification of Ebstein's anomaly. *Am Heart J* 1978;95:154–162.

16. Freedom RM, Benson LN. Neonatal expression of Ebstein's anomaly. *Prog Pediatr Cardiol* 1993;2:22–27.

17. Watson H. The natural history of Ebstein's anomaly in childhood and adolescence. A preliminary report on the first 100 cases. *Proc Assoc Eur Cardiol* 1970;6:35–39.

18. Rao PS, Jue KL, Isabel-Jones J, Ruttenberg HD. Ebstein's malformation of the tricuspid valve with atresia. Differentiation from isolated tricuspid atresia. *Am J Cardiol* 1973;32:1004–1009.

19. Gerlis LM, Anderson RH. Cor triatriatum dexter with imperforate Ebstein's anomaly. *Br Heart J* 1976;38:108–111.

20. Anderson RH, Wilkinson JE, Becker AE. The bulbus cordis—A misunderstood region of the developing human heart. Its significance to the classification of congenital cardiac malformation. In: Rosenquist GC, Bergsma D, eds. *Morphogenesis and Malformation of the Cardiaovascular System.* New York: Alan R. Liss, Inc; 1978, Birth Defects, 14(7):1–22.

21. Genton E, Blount SGJ. The spectrum of Ebstein's anomaly. *Am Heart J* 1967;73:395–425.

22. Giuliani ER, Fuster V, O BR, Mair DD. The clinical features and natural history of Ebstein's anomaly of the tricuspid valve. *Mayo Clin Proc* 1979;54:163–173.

23. Kumar AE, Fyler DC, Miettinen OS, Nadas AS. Ebstein's anomaly: Clinical profile and natural history. *Am J Cardiol* 1971;28:84–95.

24. Leung MP, Baker EJ, Anderson RH, Zuberbuhler JR. Cineangiographic spectrum of Ebstein's malformation: Its relevance to clinical presentation and outcome. *J Am Coll Cardiol* 1988;11:154–161.

25. Celermajer DS, Cullen S, Sullivan ID, Spiegelhalter DJ, Wyse RKH, Deanfield JE. Outcome in neonates with Ebstein's anomaly. *J Am Coll Cardiol* 1992;19:1041–1046.

26. Mair DD. Comment on: Celermajer DS, Cullen S, Sullivan ID, Spiegelhalter DJ, Wyse RKH, Deanfield JE. Outcome in Neonates with Ebstein's Anomaly. *J Am Coll Cardiol* 1992;19:1041–1046. *J Am Coll Cardiol* 1992;19:1047–1048.

27. Edwards WD. Embryology and pathologic features of Ebstein's anomaly. *Prog Pediatr Cardiol* 1993;2:5–15.

28. Kirklin JW, Barratt-Boyes BG. *Cardiac Surgery.* Second Edition. New York: Churchill Livingstone; 1993, pp. 1105–1130.

28a. Munoz-Castellanos L, Barros W, Garcia F, Salinas CH, Kuri M. Estudio patologia de la displasia y el adosamiento valvulares en la anomalia de Ebstein. *Arch Inst Cardiol Mex* 1993;63:101–109.

29. Becker AE, Becker MJ, Edwards JE. Pathologic spectrum of dysplasia of the tricuspid valve. Features in common with Ebstein's malformation. *Arch Pathol* 1971;91:167–178.

30. Huhta JC, Edwards WD, Tajik AJ, Mair DD, Puga FJ, Ritter DG. Pulmonary atresia with intact ventricular septum, Ebstein's anomaly of hypoplastic tricuspid valve, and double-chamber right ventricle. *Mayo Clin Proc* 1982;57:515–519.

31. Freedom RM, Culham JAG, Moes CAF. *Angiocardiography of Congenital Heart Disease.* New York: Macmillan Publishing Company; 1984, pp. 111–118.

32. Uhl HSM. A previously undescribed congenital malformation of the heart: Almost total absence of the myocardium of the right ventricle. *Bull Hopkins Hosp* 1952;91:197–205.

32a. Uhl HSM. Uhl's anomaly revisited. *Circulation* 1996;1483–1484.

32b. James TN, Nichols MM, Sapire DW, DiPatre PL, Lopez SM. Complete heart block and fatal right ventricular failure in an infant. *Circulation* 1996;93:1588–1600.

33. Anderson KR, Lie JT. The right ventricular myocardium in Ebstein's anomaly. A morphometric histopathologic study. *Mayo Clin Proc* 1979;54:181–184.

34. Cumming GC, Bowman JM, Whytehead L. Congenital aplasia of the myocardium of the right ventricle. *Am Heart J* 1965;70:671–676.

35. Zuberbuhler JR, Blank E. Hypoplasia of right ventricular myocardium (Uhl's disease). *AJR* 1970;110:491–496.

36. Arcilla R and Gasul BM. Congenital aplasia or marked hypoplasia of the myocardium of the right ventricle (Uhl's anomaly). *J Pediatr* 1961;58:381–388.

37. Kaul U, Arora R, Rani S. Uhl's anomaly with rudimentary pulmonary valve leaflets: A clinical, hemodynamic, angiographic, and pathologic study. *Am Heart J* 1980;100:673–677.

38. Kinare SG, Panday SR, Deshmukh SM. Congenital aplasia of the right ventricular myocardium (Uhl's anomaly). *Chest* 1969;55:429–431.

39. Perez Diaz L, Quero Jiminez M, Moreno Granadas F, Perez Martinez V, Merino Batres G. Congenital absence of myocardium of right ventricle: Uhl's anomaly. *Br Heart J* 1973;35:570–572.

40. Perrin EV and Mehrizi A. Isolated free-wall hypoplasia of the right ventricle. *Am J Dis Child* 1965;109:558–566.

41. Monibi AA, Neches WH, Lenox CC, Park SC, Mathews RA, Zuberbuhler JR. Left ventricular anomalies associated with ebstein's malformation of the tricuspid valve. *Circulation* 1978;57:303–306.

42. Sharma S, Rajani M, Mukhopadhyay S, Aggarwal S, Shrivastsva S, Tandon R. Angiographic abnormalities of the morphologically left ventricle in the presence of Ebstein's. *Int J Cardiol* 1989;22:109–113.

43. Gerlis LM, Ho SY, Sweeney AE. Mitral valve anomalies associated with Ebstein's malformation of the tricuspid valve. *Am J Cardiovasc Pathol* 1993;4:294–301.

43a. da Silveira WL, Leite AD, Fernandes RL, de Oliviera VG, de Mesquita AO, Melo JCG, Machado WAT, da Silva MA. Ebstein's anomaly associated with interventricular septal defect. *ArqBras Cardiol* 1993;60:421–423.

43b. Franke A, Muhler EG, Hugel W. Ebstein's malformation with covered defect of the ventricular septum. *Cardiol Young* 1996;6:341–343.

44. Celermajer DS, Dodd SM, Greenwald SE, Wyse RKH, Deanfield JE. Morbid anatomy in neonates with Ebstein's anomaly of the tricuspid valve: Pathophysiologic and clinical implications. *J Am Coll Cardiol* 1992;19:1049–1053.

45. Sahn DJ, Heldt GP, Reed KL, Kleinman CS, Meijboom EJ. Fetal heart disease with cardiomegaly may be associated with lung hypoplasia as a determinant of poor prognosis (abstract). *J Am Coll Cardiol* 1988;11:9A.

45a. Duran M, Gomez I, Palacio A . Anomalia de Ebstein con hipoplasia pulmonar. Diagnostico mediante ecocardiografia Doppler color en el feto. *Rev Esp Cardiol* 1992;45:541–542.

46. Hornberger LK, Sahn DJ, Kleinman CS, Copel JA, Reed KL. Tricuspid valve disease with significant tricuspid insufficiency in the fetus: Diagnosis and outcome. *J Am Coll Cardiol* 1991;17:167–73.

46a. Chaoui R, Bollmann R, Goldner B, Heling KS, Tennstedt C. Fetal cardiomegaly: Echocardiographic findings and outcome in 19 cases. *Fetal Diagn Ther* 1994;9:92–104.

47. Roberson DA, Silverman NH. Ebstein's anomaly: Echocardiographic and clinical features in the fetus and neonate. *J Am Coll Cardiol* 1989;14:1300–1307.

48. Lang D, Oberhoffer R, Cook A, Sharland G, Allan L, Fagg N, Anderson RH. Pathologic spectrum of malformations of the tricuspid valve in prenatal and neonatal life. *J Am Coll Cardiol* 1991;17(5):1161–1167.

49. Allan LD, Crawford DC, Tynan MJ. Pulmonary atresia in prenatal life. *J Am Coll Cardiol* 1986;8:1131–1136.

50. Allan LD and Cook A. Pulmonary atresia with intact ventricular septum in the fetus. *Cardiol Young* 1992;2:367–376.

51. Rowe RD, Freedom RM, Mehrizi A. *The Neonate with Congenital Heart Disease*. Second Edition. New York: WB Saunders Company; 1981, pp. 515–528.

52. Fyler DC. Report of the New England Regional Infant Cardiac Program. *Pediatrics* 1980;65(No. 2, Part 2):453.

53. Perry LW, Neill CA, Ferencz C, Rubin JD, Loffredo CA. Infants with congenital heart disease: The cases. In: Ferencz C, Rubin JD, Loffredo CA, Magee CA, eds. *Epidemiology of Congenital Heart Disease. The Baltimore-Washington Infant Study 1981–1989. In, Perspectives in Pediatric Cardiology*. Volume 4. Mt. Kisco, NY: Futura Publishing Company, Inc; 1993, pp. 33–62.

53a. Correa-Villasenor A, Ferencz C, Neill CA, Wilson PD, Boughman JA. Ebstein's malformation of the tricuspid valve: Genetic and environmental factors. The Baltimore-Washington Infant Study Group. *Teratology* 1994;50:137–147.

54. Allan LD, Desai G, Tynan MJ. Prenatal echocardiographic screening for Ebstein's anomaly for mothers on lithium therapy. *Lancet* 1982;2:875–876.

55. Weinstein MR, Goldfield MD. Cardiovascular malformations with lithium use during pregnancy. *Am J Psych* 1975;132:529–531.

56. Long WA and Willis PW. Maternal lithium and neonatal Ebstein's. *Am J Perinatol* 1984;1:182–184.

57. Radford DJ, Graff RF, Neilson GH. Diagnosis and natural history of Ebstein's anomaly. *Br Heart J* 1985;36:517–522.

58. Zalzstein E, Koren G, Einarson T, Freedom RM. A case-control study on the association between first trimester exposure to lithium and Ebstein's anomaly. *Am J Cardiol* 1990;65:817–818.

59. Van Praagh R, Ando M, Van Praagh S, Senno A, Hougen TJ, Novak G, Hastreiter AR. Pulmonary atresia: Anatomic considerations. In: *The Child With Congenital Heart Disease After Surgery*. Mt. Kisco, NY: Futura Publishing Company, Inc; 1976, pp. 103–135.

60. Bharati S, McAllister HAJ, Chiemmongkoltip P, Lev M. Congenital pulmonary atresia with tricuspid insufficiency: Morphologic study. *Am J Cardiol* 1977;40:70–75.

61. Freedom RM, Dische MR, Rowe RD. The tricuspid valve in pulmonary atresia and intact ventricular septum. *Arch Patholol Lab Med* 1978;102:28–31.

62. Freedom RM, Perrin D. The tricuspid valve: Morphologic considerations. In: Freedom RM. *Pulmonary Atresia and Intact Ventricular Septum*. Mt. Kisco, NY: Futura Publishing Company, Inc; 1989, pp. 37–52.

63. Freedom RM, Perrin D. The right ventricle: Morphologic considerations. In: Freedom RM. *Pulmonary Atresia and Intact Ventricular Septum*. Mt. Kisco, NY: Futura Publishing Company, Inc; 1989, pp. 53–74.

64. Stellin G, Santini F, Thiene G, Bortolotti U, Daliento L, Milanesi O, Sorbara C, Mazzucco A, Casarotto D. Pulmonary atresia, intact ventricular septum, and Ebstein anomaly of the tricuspid valve. *J Thorac Cardiovasc Surg* 1993;106:255–261.

65. Caruso G, Losekoot TG, Becker AE. Ebstein's anomaly in persistent common atrioventricular canal. *Br Heart J* 1978;40:1275–1279.

66. Roach RM, Tandon R, Moller JH, Edwards JE. Ebstein's anomaly of the tricuspid valve in persistent common atrioventricular canal. *Am J Cardiol* 1984;53:640–642.

67. Davido A, Maarek M, Jullien JL, Corone P. Maladie d'Ebstein associee a une tetralogie de Fallot. A propos d'une observation familiale, revue de la litterature, implication embryologique et genetique. *Arch Mal Coeur Vaiss* 1985;78:752–756.

68. Sahai S, Kothari SS, Wasir HS. Tetralogy of Fallot with Ebstein's anomaly of the tricuspid valve. *Indian Heart J* 1994;46:53–54.

69. Gussenhoven EJ, Essed CE, Bos E, de Villeneuve VH. Echocardiographic Diagnosis of Overriding Tricuspid Valve in a Child with Ebstein's Anomaly. *Pediatr Cardiol* 1984;5:209–212.

70. Hanley FL, Sade RM, Blackstone EH, Kirklin JW, Freedom RM, Nanda NC. Outcomes in neonatal pulmonary atresia with intact ventricular septum. *J Thorac Cardiovasc Surg* 1993;105:406–427.

71. Guzzo D, Castellano C, Munoz-Castellanos L, de Rubens J, Calderon J, Attie F. Atresia pulmonar con septum interventricular intacto y anomalia de Ebstein de la valvula tricuspide. *Arch Inst Cardiol Mex* 1989;59:133–138.

72. Yamaguchi M, Tachibana H, Hosokawa Y, Ohoshi H, Oshima Y, Obo H. Ebstein's anomaly and partial atrioventricular canal associated with double orifice mitral valve. *J Cardiovasc Surg* 1989;30:790–792.

73. Seo J-W, Jung WH, Park YW. Imperforate Ebstein's malformation in atrioventricular septal defect. *Cardiol Young* 1991;1:152–154.

74. Van Praagh S, Vangi V, Sul JH, Metras D, Parness I, Castaneda AR, Van Praagh R. Tricuspid atresia or severe stenosis with partial common atrioventricular canal: Anatomic data, clinical profile and surgical considerations. *J Am Coll Cardiol* 1991;17:932–943.

75. Handler JB, Berger TJ, Miller RH, Hagan AD, Peniston RL, Vieweg WVR. Partial atrioventricular canal in association with Ebstein's anomaly. Echocardiographic diagnosis and surgical correction. *Chest* 1981;80:515–517.

76. Hartyanszky IL, Lozsadi K, Kadar K, Huttl T, Kiraly L. Ebstein's anomaly and intermediate-form atrioventricular septal defect with double-orifice mitral valve (letter). *J Thorac Cardiovasc Surg* 1992;104:1496–1497.

77. Miyamura H, Matsukawa T, Maruyama Y, Nakazawa S, Eguchi S. (Duplication of the tricuspid valve with Ebstein anomaly. *Jpn Circ J (Japan)* 1984;48:336–338.

78. Bashour TT, Saalouke M, Yazji ZI. Apical left ventricular diverticulum with Ebstein malformation. *Am Heart J* 1988;115:1332–1334.

79. Kanjuh VI, Stevenson JE, Amplatz K, Edwards JE. Congenitally unguarded tricuspid orifice with coexistent pulmonary atresia. *Circulation* 1964;30:911–917.

80. Gussenhoven EJ, Essed CE, Bos E. Unguarded tricuspid Orifice with two-chambered right ventricle. *Pediatr Cardiol* 1986;7:175–177.

81. Anderson RH, Silverman NH, Zuberbuhler JR. Congenitally unguarded tricuspid orifice: Its differentiation from Ebstein's malformation in association with pulmonary atresia and intact ventricular septum. *Pediatr Cardiol* 1990;11:86–90.

82. Munoz Castellanos L, Salinas CH, Kuri Nivon M, Garcia Arenal F. Ausencia de la valvula tricuspide. Informe de un caso. *Arch Inst Cardiol Mex* 1992;62:61–67.

83. Rusconi PG, Zuberbuhler JR, Anderson RH, Rigby ML. Morphologic-echocardiographic correlates of Ebstein's malformation. *Eur Heart J* 1991;12:784–790.

84. Russo PA, Wyse RKH, Triumbari F, Dodd S, de Leval MR. Ebstein's anomaly in the first year of life: Factors affecting mortality (abstract). *Br Heart J* 1988;59:135.

84a. Enriquez MM, Attie F, Castellanos LM, Barron JV. Anomalia de Ebstein en el lactante. *Arch Inst Cardiol Mex* 1986;56:417–420.

85. Gussenhoven EJ, Essed CE, Bos E, de Villeneuve VH. Echocardiographic diagnosis of overriding tricuspid valve in a child with Ebstein's anomaly. *Pediatr Cardiol* 1984;5:209–212.

86. Gussenhoven WJ, Spitaels SEC, Bom N, Becker AE. Echocardiographic criteria for Ebstein's anomaly of tricuspid valve. *Br Heart J* 1980;43:31–37.

87. Gussenhoven EJ, Stewart PA, Becker AE, Essed CE, Ligtvoet KM, de Villeneuve VH. "Offsetting" of the septal tricuspid leaflet in normal hearts and in hearts with Ebstein's anomaly. *Am J Cardiol* 1984;54:172–181.

88. Berman WJ, Whitman V, Stanger P, Rudolph AM. Congenital tricuspid incompetence simulating pulmonary atresia with intact ventricular septum: A report of two cases. *Am Heart J* 1978;96:655–661.

89. Freedom RM, Culham G, Moes F, Olley PM, Rowe RD. Differentiation of functional and structural pulmonary atresia: Role of aortography. *Am J Cardiol* 1978;41:914–920.

90. Freedom RM, Olley PM, Rowe RD. The angiocardiography and morphology of ductal-dependent congenital heart disease: Selected topics with reference to the clinical application of E-type prostaglandins. In: Gallucci V, Bini RM, Thiene G, eds. *Selected Topics in Cardiac Surgery*. Bologna: Casa Editrice Bologna; 1980, pp. 109–143.

91. Haworth SG, Shinebourne EA, Miller GAH. Right-to-left interatrial shunting with normal right ventricular pressure. A puzzling haemo-dynamic picture associated with some rare congenital malformations of the tricuspid valve and right ventricle. *Br Heart J* 1975;37:386–391.

92. Newfeld EA, Cole RB, Paul MH. Ebstein's malformation of the tricuspid valve in the neonate. Functional and anatomic pulmonary outflow tract obstruction. *Am J Cardiol* 1967;19:727–731.

93. Schire V, Sutin GL, Barnard CN. Organic and functional pulmonary atresia with intact ventricular septum. *Am J Cardiol* 1961;8:100–108.

94. Shiina A, Seward JB, Edwards WD, Hagler DJ, Tajik AJ. Two-dimensional echocardiographic spectrum of Ebstein's anomaly: Detailed anatomic assessment. *J Am Coll Cardiol* 1984;3:356–370.

95. Shiina A, Seward JB, Tajik AJ, Hagler DJ, Danielson GK. Two-dimensional echocardiographic-surgical correlation in Ebstein's anomaly: Preoperative determination of patients requiring tricuspid valve plication vs. replacement. *Circulation* 1983;68:534–544.

96. Smallhorn JF, Izukawa T, Benson L, Freedom RM. Noninvasive recognition of functional pulmonary atresia by echocardiography. *Am J Cardiol* 1984;54:925–926.

97. Hagler DJ. Echocardiographic assessment of Ebstein's anomaly. *Prog Pediatr Cardiol* 1993;2:28–37.

97a. Nihoyannopoulos P, McKenna WJ, Smith G, Foale R. Echocardiographic assessment of the right ventricle in Ebstein's anomaly: Relation to clinical outcome. *J Am Coll Cardiol* 1986;8:627–635.

98. Weinhaus L, Jureidini S, Nouri S, Connors RH. Functional pulmonary atresia: Color flow recognition and treatment with extracorporeal membrane oxygenation. *Am Heart J* 1990;119:980–982.

99. Umebayashi Y, Arikawa K, Chosa N, Kinjo T, Nishida S, Tabata D, Haraguchi T, Aihoshi S, Seki S, Umemoto K, et al. [Functional pulmonary atresia: a case report]. *Kyobu Geka (Japan)* 1992;45:644–646.

100. Silberbach GM, Ferrara B, Berry JM, Einzig S, Bass JL. Diagnosis of functional pulmonary atresia using hyperventilation and Doppler ultrasound. *Am J Cardiol* 1987;59:709–711.

101. Choi YH, Park JH, Choe YH, Yoo SJ. MR imaging of Ebstein's anomaly of the tricuspid valve. *AJR* 1994;163:539–543.

102. Soto B, Pacifico AD. *Angiocardiography in Congenital Heart Malformations*. Mt. Kisco, NY: Futura Publishing Company, Inc; 1990, pp. 185–196.

103. Deutsch V, Wexler L, Blieden LC, Yahini JH, Neufeld HN. Ebstein's anomaly of the tricuspid valve: Critical review of roentgenological features and additional angiographic signs. *AJR* 1975;125:395–411.

104. Elliott LP, Hartmann AFJ. The right ventricular infundibulum in Ebstein's anomaly of the tricuspid valve. *Radiology* 1967;89:694–700.

105. Ellis K, Griffiths SP, Burris JO, Ramsay GC, Fleming RJ. Ebstein's anomaly of the tricuspid valve. Angiocardiographic considerations. *AJR* 1964;92:1338–1352.

106. Amplatz K, Moller JH. *Radiology of Congenital Heart Disease*. St. Louis, MO: Mosby Year Book; 1993, pp. 652–654.

107. Yoo S-J, Choi Y-H. *Angiocardiograms in Congenital Heart Disease. Teaching File of Sejong Heart Institute*. Oxford: Oxford Medical Publications; 1991, pp. 83–90.

108. Freedom RM, Benson LN. Ebstein's malformation of the tricuspid valve. In: Freedom RM, Benson LN, Smallhorn JF, eds. *Neonatal Heart Disease*. London: Springer-Verlag; 1992, pp. 471–483.

109. Leung MP, Lee J, Lo RNS, Mok CK. Modified Fontan procedure for severe Ebstein's malformation with tricuspid stenosis. *Ann Thorac Surg* 1992;54:523–527.

110. Fasoli G, Scognamiglio R, Daliento L. Uncommon pattern of tricuspid stenosis in Ebstein's anamoly. *Int J Cardiol* 1985;9:488–492.

111. Marcelletti C, Mazzera E, Olthof H, et al. Fontan's operation: An expanded horizon. *J Thorac Cardiovasc Surg* 1980;80:764–769.

112. Castaneda-Zuniga W, Nath HP, Moller JH, Edwards JE. Left-sided anomalies in Ebstein's malformation of the tricuspid valve. *Pediatr Cardiol* 1982;3:181–183.

113. Graham TP Jr, Smith CW. Aneurysmal dilatation of the right ventricular outflow tract in infancy: Severe form of Uhl's anomaly. *Cathet Cardiovasc Diagn* 1977; 3:397–400.

114. Eichhorn P, Ritter M, Suetsch G, von Segesser LK, Turina M, Jenni R. Congenital cleft of the anterior tricuspid leaflet with severe tricuspid regurgitation in adults. *J Am Coll Cardiol* 1992;20:1175–1179.

115. Mohan JC, Tatke M, Arora R. Rudimentary dysplastic valvar tissue guarding the tricuspid orifice with dilatation of the right ventricle and a patent outflow tract. *Int J Cardiol* 1989;25:136–139.

116. Eshaghour E, Olley PM, Collins GFN. Idiopathic right atrial enlargement in childhood. *Am Heart J* 1969;78: 373–376.

117. Actis-Dato A, Milocco I. Anomalous attachment of the mitral valve to the ventricular wall. *Am J Cardiol* 1966; 17:278–281.

118. Caruso G, Cifarelli A, Balducci G, Facilone F. Ebstein's malformation of the mitral valve in atrioventricular and ventriculoarterial concordance. *Pediatr Cardiol* 1987; 8:209–210.

119. Freedom RM, Benson L, Burrows P, Smallhorn JF, Perrin DG. Congenital deformities of the mitral valve (excluding atrioventricular septal defect): Echocardiographic and angiocardiographic findings and indications for surgery. In: Marcelletti C, Anderson RH, Becker AE, Corno A, di Carlo D, Mazzera E. *Paediatric Cardiology*. Volume 6. Edinburgh: Churchill Livingstone; 1986, pp. 240–261.

120. Ruschhaupt DG, Bharati S, Lev M. Mitral valve malformation of Ebstein type in absence of corrected transposition. *Am J Cardiol* 1976;38:109–112.

121. Dusmet M, Oberhaensli I, Cox JN. Ebstein's anomaly of the tricuspid and mitral valves in an otherwise normal heart. *Br Heart J* 1987;58:400–404.

122. Leung M, Rigby ML, Anderson RH, Wyse RK, Macartney FJ. Reversed offsetting of the septal attachments of the atrioventricular valves and Ebstein's malformation of the morphologically mitral valve. *Br Heart J* 1987;57: 184–187.

123. Ferreira SM, Ebaid M, Aiello VD. Ebstein's malformation of the tricuspid and mitral valves associated with hypoplasia of the ascending aorta. *Int J Cardiol* 1991;33: 170–172.

Chapter 15

Abnormalities of the Tricuspid Valve
Straddling, Stenosis, or Congenital Regurgitation

With the exception of the Ebstein's anomaly of the tricuspid valve, most anomalies of the tricuspid valve do not occur in isolation (see Chapter 14). Rather they are found in and may significantly influence the management and course of those conditions in which they participate. Abnormalities of the morphologically tricuspid valve are particularly common in those with pulmonary atresia and intact ventricular septum (see Chapter 23); superoinferior ventricles and crossed atrioventricular connections (see Chapter 44), and complete transposition of the great arteries with ventricular septal defect and/or left ventricular outflow tract obstruction (see Chapter 35). In those patients with discordant atrioventricular connections whether or not the ventriculoarterial connection is also discordant, one should also anticipate abnormalities of the morphologically systemic (tricuspid) valve (see Chapters 36 and 42). Suffice it to say that abnormalities of the atrioventricular junction, whether tricuspid or mitral, are best defined anatomically as well as functionally by the application of cross-sectional echocardiography with Doppler and color-flow assessment. The anatomy of the normal tricuspid valve in the human and the surgical anatomy of the tricuspid valve have received considerable attention.[1-5] An imperforate tricuspid valve must be distinguished from an absent atrioventricular connection (see Chapters 14 and 39). The peculiar developmental complex of an imperforate tricuspid valve, an intact ventricular septum, and absent pulmonary valve with its unusual myocardium is considered in Chapter 22.

Tricuspid Valve Abnormalities Producing Right Ventricular Outflow Tract Obstruction

It is well known that one of the expressions of Ebstein's anomaly of the tricuspid valve is a degree of right ventricular outflow tract obstruction reflecting attachment of the anterosuperior of the tricuspid valve leaflet to the infundibulum (Figs. 15-1 and 15-2). This is discussed fully in Chapter 14. The tricuspid valve may normally be considered as comprising membranous leaflets attached proximally to the ventricular wall and distally to the tension apparatus of tendinous cords and papillary muscles.[6] Viewed then in the context of a departure from the normal tricuspid valve, there are a number of abnormalities of the tricuspid valve with or without displacement promoting right ventricular outflow tract obstruction.[6-12] Such abnormalities include a pouch-like diverticulum of the septal leaflet that protrudes into the right ventricular outflow tract. As pointed out by Gerlis and colleagues,[6] this malformation has also been described as an aneurysm of the tricuspid valve, but this must be differentiated from a true aneurysm of the membranous septum.[13-18] In the consideration of a pouch-like or windsock deformity of the tricuspid valve are an ectopic tricuspid valve or leaflet that has its proximal attachment to the

From: Freedom RM, Mawson JB, Yoo SJ, Benson LN: *Congenital Heart Disease: Textbook of Angiocardiography.* Armonk NY, Futura Publishing Co., Inc. ©1997.

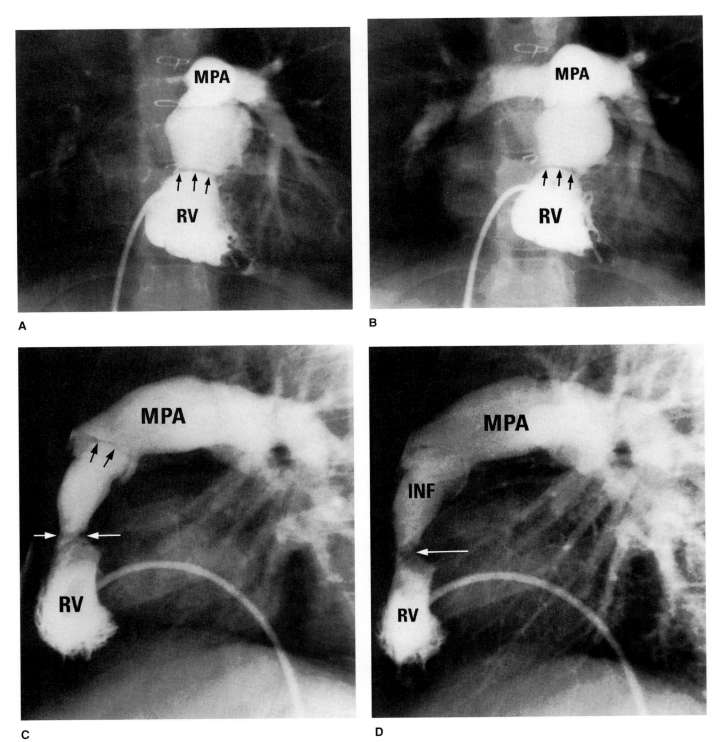

Fig. 15-1: A divided right ventricle secondary to a malattached tricuspid valve, right ventricular hypoplasia, and pulmonary stenosis.
A and B: Two frames from frontal right ventriculography show an underdeveloped right ventricle with attenuation of apical trabecular zone and a linear density (arrows) dividing the right ventricle. **C and D:** Two lateral frames from right ventriculography show the participation of the tricuspid valve (white arrows), as well as the pulmonary valve stenosis (black arrows).

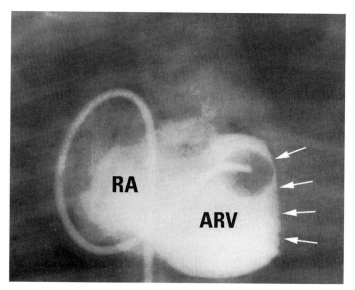

Fig. 15-2: A patient with an imperforate form of Ebstein's malformation of the tricuspid valve producing tricuspid atresia and clearly dividing the right ventricle.
Frame from frontal angiocardiography performed in the atrialized right ventricle. The linear distal attachments divide the right ventricle at the junction between the smooth inlet and apical trabecular zones.

ventricular wall of the infundibulum instead of the atrioventricular junction. In other patients linear malattachment of the tricuspid valve may divide the right ventricle (Fig. 15-1). These abnormalities of the tricuspid valve, which are really quite uncommon, contribute to the variations of a divided right ventricle (see Chapter 17), although these mechanisms are related to abnormalities of the atrioventricular valve, not muscular (see Chapter 14).

One can define a number of anomalies of the tricuspid valve that do not necessarily participate in a functional disturbance either of the valve itself or secondarily. Some of these may be found during investigation or surgery for other conditions. These include double-orifice of the tricuspid valve, frank duplication, accessory papillary muscles, endodermal cyst, etc.[19-22]

Straddling and Overriding Tricuspid Valve

Straddling of an atrioventricular valve is an anomaly that may confound a biventricular repair. This condition must be differentiated from overriding of an atrioventricular valve annulus (see Chapter 3, Fig. 3-21).[23-53] Straddling of an atrioventricular valve indicates implies that tension apparatus of atrioventricular valve has biventricular insertions. Anderson and colleagues[23,24] define straddling of an atrioventricular valve as when its tension apparatus is attached to both sides of the ventricular septum. Overriding refers to that situation when the atrioventricular valve annulus is connected to ventricles on both sides of a septal structure. Thus, an atrioventricular valve can straddle a

septal structure, may override it, or may straddle and override. Straddling and overriding of the atrioventricular valve can occur when one atrioventricular connection is either absent or imperforate, and rarely, both atrioventricular valves can straddle the ventricular septal defect.[23,24,28,30,32,39,45] Straddling and overriding of an atrioventricular valve implies the presence of a ventricular septal defect.[23,24,27,30-32,36-39,47-49] In this regard, however, Isomatsu and colleagues[54] recently reported a patient with a straddling tricuspid valve without a ventricular septal defect. In this patient with pulmonary atresia, the straddling and overriding tricuspid valve had two orifices connecting to the right and left ventricles. Valve tissue separated both orifices, and by virtue of firm attachments to the crest of the ventricular septum, sealed off the anticipated interventricular communication.

An extensive literature is devoted to the morphology of the straddling and overriding atrioventricular valves, and the types of hearts in which these anomalies occur.[23-54] Straddling of the morphologically tricuspid valve implies a posterior inlet ventricular septal defect and a septum not extending to the crux of the heart, while straddling of the mitral valve necessitates an anteriorly positioned ventricular septal defect and a ventricular septum that does extend to the crux (Fig. 15-3).[23-53] The straddling of the tricuspid valve occurs with a malaligned inlet septum, the posterior part of which is displaced rightward from the crux cordis. When the straddling is pronounced, then a double-inlet connection to the left ventricle results. This is in contrast to the straddling mitral valve that occurs with a leftward malalignment of the anterior part of the interventricular septum. As the malalignment involves the anterior part of the septum and is away from the outlet, the posterior inlet septum reaches the crux cordis. Straddling of the mitral valve (see Chapter 25) is commonly seen in patients with double-outlet right ventricle (see Chapter 37). When the straddling of the mitral valve is pronounced, a double-inlet connection to the right ventricle results. Categorization of the degree of atrioventricular valve straddling has been provided by the Mayo Clinic.[33] Type A straddling indicates relatively minor straddling with chordae inserting into the contralateral ventricle near the crest of the ventricular septum. When the chordae insert onto the contralateral ventricular septum, this is considered type B. The most severe form of straddling is characterized by chordal attachments into the contralateral ventricular free wall or its papillary muscles. Clearly, any degree of straddling of an atrioventricular valve that is more than mild or trivial usually obviates a biventricular repair, and patients with straddling atrioventricular valves will only be candidates for Fontan's procedure or one of its many modifications (see Chapter 39). Today, with a systematic approach to cross-sectional echocardiography, it is quite straightforward to recognize straddling of an atrio-

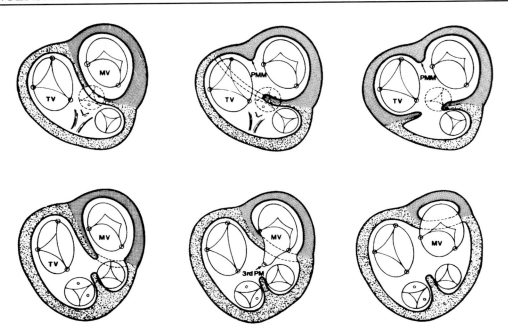

Fig. 15-3: Diagrams showing differences between straddling of tricuspid and mitral valves.
Upper panel: Diagrams showing the pathology of straddling of the tricuspid valve in situs solitus with a right ventricle having a right hand pattern of ventricular organization. The straddling tricuspid valve occurs through an inlet ventricular septal defect. From left to right: The inlet septum is malaligned from the atrial septum and the crux cordis towards the right side. The embryological remnant dividing the ventricular inlet below the right and left atrioventricular valves may be seen in the posterior aspect of the left ventricle at the crux cordis. This is designated the posteromedian muscle (PMM). When the malalignment is sever, the major part or indeed all of the tricuspid valve as well as the mitral valve are committed to the morphologically left ventricle, and the pathology of a double-inlet left ventricle ensues. **Lower panel:** Diagrams illustrating straddling of the mitral valve in situs solitus, concordant atrioventricular connection (to begin with), and double-outlet right ventricle of the Taussig-Bing type with a right-hand pattern of ventricular organization. The straddling mitral valve occurs through an anterior ventricular septal defect. The anterior part of the ventricular septum is malaligned from the anterior free wall towards the left side. The inlet component of the ventricular septum is in contact with the crux cordis. The straddling component of the mitral valve is supported by the third papillary muscle (3rd PM) in the right ventricle. When the malalignment is severe, the major part or all of the mitral valve as well as the tricuspid valve may be committed to the morphologically right ventricle, and the pathology, Indeed, the atrioventricular connection of double-inlet right ventricle ensues.

ventricular valve, or overriding prior to cardiac catheterization and angiocardiography and surgery. Among those conditions promoting a double-outlet right atrium, straddling and overriding of the tricuspid valve, a double-orifice tricuspid valve, and atrial septal malalignment are other conditions that must be brought into this differential (Fig. 15-4). A malaligned atrial septum is more commonly found in patients with an atrioventricular septal defect (see Chapter 5).

There are certain conditions where one should anticipate or at least exclude that a straddling and/or overriding tricuspid valve as straddling and/or overriding an atrioventricular valve will lead to underfilling of the ipsilateral ventricle. These conditions include any patient with a hypoplastic morphologically right ventricle; superoinferior ventricles; crossed atrioventricular connections; transposition of the great arteries with a small right ventricle; tetralogy of Fallot with a hypoplastic right ventricle; double-outlet right or left ventricle with a small right ventricle, and mitral atresia with a normal-sized left ventricle. Finally, straddling and overriding of the tricuspid valve are more likely to be ascertained in those patients with an abnormal ven-

triculoarterial connection, than in those with a concordant connection (Figs. 15-5 through 15-8).

Congenital Tricuspid Regurgitation

Isolated congenital tricuspid regurgitation is very uncommon, excluding those patients with Ebstein's malformation of the tricuspid valve. The etiologies of tricuspid regurgitation are diverse, reflecting physiological tricuspid regurgitation to primary tumorous involvement.[55–57] Dysplasia of the tricuspid valve, so-called polyvalvular disease, deficient leaflets, extra leaflets, and prolapse are but some of those conditions producing or associated with tricuspid regurgitation.[58–67] Eichhorn and colleagues[68] provided a classification of tricuspid regurgitation that has been modified for this publication (Table 15-1).

Tricuspid regurgitation may have its basis in an altered valvular morphology, or a functional disturbance of tricuspid valve function may result from a disturbed transitional circulation in the newborn and neonate resulting in transient myocardial ischemia.[56–81] Rarely an altered tricuspid valve function may accompany a pri-

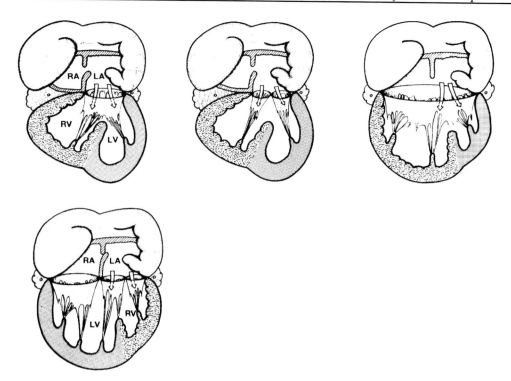

Fig. 15-4: The varying morphologies contributing to a double-outlet right atrium.
Top left: Straddling and overriding tricuspid valve. **Top center:** Double-orifice tricuspid valve with one orifice straddling and overriding. **Top right:** Common atrioventricular orifice with leftward malaligned atrial septum.

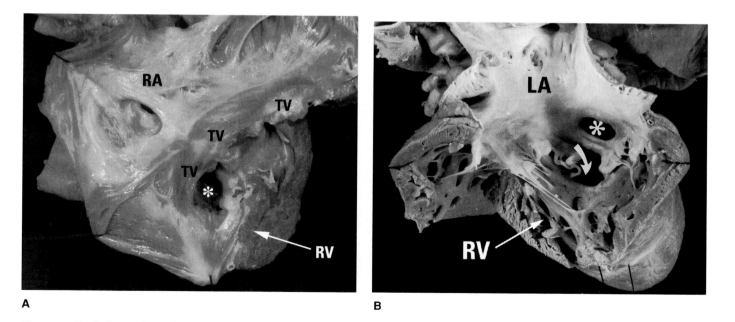

A   B

Fig. 15-5: Pathology of straddling tricuspid valve.
A: In a patient with concordant connections viewed from right ventricular aspect. The mural leaflet of the tricuspid valve straddles and overrides an inlet ventricular septal defect (✻). **B:** In a patient with discordant connections viewed from right ventricular aspect. The tricuspid valve straddles and overrides (arrow) an inlet ventricular septal defect; in addition there is an accessory orifice (✻) that also straddles.

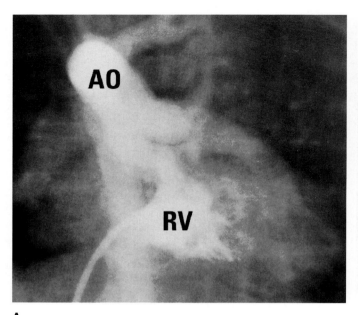

A

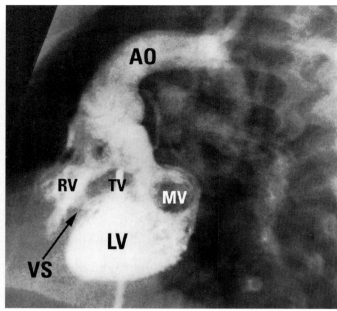

B

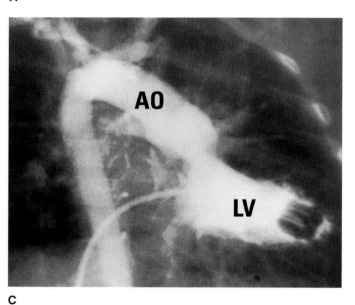

C

Fig. 15-6: Straddling and overriding tricuspid valve in a patient with right ventricular hypoplasia, ventricular septal defect, and single-outlet aorta from right ventricle with pulmonary atresia.
A: The right ventriculogram shows this chamber to be small, with opacification of the aorta. **B:** This long axial oblique view shows the overriding and straddling tricuspid valve relative to the ventricular septum, and the anterior aorta. **C:** The left ventricle is of normal size as demonstrated by this right anterior oblique left ventriculogram.

mary disorder of the right ventricular myocardium, Uhl's anomaly of the right ventricle, in which the myocardium of the right ventricle is absent, or nearly so.[82-90] A deficiency of the right ventricular myocardium, or a profoundly thinned right ventricular myocardium is particularly common in some forms of pulmonary atresia and intact ventricular septum (see Chapter 23).

Anatomic abnormalities of the tricuspid valve are uncommon in isolation. In the neonatal period, tricuspid regurgitation usually accompanies severe right ventricular outflow tract obstruction with an intact ventricular septum (critical pulmonary stenosis or atresia) (see Chapter 23); Ebstein's anomaly of the tricuspid valve (see Chapter 14), or an atrioventricular septal de-

fect (see Chapter 5). An unguarded tricuspid orifice results in tricuspid regurgitation, but again this entity, very rare, has usually been observed in the patient with pulmonary atresia and intact ventricular septum and in the patient with a double-chambered right ventricle.[60,61,91-94] An almost completely unguarded tricuspid valve has only rarely been mentioned.[59,60] Whereas isolated clefts of the tricuspid valve have been described and may be responsible for tricuspid regurgitation,[68] more likely a dysplastic tricuspid valve will be the morphological culprit.[58-60,63,65-67] An anomalous arcade first described as a cause of congenital mitral insufficiency has been identified in an infant with an arcade deformity of both atrioventricular valves and severe insufficiency of both atrioventricular valves.

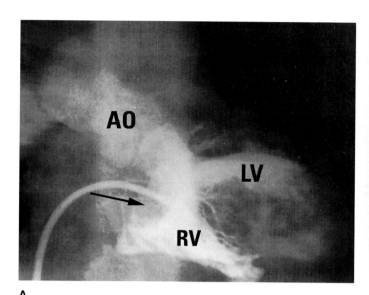
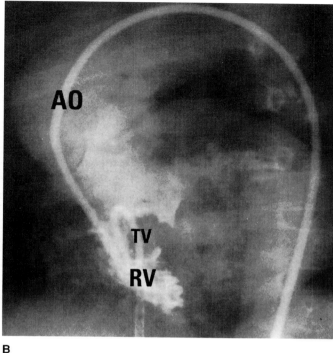

A **B**

Fig. 15-7: Single-outlet aorta with pulmonary atresia, a small right ventricle, and tricuspid annular override.
A: Frontal right ventriculogram shows a small right ventricle and tricuspid valve with a single-outlet aorta. **B:** The overiding tricuspid valve is seen in this hepatoclavicular projection.

Transient myocardial ischemia of the newborn may result in tricuspid regurgitation. Today this entity is well accepted, but there was considerable skepticism surrounding this entity in the early 1970s when it was first described clinically by Rowe and Hoffman.[79] A wealth of pathological, clinical, biochemical, and scintigraphic evidence has now firmly established this disorder.[69–81] Transient myocardial ischemia results from a disturbed transitional circulation, and its impact may be focused on either right or left subendomyocardial perfusion.[79,80] There is ample histopathologic evidence of myocardial ischemia in stressed neonates and the clinical, electrocardiographic, and echocardiographic correlates of disturbed myocardial perfusion are represented. The baby with little or no prenatal care, the infant of a diabetic mother, the product of a precipitous delivery or a delivery complicated by placenta previa or abruption is a candidate for a disturbed transitional circulation and myocardial ischemia. Yet in some neonates without structural heart disease and without evidence of a disturbed transitional circulation or fetal closure of the arterial duct, Doppler interrogation will demonstrate tricuspid insufficiency.[80a]

Eichhorn and colleagues[68] have reported as the etiology of tricuspid regurgitation in the adult so-called clefts in the anterior leaflet. Others have reported the tricuspid valve with six leaflets;[64] a myxoma of the tricuspid valve including a patient with coronary artery aneurysms secondary to Kawasaki disorder,[56,57] and tri-

cuspid regurgitation after cardiac surgery or myocardial biopsy in the monitoring of cardiac rejection.[95,96] Traumatic disruption of the tricuspid valve, infective endocarditis, especially in those with a history of intravenous substance abuse, those with pulmonary artery hypertension in mitral stenosis, primary pulmonary vascular obstructive disease, or cardiac muscle disorder; the failing right ventricle after conventional cardiac surgery (ie, repair of tetralogy of Fallot; the systemic right ventricle after Mustard's or Senning's atrial repair of transposition of the great arteries) are other conditions causing tricuspid regurgitation.[2,4,5] Burrows and colleagues[96a] have reviewed those features of the tricuspid valve contributing to left ventricular-to-right atrial shunting in a perimembranous ventricular septal defect.[96a] This only infrequently indicates a primary abnormality of the tricuspid valve.

The application of cross-sectional echocardiography with Doppler and color-flow imaging should readily differentiate a functional disturbance from a pathological anomaly of the tricuspid valve. It may be necessary in some of these babies to differentiate functional from organic pulmonary atresia. Some years ago we advocated prostaglandin-enhanced retrograde aortography as one method to establish the basis of the pulmonary atresia.[97] Today the application of Doppler and color-flow echocardiographic imaging should distinguish between functional and organic pulmonary atresia.[98–100] In the patient with functional pulmonary atre-

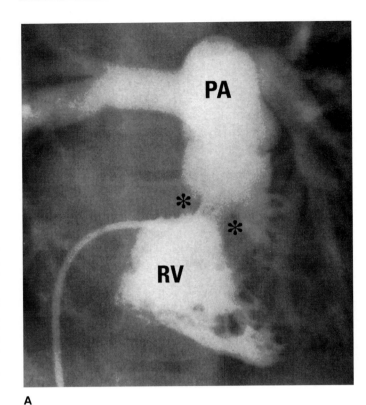

A

Fig. 15-8: Straddling and overriding tricuspid valve in a patient with a divided right ventricle that is hypoplastic.
A: Frontal right ventriculogram shows a small ventricle divided by anomalous muscle bundles (✳) at the os infundibulum. **B and C:** Frames from a left ventriculography filmed in the hepatoclavicular projection demonstrating the straddling and overriding tricuspid valve (✳).

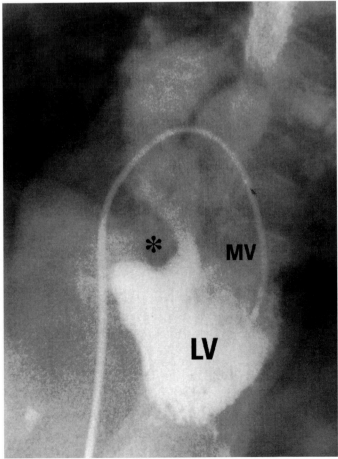

B

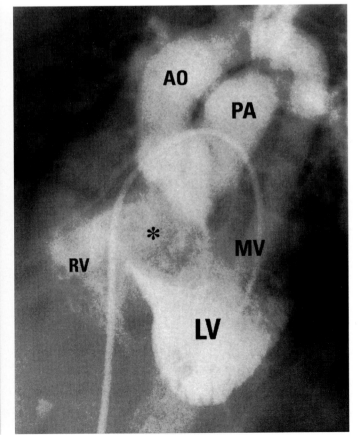

C

Table 15-1

Etiology of Tricuspid Regurgitation

1. Physiological tricuspid regurgitation

2. Secondary tricuspid regurgitation
   (reflecting pulmonary artery hypertension)

3. Acquired tricuspid regurgitation

   Infective endocarditis
   Rheumatic heart disease
   Trauma
   Tumor
   Sequelae of surgery
   Transient myocardial ischemia

4. Primary or congenital tricuspid regurgitation

   Ebstein's anomaly
   Dysplasia of the tricuspid valve
   Abnormal number of leaflets
   Supernumerary leaflet
   Windsock deformity
   Tricuspid valve prolapse
   Specific types of congenital heart disease
      Pulmonary atresia and intact ventricular septum
      Atrioventricular septal defect
      Critical pulmonary stenosis
      Unguarded tricuspid orifice
      Congenitally corrected transposition of the great arteries
      etc.

sia despite an anatomically normal pulmonary outflow tract, pulmonary regurgitation is seen in diastole. This observation, documented fully by prostaglandin-enhanced retrograde aortography, is now fully recognizable by application of Doppler and color-flow echocardiographic imaging.

Congenital Tricuspid Stenosis

Isolated congenital stenosis is distinctly uncommon. Rather, stenosis of the tricuspid valve and associated annular hypoplasia are well known to accompany a panoply of congenital heart malformations (Fig. 15-9) (see also Chapters 5, 16, 17, and 23). A stenotic expression of Ebstein's malformation of the tricuspid valve has been well described (see Chapter 14, Figs. 14-12 through 14-15) (Fig. 15-2). The inlet of the right ventricle has been thoroughly examined in the patient with pulmonary atresia and intact ventricular septum, and annular hypoplasia as well as abnormalities of virtually all aspects of the tricuspid valve, its free-valve margin, and support apparatus has been described and these data are discussed in Chapter 23.[100–107]

Isolated congenital tricuspid valve stenosis has been described in a number of patients, but recognition of this condition is extremely uncommon in the pediatric age group.[108–114] Hypoplasia of the tricuspid valve with or without stenosis of the free-valve margin and

tension apparatus is often observed in those patients with so-called isolated right ventricular hypoplasia (see Chapter 16). Many of the reports of isolated congenital tricuspid valve stenosis fail to distinguish between hypoplasia of a normally formed tricuspid valve and its annulus from annular hypoplasia and stenosis of the free-valve margin and support apparatus. The routine assessment of any form of complex congenital heart disease should include scrutiny of the right and left atrioventricular junction, comparison of annular diameters by cross-sectional echocardiography, and calculation of a tricuspid Z-value.[107] In the presence of right ventricular hypoplasia, it is essential that an abnormality of the ipsilateral atrioventricular junction be excluded. But because of the all-too-frequently associated ventricular septal defect, the size and development of the ventricle (ie, normal or nearly so) will not focus attention on its inlet. That is why discipline and consistency are required to compare the tricuspid and mitral valves with cross-sectional echocardiography.

Tricuspid valve stenosis has been identified in a wide variety of congenitally malformed hearts including tetralogy of Fallot (see Chapter 20); pulmonary atresia and intact ventricular septum (see Chapter 23); complete (see Chapter 35) or corrected transposition of the great arteries (see Chapter 36), and double-outlet right (see Chapter 37) or left (see Chapter 38) ventricle. Tricuspid stenosis has also been described in the patient with anatomically corrected malposition of the great arteries (see Chapter 43) and a hypoplastic tricuspid valve is well recognized in those patients with super-

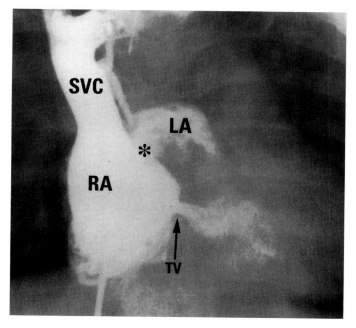

Fig. 15-9: Congenital stenosis of the tricuspid valve in a patient with concordant connections, a ventricular septal defect, and pulmonary stenosis.
This frontal right atriogram shows the very small tricuspid valve with right-to-left atrial shunting (✱)

oinferior ventricles with or without crossed or twisted atrio-ventricular connections (see Chapter 44). Obstruction of the tricuspid valve by cardiac tumors, particularly the rhabdomyoma is also well documented (see Chapter 49). Finally, tricuspid stenosis may be encountered in those with congenital polyvalvular disease, and thus trisomy 13–15 and 18.[65–67] In these patients the valve tissue is very primitive, the commissures are poorly delineated, and the valve is very thickened, fleshy, and bulky. The histopathologic correlates to these gross abnormalities include proliferation of the spongiosa and hypoelastification and disruption of the normal valvular architecture.[65]

The Tricuspid Valve and the Infundibular Septum

Attachment of the tricuspid valve to the infundibular septum probably in itself does not convey any functional disturbance.[115,116] However, resection of the infundibular septum as part of the surgical repair of any complex cardiac malformation has the potential for disruption of the tricuspid valve tension apparatus, and the sequelae of iatrogenic tricuspid regurgitation. Resection of the infundibular septum may be required in the repair of many forms of abnormal ventriculoarterial connection including transposition of the great arteries, ventricular septal defect, and left ventricular outflow tract obstruction; double-outlet right ventricle with restrictive ventricular septal defect, etc.[115–125] It is within the domain of cross-sectional echocardiography to recognize the attachment of the tricuspid valve tension apparatus to the infundibular septum.[115,116]

The Systemic Atrioventricular Valve in Discordant Atrioventricular Connections

Those abnormalities of the systemic atrioventricular valve in discordant atrioventricular connections are discussed in Chapters 36 and 42.

Imaging of Abnormalities of the Morphologically Tricuspid Valve

It has been stated several times in this chapter that abnormalities of the tricuspid valve, its form, annular dimension, and its function are best assessed by cross-sectional echocardiography, Doppler, and color-flow interrogation.

Those abnormalities of the tricuspid valve producing right ventricular outflow tract obstruction including the windsock deformity or pouch, ectopic or accessory leaflet, etc. are most uncommon.[6–12] Some of these abnormalities will be attached or fixed to the infundibulum. From frontal and lateral right ventricular cineangiocardiography these abnormalities will often demonstrate a phasic motion commensurate with the

cardiac cycle. These windsock or pouch-like abnormalities will appear as a curvilinear density protruding into the right ventricular inlet.

With rare exception,[54] a straddling and overriding tricuspid valve necessitates the presence of a posterior muscular inlet ventricular septal defect, usually large. Today all degrees of straddling of the right atrioventricular valve should be recognized from cross-sectional echocardiography (Figs. 15-5 through 15-9).[24,25,33–35,38,44,52,126] Indeed, minor degrees of straddling where tension apparatus of the tricuspid valve is attached to the crest of the interventricular septum will not be detected from cineangiocardiography. Virtually all angiographic techniques pale in comparison to cross-sectional echocardiography in the definition of this abnormality. We and others have advocated right atrial angiocardiography in frontal, lateral, and hepato-clavicular four-chamber projections to demonstrate two streams of contrast passing forward into the right and left ventricle.[25,29,36,38,48,49,51,52] The particular direction of the two streams of contrast will be determined in large part by the spatial orientation of the ventricular inlets. This technique can be used to advantage when the atrial septum is intact or nearly so. When a large interatrial communication is present, then right-to-left shunting at atrial level may confound this approach. Demonstration of the straddling tricuspid valve may also be facilitated by injection of contrast material into the morphologically left ventricle using the hepatoclavicular four-chamber projection (Figs. 15-7 through 15-9). This should profile the posterior muscular ventricular septal defect, and the unopacified contrast from the right atrium entering the left ventricle. It has been unusual for selective right ventriculography to demonstrate the straddling and overriding tricuspid valve. Nonetheless information from this injection will be helpful in determining the size of this chamber.

Right ventriculography in frontal and lateral projections will define the size of this chamber, and in the absence of ventricular ectopy, the presence and severity of tricuspid regurgitation. The catheter should not be wedged, but should move freely within the right ventricle, and it should be positioned so as not to deform the tricuspid valve. In those patients with very severe tricuspid regurgitation, both the right ventricle and the right atrium will become very dilated. With the catheter through the tricuspid valve there is always the possibility, indeed the reality, that the presence and severity of tricuspid regurgitation may be exaggerated. The tricuspid valve tissue may appear quite thickened.

Hypoplasia and/or stenosis of the tricuspid valve is uncommon in isolation, and we have listed elsewhere in this chapter those anomalies associated with congenital tricuspid valve stenosis. Again, the demonstration of a congenitally stenotic tricuspid valve is best afforded by cross-sectional echocardiographic techniques, with derivation of the Z-value. When the morphologically right ventricle is underdeveloped, then the inlet to this ventricle, the tricuspid valve, its annulus, and subvalvular apparatus must be carefully examined. Appreciation of a small tricuspid valve annulus from the contour of unopacified blood entering the right ventricle has led us to re-examine the cross-sectional echocardiogram, performing after the fact those so important measurements that should have been performed before the patient ever entered the cardiac catheterization facility. While the angiocardiographic correlates to a parachute mitral valve have been fully documented,[127,128] the parachute deformity of the tricuspid valve has only been recognized at autopsy as has the tricuspid anomalous arcade.[129,130] Those specific abnormalities of the atrioventricular junction in patients with double-inlet ventricle will be addressed fully in Chapter 40. In those forms of malformed hearts we will use the terminology of right and left atrioventricular valve as advocated by Restivo and colleagues.[131]

Tricuspid Valve Disease with Severe Tricuspid Regurgitation in the Fetus

Considerable data have been accumulated indicating that the fetus does not tolerate severe tricuspid regurgitation.[132–142] This results in right heart dilatation, cardiac failure, fetal hydrops and/or atrial flutter in some, and lung hypoplasia in many, with fetal death.

Excellent correlation has been found between echocardiographic and morphological investigations of those lesions of the tricuspid valve recognized during fetal life.[134,137,141,142] It should be remembered that fetal tricuspid regurgitation does not always imply a structural abnormality of the tricuspid valve and/or functional or anatomic pulmonary outflow tract obstruction.[143] Respondek and colleagues[143] defined the prevalence of fetal tricuspid regurgitation retrospectively in a group of 733 singleton fetuses referred for routine fetal echocardiography. The prevalence of this abnormality was 6.8%. Tricuspid valve regurgitation was most frequent in the group referred for fetal echocardiography for the evaluation of indomethacin exposure, followed by maternal diabetes. Factors associated with tricuspid valve regurgitation in these patients included fetal ductal constriction, abnormal heart rhythm, atrial septal aneurysm, congestive heart failure, pericardial effusion, myocardial hypertrophy, and extracardiac malformations. Fetal tricuspid valve regurgitation was considered trivial in 80% and significant in 20%.

Tricuspid Valve Prolapse: See Chapter 25.

The Imperforate Tricuspid Valve: See Chapter 22.

References

1. Silver MD, Lam JHC, Ranganathan N, Wigle ED. Morphology of the human tricuspid valve. *Circulation* 1971; 43:333–348.
2. Virmani R. The tricuspid valve. *Mayo Clin Proc* 1988;63: 943–946.
3. Victor S, Nayak VM. The tricuspid valve is bicuspid. *J Heart Valve Dis* 1994;3:27–36.
4. Hauck AJ, Freeman DP, Ackermann DM, Danielson GK, Edwards WD Surgical pathology of the tricuspid valve: A study of 363 cases spanning 25 years. *Mayo Clin Proc* 1988;63:851–863.
5. Pasque M, Williams WG, Coles JG, Trusler GA, Freedom RM. Tricuspid valve replacement in children. *Ann Thorac Surg* 1987;44:164–168.
6. Gerlis LM, Ho SY, Rigby ML. Right ventricular outflow obstruction by anomalies of the tricuspid valve: Report of a windsock diverticulum. *Pediatr Cardiol* 1992;13: 59–62.
7. Ehrenhaft JL, Theilen EO, Fisher J. Ectopic tricuspid leaflet producing symptoms of infundibular pulmonary stenosis. *Ann Surg* 1959;150:249–251.
8. Pate JW, Ainger LE, Butterick OD. A new form of right ventricular outflow tract obstruction. Case report. *Am Heart J* 1964;68:249–253.
9. Pate JW, Richardson RL, Giles HH. Accessory tricuspid leaflet producing right ventricular outflow obstruction. *N Engl J Med* 1968;279:867–868.
10. Flege JB, Vlad P, Ehrenhaft JL. Aneurysm of tricuspid valve causing infundibular obstruction. *Ann Thorac Surg* 1967;3:446–448.
11. Monterroso J, Fonseca MC, Cunha D, Ramalhao C.

12. La Corte MA, Boxer RA, Singh S, Parnell V Jr, Goldman M. Echocardiographic features of tetralogy of Fallot with an accessory tricuspid valve leaflet. *Am Heart J* 1985; 110:1297–1299.
13. Chesler E, Korns ME, Edwards JE. Anomalies of the tricuspid valve, including pouches, resembling aneurysms of the membranous ventricular septum. *Am J Cardiol* 1968;21:661–668.
14. Anderson RH, Lenox C, Zuberbuhler J. Mechanisms of closure of perimembranous ventricular septal defect. *Am J Cardiol* 1983;52:341–345.
15. Das JK, Jahnke EJ, Walker WJ. Aneurysm of membranous septum with interventricular septal defect producing right ventricular outflow tract obstruction. *Circulation* 1964;30:429–433.
16. Freedom RM, White RD, Pieroni DR, Varghese JP, Krovetz LJ, Rowe RD. The natural history of the so-called aneurysm of the membranous ventricular septum in childhood. *Circulation* 1974;49:375–384.
17. Ignaszewski AP, Collins-Nakai RL, Kasza LA, Gulamhussein SS, Penkoske PA, Taylor DA. Aneurysm of the membranous ventricular septum producing subpulmonic outflow tract obstruction. *Can J Cardiol* 1994;10: 67–70.
18. Bonvicini M, Piovaccari G, Picchio F. Severe subpulmonary obstruction caused by aneurysmal tissue tag complicating an infundibular perimembranous ventricular septal defect. *Br Heart J* 1982;48:189–191.
19. Yoo S-J, Houde C, Moes CAF, Perrin DG, Freedom RM,

Burrows PE. A case report of double-orifice tricuspid valve. *Int J Cardiol* 1993;39:85–87.

20. Cascos AS, Rabago P, Sokolowski M. Duplication of the tricuspid valve. *Br Heart J* 1967;29:943–946.

21. Machens G, Vahl CF, Hofmann R, Wolf D, Hagl S. Entodermal inclusion cyst of the tricuspid valve. *Thorac Cardiovasc Surg* 1991;39:296–298.

22. Prayson RA, Ratliff NB. Two unusual congenital anomalies of the tricuspid valve. *Am J Cardiovasc Pathol* 1990;3:189–194.

23. Anderson RH. Straddling and overriding valves. *Int J Cardiol* 1985;9:323–326.

23a.Serraf A, Nakamura T, Lacour-Gayet F, Piot D, Bruniaux J, Touchot A, Sousa-Uva M, Houyel L, Planche C. Surgical approaches for double-outlet right ventricle or transposition of the great arteries associated with straddling atrioventricular valves. *J Thorac Cardiovasc Surg* 1996; 111:527.

24. Anderson RH, Macartney FJ, Shinebourne EA, Tynan M. *Paediatric Cardiology*. Volume 2. Edinburgh: Churchill Livingstone; 1987, pp. 697–709.

25. Aziz KU, Paul MH, Muster AJ, Idriss FS. Positional abnormalities of atrioventricular valves in transposition of the great arteries including double outlet right ventricle, atrioventricular valve straddling and malattachment. *Am J Cardiol* 1979;44:1135–1145.

26. Becker AE, Ho SY, Caruso G, Milo S, Anderson RH. Straddling right atrioventricular valves in atrioventricular discordance. *Circulation* 1980;61:1133–1141.

27. Bharati S, McAllister HA Jr, Lev M. Straddling and displaced atrioventricular orifices and valves. *Circulation* 1979;60:673–684.

28. Bini RM, Pellegrino PA, Mazzucco A, Gallucci V, Milanesi O, Maddalena F, Thiene G. Tricuspid atresia with double-outlet left atrium. *Chest* 1980;78:109–111.

29. Freedom RM, Culham G, Rowe RD. The criss-cross and superoinferior ventricular heart: An angiocardiographic study. *Am J Cardiol* 1978;42:620–628.

30. Ho SY, Milo S, Anderson RH, Macartney FJ, Goodwin A, Becker AE, Wenink ACG, Gerlis LM, Wilkinson JL. Straddling atrioventricular valve with absent atrioventricular connection: Report of 10 cases. *Br Heart J* 1982; 47:344–352.

31. Liberthson RR, Paul MH, Muster AJ, Arcilla RA, Eckner FAO, Lev M. Straddling and displaced atrioventricular orifices and valves with primitive ventricles. *Circulation* 1971;43:213–226.

32. Milo S, Ho Yen S, Macartney FJ, Wilkinson JL, Becker AE, Wenink ACG, Gittenberger-de Groot AC, Anderson RH. Straddling and overriding atrioventricular valves: Morphology and classification. *Am J Cardiol* 1979;44: 1122–1134.

33. Rice MJ, Seward JB, Edwards WD, Hagler DJ, Danielson GK, Puga FJ, Tajik AJ. Straddling atrioventricular valve: Two-dimensional echocardiographic diagnosis, classification and surgical implications. *Am J Cardiol* 1985;55: 505–513.

34. Sieg K, Hagler DJ, Ritter DG, McGoon DC, Maloney JD, Seward JB, David GD. Straddling right atrioventricular valve in criss-cross atrioventricular relationship. *Mayo Clin Proc* 1977;52:561–568.

35. Smallhorn JF, Tommasini G, Macartney FJ. Detection and assessment of straddling and overriding atrioventricular valves by two dimensional echocardiography. *Br Heart J* 1981;46:254–262.

36. Soto B, Ceballos R, Nath PH, Bini RM, Pacifico AD, Bargeron LM Jr. Overriding atrioventricular valves. An angiographic-anatomical correlate. *Int J Cardiol* 1985; 9:327–339.

37. Wenink ACG and Gittenberger-de Groot AC. Straddling mitral and tricuspid valves: Morphologic differences and developmental backgrounds. *Am J Cardiol* 1982;49: 1959–1977.

38. Freedom RM. Supero-Inferior Ventricles, Criss-cross atrioventricular connections, and the straddling atrioventricular valve. In: Freedom RM, Benson LN, Smallhorn JF, eds. *Neonatal Heart Disease*. London: Springer Verlag; 1992, pp. 667–678.

39. Coto EO, Calabro R, Marsico F, Arranz JSL. Right atrial outlet atresia with straddling left atrioventricular valve: A form of double-outlet atrium. *Br Heart J* 1981;45: 317–324.

40. Danielson GK, Tabry IF, Ritter DG, Fulton RE. Surgical repair of criss-cross heart with straddling atrioventricular valve. *J Thorac Cardiovasc Surg* 1979;77:847–851.

41. de Vivie R, Van Praagh S, Bein G, Eigster G, Vogt J, Van Praagh R. Transposition of the great arteries with straddling tricuspid valve. Report of two cases with acquired subaortic stenosis after main pulmonary artery banding. *J Thorac Cardiovasc Surg* 1989;98:205–213.

42. Freedom RM. Supero-inferior ventricle and criss-cross atrioventricular connections: An analysis of the myth and mystery. In: Belloli GP, Squarcia U, eds. *Modern Problems in Paediatrics. Pediatric Cardiology and Cardiosurgery*. Basel: Karger; 1983, pp. 48–62.

43. Pugliese P, Speroni F, Verunelli F, Tommasini G, Macri R, Eufrate S. Valvola tricuspide a cavaliere isolata. Presentazione di due casi operati con successo. *G Ital Cardiol* 1984;14:609–613.

44. Barron JV, Sahn DJ, Valdes-Cruz LM, Lima CO, Grenadier E, Allen HD, Goldberg SJ. Two-dimensional echocardiographic evaluation of overriding and straddling atrioventricular valves associated with complex congenital heart disease. *Am Heart J* 1984;107: 1006–1014.

45. Aiello V, Ho SY, Anderson RH. Absence of one atrioventricular connection associated with straddling atrioventricular valve: Distinction of a solitary from a common valve and further considerations on the diagnosis of ventricular topology. *Am J Cardiovasc Pathol* 1990; 3:107–113.

46. Ottenkamp J, Wenink AC, Rohmer J, Gittenberger-de Groot A. Tricuspid atresia with overriding imperforate tricuspid membrane: An anatomic variant. *Int J Cardiol* 1984;6:599–613.

47. Anderson RH, Wilcox BR. The surgical anatomy of ventricular septal defects associated with overriding valvar orifices. *J Card Surg* 1993; 8:130–142.

48. Freedom RM, Culham JAG, Moes CAF. *Angiocardiography of Congenital Heart Disease*. New York: McMillan Publishing Company; 1984, pp. 99–110.

49. Soto B, Pacifico AD. *Angiocardiography in Congenital Heart Malformations*. Mt. Kisco, NY: Futura Publishing Company, Inc; 1990, pp. 273–290.

50. Rosenquist GC. Overriding right atrioventricular valve with mitral atresia. *Am Heart J* 1974;87:26–30.

50a. Scheff D, Christianson SD, Rosenquist GC. Overriding right atrioventricular valve with ventricular septal defect. *Johns Hopkins Med J* 1972;130:259–264.

51. Freedom RM, Duncan WJ, Rowe RD. The straddling and overriding atrioventricular valve: Morphological and diagnostic features. In: Gallucci V, Bini RM, Thiene G, eds. *Selected Topics in Cardiac Surgery*. Bologna: Patron Editore Bologna; 1980, pp. 297–322.

52. LaCorte MA, Fellows KE, Williams RG. Overriding tri-

cuspid valve: Echocardiographic and angiocardiographic features. *Am J Cardiol* 1976;37:911–915.

53. Tandon R, Becker AE, Moller JH, Edwards JE. Double inlet left ventricle: Straddling tricuspid valve. *Br Heart J* 1974;36:747–751.

54. Isomatsu Y, Kurosawa H, Imai Y. Straddling tricuspid valve without a ventricular septal defect. *Br Heart J* 1989;62:222–224.

55. Choong CY, Abascal VM, Weyman J, et al. Prevalence of valvular regurgitation by Doppler echocardiography in patients with structurally normal hearts by two-dimensional echocardiography. *Am Heart J* 1989;117:636–642.

56. Pessotto R, Santini F, Piccin C, Consolaro G, Faggian G, Mazzucco A. Cardiac myxoma of the tricuspid valve: Description of a case and review of the literature. *J Heart Valve Dis* 1994;3:344–346.

57. Togo T, Hata M, Sai S, Ito T, Sato N, Haneda K, Mohri H. Tricuspid valve myxoma in a child with coronary artery occlusion and aneurysms. *Cardiovasc Surg* 1994;2:418–419.

58. Becker AE, Becker MJ, Edwards JE. Pathologic spectrum of dysplasia of the tricuspid valve: Features in common with Ebstein's malformation. *Arch Pathol* 1971;91:167–178.

59. Mohan JC, Tatke M, Arora R. Rudimentary dysplastic valvar tissue guarding the tricuspid orifice with dilation of the right ventricle and a patent outflow tract. *Int J Cardiol* 1989;25:136–139.

60. Magotra RA, Agrawal NB, Mall SP, Parikh SJ. Severe dysplasia of the tricuspid valve (unguarded tricuspid anulus): Clinical presentation and surgical treatment (letter). *J Thorac Cardiovasc Surg* 1990;99:174–175.

61. Gussenhoven EJ, Essed CE, Bos E. Unguarded tricuspid orifice with two-chambered right ventricle. *Pediatr Cardiol* 1986;7:175–177.

61a. Agarwala B, Waldman JD, Carbone M. Unguarded tricuspid orifice with Uhl's malformation. *Cardiol Young* 1996;6:177–180.

62. Raichlen JS, Brest AN. Tricuspid valve prolapse. *Cardiovasc Clin* 1987;17:97–109.

63. Daliento L, Nava A, Fasoli G, Mazzucco A, Thiene G. Dysplasia of the atrioventricular valves associated with conduction system anomalies. *Br Heart J* 1984;51:243–251.

64. Ikegaya T, Kurata C, Hayashi H, Kobayashi A, Muro H, Yamazaki N. A case of congenital tricuspid valve abnormality showing six leaflets. *Eur Heart J* 1991;12:94–95.

65. Bharati S, Lev M. Congenital polyvalvular disease. *Circulation* 1973;47:575–586.

66. Musewe NN, Alexander DJ, Teshima I, Smallhorn JF, Freedom RM. Echocardiographic evaluation of the spectrum of cardiac anomalies associated with trisomy 13 and trisomy 18. *J Am Coll Cardiol* 1990;15:673–677.

66a. Balderston SM, Shaffer EM, Washington RL. Congenital poly-valvular disease in trisomy 18: Echocardiographic diagnosis. *Pediatr Cardiol* 1990;11:138–142.

67. Van Praagh S, Truman T, Firpo A, Bano-Rodrigo A, Fried R, McManus B, Engle MA, Van Praagh R. Cardiac malformations in Trisomy-18: A study of 41 postmortem cases. *J Am Coll Cardiol* 1989;13:1586–1597.

68. Eichhorn P, Ritter M, Suetsch G, von Segesser LK, Turina M, Jenni R. Congenital cleft of the anterior tricuspid leaflet with severe tricuspid regurgitation in adults. *J Am Coll Cardiol* 1992;20:1175–1179.

69. Berman WJ, Whitman V, Stanger P, Rudolph AM. Congenital tricuspid incompetence simulating pulmonary atresia with intact ventricular septum: A report of two cases. *Am Heart J* 1978;96:655–661.

70. Boucek RJJ, Graham TPJ, Morgan JP, Atwood GF, Boerth RC. Spontaneous resolution of massive tricuspid insufficiency. *Circulation* 1976;54:795–800.

71. Bucciarelli RL, Nelson RM, Eitzman DV, Egan EAI, Gessner IH. Transient tricuspid insufficiency of the newborn: A form of myocardial dysfunction in stressed newborns. *Pediatrics* 1977;59:330–337.

72. Desa DJ. Myocardial changes in immature infants requiring prolonged ventilation. *Arch Dis Child* 1977;52:138–147.

73. Desa DJ. Myocardial necrosis in the newborn. *Perspect Pediatr Pathol* 1984;8:295–312.

74. Donnelly WH, Bucciarelli RL, Nelson RM. Ischemic papillary muscle necrosis in stressed newborn infants. *J Pediatr* 1980;96:295–300.

75. Esterly JR, Oppenheimer EH. Some aspects of cardiac pathology in infancy and childhood. I. Neonatal myocardial necrosis. *Bull Johns Hopkins Hosp* 1966;119:191–199.

76. Finley JP, Howman-Giles RB, Gilday DL, Bloom KR, Rowe RD. Transient myocardial ischemia of the newborn infant demonstrated by thallium myocardial imaging. *J Pediatr* 1979;94:263–268.

77. Nelson RM, Bucciarelli RL, Eitzman DV, Egan EAI, Gessner IH. Serum creatine phosphokinase MB fraction in newborns with transient tricuspid insufficiency. *N Engl J Med* 1978;298:146–149.

78. Reller MD, Rice MJ, McDonald RW. Tricuspid regurgitation in newborn infants with respiratory distress: Echo-Doppler study. *J Pediatr* 1987;110:760–764.

79. Rowe RD, Hoffman T. Transient myocardial ishemia of the newborn infant: A form of severe cardiorespiratory distress in full-term infants. *J Pediatr* 1972;81:243–250.

80. Rowe RD, Finley JP, Gilday DL, Dische MR, Jimenez CL, Chance GL. Myocardial ischemia in the newborn. In: *Paediatric Cardiology. Volume 2. Heart Disease in the Newborn.* Edinburgh: Churchill Livingstone; 1979, pp. 87–114.

80a. Senocak F, Ozkutlu S. Neonatal tricuspid insufficiency—a Doppler echocardiographic study of 49 cases. *Cardiol Young* 1995;5:172–175.

81. Setzer E, Ermocilla R, Tonkin I, John E, Sansa M, Cassady G. Papillary muscle necrosis in a neonatal autopsy population: Incidence and associated clinical manifestations. *J Pediatr* 1980;96:289–294.

82. Uhl HMS. Previously undescribed congenital malformation of the heart: Almost total absence of the myocardium of the right ventricle. *Bull Johns Hopkins Hosp* 1953;91:197–202.

83. Arcilla RA and Gasul BM. Congenital aplasia or marked hypoplasia of the myocardium of the right ventricle (Uhl's anomaly). *Pediatrics* 1961;58:381–388.

84. Cumming GR, Bowman JM, WhyteHead L. Congenital aplasia of the myocardium of the right ventricle (Uhl's anomaly). *Am Heart J* 1965;70:671–676.

85. Kaul U, Arora R, Rani S. Uhl's anomaly with rudimentary pulmonary valve leaflets: A clinical, hemodynamic, angiographic, and pathologic study. *Am Heart J* 1980;100:673–677.

86. Kinare SG, Panday SR, Deshmukh SM. Congenital aplasia of the right ventricular myocardium (Uhl's anomaly). *Chest* 1969;55:429–431.

87. Perrin EV, Mehrizi A. Isolated Free-Wall Hypoplasia of the Right Ventricle. *Am J Dis Child* 1965;109:558–566.

88. Reeve R and MacDonald D. Partial absence of the right ventricular musculature: Partial parchment heart. *Am J Cardiol* 1964;14:415–419.

89. Zuberbuhler JR, Blank E. Hypoplasia of right ventricular myocardium (Uhl's disease). *AJR* 1970;110:491–496.

90. Perez Diaz L, Quero Jiminez M, Moreno Granadas F, Perez Martinez V, Merino Batres G. Congenital absence of myocardium of right ventricle: Uhl's anomaly. *Br Heart J* 1973;35:570–572.

91. Kanjuh VI, Stevenson JE, Amplatz K, Edwards JE. Congenitally unguarded tricuspid orifice with coexistent pulmonary atresia. *Circulation* 1964;30:911–917.

92. Anderson RH, Silverman NH, Zuberbuhler JR. Congenitally unguarded tricuspid orifice: Its differentiation from Ebstein's malformation in association with pulmonary atresia and intact ventricular septum. *Pediatr Cardiol* 1990;11:86–90.

93. Munoz Castellanos L, Salinas CH, Kuri Nivon M, Garcia Arenal F. Ausencia de la valvula tricuspide. Informe de un caso. *Arch Inst Cardiol Mex* 1992;62:61–67.

94. Freedom RM, Perrin D. The tricuspid valve: Morphologic considerations. In: Freedom RM, ed. *Pulmonary Atresia and Intact Ventricular Septum.* Mt. Kisco, NY: Futura Publishing Company, Inc; 1989, pp. 37–52.

95. Bol-Raap G, Bogers AJ, Boersma H, De Jong PL, Hess J, Bos E. Temporary tricuspid valve detachment in closure of congenital ventricular septal defect. *Eur J Cardiothorac Surg* 1994;8:145–148.

96. Huddleston CB, Rosenbloom M, Goldstein JA, Pasque MK. Biopsy-induced tricuspid regurgitation after cardiac transplantation. *Ann Thorac Surg* 1994;57: 832–836; discussion 836–837.

96a. Burrows PE, Fellows K, Keane J. Cineangiography of the perimembranous ventricular septal defect with left ventricular-right atrial shunt. *J Am Coll Cardiol* 1983; 1:1129–1134.

97. Freedom RM, Culham G, Moes F, Olley PM, Rowe RD. Differentiation of functional and structural pulmonary atresia: Role of aortography. *Am J Cardiol* 1978;41: 914–920.

98. Smallhorn JF, Izukawa T, Benson L, Freedom RM. Non-invasive recognition of functional pulmonary atresia by echocardiography. *Am J Cardiol* 1984;54:925–926.

99. Musewe N, Smallhorn JF. Echocardiographic evaluation of pulmonary atresia with intact ventricular septum. In: Freedom RM, ed. *Pulmonary Atresia and Intact Ventricular Septum.* Mt. Kisco, NY: Futura Publishing Company, Inc; 1989, pp. 133–155.

100. Silberbach GM, Ferrara B, Berry JM, Einzig S, Bass JL. Diagnosis of functional pulmonary atresia using hyperventilation and Doppler ultrasound. *Am J Cardiol* 1987; 59:709–711.

101. Elliott LP, Adams PJ, Edwards JE. Pulmonary atresia with intact ventricular septum. *Br Heart J* 1963;25: 489–501.

102. Anderson RH, Macartney FJ, Shinebourne EA, Tynan M. *Paediatric Cardiology.* Edinburgh: Churchill Livingstone; 1987, pp. 711–720.

103. Van Praagh R, Ando M, Van Praagh S, Senno A, Hougen TJ, Novak G, Hastreiter AR. Pulmonary atresia: Anatomic considerations. In: *The Child With Congenital Heart Disease After Surgery.* Mt. Kisco, NY: Futura Publishing Company, Inc; 1976, pp. 103–135.

104. Bharati S, McAllister HAJ, Chiemmongkoltip P, Lev M. Congenital pulmonary atresia with tricuspid insufficiency: Morphologic study. *Am J Cardiol* 1977;40: 70–75.

105. Freedom RM, Dische MR, Rowe RD. The tricuspid valve in pulmonary atresia and intact ventricular septum. *Arch Pathol Lab Med* 1978;102:28–31.

106. Freedom RM, Perrin D. The tricuspid valve: Morphologic considerations. In: Freedom RM, ed. *Pulmonary Atresia and Intact Ventricular Septum.* Mt. Kisco, NY: Futura Publishing Company, Inc; 1989, pp. 37–52.

107. Hanley FL, Sade RM, Blackstone EH, Kirklin JW, Freedom RM, Nanda NC. Outcomes in neonatal pulmonary atresia with intact ventricular septum. *J Thorac Cardiovasc Surg* 1993;105:406–427.

108. Calleja HB, Hosier DM, Kissane RW. Congenital tricuspid stenosis. The diagnostic value of cineangiocardiography and hepatic pulse tracing. *Am J Cardiol* 1960; 6:821–825.

109. Dimich I, Goldfinger P, Steinfeld L, Lukban SB. Congenital tricuspid stenosis. Case treated by heterograft replacement of the tricuspid valve. *Am J Cardiol* 1973;31: 89–92.

110. Keefe JW, Wolk MJ, Levine HJ. Isolated tricuspid valvular stenosis. *Am J Cardiol* 1970;25:252–256.

111. Svane S. Congenital tricuspid stenosis. A report on six autopsied cases. *Scand J Thorac Cardiovasc Surg* 1971; 5:232–239.

112. Chuah SY, Hughes-Nurse J, Rowlands DB. A successful pregnancy in a patient with congenital tricuspid stenosis and a patent oval foramen. *Int J Cardiol* 1992;34: 112–144.

113. Lokhandwala YY, Rajani RM, Dalvi BV, Kale PA. Successful balloon valvotomy in isolated congenital tricuspid stenosis. *Cardiovasc Intervent Radiol* 1990;13: 354–356.

114. Cohen ML, Spray T, Gutierrez F, Barzilai B, Bauwens D. Congenital tricuspid valve stenosis with atrial septal defect and left anterior fascicular block. *Clin Cardiol* 1990; 13:497–499.

115. Huhta JC, Edwards WD, Danielon GK, Feldt RH. Abnormalities of the tricuspid valve in complete transposition of the great arteries with ventricular septal defect. *J Thorac Cardiovasc Surg* 1982;83:569–576.

116. Deal BJ, Chin AJ, Sanders SP, Norwood WI, Castaneda AR. Subxiphoid two-dimensional echocardiographic identification of tricuspid valve abnormalities in transposition of the great arteries with ventricular septal defect. *Am J Cardiol* 1985;55:1146–151.

117. Borromee L, Lecompte Y, Batisse A, Lemoine G, Vouhe P, Sakata R, Leca F, Zannini L, Neveux JY. Anatomic repair of anomalies of ventriculoarterial connection associated with ventricular septal defect. II. Clinical results in 50 patients with pulmonary outflow tract obstruction. *J Thorac Cardiovasc Surg* 1988;95:96–102.

118. Lecompte Y, Zannini L, Hazan E, et al. Anatomic correction of transposition of the great arteries: New technique without the use of a prosthetic conduit. *J Thorac Cardiovasc Surg* 1981;82:629–631.

119. Lecompte Y, Bex JP. Repair of transposition of the great arteries with ventricular septal defect and left ventricular outflow tract obstruction. *J Thorac Cardiovasc Surg* 1985;90:151–154.

120. Lecompte Y. Reparation a l'etage ventriculaire-the REV procedure: Technique and clinical results. *Cardiol Young* 1991;1:63–70.

121. Lecompte Y, Batisse A, Di Carlo D. Double-outlet right ventricle: A surgical synthesis. *Adv Card Surg* 1993; 4:109–136.

122. Rubay J, Lecompte Y, Batisse A, Durandy Y, Dibie A, Lemoine G, Vouhe P. Anatomic repair of anomalies of ventriculo-arterial connection (REV). Results of a new technique in cases associated with pulmonary outflow tract obstruction. *Eur J Cardiothorac Surg* 1988; 2:305–311.

123. Sakata R, Lecompte Y, Batisse A, Borromee L, Durandy

Y. Anatomic repair of anomalies of ventriculoarterial connection associated with ventricular septal defect. I. Criteria of surgical decision. *J Thorac Cardiovasc Surg* 1988;95:90–95.

124. Kurosawa H and Van Mierop LHS. Surgical anatomy of the infundibular septum in transposition of the great arteries with ventricular septal defect. *J Thorac Cardiovasc Surg* 1986;91:123–132.

124a. Niinami H, Imai Y, Sawatari K, Hoshino S, Ishihara K, Aoki M. Surgical management of tricuspid malinsertion in the Rastelli operation: Conal flap method. *Ann Thorac Surg* 1995;59:1476–1480.

125. Kurosawa H, Imai Y, Takanashi Y, Hoshino S, Sawatari K, Kawada M, Takao A. Infundibular septum and coronary anatomy in Jatene operation. *J Thorac Cardiovasc Surg* 1986;91:572–583.

126. Seward JB, Tajik AJ, Ritter DG. Echocardiographic features of straddling tricuspid valve. *Mayo Clin Proc* 1975; 50:427–434.

127. Macartney FJ, Bain HH, Ionescu MI, Deverall PB, Scott O. Angiocardiographic/pathologic correlations in congenital mitral valve anomalies. *Eur J Cardiol* 1976; 4:191–211.

128. Freedom RM, Benson L, Burrows P, Smallhorn JF, Perrin DG. Congenital deformities of the mitral valve (excluding atrioventricular septal defect): Echocardiographic and angiocardiographic findings and indications for surgery. In: Marcelletti C, Anderson RH, Becker AE, Corno A, di Carlo D, Mazzera E, eds. *Paediatric Cardiology*. Volume 6. Edinburgh: Churchill Livingstone; 1986, pp. 240–261.

129. Matsushima AY, Park J, Szulc M, Poon E, Bierman FZ, Ursell PC. Anomalous atrioventricular valve arcade. *Am Heart J* 1991;121:1824–1826.

130. Milo S, Stark J, Macartney FJ, Anderson RH. Parachute deformity of the tricuspid valve. *Thorax* 1979;34: 543–544.

131. Restivo A, Ho SY, Anderson RH, Cameron H, Wilkinson JL. Absent left atrioventricular connection with right atrium connected to morphologically left ventricular chamber, rudimentary right ventricular chamber, and ventriculoarterial discordance. Problem of mitral versus tricuspid atresia. *Br Heart J* 1982;48:240–248.

132. Sahn DJ, Heldt GP, Reed KL, Kleinman CS, Meijboom EJ.

Fetal heart disease with cardiomegaly may be associated with lung hypoplasia as a determinant of poor prognosis (abstract). *J Am Coll Cardiol* 1988;11:9A.

133. Duran M, Gomez I, Palacio A. Anomalia de Ebstein con hipoplasia pulmonar. Diagnostico mediante ecocardiografia Doppler color en el feto. *Rev Esp Cardiol* 1992;45: 541–542.

134. Hornberger LK, Sahn DJ, Kleinman CS, Copel JA, Reed KL. Tricuspid valve disease with significant tricuspid insufficiency in the fetus: Diagnosis and outcome. *J Am Coll Cardiol* 1991;17:167–173.

135. Chaoui R, Bollmann R, Goldner B, Heling KS, Tennstedt C. Fetal cardiomegaly: Echocardiographic findings and outcome in 19 cases. *Fetal Diagn Ther* 1994; 9:92–104.

136. Roberson DA and Silverman NH. Ebstein's anomaly: Echocardiographic and clinical features in the fetus and neonate. *J Am Coll Cardiol* 1989;14:1300–1307.

137. Lang D, Oberhoffer R, Cook A, Sharland G, Allan L, Fagg N, Anderson RH. Pathologic spectrum of malformations of the tricuspid valve in prenatal and neonatal life. *J Am Coll Cardiol* 1991;17:1161–1167.

138. Allan LD, Crawford DC, Tynan MJ. Pulmonary atresia in prenatal life. *J Am Coll Cardiol* 1986;8:1131–1136.

139. Allan LD and Cook A. Pulmonary atresia with intact ventricular septum in the fetus. *Cardiol Young* 1992; 2:367–376.

140. Silverman NH, Kleinmann CS, Rudolph AM, Copel JA, Weinstein EM, Enderlein MA, Golbus M. Fetal atrioventricular valve insufficiency associated with nonimmune hydrops. *Circulation* 1985;72:825–832.

141. Sharland GK, Chita SK, Allan LD. Tricuspid valve dysplasia or displacement in intrauterine life. *J Am Coll Cardiol* 1991;17:944–949.

142. Oberhoffer R, Cook AC, Lang D, Sharland G, Allan LD, Fagg NLK, Anderson RH. Correlation between echocardiographic and morphologic investigations of lesions of the tricuspid valve diagnosed during fetal life. *Br Heart J* 1992;68:580–585.

143. Respondek ML, Kammermeier M, Ludomirsky A, Weil SR, Huhta JC. The prevalence and clinical significance of fetal tricuspid valve regurgitation with normal heart anatomy. *Am J Obstet Gynecol* 1994;171:1265–1270.

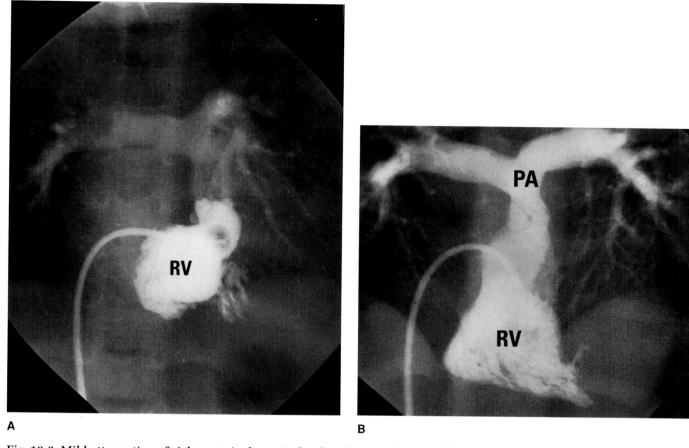

Fig. 16-2: Mild attenuation of right ventricular apical trabecular zone in two different patients.
A and B: The frontal right ventriculograms show mild attenuation of the right ventricular apical trabecular zone in these patients.

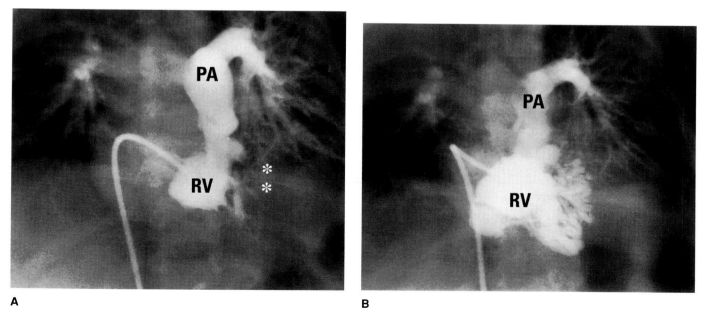

Fig. 16-3: Moderate generalized right ventricular hypoplasia with mild attenuation of apical trabecular component (✳).
A: Systole; **B:** Diastole.

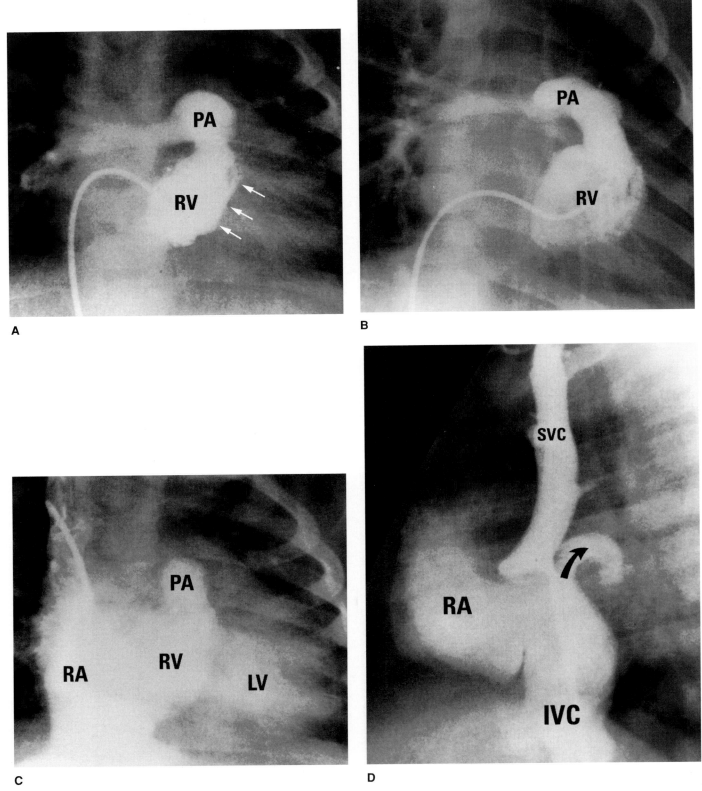

Fig. 16-4: Significant attenuation of right ventricular apical trabecular component of right ventricle with right-to-left shunting at atrial level.
A and B: Frontal and right anterior oblique right ventriculograms demonstrate important attenuation of apical trabecular component (arrows). **C and D:** Frontal and lateral right atrial angiograms showing right-to-left atrial shunting (arrow in D). In D, note the opacification of the left ventricle that constitutes the apex of the heart.

(continued on next page)

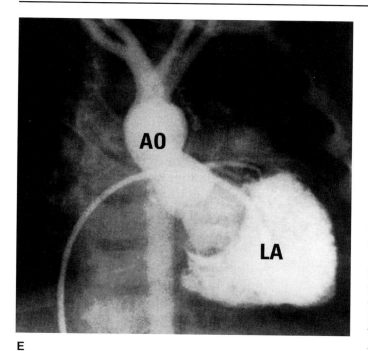

E

Fig. 16-4: *(continued)*
E: Frontal left ventriculogram demonstrates a morphologically normal chamber and absence of intracardiac shunting.

ular zone except in that patient with an imperforate Ebstein's form of tricuspid valve (see Chapter 14) (Fig. 16-2B). Rather it is more likely that the inlet and trabecular portions of the right ventricle are obviously less well developed compared with normal (Figs. 16-2 through 16-4). Volumetric analyses have been performed in these patients with varying calculations of right ventricular volume.[21] Right-to-left shunting at the atrial level may reflect either reduced right ventricular compliance or some degree of tricuspid valve hypoplasia/stenosis, or both (Fig. 16-4). The left ventricle is usually normal (Fig. 16-4E), although we have seen one patient with modest right ventricular hypoplasia and a very restrictive perimembranous ventricular septal defect.

It is also important to define the nature of the systemic venous connections as one form of therapy may take the form of a bidirectional cavopulmonary connection combined with closure of the atrial septal defect (see also Chapter 12).[19,22–24] This form of therapy may be particularly effective in unloading the right side of the heart when there is significant inlet obstruction (Fig. 16-5). Spontaneous improvement in the magnitude of right-to-left shunting has also been observed.[25]

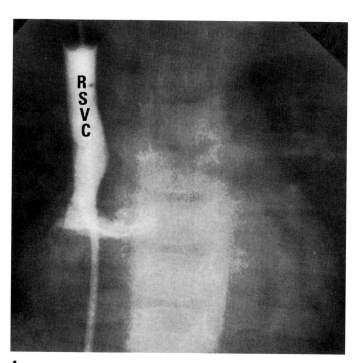

A

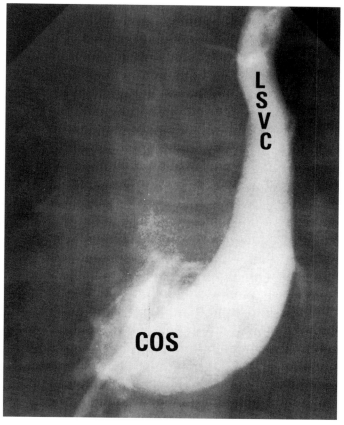

B

Fig. 16-5: Systemic venous connections in one patient considered for bilateral bidirectional cavopulmonary connections.
A: Small right superior vena cava. **B:** Larger left superior vena cava connecting to coronary sinus without a bridging brachiocephalic vein (see also Chapter 12)

References

1. Anderson RH, Wilkinson JE, Becker AE, The bulbus cordis—A misunderstood region of the developing human heart: Its significance to the classification of congenital cardiac malformation. In: Rosenquist GC, Bergsma D, eds. *Morphogenesis and Malformation of the Cardiovascular System.* New York: Alan R. Liss; 1978, pp. 1–16.

2. Freedom RM, Smallhorn JF. Ebstein's malformation of the morphologically tricuspid valve: A consideration of regurgitant and obstructive forms in patients with concordant and discordant atrioventricular connections. In: Anderson RH, Neches WH, Park SC, Zuberbuhler JR, eds. *Perspectives in Pediatric Cardiology.* Volume 1. Mt. Kisco, NY: Futura Publishing Company, Inc; 1981, pp. 127–146.

3. Freedom RM, Benson LN, Smallhorn JF, eds. *Neonatal Heart Disease.* London: Springer-Verlag; 1992, pp. 471–484.

4. Freedom RM, Culham JAG, Moes CAF. *Angiocardiography of Congenital Heart Disease.* New York: McMillan Publishing Company; 1984, pp. 119–125.

5. Freedom RM. *Pulmonary Atresia and Intact Ventricular Septum.* Mt. Kisco, NY: Futura Publishing Company, Inc; 1989, pp. 262.

6. Restivo A, Cameron AH, Anderson RH, Allwork SP. Divided right ventricle: A review of its anatomical variables. *Pediatr Cardiol* 1984;5:197–204.

7. Becker AE, Becker MJ, Moller JH, Edwards JE. Hypoplasia of the right ventricle and tricuspid valve in three siblings. *Chest* 1971;60:273–277.

8. Freedom RM, Moes CAF. The hypoplastic right heart complex. *Semin Roentgenol* 1985;20:169–183.

9. Freedom RM, Harder J, Culham JAG, Trusler GA, Rowe RD. Ventricular hypoplasia: Angiocardiography and surgical implications. In: Godman MJ, ed. *Paediatric Cardiology.* Volume 4. Edinburgh: Churchill Livingstone; 1981. pp. 117.

10. Horne MK III, Rowlands DT Jr. Case report. Hypoplastic right heart complex in a 46-year-old woman. *Br Heart J* 1971;33:167–168.

11. Karalis DG, Chandrasekaran K, Victor MF, Mintz GS. Prolonged survival despite severe cyanosis in an adult with right ventricular hypoplasia and atrial septal defect. *Am Heart J* 1990;120:701–703.

12. Medd WE, Neufeld HN, Weidman WH, Edwards JE. Isolated right ventricular hypoplasia and tricuspid valve in siblings. *Br Heart J* 1961;23:25–30.

13. Okin JT, Vogel JHK, Pryor R, Blount SG Jr. Isolated right ventricular hypoplasia. *Am J Cardiol* 1969;24:135–140.

14. Prasad K, Singh M, Radhakrishnan S. Hypoplastic right ventricle with mild pulmonary stenosis in an adult. *Int J Cardiol* 1992;37:260–262.

15. Raghib G, Amplatz K, Moller JH, Jue KL, Edwards JE. Clinical pathologic conference. *Am Heart J* 1965;70:806–812.

16. Sackner MA, Robinson MJ, Jamison WL, Lewis DH. Isolated right ventricular hypoplasia with atrial septal defect or patent foramen ovale. *Circulation* 1961;24:1388–1402.

17. Van der Hauwaert LG, Michaelsson M. Isolated right ventricular hypoplasia. *Circulation* 1971;44:466–474.

17a. Thatai D, Kothari SS, Wasir HS. Right to left shunting in atrial septal defect due to isolated right ventricular hypoplasia. *Indian Heart J* 1994;46:177–178.

18. Hanley FL, Sade RM, Blackstone EH, Kirklin JW, Freedom RM, Nanda NC. Outcomes in neonatal pulmonary atresia with intact ventricular septum. *J Thorac Cardiovasc Surg* 1993;105:406–427.

19. Alvarado O, Sreenam N, McKay R, Boyd IM. Cavopulmonary connection in repair of atrioventricular septal defect with small right ventricle. *Ann Thorac Surg* 1993;55:729–736.

20. Oldershaw P, Ward D, Anderson RH. Hypoplasia of the apical trabecular component of the morphologically right ventricle. *Am J Cardiol* 1985;55:862–864.

21. Ino T, Benson LN, Mikailian H, Freedom RM, Rowe RD. Biplane ventricular volumetry in infants and children. Right heart angiographic-cast correlations. *Am J Cardiol* 1988;61:161–165.

22. Haneda K, Togo T, Ito Y, Ogata H, Horiuchi T, Mohri H. Surgical treatment for isolated hypoplasia of the right ventricle. *J Cardiovasc Surg* 1992;33:496–501.

23. Gentles TL, Keane JF, Jonas RA, Marx GE, Mayer JE Jr. Surgical alternatives to the Fontan procedure incorporating a hypoplastic right ventricle. *Circulation* 1994;90(Part 2):II-1–II-6.

24. Van Arsdell GS, Williams WG, Maser CM, Streitenberger KS, Rebeyka IM, Coles JG, Freedom RM. Superior vena cava to pulmonary artery anastomosis: An adjunct to biventricular repair. *J Thorac Cardiovasc Surg* In press.

25. De Wolf D, Naeff MS, Losekoot G. Right ventricular hypoplasia: Outcome after conservative perinatal management. *Acta Cardiol* 1994;49:267–73.

Chapter 17

The Divided Right Ventricle
Anomalous Right Ventricular Muscle Bundles and Other Entities

Obstruction to pulmonary blood flow can result from infundibular septal malalignment (ie, tetralogy of Fallot) (see Chapter 20); valvular pulmonary stenosis (see Chapter 18); from tissue derived from perimembranous septum and/or septal leaflet of the tricuspid valve (see Chapter 6); the obstructive or imperforate form of Ebstein's tricuspid valve deformity (see Chapter 14); accessory tricuspid valve leaflet (see Chapter 15); a windsock deformity of the tricuspid valve (see Chapter 15) and contiguous tissues; from muscular division within the right ventricle; from neoplastic obstruction to the right ventricular outlet (see Chapter 49); from hypertrophic obstructive cardiomyopathy (see Chapter 28); neurofibromatosis; or from combinations of the above.[1-32]

The so-called double-chambered or divided right ventricle describes those conditions in which the morphologically right ventricle is divided or septated by muscular or fibrous structures (Fig. 17-1). The majority of reported cases of the divided right ventricle are characterized by muscular obstruction, which usually but not invariably produces some degree of obstruction within and between the component parts of the right ventricle. Division of the right ventricle can occur at the junction between the inlet and trabecular components of the right ventricle, or more distal at the level of the infundibulum.[1-15,31,32] It has been suggested elsewhere that the morphologically right ventricle is a tripartite structure with confluent inlet, apical trabecular, and infundibular or outlet components (see also Chapters 3 and 16).[33-36] Anderson and colleagues[35] have persuasively argued that a number of congenitally malformed hearts including those with isolated right ventricular hypoplasia, Ebstein's malformation with or without atresia, and divided right ventricle support the concept of the right ventricle as tripartite, not bipartite (see Chapter 14, Figs. 14-12 through 14-17). This view is not universally championed,[37] but it has been assimilated into common use.[38-41]

Restivo and colleagues[42] have thoroughly reviewed these forms of divided right ventricle, reminding us that anomalous muscle bundles of the right ventricle are but one of several conditions producing division of the right ventricle, and that an anomalous muscle band does not invariably produce a double-chambered ventricle. Among those conditions producing a divided right ventricle in the review by Restivo et al[42] are the anomalous septoparietal band; anomalous apical shelf, a condition resulting from an abnormal septoparietal band and hypertrophy of apical trabeculations; anomalous apical shelf with Ebstein's anomaly; an apical shelf confluent with the outlet septum in a heart with a two-chambered right ventricle giving the impression of a two-chambered left ventricle[43]; and sequestration of the outlet portion of the ventricle from a circumferential muscular diaphragm in a patient with tetralogy of Fallot. Indeed, the morphological and angiocardiographic findings of muscular division of the right ventricle are quite diverse. The obstruction may be localized to the os infundibulum or the obstruction may be proximal to that level. In some patients both muscular and fibrous elements contribute to the division of the right ventricle. The divided right ventricle may occur in isolation; with ventricular septal defect and/or left ven-

From: Freedom RM, Mawson JB, Yoo SJ, Benson LN: *Congenital Heart Disease: Textbook of Angiocardiography.* Armonk NY, Futura Publishing Co., Inc. ©1997.

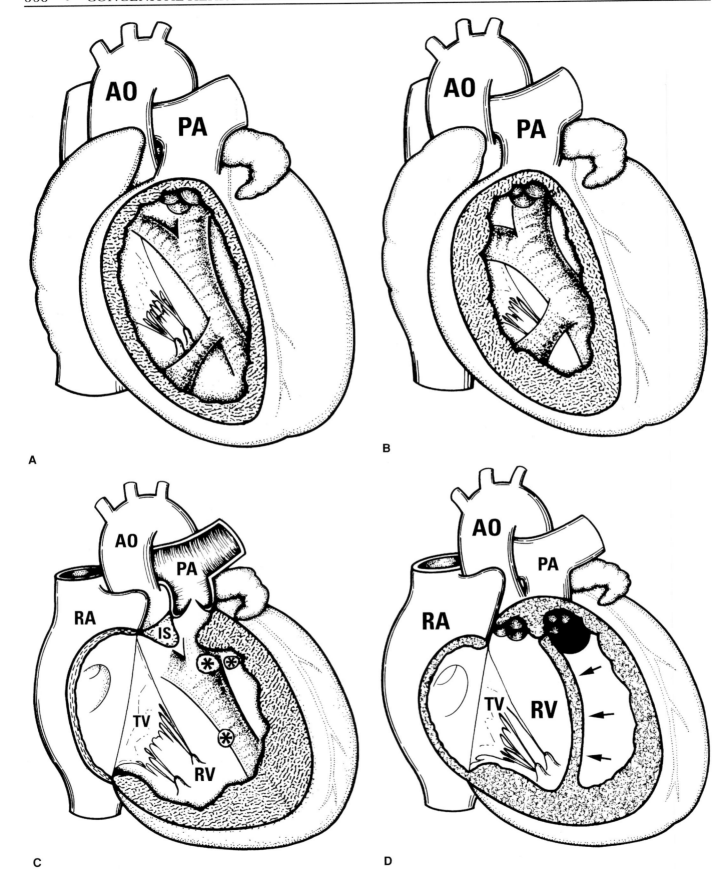

A

B

C

D

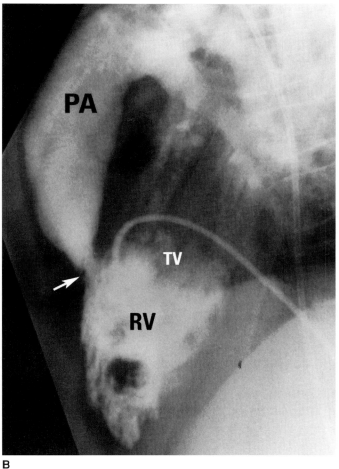

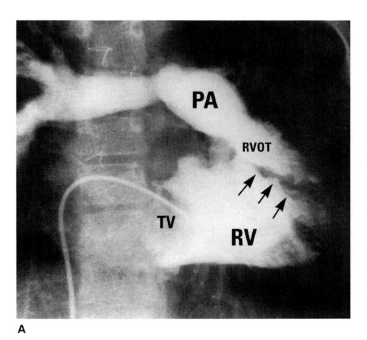

A   B

Fig. 17-2: Fibromuscular division of the right ventricle.
A: Frontal right ventriculogram shows the fibromuscular partition (arrows) promoting a divided right ventricle. **B:** Lateral right ventriculogram from another patient shows concentric narrowing of the so-called os infundibulum. *(continued on next page)*

tricular outflow tract obstruction; in complete or corrected transposition of the great arteries; in double-outlet right ventricle and in patients with pulmonary atresia and intact ventricular septum (Figs. 17-2 through 17-6).

In patients with Ebstein's anomaly of the tricuspid valve, distal attachment of the anterosuperior and/or mural leaflets to the junction between the inlet and trabecular components of the right ventricle may exhibit what Zuberbuhler and Anderson[30] characterize as linear attachments (see Chapter 14, Figs. 14-12 through 14-17). When such linear attachments are extensive, this may result in functional tricuspid stenosis.[44,45] The most florid manifestation of these linear attachments is the so-called imperforate type of Ebstein's anomaly, in effect producing functional tricuspid atresia.[26–30,44–46] This type of tricuspid atresia is very different from the classic expression of tricuspid atresia with its absent atrioventricular connection (see Chapter 39). For the majority of affected patients, however, the displace-

Fig. 17-1: Diagrams show interior of normal right ventricle and various types of pathologies promoting a divided right ventricle.
A: Interior of normal right ventricle showing disposition of the trabecula septomarginalis and moderator band. **B:** Division of right ventricle due to hypertrophy of the trabecula septomarginalis and moderator band. **C:** Division of right ventricle due to hypertrophied muscle bundles and concentric muscular hypertrophy of the os infundibuli. **D:** Division of right ventricle due to a sheet of muscle in double outlet right ventricle and subpulmonary ventricular septal defect. Note that the proximal chamber leads to the aorta, and that the distal chamber receives the blood from the left ventricle through the ventricular septal defect and leads to the pulmonary artery. Thus, the hemodynamic physiology mimicks that of complete transposition of the great arteries.

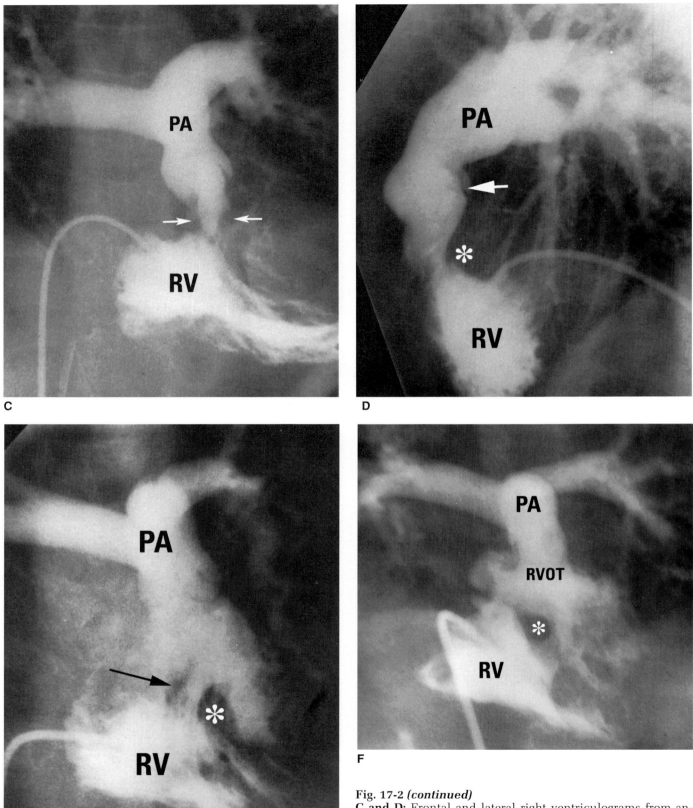

Fig. 17-2 *(continued)*
C and D: Frontal and lateral right ventriculograms from another patient with a divided right ventricle. The muscular obstruction is relatively distal (arrows in Fig. 17-2C). Arrow in Fig.17-2D indicates the thickened pulmonary valve. **E and F:** Frontal right ventriculograms from two different patients with muscular division and obstruction.

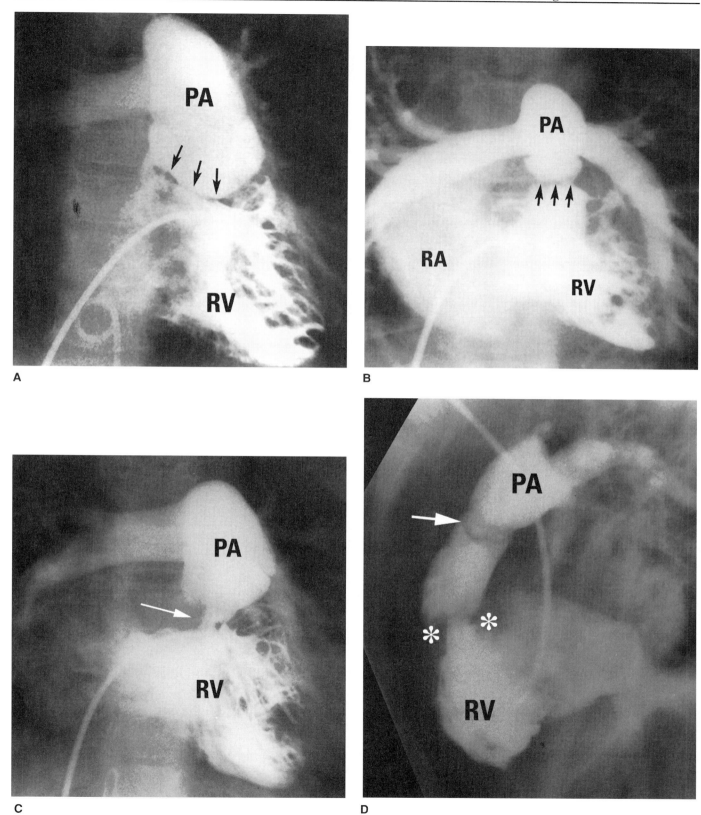

Fig. 17-3: Fibromuscular obstruction and division of the right ventricle.
A: Fibrous obstruction and division (arrows) of the right ventricle. **B:** Fibrous division of the right ventricle (arrows). **C:** Muscular division and obstruction (arrow) of the right ventricle. **D:** Muscular division and obstruction (✳) together with pulmonary valve stenosis (arrow) as demonstrated by this lateral right ventriculogram.

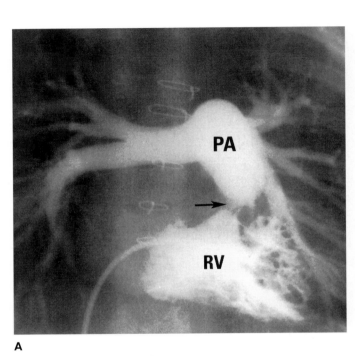

A

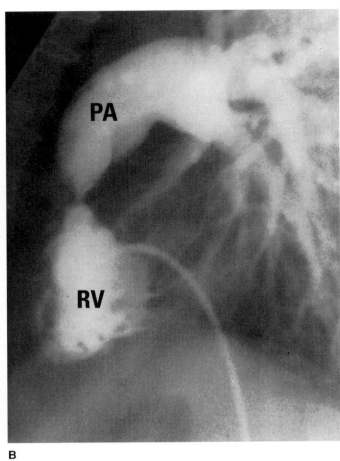

B

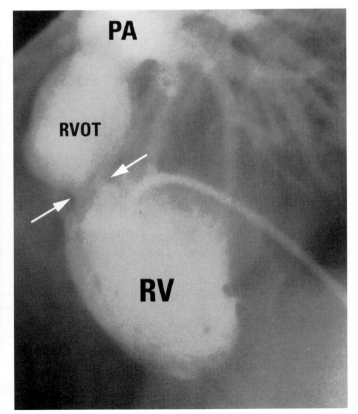

C

D

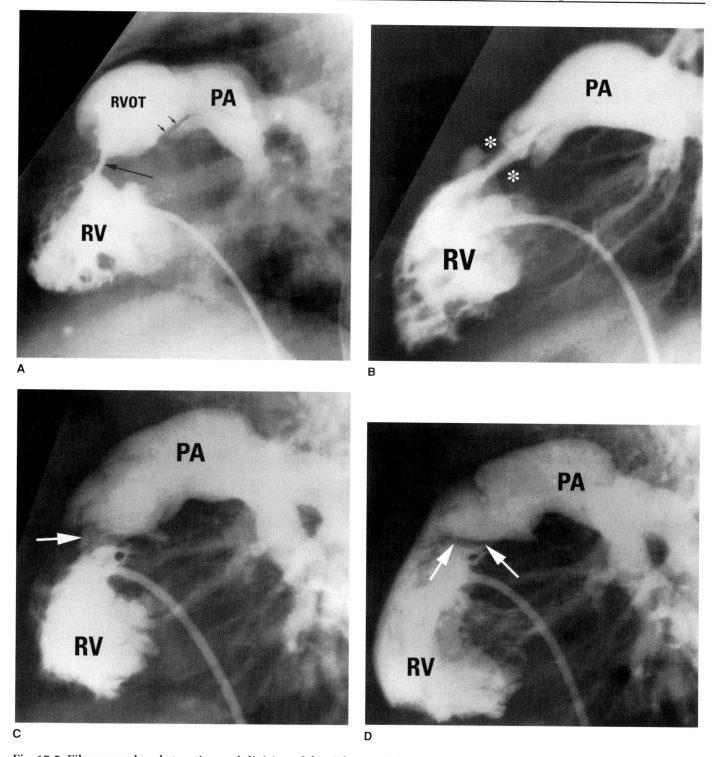

Fig. 17-5: Fibromuscular obstruction and division of the right ventricle.
A and B: Two different patients with fibromuscular obstruction (long arrow in Fig.17-5A and ✳ in Fig.17-5B) and division of the right ventricle as demonstrated by lateral right ventriculography. Pulmonary valve stenosis (arrows) is associated in Fig.17-5A. **C and D:** Lateral frames from another patient showing distal fibromuscular obstruction (arrows).

Fig. 17-4: Fibromuscular obstruction and division of the right ventricle.
A and B: Distal muscular obstruction and division (arrows) of the right ventricle as demonstrated by frontal and lateral right ventriculography. **C and D:** A different patient with muscular obstruction and division (arrows) of the right ventricle.

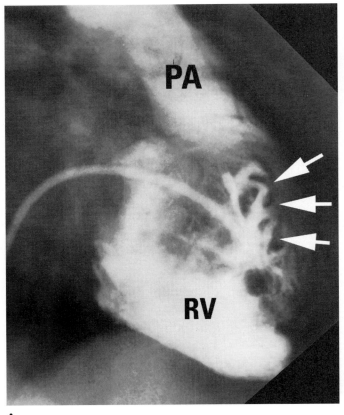

A

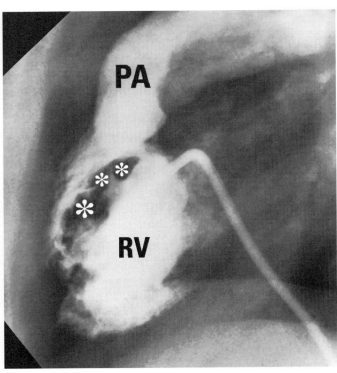

B

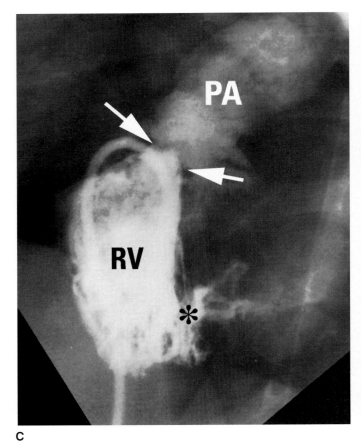

C

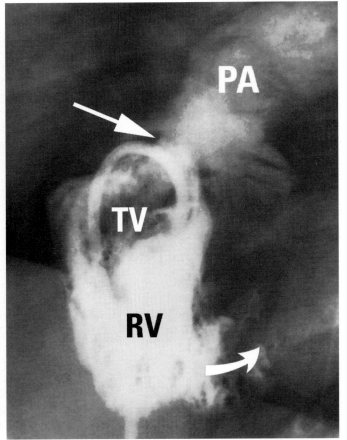

D

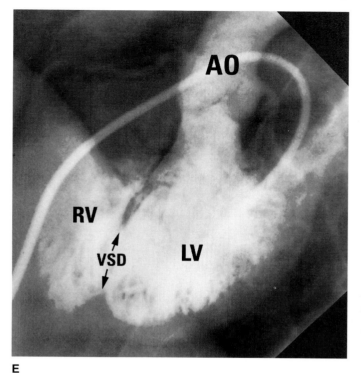

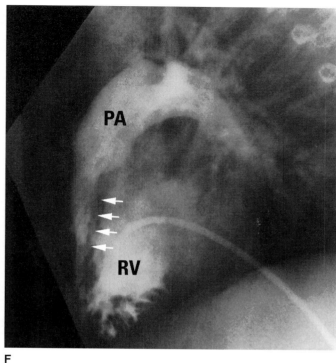

Fig. 17-6: Other examples of a divided right ventricle.
A through E: Anomalous muscle bundles dividing the right ventricle and mid- and apical muscular ventricular septal defects. **A:** Right ventriculogram in right anterior oblique projection showing severely obstructive anomalous muscle bundles (arrows) dividing the right ventricle. **B:** Lateral right ventriculogram shows the dense bar of muscle (✱) dividing the right ventricle. **C** and **D:** Lateral right ventriculograms showing the distal outflow obstruction (arrows) and the right-to-left ventricular shunting (✱ in Fig. 17-6C and curved arrow in Fig. 17-6D). **E:** Long axial oblique left ventriculogram shows the confluent apical and mid-trabecular muscular ventricular septal defects. **F:** A different patient with a peculiar linear fibromuscular obstruction and division of the right ventricle. The lateral right ventriculogram shows the linear and verticle fibromuscular obstruction and division (arrows) of the right ventricle.

---

ment of the tricuspid valve, the characteristic dysplasia, and abnormal distal attachments produce a valve that is regurgitant, and the most conspicuous alteration resulting from displacement is atrialization of a portion of the right ventricle, a process that reduces the size of the functional right ventricle.

The Divided Right Ventricle and Ventricular Septal Defect

The divided morphologically right ventricle on the basis of abnormal muscle bundles can occur in isolation, but it is more commonly associated with a perimembranous ventricular septal defect (Fig. 17-7 through 17-12).[1,2,6–8,11,12,22,31,32,42] While the perimembranous defect can be large, it tends to be moderate in size or smaller, and thus it is not surprising that the ventricular septal defect in patients with anomalous right ventricular muscle bundles tends to become smaller, or even close. When this occurs and if the

anomalous muscle bundles are severe, right ventricular pressure will become suprasystemic. The perimembranous ventricular septal defect is usually below the level of muscular division of the right ventricle, and thus the magnitude of the left-to-right shunt at ventricular level is usually hemodynamically independent of the muscular obstruction, and related to the size of the ventricular septal defect. We have commented elsewhere that the classic morphological features of tetralogy of Fallot may be complicated by more proximal muscular division of the right ventricle (see Chapter 20). It is less common for the ventricular septal defect to be muscular, malalignment, or apical (Fig. 17-6).[42a]

Mechanism of Acquired Right Ventricular Outflow Tract Obstruction in Ventricular Septal Defect

The development of right ventricular outflow tract obstruction is an important event in the patient with

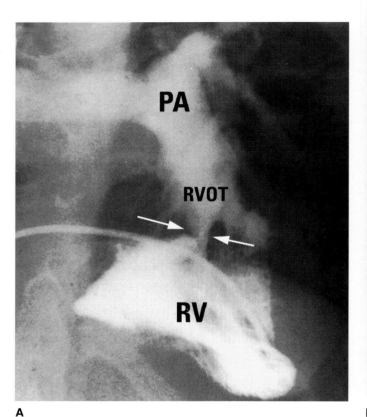

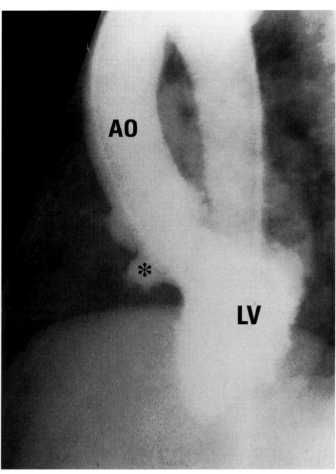

Fig. 17-7: The divided right ventricle and ventricular septal defect.
A: Right anterior oblique right ventriculogram shows the muscular division and obstruction (arrows) of the right ventricle. **B:** Long axial oblique left ventriculogram shows the nearly sealed (✱) perimembranous ventricular septal defect.

ventricular septal defect and may irrevocably alter the natural history. It has been suggested that between 3% and 7% of patients with ventricular septal defect will acquire pulmonary outflow tract obstruction, usually within the first few years of life.[47–49] Those mechanisms responsible for the development of right ventricular outflow tract obstruction are diverse and have been summarized elsewhere.[48–51] However, since the report by Gasul and colleagues[50] four decades ago of the development of infundibular obstruction in the patient with ventricular septal defect and transformation of an acyanotic patient into a cyanotic one, there has been the inference that the anatomy responsible for this change was related to tetralogy of Fallot. We addressed the mechanism(s) responsible for acquired right ventricular outflow tract obstruction in 20 patients with ventricular septal defect undergoing serial catheter studies, acquiring a pressure gradient of more than 25 mm Hg over a period of nearly 4 years.[51] Of the 20 patients in this study, the mechanism of acquired right ventricular outflow tract obstruction was related to progressive hypertrophy and obstruction from anomalous right ventricular muscle bundles in 19, and hypertrophy of a malaligned infundibular septum in only 1 patient (Fig. 17-4). The presence of a right-sided aortic arch in the patient with ventricular septal defect may be the harbinger of right ventricular outflow tract obstruction, but this does not invariably conclude in classic tetralogy.[47,52] Tyrrell and colleagues[53] have suggested that a right ventricular outflow tract more horizontal than normal is suggestive of the patient who will acquire the hemodynamics and morphology of tetralogy of Fallot. These observations do not exclude the reality that some patients with the morphology of tetralogy of Fallot have initially only mild right ventricular outflow tract obstruction that may worsen with time (see Chapter 20).

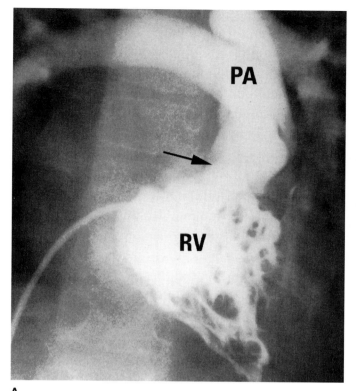

A

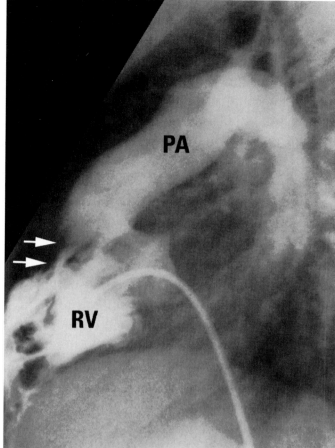

B

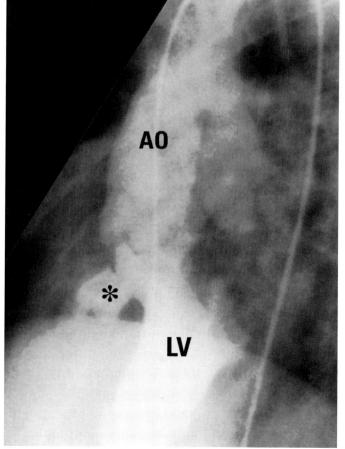

C

Fig. 17-8: The divided right ventricle and ventricular septal defect.
A and B: Frontal and lateral right ventriculograms demonstrate the muscular obstruction (arrows) in the right ventricle. **C:** The lateral left ventriculogram shows the partially sealed-off (✱) perimembranous ventricular septal defect from the adherent tricuspid valve.

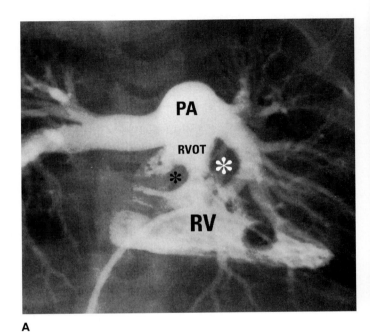

A

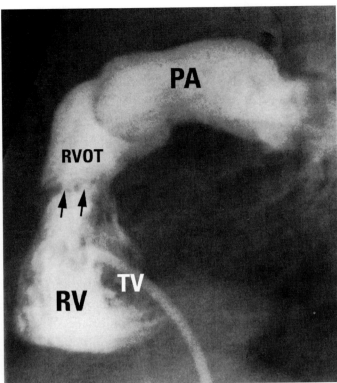

B

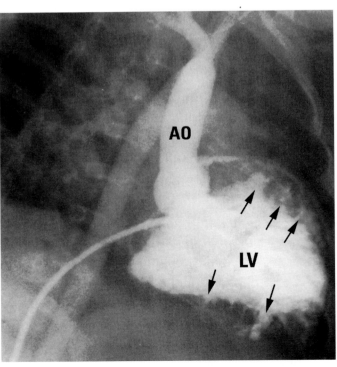

C

Fig. 17-9: The divided right ventricle and multiple ventricular septal defects.
A and B: Frontal and lateral right ventriculograms show the muscular division of the right ventricle (✳ in frontal; arrows in lateral). **C:** Right anterior oblique left ventriculogram shows the multiple muscular ventricular septal defects (arrows).

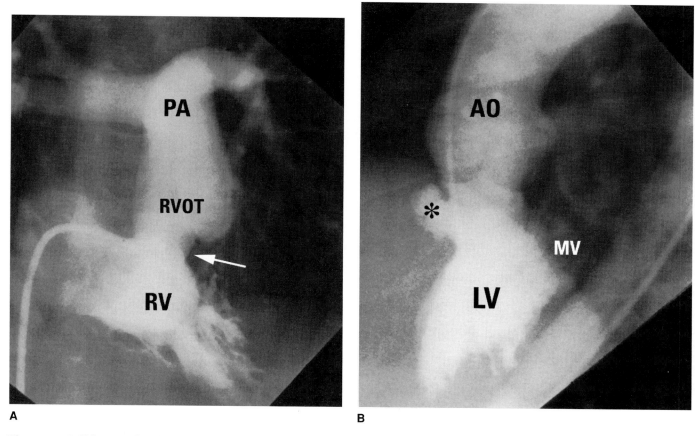

Fig. 17-10: Mild muscular division of the right ventricle and sealed ventricular septal defect.
A: Frontal right ventriculogram shows mild division (arrow) of the right ventricle. **B:** The perimembranous ventricular septal defect is closed by adherent tricuspid valve tissue (✱).

The Divided Right Ventricle and Subaortic Stenosis

A well-known relationship has been established in patients with a perimembranous ventricular septal defect, right ventricular anomalous muscle bundles, and a subaortic abnormality (see also Chapter 29, Figs. 29-28 and 29-29).[54-58] We have addressed in an echocardiographic study this association in 36 patients with perimembranous ventricular septal defect and right ventricular anomalous muscle bundles.[55] Eighty-eight percent of these patients had echocardiographic evidence of an associated subaortic abnormality, and in a number of these patients, Doppler evidence of progression of the left ventricular outflow tract gradient was provided. We have observed progression of a subaortic deformity initially producing no obstruction, to some years later severe left ventricular outflow tract obstruction after surgical closure of a ventricular septal defect and/or resection of anomalous muscle bundles of the right ventricle. Others in their cataloguing of patients with ventricular septal defect and left ventricular outflow tract obstruction have commented on the association with anomalous right ventricular muscle bundles.[55a] While in Toronto, Vogel[56] reported on 41 patients with ventricular septal defect and subaortic stenosis, 6 of them having anomalous right ventricular muscle bundles. From clinical experience, it has become clear that the subaortic abnormality may progress to severe left ventricular outflow tract obstruction, prior to closure of the ventricular septal defect and resection of the right ventricular muscle bundles, or after.[59] For this reason, we recommend that at the time of surgical repair of ventricular septal defect and right ventricular muscle bundles the subaortic abnormality be addressed and resected.

Imaging

The echocardiographic features of the divided right ventricle have been reviewed elsewhere, and these findings in isolation can be distinguished from the classic infundibular malalignment of the tetralogy type.[60-61a] It may be difficult to differentiate muscular

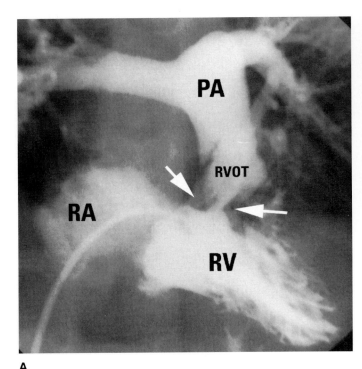

A

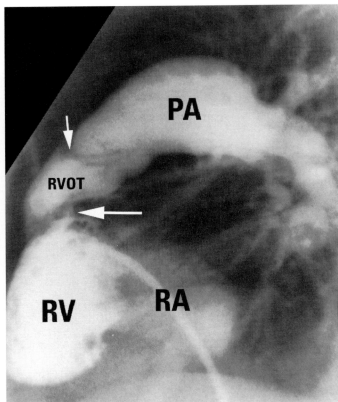

B

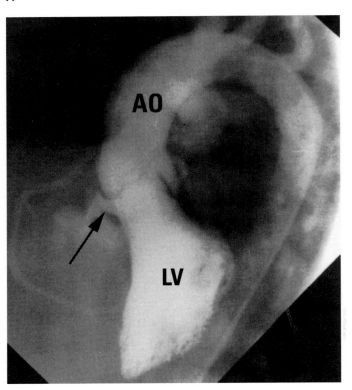

C

Fig. 17-11: Severe muscular division of the right ventricle and very restrictive perimembranous ventricular septal defect.
A and B: Frontal and lateral right ventriculograms show severe muscular obstruction (arrows) of the right ventricle. In B, the distal smaller arrow notes the level of the pulmonary valve. **C:** A small perimembranous ventricular septal defect (arrow) is demonstrated by left ventriculography in the long axial oblique.

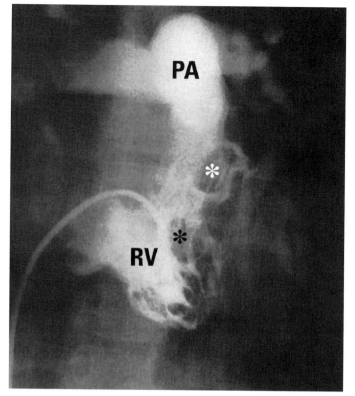

A

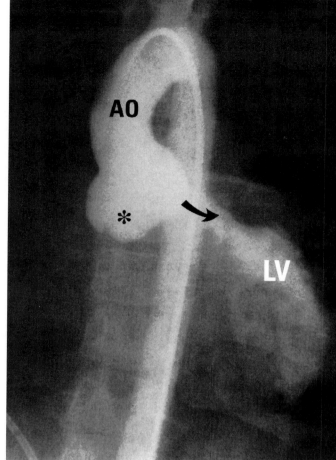

B

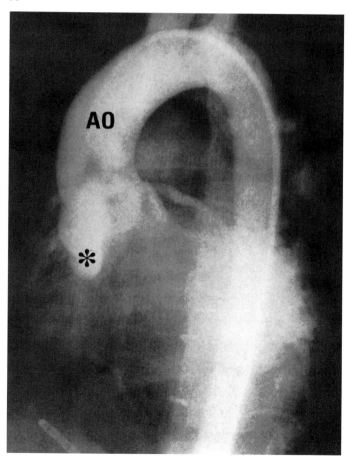

C

Fig. 17-12: Mild muscular division of the right ventricle, aortic valve prolapse and aortic regurgitation in a patient with a perimembranous ventricular septal defect.

A: Frontal right ventriculogram shows mild muscular obstruction (✳) within the right ventricle. B and C: Frontal and long axial oblique aortograms show deformity of right aortic cusp (✳) due to prolapse and aortic regurgitation (arrow) into the left ventricle.

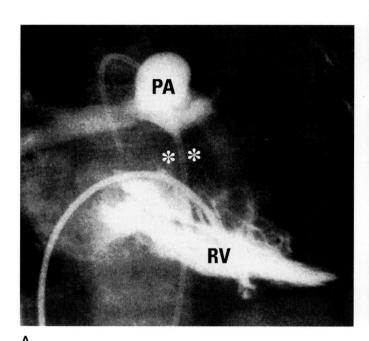

A

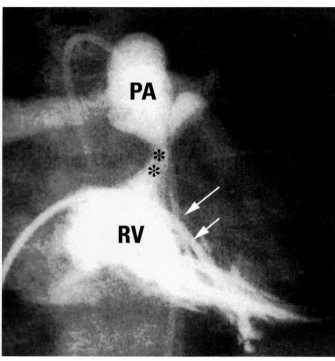

B

Fig. 17-13: Hypertrophic obstructive cardiomyopathy with severe right ventricular outflow tract obstruction.
A and B: Frontal and lateral right ventriculograms show attenuation of right ventricular outflow tract (✳). Note the septal bulge (arrows) in panel A.

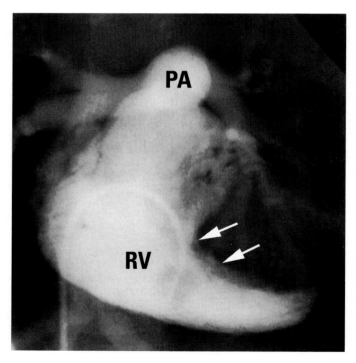

Fig. 17-14: Frontal right ventriculogram shows distorsion of right ventricle by distal septal bulge (arrows) in a patient with left-sided midventricular hypertrophic obstructive cardiomyopathy.

hypertrophy of normal septal and anterior free-wall trabeculations from hypertrophy of pathological muscular structures. There is at present relatively little information on the role of magnetic resonance imaging in the recognition of anomalous muscle bundles of the right ventricle.[62] Fetal recognition of a divided right ventricle and ventricular septal defect has been achieved.[61a] Relatively little information about the magnetic resonance features of the divided right ventricle have been published.[61b]

Angiocardiographic Imaging

The basic abnormality resides in the morphologically right ventricle. It is important that both proximal and distal chambers of the divided right ventricle be imaged, and thus it is important to be certain the catheter is not just positioned in the more distal and subpulmonary chamber. Ideally, the catheter should be positioned in the apex of the right ventricle. The right ventriculogram should be filmed in both frontal and lateral projections, with craniocaudal angulation.[62–67] The features of the obstructive forms of Ebstein's abnormality can be seen in Chapter 14. Unless there is right-to-left shunting with obscuring of the proximal pulmonary artery bifurcation, the tilted right ventriculogram should profile the right and left pulmonary arteries and their bifurcation. If the pulmonary arteries are not clearly and precisely imaged from the right ventriculogram, ideally an angiocardiogram should be performed in the main pulmonary trunk. In some patients with critically severe right ventricular outflow tract obstruction, it may be difficult or risky, or both to enter the main pulmonary trunk. The right ventriculogram will demonstrate any abnormality of the pulmonary valve, or associated tandem obstruction at the level of the os infundibulum (Figs. 17-2 through 17-14).

Left ventriculography should usually (always?) be performed in those patients undergoing angiographic investigation. While the ventricular septal defect can theoretically occupy any position within the ventricular septum, it is usually perimembranous, and thus it should be profiled in the left long axial oblique projection. The complementary right axial oblique projection should demonstrate the usually normal distal right ventricular infundibulum. These projections should demonstrate the character of the left ventricular subaortic abnormality. Similarly, in those patients with echocardiographic evidence of aortic valve prolapse, aortography should be performed (Fig. 17-12). Right ventricular obstruction may reflect right-sided hypertrophic obstructive cardiomyopathy (Fig. 17-13; see also Chapter 28). The contour of the right ventricular septal curvature may be altered by septal hypertrophy in the setting of obstructive cardiomyopathy (Fig. 17-14). When the ventricular septal defect is proximal to the obstruction, right ventriculography in the right anterior oblique projection may demonstrate right-to-left shunting through the ventricular septal defect as in tetralogy of Fallot.

Although surgical repair of divided right ventricle is usually accomplished through the right atrium and tricuspid valve, it may become necessary to perform a limited right ventriculotomy.[68,69] Thus, as in the patient with classic tetralogy of Fallot, it is advisable to image the coronary arteries to define those major vessels crossing the right ventricular outflow tract.[70,71] Finally, we have had no experience with balloon dilatation of right ventricular outflow tract obstruction secondary to anomalous muscle bundles.[72] One should also note the potential for the development of right ventricular outflow tract obstruction after double-lung transplantation for primary pulmonary hypertension.[73]

References

1. Rocchini AP, Emmanoulides GC. Pulmonary Stenosis. In: Emmanouilides GC, Allen HD, Riemenschneider TA, Gutgesell HP. *Moss and Adams' Heart Disease in Infants, Children, and Adolescents, Including the Fetus and Young Adult.* Baltimore: Williams and Wilkins; 1995, pp. 930–962.
2. Li MD, Coles JC, McDonald AC. Anomalous muscle bundle of the right ventricle. Its recognition and surgical treatment. *Br Heart J* 1978;40:1040–1045.
3. Bashour TT, Kabbani S, Sandouk A, Cheng TO. Double-chambered right ventricle due to fibromuscular diaphragm. *Am Heart J* 1984;107:792–794.
4. Wong PC, Sanders SP, Jonas RA, Colan SD, Parness IA, Geva T, Van Praagh R, Spevak PJ. Pulmonary valve-moderator band distance and association with development of double-chambered right ventricle. *Am J Cardiol* 1991;68:1681–1686.
5. Barnes RJ, Kwong KH, Cheung ACS. Aberrant muscle bundle of the right ventricle. *Br Heart J* 1971;33:546–551.
6. Hartmann AF Jr, Goldring D, Ferguson TB, Buford TH, Smith CH, Kissane JM, Frech RS. The course of children with the two-chambered right ventricle. *J Thorac Cardiovasc Surg* 1970;60:72–83.
7. Hartmann AF Jr, Tsifutis AA, Arvidsson H, Goldring D. The two-chambered right ventricle. Report of nine cases. *Circulation* 1962;26:279–287.
7a. Cil E, Saraclar M, Ozkutlu S, Ozme S, Bilgic A, Ozer S, Celiker A, Tokel K, Demircin M. Double-chambered right ventricle: Experience with 52 cases. *Int J Cardiol* 1995;50:19–29.
7b. Cabrera A, Martinez P, Rumoroso JR, Alcibar J, Arriola J, Pastor E, Galdeano JM. Double-chambered right ventricle. *Eur Heart J* 1995;16:682–686.
8. Rowland TW, Rosenthal A, Castaneda AR. Double-chamber right ventricle: Experience with 17 cases. *Am Heart J* 1975;89:455–462.
9. Folger GM Jr. Right ventricular outflow pouch associated with double-chambered right ventricle. *Am Heart J* 1985;109:1044–1049.
10. Folger GM Jr. The right ventricular pouch: A proposed explanation for the electro-vectorcardiographic pattern of double chambered right ventricle. *Angiology* 1986;37:483–486.
11. Lucas RV Jr, Varco RI, Lillehei CW, Adams P Jr, Anderson RC, Edwards JE. Anomalous muscle bundle of the right ventricle. *Circulation* 1962;25:443–455.
12. Patel R, Astley R. Right ventricular obstruction due to anomalous muscle bands. *Br Heart J* 1973;35:890–893.
13. Kurosawa H; Becker AE. Surgical anatomy of the atrioventricular conduction bundle in anomalous muscle bundle of the right ventricle with subarterial ventricular septal defect. *Pediatr Cardiol* 1985;6(3):157–160.
14. Moreno F, Calvo C, Rey C, Rubio D, Fernandez A, Zafra M, Cordovilla G. Ventriculo derecho bicameral por banda anomala. *Rev Esp Cardiol* 1992;45:339–345.
15. Pena R, Cabrera A, Pastor E, Galdeano JM, Pena N, Martinez P, Alcibar J, Sanchez J. Ventriculo derecho bicameral: Resultados quirurgicos de 28 casos. *Rev Esp Cardiol* 1992;45:183–187.
16. Gerlis LM, Ho SY, Rigby ML. Right ventricular outflow obstruction by anomalies of the tricuspid valve: Report of a windsock diverticulum. *Pediatr Cardiol* 1992;13:59–62.
17. Cosio FG, Wang Y, Nicoloff DM. Membranous right ventricular outflow obstruction. *Am J Cardiol* 1973;32:1000–1004.
18. Flege JB, Vlad P, Ehrenhaft JL. Aneurysm of tricuspid valve causing infundibular obstruction. *Ann Thorac Surg* 1967;3:446–448.

19. Pate JW, Richardson RL, Giles HH. Accessory tricuspid leaflet producing right ventricular outflow obstruction. *N Engl J Med* 1968;279:867–868.
20. Pate JW, Ainger LE, Butterick OD. A new form of right ventricular outflow tract obstruction. *Am Heart J* 1964;68: 249–251.
21. Carter JB, Van Tassel RA, Moller JH, Amplatz K, Edwards JE. Congenital diverticulum of the right ventricle. Association with pulmonary stenosis and ventricular septal defect. *Am J Cardiol* 1971;28:478–482.
22. Shepherd RL, Glancy RL, Jaffe RB, Perloff JK, Epstein SE. Acquired subvalvular right ventricular outflow obstruction in patients with ventricular septal defect. *Am J Cardiol* 1972;53;446–455.
23. Rosenquist GC, Krovetz LJ, Haller JA, Simon AL, Bannagan GA. Acquired right ventricular outflow tract obstruction in a child with neurofibromatosis. *Am Heart J* 1970; 79:103–108.
24. Anderson KR, Zuberbuhler JR, Anderson RH, Becker AE, Lie JT. Morphologic spectrum of Ebstein's anomaly of the heart. A review. *Mayo Clin Proc* 1979;54:174–180.
25. Huhta JC, Edwards WD, Tajik AJ, Mair DD, Puga FJ, Ritter DG. Pulmonary atresia with intact ventricular septum, Ebstein's anomaly of the hypoplastic tricuspid valve, and double-chamber right ventricle. *Mayo Clin Proc* 1982;57: 515–519.
26. Freedom RM, Smallhorn JF. Ebstein's malformation of the morphologically tricuspid valve: A consideration of regurgitant and obstructive forms in patients with concordant and discordant atrioventricular connections. In: Anderson RH, Neches WH, Park SC, Zuberbuhler JR, eds. *Perspectives in Pediatric Cardiology*, Volume 1. Mt. Kisco, NY: Futura Publishing Company, Inc; 1981, pp. 127–146
27. Gerlis LM, Anderson RH. Cor triatriatum dexter with imperforate Ebstein's anomaly. *Br Heart J* 1976;38:108–111.
28. Gussenhoven EJ, Essed CE, Bos E. Unguarded tricuspid orifice with two-chambered right ventricle. *Pediatr Cardiol* 1986;7:175–177.
29. Rao PS, Jue KL, Isabel-Jones J, Ruttenberg HD. Ebstein's malformation of the tricuspid valve with atresia. Differentiation from isolated tricuspid atresia. *Am J Cardiol* 1973;32:1004–1009.
30. Zuberbuhler JR, Anderson RH. Ebstein's malformation of the tricuspid valve: Morphology and natural history. In: Anderson RH, Neches WH, Park SC, Zuberbuhler JR, eds. *Perspectives in Pediatric Cardiology*, Volume 1. Mt. Kisco, NY: Futura Publishing Company, Inc; 1988, pp. 99–112.
31. Forster JW, Humphries JO. Right ventricular anomalous muscle bundle. Clinical and laboratory presentation and natural history. *Circulation* 1971;43:115–127.
32. Lintermans JP, Roberts DB, Guntheroth WG, Figley MM. Two-chambered right ventricle without outflow obstruction in ventricular septal defect. A case of spontaneous resolution. *Am J Cardiol* 1968;21:582–587.
32a. Ignaszewski AP, Collins-Nakai RL, Kasza LA, Gulamhussein SS, Penkoske PA, Taylor DA. Aneurysm of the membranous ventricular septum producing subpulmonic outflow tract obstruction. *Can J Cardiol* 1994;10:67–70.
33. Goor DA, Lillehei CW. *Congenital Malformations of the Heart*. New York: Grune and Stratton; 1975, pp. 3–13.
34. Wenink ACG, Gittenberger de Groot AC. Left and right ventricular trabecular patterns: Consequence of ventricular septation and valve development. *Br Heart J* 1982;48: 462–468.
35. Anderson RH, Wilkinson JE, Becker AE. The bulbus cordis-A misunderstood region of the developing human heart. Its significance to the classification of congenital cardiac malformation. In: Rosenquist GC, Bergsma D. eds. *Morphogenesis and Malformation of the Cardiaovascular System*. New York: Alan R Liss, Inc; 1978; Birth Defects, 14(7):1–22.
36. Grant RP, Downey FM, McMahon H. The architecture of the right ventricular outflow tract and the normal heart and the presence of ventricular septal defect. *Circulation* 1961;24:223–231.
37. Van Praagh R, Wise JR Jr, Dahl BA, Van Praagh S. Single left ventricle with infundibular outlet chamber and tricuspid valve opening only into outlet chamber in 44-year-old man with thoracoabdominal ectopia cordis without diaphragmatic or pericardial defect: Importance of myocardial morphologic method of chamber identification in congenital heart disease. In: Van Praagh R, Takao R, eds. *Etiology and Morphogenesis of Congenital Heart Disease*. Mt. Kisco, NY: Futura Publishing Company, Inc; 1980, pp. 379–420.
38. Bull C, De Leval M, Mercanti C, Macartney FJ, Anderson RH. Pulmonary atresia and intact ventricular septum: A revised classification. *Circulation* 1982;66:266–272.
39. De Leval M, Bull C, Stark J, Anderson RH, Taylor JFN, Macartney FJ. Pulmonary atresia and intact ventricular septum: Surgical management based on a revised classification. *Circulation* 1982;66:272–280.
40. Freedom RM. Angiocardiography of the right ventricle. In: Freedom RM, ed. *Pulmonary Atresia and Intact Ventricular Septum*. Mt. Kisco, NY: Futura Publishing Company, Inc; 1989, pp. 163–206.
41. De Leval M, Bull C, Hopkins R, Rees P, Deanfield J, Taylor JFN, Gersony W, Stark J, Macartney FJ. Decision making in the definitive repair of the heart with a small right ventricle. *Circulation* 1985;72(suppl II):52–60.
42. Restivo A; Cameron AH; Anderson RH; Allwork SP. Divided right ventricle: A review of its anatomical varieties. *Pediatr Cardiol* 1984;5:197–204.
42a. Wang J-K, Wu M-H, Chang C-I, Chiu I-S, Chu S-H, Hung C-R, Lue H-C. Malalignment-type ventricular septal defect in double-chambered right ventricle. *Am J Cardiol* 1996;77:839–842.
43. Beitzke A, Anderson RH, Wilkinson JL, Shinebourne EA. Two-chambered right ventricle simulating two-chambered left ventricle. *Br Heart J* 1979;42:22–26.
44. Zuberbuhler JR, Becker AE, Anderson RH, Lenox CC. Ebstein's malformation and the embryological development of the tricuspid valve. With a note on the nature of "clefts" in the atrioventricular valves. *Pediatr Cardiol* 1984;5:289–296.
45. Zuberbuhler JR, Allwork SP, Anderson RH. The spectrum of Ebstein's anomaly of the tricuspid valve. *J Thorac Cardiovasc Surg* 1979;77:202–211.
46. Freedom RM, Benson LN. Neonatal expression of Ebstein's anomaly. *Prog Pediatr Cardiol* 1993;2:22–27.
47. Freedom RM. The natural history of ventricular septal defect with morphological considerations. In: Moss AJ, ed. *Pediatrics Update*. New York: Elsevier; 1979; pp. 251–272.
48. Weidman WH, Blount SG Jr, Dushane JW, Gersony W, Hayes CS, Nadas AS. Clinical course in ventricular septal defect. *Circulation* 1977;56(suppl 1):56–69.
49. Corone P, Doyon F, Gaudreau S, Guerin F, Vernant P, Ducam H, Rumeau-Rouquette C, Gadeul P. Natural history of ventricular septal defect. A study involving 790 cases. *Circulation* 1977;55:908–915.
50. Gasul BM, Dillon RF, Urla V, Hait G. Ventricular septal defects: Their natural transformation into those with in-

fundibular stenosis or into the cyanotic or noncyanotic types of tetralogy of Fallot. *JAMA* 1957;164:847–853.

51. Pongiglione G, Freedom RM, Cook D, Rowe RD. Mechanism of acquired right ventricular outflow tract obstruction in patients with ventricular septal defect: An angiocardiographic study. *Am J Cardiol* 1982;50:776–780.

52. Varghese PJ, Allen JR, Rosenquist GC, Rowe RD. Natural history of ventricular septal defect with right-sided aortic arch. *Br Heart J* 1970;32:537–546.

53. Tyrrell MJ, Kidd BSL, Keith JD. Diagnosis of tetralogy of Fallot in the acyanotic phase (abstract). *Circulation* 1970; 41/42(suppl III):113.

54. Baumstark A, Fellows KE, Rosenthal A. Combined double chambered right ventricle and discrete subaortic stenosis. *Circulation* 1978;57:299–303.

55. Vogel M, Smallhorn JF, Freedom RM, Coles J, Williams WG, Trusler GA. The association of ventricular septal defect and anomalous right ventricular muscle bundles with fixed subaortic stenosis. An echocardiographic study of 36 patients. *Am J Cardiol* 1988;61:857–862.

55a.Ward CJB, Culham JAG, Patterson MWH, Sandor GSS. The trilogy of double-chambered right ventricle, perimembranous ventricular septal defect and subaortic narrowing-a more common association than previously recognized. *Cardiol Young* 1995;5:140–146.

56. Vogel M, Freedom RM, Brand A, Trusler GA, Williams WG, Rowe RD. Ventricular septal defect and subaortic stenosis: An analysis of 41 patients. *Am J Cardiol* 1983; 52:1258–1263.

57. Wright GB, Keane JF, Nadas AS, Bernhard WF, Castaneda AR. Fixed subaortic stenosis in the young: Medical and surgical course in 83 patients. *Am J Cardiol* 1983;52: 830–835.

58. Chung KJ, Fulton DR, Kreidberg MB, Payne DD, Cleveland RJ. Combined discrete subaortic stenosis and ventricular septal defect in infants and children. *Am J Cardiol* 1984;53:1429–1432.

59. De Leon SY, Ilbawi MN, Arcilla RA, Thilenius OG, Quinones JA, Duffy EC, Sulayman RF. Transatrial relief of diffuse subaortic stenosis after ventricular septal defect closure. *Ann Thorac Surg* 1990;49:429–434.

60. Shimada R, Tajimi T, Koyanagi S, Orita Y, Takeshita A, Nakamura M, Hirata T. Two-dimensional echocardiographic findings in double-chambered right ventricle. *Am Heart J* 1984;108:1059–1061.

61. Silverman NH. *Pediatric Echocardiography*. Baltimore:

Williams and Wilkins; 1993, pp. 327–360.

61a.Leandro J, Dyck JD, Smallhorn JF. Intra-utero diagnosis of anomalous right ventricular muscle bundles in association with a ventricular septal defect: A case report. *Pediatr Cardiol* 1994;15:46–48.

61b.Rein AJ, Gomori JM, Gilon D. Magnetic resonance and echocardiographic imaging of double chamber right ventricle. *J Comput Assist Tomogr* 1995;19:329–330.

62. Fisher Ch, James AE Jr, Humphries JO, Forster J, White RI Jr. Radiographic findings in anomalous muscle bundle of the right ventricle. An analysis of 15 cases. *Radiology* 1971;101:35–43.

63. Fellows KE, Martin EC, Rosenthal A. Angiocardiography of obstructing muscular bands of the right ventricle. *AJR* 1977;128:249–256.

64. Freedom RM, Culham JAG, Moes CAF. *Angiocardiography of Congenital Heart Disease.* New York: Macmillan Publishing Company; 1984, pp. 111–118

65. Soto B, Pacifico AD. *Angiocardiography in Congenital Heart Malformations.* Mt. Kisco, NY: Futura Publishing Company, Inc; 1990, pp. 311–316.

66. Yoo S-J, Choi Y-H. *Angiocardiograms in Congenital Heart Disease. Teaching File of Sejong Heart Institute.* Oxford: Oxford Medical Publications; 1991, pp. 91–98.

67. Amplatz K, Moller JH. *Radiology of Congenital Heart Disease.* St. Louis, MO: Mosby Year Book; 1993, pp. 520–524.

68. Kirklin JW, Barratt-Boyes BG. *Cardiac Surgery.* Second Edition. New York: Churchill Livingstone; 1993, pp. 861–1012.

69. McGrath LB, Joyce DH. Transatrial repair of double-chambered right ventricle. *J Card Surg* 1989;4:291–298.

70. Blasetto JW, Donahoo JS, Shuck JW. Single coronary artery in association with anomalous right ventricular muscle bundles. *Am Heart J* 1988;115:1122–1124.

71. Daliento L, Grisolia EF, Frescura C, Thiene G. Anomalous muscle bundle of the sub-pulmonary outflow in tetralogy of Fallot. *Int J Cardiol* 1984;6:547–550.

72. Chandrashekhar Y, Anand IS. Balloon dilatation of primary infundibular stenosis of the right ventricular outflow tract. *Am Heart J* 1992;124:1385–1386.

73. Saylam GS, Somerville J. Development of right ventricular outflow tract obstruction after double-lung transplantation for primary pulmonary hypertension. *Cardiol Young* 1995;5:278–281.

Chapter 18

Congenital Stenosis of the Pulmonary Valve, Idiopathic Dilation of the Pulmonary Trunk, and Congenital Pulmonary Insufficiency

Congenital Stenosis of the Pulmonary Valve

Obstruction of right ventricular outflow can originate at the level of the pulmonary valve or reside above or below the valve. Subvalve and supravalve obstructive lesions, although commented upon briefly here, are detailed in Chapters 16, 17, 19, and 20, and the association with complex cardiac malformations is discussed in Chapters 35 through 38, 40, and 41 through 44.

The terms valvular and valvar both refer to "a valve" and will be used interchangeably.[1] Designations that have been used to define the stenosis as an isolated lesion include pure or uncomplicated valve stenosis and pulmonary stenosis with normal aortic root or with an intact septum. Isolated pulmonary valve stenosis is a form of an acyanotic cardiac malformation with normal or diminished pulmonary blood flow. The atrial septum is usually intact; if not, the defect is usually in the form of a patent foramen ovale, although an actual atrial septal defect may coexist.

Prevalence

The New England Regional Infant Cardiac Program found a prevalence for pulmonary valvular stenosis of 0.073 per 1000 livebirths, whereas the Baltimore-Washington Infant study found a prevalence of 0.189 per 1000 livebirths.[1a,1b] The higher prevalence in the more recent study certainly reflects the role of echocardiography in the diagnosis of the more mild expressions of the disorder.

Embryology and Anatomy

As partitioning of the truncus arteriosus comes toward completion, small tubercles, the primordia of the semilunar valves can be observed emanating from the truncal swellings. Each truncal swelling has a tubercle on the extremity of its dorsal face and one of each pair is committed to either the aortic or pulmonary channels. A third channel then develops within each channel. Normally, with further growth, these tubercles become hollowed out to assume their mature form.[2] The etiology for fusion of the cusps is not definitively known.

The malformation of pulmonary valve stenosis was originally described by John Baptist Morgagni in 1761.[3] Pulmonary obstruction at the valve level is manifest in two distinct patterns (Table 18-1), so-called typical valve stenosis, and dysplastic pulmonary valve stenosis. Typical pulmonary valve stenosis is characterized by a thin, pliant, conical or dome-shaped valve with a restricted orifice (Fig. 18-1). The valve is usually tricuspid[4,5] though it may be bicuspid[6] or four leaflets may be visible.[7]

Morphologically, in the neonatal expression of critical pulmonary stenosis, the fused leaflets extend from

From: Freedom RM, Mawson JB, Yoo SJ, Benson LN: *Congenital Heart Disease: Textbook of Angiocardiography.* Armonk NY, Futura Publishing Co., Inc. ©1997.

Table 18-1

Features of Congenital Pulmonary Valve Stenosis

	Typical Valve Stenosis	Typical Valve Dysplasia
Commissural fusion	+ + +	o
Distinct valve cusps	+/o	+ +
Annulus hypoplasia	o	+/o
Post-stenotic MPA dialation	+ +	o
Short MPA	o	+ +
Associated cardiac anomalies	+/o	+ +
Associated syndromes	+/o	+ +

Abbreviations: + = present; o = not present; MPA = main pulmonary artery.

a central opening to the pulmonary artery wall (acommissural) creating an eccentric (rarely circular) hemodynamic orifice of varying diameter, depending on the extent of commissural fusion. Angiographically, the pulmonary valve leaflets may appear thin, but at postmortem or surgery the leaflets are fused and histologically demonstrate disorganized myxomatous tissue (Fig. 18-2).[5] Secondary changes occur in the right ventricle and pulmonary artery as a result of the profoundly afterloaded ventricle. The right ventricle hypertrophies, particularly the infundibular region with encroachment on the size of the cavity. This may be quite extensive, and in the neonate gives the appearance of true hypoplasia of the chamber. However, after effective relief of the valve obstruction, few newborns require additional sources of pulmonary blood flow, as the chamber will enlarge and become more compliant with time.[8–9a] However, some babies, even with a prolonged course of prostaglandin will require some surgical maneuver to augment pulmonary blood flow despite what is seemingly adequate relief of the outflow tract obstruction. This may reflect a poorly compliant ventricle, at times aggravated by a slightly restrictive tricuspid valve annulus, with right-to-left atrial shunting. The outflow portion of the ventricle, the infundibulum, is not displaced anteriorly as in tetralogy of Fallot (see Chapter 20). The tricuspid valve is generally well formed and competent, although right atrial enlargement can develop with significant tricuspid insufficiency secondary to right ventricular hypertension. In the absence of an intrinsic tricuspid valve anomaly (dysplasia of the leaflets, clefts, abnormal chordal attachments) this too, resolves with relief of the obstruc-

tion. The tricuspid valve may be congenitally abnormal especially in the neonatal expression of the disorder, although perhaps less severely disordered than in the patient with pulmonary atresia and intact ventricular septum.[9b] Post-stenotic dilation of the main pulmonary trunk is the rule, although rarely a supravalve hourglass deformity has been described.[10] Such enlargement can be seen at all stages of disease expression, from newborn through adult (Figure 18-1 and 18-3) and pulmonary artery aneurysms, although rare have been described.[11,12] There is disproportionate dilatation of the left pulmonary artery branch (Fig. 18-4), due to the leftward orientation of the right ventricular outflow tract, and the parallel takeoff of the left pulmonary artery from the main trunk. Additionally, it is thought that the alterations in fluid dynamic forces with dispersion of the kinetic energy of the jet beyond the stenotic valve increases the systolic pressures toward the left pulmonary artery.[13] Calcification may occur within the pulmonary valve, but is exceptional in any but the adult with long-standing disease.[14–18] The aortic arch is usually but not invariably left-sided when pulmonary valve stenosis is present with an intact ventricular septum. This is in contrast to the situation in tetralogy of Fallot when a right-sided aortic arch is present in 30% of cases. A right-sided aortic arch has been reported rarely[19–21] in critical pulmonary valve stenosis. While the expression of pulmonary valve stenosis is usually but not invariably an isolated malformation, in its typical presentation when the mechanism of right ventricular outflow obstruction is due to valve dysplasia (Table 18-1), there is a greater incidence of associated cardiac and noncardiac malformations (eg, Noonan's syndrome,[22–27] William's syndrome,[28–30] and Alagille's syndrome[31,32]), although peripheral pulmonary arterial stenoses is a more prominent feature (see also Chapter 19).

The dysplastic form of pulmonary valve stenosis occurs much less frequently (about 20% of cases with pulmonary valve stenosis) than that of typical valve stenosis.[22,23,33,34] In this setting, obstruction to right ventricular outflow reflects the reduced mobility of the thickened valve leaflets with the often associated hypoplasia of the valve annulus, supravalve tethering, a small or short main pulmonary artery and frequently peripheral pulmonary artery stenosis (Fig. 18-5). The three leaflets are distinct and composed of disorganized myxomatous tissue and generally have little or no commissural fusion.[5,22,23] However, the response to balloon valvotomy would suggest that in some, a commissural element exists.[35–37] Valve thickening generally involves the entire leaflet through to the attachments to the annulus.[5,34] The expression of pulmonary valve

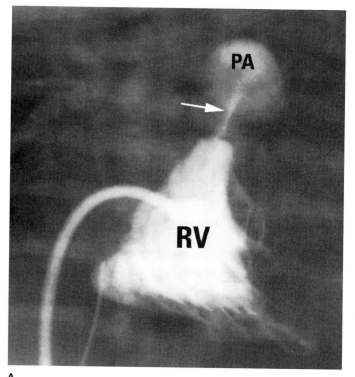

A

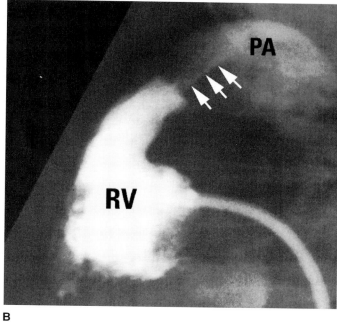

B

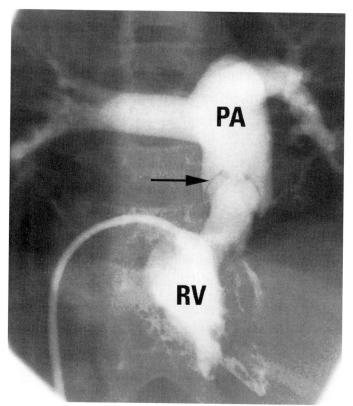

C

Fig. 18-1: Typical pulmonary valve stenosis.
Two separate patients. **A:** Cranially-tilted frontal and (**B**) lateral projections of right ventriculogram outline a well-formed tripartite chamber. The opacified jet (arrows) can be seen exiting the hemodynamic orifice and abutting the dilated main pulmonary artery. **C:** Another, slightly older patient. Cranially-tilted frontal right ventriculogram. The right ventricular cavity appears smaller due to the hypertrophy of the septal trabecular components. The domed thin pulmonary valve leaflets can be clearly seen (arrow), guarding the dilated main pulmonary artery.

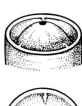

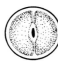

A

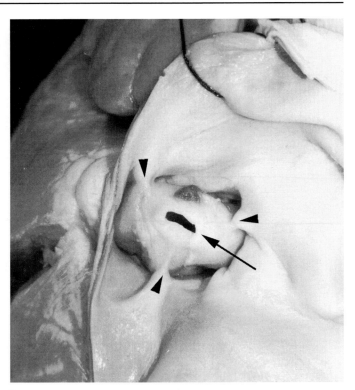

B

Fig. 18-2: Three common types of pulmonary valve stenosis.
A: Diagrammatic representation. Leftward drawings show the appearance of an acommissural leaflet with a small pinpoint orifice and primitive raphae. The thickened nodular appearance of a dysplastic pulmonary valve is seen in the middle drawings emphasizing the lack of commissural fusion, with the valve leaflets themselves the obstructive mechanism. The rightward drawings show a typical bicuspid pulmonary valve with commissural fusion and an eccentric oval shaped orifice. **B:** Postmortem specimen of a unicommissural valve. The primitive raphae are evident (arrowheads) as is the central orifice.

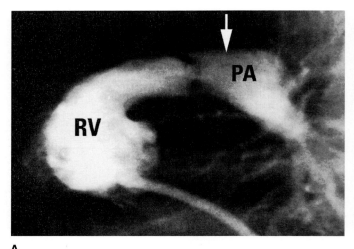

A

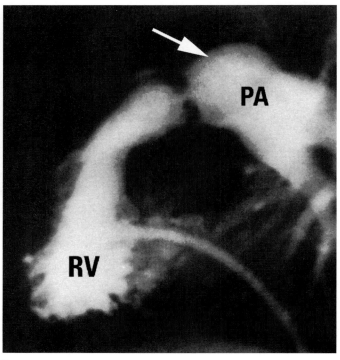

B

Fig. 18-3: Post-stenotic dilatation of main pulmonary artery.
Four patients, lateral projections of right ventriculograms. Best appreciated from the lateral right ventriculogram (or a selective main pulmonary artery injection) it is variable in extent, ranging from mild (**A**) through moderate (**B and C**) to marked (**D**) and does not correlate with hemodynamic severity.

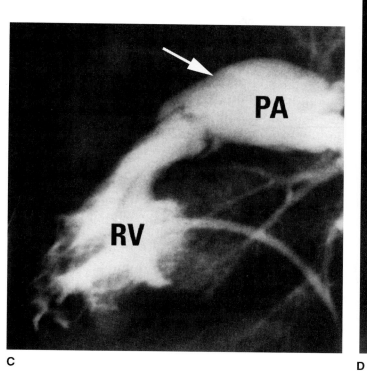

C

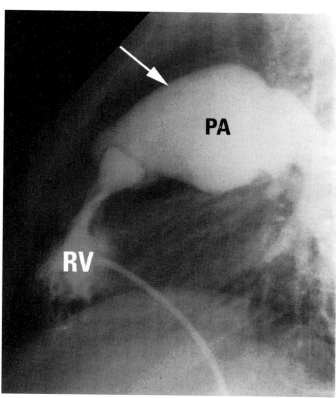

D

Fig. 18-3: *(continued)*

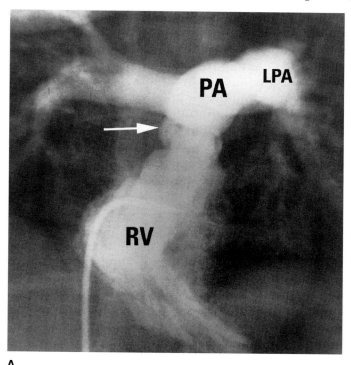

A

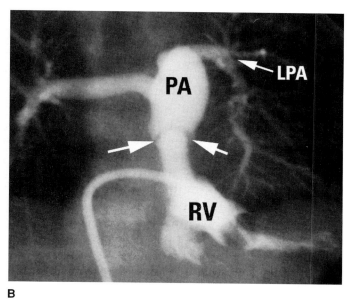

B

Fig. 18-4: Left pulmonary artery dilatation.
Two patients, cranially-tilted frontal right ventriculograms. **A:** The left pulmonary artery is generally enlarged due to the direction of the outflow jet in typical pulmonary valve stenosis. Contrast this with (**B**) where post-stenotic dilatation extends into the pulmonary ductal diverticulum, and the pulmonary arteries are hypoplastic as part of a more widespread arteriopathy. Note the doming valve leaflets (arrows).

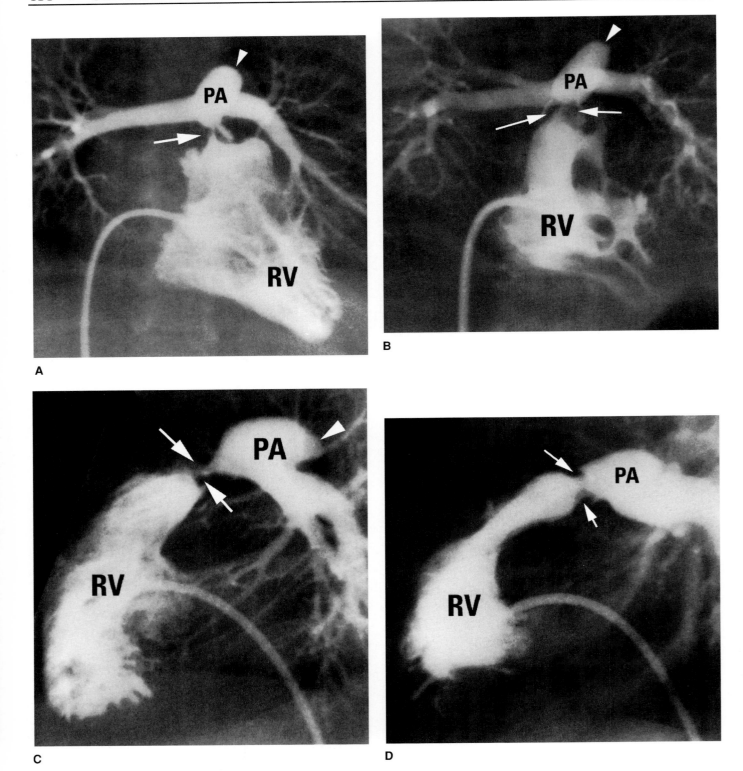

Fig. 18-5: Pulmonary valve stenosis, dysplastic leaflets.
Dysplastic pulmonary valve frequently is a component of a more diffuse cardiac lesion. Right ventriculograms in four separate patients, cranially-tilted frontal projections (**A and B**) and lateral projection (**C and D**). Well-formed chambers with varying degrees of hypertrophy are seen. The thickened pulmonary valve appears to fill the small annulii with tissue (arrows). Post-stenotic dilatation extends into the pulmonary distal diverticulum (A through C). There are normal-sized (A and D) and hypoplastic (B and C) pulmonary arteries.

stenosis in the neonate has the appearance of such dysplasia angiographically. However, medium-term studies after successful balloon dilation have documented that the valve becomes pliant, and then either with time[8,9] or spontaneously normalizes, or nearly so.[38]

Pulmonary artery stenosis may be a component of a number of more complex intracardiac anomalies, and includes those patients with anomalous muscle bundles within the right ventricular cavity (so-called divided right ventricle; see Chapter 17); obstructive anomalies within the pulmonary arteries (see Chapter 19); or other right ventricular inlet (see Chapters 14 through 16) or outlet anomalies (see Chapters 20 and 21). Diffuse infundibular obstruction within the right ventricle may also be a manifestation of a hypertrophic cardiomyopathy (see Chapter 28) as an expression of the diffuse myocardial process, particularly as seen in the young.[39]

Additional noncongenital disorders may affect the pulmonary valve and lead to its stenosis and include rheumatic heart disease,[4] infective endocarditis,[40–42] external compression from chest trauma, and most commonly carcinoid heart disease.[43–47] While these must be considered in the differential diagnosis, the congenital expression of valve obstruction accounts for over 95% of these conditions.

Angiocardiography

The pulmonary valve is best outlined by right ventriculography performed in the cranially angled (20°-30°) anteroposterior and lateral projections. As the valve points forward and downward, the anteroposterior projection without angulation will result in the outflow of the right ventricle overlapping the pulmonary valve annulus. Although not critical for defining the valve, the angulated anteroposterior projection will outline the main pulmonary trunk and branch pulmonary arteries. The stenotic pulmonary valve (typical lesion) is mildly thickened, smooth, and domes during systole (Figs. 18-1 and 18-6), although the leaflets will return to their normal position in diastole. The fused valve leaflets curve inward during systole and a jet of contrast can be identified passing across the valve. The valve annulus is usually normal in diameter, although it may be hypoplastic if the stenosis is severe, particularly in the newborn.[5] The main pulmonary artery is dilated (Fig. 18-3), and the contrast jet can frequently be identified striking the main pulmonary artery anterosuperiorly. The dilatation may extend into the left pulmonary artery, and to a lesser extent to the right branch. The degree of post-stenotic dilation is not related to the severity of obstruction.[48]

The right ventricle expresses secondary structural alterations due to the valve obstruction.[49] The trabeculae are thickened and hypertrophied, while the cavity is of normal or reduced size,[8,9] and in the absence of fixed subvalvar obstruction, the infundibular diameter will be normal in diastole. The infundibular septum is not displaced anteriorly as in tetralogy of Fallot, although due to its thickness it may seemingly encroach on the left ventricular outflow (Fig. 18-7).

The appearance of the dysplastic pulmonary valve differs from typical dome-type stenosis.[50,51] The leaflets are considerably thickened and irregular, and remain deformed during the cardiac cycle. The sinuses are narrowed and distorted, with frequently associated hypoplasia of the annulus and proximal main pulmonary trunk (Figs. 18-5 and 18-8). The post-stenotic dilation of the pulmonary trunk and systolic doming seen in typical uncomplicated pulmonary artery stenosis are not seen. When post-stenotic dilation of the main pulmonary artery is present, this suggests the presence of some degree of commissural fusion.[36] This dysplastic pulmonary valve is frequently found in association with Noonan's syndrome[22–27,52] and Leopard's syndrome.[53–55]

The levophase of the right ventricular angiogram is of value in ruling out a left-sided lesion, and can define an atrial level shunt, if one exists. The levoangiocardiogram or selective left ventriculogram may be helpful in demonstrating the association of the dysplastic pulmonary valve and Noonan's syndrome. The left ventricle in this syndrome is affected by an eccentric hypertrophy involving the septum close to the outflow tract, the superior portion of the anterior wall and/or the diaphragmatic portion of the ventricle (Fig. 18-9) (see also Chapter 28).[56–66] The right anterior oblique projection will detail a prominent indentation superolaterally and posteroinferiorly on the ventricular chamber silhouette, both systolic and diastolic. The septal hypertrophy, which bulges into the left ventricular outflow, is best visualized from the left axial oblique projection. The hypertrophy of the diaphragmatic portion of the left ventricle produces a concavity that gives a profile stylized as a "ballerina foot" deformity (Fig. 18-9).

Finally, it has been pointed out[67] that the thickened immobile dysplastic pulmonary valve may be only a part of a more widespread cardiovascular arteriopathy, noting its occurrence with myocardial dysplasia, necrosis of one or both ventricles, coronary artery occlusions and a "higgledy-piggledy" aortic wall histology. Such myocardial dysfunction, and a small, noncompliant ascending aorta should alert one to the fact that the "isolated" pulmonary lesion may indeed be a component of a more diffuse anomaly.

The neonatal expression of pulmonary valve steno-

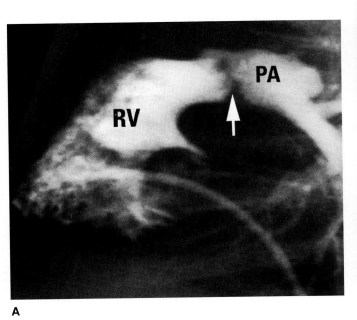

A

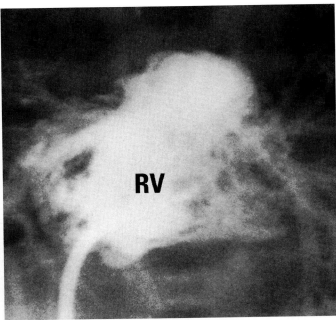

B

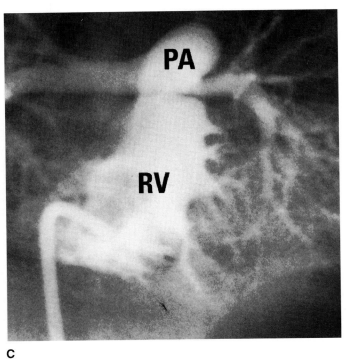

C

Fig. 18-6: Choice of angiographic projection.
Two separate right ventriculograms. **A:** The horizontal and elongated infundibulum means that the frontal projection (**B**) superimposed the outflow tract and pulmonary valve. **C:** Addition of cranial tilt to the frontal projection separates structures to better outline the anatomy.

Fig. 18-7: Angiography of pulmonary valve stenosis.
Lateral projections during systole demonstrate localized (**A**) and diffuse (**B**) dynamic subpulmonary narrowing. Subpulmonary obstruction in association with valve stenosis. Right ventriculograms in four patients. This contrasts with fixed subpulmonary obstruction (arrow) that may develop as seen on cranially-tilted frontal (**C**) and lateral (**D**) ventriculograms in two patients.

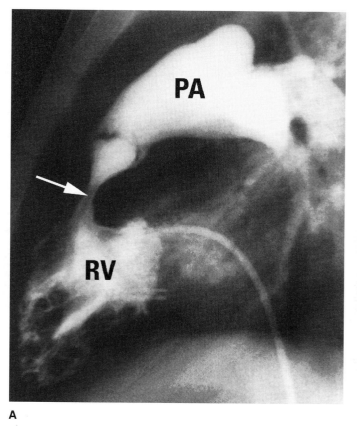

A

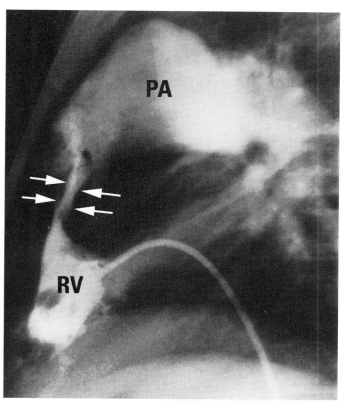

B

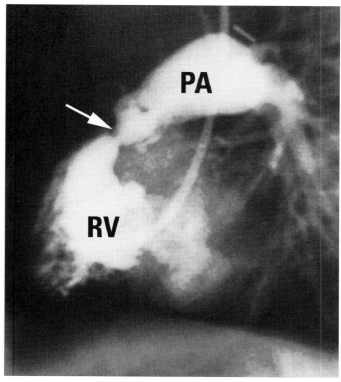

C

D

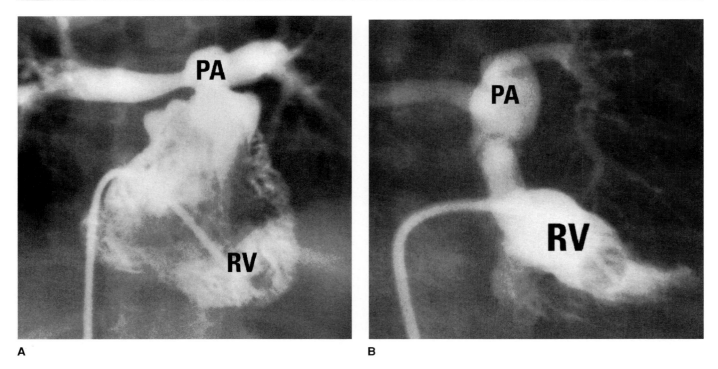

A   B

Fig. 18-8: Ventricular sizes in patients with pulmonary valve stenosis.
Two different patients. Right ventriculogram, cranially tilted frontal projections. The RV may be dilated (**A**) or (**B**) hypoplastic (same patient as in Fig. 18-4B).

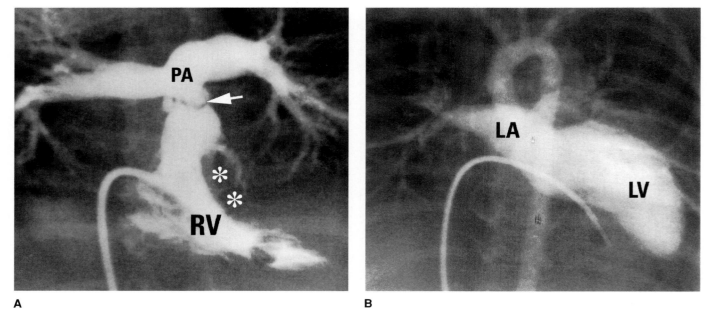

A   B

Fig. 18-9: Hypertrophic cardiomyopathy in association with pulmonary valve stenosis.
Hypertrophic cardiomyopathy frequently complicates the clinical management of the dysplastic pulmonary valve syndrome as seen in these two patients with Noonan's syndrome. (**A**) Right ventriculogram (early diastole) in cranially-tilted frontal projection shows the thickened pulmonary valve (arrow) and the substantially hypertrophied interventricular septum (✱). **B:** Levophase of right ventriculogram, in cranially tilted frontal projection reveals the typical "ballerina foot" shape to the contour of the left ventricle representing the hypertrophy of the septal wall.

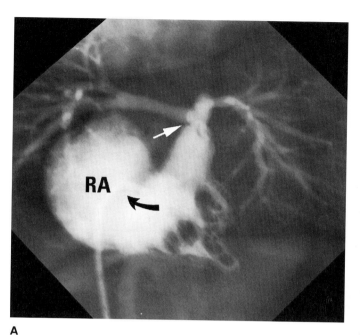

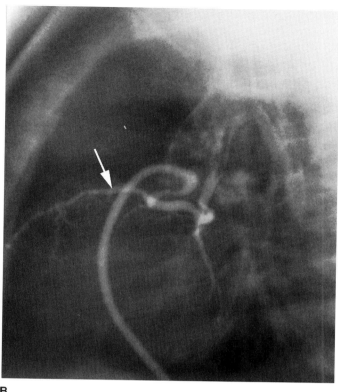

A

B

Fig. 18-10: Coronary pulmonary artery fistula in association with pulmonary valve stenosis.
A: Cranially tilted frontal right ventriculogram details annular hypoplasia valve stenosis (arrow) and pulmonary artery hypoplasia. **B:** Lateral projection. A fistula communicating from the lateral aspect of the main pulmonary artery is selectively injected, defining its communication to the left anterior descending coronary artery (arrow).

sis frequently presents with generalized cyanosis, and the patient's survival is dependent on rapid diagnosis and prompt valvotomy.[68,69] As such, reduction in right ventricular hypertension is being successfully performed in the cardiac catheterization laboratory[8,9] where angiography is critically important to define ventricular size, degree of tricuspid regurgitation if present, position of the pulmonary valve, and coexistence of ventriculocoronary connections (rare). Right ventriculography demonstrates a doming pulmonary valve during systole with a small or pinpoint orifice (Fig. 18-10). The right ventricle can be dilated, normal in size, or hypoplastic. If the cavity is small, it tends to be displaced more medially than normal, and the apex appears truncated from heavy trabeculations.[70] The tricuspid valve may also be hypoplastic.[50] This morphological constellation may mimic pulmonary atresia with intact ventricular septum (see Chapter 23). The right ventricle in critical pulmonary valve stenosis, however, rarely has

ventriculocoronary connections so frequently observed in patients with pulmonary atresia and intact ventricular septum. Dilation of the main pulmonary trunk may not be present. The right atrium is enlarged and can be outlined in the present of tricuspid regurgitation, due to extrasystoles, catheter placement or rarely an intrinsically abnormal valve. Right-to-left shunting is frequently seen in the presence of a patent oval foramen or true atrial septal defect.

Idiopathic Dilation of the Pulmonary Artery

Idiopathic dilation of the pulmonary trunk is a rare anomaly, originally described by Wessler and Jaches in 1923.[71] The lesion is characterized by dilation of the pulmonary trunk and occasionally its branches.[72] A developmental defect in the pulmonary artery elastic tissue may be the underlying fault[73,74] or disproportionate division of the primitive truncus.[75,76] This latter suggestion implies a reciprocal decrease in the dimension of the aortic root[76–78] although this is rarely found.[79]

When suspected, other causes for dilatation of the main pulmonary trunk should be considered including: 1) straight back syndrome[80]; 2) partial absence of the pericardium[81]; or 3) Marfan's syndrome, among others. A prominent main pulmonary artery trunk may also be seen in early adolescence, particularly in females.

Chest radiographs and right ventriculograms show a dilated main pulmonary trunk, but are otherwise normal. The right ventricle is of normal size, and not hypertrophied, and the pulmonary valve leaflets are thin and not stenotic. Pulmonary insufficiency may occur.[82] The normalcy of right ventricular pressure, with perhaps a trivial pulmonary artery gradient has been suggested as being the diagnostic *sine qua non* for the diagnosis of idiopathic dilation of the main pulmonary trunk.[83] The lesion is benign, and rarely may process to aneurysm formation.[11,12,84,85]

Congenital Pulmonary Valve Insufficiency

Pulmonary valve regurgitation as an isolated anomaly is a rare finding, and some patients are considered to have idiopathic dilatation of the pulmonary trunk. The current opinion is that such regurgitation is the product of a congenitally malformed pulmonary valve[86–101] or idiopathic trunk dilation.[73,75,82] One, two, or all three cusps may be involved, short and adherent to one another or rudimentary,[91,98] one absent and the remaining two rudimentary,[94] or no tissue at all.[95,96] The valve may be bicuspid[99,100] or quadricuspid[92,102] or have a moderate degree of cuspal inequality and/or a leaflet fenestrated.

Angiographic demonstration of isolated pulmonary valve insufficiency is difficult because a pulmonary artery injection is required. Placement of a catheter across the pulmonary valve in itself may cause insufficiency. It is therefore best to perform the injection with the catheter tip distal to the valve, securing

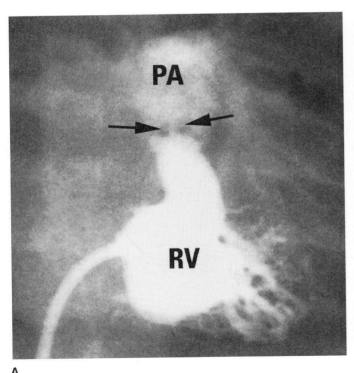

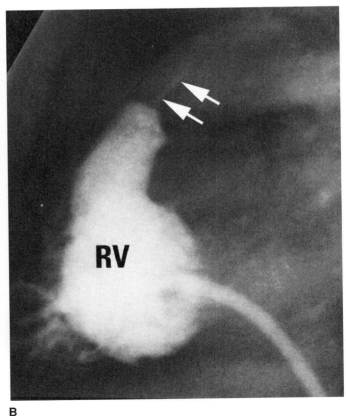

Fig. 18-11: Neonatal critical pulmonary valve stenosis. Right ventriculogram in cranially-tilted frontal and lateral projections. **A:** The right ventricle is hypertrophied, the outflow critically narrowed by the fused valve leaflets (dark arrows). **B:** The hemodynamic orifice is identified by the contrast jet (arrows), best profiled in this patient in the lateral projection.

the catheter and avoiding recoil. The main pulmonary artery will be dilated to varying degrees, depending on the severity of the regurgitation, with or without involvement of the branch vessels. The size of the right ventricle will depend on the degree of regurgitation. The valve leaflets will appear normal unless a primary anomaly is present.

Transcatheter Therapy: Balloon Dilation of Pulmonary Valve Stenosis

Rubio-Alvarez et al[103] initially described the technique by which pulmonic stenosis could be relieved by a catheter technique. Twenty-one years later Semb[104] using an inflated balloon-tipped angiographic catheter ruptured the valve when it was withdrawn from the main pulmonary artery to the right ventricle, reducing the outflow gradient. However, it was the introduction of the static balloon dilation by Kan et al[105] that fostered the application of this therapeutic modality to a greater audience. The technique has become the "treatment of choice" for pulmonary valve stenosis at any age and with any valve morphology.[106–136]

The safety and efficacy of the technique in infants, children, and adolescents has been confirmed by numerous studies summarized by McCrindle and Kan.[107] Indications for intervention in these age groups, with or without symptoms is a transvalvar gradient of >40 mm Hg in the absence of fixed subpulmonary obstruction or additional lesions that need surgical attention. It has been applied successfully in all forms of pulmonary valve obstructive morphologies (see below), after endocarditis, and in cyanotic congenital heart disease.[136a,136b]

The procedure is not technically difficult, but de-

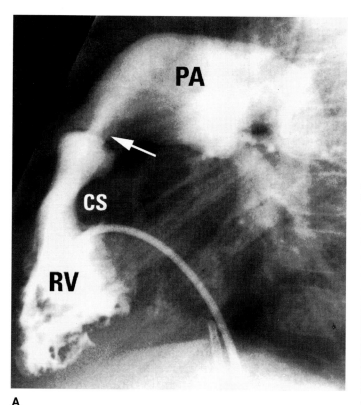

A

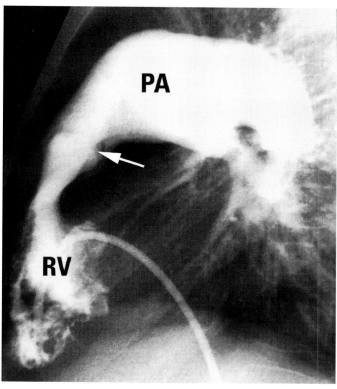

B

Fig. 18-12: Balloon valvuloplasty.
Two patients, right ventriculograms, lateral projections. **A:** Prior to and (**B**) after dilatation. There is mild dynamic subpulmonary stenosis. Note in (A), the curled doming valve (arrow) and jet of contrast hitting the anterosuperior border of the main pulmonary artery. Contrast this with (B), at the same phase of systole, where the contrast jet is wider, filling the main pulmonary artery and the excursion of the pulmonary valve (particularly the posterior leaflet) is increased (arrow). Similar observations can be seen in another child *(continued)*

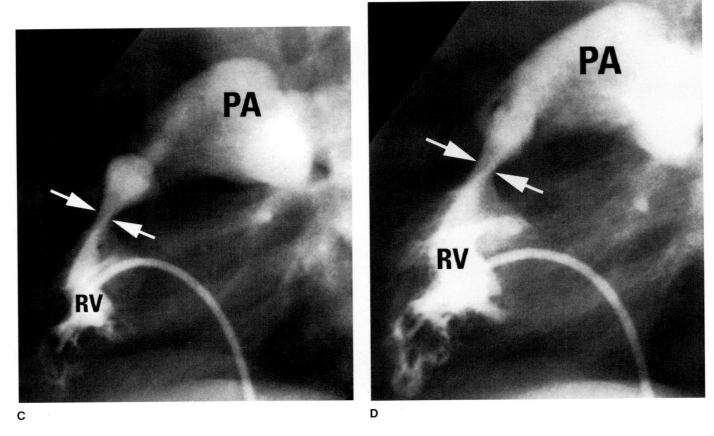

C   **D**

Fig. 18-12: *(continued)*
(C) before dilatation and **(D)** after dilatation, with considerably greater dynamic subpulmonary obstruction (arrows).

pends upon high-quality angiography for valve location and definition. A number of different protocols have been successful.[137,138] Generally, a right ventriculogram is performed using a 25° cranial tilt (we also add 10° left anterior obliquity) with 90° lateral projections (Fig. 18-1). The valve annulus is measured from the valve hinge points in the lateral projection. A 5F right coronary artery catheter is used to cross the valve with a floppy guidewire and directed to the left pulmonary artery (or through the arterial duct into the aorta in neonates). An exchange wire (0.035 inch) is placed through this catheter, over which a single balloon, 2 or 3 cm in length, is positioned to straddle the valve. The balloon diameter chosen is generally 30% to 40% larger than the measured annulus, and it is inflated several times until the "waist" of the stenotic valve is no longer visualized (Fig. 18-11). Hemodynamics and angiography are then repeated.

Morphological changes in valve mobility can be seen, as well as alterations in flow dynamics, subpul-monary valve function (dynamic subpulmonary stenosis) and the presence of any pulmonary artery tears (rare) (Fig. 18-12).[139,140] When the pulmonary valve diameter is too large (>18 mm), two "kissing" balloons, placed to straddle the valve are required (Fig. 18-13). In this case, the combined diameters of the two balloons should be 50% to 60% greater than the measured valve annulus. The balloons distort the valve in an elliptical configuration with a gap between the balloons, allowing blood to reach the pulmonary circulation. Hypotension from right ventricular outflow tract obstruction is less common in this situation, but its technical requirements (ie, a second balloon) far outweigh the marginal benefit.

Short- and long-term studies[107,108,119,120,141,142] have uniformly attested to the efficacy of the procedure with persistence of valve gradient reduction in the majority of patients to nonhemodynamically significant levels. Unsuccessful results were due to an inability to cross the pulmonary valve or the dysplastic nature of the valve leaflets (obstructive but with little commissural fusion).[106] In the latter situation, however, the degree of valve fusion is difficult to define (where its lack would predict failure).[143] In such situations, in the absence of a hypoplastic annulus (which itself is obstructive) and perhaps the finding of a dilated main pulmonary artery, dilation should be attempted.[141,144–149] Major complications outside of the neonatal period are few and have been summarized by Stanger et al[106] from the Valvuloplasty and Angioplasty of Congenital Anomalies registry.

The application of the technique in the neonate is technically more demanding. Early studies found traversing the hypoplastic infundibulum problematic,[150] but with the use of a right coronary artery curve, traversing the valve has been simplified. Additional maneuvers to help achieve the dilation include placement of the guidewire into the aorta (through the patent arterial duct) for increased guide control, and in some situations the application of graduated balloon diameters.[9,151–163] Short- and medium-term results have generally been as encouraging as in the older patient, although in some, the smaller noncompliant right ventricle may not be adequate for maintaining a normal pulmonary blood flow, requiring prolonged support with prostanoids or placement of an arterial shunt (Figure 18-14).[9] Morphological follow-up studies have confirmed that the thickened pulmonary valves mature from their dysplastic appearance, and the annulus, and right ventricular cavities grow.[9] Those newborns with the most profound (hypoplastic) right heart maldevelopment may require additional sources of pulmonary blood flow.[151,159,161]

The experience in adults similarly reflects the technical simplicity and hemodynamic improvement seen in the pediatric age group.[164–167]

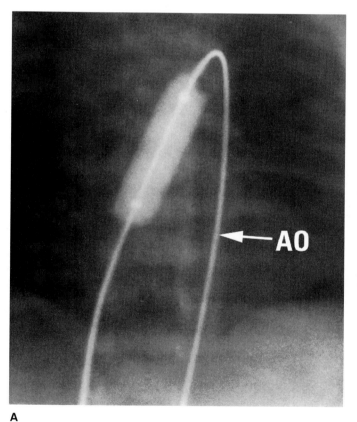

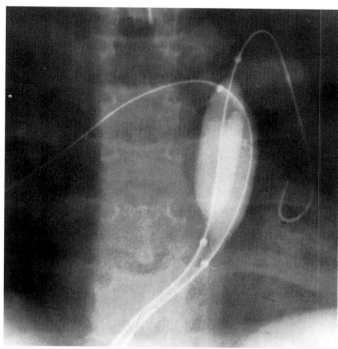

A   B

Fig. 18-13: Balloon valvuloplasty for pulmonary stenosis.
Two patients. Cranially-tilted frontal projections. **A:** Two-centimeter long balloon across the pulmonary valve annulus (same patient as Fig. 18-11). Note the guidewire in the descending aorta through the arterial duct (arrow). **B:** An older child, requiring two "kissing" balloons for dilatation. In this case, one guidewire is in each pulmonary artery branch, although a single branch may be used to position the guidewires.

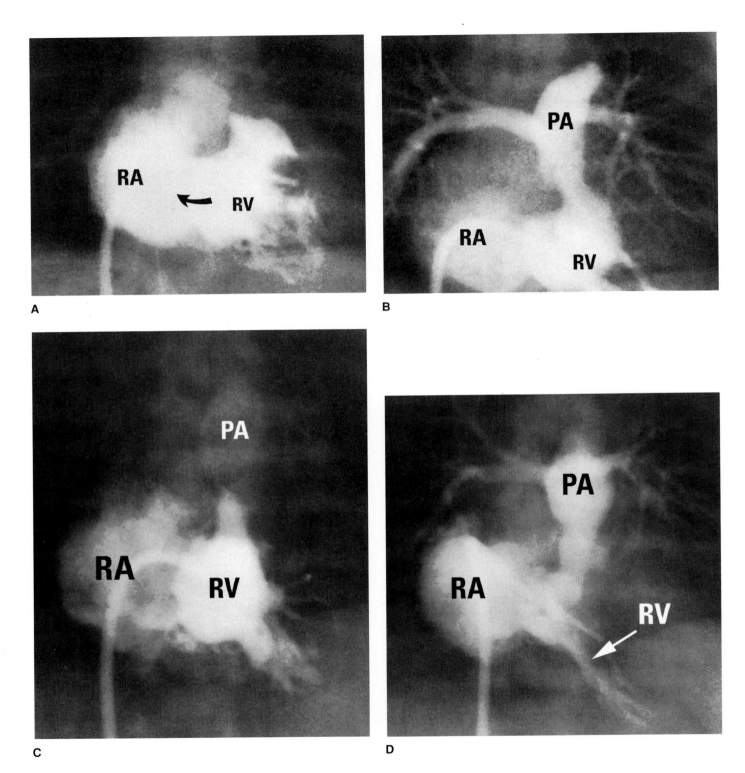

Fig. 18-14: Balloon valvuloplasty.
Cranially-tilted frontal projections from two neonates before and after balloon dilatation. (**A**) and (**C**) Predilatation, the ventricles are small due to the excessive hypertrophic process and tricuspid regurgitation of varying degrees present. Also note the well expanded infundibulum and the critical stenosis of the valve. Postdilatation (**B**) and (**D**), there are well-developed main pulmonary artery segments, small to hypoplastic pulmonary arteries and arterial duct patency.

References

1. Perloff JK. Congenital pulmonary stenosis. In: *The Clinical Recognition of Congenital Heart Disease*. Philadelphia: W.B Saunders; 1994, pp. 198–220.
2. Langman J. Medical embryology. In: *Human Development: Normal and Abnormal*. Third edition. Baltimore: Williams and Wilkins; 1975, pp. 183–204.
3. Morgagni JB. *The Seats and Causes of Diseases Investigated by Anatomy*. Padua, 1761. Translated from the Latin by Benjamin Alexander. London: Milar, Cadell, Johnson and Payne. As quoted by Perloff JK. Congenital pulmonary stenosis. In: *Clinical Recognition of Congenital Heart Disease*. Philadelphia: WB Saunders; 1994. P. 109.
4. Waller BF, Howard J, Fess S. Pathology of pulmonic valve stenosis and pure regurgitation. *Clin Cardiol* 1995; 18:45–50.
5. Gikonyo BM, Lucas RV, Edwards JE. Anatomic features of congenital pulmonary valvar stenosis. *Pediatr Cardiol* 1987;8:109–116.
6. Keith JD, Rowe RD, Vlad P. *Heart Disease in Infancy and Childhood*. Third edition. New York: MacMillan Publishing Company; 1978, pp. 762–788.
7. Edwards JE. Congenital malformations of the heart and great vessels. In: Gould SE, ed. *Pathology of the Heart*. Springfield, IL: Charles C. Thomas; 1953, pp. 94–101.
8. Colli AM, Perry SB, Lock JE, Keane JF. Balloon dilation of critical valvar pulmonary stenosis in the first month of life. *Cathet Cardiovasc Diagn* 1995;34:23–28.
9. Tabatabaei H, Boutin C, Nykanen DG, Freedom RM, Benson LN. Morphologic and hemodynamic consequences after percutaneous balloon valvotomy for neonatal pulmonary stenosis: Medium-term results. *J Am Coll Cardiol* 1996;27:473–478.
9a. Schmidt KG, Cloez Jean-L, Silverman NH. Changes in right ventricular size and function in neonates after valvotomy for pulmonary atresia or critical pulmonary stenosis and intact ventricular septum. *J Am Coll Cardiol* 1992;19:1032–1037.
10. Milo S, Fiegel A, Shem-Tov A, Neufeld HN, Goor DA. Hour-glass deformity of the pulmonary valve: A third type of pulmonary valve stenosis. *Br Heart J* 1988;60: 434–443.
11. Shindo T, Kuroda T, Watanabe S, Hojo Y, Sekiguchi H, Shimada K. Aneurysmal dilatation of the pulmonary trunk with mild pulmonic stenosis. *Intern Med* 1995;34: 199–202.
12. Tami LF, McElderry MW. Pulmonary artery aneurysm due to severe congenital pulmonic stenosis. Case report and literature review. *Angiology* 1994;45:383–390.
13. Muster JD, van Grondelle A, Paul MH. Unequal pressures in the central pulmonary arterial branches in patients with pulmonary stenosis. *Pediatr Cardiol* 1982; 2:7–13.
14. Alday LE, Morey RAE. Calcific pulmonary stenosis. *Br Heart J* 1973;35:887–889.
15. Gabriele OF, Scatliff JH. Pulmonary valve calcification. *Am Heart J* 1970;80:299–302.
16. Hardy WE, Gnoj J, Ayers SM, Giannelli S, Christianson LC. Pulmonic stenosis and associated atrial septal defects in older patients. *Am J Cardiol* 1969;24:130–134.
17. Roberts WC, Mason DT, Morrow AG, Braunwald E. Calcific pulmonic stenosis. *Circulation* 1968;37:973–978.
18. Voci G, Maniet AR, Diego JN, Baker HA III, Voci P,

Banka VS. Severe calcific pulmonic valve stenosis and restrictive ventricular septal defect in a 64-year-old man. Results of percutaneous double balloon valvuloplasty. *Cardiologia* 1994;39:863–868.
19. Freedom RM, Culham JAG, Moes CAF. Pulmonary valve stenosis. In: Freedom RM, Culham JAG, Moes CAF, eds. *Angiography of Congenital Heart Disease*. New York: MacMillan Publishing Company; 1984, pp. 222–230.
20. Bressie JF. Pulmonary valve stenosis with intact ventricular septum and ringlet aortic arch. *Br Heart J* 1964;26: 154–156.
21. Campbell M. Simple pulmonary stenosis; pulmonary valve stenosis with a closed ventricular septum. *Br Heart J* 1954;16:273–300.
22. Koretzky ED, Moller JH, Korns ME, Schwartz CJ, Edwards JE. Congenital pulmonary stenosis resulting from dysplasia of the valve. *Circulation* 1969;40:43–53.
23. Linde LM, Turner SW, Sparkes RS. Pulmonary valvular dysplasia. A cardiofacial syndrome. *Br Heart J* 1973;35: 301–304.
24. Mendez HMM, Opitz JM. Noonan syndrome: A review. *Am J Med Genet* 1985;21:493–506.
25. Sanchez-Cascos A. The Noonan syndrome. *Eur Heart J* 1983;4:223–229.
26. Noonan JA. Hypertelorism with Turner's phenotype. A new syndrome with associated congenital heart disease. *Am J Dis Child* 1968;116:373–380.
27. Sharland M, Burch M, McKenna WM, Paton MAA. A clinical study of Noonan syndrome. *Arch Dis Child* 1992;67:178–183.
28. Wessel A, Pankau R, Kececioglu D, Ruschewski W, Bursch JH. Three decades of follow-up of aortic and pulmonary vascular lesions in the Williams-Beuren syndrome. *Am J Med Genet* 1994;52:297–301.
29. Beuren AJ, Apitz J, Harmjanz D. Supravalve aortic stenosis in association with mental retardation and a certain facial appearance. *Circulation* 1962;26:1235–1240.
30. Beuren AJ, Schulze C, Eberle P, Harmjanz D, Apitz J. The syndrome of supravalvular aortic stenosis, peripheral pulmonary stenosis, mental retardation and similar facial appearance. *Am J Cardiol* 1964;13:471–483.
31. Levin SE, Zarvos P, Miller S, Schmaman A. Arteriohepatic dysplasia: Association of liver disease with pulmonary arterial stenosis as well as facial and skeletal abnormalities. *Pediatrics* 1980;66:876–883
32. Silberbach M, Lashley D, Reller MD, Kinn WF Jr, Terry A, Sunderland CO. Arteriohepatic dysplasia and cardiovascular malformations. *Am Heart J* 1994;127:695–699.
33. Patterson DF, Haskins ME, Schurr WR. Hereditary dysplasia of the pulmonary valve in beagle dogs. *Am J Cardiol* 1981;47:631–641.
34. Schneewiss A, Blieden LC, Shem-Tov A, Goor D, Milo A, Neufeld HN. Diagnostic angiocardiographic criteria in dysplastic stenotic pulmonary valve. *Am Heart J* 1983;106:761–762.
35. Marantz PM, Huhta JC, Mullins CE, Murphy DJ Jr, Nihill MR, Ludomirsky A, Yoon GY. Results of balloon valvuloplasty in typical and dysplastic pulmonary valve stenosis: Doppler echocardiographic follow-up. *J Am Coll Cardiol* 1988;12:476–479.
36. Musewe NN, Robertson MA, Benson LN, Smallhorn JF, Burrows PE, Freedom RM, Moes CA, Rowe RD. The dysplastic pulmonary valve: Echocardiographic features and results of balloon dilatation. *Br Heart J* 1987;57: 364–370.
37. DiSessa TG, Alpert BS, Chase NA, Birnbaum SE, Watson

DC. Balloon valvuloplasty in children with dysplastic pulmonary valves. *Am J Cardiol* 1987;60:405–407.

38. Kirk CR, Wilkinson JL, Qureshi SA. Regression of pulmonary valve stenosis due to a dysplastic valve presenting in the neonatal period. *Eur Heart J* 1988; 9:1027–1029.

39. Schaeffer, MS, Freedom RM, Rowe RD. Hypertrophic cardiomyopathy presenting before 2 years of age in 13 patients. *Pediatr Cardiol* 1983;4:113–119.

40. Cherukuri AK, Maloney M, O'Briain DS, Weir DG. Isolated pulmonary valve endocarditis: A rare or an underdiagnosed disease? *Ir J Med Sci* 1994;163:494–495.

41. Pontes J, Parente F, Ruas L, Isaac J, Alexandrino B, serra Silva P. Pulmonary valve endocarditis caused by Streptococcus (bovis). *Rev Port Cardiol* 1994;13;329–334.

42. Sunazawa T, Uemura S, Fukuchi S, Tsuruta Y, Murakami S, Ukita H. A case report of acute pulmonary valve endocarditis caused by fungi. *Nippon Kyobu Geka Gakkai Zasshi* 1995;43:74–77.

43. Ponte E, Valente M, Melato M. Carcinoid cardiopathy. A study of 40 cases. *Minerva Cardioangiol* 1994;42:21–25.

44. Pellikka PA, Tajik AJ, Khandheria BK, Seward JB, Callahan JA, Pitot HC, Kvols LK. Carcinoid heart disease. Clinical and echocardiographic spectrum in 74 patients. *Circulation* 1993;87:1188–1196.

45. Hargreaves AD, Pringle SD, Boon NA. Successful balloon dilatation of the pulmonary valve in carcinoid heart disease. *Int J Cardiol* 1994;45:150–151.

46. Onate A, Alcibar J, Inguanzo R, Pena N, Gochi R. Balloon dilation of tricuspid and pulmonary valves in carcinoid heart disease. *Tex Heart Inst J* 1993;20:115–119.

47. Grant SC, Scarffe JH, Levy RD, Brooks NH. Failure of balloon dilatation of the pulmonary valve in carcinoid pulmonary stenosis. *Br Heart J* 1992;67:450–453.

48. DiCruz IA, Arcilla RA, Agristsson MH. Dilatation of the pulmonary trunk in stenosis of the pulmonary valve and the pulmonary arteries in childhood. *Am Heart J* 1964; 68:612–620.

49. Rangel-Abundis A, Lopez H, Badui E, Martinez-Becerril A. Volume and function of the right ventricle before and after intraluminal pulmonary valvuloplasty. *Arch Inst Cardiol Mex* 1991;61:517–525.

50. Hanley FL, Sade RM, Freedom RM, Blackstone EH, Kirklin JW. Outcomes in critically ill neonates with pulmonary stenosis and intact ventricular septum: a multi-institutional study. Congenital Heart Surgeons Society. *J Am Coll Cardiol* 1993;22:183–192.

51. Rodriguez-Fernandez HL, Char F, Kelly DT, Rowe RD. The dysplastic valve and Noonan's Syndrome. *Circulation* 1972;46(suppl II):11–98.

52. Schieken RM, Freedman S, Pierce WS. Severe congenital pulmonary stenosis with pulmonary valvular dysplasia syndrome. *Am Thorac Surg* 1973;15:570–577.

53. Gorlin RJ, Anderson RC, Blaw M. Multiple lentigenes syndrome. *Am J Dis Child* 1969;117:652–662.

54. Watson GM. Pulmonary stenosis, "cafe-au-lait" spots and dull intelligence. *Arch Dis Child* 1967;42:303–307.

55. Hoeffel JC, Ravoult MC, Warms AM, Pernot C. Atypical pulmonary stenosis: Radiological features. *Am Heart J* 1979;98:315–320.

56. Baltaxe HA, Levin AR, Ehlers KH, Engle MA. The appearance of the left ventricle in Noonan's syndrome. *Radiology* 1973;109:155–159.

57. Pearl W. Cardiovascular anomalies in Noonan's syndrome. *Chest* 1977;71:667–679.

58. Collins E, Turner G. The Noonan syndrome—a review of the clinical and genetic features of 27 cases. *J Pediatr* 1973;83:941–950.

59. Pernot C, Marcon F, Worms AM, Cloez JL, Gilgenkrantz S, Marois L. Cardiovascular dysplasia in Noonan's syndrome. Apropos of 64 cases. *Arch Mal Coeur Vaiss* 1987; 80:434–443.

60. Burch M, Sharland M, Shinebourne E, Smith G, Patton M, McKenna W. Cardiologic abnormalities in Noonan syndrome: Phenotypic diagnosis and echocardiographic assessment of 118 patients. *J Am Coll Cardiol* 1993;22: 1189–1192.

61. Cooke RA, Chambers JB, Curry PV. Noonan's cardiomyopathy: A non-hypertrophic variant. *Br Heart J* 1994;71: 561–565.

62. Burch M, Mann JM, Sharland M, Shinebourne EA, Patton MA, McKenna WJ. Myocardial disarray in Noonan syndrome. *Br Heart J* 1992;68:586–588.

63. Doyama K, Hirose K, Fujiwara H. Asymmetric septal hypertrophy in a 41-year-old woman with Noonan's syndrome. *Chest* 1990;97:1480–1481.

64. Perrotta Scaravilli E, Pontillo D, Pennacchia F, Boccanelli A, Greco C, Lo Schiavo P. Hypertrophic cardiomyopathy associated with Noonan's syndrome and membranous aortic subvalvular stenosis associated with Turner's syndrome. Report of 2 clinical cases. *G Ital Cardiol* 1987;17:800–806.

65. Armengol AJ, Brohet CR, Lintermans JP, Vliers A. Left ventricle in Noonan's syndrome. Electro-vecto-echo and angiocardiographic aspects. *Arch Mal Coeur Vaiss* 1987; 80:445–453.

66. Shimizu A, Oku Y, Matsuo K, Hashiba K. Hypertrophic cardiomyopathy progressing to a dilated cardiomyopathy-like feature in Noonan's syndrome. *Am Heart J* 1992; 123:814–816.

67. Becu L, Somerville J, Gallo A. "Isolated" pulmonary valve stenosis is part of a more widespread cardiovascular disease. *Br Heart J* 1976;38:472–482.

67a. Shirani J, Zafari AM, Roberts WC. Sudden death, right ventricular infarction, and abnormal right ventricular intramural coronary arteries in isolated congenital valvular pulmonic stenosis. *Am J Cardiol* 1995;72: 368–370.

68. Freed MD, Rosenthal A, Bernard WF, Litwin SB, Nada AS. Critical pulmonary stenosis with a diminutive right ventricle in neonates. *Circulation* 1973;48:875–881.

69. Litwin SB, Williams WH, Freed MD, Bernard WF. Critical pulmonary stenosis in infants; a surgical emergency. *Surgery* 1973;74:880–886.

70. Williams JCP, Barratt-Boyes BG, Lowe JB. Undeveloped right ventricle and pulmonary stenosis. *Am J Cardiol* 1963;11:458–468.

71. Wessler H, Jackes L. *Clinical Reontgenology of Disease of the Chest.* Troy, NY: Southworth Company; 1923.

72. Bankl H. *Congenital malformations of the Heart and Great Vessels.* Baltimore: Urban and Schwarzenberg; 1977, pp. 229.

73. Kaplan BM, Schlichter JG, Graham G, Miller G. Idiopathic congenital dilatation of the pulmonary artery. *J Lab Clin Med* 1953;41:697–707.

74. Brenner O. Pathology of vessels of pulmonary circulation. *Arch Intern Med* 1935;56:1189–1193.

75. Goetz RH, Nellen M. Idiopathic dilatation of the pulmonary artery. *S Afr Med J* 1953;27:360–367.

76. Gold MMA. Congenital dilatation of the pulmonary arterial tree. *Arch Intern Med* 1946;78:197–209.

77. Laubry D, Routier D, Heim de Balsac R. Grosse pulmonaire. Petite aorte. Affection congenitale. *Bull et mem Soc med d'hop de Paris* 1941;56:847–850.

78. Boutin C, Davignon A, Fournier A, Houyel L, Van Does-

burg N. Idiopathic dilatation of the pulmonary artery. Echocardiographic aspects. *Arch Mal Coeur Vaiss* 1994; 86:663–666.

79. Green DG, Balwin ED, Baldwin JS, Himmelstern A, Roh CE, Cournand A. Pure congenital pulmonary stenosis and idiopathic congenital dilation of the pulmonary artery. *Am J Med* 1949;6:24–40.

80. DeLeon AC Jr, Perloff JK, Twigg H, Majd M. The straight back syndrome. *Circulation* 1965;32:193–203.

81. Nasser WK. Congenital absence of the left pericardium. *Am J Cardiol* 1970;26:466–470.

82. Brayshaw JR, Perloff JK. Congenital pulmonary insufficiency complicating idiopathic dilatation of the pulmonary artery. *Am J Cardiol* 1962;10:282–290.

83. Deskmukh M, Guvenc S, Bentivoglio L, Goldberg H. Idiopathic dilatation of the pulmonary artery. *Circulation* 1960;21:710–716.

84. Deterling RA, Clagett OT. Aneurysm of the pulmonary artery review of the literature and report of a case. *Am Heart J* 1947;34:471–491.

85. Trell E. Pulmonary artery aneurysm. *Thorax* 1973;28: 644–649.

86. Campeau L, Gilbert G, Aerichide N. Absence of pulmonary valve. *Am J Cardiol* 1961;8:113–124.

87. McCartney FJ, Miller GAM. Congenital absence of the pulmonary valve. *Br Heart J* 1970;32:483–490.

88. Chiemmongkoltip P, Replogle RL, Gongdez-Levin L, Arcilla RA. Congenital absence of the pulmonary valve with atrial septal defect surgically corrected. *Chest* 1972; 62:100–103.

89. Cortes FM, Jacoby WJ. Isolated congenital pulmonary valvular insufficiency. *Am J Cardiol* 1962;10:287–290.

90. Hambry RI, Gulotta SJ. Pulmonic valvular insufficiency: Etiology, recognition, and management. *Am Heart J* 1967;74:110–125.

91. Ito T, Engle MA, Holswade GR. Congenital insufficiency of the pulmonary valve. A rare cause of neonatal heart failure. *Pediatrics* 1961;28:712–718.

92. Kissin M. Pulmonary insufficiency with supernumerary cusp in pulmonary valve. Report of a case and review of the literature. *Am Heart J* 1936;12:206–227.

93. Sanyl SK, Hipona FA, Browne MJ, Talnea NS. Congenital insufficiency of the pulmonary valve. *J Pediatr* 1964; 64:728–734.

94. Vlad P, Widman M, Lambert EC. Congenital pulmonary regurgitation. A report of 6 autopsied cases. *Am J Dis Child* 1960;100:640–641.

95. Smith RD, DuShane JW, Edwards JE. Congenital insufficiency of the pulmonary valve. Including a case of fetal cardiac failure. *Circulation* 1959;20:554–560.

96. Pouget JM, Kelly CE, Pilz CG. Congenital absence of the pulmonary valve. Report of a case in a 73 year old man. *Am J Cardiol* 1967;19:732–734.

97. Takas S, Miyataki K, Izumi S, Okamoto M, Kinoshita N, Nakagava H, Yamamoto K, Sakakibara M, Nimura Y. Clinical implications of pulmonary regurgitation in healthy individuals. Detection by cross-sectional pulsed Doppler echocardiography. *Br Heart J* 1988;59:542–550.

98. Berman W, Fripp RR, Rowe SA, Yabek SM. Congenital isolated pulmonary valve incompetence. Neonatal presentation and early natural history. *Am Heart J* 1992; 124:248–251.

99. Ford AB, Hellerstein HK, Wood C, Kelly HB. Isolated congenital bicuspid pulmonary valve. *Am J Med* 1956; 20:474–486.

100. Dickens J, Raber GT, Goldberg H. Dynamic pulmonary regurgitation associated with a bicuspid valve. *Ann Intern Med* 1958;48:851–859.

101. Ansari A. Isolated pulmonary valvular regurgitation: Current perspectives. *Prog Cardiovasc Dis* 1991;33: 329–344.

102. Murwitz LE, Roberts WC. Quadricuspid semilunar valve. *Am J Cardiol* 1973;31:623–626.

103. Rubio-Alvarez V, Limon-Larson R, Soni J. Valvulotomias intracardiacas por medio de un cateter. *Arch Inst Cardiol Mex* 1953;23:183–192.

104. Semb BKH, Tijonneland S, Stake G. "Balloon valvulotomy" of congenital pulmonary valve stenosis with tricuspid valve insufficiency. *Cardiovasc Radiol* 1979; 2:239–241.

105. Kan SJ, White RI Jr, Mitchell SE, Gardner TJ. Percutaneous balloon valvuloplasty: A new method for treating congenital pulmonary valve stenosis. *N Engl J Med* 1982; 307:540–542.

106. Stanger P, Cassidy SC, Girod DA, Kan JS, Lababidi Z, Shapiro SR. Balloon pulmonary valvuloplasty: Results of the Valvuloplasty and Angioplasty of Congenital Anomalies Registry. *Am J Cardiol* 1990;65:775–783.

107. McCrindle B, Kan SJ. Long-term results after balloon pulmonary valvuloplasty. *Circulation* 1991:1915–1922.

108. O'Connor BK, Beekman RH, Lindaur A. Intermediate-term outcome after pulmonary balloon valvuloplasty: Comparison with a matched surgical group. *J Am Coll Cardiol* 1992;20:169–173.

109. Carminati M, Giusti S, Spadoni I, Redaelli S, Tommasini G, Bonhoeffer P, Borghi A. Pulmonary valvuloplasty. *Cardiologia* 1993;38(suppl 1):361–365.

110. Witsenburg M, Talsma M, Rohmer J, Hess J. Balloon valvuloplasty for valvular pulmonary stenosis in children over 6 months of age: Initial results and long-term follow-up. *Eur Heart J* 1993;14:1657–1660.

111. Rao PS. Transcatheter treatment of pulmonary outflow tract obstruction: A review. *Prog Cardiovasc Dis* 1992; 35:119–158.

112. Ino T, Okubo M, Akimoto K, Shimazaki S, Nishimoto K, Iwahara M, Yabuta K, Watanabe M, Hosoda Y. Intermediate-term results of balloon valvuloplasty for isolated and complicated pulmonary valve stenosis. *Jpn Circ J* 1992;56:535–453.

113. Wang JK, Lue HC, Wu MH, Young ML. Efficacy of balloon valvuloplasty in treating mild pulmonary stenosis. *Acta Cardiol* 1992;47:349–355.

114. Elliott JM, Tuzcu EM. Recent developments in balloon valvuloplasty techniques. *Curr Opin Cardiol* 1995;10: 128–134.

115. Ettedgui JA, Ho SY, Tynan M, Jones OD, Martin RP, Baker EJ, Reidy JF. The pathology of balloon pulmonary valvoplasty. *Int J Cardiol* 1987;16:285–293.

116. Lau KW, Hung JS. Controversies in percutaneous balloon pulmonary valvuloplasty: Timing, patient selection and technique. *J Heart Valve Dis* 1993;2:321–325.

117. Ali Khan MA, al-Yousef S, Moore JW, Sawyer W. Results of repeat percutaneous balloon valvuloplasty for pulmonary valvar restenosis. *Am Heart J* 1990;120: 878–881.

118. Rupprath G, Neuhaus KL. Balloon valvuloplasty of congenital pulmonary valve stenosis. *Herz* 1988;13:14–19.

119. Rao PS. Balloon pulmonary valvuloplasty: A review. *Clin Cardiol* 1989;12:55–74.

120. Miller GA. Balloon valvuloplasty and angioplasty in congenital heart disease. *Br Heart J* 1985;54:285–289.

121. McCrindle BW. Independent predictors of long-term results after balloon pulmonary valvuloplasty. Valvuloplasty and Angioplasty of Congenital Anomalies (VACA) Registry Investigators. *Circulation* 1994;89: 1751–1759.

122. Masura J, Burch M, Deanfield JE, Sullivan ID. Five-year follow-up after balloon pulmonary valvuloplasty. *J Am Coll Cardiol* 1993;21:132–136.

123. Schmaltz AA, Bein G, Gravinghoff L, Hagel K, Hentrich F, Hofstetter R, Lindinger A, Kallfelz HC, Kramer HH, Mennicken U. Balloon valvuloplasty of pulmonary stenosis in infants and children—Co-operative study of the German Society of Pediatric Cardiology. *Eur Heart J* 1989;10:967–971.

124. Becker AE, Hoedemaker G. Balloon valvuloplasty in congenital and acquired heart disease: Morphologic considerations. *Z Kardiol* 1987;76(suppl 6):73–79.

125. Rey C, Marache P, Matina D, Mouly A. Percutaneous transluminal valvuloplasty in pulmonary stenosis. Apropos of 24 cases. *Arch Mal Coeur Vaiss* 1985;78:703–710.

126. Demkow M, Ruzyllo W, Lubiszewska B, Ciszewski M, Kochman W, Ksiezycka E, Rydlewska-Sadowska W, Szaroszyk W, Wilczynski J, Kowalewska M. Percutaneous pulmonary valvuloplasty in 135 patients (in Polish). *Kardiol Pol* 1992;37:67–73.

127. Stein JI, Beitzke A, Suppan C. Percutaneous balloon valvuloplasty of pulmonary stenosis in childhood: Early hemodynamic results and long-term Doppler echocardiography results. *Z Kardiol* 1991;80:549–553.

128. Sullivan ID, Robinson PJ, Macartney FJ, Taylor JF, Rees PG, Bull C, Deanfield JE. Percutaneous balloon valvuloplasty for pulmonary valve stenosis in infants and children. *Br Heart J* 1985;54:435–441.

129. Paul T, Luhmer I, Kallfelz HC. Percutaneous intraluminal balloon dilatation of valvular pulmonary stenoses in infancy and childhood. Presentation of results with special reference to balloon size. *Z Kardiol* 1988;77:346–531.

130. Worms AM, Marcon F. Interventional catheterization in infants and neonates. *Presse Med* 1995;24:271–275.

131. Hwang B, Chen LY, Lu JH, Meng CC. A quantitative analysis of the structure of right ventricle-pulmonary artery junction for balloon pulmonary valvuloplasty in children. *Angiology* 1995;46:383–391.

132. Jaing TL, Hwang B, Lu JH, Hsieh KS, Meng CC. Percutaneous balloon valvuloplasty in severe pulmonary valvular stenosis. *Angiology* 1995;46:503–509.

133. Medina A, Bethencourt A, Olalla E, Coello I, Hernandez E, Trillo M, Goicolea J, Melian F, Laraudogoitia E, Jimenez F. Intraoperative balloon valvuloplasty in pulmonary valve stenosis. *Cardiovasc Intervent Radiol* 1989;12:199–201.

134. Melgares R, Prieto JA, Azpitarte J. Success determining factors in percutaneous transluminal balloon valvuloplasty of pulmonary valve stenosis. *Eur Heart J* 1991;12:15–23.

135. Cazzaniga M, Vagnola O, Alday L, Spillman A, Sciegata A, Faella H, Kurlat I. Balloon pulmonary valvuloplasty in infants: A quantitative analysis of pulmonary valve-annulus-trunk structure. *J Am Coll Cardiol* 1992;20:345–349.

136. Lau KW, Hung JS. Controversies in percutaneous balloon pulmonary valvuloplasty: Timing, patient selection and technique. *J Heart Valve Dis* 1993;2:321–325.

136a.Coberly LA, Harrison JK, Bashore TM. Percutaneous balloon pulmonic valvuloplasty following treated endocarditis in a patient with congenital pulmonary valve stenosis. *Cathet Cardiovasc Diagn* 1990;21:245–247.

136b.Hargreaves AD, Pringle SD, Boon NA. Successful balloon dilatation of the pulmonary valve in carcinoid heart disease. *Int J Cardiol* 1994;45:150–151.

137. Fedderly RT, Beekman RH III. Balloon valuloplasty for pulmonary valve stenosis. *J Intervent Cardiol* 1995;8:451–456.

138. Rao PS. Balloon pulmonary valvuloplasty for isolated pulmonic stenosis. In: Rao PS, ed. *Trancatheter Therapy in Pediatric Cardiology*. New York: Wiley-Liss, Inc; 1993, pp. 59–104.

139. Burrows PE, Benson LN, Moes CAF, Freedom RM. Pulmonary artery tears following balloon valvotomy for pulmonary stenosis. *Cardiovasc Intervent Radiol* 1989;12:38–42.

140. Burrows PE, Benson LN, Smallhorn JF, Moes CAF, Freedom RM, Burrows FA, Rowe RD. Angiographic features associated with percutaneous balloon valvotomy for pulmonary valve stenosis. *Cardiovasc Intervent Radiol* 1988;11:111–116.

141. Beekman RH, Rocchini AP, Rosenthal A. Therapeutic cardiac catheterization for pulmonary valve and pulmonary artery stenosis. *Cardiol Clin* 1989;7:331–340.

142. Lababidi Z, Wu JR. Percutaneous balloon pulmonary valvuloplasty. *Am J Cardiol* 1983;52:560–562.

143. Musewe NN, Robertson MA, Benson LN, Burrows PE, Freedom RM, Smallhorn JF, Rowe RD. The dysplastic pulmonary valve: Echographic features and results of balloon dilation. *Br Heart J* 1987;57:364–370.

144. Ballerini L, Mullins CE, Cifarelli A, Pasquini L, De Simone G, Giannico S, Guccione P, Di Donato R, Di Carlo D. Percutaneous balloon valvuloplasty of pulmonary valve stenosis, dysplasia, and residual stenosis after surgical valvotomy for pulmonary atresia with intact ventricular septum: Long-term results. *Cathet Cardiovasc Diagn* 1990;19:165–169.

145. David SW, Goussous YM, Harbi N, Doghmi F, Hiari A, Krayyem M, Ferlinz J. Management of typical and dysplastic pulmonic stenosis, uncomplicated or associated with complex intracardiac defects, in juveniles and adults: Use of percutaneous balloon pulmonary valvuloplasty with eight-month hemodynamic follow-up. *Cathet Cardiovasc Diagn* 1993;29:105–112.

146. Rao PS. Balloon dilatation in infants and children with dysplastic pulmonary valves: Short-term and intermediate-term results. *Am Heart J* 1988;116:1168–1173.

147. Nair M, Kaul UA, Prasad R, Arora R, Khalilullah M. Successful percutaneous pulmonary balloon valvuloplasty in Noonan's syndrome: A case report. *Indian Heart J* 1990;42:123–125.

148. Marantz PM, Huhta JC, Mullins CE, Murphy DJ Jr, Nihill MR, Ludomirsky A, Yoon GY. Results of balloon valvuloplasty in typical and dysplastic pulmonary valve stenosis: Doppler and echocardiographic follow-up. *J Am Coll Cardiol* 1988;12:476–479.

149. DiSessa TG, Alpert BS, Chase NA, Birnbaum SE, Watson DC. Balloon valvuloplasty in children with dysplastic pulmonary valves. *Am J Cardiol* 1987;66:405–407.

150. Caspi J, Coles J, Benson L, Freedom RM, Burrows P, Trusler G, Williams WW. Management of neonatal critical pulmonary stenosis in patients in the era of balloon valvotomy. *Ann Thorac Surg* 1990;49:273–278.

151. Fedderly RT, Lloyd TR, Mendelsohn AM, Beekman RH. Determinants of successful balloon valvotomy in infants with critical pulmonary stenosis or membranous pulmonary atresia with intact ventricular septum. *J Am Coll Cardiol* 1995;25:460–465.

152. Qureshi SA, Ladusans EJ, Martin RP. Dilatation with progressively larger balloons for severe stenosis of the pulmonary valve presenting in the late neonatal period and early infancy. *Br Heart J* 1989;62:311–314.

153. Ladusans EJ, Qureshi SA, Parsons JM, Arab S, Baker EJ, Tynan M. Balloon dilatation of critical stenosis of the pulmonary valve in neonates. *Br Heart J* 1990;63: 362–367.

154. Tometzki AJ, Gibbs JL, Weil J. Balloon valvoplasty of critical aortic and pulmonary stenosis in the premature neonate. *Int J Cardiol* 1991;30:248–249.

155. Walsh KP, Abrams SE, Arnold R. Arterial duct angioplasty as an adjunct to dilatation of the valve for critical pulmonary stenosis. *Br Heart J* 1993;69:260–262.

156. Burzynski JB, Kveselis DA, Byrum CJ, Kavey RE, Smith FC, Gaum WE. Modified technique for balloon valvuloplasty of critical pulmonary stenosis in the newborn. *J Am Coll Cardiol* 1993;22:1944–1947.

157. Weber HS, Cyran SE, Gleason MM, White MG, Baylen BG. Critical pulmonary valve stenosis in the neonate: A technique to facilitate balloon dilation. *Am J Cardiol* 1994;73:310–312.

158. Latson L, Cheatham J, Froemming S, Kugler J. Transductal guidewire "rail" for balloon valvuloplasty in neonates with isolated critical pulmonary valve stenosis or atresia. *Am J Cardiol* 1994;73:713–714.

159. Gournay V, Piechaud J-F, Delogu A, Sidi D, Kachaner J. Balloon valvotomy for critical stenosis or atresia of pulmonary valve in newborns. *J Am Coll Cardiol* 1995;26: 1725–1731.

160. Zeevi B, Keane JF, Fellows KE, Lock JE. Balloon dilation of critical pulmonary stenosis in the first week of life. *J Am Coll Cardiol* 1988;11:821–824.

161. Talsma M, Witsenburg M, Rohmer J, Hess J. Determinants for outcome of balloon valvuloplasty for severe pulmonary stenosis in neontes and infants up to six months of age. *Am J Cardiol* 1993;71:1246–1248.

162. Buheitel G, Hofbeck M, Singer H. Balloon dilatation of the pulmonary valve within the first 40 days of life in critical valvular pulmonary stenosis, Fallot's tetralogy and following surgical or interventional high-frequency opening of pulmonary atresia. *Z Kardiol* 1995;84:64–71.

163. Santoro G, Formigari R, Di Carlo D, Pasquini L, Ballerini L. Midterm outcome after pulmonary balloon valvuloplasty in patients younger than one year of age. *Am J Cardiol* 1995;75:637–639.

164. Kaul UA, Singh B, Tyagi S, Bhargava M, Arora R, Khalilullah M. Long-term results after balloon pulmonary valvuloplasty in adults. *Am Heart J* 1993;126: 1152–1155.

165. Goudevenos J, Wren C, Adams PC. Balloon valvotomy of calcified pulmonary valve stenosis. *Cardiology* 1990;77: 55–57.

166. Meruane J, Puccio JM, Kauffmann R, Florenzano F. Adult pulmonary stenosis: Percutaneous balloon valvuloplasty. *Rev Med Child* 1995;122:525–530

167. Portis MT, Esplugas E, Garcia del Castillo H, Jara F. Pulmonary valvuloplasty in adolescents and adults: 2 year follow-up by continuous Doppler. *Rev Esp Cardiol* 1990; 43:619–623.

Chapter 19

Abnormalities of the Pulmonary Arteries

Abnormalities of pulmonary artery branching, caliber, and origin can occur in relative isolation, may reflect a component of rubella embryopathy, an internal stigmata of generalized dysmorphism, the Silver-Russell syndrome, cutis laxa, Williams or the Alagille syndrome among others, and may reflect a component of a widespread vasculopathy, or may be an integral component of congenital cardiac anomalies. These anomalies may include tetralogy of Fallot (see Chapters 20 through 22), pulmonary atresia and ventricular septal defect (see Chapter 21), the hypogenetic right lung syndrome (see this chapter, p. 445 and also Chapter 24), and the complex heart malformations associated with right atrial isomerism (see Chapter 41) among many others. The caliber and hemodynamics of the pulmonary arteries are subject to distortion by the construction of systemic-to-pulmonary anastomosis of the classic Blalock-Taussig or modified type; from construction of a Waterston-Cooley anastomosis between the right pulmonary artery and ascending aorta; or from a Potts' shunt between the descending thoracic aorta and the left pulmonary artery; from previous pulmonary artery banding; or from any form of cardiac surgery obstructing pulmonary venous flow (ie, Mustard's or Senning's atrial repair for transposition of the great arteries; repair of partial or total anomalous pulmonary venous connections); or by alterations and redistribution of pulmonary blood flow secondary to congenital pulmonary venous obstruction (ie, unilateral pulmonary venous stenosis or hypoplasia). The pulmonary artery may be distorted by construction of a classic Glenn anastomosis or by a bidirectional cavopulmonary connection with the possibility of the development of pulmonary arteriovenous fistulae. Aneurysms of the pulmonary arteries have been observed in the patient with Marfan syndrome and alterations of functional pulmonary arterial anatomy and integrity have been observed in those with Behçet's syndrome, etc.

The Origin of the Main and Branch Pulmonary Arteries

The main pulmonary trunk and proximal right and left pulmonary arteries have different embryological origins (see also Chapter 21).[1–8] The main pulmonary trunk has its origin from truncal septation, whereas the proximal right and left pulmonary arteries are derived from the proximal sixth aortic arches (see Chapter 7). There are extremely rare malformations that lend tangible and morphological support to these embryological conclusions. Beitzke and Shinebourne[9] described a patient that, in spite of the presence of a main pulmonary artery originating from the right ventricular infundibulum and an arterial duct connecting the main pulmonary artery trunk to the descending thoracic aorta, neither right nor left branch pulmonary artery originated from the main pulmonary trunk. Instead, the pulmonary arteries arose from the ascending aorta proximal to the first brachiocephalic artery as in truncus arteriosus (see Chapter 7).[9] This patient, like those subsequently reported by Bricker, Freedom, and Aotsuka and their respective colleagues, all had an intact ventricular septum.[10–12] Aotsuka and colleagues reported a patient similar to that reported by Beitzke and Shinebourne where separation of the pulmonary arteries was accomplished surgically.[12] We reported elsewhere a 19-month-old infant in whom angiography revealed so-called normal truncal septation but with complete agenesis of the right and left pulmonary arteries.[11] In this patient, the blood flow to the lungs originated from segmental arteries arising from the descending thoracic aorta. All of these patients exhibited differential cyanosis with relatively blue toes and pinker finger tips.

Branching Pattern of the Right and Left Pulmonary Arteries

Wells and colleagues[13] have recently reviewed the branching patterns of the right pulmonary artery in the normal, as well as in various cardiovascular anomalies. Variations of the pulmonary arterial branching pattern may reflect atrial situs (see Chapters 3 and 41).[14–16] These patterns of pulmonary artery branching in patients with normal situs, situs inversus, and the indeterminate or ambiguous situs with right atrial isomerism and left isomerism are reviewed in Chapter 3. In the patient with normally lateralized atria, the branch of the right pulmonary artery supplying the right upper lobe is the first segmental branch of the right pulmonary artery.[13,17,18] In 14% to 20% of people, one or more branches of the right pulmonary artery also supply the right upper lobe.[13,17,18] The pulmonary arterial supply to the left upper lobe may be a single branch from the left pulmonary artery or a group of two to eight smaller arteries.

Diaz-Gongora and colleagues[19] have reported a unique patient with three arterial trunks, the so-called tritruncal heart (see Chapter 3, Fig. 3-23). The three arterial trunks include the aorta, the main pulmonary trunk, and an intermediate trunk (termed intermediate because it was situated between the aorta and the main pulmonary artery). The aorta and the intermediate trunk originated from the left ventricle, while the main pulmonary trunk arose from the right ventricle. The intermediate trunk continued as the right pulmonary artery, and the main pulmonary artery continued as the left pulmonary artery. The outflow tract from each ventricle was considered normal.

Peculiar orientation of the pulmonary arteries is not particularly uncommon (Fig. 19-1), and has been observed in patients with thoracic ectopia cordis, conjoined thorapagi, and in so-called 'topsy-turvy' hearts (see Chapter 44, Fig. 44-4).

Pulmonary Arterial Stenosis

Isolated pulmonary artery stenosis or that associated with systemic vascular lesions can occur in the main pulmonary artery, at its bifurcation, and at the secondary or even more distal branch points of the pulmonary artery, or such arterial stenoses may be very severe and extensive.[11,20–31a] However, isolated stenosis of the main pulmonary artery alone is uncommon. Such obstruction is usually seen as part of a generalized pulmonary vascular dysplasia associated with obstruction to the pulmonary valve or the right ventricular infundibulum. The most common site of pulmonary artery

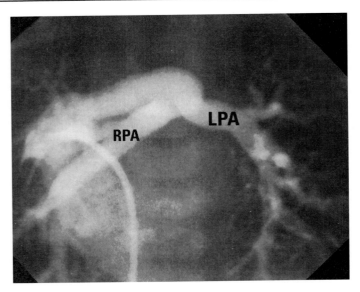

Fig. 19-1: Peculiar orientation of the pulmonary arteries in a patient with a complex cardiac malformation.

stenosis is found at the point of bifurcation of the main pulmonary artery, its right and left branches. The stenosis involves the distal main pulmonary artery and then extends a variable distance along the right and/or left pulmonary artery branch. Peripheral pulmonary artery stenosis involving the branch points of the right and/or left pulmonary artery may occur alone or associated with more proximal stenosis. Two basic forms of obstructive malformations of the pulmonary arteries can be identified: a focal and a diffuse form. The focal form of pulmonary arterial stenosis consists of a discrete obstruction preceded by a normal-sized artery and followed by post-stenotic dilatation. The more diffuse type is characterized by a small vessel that remains small distally, resembling hypoplasia, and is not amenable to surgical reconstruction by local resection (Figs. 19-2 through 19-4).[20,29,30,32]

Increasing experience has accumulated with patients with bilateral severe pulmonary hypoplasia associated with jaundice and hepatic ductular hypoplasia, the so-called Alagille syndrome.[33–44] This syndrome is an autosomal dominant disorder characterized by chronic cholestasis reflecting a paucity of intrahepatic bile ducts, typical facies, peripheral pulmonary artery stenoses, skeletal abnormalities, and ocular posterior embryotoxin.[34–35a] Pulmonary arterial stenoses may be particularly severe and diffuse in patients with this syndrome, although at least one follow-up study suggested that most such peripheral pulmonary arterial stenoses are relatively mild (Fig. 19-5).[33a] In any patient, the recognition of pulmonary arterial stenosis should raise the possibility of a more widespread vasculopathy, such as that associated with rubella, infantile hypercalcemia, cutis laxa, and Ehlers-Danlos syn-

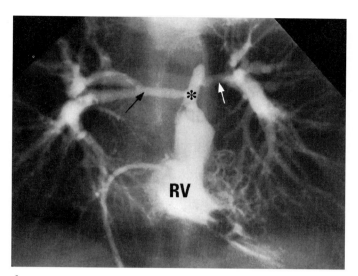

A

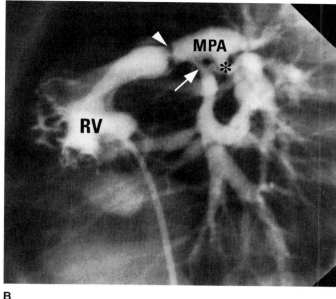

B

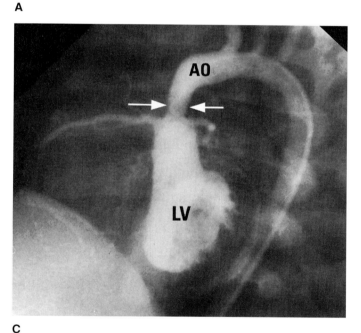

C

Fig. 19-2: Pulmonary arterial stenoses in a patient with William's syndrome and supravalvular aortic stenosis.
A and B: Cranially angled frontal and lateral pulmonary angiograms show diffusely small pulmonary arteries with extensive stenoses (arrows and *), and in the lateral, a dysplastic pulmonary valve (arrowhead); **C:** Long axial oblique shows the supravalvular aortic stenosis (arrows) (see also Chapter 29).

drome, among others.[45–52] Rodriguez and Riggs[53] have recently assessed so-called physiologic peripheral pulmonary arterial stenosis in infancy. They found that patients with physiologic peripheral pulmonary arterial stenosis have mild underdevelopment of the pulmonary artery branches, with consequent increased flow velocity and turbulent flow. This turbulent flow may be contributed to by increased cardiac output and mild anemia.

Intravascular ultrasound has been used in the investigation of the generalized arteriopathy of Williams syndrome (Fig. 19-2).[54] This study, which was conducted by Rein and colleagues, demonstrated severe wall thickening with secondary luminal obstruction. Despite these findings, and perhaps surprisingly so, clinical data support spontaneous improvement in some patients in the pulmonary arterial lesions of Williams syndrome.[55–58] The mechanisms for this spontaneous improvement have not been fully documented, nor the specific morphological/anatomic substrate in which spontaneous improvement might be anticipated. In at least one patient with Alagille syndrome and only mild pulmonary arterial stenosis, lymphatic abnormalities manifested by chylous pleural effusions have been documented.[58a] Apparently such lymphatic abnormalities had not been

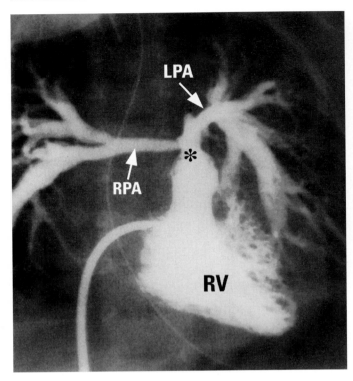

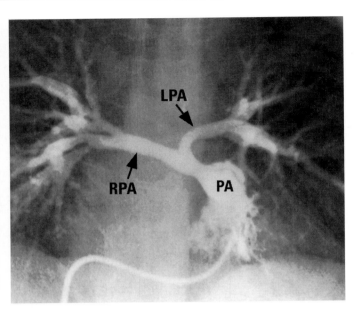

Fig. 19-4: A patient with Rubella embryopathy and severe pulmonary artery hypoplasia demonstrated by this cranially angled proximal pulmonary artery angiogram.

Fig. 19-3: Severe pulmonary artery hypoplasia is demonstrated by this cranially angled right ventriculogram.

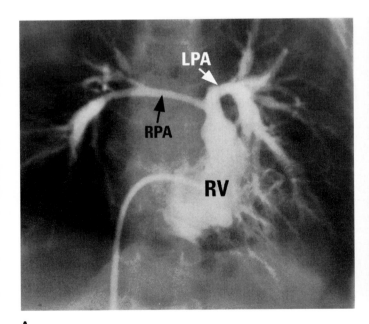

A

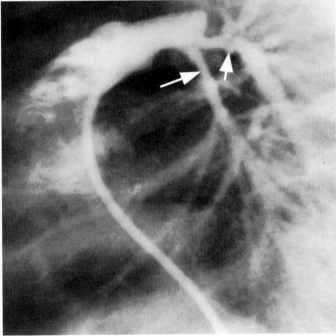

B

Fig. 19-5: Pulmonary artery hypoplasia and stenoses in a patient with the Alagille syndrome being evaluated for liver transplantation.
A and B: Cranially tilted frontal and lateral pulmonary angiogram shows severe hypoplasia of both branch pulmonary arteries.

noted previously in patients with arteriohepatic dysplasia.

Aneurysms of the Pulmonary Arteries

Aneurysms of the pulmonary arteries have been identified in patients with a wide range of systemic disorders, from those with Marfan syndrome to Behçet's syndrome. Pulmonary artery involvement in the Marfan syndrome is far less common than the well-known aortic involvement.[59–64] Aneurysms of the pulmonary arteries have been identified in those with Behçet's syndrome, a nonspecific vasculitis of unknown etiology of large and small arteries, veins, arterioles, venules, and capillaries of both the systemic and pulmonary circulations as well as in those with mucoid vasculopathy.[65–71a] Pulmonary artery stenoses and aneurysms have been observed in those patients with Takayasu's arteritis, rheumatoid arthritis, and other systemic disease processes.[72–75] Mycotic aneurysms of the pulmonary arteries have been amply recorded in those with intravenous substance abuse.[76–78] We have also seen mycotic aneurysms in the main pulmonary trunk at the site of pulmonary artery banding, and a mycotic aneurysm of the pulmonary trunk has been diagnosed and resected in a 7-year-old boy with severe valvar pulmonary stenosis probably secondary to *Staphylococcal aureus* pneumonia, septicemia, and then endarteritis and aneurysm formation.[78a]

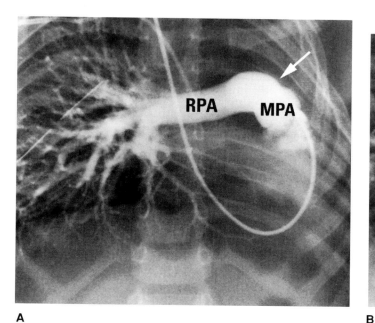

A

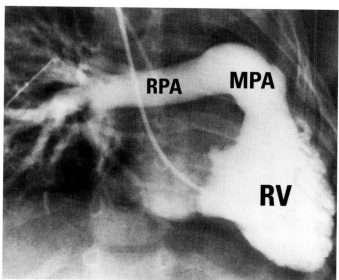

B

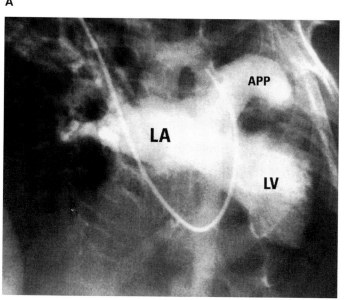

C

Fig. 19-6: Congenital absence of the left lung.
A: Cranially angled main pulmonary arteriogram in a patient with congenital absence of the left lung shows absence of origin of the left pulmonary artery (arrows). The right lung is expanded and herniated into the left thorax. Notice that the right pulmonary arterial branches cross the midline to enter the left hemithorax. **B:** Right ventriculogram in the same patient shows that the entire heart is displaced and is adjacent to the left thoracic wall. **C:** Only the right pulmonary veins can be seen entering the left atrium.

Congenital Unilateral Absence of a Pulmonary Artery

Unless the lung is congenitally absent, there must be some nutritive source of pulmonary blood flow to the lung, no matter how dysplastic or underdeveloped the lung is (Figs. 19-6 and 19-7; see also Chapter 40, Fig. 40-8).[79] Absence of the mediastinal portion of either the right or left pulmonary artery results in obligatory flow of right ventricular blood to the contralateral lung (Figs. 19-8 and 19-9).[80] There is now extensive documentation of patients in whom the sole cardiovascular abnormality is pulmonary artery nonconfluence with distal-ductal or ligamental origin of one pulmonary artery (Figs. 19-10 through 19-16).[81–104] In this condition, physiologic and then anatomic closure of the arterial duct isolates the involved pulmonary artery.[81,83,85,91, 95,99,101,102] Progressive diminution in the size of the isolated pulmonary artery, lung, and hemithorax is an inevitable consequence of this condition (Fig. 19-16). Some of these patients will develop small direct and indirect aortopulmonary collateral arteries (see also Chapter 21), while in others the arterial duct may remain patent, although tenuously so. When the arterial duct undergoes complete obliteration and the connection to the hilar pulmonary artery becomes ligamental, pulmonary vein wedge angiography may be necessary to define the size of the hilar pulmonary artery.[83,101] In distal ductal (or ligamental) origin of one pulmonary artery, it is more frequent to have the involved ductus and "absent" pulmonary artery on the side opposite the laterality of the aortic arch; thus, with a left aortic arch, distal ductal origin of the right pulmonary artery and with a right aortic arch, distal ductal origin of the left pulmonary artery (Figs. 19-12 through 19-15). So-called congenitally absent pulmonary artery from ductal closure has been recognized in the patient with tetralogy of Fallot, tetralogy of Fallot with so-called absent pulmonary valve, tetralogy with pulmonary atresia, and in the patient with complex congenital heart malformations with right isomerism among others (see Chapter 20, Figs. 20-10 through 20-12; Chapter 22, Fig. 22-8). Many but not all of the patients with distal ductal or ligamental origin of one pulmonary artery will have bilateral arterial ducts (see also Chapter 10) (Fig. 19-15).[102] In those patients with complete isolation of the pulmonary artery, the presence of a ductal diverticulum ipsilateral to the isolated pulmonary artery is evidence of this conditions pathogenesis. We have documented indirect aortopulmonary collaterals originating from the subclavian artery ipsilateral to the isolated pulmonary artery (Fig. 19-11). Rarely, the collateral circulation to the affected lung will be mediated by an anomalous collateral artery from the coronary artery.[105] Distal ductal

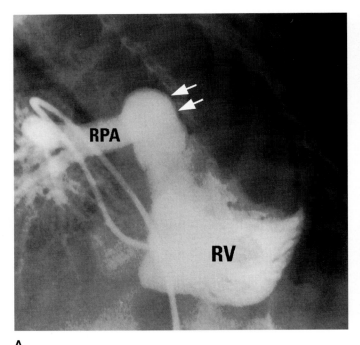

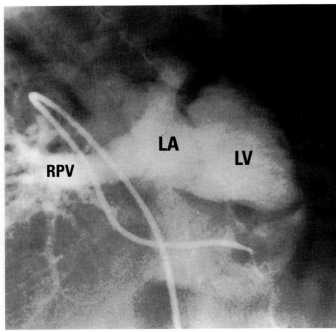

A   **B**

Fig. 19-7: A patient with azygous continuation of the inferior caval vein and congenital absence or profound hypoplasia of the left lung and pulmonary artery.
A: Cranially angled right ventriculogram via the azygous vein shows the absent mediastinal left pulmonary artery (arrows). **B:** Only the right pulmonary veins are imaged in the levophase of the right ventriculogram.

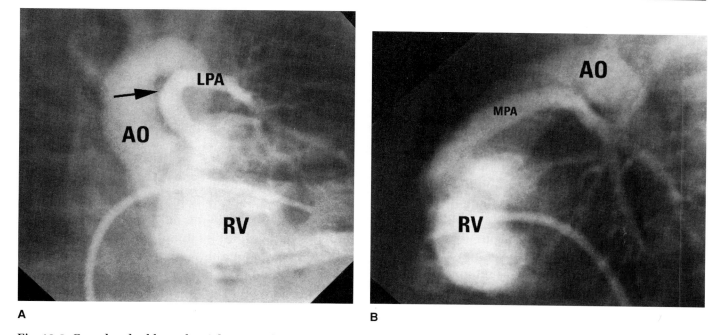

A   **B**

Fig. 19-8: Complex double-outlet right ventricle with congenitally absent right pulmonary artery.
(A) Frontal and **(B)** lateral right ventriculogram shows the main and left pulmonary artery, but not the right (arrow).

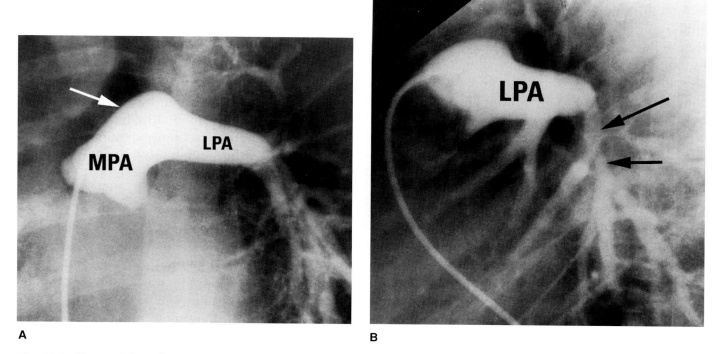

A   **B**

Fig. 19-9: Absent right pulmonary artery and multiple left pulmonary arterial stenoses.
A: The absent right pulmonary artery (arrow) is evident from the frontal main pulmonary angiogram. **B:** The left-sided peripheral pulmonary arterial stenoses (arrows) are shown in the lateral.

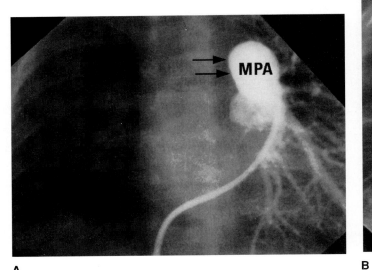

A

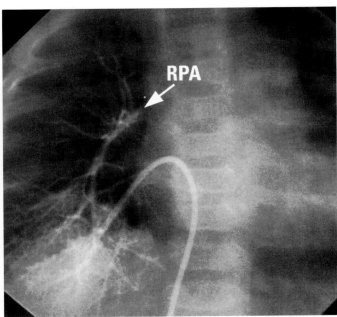

B

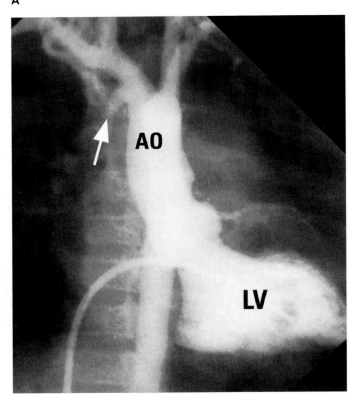

C

Fig. 19-10: Absent right pulmonary artery with a ductal diverticulun at the origin of the innominate artery.
A: Main pulmonary angiogram does not show a right pulmonary artery (arrow). **B:** Right pulmonary vein wedge angiogram defines the very small right pulmonary artery. **C:** The left ventriculogram shows the right-sided ductal diverticulum (arrow) originating from the base of the innominate artery.

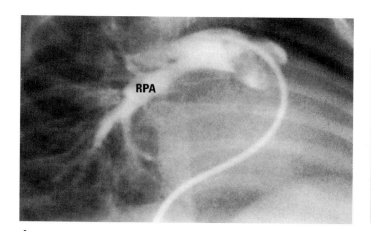

A

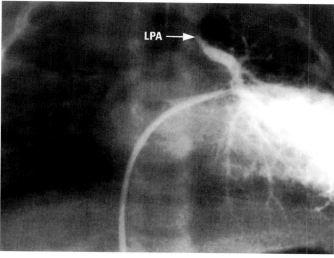

B

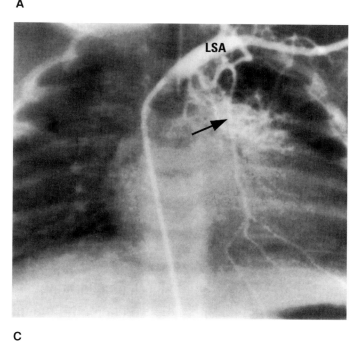

C

Fig. 19-11: Absent left pulmonary artery.
A: Only a right pulmonary artery is visualized from the main pulmonary angiogram. **B:** The left pulmonary artery is visualized by left pulmonary vein wedge angiography. The hilar left pulmonary artery is tethered superiorly. **C:** Extensive collaterals (arrow) are derived from the left subclavian artery.

or ligamental origin of the pulmonary artery may occur in isolation, but the more frequent association is with right ventricular outflow tract obstruction of the tetralogy or pulmonary atresia and ventricular septal defect types.[83,85,88,95,99,101,102] Isolation of the left pulmonary artery has been described in a neonate with a ventricular septal defect and a right aortic arch.[102a]

How does one clinically recognize so-called absence of a unilateral pulmonary artery? Once familiar with the diagnosis, it might be suspected from a chest radiograph or from an abnormal echocardiogram, the latter not demonstrating either the central or mediastinal right or left pulmonary artery. The diagnosis of congenitally absent pulmonary artery may be heralded by intractable pulmonary infection that may necessitate

pneumonectomy as in the patient reported by Canver and colleagues.[94] Indeed the clinical presentation may be subtle when this condition occurs in isolation. Hemoptysis, resulting from rupture of abundant bronchial submucosal vessels perfused by enlarged systemic collaterals supplying the affected lung has been reported in the adult.[92,93] Pneumonectomy has been recommended as definitive treatment in the adult patient presenting with hemoptysis.[93] Serial reduction of ventilation in the lung with congenital absence of pulmonary artery has been noted.[93a]

Reconstitution of the nonconfluent pulmonary arteries may require initially some form of systemic-to-pulmonary artery anastomosis.[81,83,85,89,90] We have used a modified Blalock-Taussig shunt to promote

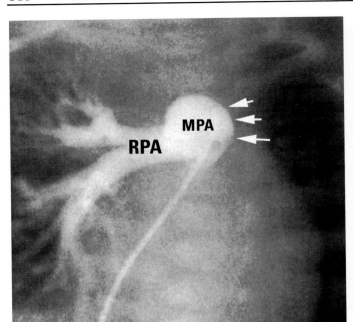

A

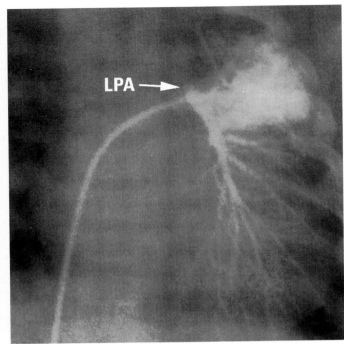

B

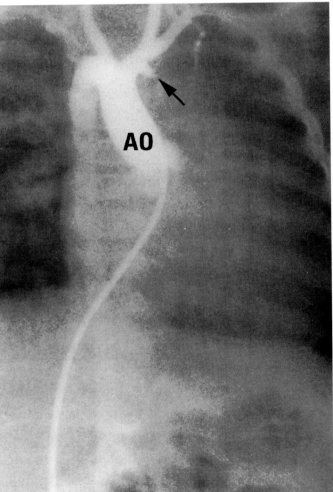

C

Fig. 19-12: Absent left pulmonary artery with a ductal diverticulum at the origin of the innominate artery in a patient with a right-sided aortic arch.
A: The main pulmonary angiogram defines only the right pulmonary artery, but not the left (arrows). **B:** The left pulmonary artery is demonstrated by left pulmonary vein wedge angiogram. **C:** The left ductal diverticulum originates from the base of the left-sided innominate artery in this patient with a right-sided aortic arch.

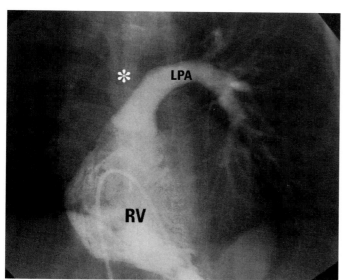

A

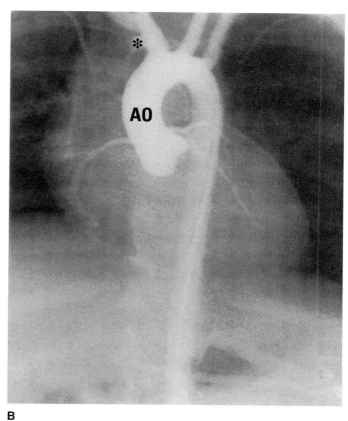

B

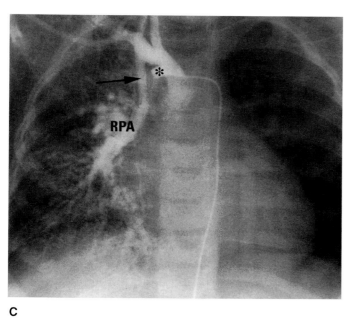

C

Fig. 19-13: Absent right pulmonary artery palliated with a modified Blalock-Taussig shunt.
A: Frontal right ventriculogram does not image the right pulmonary artery (✳). **B:** This patient's right-sided ductal diverticulum (✳) originates from the base of the innominate artery in this patient with a left aortic arch. **C:** The modified Blalock-Taussig shunt (arrows) to the hilar right pulmonary artery is imaged. The ductal diverticulum is again noted (✳).

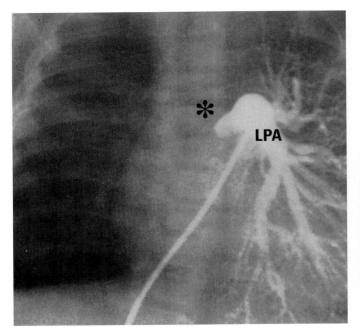

A

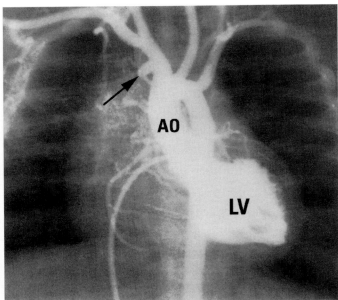

B

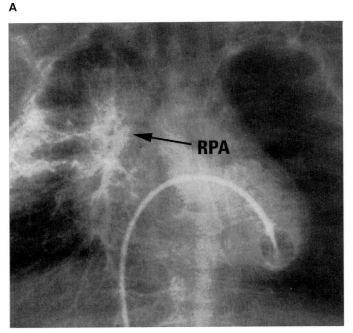

C

Fig. 19-14: Absent right pulmonary artery with opacification of intrapulmonary arteries from transpleural collateral arteries.

A: Main pulmonary angiogram does not demonstrate a right pulmonary artery (✱). **B:** This patient's right-sided ductal diverticulum (arrow) originates from the base of the innominate artery in this left aortic arch. **C:** A late frame from the left ventriculogram after opacification of multiple intercostal arteries and other chest wall collaterals provides opacification of the right pulmonary artery.

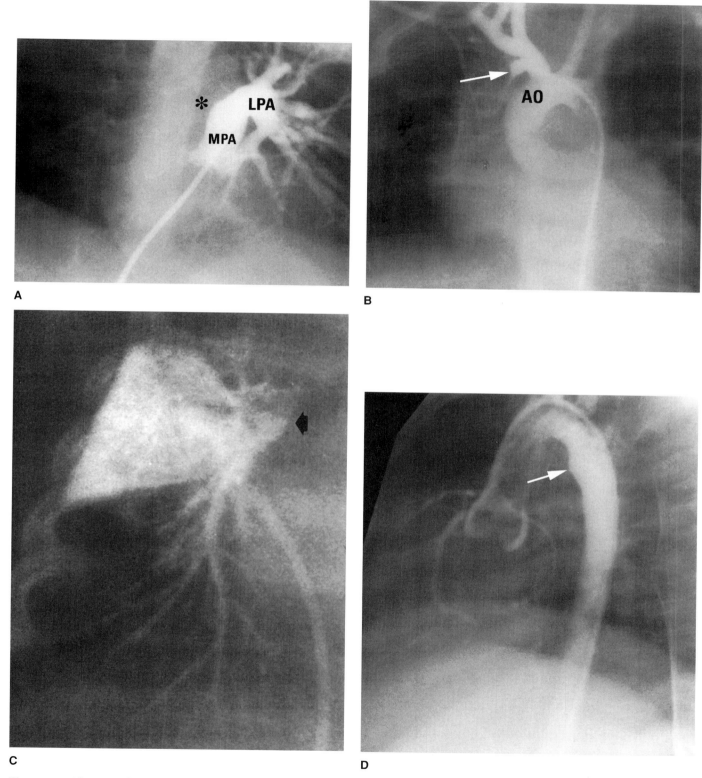

Fig. 19-15: Absent right pulmonary artery and a left-sided ductal bump: Evidence of bilateral arterial ducts.
A: Frontal main pulmonary angiogram doesn't show the filling of the right pulmonary artery (✱). **B:** Retrograde aortogram shows the typical ductal diverticulum (arrow) in a patient with a left aortic arch. **C:** Right pulmonary vein wedge angiogram shows a hilar right pulmonary artery (arrow). **D:** The descending aortogram shows the left-sided ductal bump (arrow), the remnant of the left-sided arterial duct.

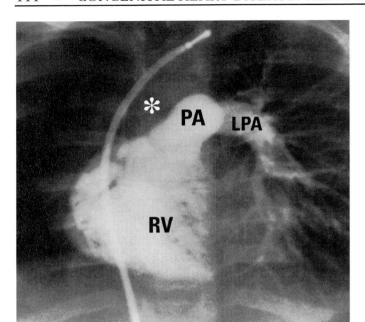

Fig. 19-16: The heart is shifted in the right chest in this patient with congenitally absent right pulmonary artery.
This frontal right ventriculogram shows the heart shifted into the right hemithorax, reflecting absence of the right (✱) pulmonary artery.

growth of a hilar pulmonary artery, while others have occasionally used an internal thoracic artery graft (see Chapter 22, Fig. 22-8).[91] Others have interposed a graft between the main pulmonary trunk and the isolated pulmonary artery at its hilum to reconstitute the pulmonary arteries. Considerable difference in size of the isolated hilar pulmonary artery has been observed, and this may influence the type of surgical repair.

One should be cognizant that nonopacification does not always imply absence or nonconfluence, but may reflect streaming, stenosis, or some combination of factors (Fig. 19-17).

Acquired Loss of the Left Pulmonary Artery

Pontius and colleagues[106] record those 'illusions' leading to surgical closure or interruption of the distal left pulmonary artery rather than the arterial duct. This complication is thought more likely to occur in the first year of life in those infants with a very large arterial duct as large as the aortic arch. Furthermore, the large duct may partially overlie the aortic arch, obscuring it from view. Additionally, Pontius' review found that surgical closure of the distal left pulmonary artery rather than the arterial duct was more likely to occur

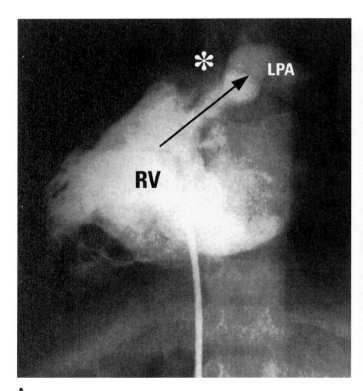

A

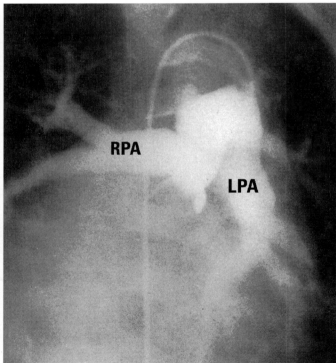

B

Fig. 19-17: Nonopacification of the right pulmonary artery in this patient with dextrocardia likely reflects maldistribution of flow to the left pulmonary artery.
A: The right ventriculogram provided opacification only of the left pulmonary artery, not the right (✱). Note the orientation of the outflow tract (arrow). **B:** After injection through a modified left-sided Blalock-Taussig shunt, there is prompt opacification of only a slightly smaller right pulmonary artery as well as the larger left pulmonary artery.

when the origin of the arterial duct was atypical and when the course of the recurrent laryngeal nerve was also atypical. The role of the arterial duct in the genesis of left pulmonary artery stenosis and later nonconfluence among patients with pulmonary atresia and ventricular septal defect is discussed in Chapters 20 and 21 (see also Chapter 35, Fig. 35-31). Reduction in flow to one lung may reflect obstruction to one or more pulmonary veins, or diaphragmatic paralysis secondary to phrenic nerve injury at the time of cardiac surgery (see Chapter 35, Fig. 35-30).[107–110]

The Hypogenetic Right Lung Complex

Hypoplasia of the right pulmonary artery of varying severity is an important component of the hypogenetic right lung complex or the scimitar syndrome (see also Chapter 24).[111–137a] In its classic expression, scimitar syndrome (Table 19-1) is characterized by dextrocardia, hypoplasia of the right pulmonary artery and underdevelopment of the right lung, abnormal connection of the right pulmonary veins to the inferior vena caval-right atrial junction (giving the scimitar appearance on the frontal chest radiograph), and anomalous systemic arterial supply to the right lung, often its basal segments (Figs. 19-18 through 19-31).

Anomalies of bronchial supply to the right lung and thus sequestration are frequently present as well. It is usually the right pulmonary artery that is underdeveloped in this syndrome, but occasionally the left lung may be underdeveloped.[137] In cataloguing those anomalies affecting the right pulmonary artery in the hypogenetic right lung syndrome, the degree of hypoplasia may be very mild, or extremely severe (Figs. 19-18 through 19-22). Indeed, congenital absence of the right pulmonary artery has also been described in this syn-

Table 19-1

The Scimitar Syndrome
(The Hypogenetic Right Lung Complex)

Dextrocardia
Right lung hypoplasia
Right pulmonary artery hypoplasia
Anomalous connection of right pulmonary veins to inferior vena cava
Anomalous systemic artery from aorta to right lung
Often pulmonary sequestration
Less common associations:
  Horseshoe lung
  Pulmonary vein stenosis

drome Fig. 19-18D).[114,129,129a] We have documented pulmonary artery stenosis in the already hypoplastic right pulmonary artery (Figs. 19-20 and 19-23).[11] Pulmonary arterial stenoses in the contralateral lung have also been observed.[115]

The so-called horseshoe lung anomaly of the right pulmonary artery, or cross-over lung anomaly is another malformation that may involve the right pulmonary artery as in the scimitar complex (Figs. 19-24 through 19-26).[138–152] The horseshoe lung, an uncommon congenital anomaly, first described by Spencer in 1962, is frequently associated with the scimitar syndrome in which the base of the right and left lungs are joined by a parenchymal isthmus posterior to the heart.[138–152] This condition is readily diagnosed by the presence of a crossing pulmonary artery branch at angiography, or by demonstration at computed tomography (CT) of fused lung tissue behind the heart.[152a] Since the horseshoe lung usually coexists with the scimitar syndrome, one should anticipate a similar

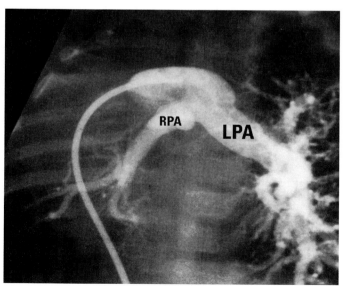

Fig. 19-18: Various expressions of right pulmonary artery hypoplasia in patients with the scimitar syndrome or hypogenetic right lung complex.
A: The heart is shifted into the right hemithorax because of pulmonary hypoplasia; note the caliber difference between right and left pulmonary arteries. **B:** A pulmonary angiogram from another patient shows a very small right pulmonary artery. The catheter was introduced retrograde from the descending thoracic aorta through the patent arterial duct into the main pulmonary trunk. **C:** The right pulmonary artery is somewhat smaller than the left pulmonary artery. **D:** Absence of the right pulmonary artery. **E:** Severe right pulmonary artery hypoplasia with profound arborization anomalies.

A

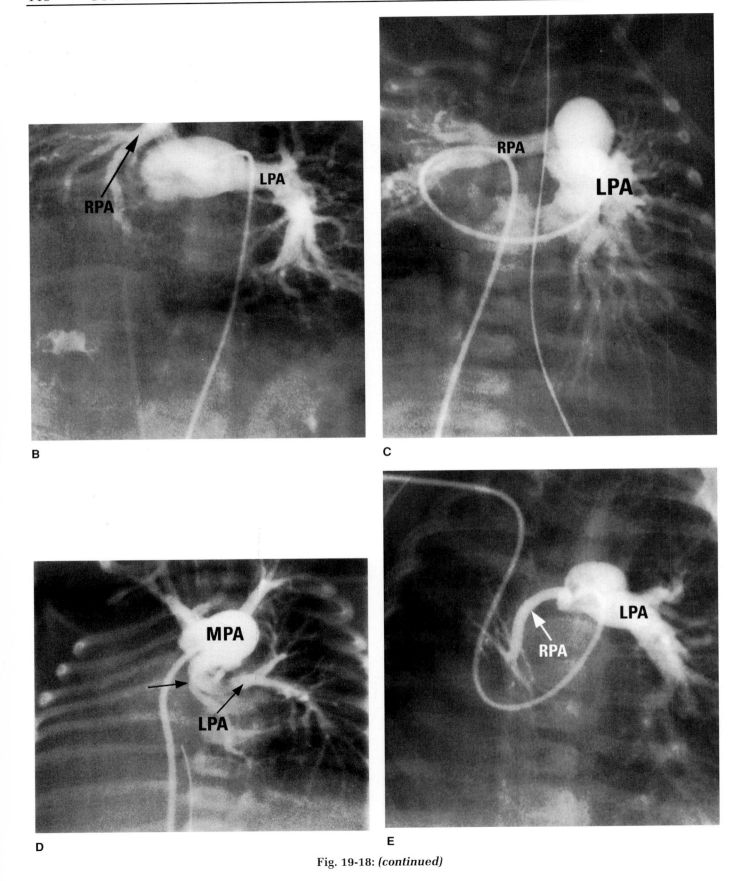

Fig. 19-18: *(continued)*

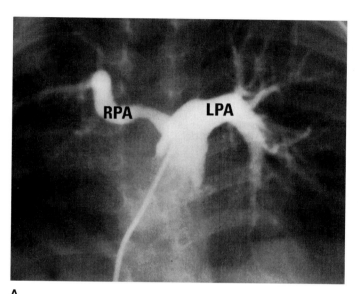

A

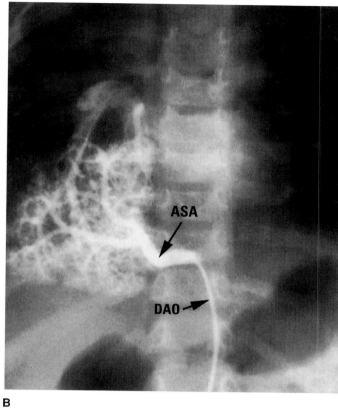

B

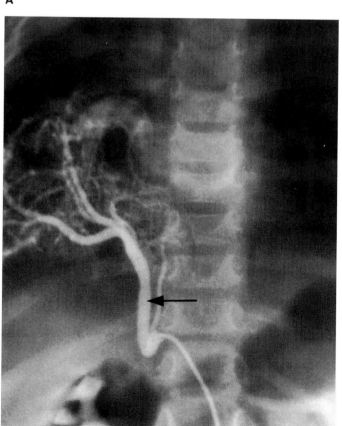

C

Fig. 19-19: The hypogenetic right lung complex.
A: Moderate hypoplasia of the right pulmonary artery. **B and C:** Two different patients with an anomalous systemic artery supplying part of the right lung. In both patients, the anomalous systemic artery (arrow) originating from the descending thoracic aorta supplying the right lower lobe is selectively injected.

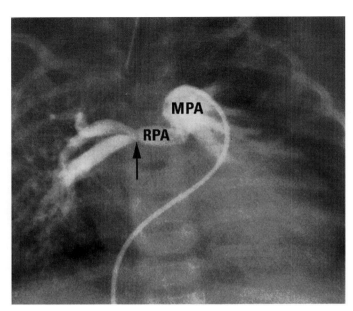

A

Fig. 19-20: Another patient with the hypogenetic right lung complex and right pulmonary artery stenosis,
A: Right pulmonary arterial stenosis (arrow) as well as right-sided pulmonary artery hypoplasia is demonstrated by this selective injection in the main pulmonary artery. **B:** The anomalous right pulmonary vein (arrow) connects in an unobstructed fashion with the inferior vena cava. **C:** The left ventricular angiogram in the frontal projection shows the anomalous systemic artery (arrow) originating from the descending thoracic aorta supplying the right lower lobe of the lung.

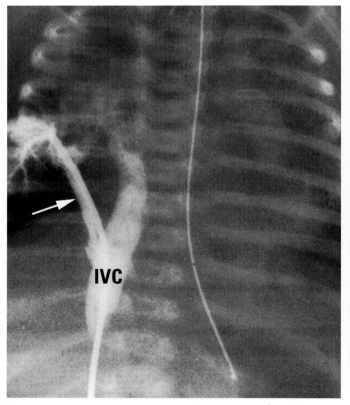

B

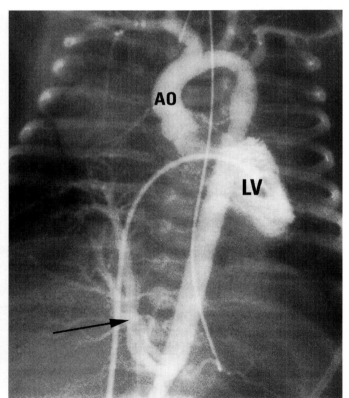

C

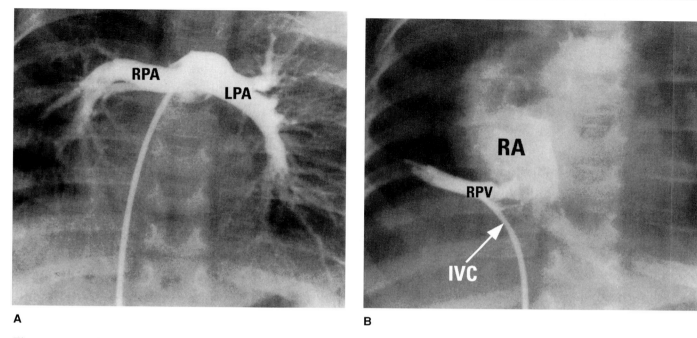

Fig. 19-21: Mild hypoplasia of the right pulmonary artery and the anomalous connection of the right pulmonary vein to the inferior caval-right atrial junction.
A: Only mild hypoplasia of the right pulmonary artery is evident. **B:** The anomalous right pulmonary vein connects to the inferior caval-right atrial junction.

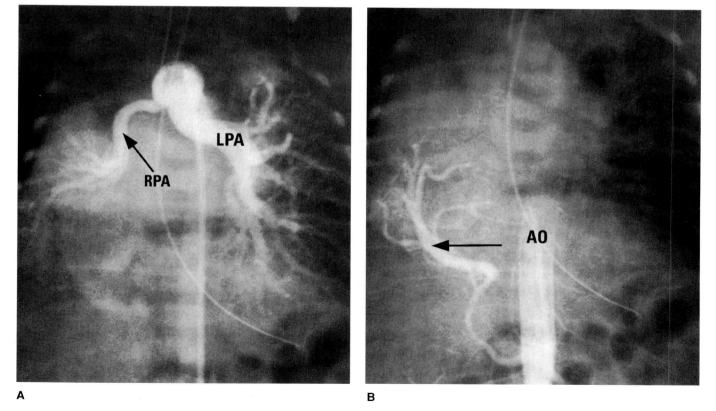

Fig. 19-22: Severe hypoplasia of the right pulmonary artery and a small, stenotic anomalous systemic artery in this patient with the scimitar syndrome.
A: Frontal pulmonary angiogram via the arterial duct and the retrograde arterial approach demonstrates the very underdeveloped right pulmonary artery. **B:** The small, stenotic anomalous systemic artery (arrow) is demonstrated by aortography.

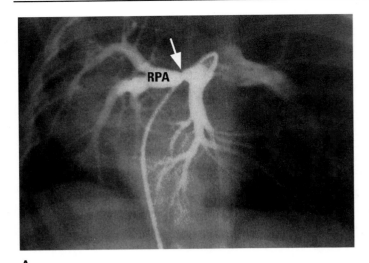

A

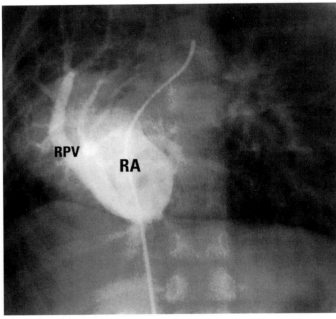

B

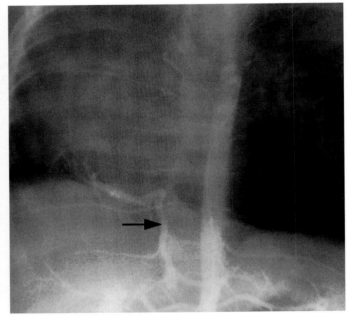

C

constellation of cardiac anomalies (see Chapter 24). Occasionally, the horseshoe lung anomaly will have anomalous pulmonary venous connections, but not pulmonary hypoplasia.[152b] One such patient in our series of patients with the hypogenetic right lung complex and horseshoe lung also had severe left pulmonary vein stenosis (Fig. 19-28).[126,144] The so-called cross-over lung or horseshoe lung does not invariably coexist with the scimitar syndrome (Fig. 19-26B and 19-26C). As we discussed in Chapter 24, anomalies of the right pulmonary veins are an integral component of scimitar syndrome, and obstruction to pulmonary venous flow so well documented in this syndrome may contribute to the ipsilateral lung and pulmonary artery hypoplasia (Fig. 19-27). Thus, patients with scimitar syndrome with or without a horseshoe lung may have extensive vascular anomalies involving their pulmonary arteries, pulmonary veins, and anomalous systemic arterial supply from the descending thoracic aorta or other systemic artery, as well as anomalies of bronchial supply.[153–171] Pulmonary artery hypertension in these patients may reflect several etiologies, including anomalous systemic arterial supply, pulmonary venous obstruction, redistribution of flow to the unaffected lung, associated cardiac malformations, or combinations of these factors.[113,114,117,120,125–127, 130,135,141,144,146] Pulmonary venous or inferior caval stenosis may occur after diversion of the right pulmonary veins to the left atrium (Fig. 19-32; see also Chapter 24, Figs. 24-31 and 24-32).

An anomalous systemic artery originating from the descending thoracic aorta may course into the affected,

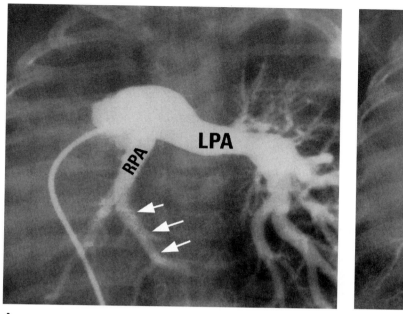

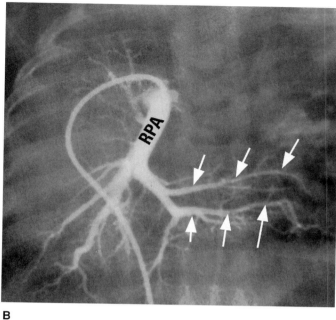

A

B

Fig. 19-24: A horseshoe lung in an infant with scimitar syndrome.
A: Frontal pulmonary angiogram shows the discrepancy in caliber between the right and left pulmonary arteries; from the right pulmonary artery a branch (arrows) that courses inferiorly and leftward arises. **B:** Selective injection of the right pulmonary artery shows the crossing pulmonary artery segments (arrows).

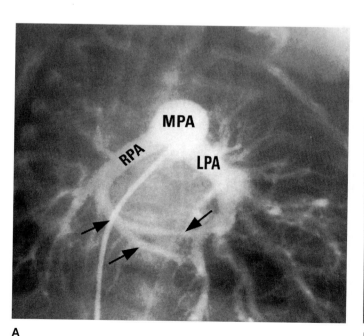

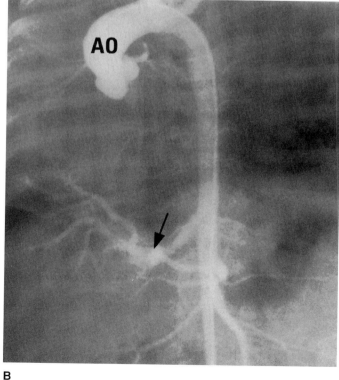

A

B

Fig. 19-25: Another infant with a horseshoe lung, a small right pulmonary artery, and an anomalous systemic artery.
A: The crossing horseshoe segments of the right pulmonary artery are seen in this frontal main pulmonary angiogram. **B:** The small systemic artery supplying a segment of the right lower lobe is seen on aortography.

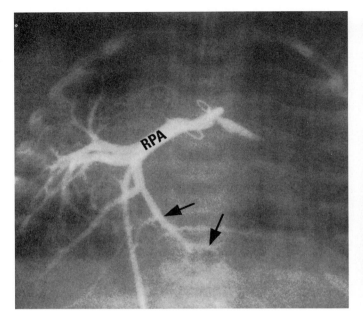

A

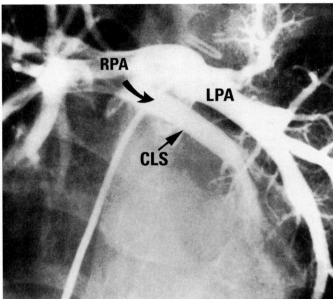

B

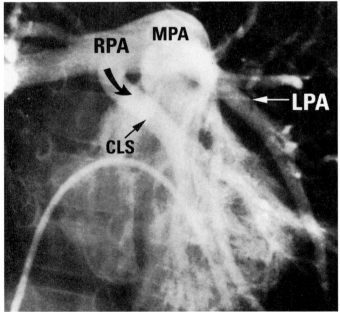

C

Fig. 19-26: A horseshoe lung or cross-over lung in two different patients.
A: Selective right pulmonary artery angiogram shows a crossover lung segment (arrows) in a patient with complex congenital heart disease treated by pulmonary artery banding. **B and C:** A different patient with a coarctation of the aorta and left ventricular outflow tract obstruction. B: The selective injection in the frontal projection shows both right and left pulmonary arteries. Originating from the posteromedial portion (curved arrow) of the right pulmonary artery is a branch that crosses the midline to supply the left lower lobe. C: The frontal right ventriculogram with some cranial tilt demonstrates with clarity that branch (curved arrow) of the right pulmonary artery crossing over to supply the left lower lobe. CLS indicates cross-over lung segment. (Figs. 19-26B and 19–26C provided by Michael Giuffre, MD, The Children's Hospital of Alberta, Calgary, Alberta, Canada.)

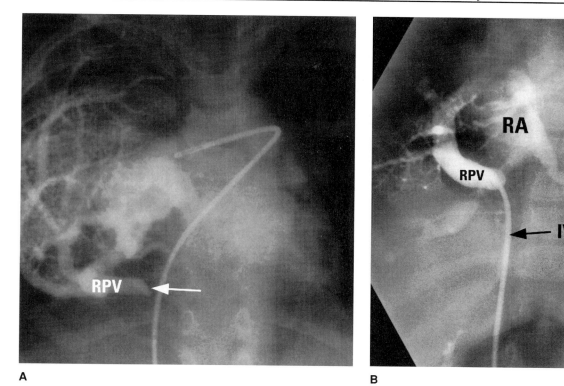

A   **B**

Fig. 19-27: Right pulmonary vein stenosis at the site of connection with the inferior vena cava is one cause for pulmonary artery hypertension in the infantile spectrum of scimitar syndrome.
A: The levophase of the pulmonary angiogram shows the severe stenosis of the right pulmonary vein. **B:** Selective injection into the anomalously connected right pulmonary vein in another patient demonstrates the severe obstruction.

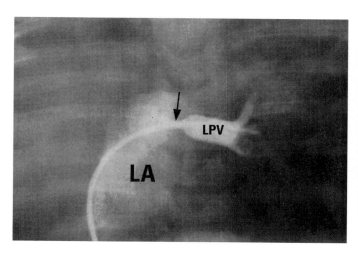

Fig. 19-28: Left pulmonary vein stenosis proved fatal in this infant with scimitar syndrome and a horseshoe lung.
Selective injection into the left pulmonary vein shows the severe stenosis (arrow).

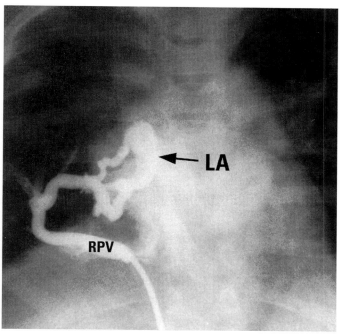

Fig. 19-29: Dual connections of the right pulmonary veins to the inferior caval vein and left atrium in this child with scimitar syndrome.
The right pulmonary veins connect both to the inferior vena cava and through a circuitous pathway to the left atrium.

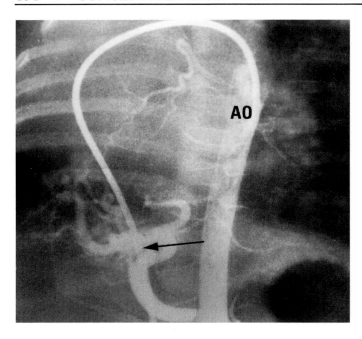

Fig. 19-30: A large systemic artery (arrow) produced heart failure in this young infant with hypogenetic right lung complex.

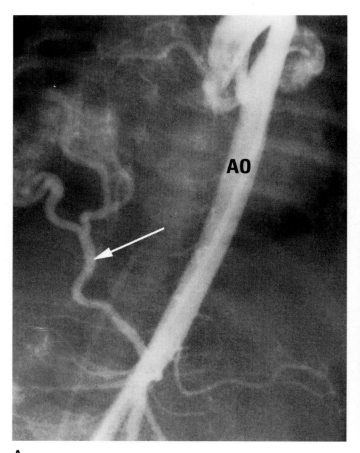

A

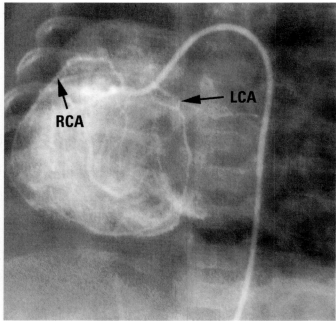

B

Fig. 19-31: This newborn had hypogenetic right lung complex with left coronary ostial atresia.
A: The aortogram shows the anomalous systemic artery and flow into the pulmonary artery via the arterial duct. B: Selective injection into the right coronary artery opacifies the entire coronary artery back to the left coronary arterial ostium at the aortic sinus.

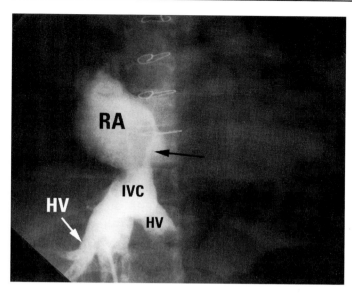

Fig. 19-32: Right pulmonary vein and caval stenosis after intra-atrial diversion of anomalously draining right pulmonary veins.
Selective injection into into the inferior vena cava shows dilated hepatic veins and jetting of blood (black arrow) in the atrial tunnel (see also Chapter 24, Figs. 24-31 and 24–32).

hypogenetic right lung.[111–137] This systemic artery, when large, causes a large left-to-right shunt, congestive heart failure, and pulmonary artery hypertension. In some patients, this anomalous systemic artery is the sole source of pulmonary blood flow, while in others it is part of dual supply (reflecting distribution of the ipsilateral pulmonary artery to the same segment of lung supplied by the anomalous systemic artery). Many of these patients should be anticipated to have anomalies of bronchial supply, also designated as sequestration.[153–171] Some patients *without* typical features of the scimitar complex may have large anomalous systemic arterial vessels which cause heart failure and pulmonary artery hypertension as the sole cardiovascular abnormality (Figs. 19-33 through 19-36).[172] The unique patient with severe pulmonary artery hypertension reported by Goldstein and colleagues[173] demonstrated severe hypoplasia of the right and left branch pulmonary arteries with a normal-sized main pulmonary trunk, bilateral infradiaphragmatic systemic arteries to the lungs, and abnormal systemic and pulmonary venous connections.

In one patient with the hypogenetic right lung complex, the prerenal segment of the inferior vena cava was

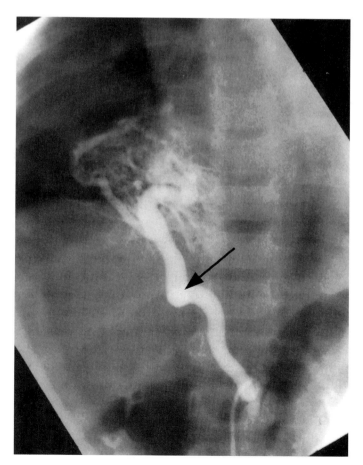

Fig. 19-33: Anomalous systemic arterial supply to the right lung with normal pulmonary venous connections and a normal caliber right pulmonary artery.
An abnormal anomalous systemic artery (arrow) was the sole abnormality in this patient with a continuous murmur over the right lower lobe of the lung. A bronchogram was normal; thus, sequestration was not present.

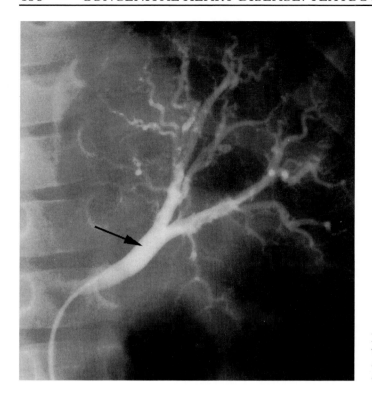

Fig. 19-34: Anomalous systemic arterial supply (arrow) to the left lung with normal pulmonary venous connections and a normal caliber and distribution of the left pulmonary artery.

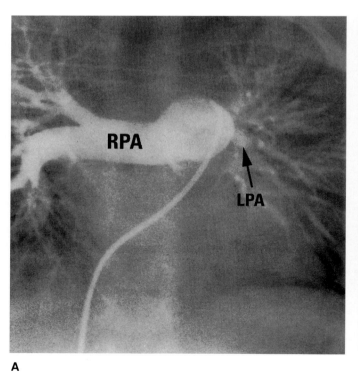

A

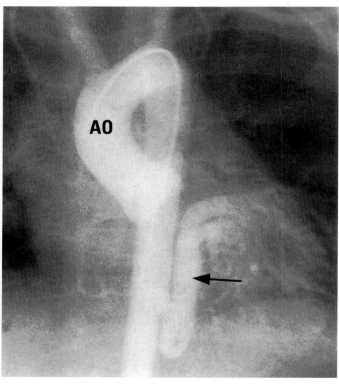

B

Fig. 19-35: Anomalous systemic arterial supply (arrow) to the left lung with normal pulmonary venous connections, but a hypoplastic caliber and distribution of the left pulmonary artery (query left-sided scimitar variant).
A: Frontal pulmonary angiogram shows the normal or enlarged right pulmonary artery and the smaller left pulmonary artery.
B: The anomalous systemic artery (arrow) to the left lung was demonstrated by aortography.

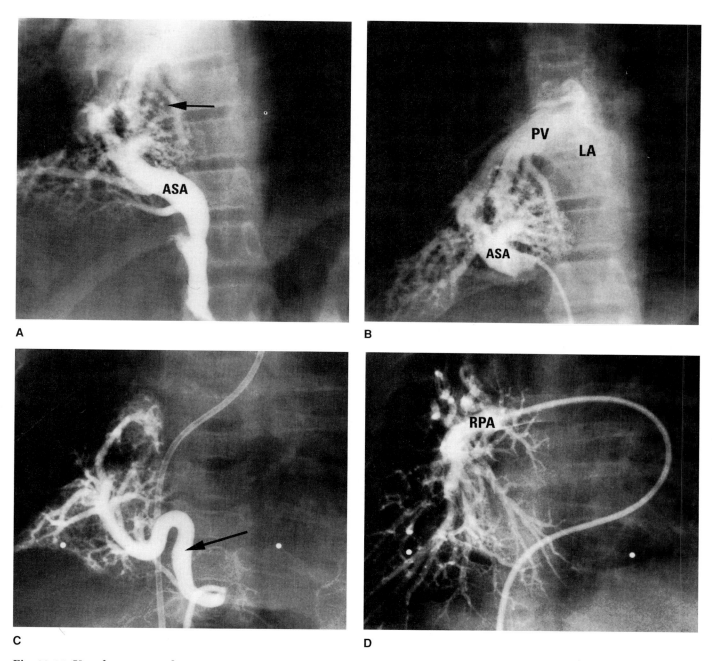

Fig. 19-36: Very large anomalous systemic artery (ASA) to the right lung with moderate pulmonary artery hypertension, but normal pulmonary venous connections and a normal caliber right pulmonary artery. The ventilation scan was also normal, probably excluding a sequestration.

A: Selective injection into the anomalous systemic artery that is seen coursing into the right lung. **B:** The levophase demonstrates the normal pulmonary venous drainage from the right lower lobe. **C and D:** Another patient with an anomalous systemic artery to the right lung and normal pulmonary venous connections. C: The aortogram shows the anomalous systemic artery coursing into the right lung. D: The right pulmonary arteriogram shows the normal distribution of the right pulmonary artery. The large anomalous systemic artery was interrrupted without incident. (Figs. 19-36C and 19–36D provided by Dr. Michael Florentine, The Children's Hospital, Grand Rapids, Michigan.)

replaced by an intrahepatic plexus of vessels draining into the right atrium and in this patient the connection between the right atrium and inferior vena caval vein was hypoplastic (see Chapter 12, Fig. 12-27).

Systemic Arterial Supply of Lung Tissue

There are a number of conditions in which lung tissue is supplied by a systemic arterial branch. These include:

1. Origin of the confluent right and left pulmonary arteries from the proximal ascending aorta in the presence of the main pulmonary trunk connected to the descending thoracic aorta via the arterial duct (see also Chapter 7).
2. Origin of one pulmonary artery from the ascending aorta and the other from the descending aorta in the presence of the main pulmonary trunk connected to the descending thoracic aorta via the arterial duct (see also Chapter 7).
3. Origin of a pulmonary artery from the aorta (See Chapters 20 and 21).
   a. from the proximal ascending aorta
   b. from the distal ascending aorta mediated by a fifth aortic arch
   c. from the arterial duct
4. Systemic arterial supply to an area of lung that is otherwise normal.
5. Systemic arterial supply to an area of lung that is sequestered from the normal tracheobronchial tree (pulmonary sequestration from the tracheobronchial tree and pulmonary artery).
6. Systemic arterial supply of lung tissue in association with tetralogy of Fallot with or without pulmonary atresia (see also Chapters 20 and 21).
7. Acquired systemic arterial supply of lung tissue through transpleural systemic-pulmonary artery anastomoses in association with pulmonary inflammation, infection, ischemia, or previous surgery.

Anomalous systemic arterial supply from the descending thoracic aorta to a normal basilar or lower lobe of a lung is a rare, congenital vascular abnormality, considered by some as part of the broad spectrum of sequestration disorders Figs. 19-33, 19-34, 19-36).[11,174–180] Pulmonary sequestration indicates that an area of lung has either no connection with the bronchial tree or an abnormal one.[153–171] In consideration of either systemic arterial supply to an area of lung that is otherwise normal or systemic arterial supply to an area of lung that is sequestered from the normal tracheobronchial tree (pulmonary sequestration from the tracheobronchial tree and pulmonary artery), the pulmonary venous connection may be either to the left atrium, to a systemic vein, or to both. In the differential diagnosis of dextrocardia and recurrent chest infection,

one must always consider Kartagener's syndrome (see Chapter 3).

Confusion may occur with acquired systemic collateral circulation into the lung, stimulated by hypoxia, inflammation, or infection. In this setting, normally present arteries undergo hypertrophy and supply the lung by myriads of small transpleural anastomoses. Although the clinical presentation is similar to sequestration, the angiographic distinction is obvious.[11,180–182]

In patients with anomalous systemic arterial supply from the descending thoracic aorta to a normal basilar or lower lobe of a lung, the involved basilar segment has its normal arterial distribution from the ipsilateral pulmonary artery, but there may be additional arterial supply from the descending thoracic aorta (Figs. 19-33, 19-34, and 19-36). This promotes a left-to-right shunt, and if the anomalous arterial vessel is large, it may promote pulmonary artery hypertension (Fig. 19-36). In those patients with normal bronchial supply to the affected lobe, interruption of the anomalous vessel, either surgically or with a catheter device, may well remedy the situation. Lobectomy may be indicated in those patients with both the anomalous systemic artery and sequestration.

Pulmonary Artery Sling
(see also Chapter 34)

This rare anomaly is well documented in the literature.[183–208b] The aberrant left pulmonary artery (pulmonary sling) is characterized by the left pulmonary artery arising from the proximal right pulmonary artery and coursing between the trachea and oesophagus to reach the left hilum. The term pulmonary sling was introduced in 1951 to differentiate this entity from vascular rings due to aortic arch anomalies.[183] More recently, the term "ring-sling complex" was introduced to emphasize the association with tracheal anomalies (Figs. 19-37 through 19-39; see also Chapter 37, Fig. 37-11).[184] The anomalous left pulmonary artery arises from the distal portion of the main pulmonary artery to the right of the trachea. This branch passes posteriorly over the proximal right bronchus, behind the trachea, and then to the left extrapericardially between the trachea and the esophagus into the left hilum. The sling that is formed may compress the right bronchus and the distal end of the trachea. There may be localized tracheomalacia at the sling level. Associated tracheal anomalies include a tracheal origin of the right upper lobe bronchus, and complete tracheal rings; this latter is associated with a high infant mortality.[184] The anomalous left pulmonary artery may be smaller than the right pulmonary artery (Fig. 19-38). Rarely, the right upper lobe branch may arise from the proximal left pulmonary artery. The anomalous vessel may supply only part of the left lung and may have an unusual course.[184a,187a]

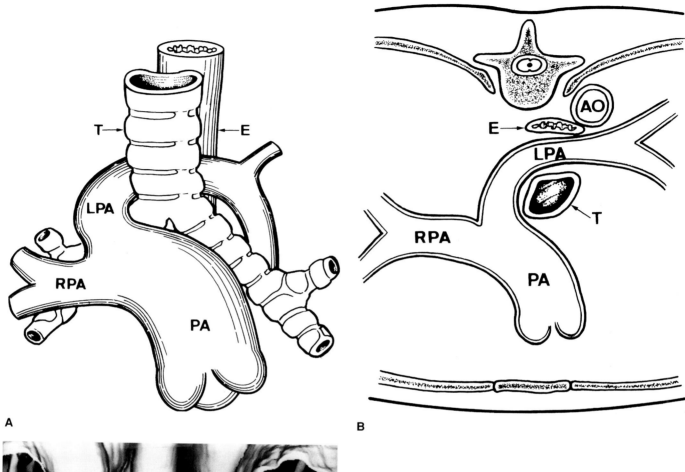

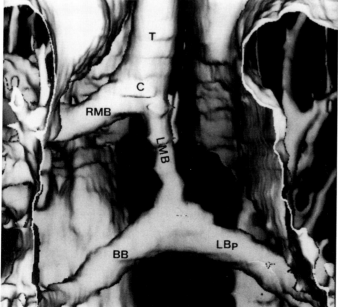

Fig. 19-37: The pulmonary artery sling and associated tracheobronchial abnormalities
A and B: Schematic diagrams showing origin of left pulmonary artery from right pulmonary artery and coursing between trachea and esophagus. **C:** Three-dimensional reconstruction of tracheobronchial anatomy in a patient with a pulmonary sling.

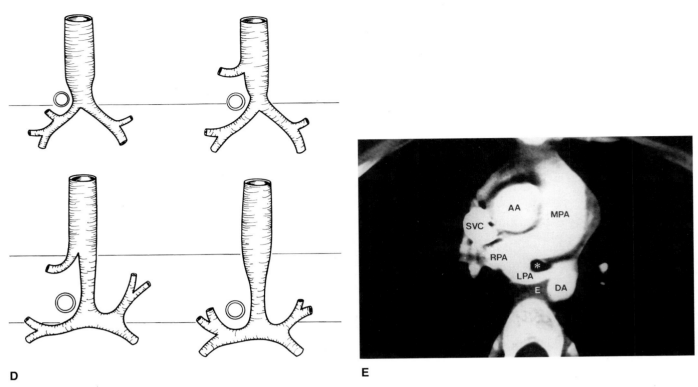

D   **E**

Fig. 19-37: *(continued)*
D: Schematic drawings showing abnormality of tracheobronchial tree in association with pulmonary artery sling. Upper left-hand panel shows stenosis of the distal trachea that has normal branching pattern. Upper right-hand panel shows the distal tracheal stenosis and the errant right upper lobar bronchus arising from midtrachea. Lower left-hand panel shows so-called bridging bronchus. The vertical segment of the left main bronchus shows diffuse narrowing. Lower right-hand panel shows that the trachea is unusually elongated and bifurcates into the right and left main bronchi at the T6–7 interspace level. Note the inverted "T" configuration of bifurcation in the two lower panels. **E:** Magnetic resonance showing the course of the left pulmonary artery.

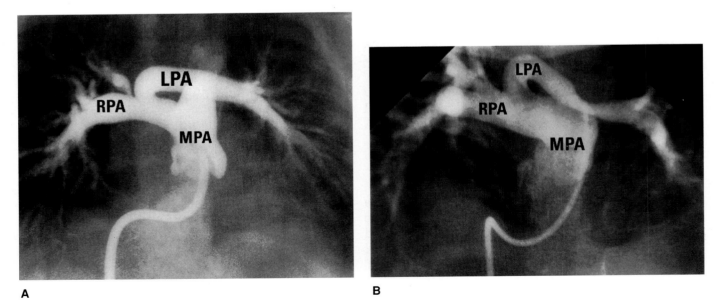

A   **B**

Fig. 19-38: Pulmonary artery sling.
A: Classic pulmonary artery sling is seen in this cranially angled main pulmonary angiogram. The left pulmonary artery originates from the right pulmonary artery. **B:** A pulmonary artery sling is shown by this cranially angled main pulmonary angiogram. The left pulmonary artery originates from the right pulmonary artery and is slightly smaller than the right pulmonary artery.

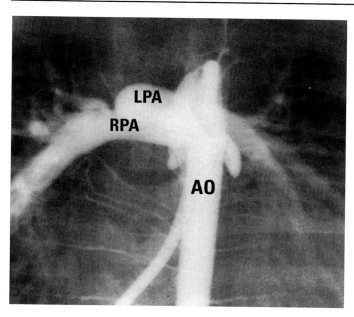

Fig. 19-39: A left-sided arterial duct led to the discovery of an asymptomatic pulmonary artery sling.

Embryologically the proximal portion of the left sixth arch that normally forms the left pulmonary artery fails to develop, or once formed, becomes obliterated at an early stage. As a result of the lack of pulmonary supply to a portion of the primitive lung bud, a branch from the pulmonary segment of the right sixth arch extends into the primitive lung tissue. With maturation and separation of the pulmonary tissue into right and left lungs, the collateral vessel elongates and grows to assume the function of the left pulmonary artery. The ductus arteriosus persists in a normal position, indicating that the distal portion of the sixth aortic arch is not involved. The surprising consistency of the malformation, both in terms of involvement of left pulmonary artery and the course, has not been explained embryologically.

In this abnormal course, the left pulmonary artery often obstructs the right bronchus or the trachea, and associated tracheal anomalies such as cartilaginous rings and long-segment tracheal stenosis are common to this disorder. The tracheobronchial tree is abnormal in most of the cases with pulmonary artery sling, with an abnormal branching pattern in about 80% of the cases. The most common pattern is an unusually long trachea that bifurcates at the level of the interspace between the sixth and seventh thoracic vertebrae, into the right and left main bronchi with the configuration of an inverted T. In about one third of the cases with an inverted T configuration of tracheal bifurcation, there is an errant bronchus arising from the trachea at the level of the interspace between the fourth and fifth thoracic vertebrae and supplying the upper part of the right lung. One may consider the site of origin of the bronchus to the right upper lung as carina, as the T4–5 interspace is the nor-

mal carinal level. Then, the vertical airway below the carina should be considered the left main bronchus instead of the distal trachea and the bronchus supplying the right lower lung is considered to arise errantly from the left main bronchus, crossing the midline to enter the right lung. The term bridging bronchus has been used to designate the errant bronchus to the right lower lung. Rarely, the trachea bifurcates at its usual T4–5 interspace level, and an errant bronchus to the right upper lung originates from the mid trachea. Regardless of the type of tracheobronchial branching pattern, the left pulmonary artery always passes over the most inferior bronchus to the right lung. The adjacent airway, whether it be lower trachea or left main bronchus, commonly demonstrates intrinsic narrowing and abnormal distribution of cartilage in its wall; the abnormality being either a complete cartilaginous ring or absence of cartilage. Patients with the pulmonary artery sling show hyperinflation of the right lung, respiratory distress, and stridor. Clinical manifestations can be observed in the newborn period, and in the particularly severely involved newborn, pneumothorax has been recorded.[185a] Initial chest films may show delayed clearing of fetal fluid from the right lung followed rarely by left air trapping as the result of compression of the proximal left bronchus by the ligamentum arteriosum or fibrosing fasciitis.[204] The symptoms tend to be respiratory in nature and are usually present at or shortly after birth. The stridor tends to be expiratory in contradistinction to inspiratory stridor noted in the aortic vascular rings. There is frequently obstruction of the right bronchus or trachea resulting in hyperinflation of the right lung. Should the obstruction become more severe, atelectasis may occur. Atelectasis or emphysema of the left lung may be present due to tracheal compression. On the lateral chest radiograph, a posterior indentation on the lower trachea may be apparent. On occasions a mass may be visible between the air filled trachea and the esophagus. An esophagram often shows an anterior indentation on the esophageal wall at the level of the tracheal bifurcation.[186,190] It should be noted however that the barium study may be normal.[204]

Angiography of the pulmonary artery filmed with cranial angulation will demonstrate the abnormal course of the left pulmonary artery (Figs. 19-37 to 19-39).[11,180,205,206] Tonkin et al[190] has advocated the use of concomitant angiography and barium esophagography in evaluation of the anomaly. The pulmonary artery sling or errant pulmonary artery may be the sole cardiovascular abnormality, but it has been identified in the patient with an arterial duct; total anomalous pulmonary venous connections; tetralogy of Fallot; double-outlet right ventricle; pulmonary atresia and intact ventricular septum, and Williams syndrome.[188,191,193,197,199,202] Tracheal or carinal stenosis or hypoplasia is well associated with the pulmonary artery sling. Indeed, in those infants and children with tracheal stenosis, a pulmonary sling must be excluded.

Other uncommon conditions that must be differentiated from the pulmonary sling include the hemitruncal sling (see Chapter 9) and the ductal sling.[209,210] Binet and colleagues[210] described a 7-week-old patient considered to have respiratory symptoms secondary to a pulmonary artery sling. At surgery, they identified an arterial duct connecting the right main pulmonary artery to the isthmic portion of the thoracic aorta, passing between the trachea and esophagus.[210] Contrast-enhanced spiral CT provides excellent definition of both the vascular and tracheobronchial anatomy.

Crossed Pulmonary Arteries

An extremely rare malformation of pulmonary artery course is crossed pulmonary arteries, where the right and left pulmonary arteries cross before entering the lung (Fig. 19-40).[211–214] This anomaly has been described in the patient with truncus arteriosus and aortic arch interruption and is also discussed in Chapter 7. Beautiful angiography of this condition can be found in the report by Wolf and colleagues.[213]

Pulmonary Artery-Left Atrial Communication

Anomalous connections can also occur directly between the pulmonary artery and left atrium.[215–223a] The hemodynamics of this malformation are similar to pulmonary arteriovenous malformation, and selective pulmonary angiography should define the lesion. In 1989, Jimenez and colleagues[222] reported a newborn with severe cyanosis with this malformation, reviewing the literature on this uncommon condition. They identified

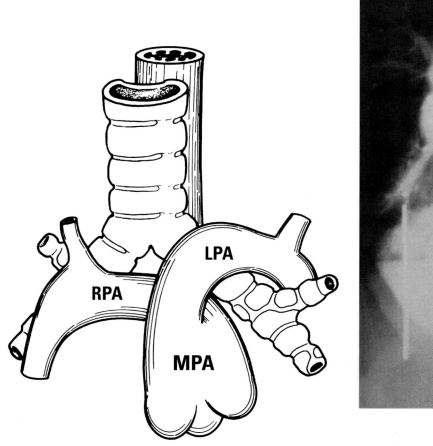

A

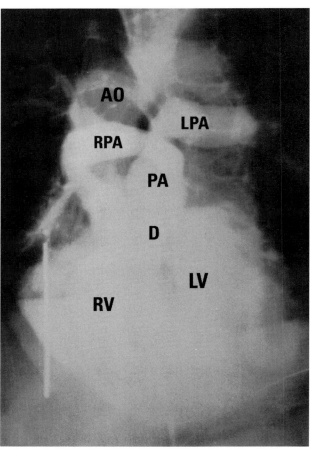

B

Fig. 19-40: Crossed pulmonary arteries.
A: Diagram showing crossed pulmonary arteries. **B:** Crossed pulmonary arteries in a patient with a ventricular septal defect (D).

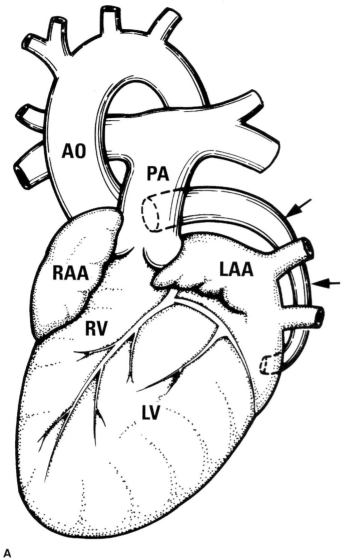

A

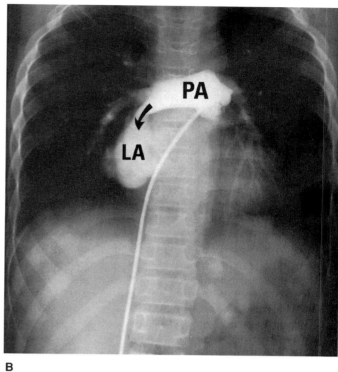

B

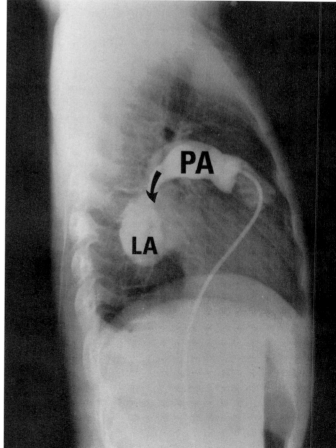

C

Fig. 19-41: Congenital pulmonary artery-left atrial communication promotes a right-to-left shunt.
A: Schematic diagram of congenital communication between pulmonary artery and left atrium. **B and C:** Frontal and lateral pulmonary angiogram. The communication between the pulmonary artery and left atrium is obvious (arrow). (Fig. 19-41B and 41C provided by Dr. M. Ando.)

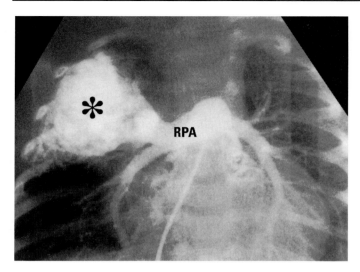

Fig. 19-42: Large, solitary pulmonary arteriovenous fistula or malformation (∗) as shown by this frontal pulmonary artery angiogram.

34 additional patients, and in all with a pulmonary artery-left atrial communication, it was the right pulmonary artery that was involved (Fig. 19-41). The opening of the communication or fistula is most frequently located at the posterior aspect of the right pulmonary artery. The communication with the left atrium can be either high or low in the left atrium. Four types of

pulmonary venous connections have been described.[218,219,222]

The review by Jimenez and colleagues[222] suggests that there are two types of presentation: 1) a neonatal form with severe hypoxemia; and 2) a milder, less severe form presenting in childhood or adulthood. The size of the communication must clearly impact on the timing of presentation. These unusual communications have been most frequently diagnosed with selective pulmonary artery angiography.

Pulmonary Arteriovenous Fistulae

Pulmonary arteriovenous fistula or malformations may be solitary, several, or many arteriovenous connections and the malformation may be localized or diffuse.[223,224] Pulmonary arteriovenous fistulae may occur in isolation as a relatively large congenital lesion, or they may be multiple and diffuse, perhaps as part of the Weber-Osler-Rendu syndrome (also known as hereditary hemorrhagic telangiectasia) (Figs. 19-42 through 19-44).[223–239] Hereditary hemorrhagic telangiectasia is an autosomal dominant disease characterized by dermal, mucosal, and visceral telangiectasia with pulmonary and cerebral malformations as well (see also Chapter 11).[228,229,234] At least half of the patients with the Weber-Osler-Rendu syndrome will demonstrate arteriovenous malformation in other areas, commonly the

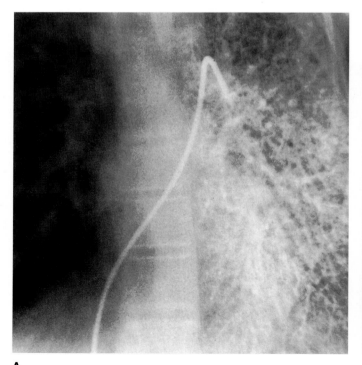

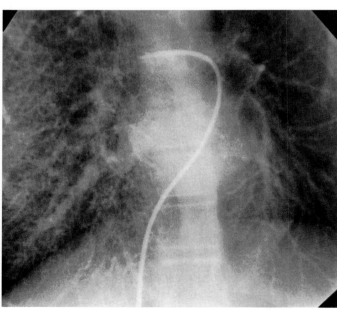

A   B

Fig. 19-43: Extremely diffuse, multiple, tiny pulmonary arteriovenous fistulae involving all lobes.
A and B: Selective pulmonary arteriography in main left and main right pulmonary arteries showing "matted" appearance of postcapillary phase consistent with the diffuse form of pulmonary arteriovenous fistulae.

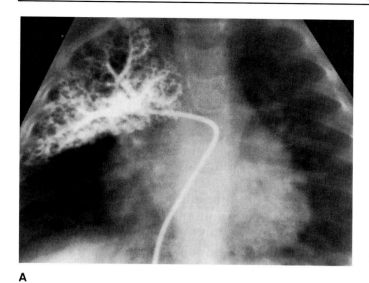

A

Fig. 19-44: Multiple, extremely diffuse, tiny pulmonary arteriovenous fistulae involving all lobes in an infant dying of progressive hypoxemia. Note the "matted" appearance of the pulmonary angiogram.

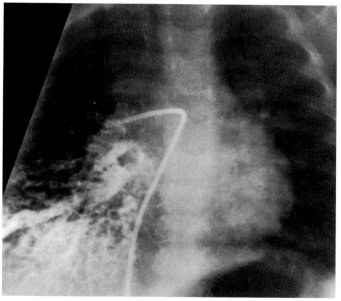

B

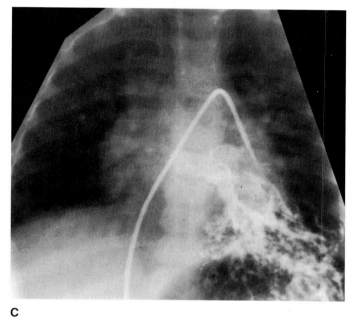

C

skin, bowel, and central nervous system.[226,228,229] These patients are at risk for brain abcess and other adverse cerebral events.[223,228–231,236] Epistaxis is a rather common presenting complaint of patients with hereditary hemorhagic telangiectasia.[237] While the majority of pulmonary arteriovenous fistulae are either congenital or associated with the Weber-Osler-Rendu syndrome, there is increasing experience with such fistulae developing in patients palliated with either a classic Glenn anastomosis, bidirectional cavopulmonary connection, Kawashima-type of total cavopulmonary bypass, or the Fontan operation (see this chapter, pp. 472 and 473). The pulmonary arteriovenous fistula, no matter what

the origin, promotes or creates a right-to-left shunt between the pulmonary arteries and veins, thus producing systemic arterial hypoxemia and polycythemia.[223] The severity of the systemic hypoxemia depends on the size and extent of the pulmonary arteriovenous fistulae.

Patients with significant pulmonary arteriovenous fistulae may be cyanotic, may have a precordial murmur, or may exhibit a pulmonary mass lesion on chest radiography. Angiography of the pulmonary arteries defines the malformation, but a thoracic aortogram is also performed to exclude systemic arterial connections to the fistula. Rarely, a massive pulmonary arteriovenous fistula will be present in the newborn; such babies are usually cyanotic and may be in heart failure.[223,225–227,232,234,235]

In recent years, some of these malformations have been successfully managed by transcatheter embolization. White and colleagues[223] and others have addressed the issue of those features of pulmonary arteriovenous malformations that lend themselves to embolotherapy.[238–248] Other patients have been treated with resection of the lobe or lobes, but in most patients redistribution of the pulmonary arteriovenous malformations occurs.[249] Armitage and colleagues[250] have transplanted patients with the diffuse form of pulmonary arteriovenous malformations. A congenital fistula between a systemic artery and a pulmonary vein may cause systemic hypoxemia as does the pulmonary arteriovenous malformation.[251–253]

The Classic Glenn or Bidirectional Cavopulmonary Connection

The classic Glenn anastomosis between the right pulmonary artery and the superior caval vein has provided excellent longterm palliation for many forms of complex congenital heart disease since its introduction in the 1950s.[254–265] The classic Glenn anastomosis is constructed between the end of the divided right pulmonary artery and the side of the superior caval vein, with ligation of the azygos vein. The superior caval vein is also ligated between the anastomosis and the right atrium to divert all superior caval return into the right pulmonary artery (Fig. 19-45). A number of factors have been implicated in late deterioration of the functionality of the Glenn anastomosis as evidenced by increasing hypoxemia and polycythemia (Figs. 19-46 through 19-48; see also Chapter 12, Figs. 12-42 and 12-43).[264–270] Isolation of the left pulmonary artery secondary to progressive closure of a ventricular septal defect or infundibular obstruction as in the patient with tricuspid atresia and normal ventriculoarterial connections previously palliated with a classic Glenn anastomosis is one anatomic reason responsible for late deterioration of the Glenn anastomosis. Other reasons for late deterioration are diminished flow through the cavopulmonary connection caused by increased vascular resistance secondary to polycythemia and hyperviscosity. In some patients development of collateral circulation from the brachiocephalic vein or one of its tributaries bypassing the lungs will lead to deterioration of the benefit from the surgical anastomosis.[264–270a] Others have suggested the decreased perfusion to the right upper and middle lobes reflecting the dependent nature of flow to the right lung characteristic of the classic Glenn anastomosis.[270] Occasionally the site of ligation of the superior caval vein at the right atrial junction may recanalize. Perhaps the most egregious cause of late failure of the classic Glenn anastomosis is the development of arteriovenous fistulae (see next section this chapter) (Fig. 19-48).

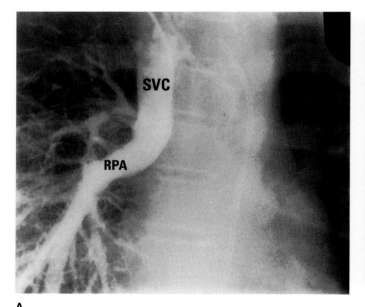

A

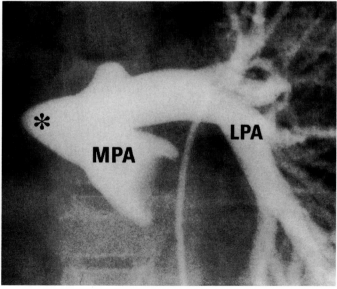

B

Fig. 19-45: The classic Glenn anastomosis.
A: The appearance of the right superior vena cava-right pulmonary artery anastomosis. **B:** After the Glenn anastomosis, flow into the left pulmonary artery is mediated either from the native pulmonary outflow tract or through a surgically created shunt, or both.

Fig. 19-46: Recanalization of the ligated superior vena cava-right atrial junction is one reason for late deterioration of the classic Glenn anastomosis.
A and B: Injection into the superior vena cava in frontal and lateral views shows the patent superior vena cava-right atrial junction (arrow).

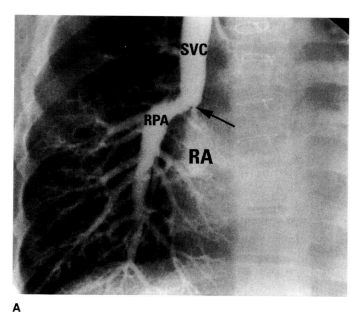

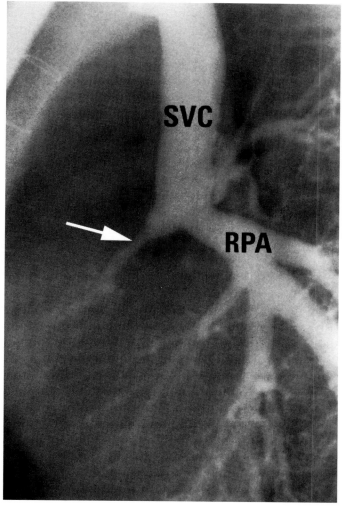

A

B

Once so-called failure of the classic Glenn anastomosis has occurred, palliation make take the form of a shunt to augment flow to the contralateral lung.[271] Others have advocated augmenting flow through the classic Glenn anastomosis by creation of an axillary artery-to-vein fistula.[272,273] We have just reported our experience with this procedure, which certainly provides excellent palliation.[274] We have augmented flow through either a classic Glenn anastomosis or bidirectional cavopulmonary connection in those patients not considered candidates for Fontan's operation (Fig. 19-49). One of the late complications of this maneuver is aneurysmal transformation of the superior caval vein (personal communication, Dr. William Hellenbrand, Yale Medical School, New Haven, CT, 1994) (see also Chapter 12, Fig. 12-8).

There is increasing experience with the so-called bidirectional cavopulmonary connection.[275–284b] This shunt uses an anastomosis between the superior vena cava and the undivided right pulmonary artery (Figs. 19-50 through 19-55). In those patients with a right and left superior vena cava but without a bridging brachiocephalic vein, it may be necessary to perform bilateral bidirectional cavopulmonary connections. In the majority of patients undergoing a bidirectional cavopulmonary connection, flow from the heart into the pulmonary trunk is interrupted, although this is not always the case as some patients are left with pulsatile flow.[283,284] The bidirectional cavopulmonary connection has some advantages over the classic Glenn anastomosis, and is being applied to ever younger infants.[275–277a,284b] First, the anastomosis is constructed in an end-to-side anastomosis, thus allowing the caliber of the superior caval vein rather than the size of the ip-

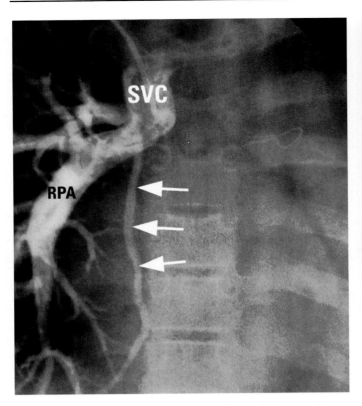

Fig. 19-47: Development of venous collaterals (arrows) may contribute to late deterioration of a classic Glenn anastomosis.

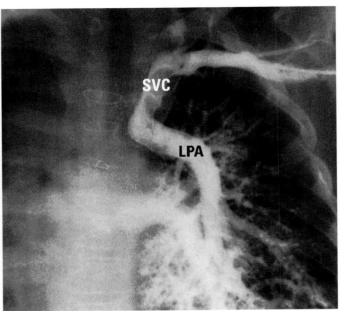

Fig. 19-48: The development of pulmonary arteriovenous fistulae after a Glenn anastomosis may contribute to late deterioration in function of this anastomosis. Once attributed to lack of pulsatile flow, the development of these fistulae are now attributed to lack of some hepatic factor.
Multiple pulmonary arteriovenous fistulae with early opacification of the pulmonary veins occurred some years after construction of this left-sided cavopulmonary connection in this patient with left atrial isomerism.

silateral pulmonary artery to define the size of the anastomosis. Second, the bidirectional cavopulmonary connection usually results in a higher oxygen saturation in young children reflecting the proportionately higher upper to lower body segment in younger children compared with older children.[278] Also, the bidirectional cavopulmonary connection provides flow to the contralateral lung without subjecting that lung to volume overloading and possibly pulmonary vascular obstructive disease from a systemic-to-pulmonary artery anastomosis to that lung, or inadequate growth and resultant hypoplasia from reduced flow. The bidirectional cavopulmonary anastomosis accomplishes these without volume-loading the ventricle, an important advantage for the patient with a univentricular atrioventricular connection.[278a,278b] Aneurysmal transformation of a left superior caval vein has been reported as a complication of a pulsatile cavopulmonary connection.[284] Mendelsohn and colleagues[275a] have studied the growth of the pulmonary arteries after a bidirectional cavopulmonary connection. Serial angiographic and hemodynamic examinations before and 17.6 +/− 1.6 months after bidirectional Glenn procedures were compared by these authors. At the follow-up study there was no significant change in diameter of the pulmonary artery ipsilateral to the bidirectional cavopulmonary

shunt. Of concern, however, was the observation of a significant decrease in the diameter of the pulmonary artery contralateral to the bidirectional cavopulmonary shunt. There was also a 32% decrease in the Nakata index of total cross-sectional pulmonary artery area after the bidirectional Glenn procedure. In addition, total pulmonary blood flow and mean pulmonary artery pressure had decreased, but arterial oxygen saturation

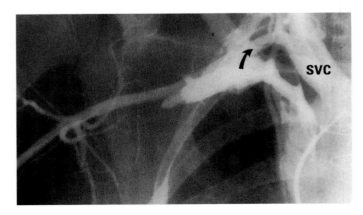

Fig. 19-49: The appearance of a surgically created axillary artery-vein fistula (arrow) to increase flow through a cavopulmonary connection (see also Chapter 12, Fig. 12-8).

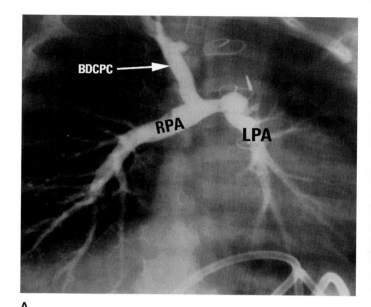

A

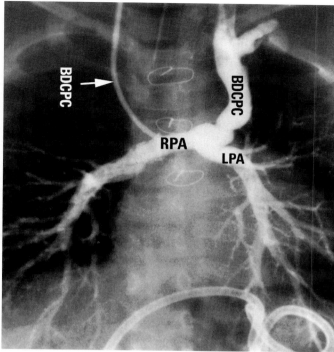

Fig. 19-51: Bilateral bidirectional cavopulmonary connections may be required in those patients with bilateral superior caval veins, but without a bridging brachiocephalic vein.

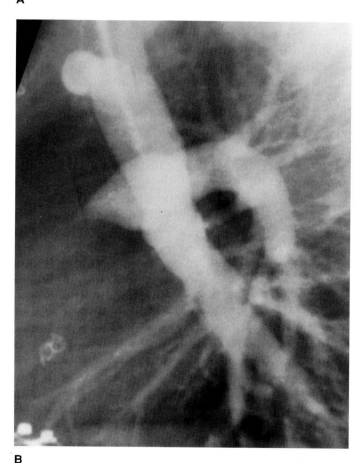

B

Fig. 19-50: The bidirectional cavopulmonary connection is now used with increasing frequency to stage to the Fontan. A and B: Frontal and axial views of the bidirectional cavopulmonary connection.

had increased at follow-up. Alejos and colleagues[284a] from their analysis of 129 patients undergoing a bidirectional cavopulmonary connection suggest that abnormal pulmonary venous drainage, a mean pulmonary artery pressure >18 mm Hg, heterotaxy syndrome, and right ventricular morphology were risk factors in predicting death or failure of the anastomosis. The study by Slavik and associates indicates that the cavopulmonary promotes growth of a small right pulmonary artery, but there is less evidence that it promotes growth of the small left pulmonary artery.[284c]

A number of studies have now addressed the influence of competitive pulmonary blood flow on the bidirectional cavopulmonary shunt.[284c-284e] The multi-institutional study of Webber and colleagues[284c] showed that competitive flow is well tolerated in the short and medium term after bidirectional cavopulmonary shunt, with improvement in early, but not late, systemic arterial oxygen saturation. These authors discuss the potential benefits of leaving some pulsatile flow including the prevention of development of pulmonary arteriovenous fistulae, and as well the potential to enhance pulmonary arterial growth. The data of Mainwaring are more cautionary in the evaluation of the role of accessory blood flow, and they state that morbidity and mortality is increased in those patients with accessory blood flow.[284d] While the analysis of

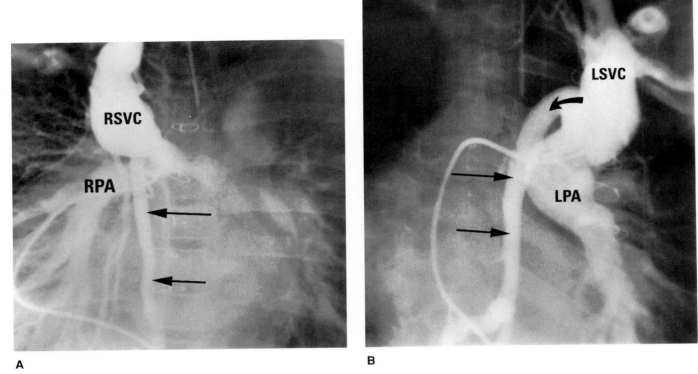

Fig. 19-52: Bilateral cavopulmonary connections with nonconfluent pulmonary arteries, both with development of systemic venous collateralization (arrows).
A: Right-sided cavopulmonary connection. **B:** Left-sided cavopulmonary connection.

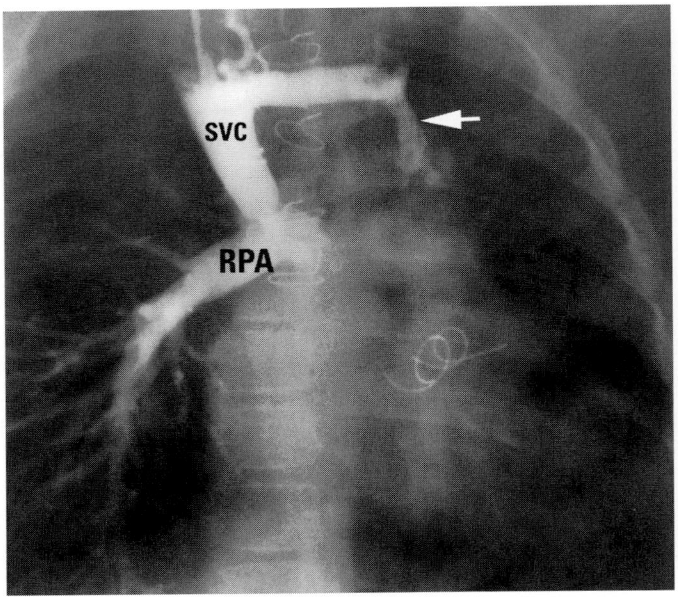

Fig. 19-53: Stenosis of the cavopulmonary connection may promote venous collateralization.
A: Frontal injection into the superior vena cava doesn't clearly demonstrate distal obstruction, despite the development of venous collaterals (arrow). **B:** A right anterior oblique view with a caudocranial angulation shows the distal stenosis (arrow).

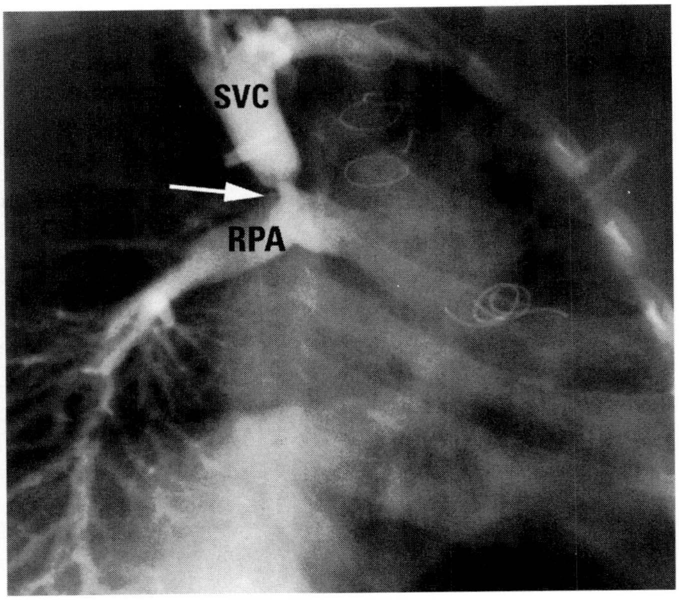

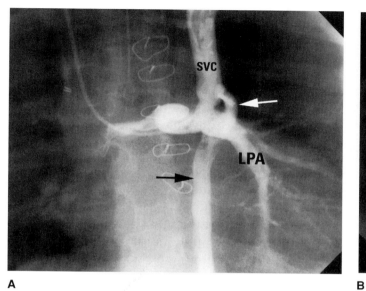

A

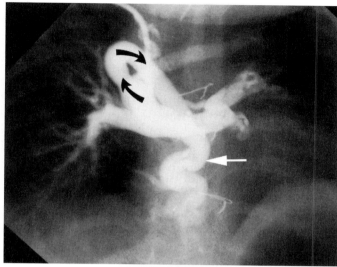

B

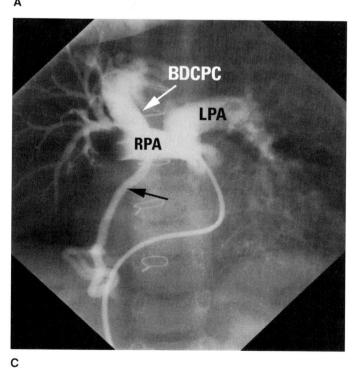

C

Fig. 19-54: Venous collateralization in a patient with bidirectional cavopulmonary connection.
A: Collateralization via the hemiazygous vein (arrows) in a patient with bilateral bidirectional cavopulmonary connection. **B:** Extensive collateralization after a bidirectional cavopulmonary connection. **C:** Peculiar venous collateral (arrow) after a bidirectional cavopulmonary connection.

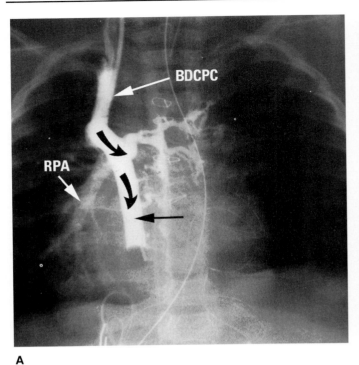
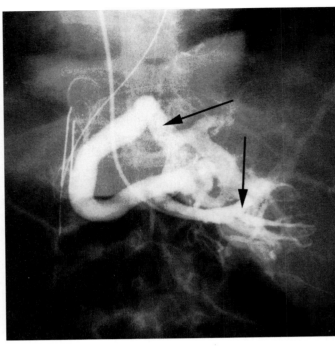

A   **B**

Fig. 19-55: Very large intra-abdominal venous collateral after a bidirectional cavopulmonary connection.
A: Retrograde flow (arrows) down the azygous vein. **B:** The very large venous channels (arrows).

Frommelt and colleagues[284e] indicates that an additional source of pulmonary blood flow in patients with a bidirectional cavopulmonary shunt may have higher oxygen saturations, their cental venous pressures are also higher, and they may be more at risk for late development of chylothorax. Finally, there is also some evidence that a staged operation to the Fontan increases the incidence of sinoatrial node dysfunction.[284f]

The Development of Pulmonary Arteriovenous Fistulae

Pulmonary arteriovenous fistulae may occur years after the construction of a classic Glenn anastomosis; after total cavopulmonary bypass as part of the Kawashima operation; after the Fontan operation; and they have been recognized in patients with polysplenia syndrome.[257,259,261,263,264,270,274,285–291c] It has been suggested that lack of pulsatile pulmonary blood flow to the basal and dependent lobes of the right lung are responsible for the development of pulmonary arteriovenous fistulae after construction of a classic Glenn anastomosis (Fig. 19-48; see also Chapter 41, Fig. 41-22).[270] Pulmonary arteriovenous malformations have subsequently been identified in the patient with polysplenia.[288–290,292] In the first such patient described, the cardiac malformations included dextrocardia, bilateral left atrial appendages, intact atrial and ventricular septa, interruption of the inferior vena cava, and connection

of all the hepatic veins to the left-sided atrium.[288] One would wonder whether the hepatic veins were isolated from the pulmonary arterial bed, a suggestion as to the etiology of the development of pulmonary arteriovenous fistulae (see Chapter 41, Figs. 41-8, 41-9, and 41-22).[292,292a] This patient also had hypoplasia of the portal vein, perhaps reminiscent of the hepatic-cirrhotic role in the genesis of pulmonary arteriovenous fistulae.[293–294a] Other such patients have now been described, and in at least one patient the hepatic venous connections were characterized as normal.[289] It is of interest, however, that reversal of cirrhosis-related pulmonary shunting has been achieved in children by orthotopic liver transplantation.[295,296] Fewtrell and colleagues[296] have fully analyzed intrapulmonary shunting in the biliary atresia/polysplenia syndrome and have demonstrated reversal after liver transplantation. Summarizing their data, 173 children, including 93 with biliary atresia, received liver grafts at Addenbrooke's Hospital between 1983 and 1993. Of these, only 7 developed cyanosis due to intrapulmonary shunting as a complication of their liver disease, and all 7 of these had biliary atresia/polysplenia syndrome. Intrapulmonary shunting was confirmed by a radioisotope scan in 4 children. Only 1 child with the syndrome did not have cyanosis when undergoing transplantation. Seven of the eight children are alive 6–54 months after transplantation, with normal pulmonary and hepatic function. Cyanosis recurred in one child who developed chronic rejection with liver failure. In conclusion: a) there is a strong association between the biliary atresia/polysplenia syndrome and cyanosis due to intrapulmonary shunting; b) intrapulmonary shunting is fully reversible after successful liver transplantation; and c) cyanosis, once present, is progressive, and these children should be considered for liver transplantation as soon as it occurs. More recently, Brodie and Mee[296a] have demonstrated reversal of acquired pulmonary arteriovenous fistulae that developed soon after after a classic Kawashima procedure. They diverted hepatic venous blood to the pulmonary arteries with a left lateral atrial tunnel. One should remember as well that pulmonary hypertension may be associated in patients with portal hypertension.[297,298] The mechanisms for this association are unclear.

Laks and colleagues[298a] have provided a modification of Fontan's procedure where the superior vena cava is connected to the left pulmonary artery and the lateral tunnel and thus the inferior caval vein and hepatic veins are diverted to the right pulmonary artery. They caution that lack of hepatic venous flow to the left lung might contribute to unilateral pulmonary arteriovenous malformations, and this is exactly what we have observed in one patient who has undergone this operation.

The Pulmonary Arteries and the Systemic-to-Pulmonary Artery Anastomosis

The era of surgical palliation for the patient with cyanotic congenital heart disease was ushered in by the benchmark contribution of Blalock and Taussig with the construction of a subclavian artery-pulmonary artery anastomosis opposite the side of the aortic arch to augment pulmonary blood flow (see Chapter 20, Fig. 20-14).[298b] The application of a Waterston-Cooley anastomosis between the right pulmonary artery and the ascending aorta, and the Potts' anastomosis between the descending thoracic aorta and the left pulmonary artery were subsequent surgical maneuvers to palliate cyanotic congenital heart disease on the basis of pulmonary oligemia. But all these surgical procedures had the potential and reality of both distorting the pulmonary artery and adversely affecting its hemodynamics.[11,299] The classic Blalock-Taussig anastomosis had the potential for obstructing the pulmonary artery, but it was uncommon for this type of shunt to result in pulmonary artery hypertension.[300–304] Scarring and retraction of the subclavian artery used in the shunt could distort by tenting up the pulmonary artery. Rarely, aneurysmal transformation of the Blalock-Taussig shunt would occur over many years, resulting in pulmonary arterial hypertension and eventually in pulmonary vascular obstructive disease.[304] With the use of Goretex as a modi-

fication of the classic Blalock-Taussig anastomosis, some of these modified shunts were complicated by seroma formation (see Chapter 37, Fig. 37-39).[305] Another complication of the modified Blalock-Taussig shunt was stenosis or interruption of the ipsilateral subclavian artery. This had the potential for promoting a vertebral or subclavian steal, with the possibility of late claudication. With small pulmonary arteries, the introduction of the Potts' shunt and the Waterston-Cooley anastomosis provided techniques to augment pulmonary blood flow, but over the years a substantial literature accumulated documenting the complications of these forms of arterial shunts. Both of these shunts are known to cause pulmonary artery stenosis and pulmonary artery hypertension, and such complications increase substantially the risk of Fontan's operation, or in fact preclude it (see also Chapter 39).[299,303,303a] Furthermore, it is quite difficult to surgically close the Potts' shunt and to rehabilitate the left lung artery from a midline stenotomy approach. Thus, with few exceptions such shunts have been abandoned over the past decade.

The Pulmonary Artery After Banding

Banding of the pulmonary main trunk has proven an effective methodology to palliate some forms of congenital heart disease (Figs. 19-56 through 19-63).[306–310] With the initiative of primary repair of congenital heart malformation whenever possible, this technique is being used with decreasing frequency. The pulmonary

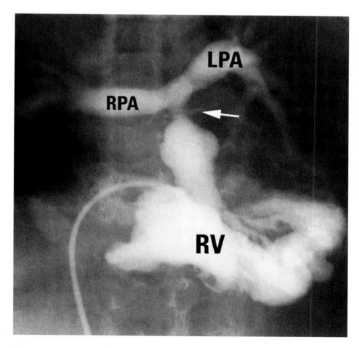

Fig. 19-56: A well-placed pulmonary artery band(arrow).

Fig. 19-57: The pulmonary artery band has slightly narrowed the right pulmonary artery (arrow).
A and B: Frontal and lateral pulmonary angiograms.

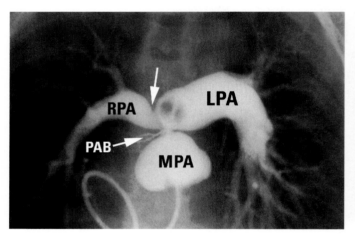

A

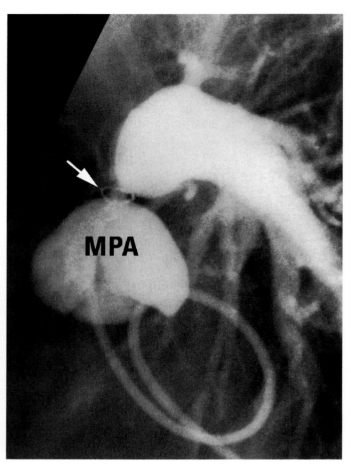

B

artery band clearly distorts the integrity of the arterial wall, can migrate distally promoting right pulmonary artery stenosis or occlusion, and in some patients distal migration of the band will severely compromise the origin of the right pulmonary artery, but not protect the vascular integrity of the contralateral pulmonary artery (Figs. 19-57 through 19-59).[11,311–312] Infective endarteritis may promote infection at the site of the band, leading to formation of a mycotic aneurysm (Figs. 19-61 through 19-63). Intraluminal disposition of the pulmonary artery band indicates erosion through the arterial wall, perhaps in response to interference with the vasa vasorum. Similarly, extrusion of the pulmonary artery band usually reflects formation of a false aneurysm. Disappearance of the pulmonary artery band reflects erosion of the band into the lumen.[311a] Unusual branching of the main pulmonary trunk into the right and left pulmonary arteries with early take-off of the right pulmonary artery might predispose this patient to narrowing of the origin of the right pulmonary artery.[311c] If hemolytic anemia occurs in a patient subsequent to pulmonary artery banding, one might suspect in the differential diagnosis intraluminal erosion of the band, and secondary mechanical hemolysis.[311b]

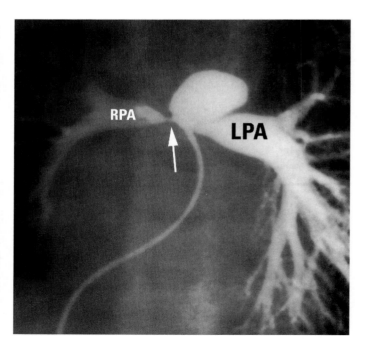

Fig. 19-58: The pulmonary artery band has severely compromised the origin of the right pulmonary artery (arrow).

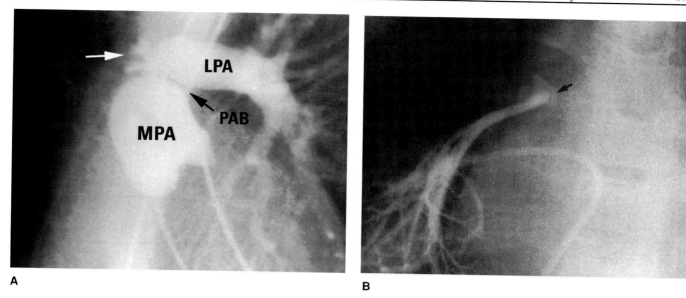

A

B

Fig. 19-59: Distal migration of the pulmonary artery band has led to complete occlusion of the right pulmonary artery.
A: Main pulmonary angiogram shows the complete occlusion of the right pulmonary artery. **B:** A right pulmonary vein wedge angiogram shows the severely hypoplastic right pulmonary artery (arrow).

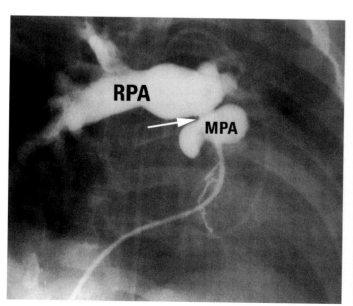

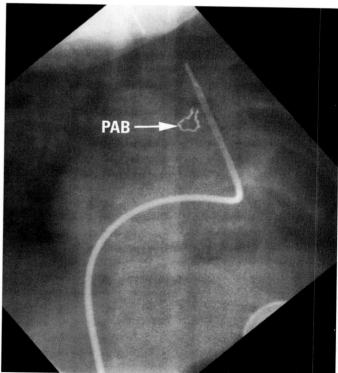

Fig. 19-60: This proximally positioned pulmonary artery band may lead to thickening of the pulmonary valve.

Fig. 19-61: Erosion of the pulmonary artery band. The catheter is in the distal main pulmonary trunk, adjacent to the band.

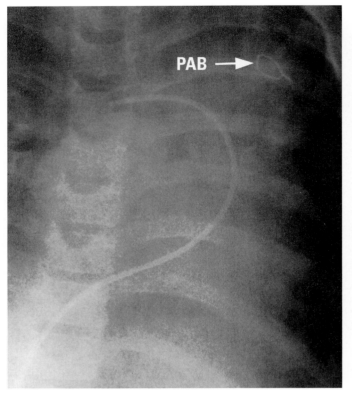

A

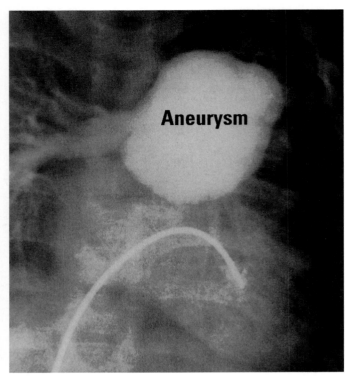

B

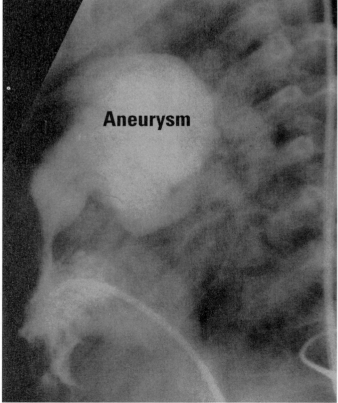

C

Fig. 19-62: A mycotic aneurysm of the pulmonary artery following banding of the main pulmonary trunk.
A: The band has been extruded as shown by the catheter and the band. **B and C:** Frontal and lateral main pulmonary angiograms demonstrate the very large mycotic aneurysm.

Fig. 19-63: Another infant with a huge mycotic aneurysm.
A: Chest radiograph shows the huge aneurysm. **B and C:** The catheter can pass on either side of the pulmonary artery band.
D: The very large mycotic aneurysm is defined by the pulmonary arteriogram.

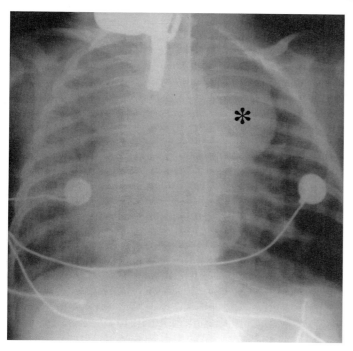

A

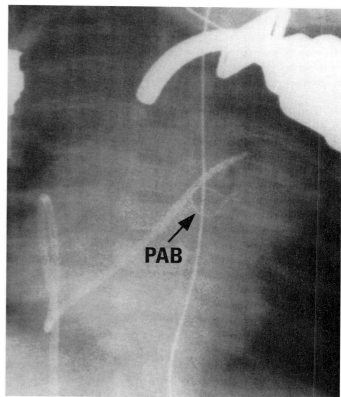

B

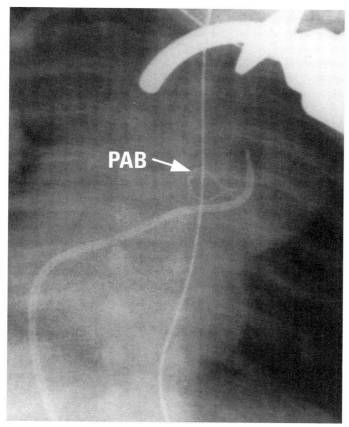

C

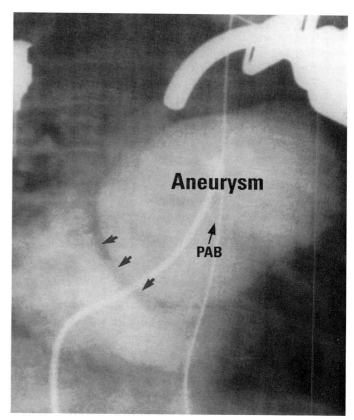

D

Hiraishi and colleagues[312] have provided data suggesting that obstruction of the proximal pulmonary artery branches following pulmonary artery banding can reflect either distal migration or placement of the band close to the bifurcation, possibly both, and that cross-sectional echocardiography can reliably assess this occurrence, and its severity.

The pulmonary artery band may be positioned just above the pulmonary valve leaflets, and turbulent flow through the band may promote vascular injury and thickening (Fig. 19-60).[11] The alteration in form and function of the pulmonary valve subsequent to pulmonary artery banding may confound the arterial switch procedure of Jatene or the integrity of a pulmonary artery-proximal aortic anastomosis of the Damus-Kaye-Stansel type (see Chapters 39 and 40).[314–323] Banding of the main pulmonary trunk, by promoting myocardial hypertrophy, may cause a significant degree of infundibular obstruction. In some patients with ventricular septal defect treated by banding of the pulmonary trunk, spontaneous diminution in size of the ventricular septal defect and progressive obstruction of the pulmonary trunk secondary to the band will lead to a hypertensive and heavily muscularized right ventricle. Finally, pulmonary artery banding has been implicated in the genesis of subaortic stenosis and myocardial hypertrophy in patients with double-inlet left ventricle, a rudimentary right ventricle and a discordant ventriculoarterial connection (see Chapter 40).[324–336] Those reasons for the development of subaortic stenosis in these patients are both complex and multifactorial, including and reflecting the initial size of the ventricular septal defect (and the tendency of a moderate-sized ventricular septal defect to spontaneous diminution in size); the role of myocardial hypertrophy to reduce the size of a ventricular septal defect; and the reduction of the ventricular end diastolic volume with remodeling of the left ventricular myocardial mass.[326–332,334–336]

Pulmonary Artery Wedge Angiography

Assessment of hemodynamics and the calculation of pulmonary vascular resistance may not be predictive of the morphologic alterations of the pulmonary vascular bed. The technique of pulmonary artery wedge angiography has been advocated to provide better information about those vascular changes, and their findings have been helpful in determining the operability in some patients and the timing of surgery in others. This technique was initially applied by Bell and colleagues in 1959, and subsequently by other investigators.[337–341] Rabinovitch and colleagues[342] have extended this technique by: 1) providing quantification of the rate of tapering of the pulmonary arteries; 2) determination of the degree of background haze with reference to standard films, and 3) calculation of the pulmonary circulation time. Furthermore, Rabinovitch and the Boston

Children's group have provided correlative data with hemodynamics and with morphometric findings from lung biopsy tissue. This technique has been used quite effectively to define the character of pulmonary venous obstruction (see also Chapter 24).

Imaging of the Pulmonary Arteries

Imaging of the pulmonary arteries has been achieved using a wide variety of methodologies including cross-sectional echocardiography, computerized tomography, magnetic resonance imaging, angiography (selective and peripheral), pulmonary vein wedge angiography, and digital subtraction techniques. We have discussed elsewhere those imaging modalities in congenital heart disease (see Chapter 1). Also Burrows, then in Toronto, and her colleagues evaluated various imaging techniques in the investigation of pulmonary artery anomalies as well as other forms of congenital heart disease.[180,343] Hernandez and colleagues[344] have performed a comparative evaluation of the pulmonary arteries in patients with right ventricular outflow tract obstructive lesions comparing the roles of CT, sonography, and cineangiocardiography. These authors concluded that these techniques tended to provide complementary information. Vick and colleagues[345] have compared the role of nuclear magnetic resonance of the pulmonary arteries, subpulmonary region and aorticopulmonary shunts with two-dimensional echocardiography and angiography. In angiographic imaging of the pulmonary arteries, clearly it is the technique of selective injection of contrast into the pulmonary artery with biplane imaging and in the appropriate projection that gives the most anatomic information. It is redundant today to emphasize how important adequate imaging of the pulmonary is in the preoperative evaluation of patients with tetralogy of Fallot, pulmonary atresia, and ventricular septal defect, as well as in all potential candidates for either a bidirectional cavopulmonary connection or any of the many modifications of Fontan's operation (see also Chapters 1, 2, 20, and 21). The role of axial angiocardiography in the demonstration of pulmonary arteries cannot be overemphasized.[346–360]

The pulmonary arteries may be imaged from ventricular angiocardiography, but all too frequently the origin of the proximal right and left pulmonary arteries and the specific anatomic detail will be obscured by contrast in the aorta. In those patients with severe pulmonary outflow tract obstruction or pulmonary atresia, access to the pulmonary arteries may be achieved through a previously constructed surgical shunt.[354–358] When there is no access to the pulmonary arteries from the heart or through a previously surgical shunt, selective injection of contrast into an arterial duct or close to it, or selective injection of aortopulmonary collateral arteries (see Chapter 21) may demonstrate the pulmonary arteries (see also Chapters 20 and 21).[354–357] Finally, the technique of pulmonary vein wedge angiography has proven very important in the visualization of the so-called absent pulmonary artery.[356–358,360–362] In this regard it is necessary to define the hemodynamics of the pulmonary artery circulation for many patients considered for reparative operations. A number of papers have addressed the correlation between direct catheter measurement of pulmonary artery pressures and indirect measurement from pulmonary vein wedge pressures.[363–365]

We have discussed in Chapters 1 and 2 those basic principles of pulmonary artery angiography that are applicable to imaging of the pulmonary arteries. In the initial investigation when it is not possible to enter the pulmonary artery, ventriculography using cranially angled projections may demonstrate the main pulmonary trunk and its branches. Forty-five degrees of axial angulation and 5% to 10% of left anterior obliquity usually elongate the main pulmonary artery, profiling as well the origins of the right and left pulmonary arteries. Arborization anomalies and obstructive lesions within the branch and parenchymal pulmonary arteries are best demonstrated by selective injections of contrast into the right and left pulmonary arteries using frontal, oblique or lateral projections. We have discussed elsewhere the role of pulmonary artery wedge angiography in demonstrating pulmonary vein stenosis (see Chapter 24) and the angiographic evaluation of the pulmonary circulation is discussed in detail in Chapter 21. Because diffuse anomalies of the pulmonary arteries may reflect a diffuse vasculopathy, a thoracic aortogram is routinely performed in our institution to image the thoracic aorta, its arch vessels, and as well an abdominal aortogram is obtained to define the origins of the coeliac, renal, and mesenteric arteries, all of which may be involved in such a diffuse process.

One can arrive at the presumptive diagnosis of a congenitally unilaterally absent pulmonary artery in a number of ways (Figs. 19-6 through 19-16).[81–105] An angiogram performed in the main pulmonary trunk will show absence of one of the pulmonary arteries. If lung tissue is present then there must be some type of arterial supply, no matter how tenuous. If the mediastinal right pulmonary artery is congenitally absent, then one might anticipate a distal ductal or ligamental origin of the parenchymal right pulmonary artery with connection of the arterial duct or its remnant to the hilar pulmonary artery. An aortogram performed in the ascending aorta may well show an arterial duct connecting to the right pulmonary artery or ductus bump or diverticulum originating from the base of the innominate artery. If the arterial duct is not patent, the presence of the ductal diverticulum ipsilateral to the presumed absent pulmonary artery is witness to the pathogenesis of the isolated pulmonary artery. It may be necessary to perform pulmonary vein wedge angiography to satis-

factorily demonstrate the caliber of the hilar pulmonary artery.[83,95,99,102,355–358,361,362] The pulmonary vein can be probed from a naturally-occurring atrial septal defect; using a transseptal technique; through an anomalously connected pulmonary vein; or from a retrograde arterial approach.[363,364] Pulmonary vein wedge pressures may be used to infer pulmonary artery pressure, remembering that there is significant scatter above a pulmonary vein wedge pressure of 20–25 mm Hg.[363–365]

Those anomalies associated with unilateral pulmonary artery hypoplasia are diverse and thus the angiographic investigation of the patient with a unilaterally hypoplastic pulmonary artery necessitates adequate imaging of the ipsilateral pulmonary veins as well as the descending thoracic aorta (Figs. 19-18 through 19-32).[111–137] Selective injection into each pulmonary artery is probably the best way to demonstrate the caliber and presence or absence of stenoses within the pulmonary arterial tree. The levophase of these selective injections must be scrutinized to determine the character of the pulmonary venous connections. If the pulmonary veins are not clearly and unequivocally imaged despite delivery of an adequate amount of contrast into the pulmonary artery, or if the transit through one or the other lung seems unduly prolonged, then one must have concern about the integrity of the pulmonary venous connection(s). The appearance of the so-called scimitar sign on the routine chest radiograph should lead one to suspect anomalies of the right pulmonary veins, and then appropriate attention will be focused on the nature of the right pulmonary veins. Hawass and colleagues[149a] have discussed the differential diagnosis of the horseshoe lung. They review the considerations of a pulmonary sling or a bridging bronchus.[366,367] Gonzales-Crussi and colleagues[366] describe the postmortem findings of an 8-week-old baby with recurrent respiratory difficulties and a bridging bronchus. The right-lower-lobe bronchus arose from the left main bronchus, crossing the mediastinum. This infant also had a patent ovale foramen and a bicuspid aortic valve. Starshak and colleagues[367] describe another infant whose right-lower-lobe bronchus also arose from the left main bronchus and bridged the mediastinum. This baby also had a hypoplastic trachea, and at postmortem, the right lung was bilobed with fusion of the upper and middle lobes, while the left lung exhibited normal lobation. In neither of these two patients did the pulmonary artery cross the mediastinum as in the cross-over lung deformity.

Pulmonary artery wedge angiography has been advocated as a technique to complement hemodynamic evaluation in the preoperative assessment of the patient with pulmonary artery hypertension and possible pulmonary vascular obstructive disease. This technique provides a morphological assessment of the pulmonary vascular bed, and using the technique published by Rabinovitch and colleagues,[342] one measures the rate of

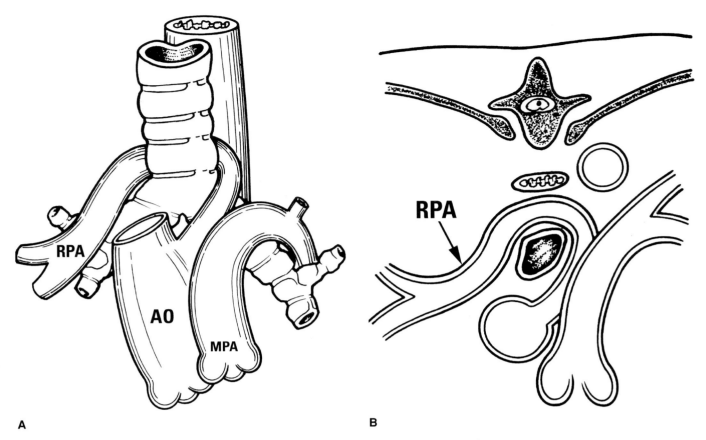

A

B

Fig. 19-64: Drawing of so-called hemitruncal sling.

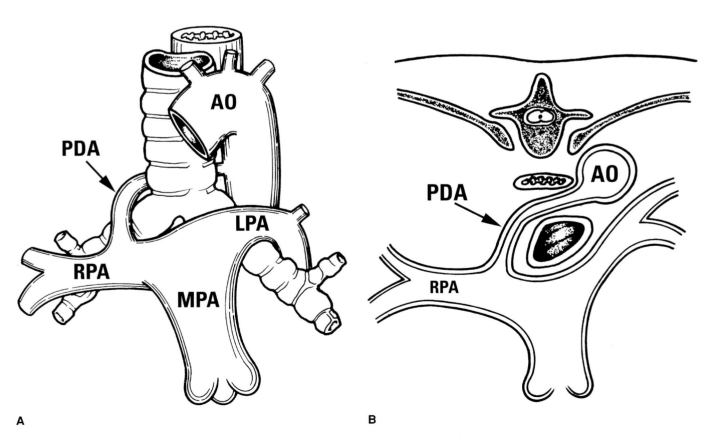

A

B

Fig. 19-65: Drawing of so-called ductal sling.

tapering of the pulmonary arteries that is indicative of vascular muscularity and tone, and the so-called background haze that provides information about the degree of filling of the small peripheral pulmonary arteries. One also can measure the pulmonary circulation time, another indicator of the status of the pulmonary vascular bed. Pulmonary vascular obstructive disease is characterized by an increased rate of tapering, a reduction in background haze, and a prolonged circulation time. Finally, we have commented earlier in this chapter on those rare anomalies producing airway obstruction, the hemitruncal sling and the ductal sling (Figs. 19-64 and 19-65).

References

1. Congdon ED. Transformation of the aortic arch system during the development of the human embryo. *Carnegie Inst Contr Embryol* 1922;14:47–110.
2. Edwards JE, McGoon DC. Absence of anatomic origin from heart of pulmonary arterial supply. *Circulation* 1973;47:393–398.
3. Sotomora RG, Edwards JE. Anatomic identification of so-called absent pulmonary artery. *Circulation* 1978;57: 624–633.
4. Haworth SG. The pulmonary circulation in congenital heart disease. *Herz* 1978;3:138–142.
5. DeRuiter MC, Gittenberger-de Groot AC, Poelmann RE, Van Iperen L, Mentink MMT. Development of the pharyngeal arch system related to the pulmonary and bronchial vessels in the avian embryo. With a concept on systemic-pulmonary collateral formation. *Circulation* 1993;87:1306–1319.
6. Huntington GS. The morphology of the pulmonary artery in the mammalia. *Anat Rec* 1919;17:165–201.
7. Manhoff LJ Jr, Howe JS. Absence of the pulmonary artery: A new classification for pulmonary arteries of anomalous origin. *AMA Arch Pathol* 1949;48:155–170.
8. Rabinovitch M, Herrera-DeLeon V, Castaneda AR, Reid L. Growth and development of the pulmonary vascular bed in patients with tetralogy of Fallot with or without pulmonary atresia. *Circulation* 1981;64:1234–1249.
9. Beitzke A, Shinebourne EA. Single origin of right and left pulmonary arteries from ascending aorta, with main pulmonary artery from right ventricle. *Br Heart J* 1980; 43:363–365.
10. Bricker DL, King SM, Edwards JE. Anomalous aortic origin of the right and left pulmonary arteries in a normally septated truncus arteriosus. *Chest* 1975;68:591–594.
11. Freedom RM, Culham JAG, Moes CAF. *Angiocardiography of Congenital Heart Disease.* New York: McMillan Publishing Company; 1984, pp. 254–273.
12. Aotsuka H, Nagai Y, Saito M, Matsumoto H, Nakamura T. Anomalous origin of both pulmonary arteries from the ascending aorta with a nonbranching main pulmonary artery arising from the right ventricle. *Pediatr Cardiol* 1990;11:156–158.
13. Wells TR, Takahashi M, Landing BH, Ritchie GW, Ang SM, Diaz JF, Mahnovski V. Branching patterns of right pulmonary artery in cardiovascular anomalies. *Pediatr Pathol* 1993;13:213–223.
14. Landing BH, Lawrence T-YK, Payne VC Jr, Wells TR. Bronchial anatomy in syndromes with abnormal visceral situs, abnormal spleen and congenital heart disease. *Am J Cardiol* 1971;28:456–462.
15. Diehl EJ, Landing BH. Syndrome of pulmonary isomerism of right lung type, congenital heart disease, pulmonary and systemic venous abnormalities and malrotation of the intestine, with a spleen or multiple spleens (m-anisosplenia): Comparison with the Ivemark syndrome. *Pediatr Pathol* 1984;2:133–138.
16. Diehl EJ, Wells TR, Landing BH, Lawrence T-YK. Three syndromes of lung isomerism, congenital heart disease, and multiple spleens (polysplenia, f-anisosplenia, and o-anisosplenia). *Pediatr Pathol* 1984;2:138–147.
17. Bloomer WE, Liebow AA, Hales MR. *Surgical Anatomy of the Bronchopulmonary Segments.* Springfield, IL: Charles C. Thomas; 1960, pp. 28–34, 143.
18. Boyden EA, Hartmann JF. An analysis of variations in the bronchopulmonary segments of the left upper lobes of fifty lungs. *Am J Anat* 1946;79:3231–360.
19. Diaz-Gongora G, Quero-Jimenez M, Espino-Vela J, Arteaga M, Bargeron L. A heart with three arterial trunks(trituncal heart). *Pediatr Cardiol* 1982; 3:293–299.
20. Gay BB, Franch RH, Shuford WH, Rogers JV Jr. The roentgenologic features of single and multiple coarctations of the pulmonary artery and branches. *AJR* 1963; 90:599–613.
20a. Kreutzer J, Landzberg MJ, Preminger TJ, Mandell VS, Treves ST, Reid LM, Lock JE. Isolated peripheral pulmonary artery stenoses in the adult. *Circulation* 1996;93: 1417–1423.
21. Guller B. Stenosis of the pulmonary arteries: Evolution and hemodynamic effects. *Chest* 1972;61:70–73.
22. Tang JS, Kauffman SL, Lynfield J. Hypoplasia of the pulmonary arteries in infants with congenital rubella. *Am J Cardiol* 1971;27:491–496.
23. Son RS, Maranhao V, Ablaza SG, Goldberg H. Coarctation of the pulmonary artery. *Dis Chest* 1966;49: 289–298.
24. Delaney TB, Nadas AS. Peripheral pulmonic stenosis. *Am J Cardiol* 1964;13:451–461.
25. Massumi RA, Donohoe RF. Congenital absence versus acquired attenuation of one pulmonary artery. *Circulation* 1965;31:436–447.
26. Massumi RA, Rios JC, Donohoe RF. The pathogenesis of angiographic nonvisualization or attenuation of a patent pulmonary artery and the role of bronchial artery-pulmonary artery anastomosis. *J Thorac Cardiovasc Surg* 1965;49:772–789.
27. Emmanouilides GC, Linde LM, Crittenden IH. Pulmonary artery stenosis associated with ductus arteriosus following maternal rubella. *Circulation* 1964;29: 514–522.
28. Luhmer I, Ziemer G. Coarctation of the pulmonary artery in neonates. *J Thorac Cardiovasc Surg* 1993;106: 889–894.
29. Franch RH, Gay BB Jr. Congenital stenosis of the pulmonary artery branches. A classification with postmortem findings in two cases. *Am J Cardiol* 1963;35: 512–517.
30. Clement JP, Pasquier J, Tulli F, Dor V. Multiple stenoses and aneurysms of the pulmonary arterial tree. *Ann Radiol* 1974;17:55–58.
31. Rocchini AP, Emmanoulides GC. Pulmonary stenosis. In: Emmanouilides GC, Allen HD, Riemenschneider TA,

Gutgesell HP, eds. *Moss and Adams' Heart Disease in Infants, Children, and Adolescents, Including the Fetus and Young Adult.* Baltimore: Williams and Wilkins; 1995, pp. 930–962.

31a. Khosroshahi HE, Uluoglu O, Olgunturk R, Basaklar C. Keutel syndrome: A report of four cases. *Eur J Pediatr* 1989;149:188–191.

32. Hoeffel JC, Henry M, Pernot C, Jimenez J. The radiological appearances of congenital stenoses of the pulmonary artery and its branches. A report of 20 cases. *Ann Radiol* 1973;16:41–44.

33. Watson GH, Miller V. Arteriohepatic dysplasia: Familial pulmonary arterial stenosis with neonatal liver diseases. *Arch Dis Child* 1973;48:459–463.

33a. Schwarzenberg SJ, Grothe RM, Sharp HL, Snover DC, Freese D. Long-term complications of arteriohepatic dysplasia. *Am J Med* 1992;93:171–176.

34. Alagille D, Odievre M, Gautier M, Estrada A, Dommergues M. Hepatic ductular hypoplasia associated with characteristic facies, vertebral malformations, retarded physical, mental, and sexual development, and cardiac murmur. *J Pediatr* 1975;86:73–81.

35. Alagille D, Estrada A, Hadchouel M, Gautier M, Odievre M, Dommergues M. Syndromic paucity of interlobar bile ducts (Alagille syndrome or arteriohepatic dysplasia: Review of 80 cases. *J Pediatr* 1987;110:195–200.

35a. Leonard NJ, Dias V, Parsons HG. Alagille syndrome: Resolution of xanthomas. *Can J Gastroenterol* 1995;9:187–190.

36. Greenwood RD, Rosenthal A, Crocker AC, Nadas AS. Syndrome of intrahepatic biliary dysgenesis and cardiovascular malformations. *Pediatrics* 1976;58:243–247.

37. Levin SE, Zarvos P, Milner S, Schmaman A. Arteriohepatic dysplasia: Association of liver disease with pulmonary arterial stenosis as well as facial and skeletal abnormalities. *Pediatrics* 1980;66:876–883.

38. Brindza D, Moodie DS, Wyllie R, Sterba R. Intravenous digital subtraction angiography to assess pulmonary artery anatomy in patients with Alagille syndrome. *Cleve Clin Q* 1984;51:493–497.

39. Ruttner JR, Bartschi J-P, Niedermann R, Schneider J. Plexogenic pulmonary arteriopathy and liver cirrhosis. *Thorax* 1980;35:133–136.

40. Kocoshis SA, Cottrill CM, O'Connor WN, Haugh R, Johnson GL, Noonan JA. Congenital heart disease, butterfly vertebrae, and extrahepatic biliary atresia: A variant of arteriohepatic dysplasia? *J Pediatrics* 1981;99:436–439.

41. Silberbach M, Lashley D, Reller MD, Kinn WF Jr, Terry A, Sutherland CO. Arteriohepatic dysplasia and cardiovascular malformations. *Am Heart J* 1994;127:695–699.

42. Riely CA, Labrecque DR, Ghent C, Horwich A, Klatskin G. A father and son with cholestasis and peripheral pulmonic stenosis. *J Pediatr* 1978;92:406–411.

43. Rosenfield NS, Kelley MJ, Jensen PS, Collier E, Rosenfield AT, Riely CA. Arteriohepatic dysplasia: Radiologic features of a new syndrome. *AJR* 1980;135:1217–1223.

44. Krowka MJ, Cortese DA. Hepatopulmonary syndrome: An evolving perspective in the era of liver transplantation. *Hepatology* 1990;11:138–142.

45. Williams JCP, Barratt-Boyes BG, Lowe JB. Supravalvular aortic stenosis. *Circulation* 1961;24:1311.

46. Beuren A, Schulze G, Eberle P, Harmjanz D, Apitz A. The syndrome of supravalvular aortic stenosis, peripheral pulmonary stenosis, mental retardation and similar facial appearance. *Am J Cardiol* 1964;13:741–745.

47. Black JA, Bonham-Carter RE. Association between aortic stenosis, peripheral pulmonary stenosis, mental retarda-

tion, and similar facial appearance. *Lancet* 1963;2:745–746.

48. Loes MH, Menashe VD, Sunderland CO, Morgan CL, Dawson PJ. Ehlers-Danlos syndrome associated with multiple pulmonary artery stenosis and tortuous systemic arteries. *J Pediatr* 1969;75:1031–1033.

49. Rowe RD. Cardiovascular disease in the rubella syndrome. *Cardiovasc Clin* 1973;4:5–11.

50. Rowe RD. Stenosis of conducting arteries in infants and children. *Birth Defects* 1972;8(5):69–74.

51. Rowe RD, Kelly DT, McCue C, Ottesen O. Unusual distribution of vascular damage as sequelae of idiopathic hypercalcemia and congenital rubella syndrome. *Birth Defects* 1974;10(4):361.

52. Hayden JG, Taler NS, Klaus SM. Cutis laxa associated with pulmonary artery stenosis. *J Pediatr* 1968;72:506–509.

53. Rodriguez RJ; Riggs TW. Physiologic peripheral pulmonic stenosis in infancy. *Am J Cardiol* 1990;66:1478–1481.

54. Rein AJJT, Preminger TJ, Perry SB, Lock JE, Sanders SP. Generalized arteriopathy in William's syndrome: An intravascular ultrasound study. *J Am Coll Cardiol* 1993;21:1727–1730.

55. Giddens NG, Finley JP, Nanton MA, Roy DL. The natural course of supravalvular aortic stenosis and peripheral pulmonary artery stenosis in Williams's syndrome. *Br Heart J* 1989;62:315–319.

56. Kececioglu D, Kotthoff S, Vogt J. Williams-Beuren syndrome: A 30-year follow-up of natural and postoperative course. *Eur Heart J* 1993;14:1458–1464.

57. Wren C, Oslizlok P, Bull C. Natural history of supravalvular aortic stenosis and pulmonary artery stenosis. *J Am Coll Cardiol* 1990;15:1625–1630.

58. Zalstein E, Moes CAF, Musewe NN, Freedom RM. Spectrum of cardiovascular anomalies in Williams-Beuren syndrome. *Pediatr Cardiol* 1991;12:219–223.

58a. Dutka DP, Cousins C, Manhire AR. Lymphatic complications in Alagille's syndrome. *Br Heart J* 1991;65:168–170.

59. Disler LJ, Manga P, Barlow JB. Pulmonary arterial aneurysms in Marfan's syndrome. *Int J Cardiol* 1988;21:79–82.

60. Gould L, Yang DC, Patel C, Patel D, Lee J, Judge D, Taddeo M. Aneurysms of the pulmonary arteries—a case report. *Angiology* 1987;38:474–478.

61. Metras D, Ouattara K, Quezzin-Coulibaly A. Aneurysm of the pulmonary artery with cystic medial necrosis and massive pulmonary valvular insufficiency. Report of two successful surgical cases. *Eur J Cardiothorac Surg* 1987;1:119–124.

62. Tanoue LT. Pulmonary involvement in collagen vascular disease: A review of the pulmonary manifestations of the Marfan syndrome, ankylosing spondylitis, Sjogren's syndrome, and relapsing polychondritis. *J Thorac Imaging* 1992;7:62–77.

63. Geva T, Sanders SP, Diogenes MS, Rockenmacher S, Van Praagh R. Two-dimensional and Doppler echocardiographic and pathologic characteristics of the infantile Marfan syndrome. *Am J Cardiol* 1990;65:1230–1237.

64. Vaideeswar P, Deshpande JR. Pulmonary arterial aneurysms. *Int J Cardiol* 1992;35:424–426.

65. Bowman S, Honey M. Pulmonary arterial occlusions and aneurysms: A forme fruste of Behcet's or Hughes-Stovin syndrome. *Br Heart J* 1990;63:66–68.

66. Numan F, Islak C, Berkmen T, Tuzun H, Cokyuksel O. Behcet disease: Pulmonary arterial involvement in 15 cases. *Radiology* 1994;192:465–468.

67. Hamuryudan V, Yurdakul S, Moral F, Numan F, Tuzun H, Tuzuner N, Mat C, Tuzun Y, Ozyazgan Y, Yazici H. Pulmonary arterial aneurysms in Behcet's syndrome: A report of 24 cases. *Br J Rheumatol* 1994;33:48–51.

68. Tunaci A, Berkmen YM, Gokman E. Thoracic involvement in Behcet's disease: Pathologic, clinical, and imaging features. *AJR* 1995;164:51–56.

69. Dennison AR, Watkins RM, Gunning AJ. Simultaneous aortic and pulmonary artery aneurysms due to giant cell arteritis. *Thorax* 1985;40:156–157.

70. Jeang MK, Adyanthaya A, Kuo L, Schweppe I, Hallman G Jr. Multiple pulmonary artery aneurysms. New use for magnetic resonance imaging. *Am J Med* 1986;81:1001–1004.

71. Gupta AK, Sandhyamani S, Ravimandalam K, Rao VR, Neelakandhan KS, Joseph S, Unni M, Rao AS. Multiple pulmonary-artery aneurysms due to mucoid vasculopathy—angiographic and histological observations. *Thorac Cardiovasc Surg* 1993;41:189–192.

71a.Kuzu MA, Ozaslan C, Koksoy C, Gurler A, Tuzuner A. Vascular involvement in Behcet's disease: 8-year audit. *World J Surg* 1994;18:948–954.

72. Iga K, Hori K, Matsumura T, Kijima K, Miyamoto T, Gen H. Multiple peripheral pulmonary artery branch stenosis in a young Japanese girl with systemic hypertension. *Chest* 1994;105:1294–1295.

73. Liu YQ, Jin BL, Ling J. Pulmonary artery involvement in aortoarteritis: An angiographic study. *Cardiovasc Intervent Radiol* 1994;17:2–6

74. Chauvaud S, Mace L, Brunewald P, Tricot JL, Camilleri JP, Carpentier A. Takayasu's arteritis with bilateral pulmonary artery stenosis. Successful surgical correction. *J Thorac Cardiovasc Surg* 1987;94:246–250.

75. Jakob H, Volb R, Stangl G, Reifart N, Rumpelt HJ, Oelert H. Surgical correction of a severely obstructed pulmonary artery bifurcation in Takayasu's arteritis. *Eur J Cardiothorac Surg* 1990;4(8):456–458.

76. Navarro C, Dickinson PC, Kondlapoodi P, Hagstrom JW. Mycotic aneurysms of the pulmonary arteries in intravenous drug addicts. Report of three cases and review of the literature. *Am J Med* 1984;76:1124–1131.

77. Vargas-Barron J, Avila-Rosales L, Romero-Cardenas A, Rijlaarsdam M, Keirns C, Buendia A. Echocardiographic diagnosis of a mycotic aneurysm of the main pulmonary artery and patent ductus arteriosus. *Am Heart J* 1992;123:1707–1709.

78. Morgan JM, Morgan AD, Addis B, Bradley GW, Spiro SG. Fatal haemorrhage from mycotic aneurysms of the pulmonary artery. *Thorax* 1986;41:70–71.

78a.Abbag F, Galal O. Mycotic aneurysm of the pulmonary trunk in a patient with with valvar pulmonary stenosis. *Cardiol Young* 1995;5:286–288.

79. Maltz D, Nadas AS. Agenesis of the lung. Presentation of eight new cases and review of the literature. *Pediatrics* 1968;42:175–188.

80. Shakibi JG, Rastan H, Nazarian I, Paydar M, Aryanpour I, Siassi B. Isolated unilateral absence of the pulmonary artery: Reviews of the world literature and guidelines for surgical repair. *Jpn Heart J* 1978;19:439.

81. Grillo R, Pipitone S, Pieri D, Spataro G, Basile G, Sperandeo V. Clinical and angiographical observation on so-called absence of a pulmonary artery branch. *G Ital Cardiol* 1986;16:1027–1031.

82. Sage MR, Brown JH. Congenital unilateral absence of a pulmonary artery. *Assist Radiol* 1972;16:228.

83. Freedom RM, Pongiglione G, Williams WG, Trusler GA, Moes CAF, Rowe RD. Pulmonary vein wedge angiography. Indications, results, and surgical correlates in 25 patients. *Am J Cardiol* 1983;51:936–941.

84. Curranino G, Williams B. Causes of congenital unilateral pulmonary hypoplasia: A study of 33 cases. *Pediatr Radiol* 1985;15:15–24.

85. Sreeram N, Asante-Korang A, Ladusans E. Distal ductal origin of the right pulmonary artery: Prospective diagnosis and primary repair in infancy. *Int J Cardiol* 1992;35:272–274.

86. Lip GYH and Dunn FG. Unilateral pulmonary artery agenesis: A rare cause of haemoptysis and pleuritic chest pain. *Int J Cardiol* 1993;40:121–125.

87. Coughlin WF, Harper RT, Hatch R, Wood BP. Radiological cases of the month. Congenital complete absence of the left pulmonary artery and hypoplastic left lung. *Am J Dis Child* 1990;144:339–340.

88. Ishizawa E, Horiuchi T, Tadokoro M, Okada Y, Suzuki Y, Tanaka S, Takamiya M, Sato T, Kano I. Diagnosis and surgical treatment of "Angiographically absent pulmonary artery syndrome". *Tohoku J Exp Med* 1978;125:1–9.

89. Moreno-Cabral RJ, McNamara JJ, Reddy VJ, Caldwell P. Unilateral absent pulmonary artery: Surgical repair with a new technique. *J Thorac Cardiovasc Surg* 1991;102:463–465.

90. Baran R, Kir A, Korap F, Kosku M. Congenital isolated unilateral absence of right pulmonary artery. *Thorac Cardiovasc Surg* 1993;41:374–376.

91. Cobanoglu A, Abbruzzese P, Brauner D, Ferre B, Issenberg H, Starr A. Therapeutic considerations in congenital absence of the right pulmonary artery. Use of internal mammary artery as a preparatory shunt. *J Cardiovasc Surg* 1984;25:241–245.

92. Cogswell TL, Singh S. Agenesis of the left pulmonary artery as a cause of hemoptysis. *Angiology* 1986;37:154–159.

93. Bekoe S, Pellegrini RV, Di Marco RF Jr, Grant KJ, Woelfel GF. Pneumonectomy for unremitting hemoptysis in unilateral absence of pulmonary artery. *Ann Thorac Surg* 1993;55:1553–1554.

93a.Lantz MM, Sziklas JJ, Diana DJ, Spencer RP. Serial reduction of ventilation in lung with congenital absence of pulmonary artery. *Clin Nucl Med* 1995;20:126–127.

94. Canver CC, Pigott JD, Mentzer RM Jr. Neonatal pneumonectomy for isolated unilateral pulmonary artery agenesis. *Ann Thorac Surg* 1991;52:294–295.

95. Presbitero P, Bull C, Haworth SG, De Leval MR. Absent or occult pulmonary artery. *Br Heart J* 1984;52:178–185.

96. Pool PE, Vogel JHK, Blount SG. Congenital unilateral absence of a pulmonary artery. *Am J Cardiol* 1962;10:706–732.

97. McKim JS and Wiglesworth FW. Absence of the left pulmonary artery: A report of six cases with autopsy finding in three. *Am Heart J* 1954;47:845–859.

98. Schneiderman LJ. Isolated congenital absence of the right pulmonary artery: A caution as to its diagnosis and a proposal for its embryogenesis. Report of a case with review. *Am Heart J* 1958;55:772–780.

99. Pfefferkorn JR, Loser H, Pech G, Toussaint R, Hilgenberg F. Absent pulmonary artery. A hint to its embryogenesis. *Pediatr Cardiol* 1982;3:283–286.

100. Cucci CE, Domle EF, Lewis EW Jr. Absence of a primary division of the pulmonary trunk: An ontogenic theory. *Circulation* 1964;29:124–131.

101. Freedom RM, Culham JAG, Moes CAF. *Angiocardiography of Congenital Heart Disease.* New York: Macmillan Publishing Company; 1984, pp. 195–210.

102. Freedom RM, Moes CAF, Pelech A, Smallhorn J, Rabinovitch M, Olley PM, Williams WG, Trusler GA, Rowe RD. Bilateral ductus arteriosus (or remnant): An analysis of 27 patients. *Am J Cardiol* 1984;53:884–891.

102a. Mianesi O, Stellin G, Zucchetta P. Isolation of the left pulmonary artery and ventricular septal defect-successful staged management. *Cardiol Young* 1995;5:180–183.

103. Moss AJ, Austin WO, O'Loughlin BJ. Congenital absence or atresia of a main branch of the pulmonary artery. *AMA J Dis Child* 1956;92:398–402.

104. Boijsen E, Kozuka T. Angiographic demonstration of systemic arterial supply in abnormal pulmonary circulation. *AJR* 1969;106:70.

105. Thompson JA, Lewis SA, Mauck HP. Absence of the left pulmonary artery: Anomalous collateral from the coronary artery to affected lung. *Am Heart J* 1986;111: 418–420.

106. Pontius RG, Danielson GK, Noonan JA, Judson JP. Illusions leading to surgical closure of the left pulmonary artery instead of the ductus arteriosus. *J Thorac Cardiovasc Surg* 1981;82:107–113.

107. Smallhorn JF, Gow R, Freedom RM, Trusler GA, Olley P, Pacquet M, Gibbons J, Vlad P. Pulsed Doppler echocardiographic assessment of the pulmonary venous pathway after the Mustard or Senning procedure for transposition of the great arteries. *Circulation* 1986;73:765–774.

108. Smallhorn JF, Pauperio H, Benson L, Freedom RM, Rowe RD. Pulsed Doppler assessment of pulmonary vein obstruction. *Am Heart J* 1985;110:483–486.

109. Smallhorn JF, Burrows P, Wilson G, Coles J, Gilday DL, Freedom RM. Two-dimensional and pulsed Doppler echocardiography in the postoperative evaluation of total anomalous pulmonary venous connection. *Circulation* 1987;76:298–305.

110. Watanabe T, Trusler GA, Williams WG, Edmonds JE, Coles JG, Hosokawa Y. Phrenic nerve paralysis after pediatric cardiac surgery. *J Thorac Cardiovasc Surg* 1987; 94:383–388.

111. Neill CA, Ferencz C, Sabiston DC, Sheldon H. The familial occurrence of hypoplastic right lung with systemic arterial supply and venous drainage "scimitar syndrome". *Bull John Hopkins Hosp* 1960;107:1–20.

112. Halasz NA, Halloran KH, Liebow AA. Bronchial and arterial anomalies with drainage of the right lung into the inferior vena cava. *Circulation* 1956;14:826–846.

113. Dupuis C, Charaf LA, Breviere GM, Abou P. "Infantile" form of the scimitar syndrome with pulmonary hypertension. *Am J Cardiol* 1993;71:1326–1330.

114. Beitzke A, Zobel G, Rigler B, Stein JI, Suppan C. Scimitar syndrome with absence of the right pulmonary artery: A case with volume-induced, reversible, left-sided pulmonary hypertension. *Pediatr Cardiol* 1992;13: 119–121.

115. Platia EV; Brinker JA. Scimitar syndrome with peripheral left pulmonary artery branch stenoses. *Am Heart J* 1984;107:594–596.

116. Blaysat G, Kachaner J, Villain E, Sidi D, Pedroni E. Le syndrome du cimeterre du nourisson. *Arch Fr Pediatr* 1987;44:245–251.

117. Boning U, Sauer U, Mocellin R, Meisner H, Schumacher G, Buhlmeyer K. Anomalous coronary drainage from the pulmonary artery with associated heart and vascular malformations: Report on 3 patients and review of the literature. *Herz* 1983;8:93–104.

117a. Lee TM, Chen WJ, Chen MF, Liau CS, Lee Yt. Anomalous origin of left circumflex artery in a scimitar syndrome. A case report. *Angiology* 1995;46:957–961.

118. Canter CE, Martin TC, Spray TL, Weldon CS, Strauss AW. Scimitar syndrome in childhood. *Am J Cardiol* 1986;58:652–654.

119. Cukier A, Kavakama J, Teixeira LR, Terra-Filho M, Vargas FH. Scimitar syndrome with normal pulmonary venous drainage and systemic arterial supply. Scimitar syndrome or bronchopulmonary sequestration? *Chest* 1994;105:294–295.

120. Dickinson DF, Galloway RM, Massey R, Sankey R, Arnold R. Scimitar syndrome in infancy. *Br Heart J* 1982; 47:468–472.

121. Everhart FJ, Korns ME, Amplatz K, Edwards JE. Intrapulmonary segment in anomalous pulmonary venous connection. Resemblance to scimitar syndrome. *Circulation* 1967;35:1163–1169.

122. Farnsworth AE and Ankeney JL. The spectrum of the scimitar syndrome. *J Thorac Cardiovasc Surg* 1974;68: 37–42.

123. Dupuis C, Charaf LAC, Breviere G-M, Abou P, Remy-Jardin M, Helmius G. The "adult" form of the scimitar syndrome. *Am J Cardiol* 1992;70:502–507.

124. Geggel RL. Scimitar syndrome associated with partial anomalous pulmonary venous connection at the supracardiac, cardiac, and infracardiac levels. *Pediatr Cardiol* 1993;14:234–237.

125. Gikonyo DK, Tandon R, Lucas RV, Edwards JE. Scimitar syndrome in neonates: Report of 4 cases and review of the literature. *Pediatr Cardiol* 1986;6:193–197.

126. Gao Y-A, Burrows PE, Benson LN, Rabinovitch M, Freedom RM. Scimitar syndrome in infancy. *J Am Coll Cardiol* 1993;22:873–882.

127. Haworth SG, Sauer U, Buhlmeyer K. Pulmonary hypertension in scimitar syndrome in infancy. *Br Heart J* 1983;50:182–189.

128. Herer B, Jaubert F, Delaisments C, Huchon G, Chretien J. Scimitar sign with normal pulmonary venous drainage and anomalous left inferior vena cava. *Thorax* 1988;43: 651–652.

129. Hollis WJ. The scimitar syndrome with absent right pulmonary artery. *Am J Cardiol* 1964;14:262–265.

129a. Dupuis C, Remy J, Remy-Jardin M, Rey C, Breviere GM, Kerkoub A. Le syndrome du cimeterre avec absence anatomique ou fonctionnelle de l'artere pulmonaire droite. A propos de quatre observations. *Arch Pediatr* 1995;2:347–352.

130. Kuiper-Oosterwal CH, Moulaert A. The scimitar syndrome in infancy and childhood. *Eur J Cardiol* 1973; 1:55–61.

131. Pearl W. Scimitar variant. *Pediatr Cardiol* 1987; 8:139–141.

132. Ferencz D. Review article: Congenital abnormalities of pulmonary vessels and their relation to malformations of the lung. *Pediatrics* 1961;28:993.

133. Thilenius OG, Ruschhaupt DG, Replogle RL, Bharati S, Herman T, Arcilla RA. Spectrum of pulmonary sequestration: Association with anomalous pulmonary venous drainage in infants. *Pediatr Cardiol* 1983;4:97–103.

134. Tumbarello R, Abbruzzese PA, Meloni G, Porcu M, Martelli V, Sanna A. A variant of the scimitar syndrome with stenosed drainage of the inferior vena cava. *Am Heart J* 1991;121:616–618.

135. Tummers RD, Lam J, Nijveld A, Marcelletti C, Losekoot TG. An infant with the scimitar syndrome and pulmonary artery hypertension: Successful surgical intervention. *Eur Heart J* 1987;8:194–197.

136. Jue KL, Amplatz K, Adams, P, Anderson RC. Anomalies of great vessels associated with lung hypoplasia. The scimitar syndrome. *Am J Dis Child* 1966;111:35.

137. Mardini MK, Sakati NA, Nyhan WL. Anomalous left pulmonary venous drainage to the inferior vena cava and through the pericardiophrenic vein to the innominate vein: Left-sided scimitar syndrome. *Am Heart J* 1981;101:860–862.

137a. Panicek DM, Heitzman ER, Randall PA, Groskin SA, Chew FS, Lane EJ Jr, Markarian B. The continuum of pulmonary developmental anomalies. *Radiographics* 1987;7:747–772.

138. Spencer H. *Pathology of the Lung.* Second Edition. Oxford: Pergamon Press; 1968, p. 73.

139. Dische MR, Teixeira ML, Winchester PH, Engle MA. Horseshoe lung associated with a variant of the "scimitar" syndrome. *Br Heart J* 1974;36:61–64.

140. Ersoz A, Soncul H, Gokgoz L, Kalaycioglu S, Tunaoglu S, Kaptanoglu M, Yener A. Horseshoe lung with left lung hypoplasia. *Thorax* 1992;47:205–206.

141. Figa FH, Yoo SJ, Burrows PE, Turner-Gomez S, Freedom RM. Horseshoe lung. A case report with unusual bronchial and pleural anomalies and a proposed new classification. *Pediatr Radiol* 1993;23:44–47.

141a. Boothroyd AE, Carty H, Arnold R Shoe, scimitar or sequestration: A shifting spectrum. *Peditatr Radiol* 1995;25:652–653.

142. Filho RIR, Cardosa CR, Rossi M. An unusual form of horseshoe lung with hypoplasia of the right pulmonary artery. *Int J Cardiol* 1991;31:259–261.

143. Frank JL, Poole CA, Rosas G. Horseshoe lung: Clinical pathologic, and radiologic features and a new plain film finding. *AJR* 1986;146:217–225.

144. Freedom RM, Burrows PE, Moes CAF. "Horseshoe" lung: Report of five new cases. *AJR* 1986;146:211–215.

145. Beitzke A. Scimitar syndrome with horseshoe lung. *ROFO* 1982;136:265–269.

146. Cerruti MM, Marmolejos F, Cacciarelli T. Bilateral intralobar pulmonary sequestration with horseshoe lung. *Ann Thorac Surg* 1993;55:509–510.

147. Cipriano P, Sweeney LJ, Hutchins GM, Rosenquist GC. Horse-shoe lung in an infant with recurrent pulmonary infections. *Am J Dis Child* 1975;129:1343–1345.

148. Clements BS, Warner JO. The crossover lung segment: Congenital malformation associated with a variant of scimitar syndrome. *Thorax* 1987;42:417–419.

149. Hawass ND, Badawi MG, Fatani JA. Horseshoe lung with multiple congenital anomalies. *Acta Radiol* 1987;28:751–754.

149a. Hawass ND, Badawi MG, Al-Muzrakchi AM, Al-Sammarai AI, Jawad AJ, Abdullah MA, Bahakim H. Horseshoe lung: Differential diagnosis. *Pediatr Radiol* 1990;20:580–584.

150. Orzan F, Angelini P, Oglietti J, Leachman RD, Cooley DA. Horseshoe lung: Report of two cases. *Am Heart J* 1986;93:501–505.

151. Purcaro A, Caruso L, Ciampani N, Inglese L. Polmone a ferro di cavallo malposizione cardiaca, Ed. Anomalie vascolari polmonari: una sindrome caratteristica. *G Ital Cardiol* 1976;6:312–316.

152. Dupuis C, Remy J, Remy-Jardin M, Coulomb M, Breviere GM, Ben Laden S. The "horseshoe" lung: Six new cases. *Pediatr Pulmonol* 1994;17:124–130.

152a. Dupuis C, Vaksmann G, Remy-Jardin M, Francart C. Horseshoe lung and scimitar syndrome in an asymptomatic child. *Eur Heart J* 1994;15:1008–1009.

152b. Corno A, Rosti L, Machado I. Horseshoe lung associated with anomalous pulmonary venous connection without pulmonary hypoplasia. *Cardiol Young* 1995;5:91–93.

153. Levine MM, Nudel DB, Gootman N, Wolpowitz A, Wisoff BG. Pulmonary sequestration causing congestive heart failure in infancy: A report of two cases and review of the literature. *Ann Thorac Surg* 1982;34:581–585.

154. Louie HW, Martin SM, Mulder DG. Pulmonary sequestration: 17-year experience at UCLA. *Am Surg* 1993;59:801–805.

155. Mortensson W, Lundstrom NR. Broncho-pulmonary vascular malformations causing left heart failure during infancy. *Acta Radiol Diagn* 1971;11:449–458.

156. Pryce DM. Lower accessory pulmonary artery with intralobar sequestration of lung: A report of seven cases. *J Pathol* 1946;58:547–567.

157. Matzinger FR, Bhargava R, Peterson RA, Shamji FM, Perkins DG. Systemic arterial supply to the lung without sequestration: An unusual cause of hemoptysis. *Can Assoc Radiol J* 1994;45:44–47.

158. Gerle RD, Jaretzki A, Ashley CA, Berne AS. Congenital bronchopulmonary foregut malformation: Pulmonary sequestration communicating with the gastrointestinal tract. *N Engl J Med* 1968;278:1413–1415.

159. Heithoff KB, Sane SM, Williams HJ, Jarvis CJ, Carter J, Kane P, Bennom W. Bronchopulmonary foregut malformation. A unifying etiological concept. *AJR* 1976;126:46.

160. Flisak ME, Chandrasekar AJ, Marsan RE, Ali MM. Systemic arterialization of lung without sequestration. *AJR* 1982;138:751.

161. Flye MW, Conle M, Silver D. Spectrum of pulmonary sequestration. *Ann Thorac Surg* 1976;22:478–482.

162. Ransom JM, Norton JB, Williams GD. Pulmonary sequestration presenting as congestive heart failure. *J Thorac Cardiovasc Surg* 1978;76:378–380.

163. Dupuis C, Rey C, Godart F, Vliers A, Gronnier P. Syndrome du cimeterre complique de stenose de la veine pulmonaire droite. A propos de 4 observations. *Arch Mal Coeur Vaiss* 1994;86:607–613.

164. Juettner FM, Pinter HH, Lammer G, Popper H, Friehs GB. Bilateral intralobar pulmonary sequestration: Therapeutic implications. *Ann Thorac Surg* 1987;43:660–662.

165. Kolls JK, Kiernan MP, Ascuitto RJ, Ross-Ascuitto NT, Fox LS. Intralobar pulmonary sequestration presenting as congestive heart failure in a neonate. *Chest* 1992;102:974–976.

166. Piccione W Jr, Burt ME. Pulmonary sequestration in the neonate. *Chest* 1990;97:244–246.

167. Bailey PV, Tracy T Jr, Connors RH, de Mello D, Lewis JE, Weber TR. Congenital bronchopulmonary malformations. Diagnostic and therapeutic considerations. *J Thorac Cardiovasc Surg* 1990;99:597–603.

168. Levi A, Findler M, Dolfin T, Di Segni E, Vidne BA. Intrapericardial extralobar pulmonary sequestration in a neonate. *Chest* 1990;98:1014–1015.

169. Chan CK, Hyland RH, Gray RR, Jones DP, Hutcheon MA. Diagnostic imaging of intralobar bronchopulmonary sequestration. *Chest* 1988;93:189–192.

170. Clements BS, Warner JO. Pulmonary sequestration and related congenital bronchopulmonary-vascular malformations: Nomenclature and classification based on anatomical and embryological considerations. *Thorax* 1987;42:401–408.

171. Clements BS; Warner JO; Shinebourne EA. Congenital bronchopulmonary vascular malformations: Clinical application of a simple anatomical approach in 25 cases. *Thorax* 1987;42:409–416.

172. Litwin SB, Plauth WH, Nadas AS. Anomalous systemic arterial supply to the lung causing pulmonary artery hypertension. *N Engl J Med* 1970;283:1098–1099.

173. Goldstein JD, Rabinovitch M, Van Praagh R, Reid L. Unusual vascular anomalies causing persistent pulmonary hypertension in a newborn. *Am J Cardiol* 1979;43: 962–968.

174. Hessel EA II, Boyden EA, Stamm SJ, Sauvage LR. High systemic origin of the sole artery to the basal segments of the left lung: Findings, surgical treatment and embryologic interpretation. *Surgery* 1970;67:624–632.

175. Hofschire PJ, Rodd EP, Varco RL, Kaplan EL, Edwards JE. Anomalous double blood supply to the lung. *Chest* 1976;69:439–441.

176. Kirks DR, Kane PE, Free EA, Taybl H. Systemic arterial supply to normal basilar segments of the left lower lobe. *AJR* 1976;126:817–822.

177. Tobin CE. The bronchial arteries and their connections with other vessels in the human lung. *Surg Gynecol Obstet* 1952;95:741–750.

178. Tao CW, Chen CH, Yuen KH, Huang MH, Li WY, Perng RP. Anomalous systemic arterial supply to normal basilar segments of the lower lobe of the left lung. *Chest* 1992;102:1583–1585.

179. Ozawa K, Sugimura S, Iriyama T, Nakamura H, Matsuta M, Mizoguchi Y. [Systemic origin of the sole artery to the basal segments of the left lung without pulmonary sequestration]. *Nippon Kyobu Geka Gakkai Zasshi* 1989; 37:529–534.

180. Burrows PE, Freedom RM, Rabinovitch M, Moes CAF. The investigation of abnormal pulmonary arteries in congenital heart disease. *Radiol Clin North Am* 1985;23: 689–717.

181. Culham JAG. Special procedures in pediatric chest radiography. *Pediatr Clin North Am* 1979;26:661–671.

182. Webb RW and Jacobs RP. Transpleural abdominal systemic artery-pulmonary artery anastomosis in patients with chronic pulmonary infection. *AJR* 1977;129: 233–235.

183. Contro S, Miller RA, White H, Potts WJ. Bronchial obstruction due to pulmonary artery anomalies. I. Vascular sling. *Circulation* 1958;17:418–427.

183a. Koopot R, Nikaidoh H, Idriss FS. Surgical management of anomalous left pulmonary artery causing tracheobronchial obstruction. Pulmonary artery sling. *J Thorac Cardiovasc Surg* 1975;69:240–245.

184. Berdon WE, Baker DH, Wung J-T, et al. Complete cartilage-ring tracheal stenosis associated with anomalous left pulmonary artery: The ring-sling complex. *Radiology* 1984;152:57–64.

184a. Baumman JL, Ward BH, Woodrum DE. Aberrant left pulmonary artery. Clinical and embryologic factors. *Chest* 1977;72:67–71.

185. Cohen SR, Landing BH. Tracheostenosis and bronchial abnormalities associated with pulmonary artery sling. *Ann Otol Rhino/Laryngol* 1976;85:582.

185a. Dohlmann C, Mantel K, Vogl TJ, Nicolai T, Schneider K, Hammerer I, Apitz J, Meisner H, Joppich I. Pulmonary sling: Morphological finding. Pre- and postoperative course. *Eur J Cardiol* 1995;154:2–14.

186. Sprague PL, Kennedy JC. Anomalous left pulmonary artery with an unusual barium swallow. *Pediatr Radiol* 1976;4:188.

187. Sade RM, Rosenthal A, Fellows K, Castaneda AR. Pulmonary artery sling. *J Thorac Cardiovasc Surg* 1975;69: 333.

187a. Vincent RN, Armstrong G, Dokler ML, Williams WH. Operative correction of subcarinal left pulmonary artery originating from the right pulmonary artery. *Am J Cardiol* 1989;64:687–688.

188. Gikonyo BM, Jue KL, Edwards JE. Pulmonary vascular sling: Report of seven cases and review of the literature. *Pediatr Cardiol* 1989;10:81–89.

189. Tester UF, Balsara RH, Niquidula FN. Aberrant left pulmonary artery (vascular sling): Report of five cases. *Chest* 1974;66:402.

190. Tonkin IL, Elliott LP, Bargeron LM Jr. Concomitant axial cineangiography and barium esophagography in the evaluation of vascular rings. *Radiology* 1980;13S:69.

191. Backer CL, Idriss FS, Holinger LD, Mavroudis C. Pulmonary artery sling. *J Thorac Cardiovasc Surg* 1992;103: 683–691.

192. Lubbers WJ, Tegelaers WHH, Losekoot TG, Becker AE. Aberrant origin of left pulmonary artery (vascular sling). Report of the clinical and anatomic features in three patients. *Eur J Cardiol* 1975;2:477.

193. Okagawa H, Kimura K, Okuno M, Hattori M, Nakagawa M. Case of Williams elfin facies syndrome with pulmonary artery sling. *Int J Cardiol* 1993;42:295–297.

194. Vogl TJ, Diebold T, Bergman C, Dohlemann C, Mantel K, Felix R, Lissner J. MRI in pre- and postoperative assessment of tracheal stenosis due to pulmonary artery sling. *J Comput Assist Tomogr* 1993;17:878–886.

195. Bertolini A, Pelizza A, Panizzon G, Moretti R, Bava CL, Calza G, Tacchino A. Vascular rings and slings. Diagnosis and surgical treatment of 49 patients. *J Cardiovasc Surg* 1987;28:301–312.

196. Gnanapragasam JP, Houston AB, Jamieson MP. Pulmonary artery sling: Definitive diagnosis by colour Doppler flow mapping avoiding cardiac catheterisation. *Br Heart J* 1990;63:251–252.

197. Hwang B. Pulmonary artery sling associated with total anomalous pulmonary venous return. A rare case report. *Jpn Heart J* 1988;29:367–370.

198. Parikh SR, Ensing GJ, Darragh RK, Caldwell RL. Rings, slings and such things: Diagnosis and management with special emphasis on the role of echocardiography. *J Am Soc Echocardiogr* 1993;6:1–11.

199. Zenati M, del Nonno F, Marino B, di Carlo DC. Pulmonary atresia and intact ventricular septum associated with pulmonary artery sling (letter). *J Thorac Cardiovasc Surg* 1992;104:1755–1766.

200. Grover FL, Norton JB, Webb GE, Trinkle JK. Pulmonary artery sling: Case report and collective review. *J Thorac Cardiovasc Surg* 1975;69:295–300.

201. Lenox CC, Crisler C, Zuberbuhler JR, Park SC, Neches WH, Mathews RA, Ricker FJ, Golding LAR. Anomalous left pulmonary artery. Successful management. *J Thorac Cardiovasc Surg* 1979;77:748.

202. Jonas RA, Spevak PJ, McGill T, Castaneda AR. Pulmonary artery sling: Primary repair by tracheal resection in infancy. *J Thorac Cardiovasc Surg* 1989;97:548–550.

203. Rheuban KS, Ayres N, Still JG, Alford B. Pulmonary artery sling: A new diagnostic tool and clinical review. *Pediatrics* 1982;69:472–475.

203a. Newman B, Meza MP, Towbin RB, Del Nido P. Left pulmonary artery sling: Diagnosis and delineation of associated tracheobronchial anomalies with MR. *Pediatr Radiol* 1996;26:661–668.

204. Williams RG, Jaffe RB, Condon VR, Nixon GW. Unusual features of pulmonary sling. *AJR* 1979;133:1065–1069.

205. Gumbiner CH, Mullins CE, McNamara DG. Pulmonary artery sling. *Am J Cardiol* 1980;45:311.

206. Capitanio MA, Ramo R, Kirkpatrick JA. Pulmonary sling. *AJR* 1971;112:28–31.

207. Ziemer G, Heinemann M, Kaulitz R, Freihorst J, Seidenberg J, Wilken M. Pulmonary artery sling with tracheal

stenosis: Primary one-stage repair in infancy. *Ann Thorac Surg* 1992;54:971–973.

208. Yeager SB, Chin AJ, Sanders SP. Two-dimensional echocardiographic diagnosis of pulmonary artery sling in infancy. *J Am Coll Cardiol* 1986;7:625–629.

208a. Pasic M, von Segesser L, Carrel T, Arbenz U, Tonz M, Niederhauser U, Vogt P, Turina M. Anomalous left pulmonary artery (pulmonary sling): Result of a surgical approach. *Cardiovasc Surg* 1993;1:608–612.

208b. Pawade A, de Leval MR, Elliott MJ, Stark J. Pulmonary artery sling. *Ann Thorac Surg* 1992;54:967–970.

209. Ben-Shachar G, Beder SD, Liebman J, Van Heeckeren D. Hemitruncal sling: A newly recognized anomaly and its surgical correction. *J Thorac Cardiovasc Surg* 1985;90:146–148.

210. Binet JP, Conso JF, Losay J, Narcy Ph, Raynaud EJ, Beaufils Fr, Dor C, Bruniaux J. Ductus arteriosus sling: Report of a newly recognised anomaly and its surgical correction. *Thorax* 1978;33:72–75.

211. Jue KL, Lockman LA, Edwards JE. Anomalous origins of pulmonary arteries from pulmonary trunk ("crossed pulmonary arteries"). *Am Heart J* 1966;71:807–812.

211a. Zimmerman FJ, Berdusis K, Wright KL, Albolaris ET. Echocardiographic diagnosis of anomalous origins of the pulmonary arteries from the pulmonary trunk (crossed pulmonary arteries). Am Heart J 1997;133:257–262.

212. Becker AE, Becker MJ, Edwards JE. Malposition of pulmonary arteries (crossed pulmonary arteries) in persistent truncus arteriosus. *Am J Radiol* 1970;110:509–514.

213. Wolf WJ, Casta A, Nichols M. Anomalous origin and malposition of the pulmonary arteries (crisscross pulmonary arteries) associated with complex congenital heart disease. *Pediatr Cardiol* 1986;6:287–291.

214. Ho SY, Wicox BR, Anderson RH, Lincoln JCR. Interrupted aortic arch: Anatomical features of surgical significance. *Thorac Cardiovasc Surg* 1983;31:199–205.

215. Tuncali T, Aytac A. Direct communication between right pulmonary artery and left atrium. Report of a case and proposal of a new entity. *J Pediatr* 1967;71:384.

216. Arendrup H. Direct communication between the pulmonary artery and left atrium. *Scand J Thorac Cardiovasc Surg* 1982;16:157–160.

217. Cheatham JP, Barnhart DA, Gutgesell HP. Right pulmonary artery to left atrium communication. An unusual cause of cyanosis in the newborn. *Pediatr Cardiol* 1982;2:149–152.

218. Ohara H, Ito K, Kohguchi N, Ohkawa Y, Akasaka T, Takarada M, Aoki H, Ogata M, Nishibatake M, Fukatsu O, Matsushima K, Sasaki Y. Direct communication between the right pulmonary artery and the left atrium. *J Thorac Cardiovasc Surg* 1979;77:742–747.

219. de Souza e Silva NA, Giuliani ER, Ritter DG, Davis GD, Pluth JR. Communication between right pulmonary artery and left atrium. *Am J Cardiol* 1974;34:857–863.

220. Nelson ASS, Giuliani EQ, Davis GD, Pluth JR. Communication between right pulmonary artery and left atrium. *Am J Cardiol* 1974;34:857–860.

221. Lucas RV Jr, Lund GE, Edwards JE. Direct communication of a pulmonary artery with the atrium: An unusual variant of pulmonary arteriovenous fistula. *Circulation* 1961;24:1409.

222. Jimenez M. Fournier A, Chossat A. Pulmonary artery to left atrium fistula as an unusual cause of cyanosis in the newborn. *Pediatr Cardiol* 1989;10:216–220.

223. Preminger TJ, Perry SB, Burrows PE. Vascular Anomalies. In: Emmanouilides GC, Allen HD, Riemenschneider TA, Gutgesell HP, eds. *Moss and Adams' Heart Disease in Infants, Children, and Adolescents, Including the Fetus and Young Adult.* Baltimore: Williams and Wilkins; 1995, pp. 791–810.

223a. Saatvedt K, Stake G, Lindberg H. Fistula between the right pulmonary artery and the left atrium—An unusual cause of cyanotic heart disease. *Cardiol Young* 1995;5:85–87.

224. Ben-Menachem Y, Kuroda K, Kyger ER, Brest AN, Copeland OP, Coan JD. The various forms of pulmonary varices: Report of three new cases and review of the literature. *AJR* 1975;125:88–91.

225. Clarke CP, Goh TH, Blackwood A, Venables A. Massive pulmonary arteriovenous fistula in the newborn. *Br Heart J* 1976;38:1092.

226. Dines DE, Arms RA, Bernatz PE, Gomes MR: Pulmonary arteriovenous fistulas. *Mayo Clin Proc* 1974;49:460.

227. Fried R, Amberson JB, O'Loughlin JE, Cruz SB, Sniderman KW, Firpo AB, Engle MA. Congenital pulmonary arteriovenous fistula producing pulmonary arterial steal syndrome. *Pediatr Cardiol* 1982;2:313.

228. Hodgson CH, Kay RL. Pulmonary arteriovenous fistula and hereditary hemorrhagic telangiectasia: A review and report of 35 cases of fistula. *Dis Chest* 1963;43:449.

229. Hodgson CH, Burchell HB, Good CA, Clagett OT. Hereditary hemorhagic telangiectasia and pulmonary arteriovenous fistula: Survey of a large family. *N Engl J Med* 1959;261:625–628.

230. Gelfand MS, Stephen DS, Howell E, Alford RH, Kaiser AB. Brain abcess: Association with pulmonary arteriovenous fistula and hereditary hemorhagic telangiectasia-report of 3 cases. *Am J Med* 1988;85:718–720.

231. Hewes RC, Auster M, White RI Jr. Cerebral embolism: First manifestation of pulmonary arteriovenous malformation in hereditary hemorrhagic telangiectasia. *Cardiovasc Intervent Radiol* 1985;8:151–155.

231a. Walder LA, Anastasia LF, Spodick DH. Pulmonary arteriovenous malformations with brain abscess. *Am Heart J* 1994;127:227–232.

232. Chilvers ER. Clinical and physiologic aspects of pulmonary arteriovenous malformations. *Br J Hosp Med* 1988;39 188–192.

233. Vase P, Holm M, Arendrup H. Pulmonary arteriovenous fistulas in hereditary hemorhagic telangiectasia. *Acta Med Scand* 1985;218:105–109.

234. Knight WB, Bush A, Busst CM, Haworth SG, Bowyer JJ, Shinebourne EA. Multiple pulmonary arteriovenous fistulas in childhood. *Int J Cardiol* 1989;23:105–116.

235. Vincent RN, Casiro OG, Pelech AN, Collins GF. Evaluation of pulmonary vascular resistance in the presence of a large pulmonary arteriovenous malformation. *J Am Coll Cardiol* 1986;7:1104–1106.

235a. Kilbride HW, Gowdamaran R, Thibeault DW. Neonatal pulmonary vascular and parenchymal changes associated with arteriovenous malformation. *Pediatr Pulmonol* 1993;16:201–206.

236. White RI Jr. Pulmonary arteriovenous malformations: How do we diagnose them and why is it important to do so? *Radiology* 1992;182:633–635.

237. AAssar OS, Friedman CM, White RI Jr. The natural history of epistaxis in hereditary hemorrhagic telangiectasia. *Laryngoscope* 1991;101:977–980.

238. Puskas JD, Allen MS, Moncure AC, et al. Pulmonary arteriovenous malformations: Therapeutic options. *Ann Thorac Surg* 1993;56:253–258.

239. Hughes JMB, Allison DJ. Pulmonary arteriovenous malformations: The radiologist replaces the surgeon. *Clin Radiol* 1990;41:297–298.

240. Terry PB, Klemens BH, Kaufman SL, White RI Jr. Balloon embolization of pulmonary arteriovenous fistulas. *N Engl J Med* 1980;302:1189.

241. White RI Jr, Kaufman SL, Barth KH, DeCaprio V, Strandberg JD. Embolotherapy with detachable silicone balloons: Technique and clinical results. *Radiology* 1979; 131:619.

242. White RI Jr., Lynch-Nyhan A, Terry P, et al. Pulmonary arteriovenous malformations: Techniques and long term outcome. *Radiology* 1988;169:663–669.

243. Rosenblatt M, Pollak JS, Fayad PB, Egglin TE, White RI Jr. Pulmonary arteriovenous malformations: What size should be treated to prevent embolic stroke? *Radiology* 1993;186:937.

244. Marin-Garcia J, Lock JE. Catheter embolization of pulmonary arteriovenous fistulas in an infant. *Pediatr Cardiol* 1992;13:41–43.

245. Barzilai B, Waggoner AD, Spessert C, Picus D, Goodenberger D. Two-dimensional contrast echocardiography in the detection and follow-up of congenital pulmonary arteriovenous malformations. *Am J Cardiol* 1991;68: 1507–1510.

246. Kirsch LR, Sos TA, Engle MA. Successful coil embolization for diffuse, multiple pulmonary arteriovenous fistulas. *Am Heart J* 1991;122:245–248.

247. White RI Jr, Pollak JS. Pulmonary arteriovenous malformations: Options for management (letter). *Ann Thorac Surg* 1994;57:519–521.

248. Grady RM, Sharkey AM, Bridges ND. Transcatheter coil embolisation of a pulmonary arteriovenous malformation in a neonate. *Br Heart J* 1994;71:370–371.

249. Mitchell RO, Austin EH III. Pulmonary arteriovenous malformation in the neonate. *J Pediatr Surgery* 1993;28: 1536–1538.

250. Armitage JM, Fricker FJ, Kurland G, Michaels M, Griffith BP. Pediatric lung transplantation: Expanding indications, 1985 to 1993. *J Heart Lung Transplant* 1993;12: 246–254.

251. Curranno G, Willis K, Miller W. Congenital fistula between an aberrant systemic artery and a pulmonary vein without sequestration. *J Pediatr* 1975;87:554.

252. Robida A, Eltohami EA, Chaikhouni A. Aberrant systemic artery-pulmonary venous fistula: Diagnosis with Doppler imaging. *Int J Cardiol* 1992;35:407–411.

253. Wolf WJ, Casta A, Swischuk L. Aberrant systemic artery-pulmonary vein fistula: Detection of an occult lesion by contrast echocardiography. *Am Heart J* 1985;110: 480–482.

254. Glenn WWL. Circulatory bypass of the right side of the heart. IV. Shunt between superior vena cava and distal right pulmonary artery-report of clinical application. *N Engl J Med* 1958;259:117–120.

255. Glenn WWL. Superior vena cava-pulmonary artery shunt. *Ann Thorac Surg* 1989;47:62–64. 256. Glenn WWL, Ordway NK, Talner NS, Call EP. Circulatory bypass of the right side of the heart. *Circulation* 1965;31: 172–189.

257. Glenn WWL. Superior vena cava-pulmonary artery anastomosis. *Ann Thorac Surg* 1984;37:9–11.

258. Pacifico AD, Kirklin JW. Take-down of cavo-pulmonary artery anastomosis (Glenn) during repair of congenital cardiac malformations. *J Thorac Cardiovasc Surg* 1975; 70:272–277.

259. Pennington DG, Nouri S, Ho J, Secker-Walker R, Patel B, Sivakoff M, Willmann VL. Glenn shunt: Long-term results and current role in congenital heart operations. *Ann Thorac Surg* 1981;31:532–539.

260. Robicsek F. An epitaph for cavopulmonary anastomosis. *Ann Thorac Surg* 1982;34:208–220.

261. Laks H, Mudd JG, Standeven JW, Fagan L, Willman VL. Long-term effect of the superior vena cava-pulmonary artery anastomosis on pulmonary blood flow. *J Thorac Cardiovasc Surg* 1977;74:253–260.

262. Mathur M, Glenn WWL. Long-term evaluation of cavapulmonary artery anastomosis. *Surgery* 1973;74: 899–916.

263. Kopf GS, Laks H, Stansel HC, Hellenbrand WE, Kleinman CS, Talner NS. Thirty-year follow-up of superior vena cava-pulmonary artery (Glenn) shunts. *J Thorac Cardiovasc Surg* 1990;100:662–671.

264. Trusler GA, Williams WG, Cohen AJ, Rabinovitch M, Moes CAF, Smallhorn JF, Coles JG, Lightfoot NE, Freedom RM. William Glenn Lecture: The cavopulmonary shunt. Evolution of a concept. *Circulation* 1990; 82(suppl IV):131–138.

265. Di Carlo D, Williams WG, Freedom RM, Trusler GA. The role of cava-pulmonary (Glenn) anastomosis in the palliative treatment of congenital heart disease. *J Thorac Cardiovasc Surg* 1982;83:437–441.

266. Bargeron LM Jr, Karp RB, Barcia A, Kirklin JW, Hunt D, Deverall PB. Late deterioration of patients after superior vena cava to right pulmonary artery anastomosis. *Am J Cardiol* 1972;30:211–216.

267. Boruchow IB, Swenson EW, Elliott LP, Bartley TD, Wheat MW Jr, Schiebler GL. Study of the mechanisms of shunt failure after superior vena cava-right pulmonary artery anastomosis. *J Thorac Cardiovasc Surg* 1970;60: 531–539.

268. Boruchow IB, Bartley TD, Elliott LP, Schiebler GL. Late superior vena cava syndrome after superior vena cava-right pulmonary artery anastomosis. *N Engl J Med* 1969; 281:646–650.

269. Gleason WA Jr., Roodman ST, Laks H. Protein-losing enteropathy and intestinal lymphangiectasia after superior vena cava-right pulmonary artery (Glenn) shunt. *J Thorac Cardiovasc Surg* 1979;77:843–846.

270. Cloutier A, Ash JM, Smallhorn JF, Williams WG, Trusler GA, Rowe RD, Rabinovitch M. Abnormal distribution of pulmonary blood flow after the Glenn shunt or Fontan procedure: Risk of development of arteriovenous fistulae. *Circulation* 1985;72:471–479.

270a. Gatzoulis MA, Shinebourne EA, Redington AN, Rigby ML, Ho SY, Shore DF. Increasing cyanosis after cavopulmonary connection caused by abnormal systemic venous channels. *Br Heart J* 1995;73:182–186.

271. Allen RG. The addition of cava pulmonary artery shunts to patients with existing systemic pulmonary artery shunts. *J Pediatr Surg* 1970;5:102–110.

272. Glenn WW, Fenn JE. Axillary arteriovenous fistula. A means of supplementing blood flow through a cava-pulmonary artery shunt. *Circulation* 1972;46:1013–1017.

273. Mitchell IM, Goh DW, Abrams LD. Creation of brachial artery-basilic vein fistula. A supplement to the cavopulmonary shunt. *J Thorac Cardiovasc Surg* 1989; 98(2):214–216.

274. Magee A, Sim E, Benson LN, Williams WG, Trusler GA, Freedom RM. Augmentation of pulmonary blood flow using an axillary arteriovenous fistula after a cavopulmonary shunt. *J Thorac Cardiovasc Surg* 1996;111: 176–180.

275. Jonas RA. Indications and timing for the bidirectional Glenn shunt versus the fenestrated Fontan circulation. *J Thorac Cardiovasc Surg* 1994;108:522–524.

275a. Mendelsohn AM, Bove EL, Lupinetti FM, Crowley DC, Lloyd TR, Beekman RH III. Central pulmonary artery growth patterns after the bidirectional Glenn procedure. *J Thorac Cardiovasc Surg* 1994;107:1284–1290.

276. Chang AC, Hanley FL, Wernovsky G, Rosenfeld HM, Wessel DL, Jonas RA, Mayer JE, Lock JE, Castaneda AR. Early bidirectional cavopulmonary shunt in young infants. Postoperative course and early results. *Circulation* 1993;88(part 2):149–158.

277. Hopkins RA, Armstrong BE, Serwer GA, Peterson RJ, Oldham HN Jr. Physiological rationale for a bidirectional cavopulmonary shunt. *J Thorac Cardiovasc Surg* 1985;90:391–398.

277a. Calderon-Colmenero J, Ramirez S, Rijlaarsdam M, Buendia A, Zabal C, Zarco-Martinez E, Attie F. Use of bidirectional cavopulmonary shunt in patients under one year of age. *Cardiol Young* 1995;5:28–30.

278. Gross GJ, Jonas RJ, Castaneda AR, Hanley FL, Mayer JE, Bridges NB. Maturational and hemodynamic factors predictive of increased cyanosis following bidirectional cavopulmonary anastomosis. *Am J Cardiol* 1994;74:705–709.

278a. Allgood NL, Alejos J, Drinkwater DC, Laks H, Williams RG. Effectiveness of the bidirectional Glenn shunt procedure for volume unloading in the single ventricle patient. *Am J Cardiol* 1994;74:834–836.

278b. Nykanen DG, Freedom RM. Variations on the theme of Fontan: Consideration of the bidirectional cavopulmonary connection or the fenestrated Fontan. *ACC Curr J Rev* 1995;4:49–52.

279. Lamberti JJ, Spicer RL, Waldman JD, Grehl TM, Thomson D, George L, Kirkpatrick SE, Mathewson JW. The bidirectional cavopulmonary shunt. *J Thorac Cardiovasc Surg* 1990;100:22–30.

280. Albanese SB, Carotti A, Di Donato RM, Mazzera E, Troconis CJ, Giannico S, Picardo S, Marcelletti C. Bidirectional cavopulmonary anastomosis in patients under two years of age. *J Thorac Cardiovasc Surg* 1992;104:904–909.

281. Bridges ND, Jonas RA, Mayer JE, Flanagan MF, Keane JF, Castaneda AR. Bidirectional cavopulmonary anastomosis as interim palliation for high-risk Fontan candidates. Early results. *Circulation* 1990;82(5 suppl IV):170–176.

282. Hawkins JA, Shaddy RE, Day RW, Sturtevant JE, Orsmond GS, McGough EC. Mid-term results after bidirectional cavopulmonary shunts. *Ann Thorac Surg* 1993;56:833–837.

283. Kobayashi J, Matsuda H, Nakano S, Shimazaki Y, Ikawa S, Mitsuno M, Takahashi Y, Kawashima Y, Arisawa J, Matsushita T. Hemodynamic effects of bidirectional cavopulmonary shunt with pulsatile pulmonary flow. *Circulation* 1991;84(5 suppl):219–225.

283a. Slavik Z, Webber SA, Lamb RK, Horvath P, et al. Influence of bidirectional superior cavopulmonary anatomosis on pulmonary arterial growth. *Am J Cardiol* 1995;76:1085–1087.

284. Teske DW, Davis JT, Allen HD. Cavopulmonary anastomotic aneurysm: A complication in pulsatile pulmonary arteries. *Ann Thorac Surg* 1994;57:1661–1664.

284a. Alejos JC, Williams WG, Jarmakani JM, Galindo AJ, Isabel-Jones JB, Drinkwater D, Laks H, Kaplan S. Factors influencing survival in patients undergoing the bidirectional Glenn anastomosis. *Am J Cardiol* 1995;75:1048–1050.

284b. Reddy VM, Liddicoat JR, Hanley FL. Primary bidirectional superior cavopulmonary shunt in infants between 1 and 4 months of age. *Ann Thorac Surg* 1995;59:1120–1126.

284c. Webber SA, Horvath P, LeBlanc JG, Slavik Z, Lamb RK, Monro JL, Reich O, Hruda J, Sandor GGS, Keeton BR, Salmon AP. Influence of competitive pulmonary blood flow on the bidirectional superior cavopulmonary shunt. A multi-institutional study. *Circulation* 1995;92(suppl II):II-279-II-286.

284d. Mainwaring RD, Lamberti JJ, Uzark K, Spicer RL. Bidirectional Glenn. Is accessory pulmonary blood flow good or bad? *Circulation* 1995;92(suppl II):II-294-II-297.

284e. Frommelt M, Frommelt PC, Berger S, Pelech AN, Lewis DA, Tweddell JS, Litwin SB. Does an additionmal source of pulmonary blood flow alter outcome after a bidirectional cavopulmonary shunt? *Circulation* 1995;92(suppl II):II-240-II-244.

284f. Manning PB, Mayer JE Jr, Wernovsky G, Fishberger SB, Walsh EP. Staged operation to Fontan increases the incidence of sinoatrial node dysfunction. *J Thorac Cardiovasc Surg* 1996;111:833–840.

285. McFaul RC, Tajik AJ, Mair DD, Danielson GK, Seward JB. Development of pulmonary arteriovenous shunt after superior vena cava-right pulmonary artery (Glenn) anastomosis. *Circulation* 1977;55:212–216.

286. Van Den Bogaert-Van Heesvelde AM, Derom F, Kunnen M, Van Egmond H, Devloo-Blancquaert. Surgery for arteriovenous fistulas and dilated vessels in the right lung after the Glenn procedure. *J Thorac Cardiovasc Surg* 1978;76:195–197.

287. Gomes AS, Benson L, George B, Laks H. Management of pulmonary arteriovenous fistulas after superior vena cava-right pulmonary artery (Glenn) anastomosis. *J Thorac Cardiovasc Surg* 1984;87:636–639.

288. Papagiannis J, Kanter RJ, Effman EL, Pratt PC, Marcille R, Browning IB III, Armstrong BE. Polysplenia with pulmonary arteriovenous malformations. *Pediatr Cardiol* 1993;14:127–129.

289. Burch M, Iacovides P, Habibi P, Celermajer D. Non-cardiac cyanosis in left isomerism-report of two cases of multiple pulmonary arteriovenous malformations. *Cardiol Young* 1993;3:64–66.

290. Amodeo A, Di Donato R, Carotti A, Marino B, Marcelletti C. Pulmonary arteriovenous fistulas and polysplenia syndrome (letter). *J Thorac Cardiovasc Surg* 1994;107:1378–1379.

291. Moore JW, Kirby WC, Madden WA, Gaither NS. Development of pulmonary arteriovenous malformations after modified Fontan operations. *J Thorac Cardiovasc Surg* 1989;98:1045–1050.

291a. Kawashima Y, Kitamura S, Matsuda H, Shimazaki Y, Nakano S, Hirose H. Total cavopulmonary shunt operation in complex cardiac anomalies. A new operation. *J Thorac Cardiovasc Surg* 1984;87:74–81.

291b. Kawashima Y, Matsuki O, Yagihara T, Matsuda H. Total cavo-pulmonary shunt operation. *Semin Thorac Cardiovasc Surg* 1994;6:17–20.

291c. Feigl A, Feigl D, Tamir A, Berant M, Bleiden L. Multiple pulmonary arteriovenous fistulae, atrial septal defect, interruption of the inferior vena cava in the polysplenia syndrome (abstract). In: *Abstracts of the Third World Congress of Pediatric Cardiology*. Bangkok: 1989, pp. 33.

292. Srivastava D, Preminger TJ, Spevak PJ, Lock JE. Development of pulmonary arteriovenous malformations following cavopulmonary anastomosis. *Circulation* 1993;88(4 part 2);I-149.

292a. Srivastava D, Preminger TJ, Lock JE, Mandell V, Keane JF, Mayer JE Jr, Kozakewich H, Spevak PJ. Hepatic venous blood and the development of pulmonary arteriovenous malformations in congenital heart disease. *Circulation* 1995;92:1217–1222.

293. Hansoti RC and Shah NJ. Cirrhosis of liver simulating congenital cyanotic heart disease. *Circulation* 1966;33:71–77.

294. Hansoti RC, Sharma S. Cirrhosis of the liver simulating congenital cyanotic heart disease. *Chest* 1989;96:843–848.

294a. Kalra S, Pandit A, Taylor PM, Prescott MC, Woodcock AA. Concealed intrapulmonary shunting in liver disease. *Respir Med* 1994;88:545–547.

295. Laberge J-M, Brandt ML, Lebecque P, Moulin D, Veykemans F, Paradis K, Pelletier L, et al. Reversal of cirrhosis-related pulmonary shunting in two children by orthotopic liver transplantation. *Transplantation* 1992;53:1135–1138.

296. Fewtrell MS, Noble-Jamieson G, Revell S, Valente J, Friend P, Johnston P, Rasmussen A, Jamieson N, Calne RY, Barnes ND. Intrapulmonary shunting in the biliary atresia/polysplenia syndrome: Reversal after liver transplantation. *Arch Dis Child* 1994;70:501–504.

296a. Knight WB, Mee RBB. A cure for pulmonary arteriovenous fistulas. *Ann Thorac Surg* 1995;59:999–1001.

297. Silver MM, Bohn D, Shawn DH, Shuckett B, Eich G, Rabinovitch M. Association of pulmonary hypertension with congenital portal hypertension in a child (clinical conference). *J Pediatr* 1992;120:321–329.

297a. Edwards BS, Weir EK, Edwards WD, Ludwig J, Dykoski RK, Edwards JE. Coexistent pulmonary and portal hypertension: Morphologic and clinical features. *J Am Coll Cardiol* 1987;10:1233–1238.

298. Land SD, Shah MD, Berman WF. Pulmonary hypertension associated with portal hypertension in a child with Williams syndrome—a case report. *Pediatr Pathol* 1994;14:61–68.

298a. Laks H, Ardehali A, Grant PW, Permut P, Aharon A, Kuhn M, Isabel-Jones J, Galindo A. Modification of Fontan procedure. Superior vena cava to left pulmonary artery connection and inferior vena cava to right pulmonary artery connection with adjustable atrial septal defect. *Circulation* 1995;91:2943–2947.

298b. Blalock A, Taussig HB. Surgical treatment of malformation of the heart in which there is pulmonary stenosis or pulmonary atresia. *JAMA* 1945;128:189–202.

299. Trusler GA, Miyamura H, Culham JAG, Fowler RS, Williams WG. Pulmonary artery stenosis following aortopulmonary anastomoses. *J Thorac Cardiovasc Surg* 1981;82:398–404.

300. Hofschire PJ, Rosenquist GC, Ruckerman RN, Moller JH, Edwards JE. Pulmonary vascular disease complicating the blalock-taussig anastomosis. *Circulation* 1977;56:125–126.

301. de Leval MR, McKay R, Jones M, Stark J, Macartney FJ. Modified Blalock-Taussig shunt. Use of subclavian artery orifice as flow regulator in prosthetic systemic-pulmonary artery shunts. *J Thorac Cardiovasc Surg* 1981;81:112.

302. Litwin SB, Fellows KE. Systemic to pulmonary arterial shunts for patients with cyanotic congenital heart disease: Current status. *Pediatr Radiol* 1973;1:41.

303. Mietus-Snyder M, Lang P, Mayer JE, Jones RA, Castaneda AR, Lock JE. Childhood systemic-pulmonary shunts: Subsequent suitability for Fontan operation. *Circulation* 1987;76(suppl 3):34–39.

303a. Levin DC, Fellows KE, Sos TA. Angiographic demonstration of complications resulting from the Waterston procedure. *AJR* 1978;131:431–437.

304. Scott WC, Zhao HX, Allen M, Kim D, Miller DC. Aneurysmal degeneration of Blalock-Taussig shunts: Identification and surgical treatment options. *J Am Coll Cardiol* 1984;3:1277–1281.

305. Leblanc J, Albus R, Williams WG, Moes CAF, Wilson G, Freedom, RM, Trusler GA. Serous fluid leakage. A complication following the modified Blalock-Taussig shunt. *J Thorac Cardiovasc Surg* 1984;83:259–261.

306. Trusler GA, Mustard WT. A method of banding the pulmonary artery for large isolated ventricular septal defect with and without transposition of the great arteries. *Ann Thorac Surg* 1972;13:351–355.

306a. Nolan SP. The origins of pulmonary artery banding. *Ann Thorac Surg* 1987;44:427–429.

307. Stewart S, Harris P, Manning, J. Pulmonary artery banding. An analysis of current risks, results, and indications. *J Thorac Cardiovasc Surg* 1980;80:431.

308. Albus RA, Trusler GA, Izukawa T, Williams WG. Pulmonary artery banding. *J Thorac Cardiovasc Surg* 1984;88:645–653.

309. Dooley KJ, Parisi-Buckley L, Fyler DC, Nadas AS. Results of pulmonary arterial banding in infancy. Survey of 5 years experience in the New England Regional Infant Cardiac Program. *Am J Cardiol* 1985;36:484–488.

310. Leblanc JG, Ashmore PG, Pineda E, Sandor GG, Patterson MW, Tipple M. Pulmonary artery banding: Results and current indications in pediatric cardiac surgery. *Ann Thorac Surg* 1987;44:628–632.

311. Robertson MA, Penkoske PA, Duncan NF. Right pulmonary artery obstruction after pulmonary artery banding. *Ann Thorac Surg* 1991;51:73–75.

311a. Danilowicz D, Presti S, Colvin S. The disappearing pulmonary artery band. *Pediatr Cardiol* 1990;11:47–49.

311b. Kutsche LM, Alexander JA, Van Mierop LH. Hemolytic anemia secondary to erosion of a Silastic band into the lumen of the pulmonary trunk. *Am J Cardiol* 1985;55:1438–1439.

311c. Galinanes M, Stanley P, Guerin R, Kratz C, Chartrand C. Pulmonary banding complicated by low origin of right pulmonary artery. *Tex Heart Inst J* 1993;20:238–240.

312. Hiraishi S, Misawa H, Agata Y, Hirota H, Horiguchi Y, Fujino N, Takeda N, Nakae, Kawada M. Obstruction of the proximal pulmonary artery branches after banding of the pulmonary trunk. *Am J Cardiol* 1995;76:842–846.

313. Carter TL, Mainwaring RD, Lamberti JJ. Damus-Kaye-Stansel Procedure: Midterm follow-up and technical considerations. *Ann Thorac Surg* 1994;56:1603–1608.

314. Damus PS. Correspondence. *Ann Thorac Surg* 1975;20:724–725.

315. Kaye MP. Anatomic correction of transposition of the great arteries. *Mayo Clin Proc* 1975;50:638–640.

316. Stansel HC Jr. A new operation for d-loop transposition of the great vessels. *Ann Thorac Surg* 1975;19:565–567.

317. Ceithaml EL, Puga FJ, Danielson GK, McGoon DC, Ritter DG. Results of the Damus-Stansel-Kaye procedure for transposition of the great arteries and for double-outlet right ventricle with subpulmonary ventricular septal defect. *Ann Thorac Surg* 1984;38:433–437.

318. Lui RC; Williams WG; Trusler GA; Freedom RM; Coles JG; Rebeyka IM; Smallhorn J. Experience with the Damus-Kaye-Stansel procedure for children with Taussig-Bing hearts or univentricular hearts with subaortic stenosis. *Circulation* 1993;88(5 Pt 2):170–176.

319. De Leon SY, Ilbawi MN, Tubeszewski K, Wilson WR Jr, Idriss FS. The Damus-Stansel-Kaye procedure: Anatomical determinants and modifications. *Ann Thorac Surg* 1991;52(3):680–687.

320. De Leon SY, Idriss FS, Ilbawi MN, Muster AJ, Paul MH, Berry TE, Duffy CE, Quinones J. The Damus-Stansel-Kaye procedure. Should the aortic valve or subaortic valve region be closed? *J Thorac Cardiovasc Surg* 1986;91:747–753.

321. Waldman JD, Lamberti JJ, George L, Kirkpatrick SE. Experience with Damus procedure. *Circulation* 1988;78(5 Pt 2):32–39.

322. Matsuno S, Yokota Y, Ando F, Okamoto F, Shimizu A, Nakayama S, Ikeda T, Ohtani S, Oda K, Murakami Y. New modification of the Damus-Kaye-Stansel operation. *Ann Thorac Surg* 1994;58(1):231–233.

323. Gates RN, Laks H, Elami A, Drinkwater DC Jr, Pearl JM, George BL, Jarmakani JM, Williams RG. Damus-Stansel-Kaye procedure: Current indications and results. *Ann Thorac Surg* 1993;56:111–119.

324. Freedom RM, Sondheimer H, Dische R, Rowe RD. Development of "subaortic stenosis" after pulmonary arterial banding for common ventricle. *Am J Cardiol* 1977; 39:78–83.

325. Freedom RM, Benson LN, Smallhorn JF, Williams WG, Trusler GA, Rowe RD. Subaortic stenosis, the univentricular heart, and banding of the pulmonary artery: An analysis of the courses of 43 patients with univentricular heart palliated by pulmonary artery banding. *Circulation* 1986;73:758–764.

326. Freedom RM. The dinosaur and banding of the main pulmonary trunk in the heart with functionally one ventricle and transposition of the great arteries: A saga of evolution and caution. *J Am Coll Cardiol* 1987;10: 427–429.

327. Caspi J, Coles JG, Rabinovitch M, Cohen D, Trusler GA, Williams WG, Wilson GJ, Freedom RM. Morphological findings contributing to a failed fontan procedure in the current era. *Circulation* 1990;82(suppl IV):IV-177-IV-182.

328. Akagi T, Benson LN, Williams WG, Freedom RM. The relation between ventricular hypertrophy and clinical outcome in patients with double inlet left ventricle after atrial to pulmonary anastomosis. *Herz* 1992;17: 220–227.

329. Freedom RM, Akagi T, Benson LN. The potentially obstructive subaortic region and pulmonary artery banding: Selected observations in the patient considered for a Fontan algorithm. *Cardiol Young* 1993;3:91–97.

330. Kirklin JK, Blackstone EH, Kirklin JW, Pacifico AD, Bargeron LM. The Fontan operation. Ventricular hypertrophy, age, and date of operation as risk factors. *J Thorac Cardiovasc Surg* 1986;92:1049–1064.

331. Seliem M, Muster AJ, Paul MH, Benson DW. Relation between preoperative left ventricular muscle mass and outcome of the Fontan procedure in patients with tricuspid atresia. *J Am Coll Cardiol* 1989;14:750–755.

332. Vogel M, Staller W, Buhlmeyer K, Sebening F. Influence of age at time of surgery on preoperative left ventricular mass and postoperative outcome of Fontan operation in children with tricuspid atresia and native pulmonary stenosis. *Herz* 1992;17:228–233.

333. O'leary PW, Driscoll DJ, Connor AR, Puga FJ, Danielson GK. Subaortic obstruction in hearts with a univentricular connection to a dominant left ventricle and an anterior subaortic outlet chamber. Results of a staged approach. *J Thorac Cardiovasc Surg* 1992;104:1231–1237.

334. Franklin RC, Sullivan ID, Anderson RH, Shinebourne EA, Deanfield JE. Is banding of the pulmonary trunk obsolete for infants with tricuspid atresia and double inlet ventricle with a discordant ventriculoarterial connection? Role of aortic arch obstruction and subaortic stenosis. *J Am Coll Cardiol* 1990;16:1455–1464.

335. Rychik J, Lieb DR, Jacobs ML, Norwood WI, Chin AJ. Acute changes in in left ventricular geometry following removal of volume overload. World Congress of Pediatric Cardiology and Pediatric Cardiac Surgery (abstract). *Cardiol Young* 1993;3(suppl 1):12.

336. Malcic I, Sauer U, Stern H, Kellerer M, Kuhlein B, Locher D, Buhlmeyer K, Sebening F. The influence of pulmonary artery banding on outcome after the Fontan operation. *J Thorac Cardiovasc Surg* 1992;104:743–747.

337. Bell ALL, Shimomura S, Guthne WJ, Hempell HF, Fitzpatrick HF, and Begg CF. Wedge pulmonary arteriography in congenital and acquired heart disease. *Radiology* 1959;73:566–560.

338. Jacobsen G. Peripheral pulmonary (wedge) angiography: A standardized technique for the single film arteriogram. *Clin Radiol* 1963;14:326–329.

339. Castellanos A, Hernandez FA, Mercado HG. Wedge pulmonary arteriography in congenital heart disease. *Radiology* 1965;85:838–841.

340. Nihill MR, McNamara DG. Magnification pulmonary wedge angio-graphy in the evaluation of children with congenital heart disease and pulmonary hypertension. *Circulation* 1978;58:1094–1099.

341. Collins-Nakai RL and Rabinovitch M. Pulmonary vascular obstructive disease. *Cardiol Clin* 1993;11:675–687.

342. Rabinovitch M, Keane JF, Fellows KE, Castaneda AR, and Reid L. Quantitative analysis of the pulmonary wedge angiogram in congenital heart defects. Correlation with hemodynamic data and morphometric findings in lung biopsy tissue. *Circulation* 1981;63:152–160.

343. Burrows PE, Moes CAF, Freedom RM. Imaging of the neonate with congenital heart disease. In: Freedom RM, Benson LN, Smallhorn JF, eds. *Neonatal Heart Disease*. London: Springer-Verlag; 1992, pp. 101–118.

344. Hernanadez RJ, Bank ER, Shaffer EM, Snider AR, Rosenthal A. Comparative evaluation of the pulmonary arteries in patients with right ventricular outflow tract obstructive lesions. *AJR* 1987;148:1189–1194.

345. Vick GW III, Rokey R, Huhta JC, Mulvagh SL, Johnston DL. Nuclear magnetic resonance imaging of the pulmonary arteries, subpulmonary region, and aorticopulmonary shunts: A comparative study with two-dimensional echocardiography and angiography. *Am Heart J* 1990;119:1103–1110.

346. Kattan KR. Angled views in pulmonary angiography. A new roentgen approach. *Radiology* 1970;94:79–82.

347. Bargeron LM Jr, Elliott LP, Soto B, Bream PR, Curry CG. Axial cineangiography in congenital heart disease. Section I. Concept, technical and anatomic considerations. *Circulation* 1977;56:1075–1083.

348. Elliott LP, Bargeron LM, Bream PR, Soto B, Curry GC (1977). Axial angiography in congenital heart disease. Section II. Specific lesions. *Circulation* 1977;56:1084–1093.

349. Soto B, Coghlan CH, Bargeron LM. Present status of axially angled angiocardiography. *Cardiovasc Intervent Radiol* 1984;7:156–165.

350. Freedom RM. Axial Angiocardiography in the critically ill infant. Indications and contraindications. *Cardiol Clin* 1983;1(3):387–411.

351. Fellows KE, Keane JF, Freed MD. Angled views in cineangiocardiography of congenital heart disease. *Circulation* 1977;56:485–490.

352. Fellows KE, Smith J, Keane JF. Preoperative angiocardiography in infants with tetralogy of Fallot. *Am J Cardiol* 1981;47:1279–1285.

353. Freedom RM, Olley PM. Pulmonary arteriography in congenital heart disease. *Cathet Cardiovasc Diag* 1976; 2:309–312.

354. Soto B, Pacifico AD, Ceballos R, Bargeron LM Jr. Tetral-

ogy of Fallot: An angiographic-pathologic correlative study. *Circulation* 1981;64:558–566.

355. Freedom RM, Benson LN. Tetralogy of Fallot. In: Freedom RM, Benson LN, Smallhorn JF, eds. *Neonatal Heart Disease.* London: Springer-Verlag; 1992, pp. 213–228.

356. Freedom RM, Smallhorn JF, Burrows PE. Pulmonary atresia and ventricular septal defect. In: Freedom RM, Benson LN, Smallhorn JF, eds. *Neonatal Heart Disease.* London: Springer-Verlag; 1992, pp. 229–256.

357. Freedom RM, Rabinovitch M. The angiography of the pulmonary circulation in patients with pulmonary atresia and ventricular septal defect. In: Tucker BL, Lindesmith GC, Takahashi M, eds. *Obstructive Lesions of the Right Heart.* Baltimore: University Park Press; 1984, pp. 191–216.

358. Soto B, Pacifico AD. *Angiocardiography in Congenital Heart Malformations.* Mt. Kisco, NY: Futura Publishing Company, Inc; 1990, pp. 3–38, 121–158, 353–376, 449–491, 517–541.

359. Garcia-Medina V, Bass J, Braunlin E, Krabill KA, Pyles L, Castaneda-Zuniga WR, Hunter DW, Amplatz K. A useful projection for demonstrating the bifurcation of the pulmonary artery. *Pediatr Cardiol* 1990;11:147–149.

360. Freedom RM, Moes CAF, Pelech A, Smallhorn J, Rabinovitch M, Olley PM, Williams WG, Trusler GA, Rowe RD. Bilateral ductus arteriosus (or remnant): An analysis of 27 patients. *Am J Cardiol* 1984;53:884–891.

361. Rao PS. Pulmonary vein wedge angiography in visualization obstructed ipsilateral pulmonary artery. *Radiology* 1978;1:151–152.

362. Rao PS. Complications of pulmonary vein angiography. *Br Heart J* 1980;43:124.

363. Hawker RE, Celermajer JM. Comparison of pulmonary artery and pulmonary venous wedge pressure in congenital heart disease. *Br Heart J* 1973;35:386–391.

364. Waldman JD, LaCorte M, Dick M II, John SA, Miettinen OS, LaFarge CG. The pulmonary venous wedge pressure in pulmonary arterial hypertension. *Cathet Cardiovasc Diagn* 1977;3:231–239.

365. Chern MS, Yeh SJ, Lin FC, Wu D, Hung JS. Estimation of pulmonary artery pressure from pulmonary vein wedge pressure. *Cathet Cardiovasc Diagn* 1994;31:277–82.

366. Gonzales-Crussi F, Padilla L-M, Miller JK, Grosfeld JL. "Bridging bronchus". A previously undescribed airway anomaly. *Am J Dis Child* 1976;130:1015–1018.

367. Starshak RJ, Sty JR, Woods G, Kreitzer FV. Bridging bronchus: A rare airway anomaly. *Radiology* 1981;140: 95–96.

Chapter 20

Tetralogy of Fallot and Pulmonary Atresia and Ventricular Septal Defect

There has been considerable evolution in our understanding of what constitutes tetralogy of Fallot. Fallot, and those who have translated his work, considered tetralogy as consisting of a ventricular septal defect, stenosis of the pulmonary outflow tract, an overriding aorta, and right ventricular myocardial hypertrophy this last feature a natural consequence of the pulmonary outflow tract obstruction.[1-4] The evolution in our understanding of the morphology is paralleled by those achievements in therapy: from palliation as the only form of therapy 50 years ago, to repair of this malformation at almost any age today.[5-19] This chapter addresses the anatomy of tetralogy of Fallot, the associated anomalies, the intracardiac anatomy of tetralogy with pulmonary atresia or pulmonary atresia and ventricular septal defect, and the relevant angiocardiographic features. The nature of the pulmonary circulation when there is not continuity between the ventricle and the pulmonary circulation and the related imaging modalities are addressed in Chapter 21. Tetralogy of Fallot with absent pulmonary valve is considered in Chapter 22.

Prevalence

The diagnostic frequency of tetralogy of Fallot of 0.214 per 1000 livebirths was provided by the New England Regional Infant Cardiac Program,[20] and data from the more recently completed Baltimore-Washington Infant Study provided a prevalence of 0.262 per 1000 livebirths.[21] The Alberta Heritage Study indicated a liveborn prevalence of 0.184 per 1000 livebirths for tetralogy of Fallot.[22]

Segmental Anatomy

The most frequent segmental anatomy of tetralogy of Fallot is levocardia, atrial situs solitus, and concordant atrioventricular and ventriculoarterial connections. Tetralogy of Fallot in situs inversus totalis is uncommon (<5%), and tetralogy of Fallot with isolated dextrocardia is also very uncommon. Tetralogy of Fallot has been infrequently diagnosed in those patients with incomplete visceral lateralization, usually left isomerism with or without polysplenia. Tetralogy of Fallot with inverted normal great arteries is an uncommon form of tetralogy. The connections between atria and ventricles and ventricles and great arteries are concordant in this variant, but with the infundibuloarterial inversion, the right coronary artery traverses the stenotic right ventricular outflow tract.[22a-22c]

The Morphology of Tetralogy of Fallot

Those morphological findings of tetralogy of Fallot include pulmonary stenosis of a specific infundibular character; a ventricular septal defect located between the anterior and posterior limbs of the trabecular septal band; overriding of the aorta; and right ventricular hypertrophy.[5-8,19,23-31] Right ventricular hypertrophy is progressive, reflecting the myocardial response to both right ventricular outflow tract obstruction and to the large, nonrestrictive ventricular septal defect. Uniting these features is anterocephalad deviation of the infundibular outlet septum, and this malalignment of the infundibular septum is now considered the essence of tetralogy of Fallot (Figs. 20-1 through 20-3). Indeed,

From: Freedom RM, Mawson JB, Yoo SJ, Benson LN: *Congenital Heart Disease: Textbook of Angiocardiography.* Armonk NY, Futura Publishing Co., Inc. ©1997.

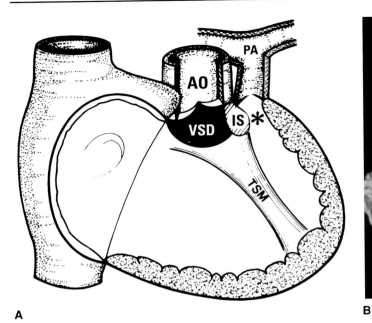

A

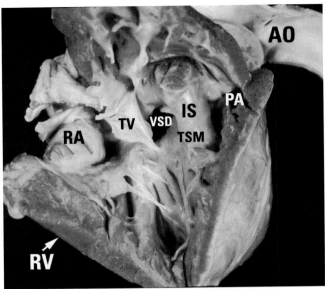

B

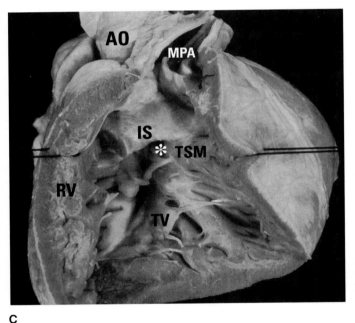

C

Fig. 20-1: Diagram shows the fundamental role of the outlet or infundibular septum in the morphogenesis of tetralogy of Fallot.
A: This diagram shows the fundamental role of the infundibular or outlet septum in the morphogenesis of tetralogy of Fallot. Displacement of the infundibular septum is indeed the essence of the "monology" of Fallot. **B and C:** Internal views of the morphologically right ventricle in two specimens from unoperated patients with tetralogy of Fallot. Note in both specimens the displaced infundibular septum produces a ventricular septal defect (✻ in C) and this displacement narrows the right ventricular outlet to the pulmonary artery.

more than two decades ago, Van Praagh and his colleagues suggested that tetralogy of Fallot is really a "monology" of Fallot resulting from this displaced infundibular or outlet septum, and that in tetralogy, the outlet septum is "too short, too narrow, and too shallow."[30,31] The leftward or septal end of the infundibular septum is displaced anteriorly, inserting in front of the left anterior division of the septal band rather than between its two divisions as in the normal heart. The rightward aspect of the infundibular septum is rotated anteriorly and passed anteriorly and inferiorly to reach the free wall of the right ventricle so that the in-

fundibular septum and its parietal extension lie almost in a sagittal plane rather than the usual frontal plane.[13] Others, while agreeing that tetralogy reflects this malalignment of the outlet septum, do not agree that invariably the outlet septum is hypoplastic.[23] Geva and colleagues[23a] have recently published a prospective longitudinal echocardiographic study of those quantitative features characteristic of progressive infundibular obstruction in tetralogy of Fallot. Their data showed that the subpulmonary infundibulum in tetralogy of Fallot, when compared with healthy infants, is characterized by a smaller volume, shorter and thicker in-

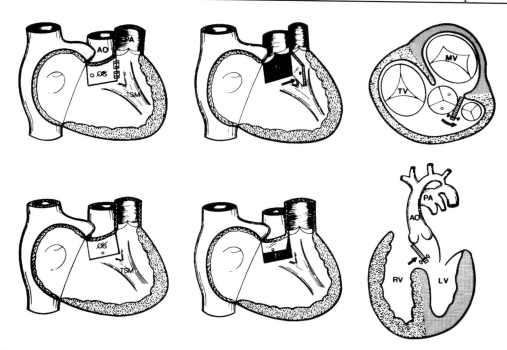

Fig. 20-2: This diagram shows that in patients with atrioventricular and ventriculoarterial concordance, anteroseptal displacement of the infundibular septum results in tetralogy of Fallot, whereas posterocaudal displacement produces left ventricular outflow tract obstruction, which is often seen in patients with interruption of the aortic arch or coarctation of the aorta.

fundibular septum, and anterosuperior deviation of the infundibular septum. Thus, the character of the pulmonary stenosis is clearly related in typical cases to this deviation of the infundibular septum, and thus this obstruction by definition is muscular and tends to be progressive. In many patients this infundibular obstruction is aggravated by a hypoplastic pulmonary valvular annulus, pulmonary valve stenosis with a bicuspid valve with thickened cusps and fused commissures, anomalous muscle bundles and varying degrees of hypoplasia of the main pulmonary trunk and its branches.[8,19,32] Those patients with absence of the outlet septum are not really examples of tetralogy of Fallot, despite similar hemodynamics.[13,19,33–36a] An overriding aorta is also consistently identified in the patient with tetralogy of Fallot, and Kirklin and Barratt-Boyes[13] indicated that the overriding varies from about 30% to 90%, with usually about 50% of the aortic orifice above the right ventricle. Kirklin and Barratt-Boyes[13] also pointed out that aortic override is associated with a variable degree of clockwise rotation of the aortic root as viewed from the ventricular apex. This rotation moves the base of the noncoronary cusp rightward and superiorly onto the posterosuperior margin of the ventricular septal defect and away from the base of the anterior or aortic leaflet

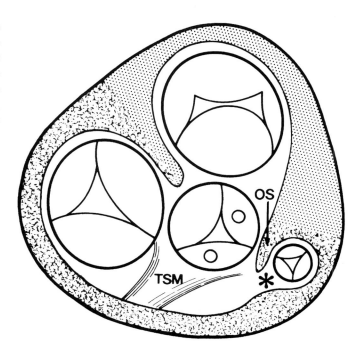

Fig. 20-3: Schematic diagram shows the relationship of the aorta, the ventricular septal defect, and the displaced infundibular septum producing right ventricular outflow tract obstruction.

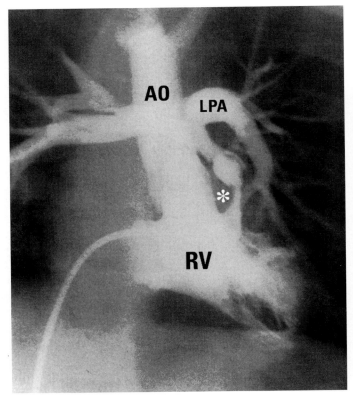

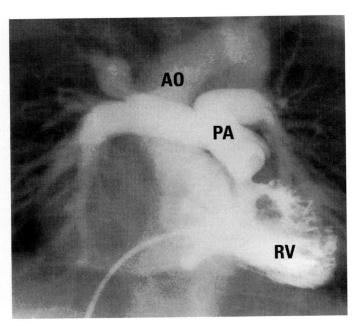

A   **B**

Fig. 20-4: The various angiographic appearances of the morphologically right ventricle and pulmonary outflow tract in tetralogy of Fallot.
A: Right ventriculogram in right anterior oblique projection with cranial angulation shows the moderately narrowed pulmonary outflow tract due to the deviated infundibular septum (✻) and the small pulmonary arteries. There is significant right-to-left shunting at the ventricular level opacifying the ascending aorta. **B:** A short-segment infundibular obstruction with excellent caliber pulmonary arteries with right-to-left shunting at ventricular level opacifying the ascending aorta. *(figure continues)*

of the mitral valve.[13,31] The rightward rotation of the left aortic cusp results in more of it becoming continuous with the anterior mitral leaflet, while the superiorly positioned right cusp moves to the left. The degree of overriding and clockwise rotation of the aortic root relates to the degree of underdevelopment or hypoplasia of the right ventricular outflow tract and to malalignment of the infundibular septum.[13,31]

What are those morphological features proximal to the pulmonary arteries contributing to pulmonary outflow obstruction in tetralogy of Fallot? While the essence of tetralogy of Fallot may be the anterosuperior deviation of the infundibular septum, there is disagreement whether the infundibular septum is hypoplastic.[5–8,23,37] It certainly becomes hypertrophied with time; the subpulmonary outflow tract appears elongated, and anterior muscle bundles on the free or parietal wall of the right ventricle contribute to the infundibular obstruction. In addition, hypertrophied septoparietal bands course from the septum anteroinfe-

riorly to the parietal wall, and these contribute to the subinfundibular obstruction.[32] In his recent review of tetralogy of Fallot, Zuberbuhler[19] suggested that anomalous right ventricle muscles also contribute to right ventricular outflow muscular obstruction, recognized in 11% of operated patients in the Pittsburgh series. The pulmonic valve is abnormal and stenotic in three-quarters of patients with tetralogy of Fallot. At least two-thirds of the stenotic pulmonary valves in the tetralogy malformation are bicuspid.[13,19,38,39]

The right ventricle is almost always of normal size in patients with tetralogy of Fallot, but we as well as others have recognized right ventricular hypoplasia with tricuspid valve hypoplasia/stenosis and attenuation of the right ventricular apical trabecular zone in about 1% to 2% of patients (Fig. 20-4).[13,40,41] The patient who was reported by Garcia and colleagues[41] should be considered a variant of pulmonary atresia and intact ventricular septum rather than tetralogy of Fallot (see Chapter 23). Closely related to tetralogy of Fallot is that variant

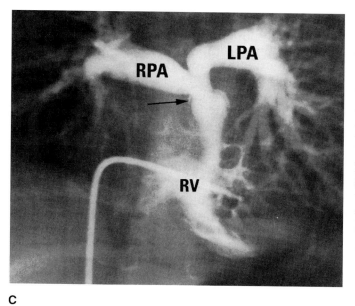

C

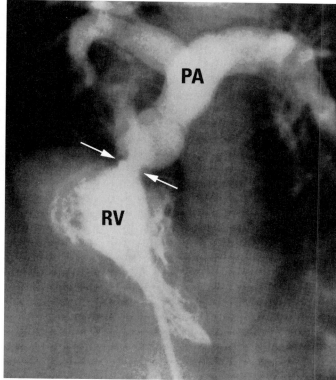

E

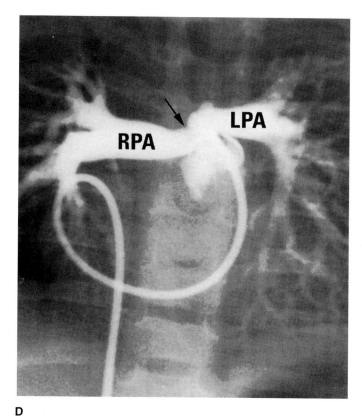

D

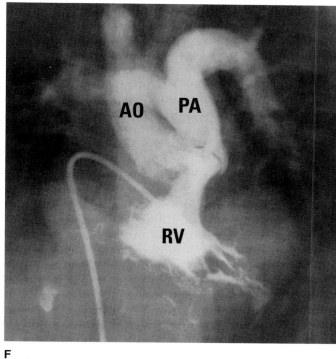

F

Fig. 20-4: *(continued)*
C and D: Cranially angled frontal right ventriculogram and pulmonary angiogram. The right ventricular outflow tract is diffusely narrowed with pulmonary valvular and supravalvular stenosis as well; mild narrowing of the origins of both pulmonary arteries can be seen both from the right ventriculogram and the pulmonary angiogram. **E:** Right ventriculogram in hepatoclavicular view shows nicely the infundibular obstruction (between arrows). **F:** Frontal cranially-angled right ventriculogram shows moderate infundibular obstruction, but severe pulmonary valvular stenosis. *(figure continues)*

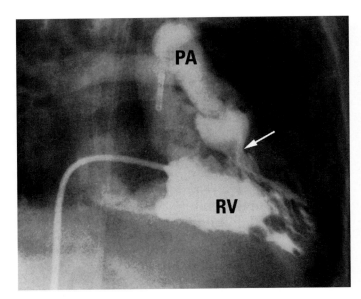

G

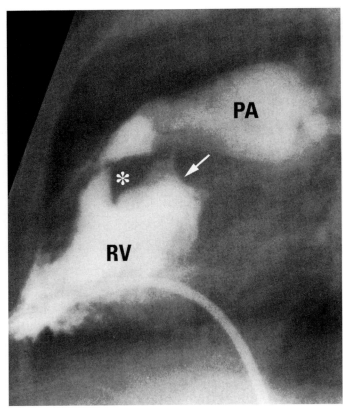

H

I

Fig. 20-4: *(continued)*
G and H: Frontal and lateral right ventriculogram of a patient with both infundibular displacement and anterior wall muscle bundles (✱) obstructing the outlet to the right ventricle. **G:** Note the subpulmonary obstruction with contributions from the right ventricular free wall (arrow). **H:** Anterocephalad displacement of the infundibular septum (✱) is nicely seen in this lateral right ventriculogram. The aortic valve is seen (arrow). **I:** The anterior wall muscle encroaches (✱) on the right ventricular outflow tract.

with the subpulmonary or doubly committed subarterial ventricular septal defect (Fig. 20-5).

The ventricular septal defect in typical tetralogy is large, subaortic, and reflects in its very nature the deviation of the outlet septum.[28] As pointed out by Anderson and Tynan, their colleagues and others,[5-8,13,19] such defects are also perimembranous, and the roof of the left ventricular margin of the ventricular septal defect is formed by the area of fibrous continuity between the leaflets of the aortic and mitral valves (Fig. 20-6).[42,43] The ventricular septal defect of tetralogy of Fallot may be confluent with a large perimembranous defect, muscular inlet type, or ventricular septal defect of the atrioventricular septal or canal type. Soto and Pacifico suggest that three types of ventricular septal defect have been identified in the patient with tetralogy of Fallot: 1) perimembranous; 2) muscular infundibular, and 3) subarterial.[42] We would agree that the typical malalignment defect has its perimembranous component, and may extend to the site of attachment of the tricuspid

valve annulus to the central fibrous body. Soto and Pacifico distinguish the perimembranous type of ventricular septal defect in tetralogy from the muscular infundibular type. The muscular infundibular ventricular septal defect is similar to the perimembranous defect but in the muscular infundibular ventricular septal defect, the ventricular septal defect and tricuspid annulus are not in fibrous continuity. They are separated by a muscular bar representing the posterior limb of the trabecula septomarginalis at its junction with the ventriculoinfundibular fold. Although Soto and Pacifico indicated that the subarterial ventricular septal defect is the third type of ventricular septal defect in tetralogy of Fallot, they appropriately question whether hearts with the subarterial ventricular septal defect should be considered as belonging to the tetralogy family. The infundibular septum in this variety is either atretic or severely hypoplastic, and thus infundibular septal malalignment is not responsible for the right ventricular outlet obstruction.[13,19,33-36a]

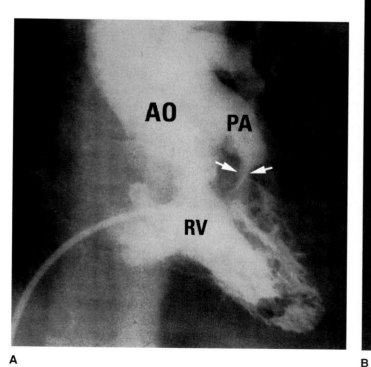

A

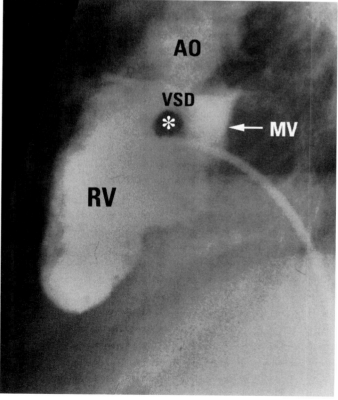

B

Fig. 20-5: So-called tetralogy of Fallot with doubly committed subarterial or subpulmonary ventricular septal defect.
A: Frontal right ventriculogram shows muscular obstruction to the right ventricular outflow tract. **B:** The lateral right ventriculograms from two different patients show the subpulmonary ventricular septal defect roofed by the aortic valve as well. The infundibular septum is either absent or grossly deficient. *(figure continues)*

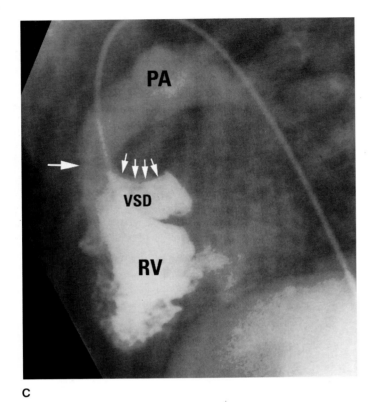

C

Fig. 20-5: *(continued)*
C: The lateral right ventriculograms from two different patients show the subpulmonary ventricular septal defect roofed by the aortic valve as well. The infundibular septum is either absent or grossly deficient. **D:** A different patient with significant valve and subvalve (arrows) right ventricular outflow tract obstruction and (**E**) a right aortic arch with aberrant left subclavian artery.

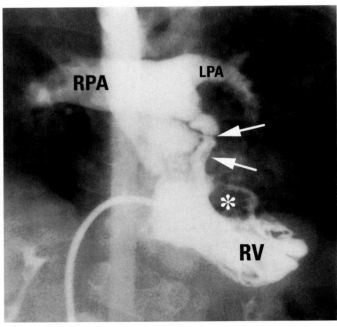

D

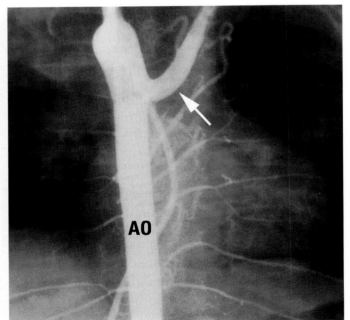

E

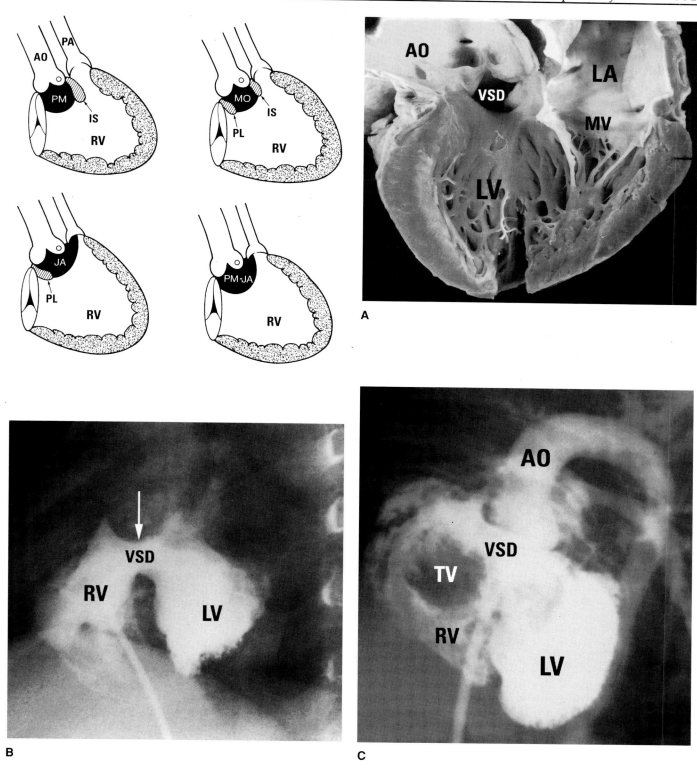

Fig. 20-6: The ventricular septal defect in tetralogy of Fallot. Diagram shows the various types of ventricular septal defects in tetralogy of Fallot.

A: Internal view of morphologically left ventricle and aortic outflow tract in a patient with severe tetralogy of Fallot. Note that the overriding aortic valve roofs the ventricular septal defect and that aortic valve-mitral valve fibrous continuity is present. **B through E:** The large ventricular septal defect of typical tetralogy is profiled in these long axial oblique left ventriculograms in four different patients; note in E the marked aortic override. **F:** The ventricular septal defect is beneath the displaced infundibular septum as shown in this lateral right ventriculogram. **G and H:** The right anterior oblique left ventriculograms clearly show the displaced infundibular septum (✳ in G) narrowing the right ventricular outflow tract in these two patients. *(figure continues)*

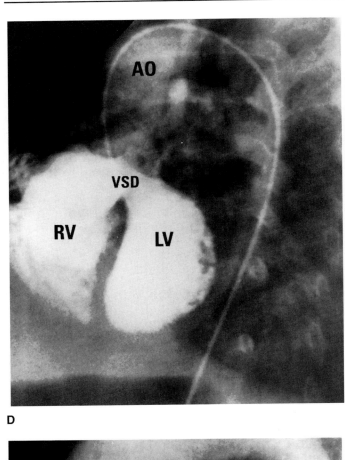

D

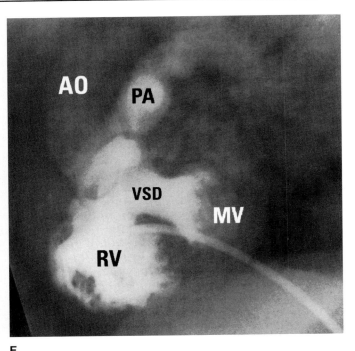

F

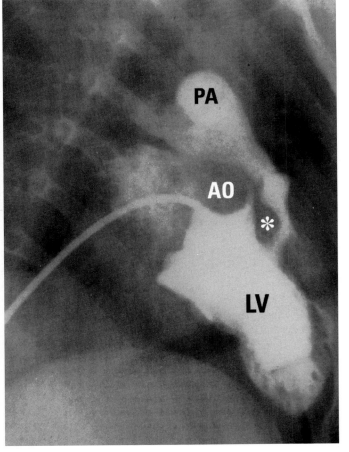

E

G

Fig. 20-6 *(continued)*

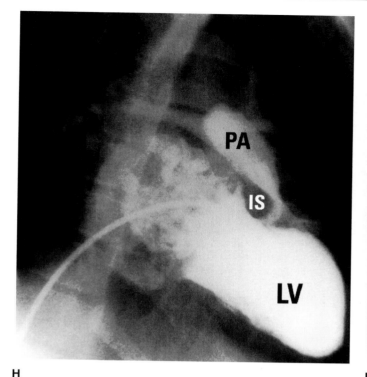

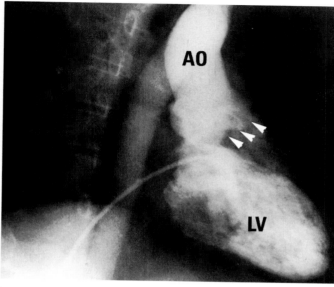

H   I

Fig. 20-6: *(continued)*
I: This right anterior oblique left ventriculogram demonstrates considerable aortic override (arrows).

The ventricular septal defect may be obstructive in the patient with tetralogy of Fallot (Fig. 20-7).[44–50] This has rarely been recognized in the neonate with tetralogy of Fallot, but has been diagnosed with increasing frequency in the older infant and child with tetralogy. The clinical presentation and hemodynamic recordings are similar to the patient with pulmonary stenosis.[44] While there are several mechanisms responsible for occlusion of the ventricular septal defect in tetralogy of Fallot, the most common mechanism is related to mobile tricuspid valve tissue associated with its septal leaflet. Less commonly, muscular obstruction may contribute to the restriction at ventricular septal defect level.[28] Similar mechanisms have been identified in the patient with pulmonary atresia and ventricular septal defect (see Chapter 21).

Overriding of the aorta relative to the trabecular septum is an essential component of the tetralogy of Fallot.[5–8,13,19,51] The degree of overriding can vary considerably, and in some patients both great arteries may have their origin primarily from the morphologically right ventricle. One might then ask can tetralogy of Fallot and double-outlet right ventricle coexist?[8,52] Taking the position that tetralogy represents an anomaly of the outlet septum and that double-outlet right ventricle describes an abnormal ventriculoarterial connection, then these two conditions can and do coexist.[26,27,53] The aortic valve cusps are abnormally positioned in tetralogy of Fallot, with the noncoronary cusp positioned more anteriorly and to the right than in the normal heart.[13] The quantitative anatomy of cyanotic tetralogy of Fallot has been previously assessed,[26,27] and Rao and Ed-

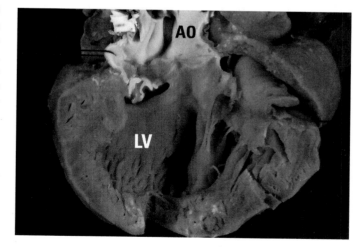

Fig. 20-7: The morphology of the restrictive ventricular septal defect in either tetralogy of Fallot or pulmonary atresia and ventricular septal defect.
Internal view of the morphologically left ventricle shows the ventricular septal defect partially occluded by tricuspid valve tissue.

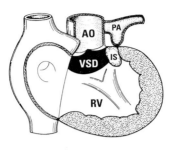
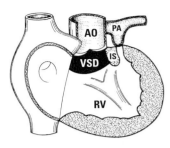

Fig. 20-8: The right ventricle in the patient with pulmonary atresia and ventricular septal defect, so-called tetralogy with pulmonary atresia.
Diagram shows infundibular atresia in **left panel** and a patent infundibulum in **right panel** with pulmonary valvar atresia. **A:** Frontal right ventriculogram doesn't show evidence of infundibular septation. **B:** Some attenuation of the apical trabebular zone. **C:** Evidence of infundibular septation in a patient with multiple aortopulmonary collaterals. **D:** Frontal right ventriculogram in a patient with complex pulmonary arterial anatomy. *(figure continues)*

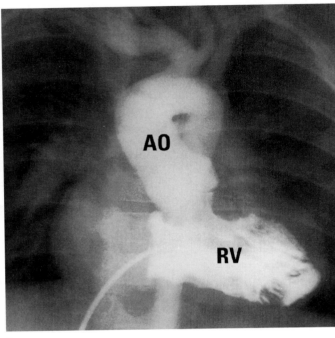

A

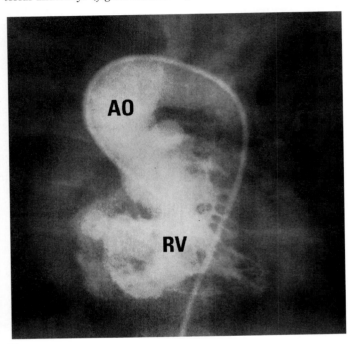

B

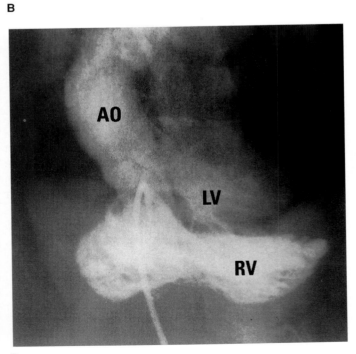

C

D

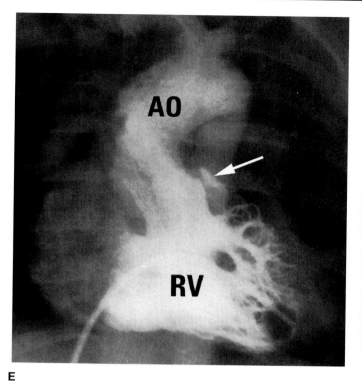

E

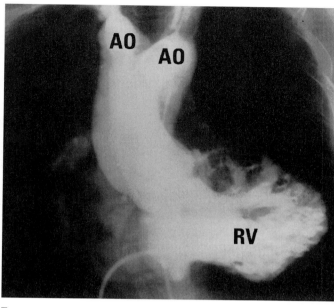

F

Fig. 20-8: *(continued)*
E: Some infundibular septation (arrow) in a patient with no evidence of mediastinal pulmonary arteries. **F:** A double aortic arch in a patient with pulmonary atresia and ventricular septal defect and no evidence of infundibular septation. (Fig. 20-8F was provided by Dr. Gordon Cumming, Children's Health Center, Winnipeg, Manitoba.)

wards[54] have reviewed those conditions that must be differentiated from tetralogy of Fallot.

The intracardiac anatomy of tetralogy of Fallot with pulmonary atresia is similar in many respects to tetralogy of Fallot with a perforate outflow tract. Infundibular septation may or may not be conspicuous. (Fig. 20-8).[5–9,13,19,55–61] The degree of infundibular septation found either clinically or at postmortem does not convey specific information about the pulmonary circulation. That is, evidence of infundibular septation does not and should not lead to the conclusion that the pulmonary circulation is mediated by an arterial duct. Conversely, the absence of recognizable infundibular septation does not imply a more primitive (ie, from aortopulmonary collaterals, either direct or indirect; see Chapter 21) pulmonary circulation.

The Pulmonary Arteries in Tetralogy of Fallot

The pulmonary artery circulation in patients with tetralogy of Fallot has undergone particular scrutiny (Figs. 20-4A through 20-4F and Figs. 20-9 through 20-12).[5–8,13–15,19,62–89] Tremendous variability in pul-

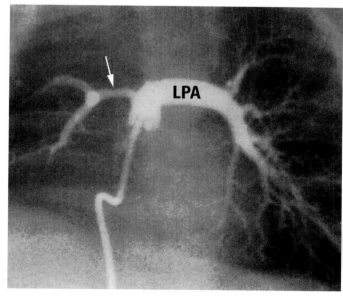

A

Fig. 20-9: Confluent pulmonary arteries in tetralogy of Fallot. A: Marked hypoplasia of the right pulmonary artery (arrow). *(figure continues)*

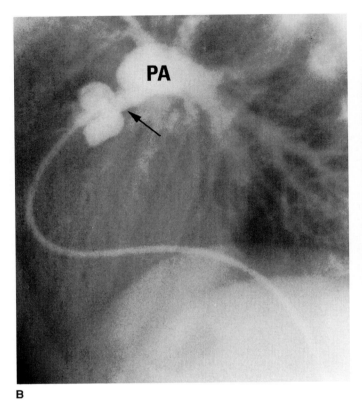

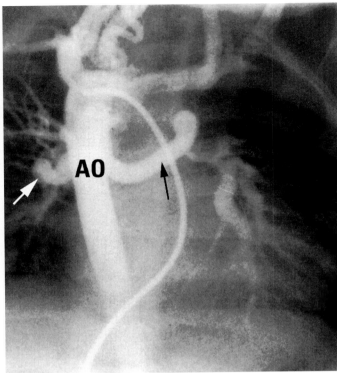

Fig. 20-9: *(continued)*
B: Stenosis of the main pulmonary artery (arrow). **C and D:** A patient with confluent pulmonary arteries and direct aortopulmonary collaterals. C: Frontal right ventriculogram shows very underdeveloped pulmonary arteries, especially the right pulmonary artery (arrow). D: From the descending aorta of this right aortic arch arise direct aortopulmonary collateral arteries (arrows).

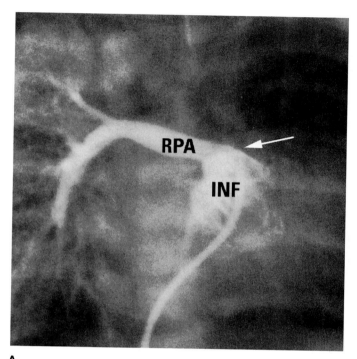

A

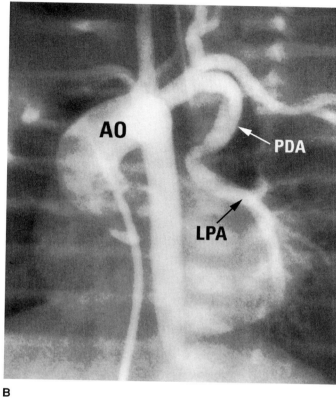

B

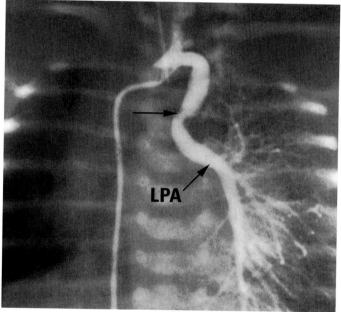

C

Fig. 20-10: Nonconfluent pulmonary arteries in tetralogy of Fallot with a distal ductal origin of the left pulmonary artery. A: Injection into the right ventricular infundibulum of a newborn on E-type prostaglandin shows a small right pulmonary artery, without opacification of a left pulmonary artery (arrow). **B:** Selective aortogram shows the left pulmonary artery originates from a left-sided arterial duct. **C:** Injection into the origin of the arterial duct (arrow) confirms the ductal origin of the left pulmonary artery with a widely patent arterial duct. *(figure continues)*

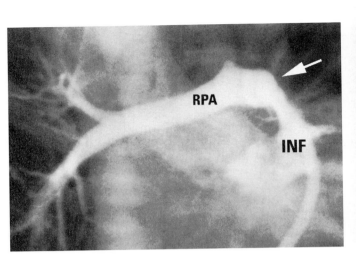

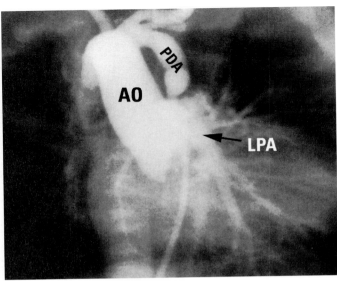

D

E

Fig. 20-10: *(continued)*
D and E: Another newborn with ductal origin of the left pulmonary artery. **D:** Injection into the right ventricular infundibulum shows opacification only of the right pulmonary artery, with no visualization of a proximal left pulmonary artery (arrow). **E:** The aortogram demonstrates a large left-sided arterial duct connected to the left pulmonary artery.

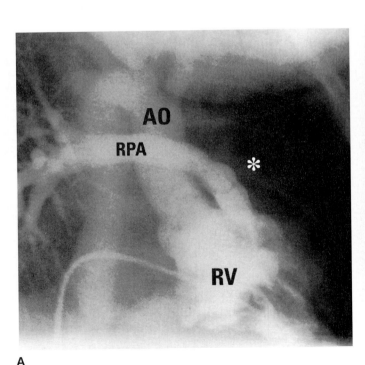

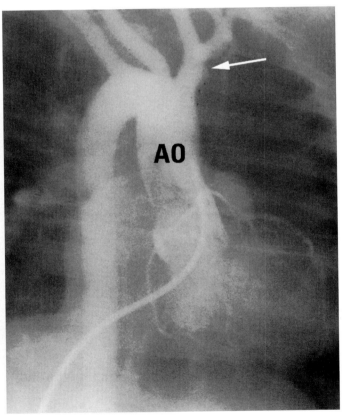

A

B

Fig. 20-11: Nonconfluent pulmonary arteries in tetralogy of Fallot with a distal ligamental origin of the left pulmonary artery.
A: Frontal right ventriculogram shows a right pulmonary artery opacifying from this ventriculogram, with right-to-left shunting at ventricular level and opacification of a the right-sided aortic arch. **B:** The aortogram shows a left-sided ductal diverticulum (arrow) originating from the base of the left innominate artery. *(figure continues)*

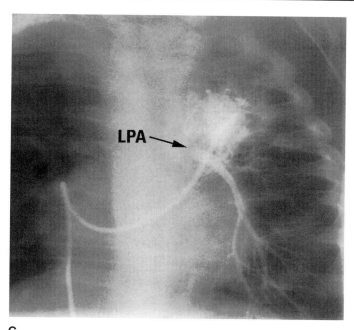

C

Fig. 20-11: *(continued)*
C: The left pulmonary vein wedge angiogram confirms the presence of a left pulmonary artery.

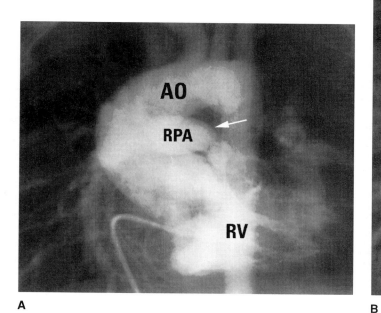

A

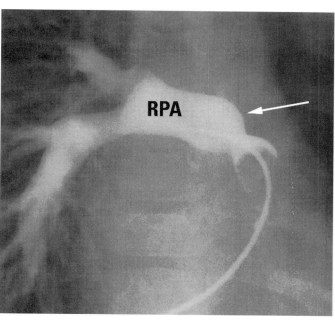

B

Fig. 20-12: Pulmonary vein wedge angiography demonstrates a small left pulmonary artery in a patient with tetralogy of Fallot and distal ligamental origin of the left pulmonary artery.
A: Frontal right ventriculogram demonstrates a well-formed right pulmonary artery with no visualization of the left pulmonary artery (arrow); right-to-left shunting at ventricular level is reflected by opacification of the left aortic arch. **B:** Selective injection in the main pulmonary trunk in the frontal projection confirms the 'absent' left pulmonary artery (arrow) and pulmonary valvular stenosis with a doming valve. **C:** Left-sided pulmonary vein wedge angiogram shows a very small hilar left pulmonary artery, seemingly retracted superiorly. **D:** After construction of a modified Blalock-Taussig shunt into the hilar left pulmonary artery (see also Chapter 22, Fig. 22-8) *(figure continues)*

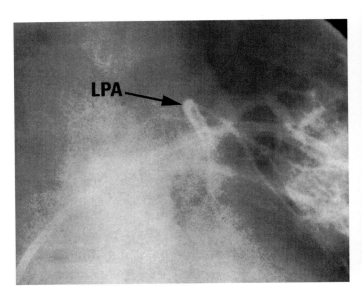

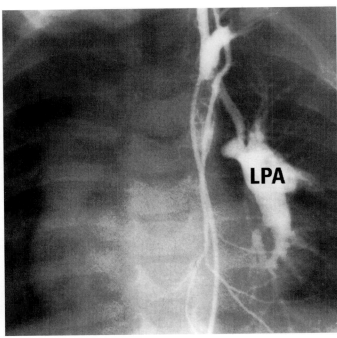

C

D

Fig. 20-12 *(continued)*

monary artery size is evident in any large cohort of patients with tetralogy of Fallot. The smallest confluent pulmonary arteries (1.0 mm in diameter) are seen in those patients with tetralogy of Fallot and pulmonary atresia. That even very small arteries reflect underfilling because of severe outflow tract obstruction is supported by results of surgical repair of tetralogy of Fallot in the first months of life. Multiple diffuse caliber abnormalities, arterial stenoses, the so-called arborization abnormalities, can be evident in the patient with tetralogy of Fallot and a perforate outflow tract, but these are much more common in the patient with pulmonary atresia and multiple aortopulmonary collaterals (see Chapter 21). Left pulmonary stenosis at the site of ductal insertion has been observed with increasing frequency in patients with tetralogy of Fallot, although the initial observations were in patients with pulmonary atresia and ventricular septal defect.[67,68,70,80,80A,81,88] Despite perforate continuity of the right ventricular outflow tract with the main pulmonary trunk, the right and left pulmonary arteries may be nonconfluent (Figs. 20-10 through 20-13). One pulmonary artery, usually the left may originate from the ascending aorta, or may have a ductal origin.[62,65,68,70,75,76,78,82] Significant naturally occurring multiple aortopulmonary collaterals are uncommon in tetralogy of Fallot with confluent pulmonary arteries, but we and others have described their coexistence in

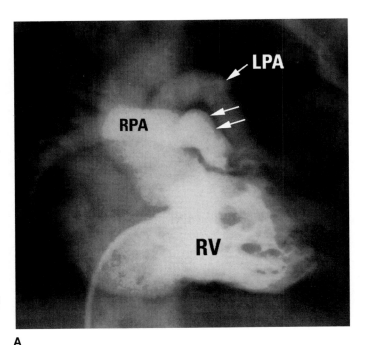

A

Fig. 20-13: Nonconfluent pulmonary arteries in tetralogy of Fallot with an aortic origin of the left pulmonary artery.
A: A disparity in opacification between the right and left pulmonary arteries is seen on the frontal right ventriculogram; the left pulmonary artery does not seem to have its normal origin from the main pulmonary trunk (arrows). *(figure continues)*

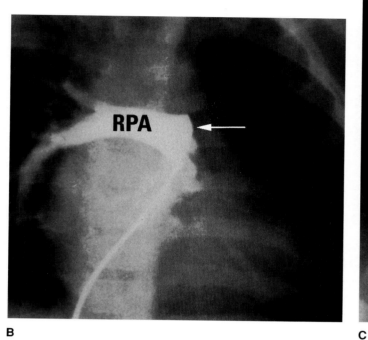

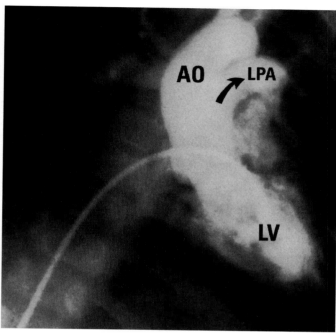

B

C

D

Fig. 20-13: *(continued)*
B: Selective injection in the main pulmonary trunk in the frontal projection confirms the 'absent' left pulmonary artery. **C:** The left ventriculogram demonstrates the proximal aortic origin of the left pulmonary artery (see also Chapter 22, Fig. 22-9). **D-F:** A different patient with tetralogy of Fallot and ascending aortic origin of the left pulmonary artery. **D and E:** Two frames from a frontal right ventriculogram demonstrates the infundibular obstruction and the white arrow indicates the anticipated position of the left pulmonary artery; **F:** The frontal aortogram shows the right-sided aortic arch, and the slightly narrowed (arrow) ascending aortic origin of the left pulmonary artery. *(figure continues)*

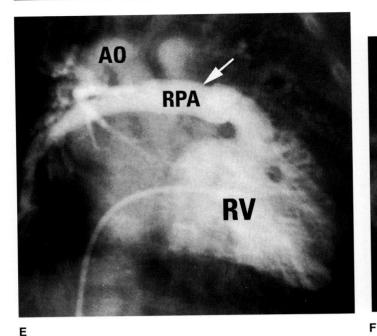

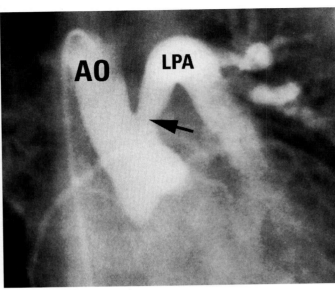

E

F

Fig. 20-13 *(continued)*

classic tetralogy as well as in the absent pulmonary valve variant (see Chapter 22).[62,74,84,89] Origin of the left pulmonary artery from the right pulmonary artery (so-called pulmonary sling) has been seen in the patient with tetralogy of Fallot (see also Chapter 19).[80,83] This may result in tracheal obstruction. The hypoge-

netic right lung complex with right pulmonary artery hypoplasia and abnormal connection of the right pulmonary veins has been seen in the patient with tetralogy of Fallot. The pulmonary arteries may be distorted by surgically created shunts to augment pulmonary blood flow (Fig. 20-14).

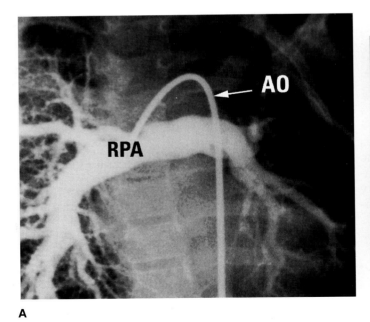

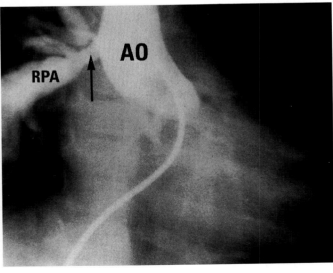

A

B

Fig. 20-14: The pulmonary arteries may be distorted by an arterial shunt.
A: An excellent Waterston shunt without significant distortion. **B:** Significant stenosis of the right pulmonary artery (arrow) from the Waterston shunt. *(figure continues)*

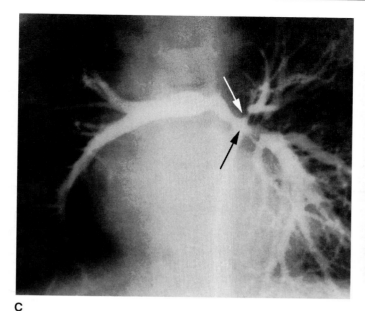

C

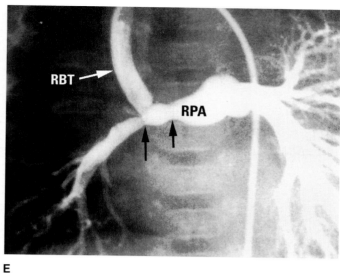

E

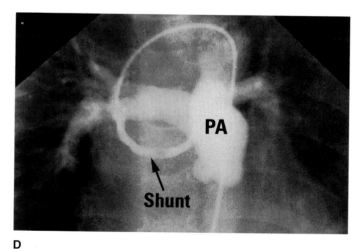

D

Fig. 20-14: *(continued)*
C: Significant left pulmonary artery stenoses (arrows) from a Potts' shunt. **D:** A central Goretex shunt promoted excellent growth of the pulmonary arteries. **E:** Mild stenosis (arrows) of the right pulmonary artery after a modified Blalock-Taussig shunt.

The Left Ventricle and Aortic Valve

The left ventricle is usually of normal thickness and size in tetralogy of Fallot, although uncommonly it is considered hypoplastic.[5,7,8,13,19] In those patients with severe forms of tetralogy of Fallot, almost always nonshunted, the left ventricular end-diastolic volume is normal or somewhat small.[90–93] Rarely, the left ventricle end diastolic volume will be prohibitively small.[93] Abnormalities of left ventricular inflow including mitral stenosis and supravalvular stenosing mitral ring have been recognized in the patient with tetralogy of Fallot.[94,95] A bicuspid aortic valve, aortic valve stenosis, and aortic regurgitation have all been observed in the patient with tetralogy of Fallot.[96–98] Aortic regurgitation is uncommon in early infancy, developing later in adolescence or young adults, primarily in those with uncorrected tetralogy, perhaps reflecting progressive aortic annular dilatation.[19]

Left ventricular outflow tract obstruction has been observed prior to repair of tetralogy of Fallot, but, more commonly is seen postoperatively.[30,99,99a,99b,100] The mechanism of left ventricular outflow tract obstruction prior to repair has been related both to fibrous-fibromuscular obstruction, as well as to anomalous attachment of the mitral valve.[30,101]

The Aortic Arch and Arterial Duct

A left aortic arch is seen in about 75% of patients with tetralogy of Fallot, and in these patients the arch branching pattern is usually normal, although one should always exclude aberrant origin of the right subclavian artery.[5–8,13,14,18,19] Twenty-five percent of patients with tetralogy of Fallot will have a right-sided aortic arch (Figs. 20-4A, 20-4F, 20-9C, 20-9D, 20-10, and 20-11). In the patient with a right-sided aortic arch and an aberrant left subclavian artery, the anomalous subclavian artery almost always originates directly from the descending aorta, not from an aortic diverticulum (Fig. 20-15).[13,19,102,103] In classic tetralogy of Fallot, an arterial duct is usually present, but closes physio-

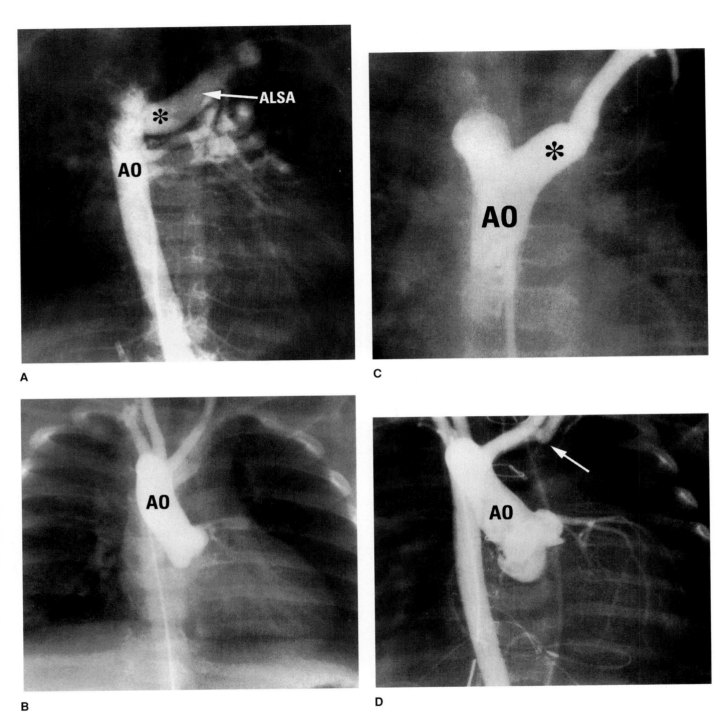

Fig. 20-15: Two patterns of right aortic arch with an aberrant left subclavian artery.
A: This patient has tetralogy of Fallot with absent pulmonary valve and aortopulmonary collaterals. The aortogram demonstrates the aberrant left subclavian artery (✱) not originating from a diverticulum. **B and C:** The left subclavian artery originates from a diverticulum. This patient does not have tetralogy of Fallot, but was investigated for the mucocutaneous lymph node syndrome of Kawasaki. B: Frontal aortogram showing the right aortic arch. C: The descending aorta shows the origin of the left subclavian artery from the diverticulum (✱). **D:** A right aortic arch with an an aberrant left subclavian artery in a patient with tetralogy of Fallot. A left ligamentum arteriosus closed a vascular ring. The tethered position (arrow) of the aberrant left subclavian artery is inferential of a left ductal ligamentum and this was confirmed at surgery.

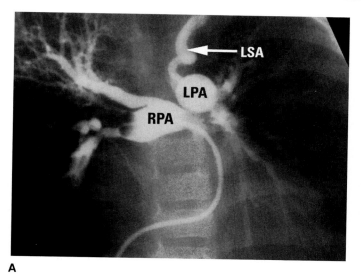

A

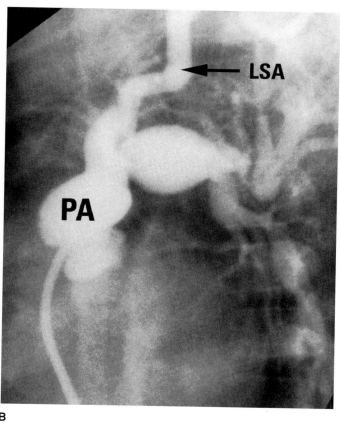

Fig. 20-16: Origin of the left subclavian artery from the left pulmonary artery in a patient with tetralogy of Fallot.
Selective pulmonary arteriograms in frontal (**A**) and lateral (**B**) projections show the left subclavian artery originating from the left pulmonary artery, with a stenosis at the origin of the left pulmonary artery.

B

logically as in the normal individual. The arterial duct may be absent in those patients whose pulmonary arterial supply is mediated by aortopulmonary collaterals (see Chapter 21), or in those patients with so-called absent pulmonary valve (see Chapter 22). The left subclavian artery may be isolated from its normal aortic arch origin, having instead its origin from the left pulmonary artery (Fig. 20-16).[103–105] With closure of the left arterial duct the left subclavian artery will be isolated, filling from a left vertebral steal. Bilateral arterial ducts have been diagnosed in the patient with tetralogy of Fallot.[103–108] Isolation of the right subclavian artery is far less common than isolation of the left subclavian artery.[108a] Rarely coarctation of the aorta or interruption of the aortic arch have been described in the patient with tetralogy of Fallot.[109–112a] A cervical aortic arch, double aortic arch, vascular ring with and without bronchial compression have all been observed in the patient with tetralogy of Fallot (Fig. 20-8).[113–117] The rotation of the aortic root is responsible for the abnormal orientation of the aortic sinus and coronary artery course seen on aortograms in patients with tetralogy of Fallot (Fig. 20-17). Thus, one should be cautious in depicting the coronary artery pattern in tetralogy of Fallot and should take this abnormal orientation into consideration.

The Coronary Arteries

Coronary artery anomalies assume importance in tetralogy of Fallot because of their potential for interruption or damage at the time of right ventriculotomy.[5–8,13,14,19,118–137] Coronary artery anomalies are not uncommon in patients with tetralogy of Fallot (Figs. 20-18 and Fig. 20-19). The most common abnormality complicating repair of tetralogy of Fallot is origin of the left anterior descending coronary artery from the right coronary artery, occurring in about 5% of patients.[13] In this situation, the anterior descending coronary artery crosses the right ventricular outflow tract a variable distance from the pulmonary valve. We have seen an accessory anterior descending originating from the right coronary artery in about 2.5% of patients with tetralogy of Fallot. Less common are instances of a single right or left coronary artery, anomalous origin of the left coronary artery or the anterior descending coronary artery from the main pulmonary trunk, origin of both coronary arteries from the pulmonary trunk; or multiple coronary artery-cameral fistulae (Fig. 20-20).[42,128] In the rare variant of tetralogy of Fallot with infundibuloarterial inversion, the stenotic pulmonary outflow tract is to the right of the aorta. Thus, the right coronary artery must cross

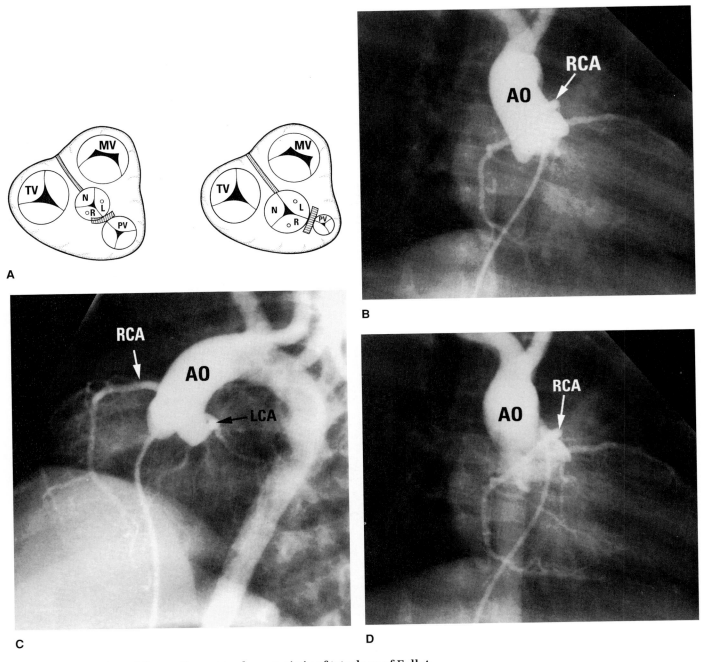

Fig. 20-17: Rotation of the aortic root is characteristic of tetralogy of Fallot.
A: Diagram shows rotation of aortic root typical of tetralogy of Fallot; left-hand panel, normal; right-hand panel, tetralogy of Fallot; **B and C:** Two frames from right anterior oblique aortogram. The right coronary sinus of the aortic valve locates more anteriorly and to the left than the left coronary sinus in this projection. Thus, the right coronary artery has an unusual sharp hair-pin turn after its origin from the right coronary sinus. This abnormal orientation of the aortic root and sinuses is commonly seen in tetralogy of Fallot because of so called "dextroposition" or "dextrorotation" of the aorta. Normally, in this projection, the right and left coronary sinuses should be superimposed on each other. **D:** Long axial aortogram also shows an abnormal orientation of the aortic sinuses. The right coronary sinus together with its right coronary artery is projected posteriorly, relative to the non-coronary sinus that locates more anteriorly than that seen in normal heart in this long axial oblique view.

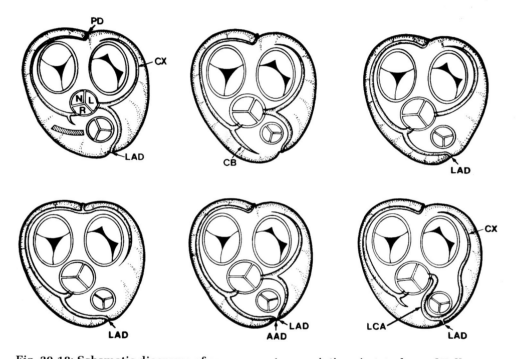

Fig. 20-18: Schematic diagrams of coronary artery variations in tetralogy of Fallot.

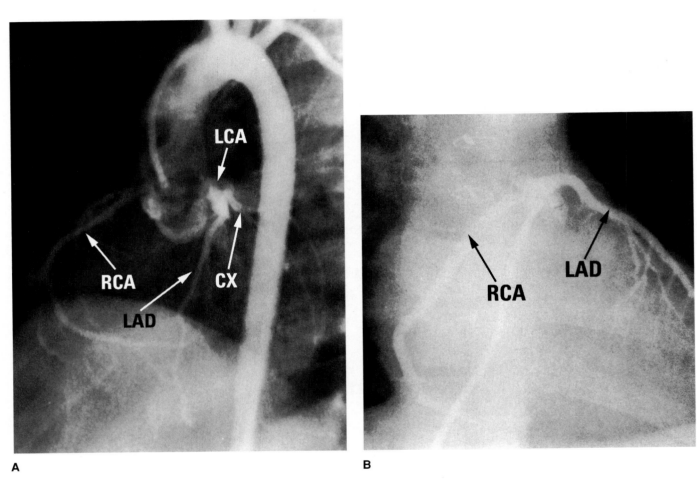

Fig. 20-19: Angiographic findings of coronary artery variations in tetralogy of Fallot.
A: Long axial oblique aortogram shows normal distribution of coronary arteries in a patient with tetralogy of Fallot. **B and C:** Anterior descending coronary artery from right coronary artery. Selective injection into right coronary artery opacifies the right coronary artery proper and the left anterior descending artery crossing the right ventricular outflow tract. **D and E:** Single right coronary artery: ascending aortogram. **D:** RAO projection shows a vessel arising from RCA and coursing to supply anterior myocardium with a cranial loop to its proximal course (arrowheads). **E:** LAO projection demonstrates this vessel to have an RV free wall course (great arteries nearly side by side). The long left main branches into a modest-sized LAD and a small circumflex.

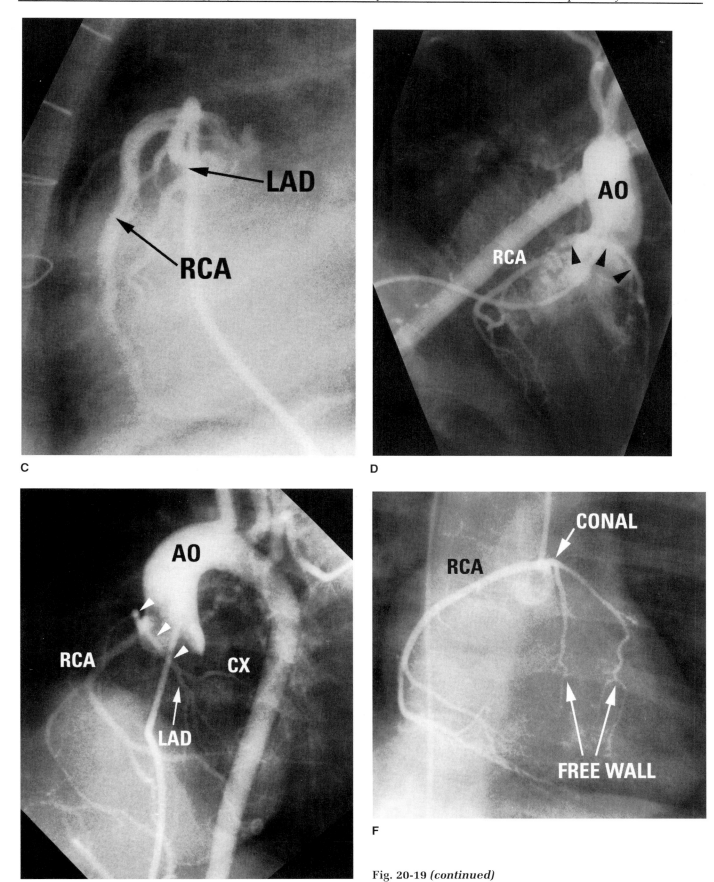

Fig. 20-19 *(continued)*

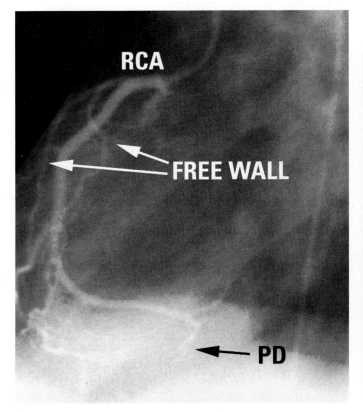

G

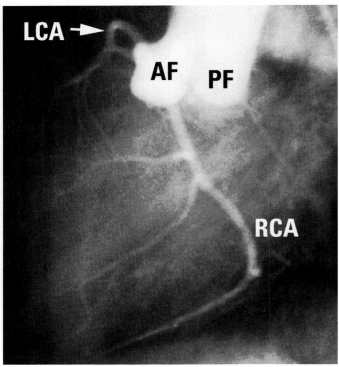

I

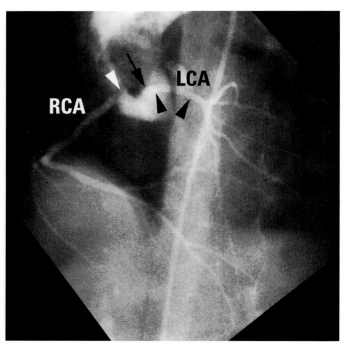

H

Fig. 20-19: *(continued)*
F and G: Right ventricular free wall supply from right coronary artery. Selective right coronary injection. **F:** The RAO projection demonstrates a very good sized RCA but shows a proximal branch extending across the RV free wall. **G:** These free-wall branches never come close to the plane of the interventricular septum as indicated by the course of the posterior descending (PD), and thus do not represent vessels extending to the anterior interventricular groove to supply high anterior septum which would complicate tetralogy repair. **H and I:** Anomalous left coronary artery from anterior facing sinus. Retrograde aortogram. **H:** Shallow LAO projection shows two coronaries arising from the anterior facing sinus. The RCA arises normally (white arrowhead). The anomalous LCA arises separately (black arrow) and has a proximal cranial course (black arrowheads). **I:** With the great arteries side by side, this end-on LCA is well seen (arrow) remaining anterior and thus having an RV free wall course. No vessel arises from the posterior facing sinus. The RCA is dominant. *(figure continues)*

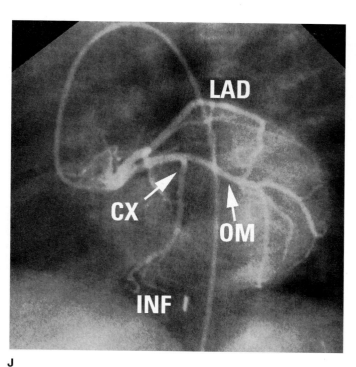

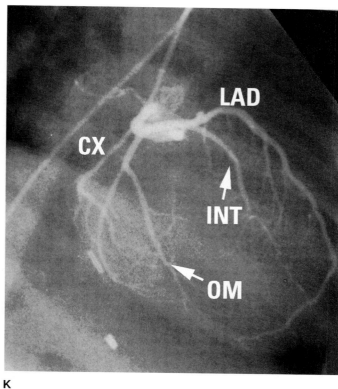

J

K

Fig. 20-19: *(continued)*
J and K: Dominant left coronary artery with unusual ventricular orientation. **J:** Left ventriculogram in shallow LAO projection demonstrates the LV in profile, rotated leftward by the enlarged RV. Note the markedly elevated LV apex. **K:** Selective LCA injection. RAO projection. All the LV and septal myocardium is supplied by branches of LCA.

the right ventricular outflow tract to reach the right atrioventricular groove, positioning this artery in a disadvantageous way.[22a-22c] Sharma and colleagues addressed collateral arteries originating from the coronary arteries in tetralogy of Fallot.[137] Semiselective aortic root and some selective coronary angiographic studies were performed in 330 patients with tetralogy of Fallot over a period of 4 years. Collateral vessels arising from the coronary arteries were found in 11 cases and a direct communication between the coronary artery and pulmonary arteries in one case (3.6%). Tetralogy of Fallot with anomalous origin of the right

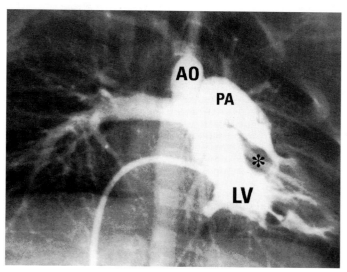

A

Fig. 20-20: Multiple coronary artery-cameral fistulae originating from both coronary arteries in a patient with tetralogy of Fallot.
A: Frontal right ventriculogram shows typical tetralogy anatomy with a right aortic arch. *(figure continues)*

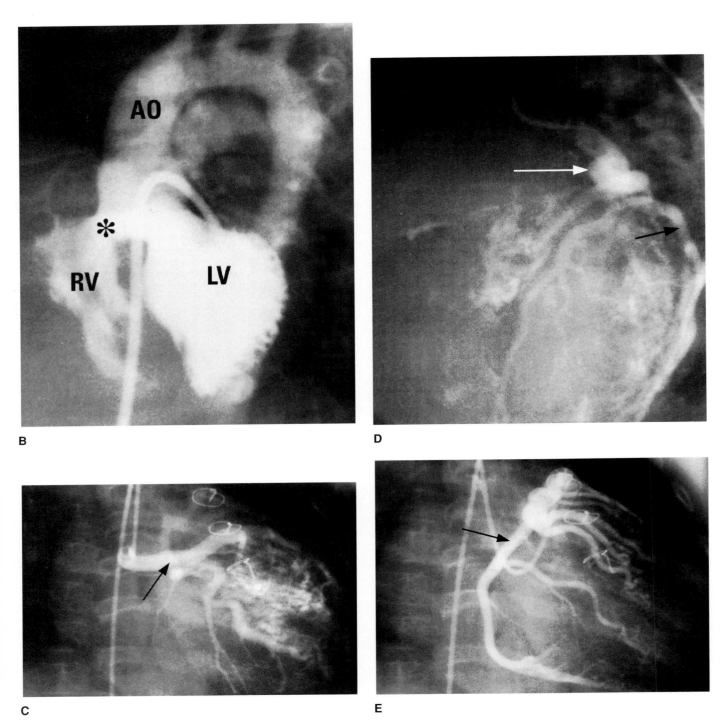

Fig. 20-20: *(continued)*
B: The long axial oblique left ventriculogram shows the large ventricular septal defect and the overriding aorta. **C through E:** Selective coronary arteriograms show coronary-cameral fistulae.

coronary artery has been described by Moss and colleagues.[137a] In this 8-year-old child, the right coronary artery did not have an aortic origin. Rather, it originated from the right anterior sinus of the pulmonary artery. Flow from the left coronary artery was to the right coronary artery and then into the main pulmonary artery, and this connection was the sole source of pulmonary blood flow. Among patients with pulmonary atresia and ventricular septal defect, a coronary artery-pulmonary artery communication may be the sole source of pulmonary blood supply (see Chapter 21).

Aortopulmonary Collateral Circulation

Small indirect aortopulmonary collaterals and enlarged bronchial arteries are easily identified in the older infant and child, reflecting increasing hypoxemia and polycythemia. It is uncommon to identify large direct aortopulmonary collateral vessels originating from the descending thoracic aorta in the patient with 'uncomplicated' tetralogy of Fallot, but like the observations of Ramsay and colleagues,[89] we have identified a number of such patients (Figs. 20-9 and 20-21) (see also Chapter 22, Figs. 22-6 and 22-7).

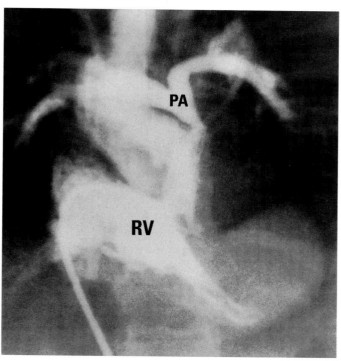

A

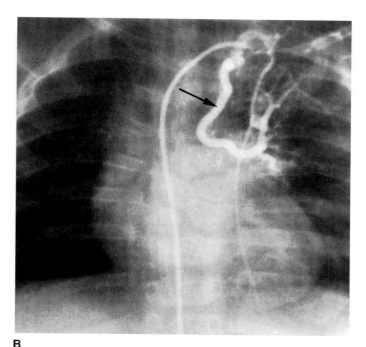

B

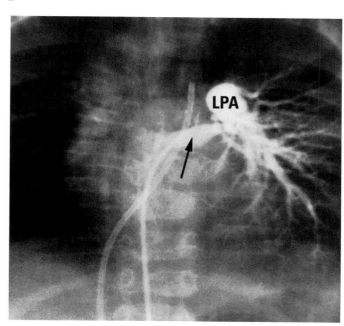

C

Fig. 20-21: Indirect and direct aortopulmonary collateral vessels in a patient with tetralogy of Fallot.
A: Frontal cranially-angled right ventriculogram demonstrates anatomy characteristic of tetralogy of Fallot. **B:** indirect aortopulmonary collateral originating from left subclavian artery. **C:** Direct aortopulmonary collateral originating from descending aorta and connecting with hilar left pulmonary artery.

Associated Anomalies

Associated anomalies are particularly common in tetralogy of Fallot, and these have been amply and widely catalogued. These include a patent ovale foramen or true atrial septal defect, the latter being found in about 5% of patients with tetralogy (designated by some pentalogy of Fallot); left superior vena cava with unroofed coronary sinus; anomalies of the tricuspid valve including Ebstein's anomaly, cleft, straddling and overriding, as well as tricuspid valve hypoplasia or stenosis; right ventricular hypoplasia; anomalies of pulmonary venous connections including partial and total anomalous pulmonary venous connections; mitral valve anomalies including isolated cleft; mitral stenosis and supravalvular stenosing mitral ring; multiple ventricular septal defects; atrioventricular septal defect, usually type C (see Chapter 5); left ventricular outflow tract obstruction; asymmetric septal hypertrophy double-outlet right ventricle; and aorticopulmonary window; omphalocele with cardiac diverticulum (Figs. 20-22, 20-23, and 20-24).[5,7,13,14,18,19,26,29,30,32,38,138–153a]

Imaging in Tetralogy of Fallot

The echocardiographic features of tetralogy of Fallot have been thoroughly reviewed, and there is now increasing experience with both palliation and repair based solely on echocardiographic examination.[7,14,19,46–51,62,91,94,99,150,154–165] We have summarized elsewhere those echocardiographic features permitting palliation without angiocardiography in our institution. We are still performing angiocardiography prior to reparative surgery for patients with tetralogy of Fallot. Hornberger and colleagues[165a] have documented fetal progression of tetralogy with forward pulmonary blood flow to pulmonary atresia, and they have also documented pulmonary artery and aortic growth in tetralogy of Fallot.

Angiocardiography in Tetralogy of Fallot

The angiocardiographic features of tetralogy of Fallot have been fully reviewed elsewhere.[7,18,19,29,30,35,42,59,62,64,88,89,106,119,120,124,126,129,134–137,149,150,152,166–185] The complete angiocardiographic imaging in tetralogy of Fallot requires biplane right ventricular angiocardiography (Figs. 20-4, 20-5, and 20-8); biplane left ventricular angiocardiography (Figs. 20-6 and 20-7); imaging of the pulmonary arteries (Figs. 20-9 through 20-14); and assessment of the coronary arteries (Figs. 20-18 through 20-20). In addition, the aorta should be imaged to exclude significant aortopulmonary collateral arteries that could compromise cardiopulmonary bypass (Figs. 20-9 and 20-21).

Right ventricular angiocardiography will differentiate the anatomy of tetralogy of Fallot from anomalous bundles of the right ventricle, realizing that these diag-

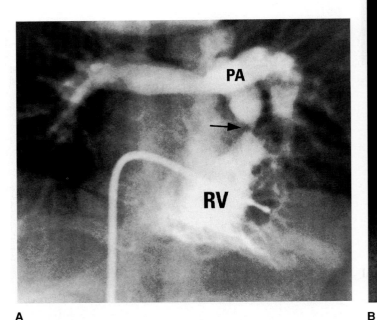

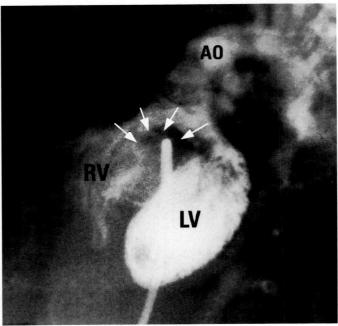

A **B**

Fig. 20-22: Tetralogy of Fallot with complete form of atrioventricular septal defect.
A: Frontal right ventriculogram shows tetralogy of Fallot anatomy. **B:** Long axial oblique left ventriculogram shows a common atrioventricular orifice (arrows) (see also Chapter 5, Figs. 5-41 and 5–42).

noses are not mutually exclusive.(Figs. 20-4, 20-5, and 20-8).[19,32,149,150,181] Prior to complete repair it is important to image both ventricles, the aortic root (to define the origin and epicardial distribution of the coronary arteries) (Figs. 20-18 through 20-20) and aortic arch. It may be important to image the descending thoracic aorta to define the character of the aortopulmonary collateral circulation in those uncommon situations where tetralogy and major direct aortopulmonary collaterals are both present (Figs. 20-9 and 20-21).

The right ventriculogram should be filmed using biplane angiocardiography (Figs. 20-4, 20-5, and 20-8). Caudocranial angulation should image the right ventricle and pulmonary arteries. Cranially angulated pulmonary arteriography may be necessary if the right ventriculogram does not completely define the distribution and caliber of the pulmonary arteries (Figs. 20-9 through 20-14). If the patient has had a previous palliative shunt it is essential to obtain appropriate hemodynamic recordings to exclude pulmonary artery hypertension. The pulmonary artery can be entered from the

right ventricle, or through the previously constructed pulmonary artery anastomosis (Fig. 20-14). If the pulmonary artery can not be entered, recording of right and left pulmonary vein wedge pressures will give important information about the status of the pulmonary vascular bed. Right-to-left shunting at the ventricular level and subsequent opacification of the ascending aorta may obscure some of the pulmonary arteries. It is always important to follow the flow of contrast material through the lungs, both to define normal pulmonary venous connections, as well as to exclude asymmetric pulmonary venous flow which could indicate stenosis of one or more individual pulmonary veins (see Chapter 24). The classic scimitar syndrome has been identified in the patient with tetralogy of Fallot. The hypoplastic pulmonary artery is particularly predisposed to distortion by a systemic-to-pulmonary artery anastomosis; a Waterston-Cooley shunt between the ascending aorta and right pulmonary artery, or from the Potts' shunt between the left pulmonary artery and the descending thoracic aorta. Soto and Pacifico[42] advocate

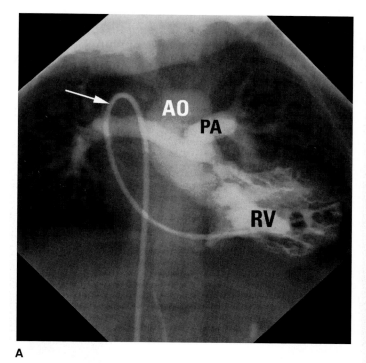

A

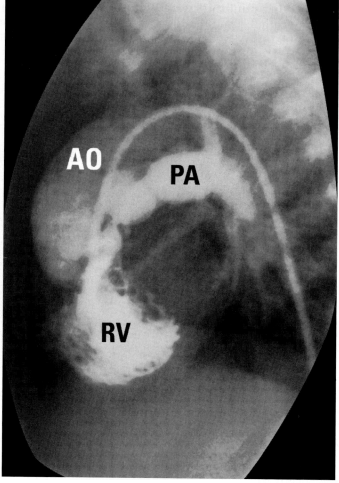

B

Fig. 20-23: Tetralogy of Fallot with an azygous continuation of the right inferior caval vein and presumed left atrial isomerism.
A and B: Frontal and lateral right ventriculograms with catheter advanced via the azygous continuation of the right inferior caval vein (arrow) show severe tetralogy of Fallot.

the long axial view as well as standard frontal, lateral, or left anterior oblique projections to image the pulmonary arteries.

Left ventriculography in the long axial oblique projections will demonstrate the perimembraneous-outlet ventricular septal defect and the degree of aortic override (Fig. 20-6). The right oblique will demonstrate the displaced infundibular septum and will profile any anterior trabecular ventricular septal defects. The severity of the pulmonary outflow tract obstruction is often nicely visualized in this projection. Also this view is very helpful in demonstrating the absence or profound attenuation of the infundibular septum in the patient with the subarterial ventricular septal defect in tetralogy of Fallot (Figs. 20-5 and 20-6). A left ventricular angiocardiogram using the hepatoclavicular projection may be necessary to exclude associated inlet and posterior muscular ventricular septal defects. The degree of aortic overriding is best obtained from either the right or left ventriculogram performed in the long axial oblique projection.

The assessment of the coronary arteries is particularly important in the preoperative assessment of the patient with tetralogy of Fallot, and this can be accomplished in a number of ways. If the neonate or young infant is catheterized, balloon occlusion via the venous route can ideally demonstrate the coronary arteries.

Aortography performed in the aortic root, selective coronary arteriography, orifice view coronary angiography have all been advocated as a methodology to define the origin and epicardial distribution of the coronary arteries in tetralogy of Fallot. From its anomalous origin from the right coronary artery, the left anterior descending coronary artery crosses the right ventricular outflow tract over its anterior wall, coursing towards the anterior interventricular sulcus. Soto and Pacifico caution us that this anomaly must not be confused with the frequent enlargement of the first right marginal artery (the conus artery) which usually takes a peculiar left position, supplying the anterior wall of the right ventricular infundibulum. In about 4% of patients with tetralogy of Fallot, one can identify a single coronary artery, either a single right or left coronary artery. If there is any concern about the origin and epicardial distribution of the coronary arteries, then selective coronary arteriography should be performed. Aortic root angiography will demonstrate (or more likely exclude) the rare association with an aorticopulmonary septal defect, and should demonstrate as well any collateral circulation between the coronary arteries and bronchopulmonary circulation. Aortography performed in the descending thoracic aorta should show the presence and extent of any significant direct aortopulmonary collaterals. It may be necessary to selectively

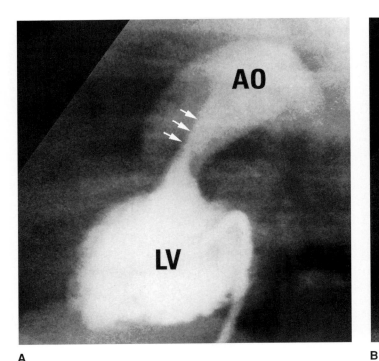

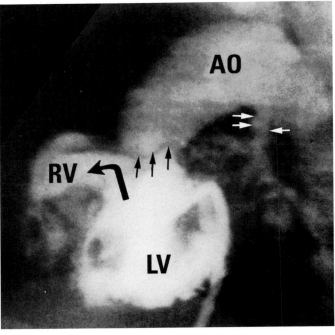

A   **B**

Fig. 20-24: Severe aortic stenosis in a patient with pulmonary atresia, a ventricular septal defect, and a left-sided arterial duct supplying confluent pulmonary arteries.
A: Early frame from lateral left ventriculogram shows jetting (arrows) of contrast medium through the stenotic aortic valve. **B:** A slightly later frame shows the left-to-right shunting at ventricular level (curved arrow), the thickened aortic valve (black arrows) and the narrowed arterial duct (white arrows).

inject either the right or left subclavian artery to define the presence and extent of so-called indirect aortopulmonary collaterals (see Chapter 21) (Fig. 20-21).

Transcatheter Therapy: Balloon Dilation of the Right Ventricular Outflow Tract in Tetralogy of Fallot

The first reported attempts to relieve outflow tract obstruction in the setting of Fallot's tetralogy was by Labadidi and colleagues in 1983.[186,187] Concern over induced avulsion of the pulmonary valve leaflets after dilation damped the initial enthusiasm for this form of palliation. However, a number of subsequent investigations into the clinical impact of this form of intervention,[188–199] has established this approach as effective in providing improvement in pulmonary blood flow, such that early surgical palliation can be avoided or postponed.

The dilation is approached in the same manner as that for critical pulmonary valve stenosis (with intact ventricular septum) in the newborn. Initial angiography is best accomplished in the right ventricle, in the cranial projection (about 25° in the anteroposterior tube) and 10° left anterior oblique. This will outline the position of the right ventricular outflow tract in the left-right orientation and identify any additional pulmonary arterial lesions (proximal branch hypoplasia, distal pulmonary artery stenosis) which may be addressed with angioplasty at the same procedure. Due to intracardiac shunting and the more horizontal orientation of the valve and outflow tract, it is at times difficult to outline the details of the valve annulus, from this projection. The valve leaflets and annular dimensions however, can be visualized from the lateral projection. Selective injections into the right ventricular outflow tract or main pulmonary artery can also detail such anatomic information. After the orientation, position and dimensions of the annulus are identified, a right coronary artery catheter can be used to cross the valve, with a guide wire. Frequently, due to the rightward and anterior orientation of the aorta, the catheter will, with clockwise rotation, enter the aorta. In this situation, counterclockwise catheter rotation will position the catheter more anterosuperiorly into the right ventricular outflow tract, allowing cannulation of the infundibulum, and crossing of the pulmonary valve. If the arterial duct is patent, the wire can be positioned in the aorta to allow better traction of the balloon across the outflow tract and valve. Complications unique to this catheterization procedure include pulmonary artery tears and annular tears with cardiac tamponade.[197,200] Temporary arterial desaturation occurs during balloon inflation, but generally rapidly recovers. Maintenance of arterial blood pressure and circulating blood volume helps modify the extent of right to left shunting.[192] The use of general anesthesia during the procedure may give better overall procedural control and patient stability.

The impact on the clinical course has been encouraging with a majority of patients attaining and maintaining an increase in arterial oxygen saturation and avoiding a surgical aortopulmonary shunt. Alterations in outflow tract morphology have been more variable, ranging from no change in annular dimensions or pulmonary artery sizes[195] to significant improvements[193,194,196] in follow-up. Similarly, the need for transannular patch outflow tract reconstruction also varied, among the series reported. There appears to be no relation with outcome (ie, annular or pulmonary artery growth) with dilating balloon diameter or initial anatomic substrate. With such varied results, institutional prerogatives and operator related variables have a strong impact on outcome results. The application of such techniques to a wide variety of pulmonary outflow tract obstruction lesions can in many avoid surgical palliation (shunts), if the patient is not a candidate for primary repair.

References

1. Fallot A. Contribution a l'anatomie pathologique de la maladie bleue (cyanose cardiaque). *Marseille Med* 1888; 25:377–403.
2. Anderson RH,. Becker AE. Etienne-Louis Arthur Fallot and his tetralogy: A new translation of Fallot's summary and a modern reassessment of this anomaly. *Eur J Cardiothorac Surg* 1990;4:229–232.
3. Van Praagh R. Etienne-Louis Arthur Fallot and his tetralogy: A new translation of Fallot's summary and a modern reassessment of this anomaly. *Eur J Cardiothorac Surg* 1989;3:381–386.
4. Allwork SP. Tetralogy of Fallot: The centenary of the name. A new translation of the first of Fallot's papers. *Eur J Cardiothorac Surg* 1988;2:386–392.
5. Anderson RH, Allwork SP, Ho SY, Lenox CC, Zuberbuh-ler JR. Surgical anatomy of tetralogy of Fallot. *J Thorac Cardiovasc Surg* 1981;81:887–896.
6. Anderson RH, Becker AE. The surgical anatomy of Fallot's tetralogy. *The Current Status of Cardiac Surgery.* Lancaster: MTP; 1975, pp. 11–19.
7. Anderson RH, Macartney FJ, Shinebourne EA, Tynan M. *Paediatric Cardiology.* Edinburgh: Churchill Livingstone; 1987, pp. 765–798.
8. Anderson RH, Tynan M. Tetralogy of Fallot—A centennial review. *Int J Cardiol* 1988;21:219–232.
9. Bertranou EG, Blackstone EH, Hazelrig JB, Turner ME Jr, Kirklin JW. Life expectancy without surgery in tetralogy of Fallot. *Am J Cardiol* 1978;42:458–466.
10. Blalock A, Taussig HB. The surgical treatment of malformations of the heart in which there is pulmonary stenosis or pulmonary atresia. *JAMA* 1945;128: 189–192.

11. Castaneda AR. Repair of tetralogy of Fallot. *Curr Opin Cardiol* 1987;2:847–853.

12. Castaneda AR. Tetralogy of Fallot: Advantages of early repair. *Saudi Heart Bull* 1989;1:24–26.

13. Kirklin JW, Barratt-Boyes BG. *Cardiac Surgery.* Second edition. New York: Churchill Livingstone; 1993, pp. 861–1012

14. Fyler DC. Tetralogy of Fallot. In: Fyler DC, ed. *Nadas' Pediatric Cardiology.* St. Louis: Mosby Year Book Inc.; 1992, pp. 471–491.

15. Di Donato RM, Jonas RA, Lang P, Rome JJ, Mayer JE Jr, Castaneda AR. Neonatal repair of tetralogy of Fallot with and without pulmonary atresia. *J Thorac Cardiovasc Surg* 1991;101:126–131.

16. Kirklin JW, Blackstone E, Kirklin JK, Pacifico AD, Aramendi J, Bargeron Jr LM. Surgical results and protocols in the spectrum of tetralogy of Fallot. *Ann Surg* 1983; 198:251–261.

17. Kirklin JW, Blackstone EH, Pacifico AD, Kirklin JK, Bargeron LM Jr. Risk factors of early and late failure after repair of tetralogy of Fallot, and their neutralization. *Thorac Cardiovasc Surg* 1984;32:208–214.

18. Mair DD, Edwards WD, Hagler DJ, Julsrud PR, Puga FJ. Tetralogy of Fallot and pulmonary atresia with ventricular septal defect. In: Moller JH, Neal WA, eds. *Fetal, Neonatal, and Infant Cardiac Disease.* Norwalk, CT: Appleton and Lange; 1989, pp. 639–669.

19. Zuberbuhler JR. Tetralogy of Fallot. In: Emmanouilides GC, Allen HD, Riemenschneider TA, Gutgesell HP, eds. *Moss and Adams' Heart Disease in Infants, Children, and Adolescents. Including the Fetus and Young Adult.* Baltimore: Williams and Wilkins; 1995, pp. 998–1018.

20. Fyler DC. Report of the New England Regional Infant Cardiac Program. *Pediatrics* 1980;65(suppl):376–461.

21. Ferencz C, Rubin JD, McCarter RJ, Brenner JI, Neill CA, Perry LW, Hepner SI, Downing JW. Congenital heart disease: Prevalence at livebirth. The Baltimore-Washington Infant Study. *Am J Epidemiol* 1985;121:31–36.

22. Grabitz RG, Joffres MR, Collins-Nakai RL. Congenital heart disease: Incidence in the first year of life. The Alberta Heritage Pediatric Cardiology Program. *Am J Epidemiol* 1988;128:381–388.

22a. Foran RB, Belcourt C, Nanton MA, Murphy DA, Weinberg AG, Liebman J, Castaneda AR, Van Praagh R. Isolated infundibuloarterial inversion (S,D,I): A newly recognized form of congenital heart disease. *Am Heart J* 1988;116:1337–1350.

22b. Santini F, Jonas RA, Sanders SP, Van Praagh R. Tetralogy of Fallot {S,D, I}: Succesful repair without a conduit. *Ann Thorac Surg* 1995;59:747–749.

22c. Anderson RH. What is meant by Tetralogy of Fallot {S, D, I}?. *Ann Thorac Surg* 1995;59:562–564.

23. Becker AE, Connor M, Anderson RH. Tetralogy of Fallot: A morphometric and geometric study. *Am J Cardiol* 1975;35:402–412.

23a. Geva T, Ayres NA, Pac FA, Pignatelli R. Quantitative morphometric analysis of progressive infundibular obstruction in tetralogy of Fallot. A prospective longitudinal echocardiographic study. *Circulation* 1995;92: 886–892.

24. Dickinson DF, Wilkinson JL, Smith A, Hamilton DI, Anderson RH. Variations in the morphology of the ventricular septal defect and disposition of the atrioventricular conduction tissues in tetralogy of Fallot. *Thorac Cardiovasc Surg* 1982;5:243–249.

25. Goor DA, Lillehei CW, Edwards JE. Ventricular septal defects and pulmonic stenosis with and without dex-

troposition. Anatomic features and embryologic implications. *Chest* 1971;60:117–128.

26. Lev M and Eckner FAO. The pathologic anatomy of tetralogy of Fallot and its variants. *Dis Chest* 1964;45: 251–261.

27. Lev M, Rimoldi JA, Rowlatt UF. The quantitative anatomy of cyanotic tetralogy of Fallot. *Circulation* 1964;30:531–538.

28. Rosenquist GC, Sweeney LJ, Stemple DR, Christianson SD, Rowe RD. Ventricular septal defect in tetralogy of Fallot. *Am J Cardiol* 1973;31:749–754.

29. Soto B, Pacifico AD, Ceballos R, Bargeron LM Jr. Tetralogy of Fallot: An angiographic-pathologic correlative study. *Circulation* 1981;64:558–566.

30. Van Praagh R, Corwin RD, Dahlquist E, Freedom RM, Matioli L, Nebesar RA. Tetralogy of Fallot with severe left ventricular outflow tract obstruction due to anomalous attachment of the mitral valve to the ventricular septum. *Am J Cardiol* 1970;26:95–101.

31. Van Praagh R, Van Praagh S, Nebesar RA, Muster AJ, Sinha SN, Paul MH. Tetralogy of Fallot: Underdevelopment of the pulmonary infundibulum and its sequelae. *Am J Cardiol* 1970;26:25–33.

32. Daliento L, Grisolia EF, Frescura C, Thiene G. Anomalous muscle bundle of the sub-pulmonary outflow in tetralogy of Fallot. *Int J Cardiol* 1984;6:547–550.

33. Ando M. Subpulmonary ventricular septal defect with pulmonary stenosis (letter to the editor). *Circulation* 1974;50:412.

34. Neirotti R, Galindez E, Kreutzer G, Coronel AR, Pedrini M, Becu L. Tetralogy of Fallot with sub-pulmonary ventricular septal defect. *Ann Thorac Surg* 1978;25:51–56.

35. Vargas FJ, Kreutzer GO, Pedrini M, Capelli H, Rodriguez Coronel A. Tetralogy of Fallot with subarterial ventricular septal defect. Diagnostic and surgical considerations. *J Thorac Cardiovasc Surg* 1986;92:908–912.

36. Capelli H, Somerville J. Atypical Fallot's Tetralogy with doubly committed subarterial ventricular septal defect. *Am J Cardiol* 1983;51:282–285.

36a. Okita Y, Miki S, Ueda Y, Tahata T, Sakai T, Matsuyama K, Matsumura M, Tamura T. Early and late results of repair of tetralogy of Fallot with subarterial ventricular septal defect. A comparative evaluation of tetralogy with perimembranous ventricular septal defect. *J Thorac Cardiovasc Surg* 1995;110:180–185.

37. Howell CE, Ho SY, Anderson RH, Eliott MJ. Variations within the fibrous skeleton and ventricular outflow tracts in tetralogy of Fallot. *Ann Thorac Surg* 1990;50: 450–457.

38. Nagao GI, Daoud GI, McAdams AJ, Scwartz DC, Kaplan S. Cardiovascular anomalies associated with tetralogy of Fallot. *Am J Cardiol* 1967;20:206–211.

39. Rao BNS, Anderson RC, Edwards JE. Anatomic variations in the tetralogy of Fallot. *Am Heart J* 1971;81: 361–371.

40. Muster AJ, Zales VR, Ilbawi MN, Backer CL, Duffy CE, Mavroudis C. Biventricular repair of hypoplastic right ventricle assisted by pulsatile bidirectional cavopulmonary anastomosis. *J Thorac Cardiovasc Surg* 1993; 105:112–119.

41. Garcia OL, Gelband H, Tamer DF, Fojaco RM. Exclusive origin of both coronary arteries from a hypoplastic right ventricle complicating an extreme tetralogy of Fallot: Lethal myocardial infarction following a palliative shunt. *Am Heart J* 1988;115:198–201.

42. Soto B, Pacifico AD. Tetralogy of Fallot. In: *Angiocar-*

diography in Congenital Heart Malformations. Mt. Kisco, NY: Futura Publishing Company, Inc; 1990, pp. 353–375.

43. Suzuki A, Ho SY, Anderson RH, Deanfield JE. Further morphologic studies on tetralogy of Fallot, with particular emphasis on the prevalence and structure of the membranous flap. *J Thorac Cardiovasc Surg* 1990;99: 528–535.

44. Hoffman JIE, Rudolph AM, Nadas AS, Gross RE. Pulmonic stenosis, ventricular septal defect and right ventricular pressure above systemic level. *Circulation* 1960; 22:405–411.

44a. Neufeld HN, McGoon DC, DuShane JW, Edwards JE. Tetralogy of Fallot with anomalous tricuspid valve simulating pulmonary stenosis with intact septum. *Circulation* 1960;22:1083–1086.

45. Faggian G, Frescura C, Thiene G, Bortolotti U, Mazzucco A, Anderson RH. Accessory tricuspid valve tissue causing obstruction of the ventricular septal defect in tetralogy of Fallot. *Circulation* 1983;49:324–327.

46. Monterroso J, Fonseca MC, Cunha D, Ramalhao C. Tetralogy of Fallot with accessory tricuspid valve tissue obstructing the ventricular septal defect. The need of its early recognition by noninvasive methods. *Acta Cardiol* 1991;46:33–37.

47. Flanagan MF, Foran RB, Van Praagh R, Jonas R, Sanders SP. Tetralogy of Fallot with obstruction of the ventricular septal defect: Spectrum of echocardiographic findings. *J Am Coll Cardiol* 1988;11:386–395.

48. Glaser J, Rosenmann D, Balkin J, Zion MM. Acquired obstruction of the ventricular septal defect in tetralogy of Fallot. *Cardiology* 1989;76:309–311.

49. Johnson GL, O'Connor WN, Verble SM, Cottrill CM, Noonan JA. Ventricular septal defect with mobile tricuspid valve pouch mimicking tetralogy of Fallot. *Pediatr Cardiol* 1986;7:53–56.

50. Musewe NN, Smallhorn JF, Moes CAF, Freedom RM, Trusler GA. Echocardiographic evaluation of obstructive mechanism of tetralogy of Fallot with restrictive ventricular septal defect. *Am J Cardiol* 1988;61:664–668.

51. Isaaz K, Cloez JL, Marcon F, Worms AM, Pernod C. Is the aorta truly dextroposed in tetralogy of Fallot? A two-dimensional echocardiographic answer. *Circulation* 1986; 73:892–899.

52. Edwards WD. Double-outlet right ventricle and tetralogy of Fallot: Two distinct but not mutually exclusive entities. *J Thorac Cardiovasc Surg* 1981;82:418–422.

53. Lev M, Bharati S, Meng CCL, Liberthson RR, Paul NH, Idriss F. A concept of double-outlet right ventricle. *J Thorac Cardiovasc Surg* 1972;64:271–281.

54. Rao BNS, Edwards JE. Conditions simulating the tetralogy of Fallot. *Circulation* 1974;49:173–178.

55. Anderson RH, Devine WA, del Nido P. The surgical anatomy of tetralogy of Fallot with pulmonary atresia rather than pulmonary stenosis. *J Card Surg* 1991; 6:41–59.

56. Bharati S, Paul MH, Idriss FS, Potkin RT, Lev M. The surgical anatomy of pulmonary atresia with ventricular septal defect: Pseudotruncus. *J Thorac Cardiovasc Surg* 1975;69:713–721.

57. Davis GD, Fulton RE, Ritter DG, Mair DD, McGoon DC. Congenital pulmonary atresia with ventricular septal defect: Angiographic and surgical correlates. *Radiology* 1978;128:133–144.

58. Macartney FJ, Haworth SG. Pulmonary Atresia with VSD: Investigation of pulmonary atresia with ventricu-

lar septal defect. In: Anderson RH, Macartney FJ, Shinebourne EA, Tynan M, eds. *Paediatric Cardiology.* Volume 5. Edinburgh: Churchill Livingstone; 1983, pp. 111–125.

59. Soto B, Pacifico AD, Luna RF, Bargeron LM Jr. A radiographic study of congenital pulmonary atresia with ventricular septal defect. *AJR* 1977;129:1027–1037.

60. Thiene G, Anderson RH. Pulmonary atesia with VSD: Anatomy. In: Anderson RH, Macartney FJ, Shinebourne EA, Tynan M, eds. *Paediatric Cardiology.* Volume 5. Edinburgh: Churchill Livingstone; 1983, pp. 81–101.

61. Thiene G, Bortolotti U, Gallucci V, Valente ML, Volta SD. Pulmonary atresia with ventricular septal defect. *Br Heart J* 1977;39:1223–1233.

62. Burrows PE, Freedom RM, Rabinovitch M, Moes CAF. The investigation of abnormal pulmonary arteries in congenital heart disease. *Radiol Clin North Am* 1985;23: 689–717.

63. Rabinovitch M, Herrera-DeLeon V, Castaneda AR, Reid L. Growth and development of the pulmonary vascular bed in patients with tetralogy of Fallot with or without pulmonary atresia. *Circulation* 1981;64:1234–1249.

64. Freedom RM, Pongiglione G, Williams WG, Trusler GA, Rowe RD. Palliative right ventricular outflow tract construction for patients with pulmonary atresia, ventricular septal defect, and hypoplastic pulmonary arteries. *J Thorac Cardiovasc Surg* 1983;86:24–36.

65. Presbitero P, Bull C, Haworth SG, De Leval MR. Absent or occult pulmonary artery. *Br Heart J* 1984;52: 178–185.

66. Matsuda H, Kuratani T, Shimizaki Y, Kadoba K, Kobayashi J, Ohtake S, Nakayama M, Nakada T. Deposition of collagen in the alveolar wall of lungs from patients with tetralogy of Fallot and pulmonary atresia with major aortopulmonary collateral arteries—an ultrastructural study. *Cardiol Young* 1994;4:277–284.

67. Elzenga NJ, Gittenberger-de Groot AC. The ductus arteriosus and stenoses of the pulmonary arteries in pulmonary atresia. *Int J Cardiol* 1986;11:195–208.

68. Judeikin R, Rheuban KS, Carpenter MA. Ductal origin of the left pulmonary artery in severe tetralogy of Fallot: Problems in management. *Pediatr Cardiol* 1984; 5:323–326.

69. Laas J, Engeser U, Meisner H. Tetralogy of Fallot. Development of the hypoplastic pulmonary arteries after palliation. *J Cardiovasc Surg* 1984;32:133–138.

70. Gerlis LM, Yen Ho S, Smith A, Anderson RH. The site of origin of nonconfluent pulmonary arteries from a common arterial trunk or from the ascending aorta: Its morphological significance. *Am J Cardiovasc Pathol* 1990; 3:115–120.

71. Hislop A, Reid L. Structural changes in the pulmonary arteries and veins in tetralogy of Fallot. *Br Heart J* 1973; 35:1178–1183.

72. Shimazaki Y, Maehara T, Blackstone EH, Kirklin JW; Bargeron LM Jr. The structure of the pulmonary circulation in tetralogy of Fallot with pulmonary atresia. A quantitative cineangiographic study. *J Thorac Cardiovasc Surg* 1988;95:1048–1058.

73. Barbero-Marcial M, Jatene AD. Surgical management of the anomalies of the pulmonary arteries in the tetralogy of Fallot with pulmonary atresia. *Semin Thorac Cardiovasc Surg* 1990;2:93–107.

74. Magnier S, Legendre T, Casasoprana A, Bloch G, Le Van Than N, Vernant P. La circulation pulmonaire de suppleance dans la tetralogie de Fallot. *Arch Mal Coeur Vaiss* 1985;78:917–923.

74a. Pahl E, Muster AJ, Ilbawi MN, DeLeon SY. Tetralogy of Fallot with absent ductus arteriosus and absent collateral pulmonary circulation: Diagnostic and surgical implications during the neonatal period. *Pediatr Cardiol* 1988;9:45–49.

75. Yen Ho S, Catani G, Seo J-W. Arterial supply to the lungs in tetralogy of Fallot with pulmonary atresia or critical stenosis. *Cardiol Young* 1992; 2:65–72.

76. Fong LV, Anderson RH, Siewers RD, Trento A, Park SC. Anomalous origin of one pulmonary artery from the ascending aorta: A review of echocardiographic, catheter, and morphological features. *Br Heart J* 1989;62:389–395.

77. Canter CE, Gutierresz FR, Mirowitz SA, Martin EC, Hartmann AF Jr. Evaluation of pulmonary arterial morphology in cyanotic congenital heart disease by magnetic resonance imaging. *Am Heart J* 1989;118:347–351.

78. Py A, Lazarus A, Spaulding C, Toussaint M, Planche C, Duboc D, Fouchard J, Guerin F. Artere pulmonaire gauche naissant de l'aorte ascendante dans une tetralogie de Fallot. Strategie therapeutique. *Arch Mal Coeur Vaiss* 1993;86:1069–1072.

79. Rome JJ, Mayer JE, Castaneda AR, Lock JE. Tetralogy of Fallot with pulmonary atresia. Rehabilitation of diminutive pulmonary arteries. *Circulation* 1993;88:1691–1698.

80. Murdison KA; Weinberg PM. Tetralogy of Fallot with severe pulmonary valvar stenosis and pulmonary vascular sling (anomalous origin of the left pulmonary artery from the right pulmonary artery). *Pediatr Cardiol* 1991; 12:189–191.

80a. Waldman JD, Karp RB, Gittenberger-de Groot AC, Agarwala B, Glagov S. Spontaneous acquisition of discontinuous pulmonary arteries. Ann Thorac Surg 1996; 62:161–168.

81. Momma K, Takao A, Ando M, Nakazawa M, Satomi G, Imai Y, Takanashi Y, Kurosawa H. Juxtaductal left pulmonary artery obstruction in pulmonary atresia. *Br Heart J* 1986;55:39–44.

82. Morgan JR. Left pulmonary artery from ascending aorta in tetralogy of Fallot. *Circulation* 1972;45:653–655.

83. Gikonyo BM, Jue KL, Edwards JE. Pulmonary vascular sling: Report of seven cases and review of the literature. *Pediatr Cardiol* 1989;10:81–89.

84. Magnier S, Legendre T, Casasoprana A, Bloch G, Le Van Than N, Vernant P. La circulation pulmonaire de suppleance dans la tetralogie de Fallot. *Arch Mal Coeur Vaiss* 1985;78:917–923.

85. Turinetto B, Coli G, Donati A, et al. Absent right pulmonary artery complicating tetralogy of Fallot. *J Cardiovasc Surg* 1975;16:322–326.

86. Pahl E, Fong L, Anderson RH, Park SC, Zuberbuhler JR. Fistulous communications between a solitary coronary artery and the pulmonary arteries as the primary source of pulmonary blood supply in tetralogy of Fallot with pulmonary valve atresia. *Am J Cardiol* 1989;63:140–143.

87. Groh MA, Meliones JN, Bove EL, Kirklin JW, Blackstone EH, Lupinetti FM, Snider AR, Rosenthal A. Repair of tetralogy of Fallot in infancy. Effect of pulmonary artery size on outcome. *Circulation* 1991;84(5 suppl):III-206-III-212.

88. Pfefferkorn JR, Loser H, Pech G, Toussaint R, Hilgenberg F. Absent pulmonary artery. A hint to its embryogenesis. *Pediatr Cardiol* 1982;3:283–286.

89. Ramsay JM, Macartney FJ, Haworth SG. Tetralogy of Fallot with major aortopulmonary collateral arteries. *Br Heart J* 1985;53:167–172.

90. Naito Y, Fujita T, Yagihara T, Isobe F, Yamamoto F, Tanaka K, Manabe H, Takahashi O, Kamiya T. Usefulness of left ventricular volume in assessing tetralogy of Fallot for total correction. *Am J Cardiol* 1985;56:356–359.

91. Oberhansli I, Friedli B. Cross sectional echocardiographic assessment of left ventricular volume and ejection fraction in patients with tetralogy of Fallot. Comparison with biplane angiographic measurements. *Br Heart J* 1984;52:191–197.

92. Nomoto S, Muraoka R, Yokota M, Aoshima M, Kyoku I, Nakano H. Left ventricular volume as a predictor of postoperative hemodynamics and a criterion for total correction of tetralogy of Fallot. *J Thorac Cardiovasc Surg* 1984;88:389–394.

93. Graham TP Jr, Faulkner S, Bender H Jr, Wender CM. Hypoplasia of the left ventricle: Rare cause of postoperative mortality in tetralogy of Fallot. *Am J Cardiol* 1977;40:454–457.

94. Nagata S, Park YD, Nakanishi N, Beppu S, Sakakibara H, Nimura Y. Mitral valve abnormalities in patients with right ventricular pressure overload. Analysis by real time cross sectional echocardiography. *Br Heart J* 1984;52:186–190.

95. Hohn AR, Jain KK, Tamer DM. Supravalvular mitral stenosis in tetralogy of Fallot. *Am J Cardiol* 1968;22:733–737.

96. Ino T, Yabuta K, Okada R. Rare association of tetralogy of Fallot and aortic valve stenosis. Autopsy findings after failed balloon aortic valvuloplasty. *Jpn Heart J* 1992;33(1):125–130.

97. Glancy DI, Morrow AG, Roberts WC. Malformations of the aortic valve in patients with the tetralogy of Fallot. *Am Heart J* 1968;76:755–759.

98. Capelli H, Ross D, Somerville J. Aortic regurgitation in tetralogy of Fallot and pulmonary atresia. *Am J Cardiol* 1982;49:1979–1981.

99. Radhakrishnan S, Shrivastava S. Tetralogy of Fallot with discrete subaortic shelf: Cross-sectional echocardiographic and Doppler diagnosis of a rare association. *Int J Cardiol* 1989;23:413–414.

99a. Sanders JH, Van Praagh R, Sade RM. Tetralogy of Fallot with discrete fibrous subaortic stenosis. *Chest* 1976;69:543–544.

99b. Vogel M, Freedom RM, Brand A, Trusler GA, Williams WG, Rowe RD. Ventricular septal defect and subaortic stenosis: An analysis of 41 patients. *Am J Cardiol* 1983;52:1258–1263.

100. Smolinsky A, Ziskind Z, Ruvolo G, Goor DA. Staged surgical treatment of early bacterial endocarditis after surgical repair of tetralogy of Fallot and discrete subaortic stenosis: Report of a case. *J Thorac Cardiovasc Surg* 1985;90:788–789.

101. Cicini MP, Giannico S, Marino B, Iorio FS, Corno A, Marcelletti C. "Acquired" subvalvular aortic stenosis after repair of a ventricular septal defect. *Chest* 1992;101:115–118.

102. Velasquez G, Nath PH, Castaneda-Zuniga WR, Amplatz K. Aberrant left subclavian artery in tetralogy of Fallot. *Am J Cardiol* 1980;45:811–818.

102a. Hastreiter AR, D'Cruz IA, Cantez T. Right-sided aorta. *Br Heart J* 1966;28:722–739. 102b. Knight L, Edwards JE. Right aortic arch. Types and associated cardiac anomalies. *Circulation* 1974;50:1047–1051.

103. Nakajima Y, Nishibatake M, Ikeda K, Takao A, Terai M. Abnormal development of fourth aortic arch derivatives in the pathogenesis of tetralogy of Fallot. *Pediatr Cardiol* 1990;11:69–71.

104. Rodriguez L, Izukawa T, Moes CAF, Trusler GA, Williams WG. Surgical implications of right aortic arch with isolation of left subclavian artery. *Br Heart J* 1975; 37:931–933.

104a.Smith JA, Hirschklau MJ, Reitz BA. An unusual presentation of isolation of the right subclavian artery. *Cardiol Young* 1994;4:181–183.

105. Luetmer PH, Miller GM. Right aortic arch with isolation of the left subclavian artery: Case report and review of the literature. *Mayo Clin Proc* 1990;65:407–413.

106. Freedom RM, Moes CAF, Pelech A, Smallhorn J, Rabinovitch M, Olley PM, Williams WG, Trusler GA, Rowe RD. Bilateral ductus arteriosus (or Remnant): An analysis of 27 patients. *Am J Cardiol* 1984;53:884–891.

107. Lenox CC, Neches WH, Zuberbuhler JR, Park SC, Mathews RA, Siewers RD, Lerberg DG, Bahnson HT. Management of bilateral ductus arteriosus in complex cyanotic heart disease. *J Thorac Cardiovasc Surg* 1977;74: 607–613.

108. Todd EP, Lindsay WG, Edwards JE. Bilateral ductal origin of the pulmonary arteries. Systemic-pulmonary arterial anastomosis as first stage in planned total correction. *Circulation* 1976;54:834–836.

108a.Baudet E, Roques XF, Guibaud J-P, Laborde N, Choussat A. Isolation of the right subclavian artery. *Ann Thorac Surg* 1992;53:501–503.

109. Gunthard J, Murdison KA, Wagner HR, Norwood WI Jr. Tetralogy of Fallot and coarctation of the aorta: A rare combination and its clinical implications. *Pediatr Cardiol* 1992;13:37–40.

110. Bullaboy CA, Derkac WM, Johnson DH, Jennings RB Jr. Tetralogy of Fallot and coarctation of the aorta: Successful repair in an infant. *Ann Thorac Surg* 1984;38: 400–401.

111. Korula RJ, Bais A, Lal N, Jairaj PS. Interrupted aortic arch with tetralogy of Fallot. A report of an unsuccessful surgically treated case. *J Cardiovasc Surg* 1991;32: 541–543.

112. Rey C, Coeurderoy A, Dupuis C. Coarctation de l'aorte et tetralogie de fallot. A propos de deux observations. *Arch Mal Coeur Vaiss* 1984;77:526–533.

112a.Yoshigi M, Momma K, Imai Y. Tetralogy of Fallot and coarctation of the aorta. *Cardiol Young* 1994;4:75–78.

113. Husseini ZM, Slim MS, Kutayli FN, Hatem JN. Tetralogy of Fallot with double aortic arch: Successful staged repair. Case report and review of literature. *J Cardiovasc Surg* 1987;28:339–340.

114. Virdi IS, Keeton BR, Shore DF, Monro JL. Surgical management in tetralogy of Fallot and vascular ring. *Pediatr Cardiol* 1987;8:131–134.

115. Patel KR, Hurwitz JL, Clauss RH. Cervical aortic arch associated with tetralogy of Fallot. *Cardiovasc Surg* 1993: 1:602–604.

116. Kramer LA, Horowitz D, Ilkiw R. Rare case of double aortic arch with hypoplastic right dorsal segment and associated tetralogy of Fallot: MR findings. *Magn Reson Imaging* 1993;11:1217–1221.

117. Anderson RH. Tetralogy of Fallot and the fifth aortic arch (letter). *Int J Cardiol* 1994;44:104.

118. Dabizzi RP, Caprioli G, Aiazzi L. Distribution and anomalies of the coronary arteries in tetralogy of Fallot. *Circulation* 1980;61:95–102.

119. Dabizzi RP, Teodori G, Barletta GA, Caprioli G, Baldrighi G, Baldrighi V. Associated coronary and cardiac anomalies in the tetralogy of Fallot. An angiographic study. *Eur Heart J* 1990;11:692–704.

120. Fellows KE, Freed MD, Keane JF, Van Praagh R, Bernhard W, Castenada AC. Results of routine preoperative coronary angiography in tetralogy of Fallot. *Circulation* 1975; 51: 561–566.

121. Heuser RR, Achuff SC, Brinker JA. Inadvertent division of an anomalous left anterior descending coronary artery during complete repair of tetralogy of Fallot: 22-year follow-up. *Am Heart J* 1982;103:430–432.

122. Humes RA, Driscoll DJ, Danielson GK, Puga FJ. Tetralogy of Fallot with anomalous origin of left anterior descending coronary artery. Surgical options. *J Thorac Cardiovasc Surg* 1987;94:784–787.

123. Longnecker CG, Reemtsma K, Creech O Jr. Anomalous coronary artery distribution associated with tetralogy of Fallot: A hazard in open cardiac repair. *J Thorac Cardiovasc Surg* 1961;42:258–262.

124. McManus BM, Waller BF, Jones M, Epstein SE, Roberts WC. The case for preoperative coronary angiography in patients with tetralogy of Fallot and other complex congenital heart disease. *Am Heart J* 1982;103:451–456.

125. Meng CC, Eckner FAO, Lev M. Coronary artery distribution in tetralogy of Fallot. *Arch Surg* 1965;90:363–396.

125a.Berry BE and McGoon DC. Total correction for tetralogy of Fallot with anomalous coronary artery. *Surgery* 1973; 74:894–898.

126. White RI Jr, French RS, Castaneda A, Amplatz K. The nature and significance of anomalous coronary arteries in tetralogy of Fallot. *AJNR* 1972;114:350–354.

127. Bhutani AK, Koppala MM, Abraham KA, Balakrishnan KR, Desai RN. Inadvertent transection of anomalously arising left anterior descending artery during tetralogy of Fallot repair: Bypass grafting with left internal mammary artery (letter). *J Thorac Cardiovasc Surg* 1994;108: 589–590.

128. Heifetz SA, Robinowitz M, Mueller KH, Virmani R. Total anomalous origin of the coronary arteries from the pulmonary artery. *Pediatr Cardiol* 1986;7:11–18.

129. Honnekeri ST, Lokhandwala YY, Tendolkar AG. A pitfall of selective coronary angiography—dual anterior descending arteries in tetralogy of Fallot. *Indian Heart J* 1991;43:113–115.

130. Landolt CC, Anderson JE, Zorn-Chelton S, Guyton RA, Hatcher CR Jr, Williams WH. Importance of coronary artery anomalies in operations for congenital heart disease. *Ann Thorac Surg* 1986;41:351–355.

131. Gutierrez Escalada B, Calderon Colmenero J, Attie F, Ramirez S, Lopez Soriano F, Buendia A. Tetralogia de Fallot asociada a anomalias de las arterias coronarias. *Arch Inst Cardiol Mex (Mexico)* 1990;60:301–304.

132. di Carlo D, De Nardo D, Ballerini L, Marcelletti C. Injury to the left coronary artery during repair of tetralogy of Fallot: Successful aorta-coronary polytetrafluoroethylene graft. *J Thorac Cardiovasc Surg* 1987;93:468–470.

133. Yamaguchi M, Tsukube T, Hosokawa Y, Ohashi H, Oshima Y. Pulmonary origin of left anterior descending coronary artery in tetralogy of Fallot. *Ann Thorac Surg* 1991;52:310–312.

134. O'Sullivan J, Bain H, Hunter S, Wren C. End-on aortogram: Improved identification of important coronary artery anomalies in tetralogy of Fallot. *Br Heart J* 1994; 71:102–106.

135. Carvalho JS, Silva CM, Rigby ML, Shinebourne EA. Angiographic diagnosis of anomalous coronary artery in tetralogy of Fallot. *Br Heart J* 1993;70:75–78.

136. Shrivastava S, Mohan JC, Mukhopadhyay S, Rajani M, Tandon R. Coronary artery anomalies in tetralogy of Fallot. *Cardiovasc Intervent Radiol* 1987;10:215–218.

136a.Saxena A, Sharma S, Shrivastava S. Coronary arteriovenous fistula in tetralogy of Fallot: An unusual association. *Int J Cardiol* 1990;28:373–374.

137. Sharma S, Rajani M, Mukhopadhyay S, Shrivastava S, Tandon R. Collateral arteries arising from the coronary circulation in tetralogy of Fallot. *Int J Cardiol* 1988;19:237–243.

137a.Moss RL, Backer CL, Zales VR, Florentine MS, Mavroutis C. Tetralogy of Fallot with anomalous origin of the right coronary artery. *Ann Thorac Surg* 1995;59:229–231.

138. Sahai S, Kothari SS, Wasir HS. Tetralogy of Fallot with Ebstein's anomaly of the tricuspid valve. *Indian Heart J* 1994;46:53–54.

139. Abdallah HI, Marks LA, Balsara RK, Davis DA, Russo PA. Staged repair of pentalogy of Cantrell with tetralogy of Fallot. *Ann Thorac Surg* 1993;56:979–980.

140. Grinneiser D, Bourlon F, Redjimi M. Une association pathologique rare: Tetralogie de Fallot et hypertrophie septale asymetrique. *Arch Mal Coeur Vaiss* 1984;77:577–580.

141. Kothari SS, Rajani M, Shrivastava S. Tetralogy of Fallot with aorto-pulmonary window. *Int J Cardiol* 1988;18:105–108.

141a.Bhagwat AR, Pinto RJ, Sharma S. Tetralogy of Fallot with pulmonary atresia associated with aortopulmonary window and major aortopulmonary collaterals. *Cardiol Young* 1995;5:289–290.

142. Vogel M, Sauer U, Buhlmeyer K, Sebening F. Atrioventricular septal defect complicated by right ventricular outflow tract obstruction. Analysis of risk factors regarding surgical repair. *J Cardiovasc Surg* 1989;30:34–39.

143. Redington AN, Raine J, Shinebourne EA, Rigby ML. Tetralogy of Fallot with anomalous pulmonary venous connections: A rare but clinically important association. *Br Heart J* 1990;64:325–328.

144. Carminati M, Borghi A, Valsecchi O, Quattrociocchi M, Balduzzi A, Rusconi P, Russo MG, Festa P, Preda L, Tiraboschi R. Aortopulmonary window coexisting with tetralogy of Fallot: Echocardiographic diagnosis. *Pediatr Cardiol* 1990;11:41–43.

145. Gatzoulis MA, Shore D, Yacoub M, Shinebourne EA. Complete atrioventricular septal defect with tetralogy of Fallot: Diagnosis and management. *Br Heart J* 1994;71:579–583.

146. Piot JD, Leriche H, Losay J, Touchot A, Piot C, Worms AM, Planche C, Pernot C, Binet JP. Malformations de la valve tricuspide associees a la tetralogie de Fallot. A propos d'une serie de 224 tetralogies de Fallot operees. *Arch Mal Coeur Vaiss* 1985;78:757–761.

147. Vargas FJ, Coto EO, Mayer JE Jr, Jonas RA, Castaneda AR. Complete atrioventricular canal and tetralogy of Fallot: Surgical considerations. *Ann Thorac Surg* 1986;42:258–263.

148. Castaneda A and Kirklin JW. Tetralogy of Fallot with aorticopulmonary window. Report of two surgical cases. *J Thorac Cardiovasc Surg* 1977;74:467–470.

149. Freedom RM, Culham JAG, Moes CAF. *Angiocardiography of Congenital Heart Disease.* New York: Macmillan Publishing Co; 1984, pp. 173–213.

150. Freedom RM, Benson LN, Smallhorn JF. *Neonatal Heart Disease.* London: Springer-Verlag; London, 1992, pp. 213–228.

151. Gerlis LM, Fiddler GI, Pearse RG. Total anomalous pulmonary venous drainage associated with tetralogy of Fallot: report of a case. *Pediatr Cardiol* 1984;4:297–300.

152. Nath PH, Soto B, Bini RM, Bargeron Jr LM, Pacifico AD. Tetralogy of Fallot with atrioventricular canal. An an-

giographic study. *J Thorac Cardiovasc Surg* 1984;87:421–430.

153. Rowe RD, Freedom RM, Mehrizi A. *The Neonate with Congenital Heart Disease.* New York: WB Saunders Co; 1981, pp. 286–300.

153a.Bharati S, Kirklin JW, Mcallister HA Jr, Lev M. The surgical anatomy of common atrioventricular orifice associated with tetralogy of Fallot, double outlet right ventricle and complete regular transposition. *Circulation* 1980;61:1142–1149.

154. Marino B, Corno A, Carotti A, Pasquini L, Giannico S, Guccione P, Bevilacqua M, De Simone G, Marcelletti C. Pediatric cardiac surgery guided by echocardiography. Established indications and new trends. *Scand J Thorac Cardiovasc Surg* 1990;24:197–201.

155. Santoro G, Marino B, DiCarlo D, Formigari R, de Zorzi A, Mazzera E, Rinelli G, Marcelletti C, De Simone G, Pasquini L. Echocardiographically guided repair of tetralogy of Fallot. *Am J Cardiol* 1994;73:808–811.

156. Jureidini SB, Appleton RS, Nouri S. Detection of coronary artery abnormalities in tetralogy of Fallot by two-dimensional echocardiography. *J Am Coll Cardiol* 1989;14:960–967.

157. Saraclar M, Ozkutlu S, Ozme S, Bozer AY, Yurdakul Y, Pasaoglu I, Demircin M, Baysal K, Cil E. Surgical treatment in tetralogy of Fallot diagnosed by echocardiography. *Int J Cardiol* 1992;37;29–35.

158. McConnell ME. Echocardiography in classical tetralogy of Fallot. *Semin Thorac Cardiovasc Surg* 1990;2:2–11.

159. Berry JM Jr, Einzig S, Krabill KA, Bass JL. Evaluation of coronary artery anatomy in patients with tetralogy of Fallot by two-dimensional echocardiography. *Circulation* 1988;78:149–156.

160. Marino B, Ballerini L, Marcelletti C, Piva R, Pasquini L, Zacche C, Giannico S, De Simone G. Right oblique subxiphoid view for two-dimensional echocardiographic visualization of the right ventricle in congenital heart disease. *Am J Cardiol* 1984;54:1064–1068.

161. Hagler DJ, Tajik AJ, Seward JB, Mair DD, Ritter DG. Wide-angle two-dimensional echocardiographic profiles of conotruncal abnormalities. *Mayo Clin Proc* 1980;55:73–82.

162. Huhta JC, Gutgesell HP, Latson LA, Huffines FD. Two-dimensional echocardiographic assessment of the aorta in infants and children with congenital heart disease. *Circulation* 1984;70:417–424.

163. Huhta JC, Piehler JM, Tajik AJ, et al. Two-dimensional echocardiographic detection and measurement of the right pulmonary artery in pulmonary atresia-ventricular septal defect: Angiographic and surgical correlation. *Am J Cardiol* 1982;49:1235–1240.

163a.Isaaz K, Cloez JL, Danchin N, Marcon F, Worms AM, Pernot C. Right ventricular outflow tract assessment by two-dimensional echocardiography in children using a new subcostal view: Angiocardiographic and morphologic correlative study. *Am J Cardiol* 1985;56:539–545.

164. Sanders SP, Bierman FZ, Williams RG. Conotruncal malformations: Diagnosis in infancy using subxiphoid 2–dimensional echocardiography. *Am J Cardiol* 1982;50:1361–1367.

165. Silove ED, de Giovanni JV, Shiu MF, Yi MM. Diagnosis of right ventricular outflow obstruction by cross-sectional echocardiography. *Br Heart J* 1983;50:416–420.

165a.Hornberger LK, Sanders SP, Sahn DJ, Rice MJ, Spevak PJ, Benacerraf BR, McDonald RW, Colan SD. In utero pulmonary artery and aortic growth and potential for progression of pulmonary outflow tract obstruction in tetralogy of Fallot. *J Am Coll Cardiol* 1995;25:739–745.

166. Baron MG. Radiologic notes in cardiology-angiographic differentiation between tetralogy of Fallot and double-outlet right ventricle. Relationship of the mitral and aortic valves. *Circulation* 1971;43:451–455.

167. Chen MR, Chiu IS, Chiu CB. Angiographic classification of ventricular septal defects in tetralogy of Fallot. *Int J Cardiol* 1994;44:115–122.

168. Ceballos R, Soto B, Bargeron Jr LM. Angiographic anatomy of the normal heart through axial angiography. *Circulation* 1981;64:351–357.

169. Deutsch V, Shem-Tov A, Yahini JH, Neufeld HN. Cardioangiographic evaluation of the relationship between atrioventricular and semilunar valves: Its diagnostic importance in congenital heart disease. *AJR* 1970;110:474–490.

170. Fellows KE, Keane JF, Freed MD. Angled views in cineangiocardiography of congenital heart disease. *Circulation* 1977;56:485–490.

171. Fellows KE, Smith J, Keane JF. Preoperative angiocardiography in infants with tetralogy of Fallot. *Am J Cardiol* 1981;47:1279–1285.

172. Freedom RM, Olley PM. Pulmonary arteriography in congenital heart disease. *Cathet Cardiovasc Diagn* 1976;2:309–312.

173. Freedom RM, Pongiglione G, Williams WG, Trusler GA, Moes CAF, Rowe RD. Pulmonary vein wedge angiography. Indications, results, and surgical correlates in 25 patients. *Am J Cardiol* 1983;51:936–941.

174. Hardy C, Wong J, Young JN, McCray J. Balloon occlusion scintigraphy of aortopulmonary collaterals. *Pediatr Cardiol* 1994;15:241–245,

175. Kattan KR. Angled views in pulmonary angiography. A new roentgen approach. *Radiology* 1970;94:79–82.

176. Lacina SJ, Hamilton WT, Thilenius OG, Bharati S, Lev M, Arcilla RA. Angiographic evidence of absent ductus arteriosus in severe right ventricular outflow tract obstruction. *Pediatr Cardiol* 1983;4:5–11.

177. Nihill MR, Mullins CE, McNamara DG. Visualization of the pulmonary arteries in pseudotruncus by pulmonary vein wedge angiography. *Circulation* 1978;58:140–147.

178. Soto B, Coghlan CH, Bargeron LM. Present status of axially angled angiocardiography. *Cardiovasc Intervent Radiol* 1984;7:156–165.

179. Taylor JFN and Chrispin AR. Interventricular septal defect shown by left ventricular cine-angiocardiography. *Br Heart J* 1971;33:285–289.

180. Vincent RN, Hawkins LE, Pelech AN, Collins GF. Balloon occlusion aortography. *Can J Cardiol* 1987;3:52–59.

181. Pongiglione G, Freedom RM, Cook D, Rowe RD. Mechanism of acquired right ventricular outflow tract obstruction in patients with ventricular septal defect: An angiocardiographic study. *Am J Cardiol* 1982;50:776–780.

182. Rao PS. Descending aortography with balloon inflation. A technique for evaluating the size of persistent ductus arteriosus in infants with large proximal left to right shunts. *Br Heart J* 1985;54:527–532.

183. Shinebourne EA, Anderson RH, Bowyer JJ. Variations in clinical presentation of Fallot's tetralogy. Angiographic and pathogenetic implications. *Br Heart J* 1975;37:946–955.

184. Strife JL. Tetralogy of Fallot. *Semin Roentgenol* 1985;20:160–168.

185. O'Sullivan J, Bain H, Hunter S, Wren C. End-on aortogram: Improved identification of important coronary artery anomalies in tetralogy of Fallot. *Br Heart J* 1994;71:102–106.

186. Labadidi Z, Wu JR. Percutaneous balloon pulmonary valvuloplasty. *Am J Cardiol* 1983;52:560–562.

187. Walls JT, Labadidi Z, Cutris JJ, Silver D. Assessment of percutaneous balloon pulmonary and aortic valvuloplasty. *J Thorac Cardiovasc Surg* 1984;88:352–356.

188. Rao PS, Brais M. Balloon pulmonary valvuloplasty for congenital cyanotic heart defects. *Am Heart J* 1988;115:1105–1110.

189. Rao PS, Wilson AD, Thapar MK, Brais M. Balloon pulmonary valvuloplasty in the management of cyanotic congenital heart defects. *Cathet Cardiovasc Diagn* 1992;25:16–24.

190. McCredie RM, Lee CL, Swinburn MJ, Warner G. Balloon dilation pulmonary valvuloplasty in pulmonary stenosis. *Aust NZ J Med* 1986;16:20–23.

191. Boucek MM, Webster HE, Orsmond GS, Ruttenberg HD. Balloon pulmonary valvotomy: Palliation for cyanotic heart disease. *Am Heart J* 1988;115:318–322.

192. Qureshi SA, Kirk CR, Lamb RK, Arnold R, Wilkinson JL. Balloon dilatation of the pulmonary valve in the first year of life in patients with tetralogy of Fallot: A preliminary study. *Br Heart J* 1988;60:232–235.

193. Sreeram N, Saleem M, Jackson M, Peart I, McKay R, Arnold R, Walsh K. Results of balloon pulmonary valvuloplasty as a palliative procedure in tetralogy of Fallot. *J Am Coll Cardiol* 1991;18:159–165

194. Parsons JM, Ladusans EJ, Qureshi SA. Growth of the pulmonary artery after neonatal balloon dilatation of the right ventricular outflow tract in an infant with the tetralogy of Fallot and atrioventricular septal defect. *Br Heart J* 1989;62:65–68.

195. Battistessa SA, Robles A, Jackson M, Miyamoto S, Arnold R, McKay R. Operative findings after percutaneous pulmonary balloon dilatation of the right ventricular outflow tract in tetralogy of Fallot. *Br Heart J* 1990;64:321–324.

196. Matsuoka S, Ushiroguchi Y, Kubo M, Tatara K, Kitagawa T, Katoh I, Kuroda Y. Balloon pulmonary valvuloplasty for infants with severe tetralogy of Fallot. *Jpn Heart J* 1993;34:643–651.

197. Piechaud JF, Delogu AB, Iserin L, Aggoun Y, Cohen L, Sidi D, Kachaner J. Palliative treatment of tetralogy of Fallot by percutaneous dilatation of the right ventricular outflow tract. 40 cases. *Arch Mal Coeur Vaiss* 1994;86:573–579.

198. Buheitel G, Hofbeck M, Singer H. Balloon dilatation of the pulmonary valve within the first 40 days of life in critical valvular pulmonary stenosis, Fallot's tetralogy and following surgical or interventional high-frequency opening of pulmonary atresia. *Z Kardiol* 1995;84:64–71.

199. Sluysmans T, Neven B, Rubay J, Lintermans J, Ovaert C, Mucumbitsi J, Shango P, Stijns M, Vliers A. Early balloon dilatation of the pulmonary valve in infants with tetralogy of Fallot. Risks and benefits. *Circulation* 1995;91:1506–1511.

200. Lamb RK, Qureshi SA, Arnold R. Pulmonary artery tear following balloon valvoplasty in Fallot's tetralogy. *Int J Cardiol* 1987;15:347–349.

Chapter 21

The Pulmonary Circulation in Pulmonary Atresia

Among hearts with tetralogy of Fallot and pulmonary atresia or pulmonary atresia and ventricular septal defect, fundamental to management and prognosis is the source and arrangement of pulmonary arterial supply.[1–12] Remarkable surgical advances have been recorded in the past decade in the treatment of patients with complex forms of pulmonary atresia, achieving in some a biventricular repair, and in others a one-ventricle or Fontan repair.[13–58] The pulmonary arterial supply in patients with pulmonary atresia and ventricular septal defect is for the most part via the arterial duct or from collateral arteries originating directly or indirectly from the aorta. The surgical challenges in these patients are many, but much of the challenge rests with the ability to define, recruit, and rehabilitate the pulmonary arteries. This is achieved in part by resolution of the following questions: 1) How is blood conducted into the lungs and 2) How does one define those source(s) of pulmonary blood supply to each of the bronchopulmonary segments? The answers to these questions are very simple in those patients with ventriculopulmonary artery imperforate continuity, confluent pulmonary arteries, and absence of major or significant collateral vessels originating from the descending thoracic aorta or any of the arch or other conducting arteries. However, for those patients with pulmonary atresia, diminutive pulmonary arteries, and multiple large and small aortopulmonary collaterals, definition of the source or sources of blood supply to each of the bronchopulmonary segments may prove vexatious, and methodologies complex. One of the conundrums in the assessment and consideration for surgical treatment of these patients is whether the patient with a complex pulmonary circulation will be substantially improved by surgery, or whether such intervention should be eschewed because of the potential and reality for compromising the often fragile pulmonary circulation.[59–64] Using data from Bertranou,[64] much progress has been made for many patients with tetralogy of Fallot with pulmonary atresia. This is also true for many, but not all patients with pulmonary atresia and ventricular septal defect.[28,31,59–60]

Intracardiac Anatomy

The intracardiac anatomy and pertinent angiocardiographic features of tetralogy of Fallot and pulmonary atresia and ventricular septal defect were presented in Chapter 20.[3–5,7–9,12–14,26–28] Suffice it to say that some patients with anatomy typical of tetralogy of Fallot may have a significant collateral circulation to the lungs (see Chapter 20, Fig. 20-21).[65] This is true as well for that variant of tetralogy with absent pulmonary valve (see Chapter 22, Fig. 22-6). The process and methodology to define the nature of the collateral circulation to the lungs is really independent of the type of underlying congenital heart malformation; ie, tetralogy of Fallot; pulmonary atresia and ventricular septal defect; or hearts with visceral heterotaxy and right atrial isomerism (see Chapter 41). Indeed, pulmonary atresia with an extensive collateral circulation or a duct-mediated pulmonary circulation has been described in hearts with a discordant atrioventricular connection (see Chapter 36); classic tricuspid atresia (see Chapter 39); or hearts with other forms of univentricular atrioventricular connection (see Chapter 40). The presence of infundibular septation in those patients with tetralogy of Fallot and pulmonary atresia is not

From: Freedom RM, Mawson JB, Yoo SJ, Benson LN: *Congenital Heart Disease: Textbook of Angiocardiography.* Armonk NY, Futura Publishing Co., Inc. ©1997.

predictive of the type of pulmonary circulation.[7-9] Similarly, even in those patients with right atrial isomerism, the pulmonary arteries may be confluent and mediated by a unilateral arterial duct, or the pulmonary arteries may be nonconfluent with an extensive aortopulmonary collateral circulation (see also Chapter 41).[11,66,67] Among those biventricular hearts with pulmonary atresia and ventricular septal defect, the ventricular septal defect may be obstructed, analogous to the situation in tetralogy of Fallot.[7,12,68] Aortic valve stenosis is also well known in the patient with pulmonary atresia and ventricular septal defect.[12,69,70] Another confounding issue that may require resolution in patients with pulmonary atresia are obstructed pulmonary venous connections, often masked by the profoundly reduced pulmonary blood flow (see also Chapters 24, 40, and 41).[71-74]

Prevalence

Data from the New England Regional Infant Cardiac Program provided a frequency of 0.042 per 1000 livebirths for tetralogy with pulmonary atresia,[75] while that of the more recently completed Baltimore-Washington Infant Study did not specifically mention pulmonary atresia with ventricular septal defect.[76] Among neonates presenting with cyanosis and cardiac hypoxemia, pulmonary atresia with ventricular septal defect is a frequent diagnosis, included with transposition of the great arteries and pulmonary atresia and intact ventricular septum.

Morphogenesis

The morphogenesis of pulmonary atresia and the particular cardiac malformation is complex.[77-83] Kutsche and Van Mierop[83] have studied the morphology of hearts exhibiting pulmonary atresia with and without ventricular septal defect. Addressing the morphology of the pulmonary valve, the diameter of the main pulmonary trunk, and the morphology and topography of the ductus arteriosus, they conclude that hearts exhibiting pulmonary atresia and ventricular septal defect reflect a maturational arrest that is considerably earlier than that of pulmonary atresia and intact ventricular septum (see Chapter 19). That specific embryological factor involved in the etiology of pulmonary atresia and ventricular septal defect may be related to an abnormality of mesenchymal and/or neural crest migration.

Embryological Origin of the Main, Right, and Left Pulmonary Arteries and the Intrapulmonary Arteries

The ability to answer those fundamental questions asked in the first paragraph of this chapter necessitates understanding the origins of the main and branch pulmonary arteries, as well as the complex nature of the collateral circulation to the lungs. The main pulmonary trunk clearly originates from the process of truncal septation (Fig. 21-1).[78,80,83-87] Although this has been determined from the study of human and avian embryos, there are now a number of reports of hearts demonstrating normal truncal septation, but with the branch pulmonary arteries originating from the aorta.[84-87] These very unusual hearts are characterized by a main pulmonary trunk originating above a right ventricular infundibulum and connected to the descending aorta through a patent arterial duct, but without branch pul-

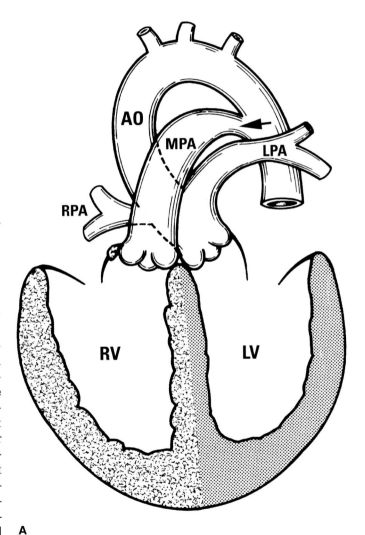

A

Fig. 21-1: The morphogenesis of the pulmonary arteries. The main pulmonary trunk is derived from truncal septation and the proximal right and left pulmonary arteries from the sixth aortic arch. There are several varieties of so-called "normal" truncal septation as depicted in these drawings.
A: The main pulmonary artery is connected to the descending aorta via an arterial duct; the right and left pulmonary arteries originate from the ascending aorta. *(figure continues)*

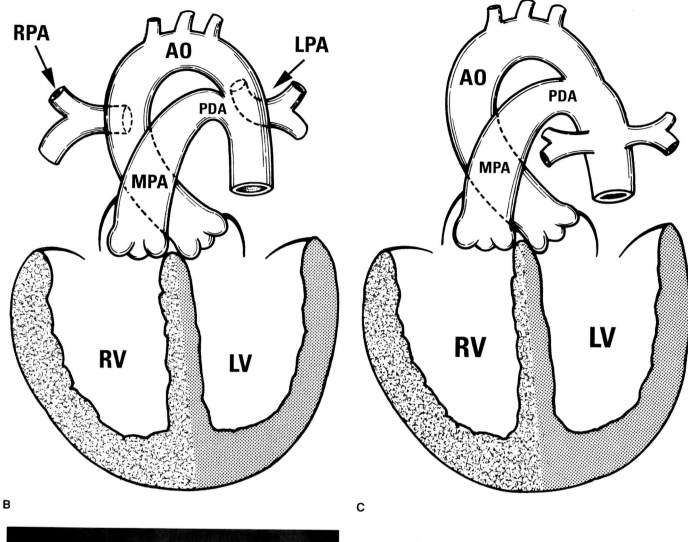

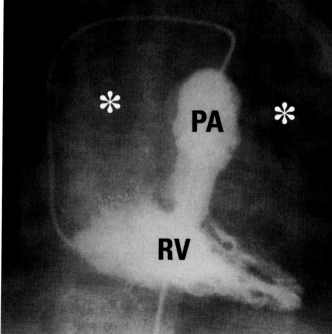

Fig. 21-1: *(continued)*
 B: The main pulmonary artery is connected to the descending aorta via an arterial duct; the right pulmonary artery originates from the ascending aorta; the left pulmonary artery originates from a collateral artery. **C:** The main pulmonary artery is connected to the descending aorta via an arterial duct; the branch pulmonary arteries are derived from persistence of primitive intersegmental arteries. **D through G:** This patient with normal truncal septation had a main pulmonary trunk, but the branch pulmonary arteries were derived from persistence of primitive intersegmental arteries. **D:** The right ventriculogram in the frontal projection shows a main pulmonary trunk, but no branches (✱). *(figure continues)*

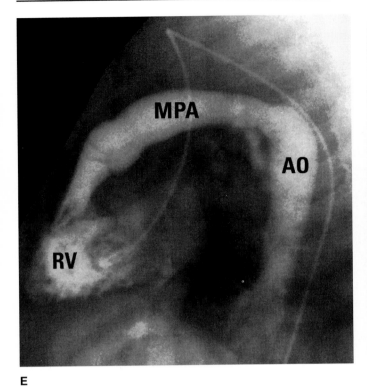

E

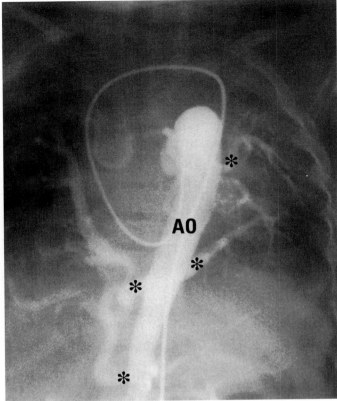

G

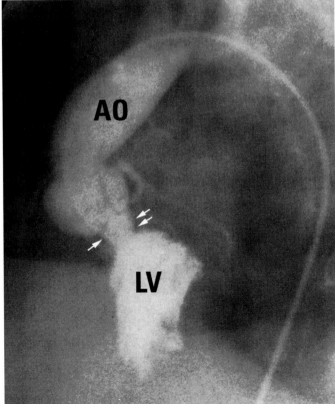

F

Fig. 21-1: *(continued)*
E through G: This patient with normal truncal septation had a main pulmonary trunk, but the branch pulmonary arteries were derived from persistence of primitive intersegmental arteries. **E:** The main pulmonary trunk is continuous with the descending aorta via an arterial duct. **F:** The retrograde left ventriculogram shows modest subaortic narrowing (arrows). **G:** The only source of pulmonary blood supply is via the persistence of the primitive intersegmental arteries, persisting as direct aortopulmonary collateral arteries as seen on this frontal descending thoracic aortogram. *(figure continues)*

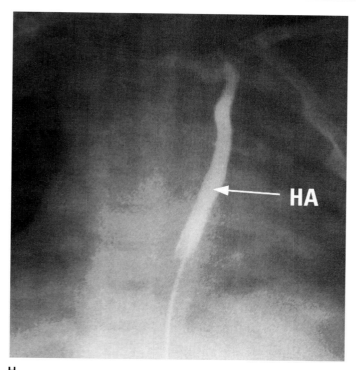

H

Fig. 21-1: *(continued)*
H: Access to the right ventricle was via the left-sided hemi-azygous vein (HA).

monary arteries originating from the main pulmonary trunk. The right and left pulmonary arteries in these extremely rare cases may originate from the ascending aorta or from the descending thoracic aorta (representing persistence of primitive intersegmental arteries). The normal right and left pulmonary arteries are the central pulmonary arteries that are located within the mediastinum that enter the respective lungs and are considered that arise from the proximal sixth aortic arches. Indeed, the definitive branch pulmonary arteries originate from the aortic sac, often before the sixth aortic arches are completely formed.[77,80,81] The intrapulmonary arteries, the arteries within the lung parenchyma, are derived from the vascular plexus of the embryological lung buds arising from the foregut.[77,79,80]

Anatomy of the Pulmonary Arteries and Source of Blood Supply

The right and left pulmonary arteries may be confluent with or without a blind main pulmonary trunk originating from the ventricular mass.[1–6,10–12,25,28,36,38–40,56,57] The term confluence means that the right and left pulmonary arteries are connected within the mediastinum, and usually, but not invariably so, the point or site of connection is perforate (Fig. 21-2). Sometimes, the point of conjunction between the right and left pul-

monary arteries is imperforate, or virtually so, presumably secondary to constriction of the arterial duct (Figs. 21-2 and 21-3).[12,88–91] Confluent pulmonary arteries may be supplied by a patent arterial duct; a direct aortopulmonary collateral originating from the descending thoracic aorta; less commonly from an indirect aortopulmonary collateral; by a coronary artery-pulmonary artery connection; from an aortopulmonary fenestration; or from a fifth aortic arch (Figs. 21-2 through 21-16).[92–133a] The solitary arterial duct may be right- or left-sided, or bilateral arterial ducts may be present.[92]

Only a few examples of a fifth aortic arch supporting the pulmonary circulation have been recorded (Fig. 21-14 and 21-15).[128–133] The fifth aortic arch may support the pulmonary circulation directly as a systemic-to-pulmonary artery connection, as in the patient with tricuspid and pulmonary atresia and coarctation of the aorta reported by Freedom and colleagues (Fig. 21-15).[130] In this patient, the fifth aortic arch originated from the ascending aorta well proximal to the brachio-

(text continues on p. 547)

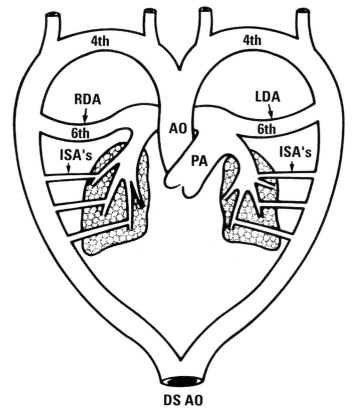

A

Fig. 21-2: A: Drawing showing right and left fourth and sixth aortic arches and intersegmental arteries (ISA). From this diagram it is possible to understand how bilateral arterial ducts may supply the entirety of the pulmonary circulation. *(figure continues)*

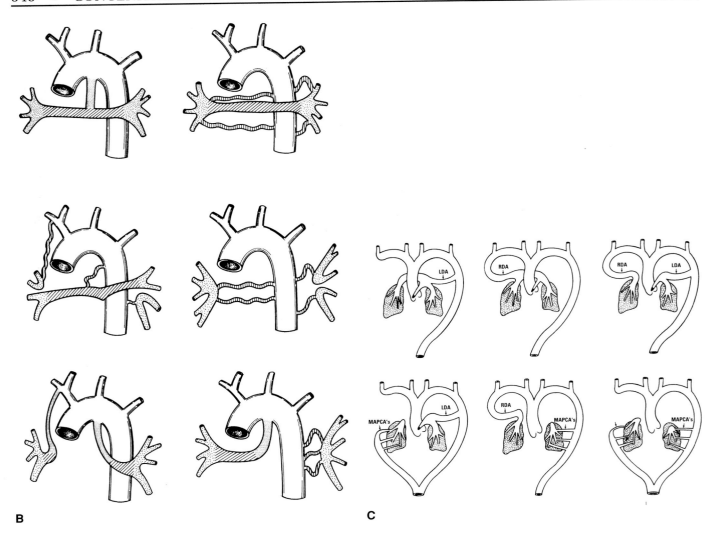

B

C

Fig. 21-2: *(continued)*
B: Some patterns of pulmonary blood supply with confluent and nonconfluent pulmonary arteries. **Top, left**: Confluent pulmonary arteries supplied by a single arterial duct. **Middle, left:** Confluent pulmonary arteries supplied by direct and indirect aortopulmonary collaterals. ***Bottom, left***: Nonconfluent pulmonary arteries supplied by bilateral arterial ducts. ***Top, right***: Confluent pulmonary arteries supplied by multiple direct aortopulmonary collaterals. ***Middle, right***: Nonconfluent pulmonary arteries supplied by multiple direct aortopulmonary collaterals. ***Bottom right***: nonconfluent pulmonary arteries supplied by left-sided arterial duct and direct aortopulmonary collaterals. **C:** Ductal and collaterals as sources of pulmonary blood supply in pulmonary atresia. **Top, left**: Left arterial duct supplying confluent pulmonary arteries. **Top, middle**: Right-sided arterial duct supplying confluent pulmonary arteries. ***Top, right***: Bilateral arterial ducts supplying nonconfluent pulmonary arteries. **Bottom, left**: Right lung supplied by multiple aortopulmonary collateral arteries and left lung via an arterial duct. ***Bottom center***: Left lung supplied by multiple aortopulmonary collateral arteries and right lung by a right-sided arterial duct. ***Bottom right***: Both lungs supplied only by multiple aortopulmonary collateral arteries.

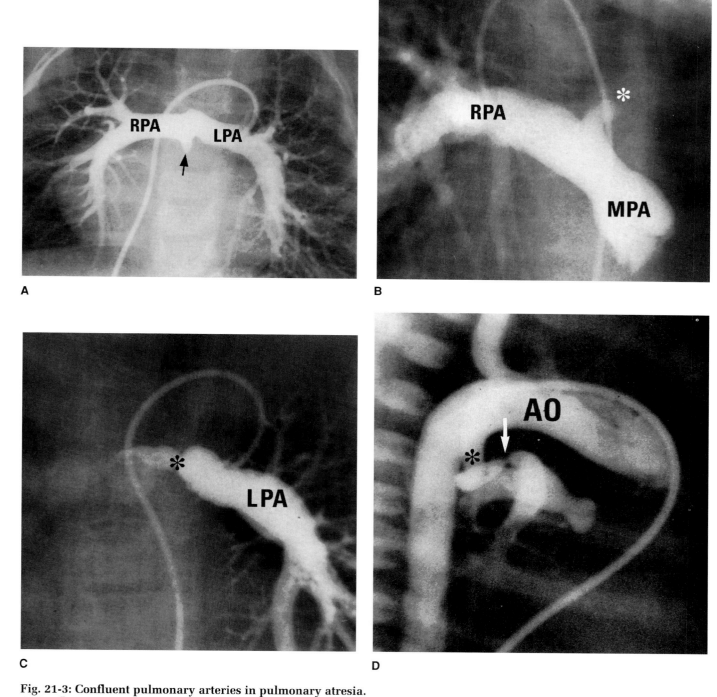

Fig. 21-3: Confluent pulmonary arteries in pulmonary atresia.
A: Confluent pulmonary arteries with a small main pulmonary artery (arrow). The catheter has been advanced through a left-sided arterial duct. **B and C:** Confluent pulmonary arteries with very severe left pulmonary artery stenosis at the site of ductal insertion. **B:** Selective right pulmonary artery injection showing no filling past stenotic (?atretic) left pulmonary artery. **C:** selective injection into left pulmonary artery shows the severe stenosis (✱). **D:** Another newborn with severe left pulmonary artery stenosis (arrow).

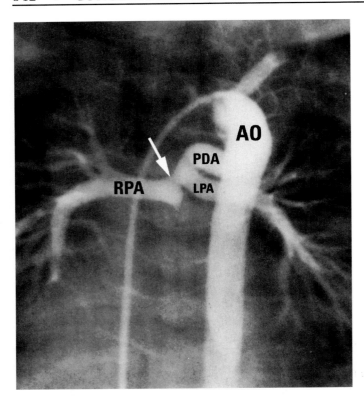

Fig. 21-4: Confluent pulmonary arteries mediated via a left-sided arterial duct in a patient with a left-sided aortic arch. The left pulmonary artery is retracted by the arterial duct. Note as well the proximal left pulmonary artery stenosis (arrow).

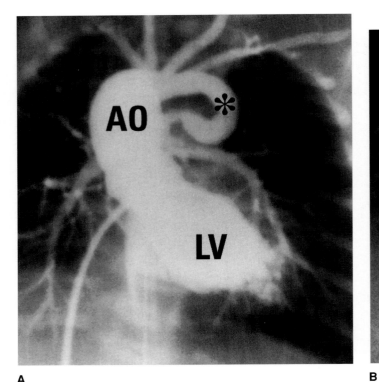

A

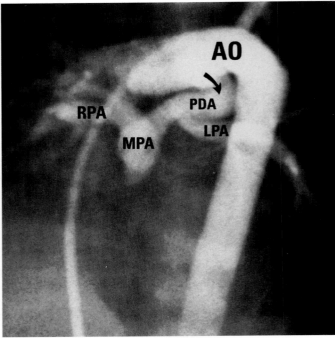

B

Fig. 21-5: Confluent pulmonary arteries mediated via a left-sided arterial duct in two different patients.
A: This frontal left ventriculogram shows the large left-sided arterial duct (*) in this patient with a right-sided aortic arch, but the overlapping aorta obscures the point of confluence. **B:** This aortogram shows a left-sided aortic arch and a large arterial duct supporting (arrow) confluent pulmonary arteries. The configuration of the arterial duct and left pulmonary artery are most peculiar, probably indicating ductal tissue involving the anterosuperior portion of the pulmonary artery wall.[90a] The angiography suggests the left pulmonary artery originates from the arterial duct.

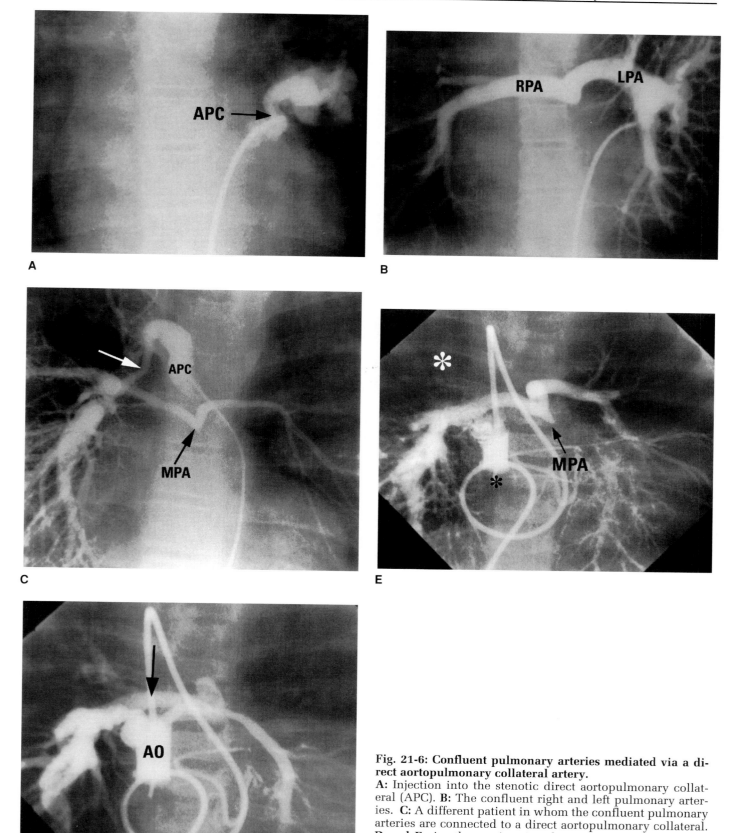

Fig. 21-6: Confluent pulmonary arteries mediated via a direct aortopulmonary collateral artery.
A: Injection into the stenotic direct aortopulmonary collateral (APC). B: The confluent right and left pulmonary arteries. C: A different patient in whom the confluent pulmonary arteries are connected to a direct aortopulmonary collateral. D and E: Another patient in whom direct aortopulmonary collaterals connect to the confluent pulmonary arteries demonstrated by this frontal balloon occlusion aortogram. Note in Fig. 21-6E, the arborization anomaly (∗).

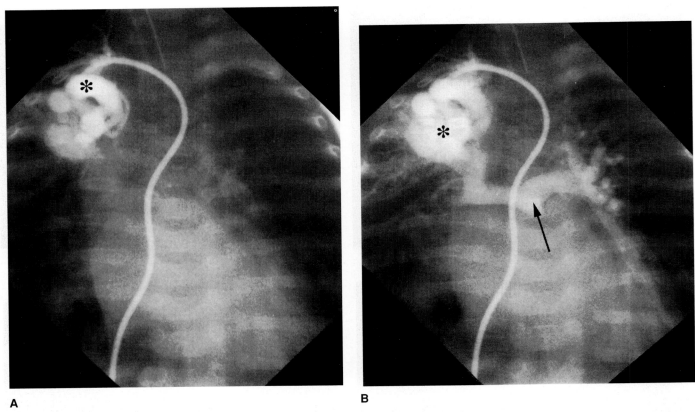

A **B**

Fig. 21-7: Confluent pulmonary arteries mediated via an indirect aortopulmonary collateral originating from the right subclavian artery.
A: Injection into the right subclavian artery shows a tortuous collateral (✱). **B:** Later in the same injection, the confluent pulmonary arteries are opacified. The arrow notes a small main pulmonary trunk.

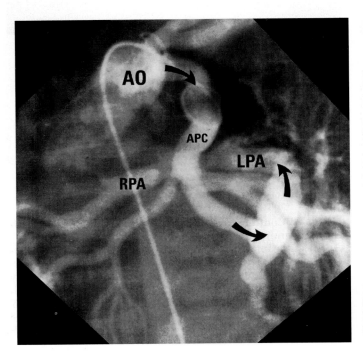

Fig. 21-8: Confluent pulmonary arteries are opacified from an aortopulmonary collateral.
Selective injection into an aortopulmonary collateral demonstrates connection with the left pulmonary artery and then there is opacification of the confluent right pulmonary artery.

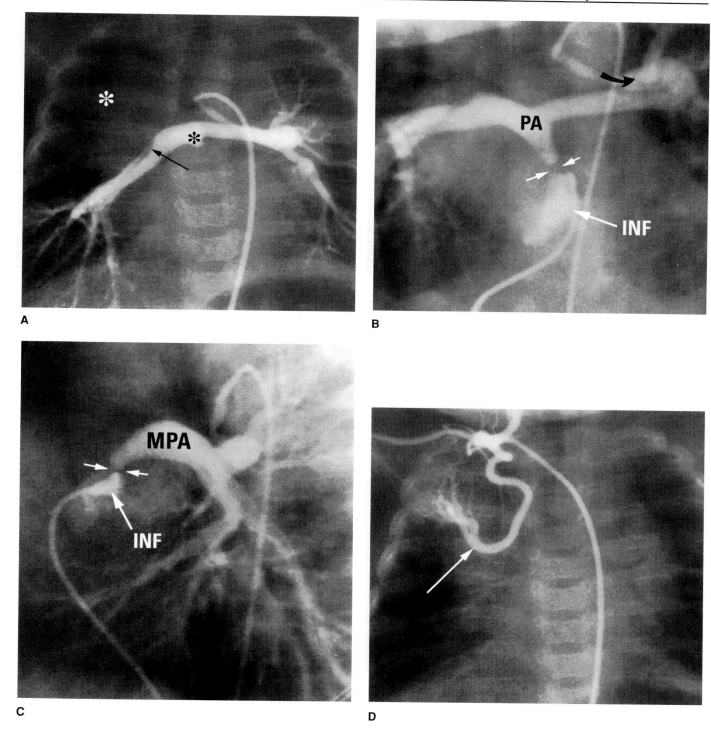

Fig. 21-9: Confluent pulmonary arteries are mediated via a left-sided arterial duct.
A: The pulmonary arteries are opacified from injection into a left-sided arterial duct. The main pulmonary artery is present (✻); note the wash-in of nonopacified blood into the right pulmonary artery (arrow). There is no right upper lobe branch pulmonary artery. **B and C:** Double-catheter technique shows short-segment infundibular atresia (arrows). **D:** Injection of contrast into the right subclavian artery shows the indirect collateral perfusing the right upper lobe of the lung.

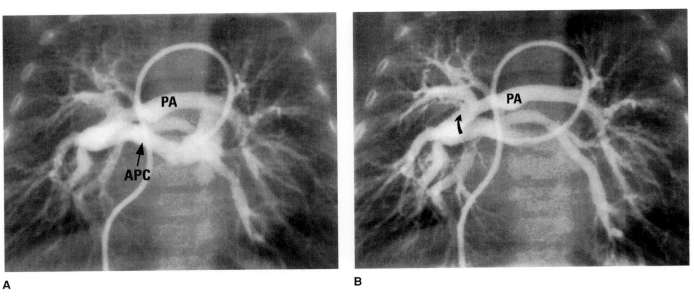

A   **B**

Fig. 21-10: Confluent pulmonary arteries connected to a large direct aortopulmonary collateral artery.
A and B: Two frames from selective injection into a large direct aortopulmonary collateral artery with opacification of 5.0 mm confluent pulmonary arteries.

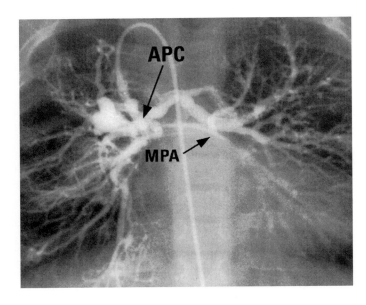

Fig. 21-11: A diminutive "seagull" confluence and its main pulmonary trunk imaged by selective injection of an indirect aortopulmonary collateral vessel.

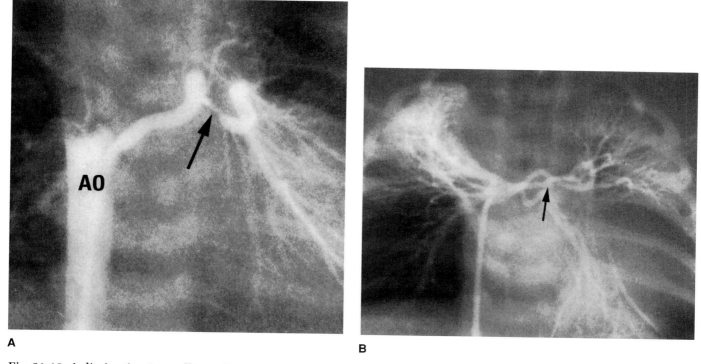

A

B

Fig. 21-12: A diminutive "seagull" confluence and a tenuous or precarious aortopulmonary collateral.
A: Selective injection into a direct aortopulmonary collateral shows a severe stenosis (arrow). **B:** The diminutive "seagull" confluence (arrow) is visualized by the injection of a direct aortopulmonary collateral.

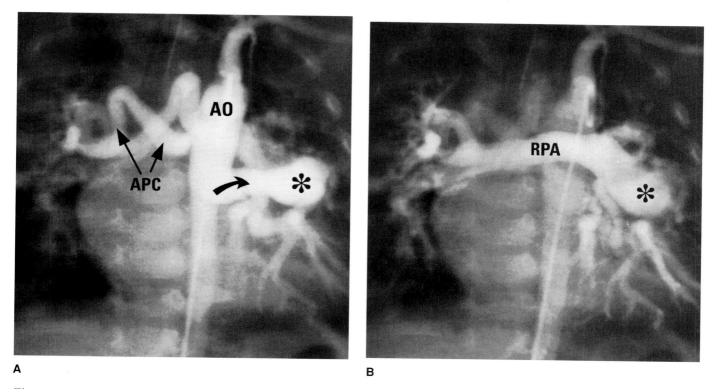

A

B

Fig. 21-13: Large confluent pulmonary arteries mediated by a large direct aortopulmonary collateral with other direct aortopulmonary collateral arteries.
A and B: Two frames from injection into the descending thoracic aorta with opacification (curved arrow) of a large direct aortopulmonary collateral (APC) artery that connects with the left pulmonary artery (✱). *(figure continues)*

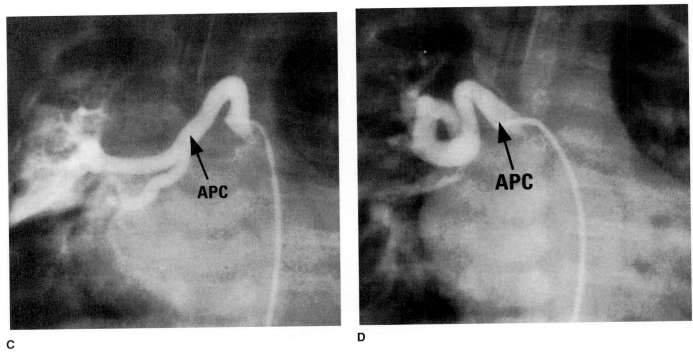

C   **D**

Fig. 21-13: *(continued)*
C and D: Two other aortopulmonary collaterals in the same patient that do not connect with the true pulmonary arteries.

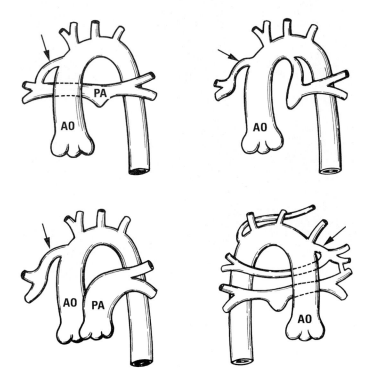

Fig. 21-14: Fifth aortic arch and pulmonary blood supply.
These diagrams depict *possible* contributions of a fifth aortic arch to pulmonary blood supply. **Top, left:** The fifth aortic arch (arrow) supplies confluent pulmonary arteries. **Bottom, left:** The fifth aortic arch (arrow) supplies only the right pulmonary artery while the main pulmonary trunk continues to the left pulmonary artery. **Top, right:** Nonconfluent pulmonary arteries with the fifth aortic arch (arrow) supplying the right pulmonary artery and the arterial duct the left pulmonary artery. **Bottom, right:** Fifth aortic arch connecting to systemic collaterals that in turn connect to the confluent pulmonary arteries.

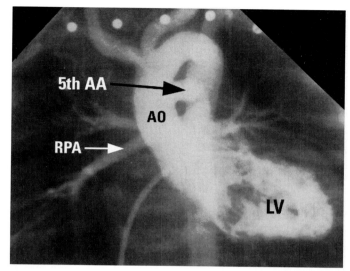

A

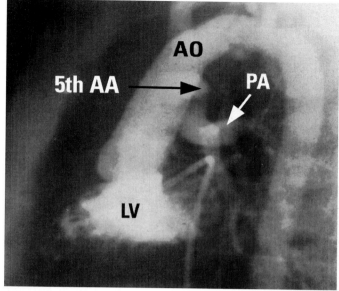

B

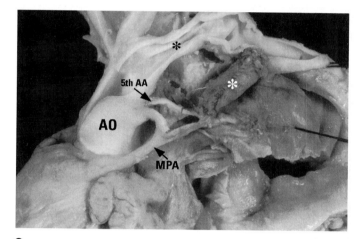

C

Fig. 21-15: Fifth aortic arch with a systemic-to-pulmonary artery connection in a patient with tricuspid and pulmonary atresia.
A and B: Frontal and lateral left ventriculogram shows the fifth aortic arch originating from the ascending aorta proximal to the brachiocephalic arteries connecting to the pulmonary arteries. **C:** Postmortem specimen. The hypoplastic aortic arch and isthmus is noted with a black (✱); the surgically created shunt with a white (✱). **D through G:** Fifth aortic arch with a systemic-to-systemic connection in a different patient with pulmonary atresia and ventricular septal defect. **D:** Aortogram shows fifth aortic arch with its systemic-systemic connection and subsequent opacification of the true main pulmonary trunk. *(figure continues)*

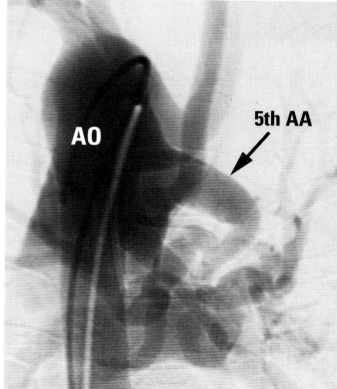

D

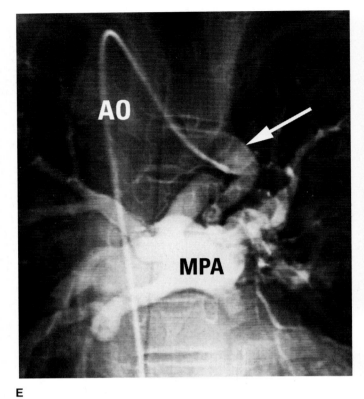

E

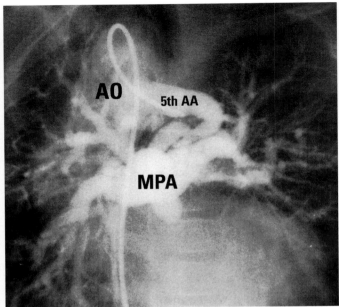

F

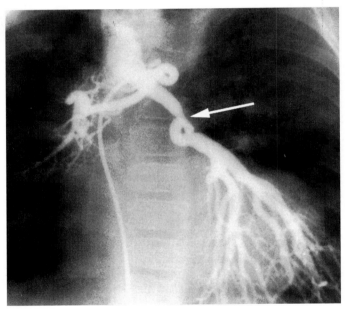

G

Fig. 21-15: *(continued)*
E and F: Selective injection of the fifth aortic arch. **G:** This same patient has tortuous, stenotic, direct aortopulmonary collateral arteries.

cephalic artery and connected directly with the pulmonary arteries. Through a systemic-to-systemic connection the fifth aortic arch may also support the pulmonary circulation indirectly as in the patient published by Yoo and his colleagues (Fig. 21-15).[129] This particular patient had pulmonary atresia and ventricular septal defect with a right-sided aortic arch. The fifth aortic arch originated from the posterolateral wall of the ascending aorta, and supplied the intrapulmonary arteries of both lungs through a bifurcating collateral artery (Fig. 21-15). The confluent pulmonary arteries were then perfused by a communicating channel from the left branch of the collateral artery. The patient reported by Hashimoto and colleagues[133] had an un-usual aortopulmonary collateral artery originating from the ascending aorta just superior to the coronary artery ostia and extending to the pulmonary trunk, reminiscent of the fifth arch anatomy reported by Freedom,[130] although the authors did not consider this peculiar vessel a fifth aortic arch.

Origins of Nonconfluent Pulmonary Arteries

Nonconfluent pulmonary arteries may reflect a congenital abnormality, or virtual nonconfluence may be acquired after surgical palliation, either purposefully (as after a classical Glenn anastomosis), or through scarring and distorsion of a pulmonary artery (Figs.

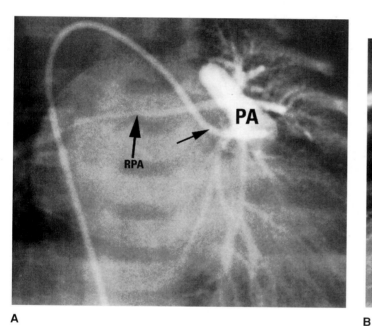

A

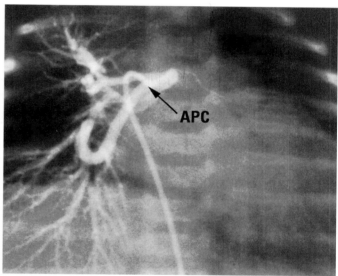

B

Fig. 21-16: Pulmonary atresia, ventricular septal defect, aortopulmonary window, and aortopulmonary collaterals.
A: The retrograde arterial catheter has been advanced across an aorto-pulmonary window (arrow) where this injection shows a reasonably well-developed left pulmonary artery, but a thread-like right pulmonary. **B:** Much of the right pulmonary artery is supplied by this aortopulmonary collateral artery. **C:** A different patient whose aortopulmonary window (APW) is demonstrated by aortic root angiography.

C

21-17 through 21-29). In addition, progressive obstruction at the site of ductal insertion or incorporation may lead to nonconfluence (Fig. 21-30). On a congenital basis and without any connection between right and left pulmonary artery branches, the pulmonary arteries may be nonconfluent, indicating a completely separate origin for the right and left pulmonary arteries.[1–6,7,9,11,12,28–30,57,67,92,94,95,98–100,106–109,116,117,119,134–149] Either the right or left pulmonary artery may originate from the ascending aorta; from an arterial duct; from direct or indirect aortopulmonary collaterals; or in some patients, mediastinal pulmonary arteries cannot be identified by any methodology. It is important to remember that in most cases the two blood sources (ie, the arterial duct and aortopulmonary collateral arteries) do not coexist in supplying the same lung (Figs. 21-31 through 21-33). There are exceptions to this reciprocal supply with the same lung being supplied by the two sources. Even in those rare cases with coexisting ductal and aortopulmonary collateral supply to the same lung, any given bronchopulmonary segment will be supplied either by an arterial duct or from an aortopulmonary collateral, not by both.[7–9,12,92,95,116,117,150,151] Those cases of part of the lung supplied by both sources are extremely rare. Thus, in some patients, nonconfluent pulmonary arteries will be supported by bilateral arterial ducts; by an arterial duct on one side and aortopulmonary collaterals to the other; or by different aortopulmonary collaterals, etc. In the older patient, the collateral circulation may involve

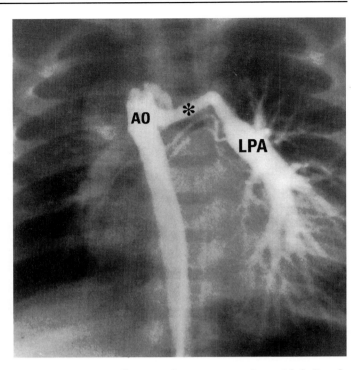

Fig. 21-18: Nonconfluent pulmonary arteries with left pulmonary artery from left arterial duct (∗) or aortopulmonary collateral.

the aortic vasa vasorum[152] and connections between the coronary arteries and bronchial arteries are well described as well (Figs. 21-34 and 21-35).[153–156] Connections between the root of the aorta (ie, aortopulmonary fenestration) or coronary artery and pulmonary trunk may support some or all of the pulmonary blood supply (Fig. 21-16).[12,28,109,110,121–127,133a,157] Schulze-Neick and colleagues[148] describe a very interesting patient with pulmonary atresia and nonconfluent pulmonary arteries. The right pulmonary artery originated from the ascending aorta close to the left coronary artery and the left pulmonary artery had a distal ductal origin. This unusual case prompted a letter from Gerlis and colleagues[158] who suggest that the unusual vessel originating from the ascending aorta represents a left fifth aortic arch. The angiographic appearance of the fifth aortic arch from the separate reports by Freedom[129] and Yoo[130] support the observations of Gerlis and colleagues[158] in this letter and in Gerlis's other reports of the fifth aortic arch (Figs. 21-14 and 21-15).[131,132]

Bilateral Arterial Ducts and Pulmonary Atresia

Formigari and colleagues[66] have reported the prevalence of bilateral patent arterial ducts in patients with different types of pulmonary atresia. They did not

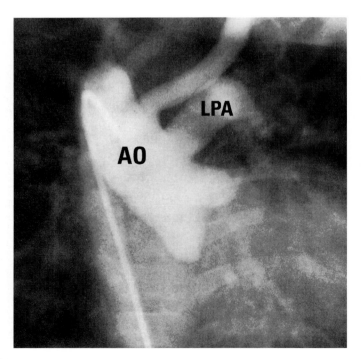

Fig. 21-17: Nonconfluent pulmonary arteries with left pulmonary artery from ascending aorta (see also Chapter 20, Fig. 20–13 and Chapter 22, Fig. 22-9).

(text continues on p. 569)

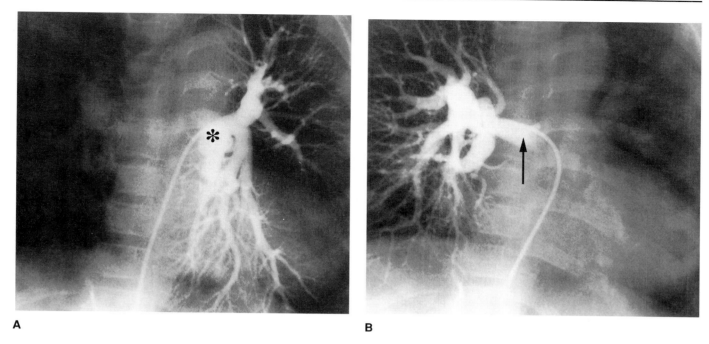

Fig. 21-19: Nonconfluent pulmonary arteries with right and left pulmonary arteries originating from direct aortopulmonary collateral arteries.
A: Selective injection into left-sided direct aortopulmonary collateral artery(✱). **B:** Selective injection into right-sided direct aortopulmonary collateral artery (arrow).

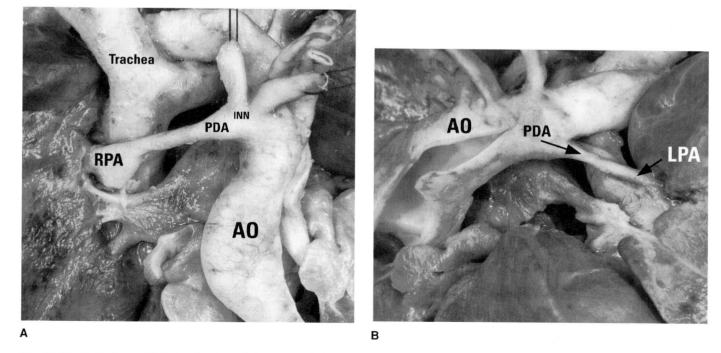

Fig. 21-20: Pathology of bilateral arterial ducts supplying nonconfluent pulmonary arteries.
A: Right-sided arterial duct connected to right pulmonary artery. **B:** Left-sided arterial duct connected to left pulmonary artery.

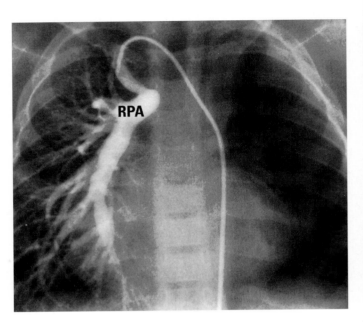

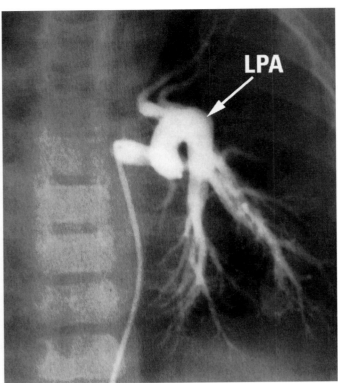

A   **B**

Fig. 21-21: Nonconfluent pulmonary arteries supported by ipsilateral arterial ducts.
A: Right-sided duct to right pulmonary artery. **B:** Left-sided duct to left pulmonary artery.

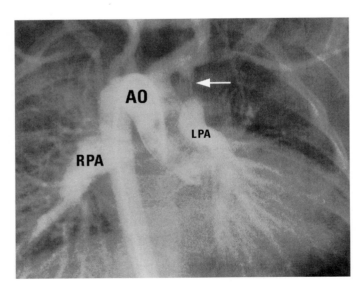

Fig. 21-22: Nonconfluent pulmonary arteries supported by ipsilateral arterial ducts in a patient with a right-sided aortic arch.
A: Right-sided duct supports the right pulmonary artery. **B:** The very narrowed left-sided arterial duct (arrow) tenuously connects to the left pulmonary artery.

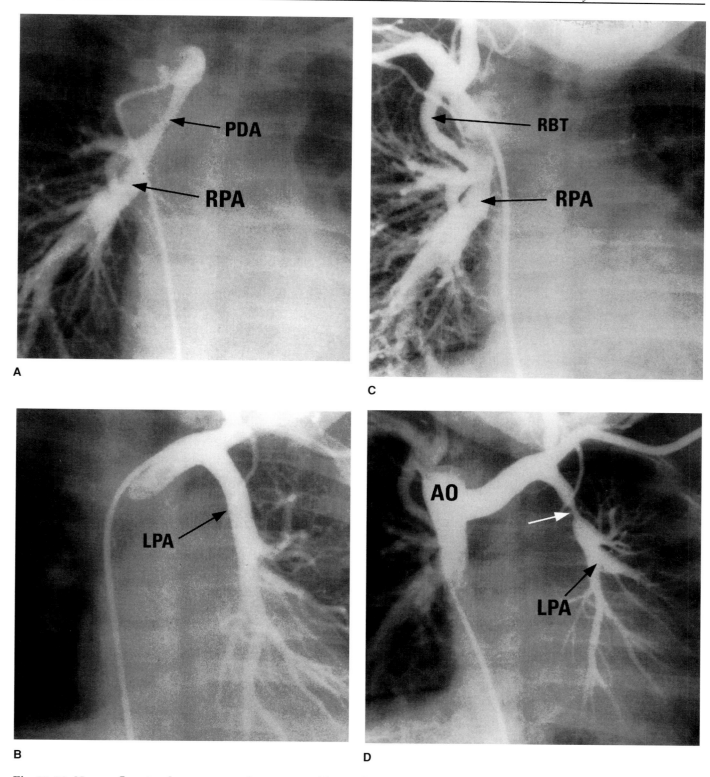

Fig. 21-23: Nonconfluent pulmonary arteries supported by ipsilateral arterial ducts before and after palliation.
A: The narrowed right-sided arterial duct. **B:** The hypertensive left-sided arterial duct and left pulmonary artery originating from an aberrant left subclavian artery. **C:** After a right-sided arterial shunt. **D:** After banding of the left arterial duct (arrow).

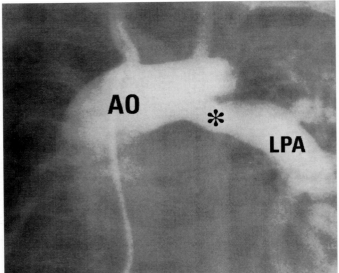
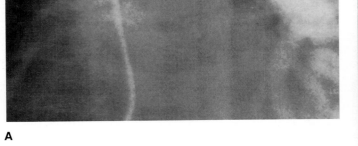

A

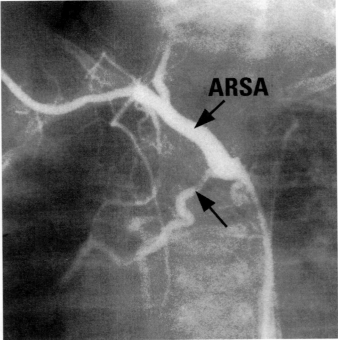

B

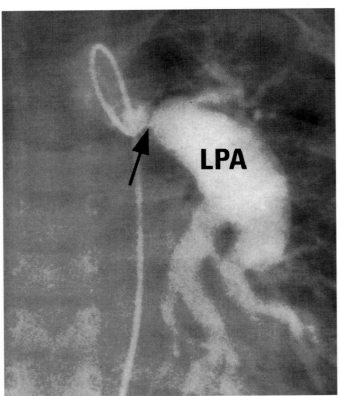

C

Fig. 21-24: Nonconfluent pulmonary arteries supported by ipsilateral arterial ducts, one very narrowed and one hypertensive.
A: The large hypertensive left-sided arterial duct (✱) and the left pulmonary artery. **B:** The very narrowed right-sided arterial duct originating from the aberrant right subclavian artery. **C:** The left-sided arterial duct-left pulmonary artery after pulmonary artery banding (arrow).

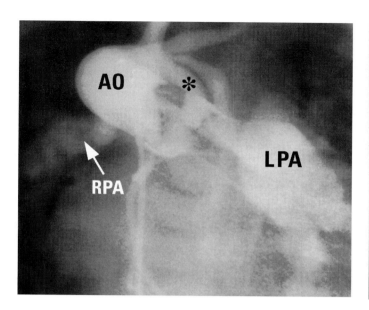

Fig. 21-25: Nonconfluent pulmonary arteries supported by ipsilateral arterial ducts in a patient with presumed left atrial isomerism palliated with a modified left-sided Blalock-Taussig shunt. The left arterial duct is noted (✳).

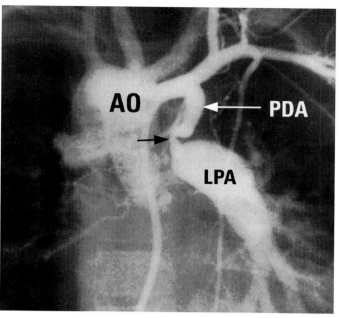

Fig. 21-27: Nonconfluent pulmonary arteries with the left pulmonary artery supported by an arterial duct and severe distal obstruction (arrow).

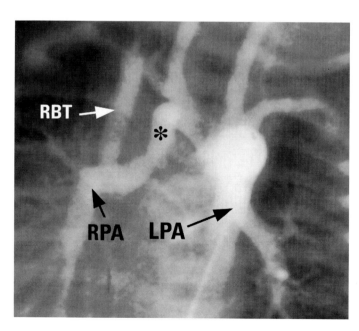

Fig. 21-26: Nonconfluent pulmonary arteries supported by ipsilateral arterial ducts with a right-sided Blalock-Taussig shunt (RBT). Note the right-sided arterial duct (✳).

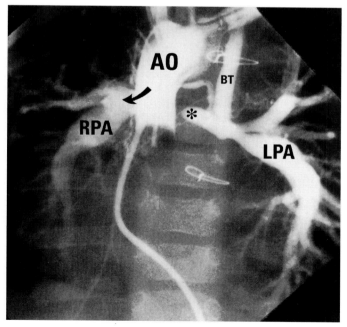

Fig. 21-28: Nonconfluent pulmonary arteries with the left pulmonary artery supported by a Blalock-Taussig (BT) shunt. Note the proximal (✳) left pulmonary artery. This figure provided by Dr. M. Legras, Children's Hospital of Western Ontario.

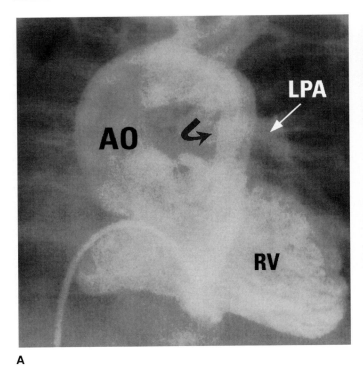

A

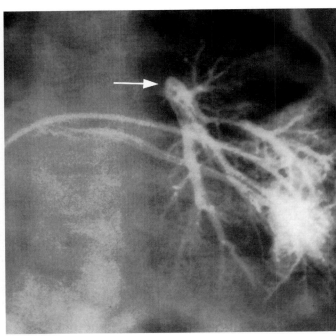

B

Fig. 21-29: Isolation of left pulmonary artery.
A: Neonatal study shows nonconfluent pulmonary arteries with the left pulmonary artery supported by its patent arterial duct (curved arrow). **B:** Some years later after closure of the arterial duct, the left pulmonary artery (arrow) could only be demonstrated by left pulmonary vein wedge angiography.

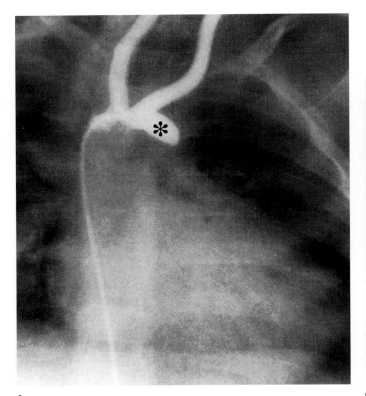

A

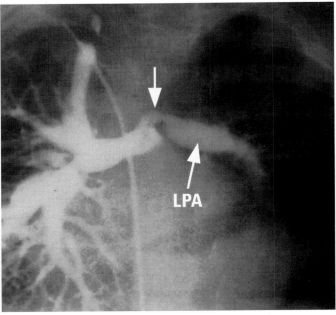

B

Fig. 21-30: Left pulmonary artery branch stenosis and the arterial duct.
A: The ductal diverticulum. **B:** Severe (arrow) left pulmonary artery branch stenosis at the site of ductal tissue. *(figure continues)*

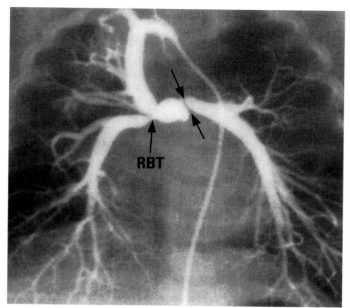

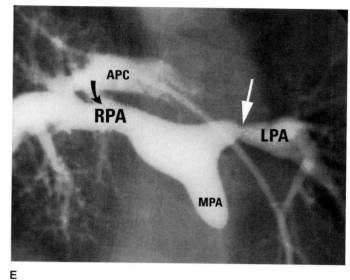

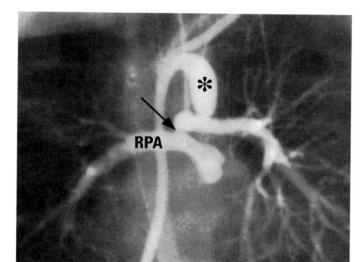

Fig. 21-30: *(continued)*
C: Another patient with severe left pulmonary artery stenosis at the site of ductal insertion (arrows); **D:** Severe proximal left pulmonary artery stenosis (arrow). **E:** Another patient with left pulmonary artery stenosis at the site of ductal (white arrow) insertion (arrows). Angiographic access to the confluent pulmonary arteries was via the direct aortopulmonary collateral (APC). *(figure continues)*

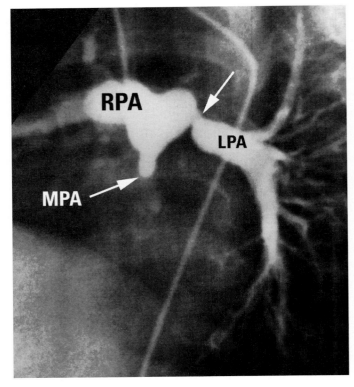

F

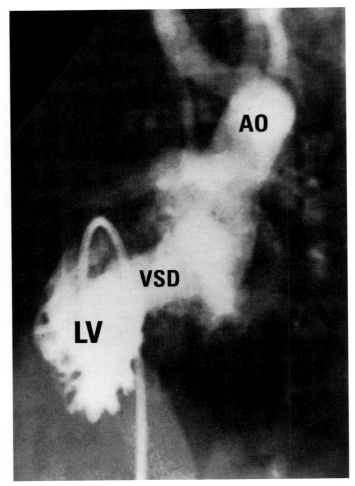

H

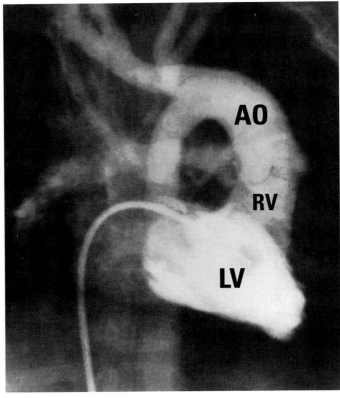

G

Fig. 21-30: *(continued)*
F: Severe left pulmonary artery stenosis (arrow) in a patient with atrioventricular discordance (**G**) and large ventricular septal defect with single-outlet aorta (**H**).

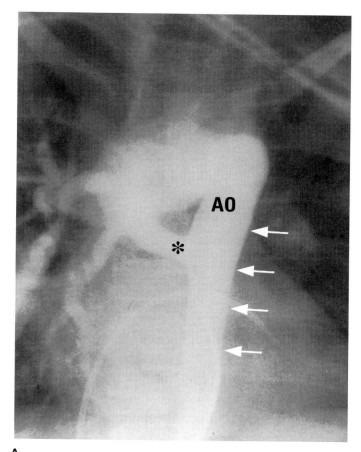

A

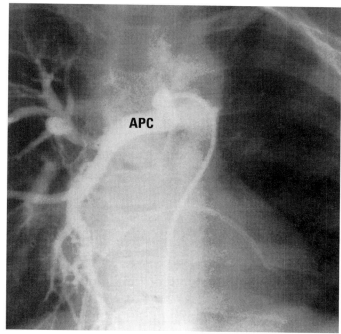

B

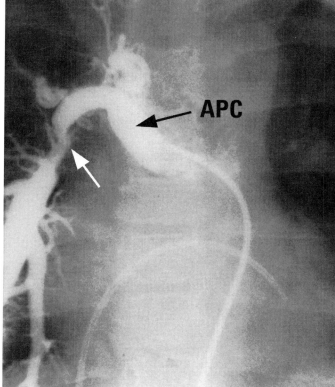

C

Fig. 21-31: The reciprocal relationship between the arterial duct and aortopulmonary collateral supply to any given bronchopulmonary segment: both usually do not supply the same bronchopulmonary segment.
A: Descending thoracic aortogram shows collateral (✳) to right lung, but no collaterals (arrows) to the left lung. **B and C:** Selective injection of collaterals to right lung. *(figure continues)*

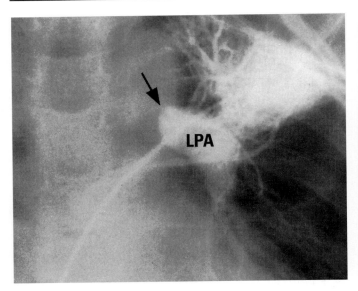

D

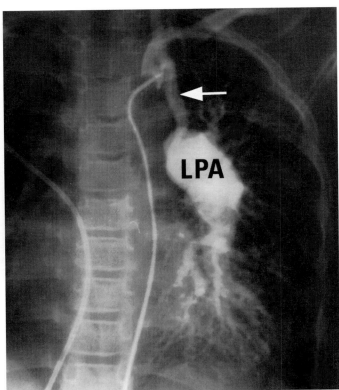

E

Fig. 21-31: *(continued)*
D: Left-sided pulmonary vein wedge injection shows a hilar left pulmonary artery (arrow). **E:** Modified Blalock-Taussig shunt was constructed into the hilar left pulmonary artery. This patient eventually underwent repair to her left lung.

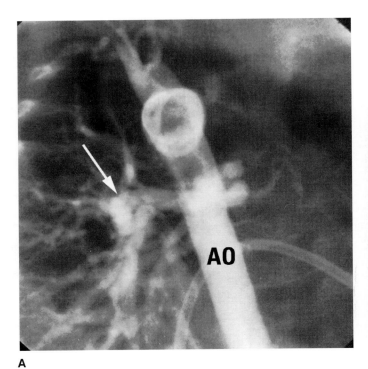

A

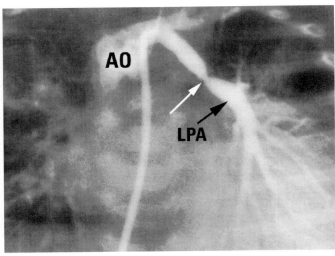

B

Fig. 21-32: Another example of the reciprocal relationship between the arterial duct and aortopulmonary collateral supply to any given bronchopulmonary segment.
A: Descending thoracic aortogram shows a collateral supplying most of the right lung. **B:** A left-sided arterial duct supplies all of the left pulmonary artery.

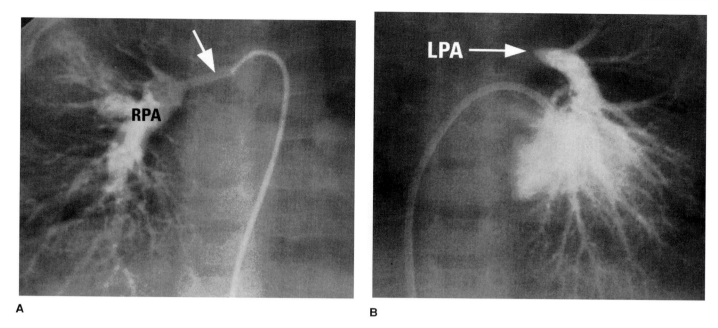

Fig. 21-33: Yet another example of the reciprocal relationship between the arterial duct and aortopulmonary collateral supply to any given bronchopulmonary segment.
A: Descending thoracic aortogram shows a collateral supplying most of the right lung. **B:** The left pulmonary artery has become isolated after ductal closure.

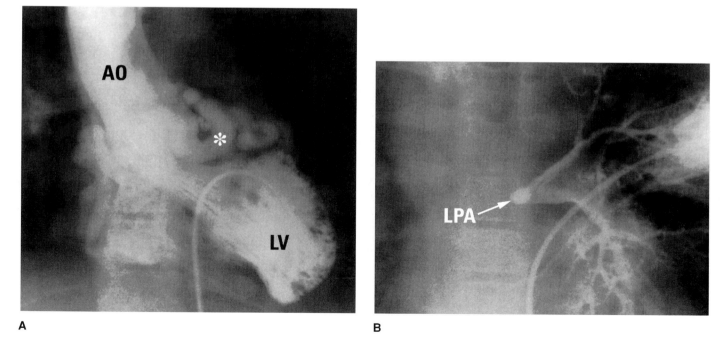

Fig. 21-34: Very much enlarged coronary arteries participating in coronary artery-bronchial artery connections in a patient with pulmonary atresia and nonconfluent pulmonary arteries.
A: Left ventriculogram in frontal projection shows enlarged tortuous coronary arteries (✳). **B:** Left pulmonary vein wedge angiogram shows the hilar left pulmonary artery.

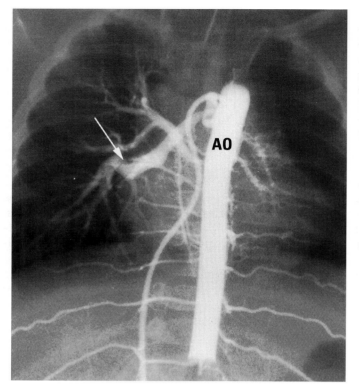

A

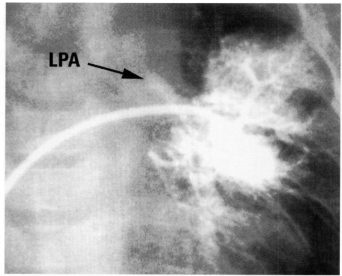

B

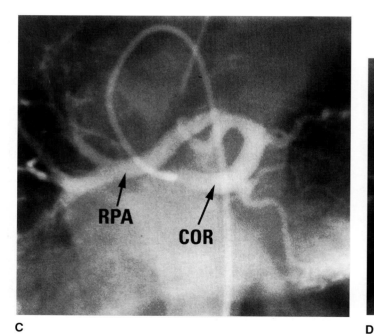

C

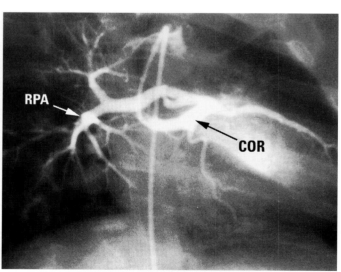

D

Fig. 21-35: The left anterior descending coronary artery supplies the right pulmonary artery in this patient with nonconfluent pulmonary arteries.
A: Descending thoracic aortogram shows small aortopulmonary collaterals to the right lung. **B:** Left pulmonary vein wedge angiography shows the hilar left pulmonary artery. **C and D:** Selective left coronary arteriography shows most of the right pulmonary artery supplied by the left anterior descending coronary artery.

identify bilateral patent arterial ducts in any patient with pulmonary atresia and intact ventricular septal defect, remembering the case report of Milanesi and colleagues,[137] nor in any patient with tricuspid atresia or single ventricle (not associated with asplenia). Of those patients with pulmonary atresia and ventricular septal defect, 2% were found to have bilateral patent arterial ducts, and bilateral patent arterial ducts were identified in 5% of patients with either complete or corrected transposition of the great arteries. The highest prevalence of bilateral patent arterial ducts was found in patients with asplenia syndrome (25%) (see also Chapter 41). Bilateral arterial ducts have been identified in a rare patient with pulmonary atresia and intact ventricular septum (see also Chapter 23, Fig. 23-3).[137] It is of interest that bilateral arterial ducts thus may support the entirety of the pulmonary circulation (Figs. 21-20 through 21-26), but may also support the entirety of the systemic circulation in those rare patients with aortic atresia and interruption of the aortic arch (see also Chapters 26 and 33).[159,160] As we and others have pointed out, isolation of a subclavian artery has been identified in patients with tetralogy of Fallot, with the subclavian artery-pulmonary artery connection mediated by an arterial duct, and in patients with interruption of the aortic arch (see also Chapters 20, Fig. 20-16 and 34).[12,92,92a]

The Nature of the Collateral Circulation in Pulmonary Atresia

The designation of those systemic arterial vessels considered collateral circulation to the lungs has changed commensurate with increased understanding of the origin and distribution of these vessels. For a long time, all collateral arteries to the lungs regardless of their sites of origin and distribution were considered and indeed designated as bronchial arteries. This was clearly incorrect, as many of these vessels did not have an appropriate anatomy, origin nor did they follow the course of the major bronchi.[78,96,156] In some patients with reasonably well-developed pulmonary arteries, one can define a group of small and tortuous systemic-to-pulmonary artery collateral arteries with a multifocal origin from the aorta and its branches. These vessels are probably acquired postnatally to achieve a greater pulmonary blood flow.[112] The other major type of systemic-to-pulmonary collateral artery are rather large arteries frequently associated with absent or hypoplastic central or mediastinal pulmonary arteries, considered congenital, and representing persistent embryonic ventral splanchnic arteries.[78,80,105,112] Rabinovitch and colleagues[94,98,151] have categorized those collateral vessels into three major types, both by their site of origin as well as from the way in which they connect to the lung. These three types are: 1) direct aortopulmonary collat-

eral; 2) indirect aortopulmonary collateral; and 3) true bronchial arteries. Direct aortopulmonary collaterals probably represent persistence of primitive intersegmental arteries that originate from the descending thoracic aorta and which have not involuted.[9,77-80,94-99,106-109,114-117,119,120,144,156,161] These direct collaterals originating from the descending thoracic aorta connect with the lung arteries at the hilum of the lung, passing either in front of or behind the bronchus (Figs. 21-1, 21-6, 21-10, 21-12, 21-13, 21-15, 21-19, and 21-36 through 21-40). They usually number from two to six in any patient. The indirect collateral arteries originate from the arch vessels, primarily the subclavian arteries or the carotid arteries, but not the bronchial arteries, with extrapulmonary anastomoses to the lungs (Figs. 21-7, 21-11, 21-40, and 21-41 through 21-45). The aortopulmonary collateral arteries of congenital nature, whether they arise directly from the aorta or indirectly from the arch vessels, enter the lung through the pulmonary hilum or the inferior pulmonary ligament. They may connect with the central or true pulmonary artery in the mediastinum or with the intrapulmonary artery at its lobar or segmental branch level. They should be differentiated from the acquired collateral arteries that have interconnections with the minute peripheral tributaries of the intrapulmonary arteries. These acquired collaterals may be either the preexisting bronchial arteries that enter the lung through the hilum or the newly formed transpleural systemic-pulmonary communications. We and others have identified indirect collateral arteries

(text continues on p. 569)

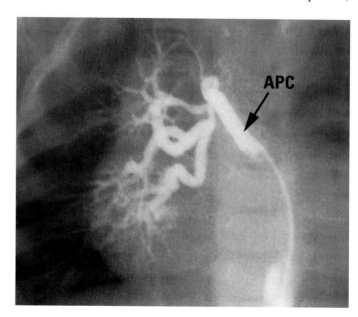

Fig. 21-36: Selective injection into a single aortopulmonary collateral demonstrates some distribution to the right upper and middle lobe segments of the lung. There are distal stenoses beyond the hilar connections of the aortopulmonary collateral.

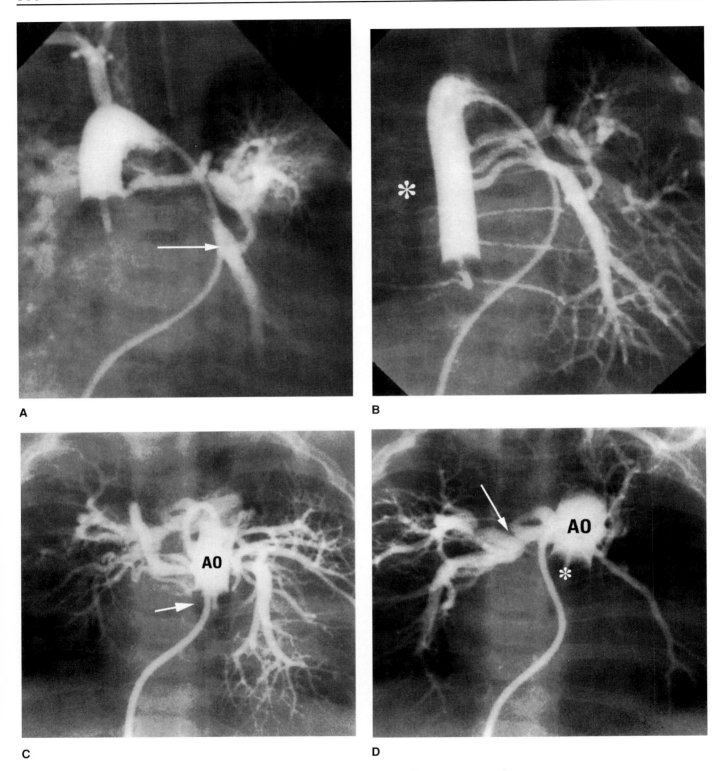

A

B

C

D

Fig. 21-37: Multiple aortopulmonary collaterals shown by balloon occlusion aortography.
A: A stenotic collateral with connection to the left pulmonary artery (arrow). **B:** Multiple collaterals to the left lung and relatively sparse vessels (✳) to the right lung. **C and D:** Two other balloon occlusion aortograms demonstrate multiple aortopulmonary collaterals.

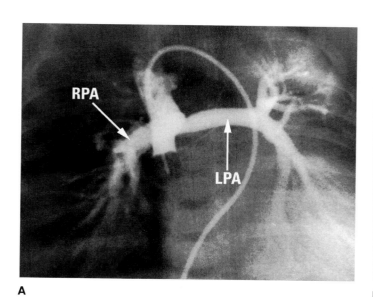

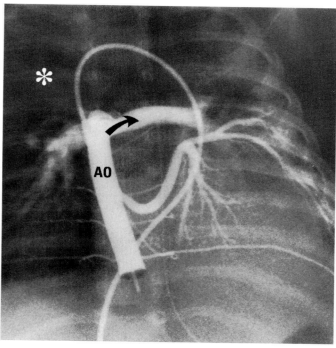

A

B

Fig. 21-38: Right and left pulmonary arteries and direct aortopulmonary collaterals shown from balloon occlusion descending aortography.
A: Right and left pulmonary arteries are demonstrated by this balloon occlusion aortogram. **B:** This selective balloon occlusion aortogram also demonstrates a left-sided direct aortopulmonary collateral (arrow) The right pulmonary artery is not distributed to the right upper lobe (✱).

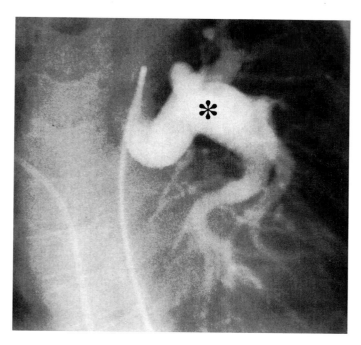

Fig. 21-39: Pulmonary vascular disease was found in this segment of lung supplied by this very large direct aortopulmonary collateral vessel. Systemic pressures were measured with an endhole catheter at this position (✱).

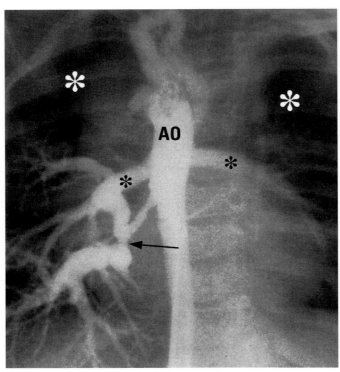

A

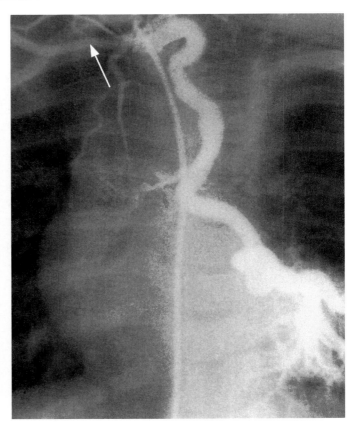

B

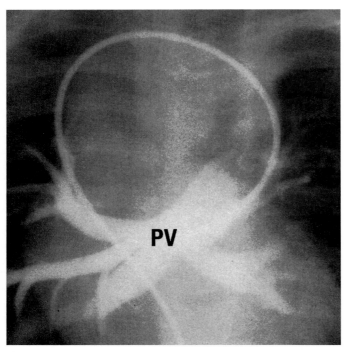

C

Fig. 21-40: Direct and indirect aortopulmonary collaterals in this patient with right atrial isomerism and anomalous pulmonary venous connections.
A: Aortogram shows several direct aortopulmonary collaterals (black ✱); the upper lobes (white ✱) are relatively underperfused. **B:** A large indirect aortopulmonary collateral originating from the right subclavian artery (arrow) courses to supply the left lower lobe. **C:** The catheter is in the pulmonary venous (PV) confluence.

originating from or adjacent to the renal arteries as well (Fig. 21-46).[12] The true bronchial arteries follow the major bronchi, have intrapulmonary connections to the lungs, and may dilate in response to a variety of challenges. The majority of direct aortopulmonary collateral arteries are narrow with stenoses, and the pathological basis for this anatomic obstruction is related to the prominence of intimal cushions as well as the resistance to flow imposed by their length as well as by their caliber.[162] With ongoing turbulent flow through the point of stenosis or narrowing within the collateral vessel and with increasing polycythemia and hyperviscosity, it is common for the obstruction within the aortopulmonary collateral to worsen, eventuating in virtual acquired absence of flow through that particular vessel.[4,5,7–9,12,94,98,151,162,162a] For this reason such collateral circulation is considered precarious. Such events rarely occur in the neonatal period, but even a mild obstruction documented in that time period may worsen. Some major direct aortopulmonary collaterals with no evidence of obstruction will perfuse its bronchopulmonary segment(s) at systemic pressure, and thus it is possible within a given lung to have some bronchopulmonary segments with and without pulmonary vascular obstructive disease (Fig. 21-39).[7–9,12,162] The development of fixed pulmonary vascular obstructive disease is usually a consideration beyond the neonatal period, although the substrate for pulmonary vascular obstruction may be unequivocally present. Indeed, the combinations for source of pulmonary blood flow and differential areas of pulmonary vascular disease are very complex, as are the sources of collateral supply, from below the diaphragm to cervical collateral arteries.[163–165] Indirect collaterals originating from the subclavian arteries are particularly common in patients with complex pulmonary atresia (Figs. 21-41 through 21-50).

Unifocal or Dual Arterial Supply of Bronchopulmonary Segment

Once one has identified the sources of blood flow to each lung, two questions must be answered: 1) How many bronchopulmonary segments are connected to the true pulmonary arteries and 2) What are the sources of arterial blood supply to each bronchopulmonary segment?[4–9,12–14,18,22,28,30,31,35,36,55,57,61,94,95,98,100,105–109,114,116,119,151,157,166,167] With thoracic situs solitus, the right lung has 10 bronchopulmonary segments and the left lung has 9 bronchopulmonary segments. Those pulmonary arteries supported by a patent arterial duct have a virtually normal segmental supply within the lung. This is far from the situation in those patients

(text continues on p. 574)

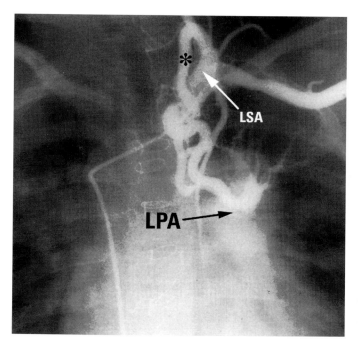

Fig. 21-41: Indirect aortopulmonary collateral connects to the left pulmonary artery.
An indirect aortopulmonary collateral artery (✳) originating from the left subclavian artery connects in a circuitous fashion to the left pulmonary artery.

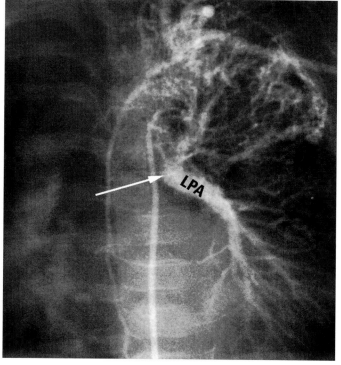

Fig. 21-42: Multiple indirect chest wall collateral arteries connect to the left pulmonary artery.

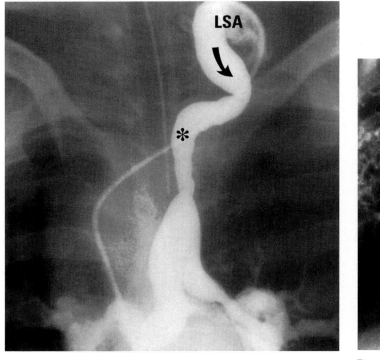

A

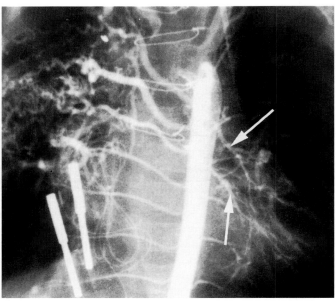

B

Fig. 21-43: A: Large indirect aortopulmonary collateral artery originating from the left subclavian artery, then bifurcating. **B:** Bronchial arterial arteries following the course of the major bronchi (arrow).

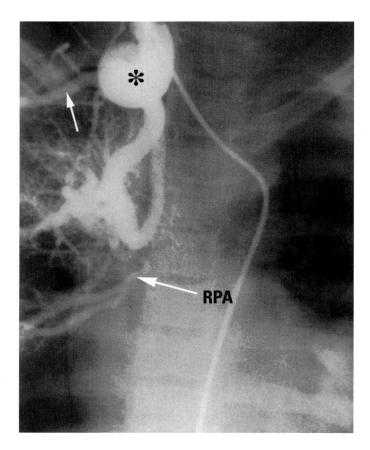

Fig. 21-44: Indirect aortopulmonary collateral artery originating from the right subclavian artery (white arrow), connecting with a small right pulmonary artery.

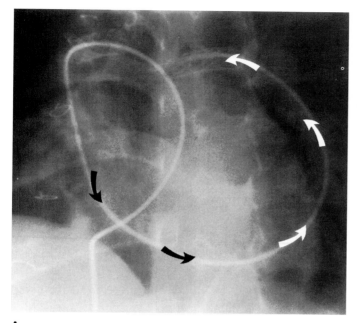

A

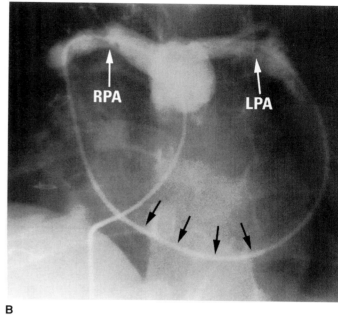

B

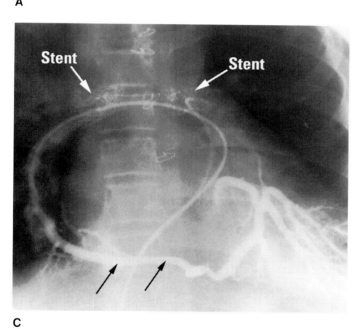

C

Fig. 21-45: Peculiar aortopulmonary collateral artery in a patient with pulmonary atresia and ventricular septal defect in whom continuity between pulmonary artery and right ventricle had been established.
A: Catheter advanced from IVC to RA to RV to MPA to RPA through collateral to distal LPA to proximal LPA. B: Angiogram shows the right and left pulmonary arteries with the angiogram performed via the peculiar connecting collateral (arrows). C: The connecting collateral (black arrows) is imaged.

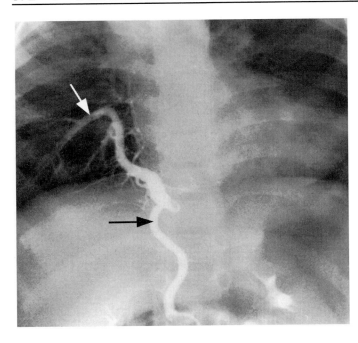

Fig. 21-46: Peculiar collateral originating from abdominal aorta adjacent to right renal artery and supplying a segment of the right lung.

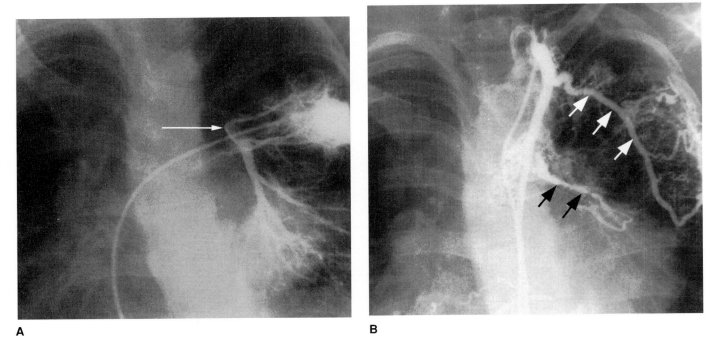

A

B

Fig. 21-47: Nonconfluent pulmonary arteries, collaterals originating from internal thoracic artery.
A: Left pulmonary vein wedge angiogram demonstrates the left pulmonary artery extending to the hilum (arrow). **B:** Large collateral arteries (arrows) arise from the left internal thoracic artery.

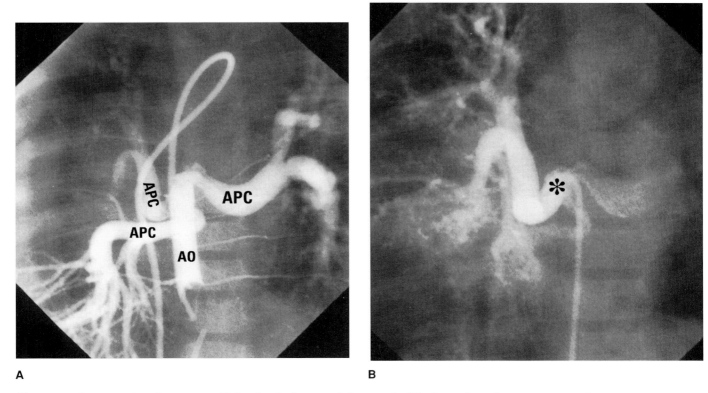

Fig. 21-48: Large aortopulmonary collateral arteries supplying most of the bronchopulmonary segments.
A: Balloon occlusion aortogram shows the direct aortopulmonary collaterals to both lungs. **B:** Selective injection of one of the right-sided collateral arteries.

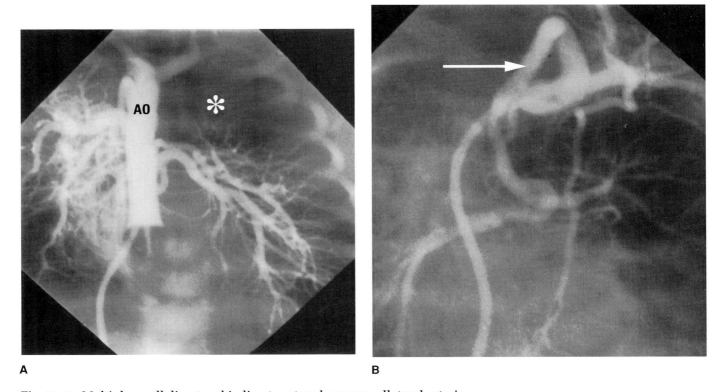

Fig. 21-49: Multiple small direct and indirect aortopulmonary collateral arteries.
A: Balloon occlusion aortography demonstrates a number of small direct aortopulmonary collaterals, with relatively little flow to the left upper lobe (✱). **B:** An indirect collateral (arrow) from the left subclavian artery connects to left and right-sided collateral arteries.

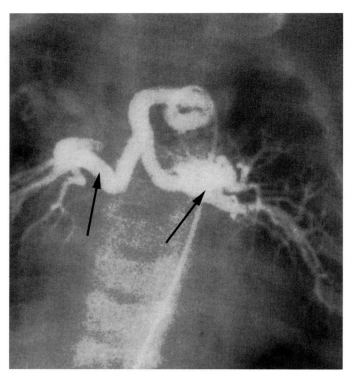

Fig. 21-50: A single aortopulmonary collateral artery originates from the upper thoracic aorta, then bifurcates (arrows).

with systemic-to-pulmonary collateral arteries (Figs. 21-51 through 21-54).

Almost always, as pointed out by Yen Ho,[119] these collateral arteries coexist with so-called central pulmonary arteries. The collateral vessels, having their origin from the systemic circulation, course to the lungs and feed the pulmonary circulation in one of two ways. The collateral artery may continue directly into the pulmonary parenchyma and support and supply a number of bronchopulmonary segments (Fig. 21-51). In other situations, the collateral runs towards the hilum of the lung, anastomosing with branches of the central pulmonary artery. In this situation, the particular collateral artery supplies the segmental area distal to its entrance to the pulmonary parenchyma, supporting all the bronchopulmonary segments fed by the central pulmonary artery. One must define for each of the bronchopulmonary segments whether it is connected to a true or central pulmonary artery, to a collateral, or both. To ask the second of these questions in terms of a therapeutic algorithm: If one identifies an aortopulmonary collateral supplying one or more bronchopulmonary segments, is it safe to interrupt this particular collateral as part of staged surgical or presurgical (ie, catheter intervention) management (Figs. 21-52, 21-53, 21-54) or

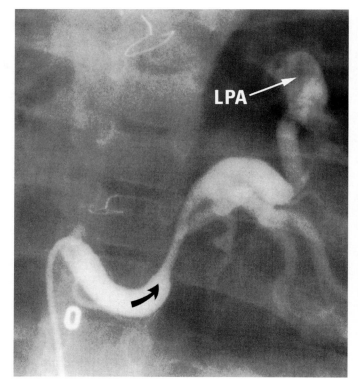

A

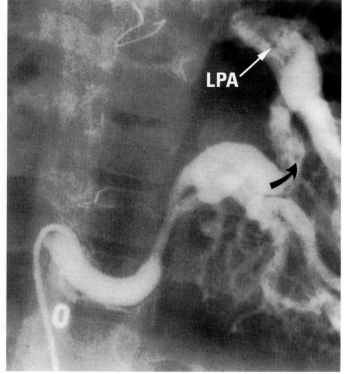

B

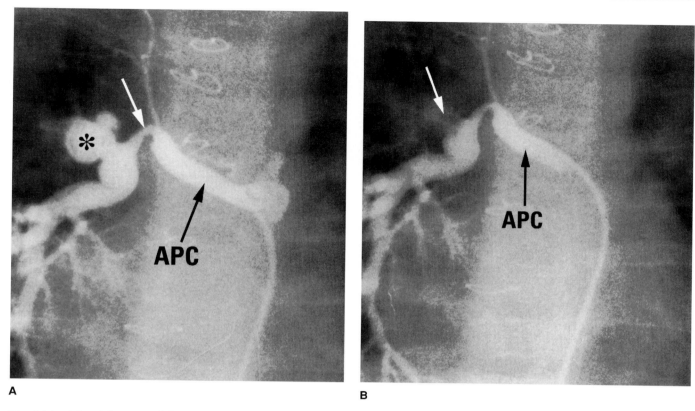

A   **B**

Fig. 21-52: The right upper lobe of lung is connected to the stenotic collateral as demonstrated by "wash-out" of contrast material.
A: Selective injection of contrast into the stenotic collateral (arrow). **B:** There is washout of contrast (white arrow) by the interconnected segment (arrow), indicating a connection between the collateral and the right upper lobe.

must that collateral be connected in some way, so-called unifocalized, directly or indirectly, to the true right or left pulmonary artery?[4–9,12–14,18,22,28,30,31,35,36,55,57,61,94,95,98,100,105–109,114,116,119,151,157,165,166] The answer rests in the nature of the blood supply to each bronchopulmonary segment. If the specific bronchopulmonary segment has a connection to the true pulmonary artery as well as arterial supply from an aortopulmonary collateral (clearly a dually supplied segment), or are clearly connected within the lung by arterial channels to other bronchopulmonary segments that are connected to the true pulmonary arteries, then it

would be prudent to interrupt the collateral. If the collateral artery is the only source of arterial supply to the given segment of lung, then interruption could lead to infarction of those segments supplied by the collateral. The impact of the appreciation of any segment as supplied only by an aortopulmonary collateral is that this segment of lung would have to be surgically connected or unifocalised to prevent infarction. Iyer and Mee have reported their extensive experience in the repair of pulmonary atresia and ventricular septal defect and major aortopulmonary collaterals, specifically focusing on the criteria for ligation of these collateral arteries.[51] Their

Fig. 21-51: This direct left-sided aortopulmonary collateral artery connects with the true left pulmonary artery as shown by "wash-in" of contrast material.
A: Selective injection into the direct left-sided aortopulmonary collateral artery fills the left pulmonary artery. **B:** A slightly later frame shows clearly the point of interconnection (curved arrow). The collateral was uneventfully interrupted.

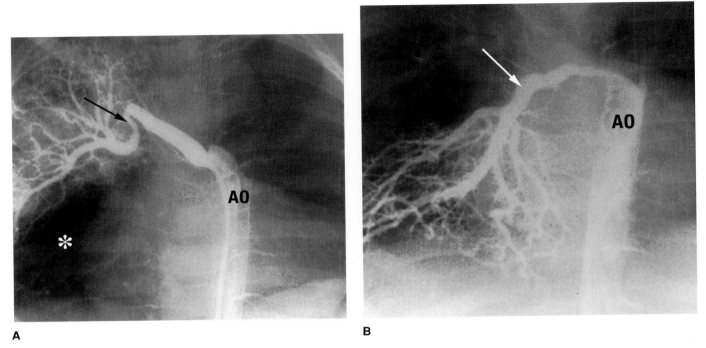

Fig. 21-53: These two collateral arteries were the only source of blood supply to their respective bronchopulmonary segments. There was neither wash-in, nor wash-out phenomenon. Note the areas of the right lung that are are not perfused by the collateral selectively injected.

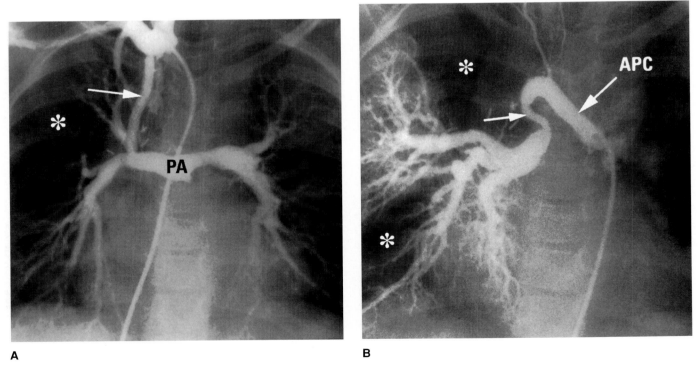

Fig. 21-54: The surgically created Blalock-Taussig shunt provides a window to the pulmonary vascular bed.
A: Note that the true pulmonary artery is not distributed to the right middle lobe (✱). **B:** The selective injection of the direct aortopulmonary collateral artery shows this vessel "fills in" those areas not provided by the true pulmonary artery.

first criterion for ligation of a major aortopulmonary collateral was that the collateral artery unequivocally duplicated supply to a segment from a central pulmonary artery. The second criteria for ligation of a collateral was the presence of wide connections between the collateral and central pulmonary arteries. Finally, duality of supply does not necessarily mean that one source of supply may be more or less precarious than the other.

Arborization Anomalies

The arborization anomalies of the intraparenchymal pulmonary arteries are another of the complex features of the pulmonary circulation in patients with pulmonary atresia and ventricular septal defect. These anomalies are characterized by abnormal distribution of arterial supply to various segments of the lung and often there are stenoses within some of the intraparenchymal arteries.[113] These may be recognized by caliber changes as well as by differing density of distribution of vessels to given segments of lung when compared with a normal pattern of distribution. Furthermore, there is increasing clinical, angiocardiographic, and histopathological data that in the setting of pulmonary atresia, involution of the ductus arteriosus is the basis of severe pulmonary artery stenosis or acquired atresia.[88–91] Acquired collateralization is uncommon in the first 3 months of life, but one is often impressed by the development of collateral vessels with the passage of time.

Laterality of the Aortic Arch

A right-sided aortic arch is identified in about 20% of patients with pulmonary atresia and ventricular septal defect, similar to that in patients with tetralogy of Fallot (Fig. 21-55; see also Chapter 20, Fig. 20-15).[3–5,12] The anatomy of the aberrant left subclavian artery in a right-sided aortic arch in a patient with tetralogy of Fallot/pulmonary atresia differs from that in persons with a normal heart. As pointed out by Velasquez and colleagues,[167a] the aberrant left subclavian artery originates directly from the aortic arch when tetralogy anatomy is present (see Chapter 20, Fig. 20-15). However, when the heart is normal, the aberrant left subclavian artery and arterial duct originate from a diverticulum. A double aortic arch and cervical aorta are well-recognized in the patient with complex pulmonary atresia.[12,151]

Bronchial Compression Syndrome and Pulmonary Atresia

Airway compromise from a vascular ring has been rarely described in the patient with tetralogy of Fallot, and double-aortic arch, left aortic arch, aberrant right subclavian artery, and a right-sided arterial duct, and a right aortic arch with aberrant left subclavian artery have been described as causal.[168–171] A so-called pulmonary vascular sling has also been reported in the patient with tetralogy of Fallot and severe airway compromise (see also Chapters 19 and 34).[172] Other even

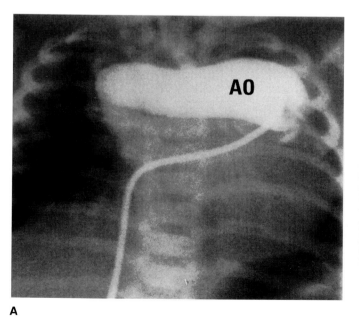
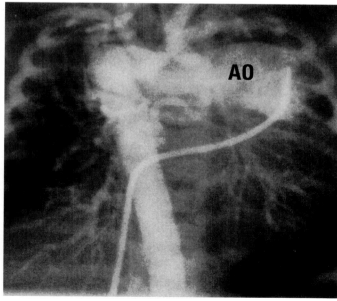

A　　　　　　　　　　　　**B**

Fig. 21-55: A right-sided aortic arch in a patient with pulmonary atresia and ventricular septal defect and multiple aortopulmonary collaterals. A and B: Two frames from frontal aortogram.

less common mechanisms for compromising the airway in the patient with complex pulmonary atresia include aneurysmal dilatation of the ascending aorta compressing the right bronchus and in another patient with pulmonary atresia and ventricular septal defect, an aneurysm of a large direct aorto-pulmonary collateral compressed the trachea, promoting respiratory distress in these patients.[173–175]

Pulmonary Atresia and Obstructive Anomalies of the Aortic Arch

Coarctation of the aorta and interruption of the aortic arch have all been described in patients with tetralogy of Fallot, despite the usual reciprocal relationship between obstruction to pulmonary blood flow and obstruction to systemic blood flow.[176–182] Such obstructive anomalies are very uncommon in the patient with tetralogy of Fallot and are even less common in the patient with pulmonary atresia. We described one of the very few cases of coarctation of the aorta in a patient with tricuspid and pulmonary atresia whose pulmonary blood flow was mediated by a fifth aortic arch (see Fig. 21-15).[130]

Prostaglandin and Pulmonary Atresia

The application and role of an E-type prostaglandin has been described in the management of the patient with pulmonary atresia and a duct-dependent pulmonary circulation.[183–185] Prostaglandin administered intravenously or orally has dramatically altered the potential for surgical intervention by preventing anatomic constriction and closure of the arterial duct in those patient whose pulmonary blood flow is in large part duct-dependent. There is considerable literature addressing the effect of prostaglandin on the histological integrity of the arterial duct.[186–190] However, there is no consensus as to those changes in the wall of the arterial duct subsequent to prostaglandin therapy, and whether these histological changes may potentially disadvantage the patient.[186–190] Silver and colleagues[189] from the Toronto Hospital for Sick Children and Teixeira and colleagues[190] examined the morphology of the arterial duct with special reference to prostaglandin therapy, and could not delineate specific changes attributable to its use. Nonetheless, aneurysmal change of the ductus arteriosus after prostaglandin E_1 administration for pulmonary atresia has been documented.[191] These alterations in the morphology of the arterial duct after prostaglandin administration may have some influence when one considers manipulation and stenting of the arterial duct.[192–194] One should also be aware of the effect of prostaglandin E_1 on the pulmonary circulation itself. Data from Haworth and colleagues[195,196] have shown that the most striking effect

of prostaglandin E_1 administration was to reduce pulmonary arterial smooth muscle, with the inference that the pulmonary vascular bed would become more compliant. There are those occasional newborn patients with pulmonary atresia who seemingly do not benefit from prostaglandin E_1 administration. In this context, there are those patients with absent ductus arteriosus and absent collateral pulmonary circulation where any effect would be on the integrity of the pulmonary vascular bed.[197]

Echocardiographic Imaging

We and others have documented the approach and indeed limitations of echocardiography in the definition of the pulmonary circulation in patients with pulmonary atresia.[4,5,12,157,198] The techniques and application of echocardiography and angiocardiography are rarely mutually exclusive in the investigation of any patients with congenital heart disease, and this is true for the patient with pulmonary atresia. That echocardiography can define the presence of some kinds of collateral circulation is well established, but the unraveling of the complexities of the pulmonary circulation in many, if not all, of these patients will unequivocally require angiocardiography.[199–207] Other methodologies including magnetic resonance imaging (MRI) have advocated in the recognition of major aortopulmonary collaterals. At the present time, this technique provides a gross perspective on the status of the collateral circulation, but MRI does not preempt angiocardiographic imaging. While initial management may be formulated in some patients from noninvasive imaging, the morbidity and pulmonary artery distortion from a systemic-to-pulmonary artery anastomosis will of course necessitate further angiographic imaging.[208–209]

Hemodynamic and Angiocardiographic Investigation

We have outlined elsewhere our investigative algorithms for the management of the neonate with pulmonary atresia.[12,157] While much of the intracardiac anatomy can be defined with contemporary echocardiographic techniques, when one is contemplating neonatal biventricular repair of pulmonary atresia and ventricular septal defect, then a complete angiographic investigation is necessary (see Chapter 20). The right ventricle will be profiled as in the patient with tetralogy of Fallot or pulmonary atresia and ventricular septal defect (see Chapter 20, Fig. 20-8). While a restrictive ventricular septal defect has been well-defined in the patient with tetralogy of Fallot,[210–218] this occurrence is less well-documented in patients with pulmonary atresia and ventricular septal defect (See Chapter 36, Fig. 36-11).[7,12,68] The usual mechanism for obstruction of the ventricular septal defect is tissue derived from the tricuspid valve.[12] Aortic valve stenosis has also been documented in the patient with pulmonary atresia (see Chapter 20, Fig. 20-24).[12,69,70] As in all patients with tetralogy-like cardiac anatomy, but even more in those where conduit reconstitution of the right ventricular outflow tract is contemplated, assessment of the coronary arterial anatomy is mandatory to define (or exclude) the presence of an anterior descending coronary artery or other large infundibular branch making such infundibular surgery potentially hazardous (see Chapter 20, Figs. 20-18, 20-19, and 20-20).[219-228] From the retrospective analysis reported by Carvalho,[227] standard frontal and lateral aortography does not provide as much information as angled views in the definition of origin and epicardial course of the coronary arteries in these conditions. Others have advocated end-on aortography as methodology to provide more information from aortography (see also Chapters 2, 20, and 35).[228] Finally such angiographic investigations are important in excluding some uncommon conditions including anomalous origin of the left coronary from the pulmonary artery or multiple coronary-cameral fistulae, both of which have been defined in the patient with tetralogy of Fallot.[229-232] Because a coronary artery-pulmonary artery communication may support the entirety or part of the pulmonary circulation, selective coronary arteriography may be necessary as well (Fig. 21-35).[121-127] These investigations may also be helpful in differentiating between an aortopulmonary fenestration as the source of pulmonary blood flow and a proximal left coronary artery connection.[104,110,233,234]

The immediate management of patients with complex forms of pulmonary atresia, however, requires definition of the source of pulmonary blood supply. When the pulmonary arteries are, from echocardiographic examination, clearly confluent, supplied by an arterial duct, and the brachiocephalic arteries clearly imaged, such patients can be sent to surgery for a systemic-to-pulmonary artery anastomosis, realizing these patients will require at a later date postshunt angiocardiographic imaging (Figs. 21-54, and 21-56 through 21-70).[204,205] Prior to repair, the intracardiac anatomy should be delineated by selective right and left ventricular angiocardiography, and the coronary arteries should be imaged, both to define their epicardial distribution, as well as to determine if there are connections to the bronchopulmonary circulation (see also Chapter 20).

The patient with complex pulmonary atresia and multiple sources of pulmonary blood supply cannot be managed either in the short- or long-term without complete definition of the nature of the pulmonary arterial supply. These patients will require a systematic approach to the angiography of the pulmonary circulation. Complementary information to aid in the angio-

graphic agenda should be provided by echocardiography (see above), and in some patients from computed tomography (CT) and MRI.[235,236] Standard imaging techniques including pulmonary vein wedge angiography[237-240] will be complemented by balloon occlusion aortography (selective or not).[241-248] While various maneuvers have been advocated to enhance angiographic imaging of the collateral circulation, including abdominal compression, we have not found these particularly necessary, nor helpful.[249,250] For a number of reasons, the pulmonary circulation cannot in any

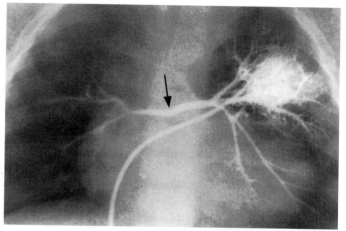

A

B

Fig. 21-56: The role of pulmonary vein wedge angiography in demonstrating a pulmonary artery confluence. A and B: The appearance of pulmonary artery confluence demonstrated by pulmonary vein wedge angiography. *(figure continues)*

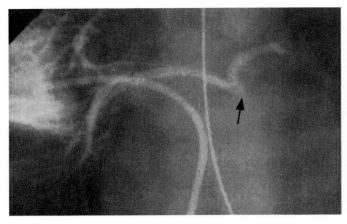

C

Fig. 21-56: *(continued)*
C and D: The appearance of pulmonary artery confluence demonstrated by pulmonary vein wedge angiography.

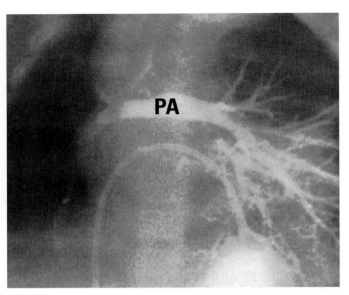

D

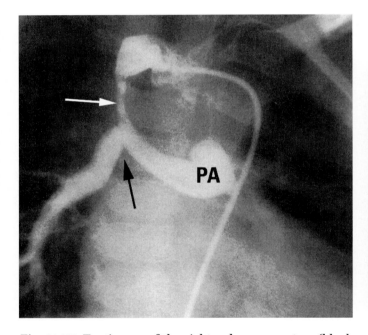

Fig. 21-57: Tenting-up of the right pulmonary artery (black arrow) by a modified Blalock-Taussig shunt (white arrow).

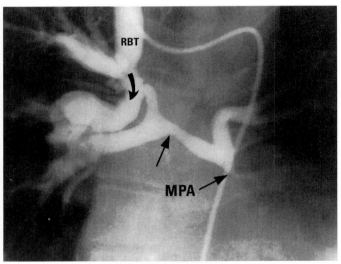

Fig. 21-58: A shunt performed to the right upper lobe pulmonary artery (curved arrow). Note the proximal right pulmonary artery stenosis (arrow).

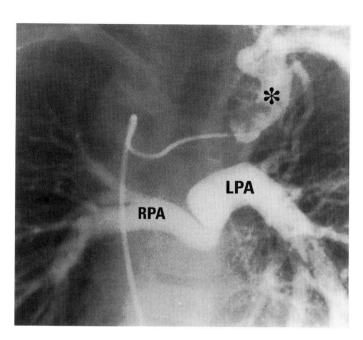

Fig. 21-59: A very narrowed left-sided modified Blalock-Taussig shunt provides access to image the pulmonary arteries. The right pulmonary artery is somewhat smaller than the left pulmonary artery,

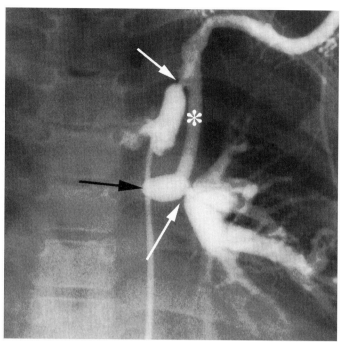

Fig. 21-61: A modified left-sided Blalock-Taussig shunt to a nonconfluent left pulmonary artery. The left subclavian artery is very narrowed (upper white arrow) just proximal to the insertion of the shunt (✱); a severe left pulmonary artery stenosis distal to the shunt is also evident (lower white arrow).

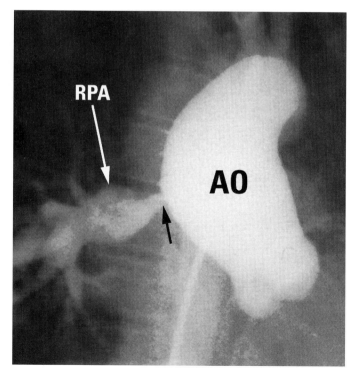

Fig. 21-60: A right pulmonary artery narrowed (arrow) by a Waterson anastomosis.

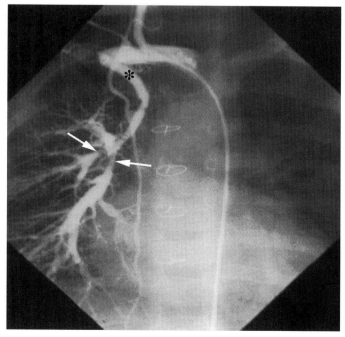

Fig. 21-62: A modified right-sided Blalock-Taussig shunt (✱)to a nonconfluent right pulmonary artery. Note the severe distal arterial stenoses (arrows).

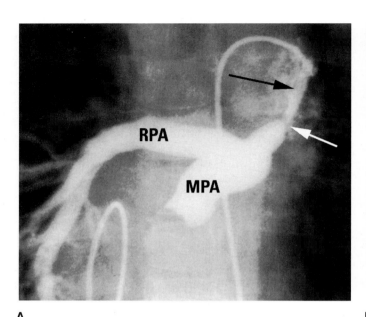

A

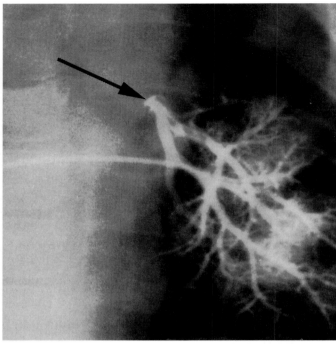

B

Fig. 21-63: Complete occlusion of the distal left pulmonary artery after a Blalock-Taussig shunt.
A: The distal left pulmonary artery is not opacified (white arrow) by this injection through the left-sided Blalock-Taussig shunt. **B:** The very small (hilar) left pulmonary artery (arrow) is demonstrated by the left pulmonary vein wedge angiogram.

way be viewed as static. The precarious nature of some aortopulmonary collaterals; the lack of obstruction in other collaterals predisposing to pulmonary vascular obstruction; those changes of polycythemia and hyperviscosity which may precipitate in situ thrombosis; those hemodynamic and morphological alterations secondary to surgically created systemic-to-pulmonary artery anastomoses all contribute to a dynamic and changing pulmonary circulation (Figs. 21-12, 21-15, 21-31, 21-37, 21-39, and 21-40).

Usually a "road-map" is required to begin to understand the nature of the pulmonary circulation in these patients. One can make the analogy of defining a "country" map, then a "city" map, followed by a "block" map, each map providing increasingly specific and more focused information, and this is what is needed to understand the pulmonary circulation. To define with anatomic and hemodynamic precision those parameters of the pulmonary circulation, one can pose a number of questions that must be answered:

1. Is the pulmonary circulation supported by a patent arterial duct or aortopulmonary collaterals (direct or indirect), or both? Is there a fifth aortic arch? And if so, is the connection systemic-to-pulmonary or systemic-to-systemic (Figs. 21-14 and 21-15)?

2. Are there connections between the aortic root, coronary artery or ascending aorta and the pulmonary arteries? If such a connection is present, where is it, and

does it support the entirety or just part of the pulmonary circulation (Figs. 21-16 and 21-34)?

3. Are the pulmonary arteries confluent or nonconfluent? If nonconfluent, is the supply to each lung via an arterial duct, aortopulmonary collaterals, or con-

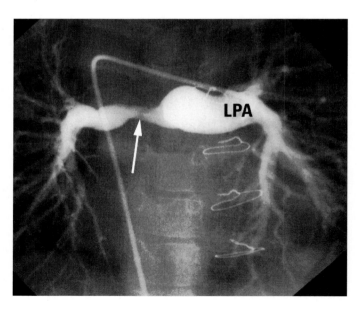

Fig. 21-64: The central shunt allows visualization of the proximal right pulmonary artery stenosis and hypoplasia (white arrow).

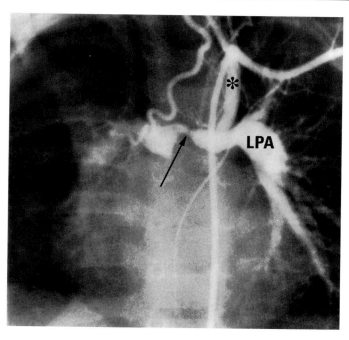

Fig. 21-65: The modified left-sided Blalock-Taussig shunt (✱) allows imaging of the pulmonary arteries and the severe right pulmonary artery stenosis (arrow) reflecting the insertion of the right-sided arterial duct.

nections from the aortic root or ascending aorta? Or from other sources?

4. Do important aortopulmonary collaterals exist in this patient?

5. Where is the origin of each aortopulmonary collateral? From the descending thoracic aorta; indirect collateral from a brachiocephalic artery; from the renal or celiac artery (Fig. 21-46)?

6. Where and how does each aortopulmonary collateral connect with the lung?

7. Does the aortopulmonary collateral artery continue directly into the pulmonary parenchyma supporting and supplying a bronchopulmonary segment(s) or does the collateral anastomose with branches of the central pulmonary artery?

8. Does a stenosis within the aortopulmonary collateral artery prevent transmission of systemic pressure to that or those segments of lung connected to the aortopulmonary collateral artery?

9. For any given aortopulmonary collateral and its bronchopulmonary segment(s), does the absence of a stenosis provide the hemodynamic basis for pulmonary artery hypertension and pulmonary vascular obstruction (Fig. 21-39)?

10. Can an aortopulmonary collateral artery be interrupted without the possibility of pulmonary infarction? That is, is there more than one source of pulmonary blood supply to that segment of lung under consideration (Figs. 21-51 through 21-53)? And how precarious are both sources of supply?

11. Are the pulmonary venous connections normal? Is there stenosis of any pulmonary vein?

The definition of the road-map concept is achieved by selective injection of contrast into the ascending and descending thoracic aorta using, when indicated, the technique of balloon occlusion.[4,5,12,21,26,27,36,40,48, 57,98,105–109,111,112,114–117,128,129,150,151,157,162,163,166,167, 184,251–263] Injection of contrast material into the ascending aorta just above the coronary arteries should define the gross status of the coronary arteries, including their origin and epicardial distribution, their participation in a coronary artery-pulmonary artery communication, the aortic origin of a right or left pulmonary artery, the origin of a fifth aortic arch with a systemic-to-pulmonary artery or systemic-to-systemic connection, or an aortopulmonary fenestration. To achieve this initial injection, the catheter may be venous, floated or advanced from the ventricle into the ascending aorta, or a retrograde arterial approach may be necessary, or at times, preferable. In addition, the brachiocephalic arteries will be imaged, and the presence or absence of indirect collaterals originating from the brachiocephalic arteries can be determined. Selective injection of contrast into the right and left brachiocephalic arteries may be required. The adult with pulmonary atresia and ventricular septal defect has a dilated aortic root, and aortic regurgitation on this basis is not uncommon; other reasons for aortic regurgitation include infective endocarditis and an intrinsically abnormal aortic

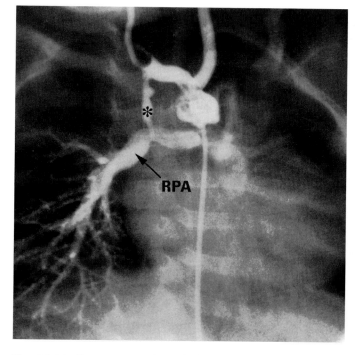

Fig. 21-66: Some narrowing of the right pulmonary artery following construction of this modified right-sided Blalock-Taussig shunt. Note the irregularity of the shunt (✱).

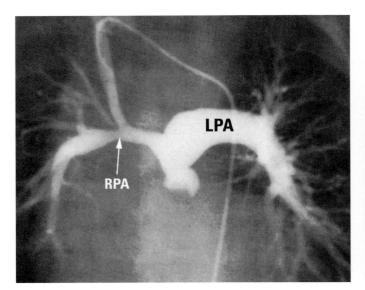

A

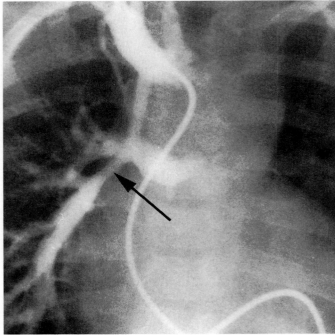

C

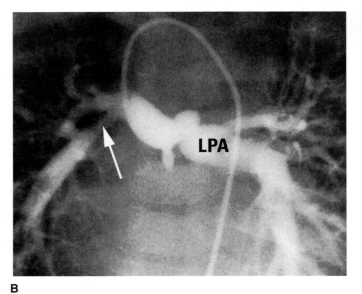

B

Fig. 21-67: The complications of the right-sided modified Blalocck-Taussig shunt. A: Diffuse hypoplasia. **B and C:** Distal stenoses.

valve.[70,264–267a] The severity of the aortic regurgitation can be assessed clinically, from echocardiographic examination, and by injection of contrast above the aortic valve (not using a catheter with an end-hole). Selective coronary artery injection is probably necessary in the adult, and if the initial ascending aortogram indicates any suggestion of a connection between coronary artery and pulmonary artery, selective injection of the coronary arteries may be helpful in improving definition. Similarly, if indirect collaterals are recognized originating from either the right or left subclavian arteries or elsewhere, selective injection of contrast will escalate the appreciation of these collaterals.

Selective opacification of the descending thoracic aorta is not always required if the initial ascending aortogram, when filmed in frontal and lateral projections, excludes direct and indirect aortopulmonary collater-

als. However, when direct collaterals are imaged or suggested by echocardiography or seen on the original ascending aortogram, then selective opacification of the descending thoracic aorta is necessary. The ascending and then the descending thoracic aorta can usually be entered using the venous catheter which can be manipulated or floated from the ventricle into the ascending aorta. We prefer to perform the initial descending thoracic aortogram in the neonate or young infant with the venous catheter at the level of the diaphragm using the balloon occlusion technique. This technique is often not applicable to the older child or adult whose descending thoracic aorta may be quite dilated. When using the arterial approach, the descending thoracic aortogram should be performed at the level of the arterial duct, or ligamentum, or just distal to the origin of the subclavian artery. The advantage of the venous ap-

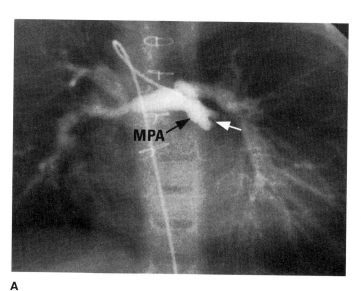

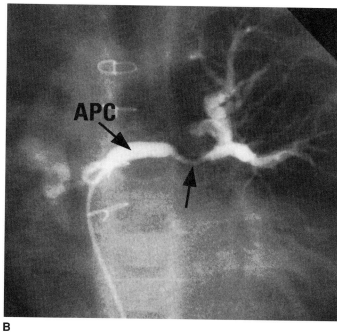

A

B

Fig. 21-68: The central shunt allows access to the pulmonary arterial tree.
A: Injection into main pulmonary trunk via the central shunt; the doming imperforate pulmonary valve (white arrow) is seen.
B: Selective injection into a direct aortopulmonary collateral shows a severe stenosis (arrow).

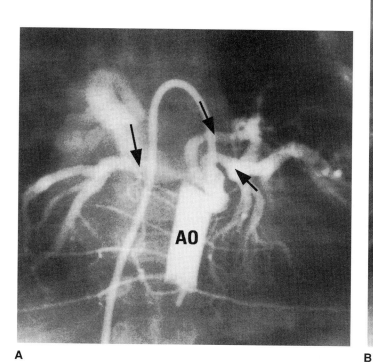

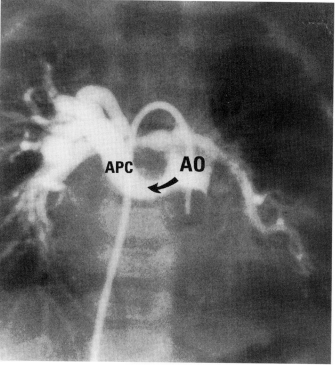

A

B

Fig. 21-69: Selective balloon occlusion aortography provides a "road-map" for more selective angiography.
A: The balloon-catheter is advanced from the venous route to the ascending aorta, and it is then inflated and advanced to the level of the diaphragm where it is inflated. Balloon occlusion aortography shows several collaterals; (arrows). **B:** The balloon catheter is withdrawn to the midthoracic aorta where it is inflated and another balloon occlusion aortogram is performed, almost selectively filling (curved arrow) a large aortopulmonary collateral.

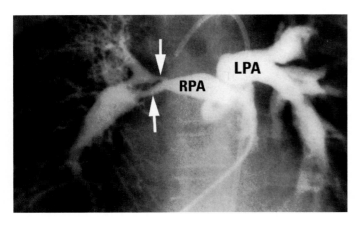

Fig. 21-70: Note the intrinsic stenoses and hypoplasia of the right pulmonary artery in this patient with a complex form of pulmonary atresia.

proach using a balloon catheter is that one can selectively balloon occlude the descending thoracic aorta at various levels, providing increasingly specific information (Figs. 21-38 and 21-69).[241] Once these initial "scouting" maps have been performed, one can see the various collaterals, direct and indirect. Selective injection of contrast into the direct aortopulmonary collaterals with prior recording of pressures with an end-hole catheter should be performed. Because stenoses are so very common in the direct and indirect aortopulmonary collaterals, it is probably wise to record for the permanent angiographic record where the specific pressure was obtained, particularly when that pressure is elevated. Usually these maneuvers will demonstrate the mediastinal pulmonary arteries, confluent or not, assuming they are present.

However, there are those patients in whom none of the preceding angiographic techniques demonstrate true pulmonary arteries. We would then utilize the technique of pulmonary vein wedge angiography to further enhance or refine our ability to define the presence or absence of true pulmonary arteries (Figs. 21-29, 21-31, 21-34, 21-36, 21-47, 21-56, and 21-63).[237–240] This technique requires wedging an endhole catheter in the pulmonary vein and injection of contrast at relatively low pressure. Entry into the pulmonary vein is via a preexisting interatrial communication; transseptal entry into the left atrium; from a retrograde arterial approach into ventricle, left atrium, and pulmonary vein; or by entry into an anomalously connected pulmonary vein from the systemic venous circulation. The wedged injection of contrast will result in retrograde flow from the pulmonary venous circulation into the capillary bed, with sequential opacification of the arteriolar bed, and then the pulmonary arteries. Sometimes the pulmonary vein wedge angiography is complicated by extravasation of contrast material into the bronchi, precipitating bronchospasm and hemoptysis with

worsening of arterial hypoxemia.[238,239] Thus these patients, sometimes precarious to begin with, should be receiving supplemental oxygen and we will usually have anesthesia stand-by. Surprisingly excellent definition of the pulmonary circulation can be achieved by this technique.[237,239,240,261,263] Often more than one pulmonary vein will have to be catheterized in order to provide enough information about the status of the pulmonary arteries. All of these angiocardiographic techniques may be utilised to define the presence or absence of mediastinal pulmonary arteries, confluent or not, but there are still questions to be answered.

Not infrequently, opacification of the descending aorta demonstrates considerable collateral flow to one lung, but no, or trivial collateral flow to the other lung. The fact that there is a lung implies intraparenchymal pulmonary arteries, but was this lung, seemingly devoid of collateral vessels connected to the arterial system, even tenuously? The absence of major collateral supply to one lung suggests that this lung was probably connected at some time to a distal sixth arch; ie, an arterial duct (see also Chapter 19). This view supports the reciprocal nature of the systemic and ductal supply to the lung, or to any given bronchopulmonary segment. This reciprocal nature of arterial supply to the lung in the patient with pulmonary atresia has been illustrated in several venues (Figs. 21-31 through 21-33).[86,95,116,117,151,157]

One of the frequent problems in the assessment of these patients is the determination if a collateral, direct or indirect, is the only source of blood supply to a given bronchopulmonary segment. Some bronchopulmonary segments will have two or more sources of nutrient vessels, while in others only one collateral is the nutrient source (Figs. 21-51 through 21-53). The other issue that must be resolved is the determination of connection of a bronchopulmonary segment to the true pulmonary artery. These issues are clearly related, and the similar methodologies are utilized to make these determinations. The so-called "wash-in and wash-out" phenomenon can provide evidence of the duality of arterial supply.[4,5,12,28,36,48,93,94,107,108,151,157,166] The dilution of contrast material in either a collateral or true pulmonary artery segment by undyed blood (washout) from an adjacent lung segment is inferential evidence of interconnection between the segments of lung. When contrast material is injected into a collateral, and there is sequential opacification of the collateral, followed by visualization of the true pulmonary artery (wash-in), this is ample evidence of dual supply to that segment of lung connected to both the collateral and the true pulmonary artery. The implication is that one can interrupt the collateral without jeopardizing the integrity of the lung. Other phenomenon can also provide evidence of vascular interconnection between the bronchopulmonary segments, and between collateral circulation and the true pulmonary artery. To make these determinations in patients with complex pulmonary atresia, it may be necessary to temporarily occlude one or more collaterals while injecting others.

Anomalously connected pulmonary veins may further complicate the situation in some patients with complex pulmonary atresia, especially but not exclusively in the patient with visceroatrial heterotaxia and right atrial isomerism (see Chapter 41) (Figs. 21-25 and 21-40). The levophase of the pulmonary artery or aortopulmonary collateral artery injection should be scrutinized for the pulmonary vein(s) and their connection to the left atrium of the systemic venous circulation.

Finally, we have studied one patient with pulmonary atresia, a ventricular septal defect, severe aortic stenosis, and multiple aortopulmonary collaterals with an aortopulmonary window providing one source of flow to the mediastinal pulmonary arteries (Fig. 21-16). Some of the features of this patient were suggestive of a truncus arteriosus (see Chapter 7). Aortic valve stenosis may also complicate pulmonary atresia and ventricular septal defect (see Chapter 20, Fig. 20-24).

References

1. Edwards JE, McGoon DC. Absence of anatomic origin from heart of pulmonary arterial supply. *Circulation* 1973;47:393–398.
2. Berry BE, McGoon DC, Ritter DG, Davis GD. Absence of anatomic origin from heart of pulmonary arterial supply. Clinical application of classification. *J Thorac Cardiovasc Surg* 1974;68:119–125.
3. Bharati S, Paul MH, Idriss FS, Potkin RT, Lev M. The surgical anatomy of pulmonary atresia with ventricular septal defect: Pseudotruncus. *J Thorac Cardiovasc Surg* 1975;69:713–721.
4. Mair DD, Edwards WD, Hagler DJ, Julsrud PR, Puga FJ. Tetralogy of Fallot and pulmonary atresia with ventricular septal defect. In: Moller JH, Neal WA, eds. *Fetal, Neonatal, and Infant Cardiac Disease*. Norwalk, CT: Appleton and Lange; 1989, pp. 639–669.
5. Mair DD, Edwards WD, Julsrud PR, Hagler DJ, Puga FJ. Pulmonary atresia and ventricular septal defect. In: Adams FH, Emmanoulides GC, Riemenschneider TA, eds. *Moss' Heart Disease in Infants, Children, and Adolescents*. Baltimore: Williams and Wilkins; 1989, pp. 289–301.
6. Anderson RH, Seo JW, Yen Ho S. The pulmonary arterial supply in tetralogy of Fallot with pulmonary atresia. *Ann Cardiac Surg* 1990–1991;77–83.
7. Thiene G, Anderson RH. Pulmonary atresia with VSD: Anatomy. In: Anderson RH, Macartney FJ, Shinebourne EA, Tynan M, eds. *Paediatric Cardiology*. Volume 5. Edinburgh: Churchill Livingstone; 1983, pp. 81–101.
8. Thiene G, Bortolotti U, Gallucci V, Valente ML, Volta SD. Pulmonary atresia with ventricular septal defect. *Br Heart J* 1977;39:1223–1233.
9. Thiene G, Frescura C, Bini RM, Valente M, Gallucci V. Histology of pulmonary arterial supply in pulmonary atresia with ventricular septal defect. *Circulation* 1979; 60:1066–1074.
10. Sotomora RG, Edwards JE. Anatomic identification of so-called absent pulmonary artery. *Circulation* 1978;57: 624–633.
11. Marino B, Calabro R, Gagliardi MG, Bevilacqua M, Ballerini L, Marcelletti C. Patterns of pulmonary arterial anatomy and blood supply in complex congenital heart disease with pulmonary atresia. *J Thorac Cardiovasc Surg* 1987;94:518–520.
12. Freedom RM. Pulmonary atresia and ventricular septal defect. In: Freedom RM, Benson LN, Smallhorn JF, eds. *Neonatal Heart Disease*. London: Springer-Verlag; 1992, pp. 229–256.
13. Castaneda AR, Mayer JE Jr, Lock JE. Tetralogy of Fallot, pulmonary atresia, and diminutive pulmonary arteries. *Prog Pediatr Cardiol* 1992;1:50–60.
14. Puga FJ. Surgical treatment of pulmonary atresia and ventricular septal defect. *Prog Pediatr Cardiol* 1992; 1:37–49.
15. Kirklin JW, Blackstone EH, Kirklin JK, Pacifico AD. Predicting the degree of relief of the pulmonary stenosis or atresia after the repair of tetralogy of Fallot. *Semin Thorac Cardiovasc Surg* 1990;2:55–60.
16. Groh MA, Meliones JN, Bove EL, Kirklin JW, Blackstone EH, Lupinetti FM, Snider AR, Rosenthal A. Repair of tetralogy of Fallot in infancy. Effect of pulmonary artery size on outcome. *Circulation* 1991;84(5 Suppl):III-206-III-212.
17. Warnes CA. Tetralogy of Fallot and pulmonary atresia/ventricular septal defect. *Cardiol Clin* 1993;11: 643–650
18. Millikan JS, Puga FJ, Danielson GK, Schaff HV, Julsrud PR, Mair DD. Staged surgical repair of pulmonary atresia, ventricular septal defect, and hypoplastic, confluent pulmonary arteries. *J Thorac Cardiovasc Surg* 1986;91: 818–825.
19. Agarwal KC. Surgical repair of pulmonary atresia with ventricular septal defect and hypoplastic pulmonary arteries: A different approach. *J Thorac Cardiovasc Surg* 1981;82:638–644.
20. Alfieri O, Blackstone EH, Kirlkin JW, Pacifico AD, Bargeron LM Jr. Surgical treatment of tetralogy of Fallot with pulmonary atresia. *J Thorac Cardiovasc Surg* 1978;76: 321–335.
21. Cotrufo M, Arciprete P, Caianiello G, Fittipaldi O, de Leva F, Violini R, Calabro R, Vosa C. Right pulmonary artery development after modified Blalock-Taussig shunt (MBTS) in infants with pulmonary atresia, VSD and confluent pulmonary arteries. *Eur J Cardiothorac Surg* 1989;3:12–15.
22. Permut LC, Laks H. Surgical management of pulmonary atresia with ventricular septal defect and multiple aortopulmonary collaterals. *Adv Card Surg* 1994;5:75–95.
23. Shimazaki Y, Iio M, Nakano S, Morimoto S, Ikawa S, Matsuda H, Kawashima Y. Pulmonary artery morphology and hemodynamics in pulmonic valve atresia with ventricular septal defect before and after repair. *Am J Cardiol* 1991;67:744–748.
24. al-Halees Z, Galal O, Wilson N. Successful repair of pulmonary atresia with ventricular septal defect without the use of a conduit: A new surgical option. Report of two cases. *Br Heart J* 1992;68:320–322.
25. Lane I, Treasure T, Leijala M, Shinebourne EA, Lincoln C. Diminutive pulmonary artery growth following right ventricular outflow tract enlargement. *Int J Cardiol* 1983; 3:175–185.
26. Rome JJ, Mayer JE, Castaneda AR, Lock JE. Tetralogy of Fallot with pulmonary atresia. Rehabilitation of diminu-

tive pulmonary arteries. *Circulation* 1993;88: 1691–1698.

27. Di Donato RM, Jonas RA, Lang P, Rome JJ, Mayer Jr JE, Castaneda AR. Neonatal repair of tetralogy of Fallot with and without pulmonary atresia. *J Thorac Cardiovasc Surg* 1991;101:126–137.

28. Kirklin JW, Barratt-Boyes BG. *Cardiac Surgery.* Second edition. New York: Churchill Livingstone; 1993, pp. 861–1012

29. Fyler DC. Tetralogy of Fallot. In: Fyler DC, ed. *Nadas' Pediatric Cardiology.* St. Louis: Mosby-Year Book Inc; 1992, pp. 471–491.

30. Barbero-Marcial M, Jatene AD. Surgical management of the anomalies of the pulmonary arteries in the tetralogy of Fallot with pulmonary atresia. *Semin Thorac Cardiovasc Surg* 1990;2:93–107

31. Kirklin JW, Blackstone EH, Shimazaki Y, Maehara T, Pacifico AD, Kirklin JK, Bargeron LM Jr. Survival, functional status, and reoperations after repair of tetralogy of Fallot with pulmonary atresia. *J Thorac Cardiovasc Surg* 1988;96:102–16.

32. Matsuda H, Hirose H, Nakano S, Shimazaki Y, Kishimoto H, Kobayashi J, Arisawa J, Kawashima Y. Management of large aortopulmonary collateral arteries in patients with ventricular septal defect and pulmonary atresia: Simultaneous ligation through median sternotomy during intracardiac repair. *Ann Thorac Surg* 1985;40:593–598.

33. Zahn EM, Lima VC, Benson LN, Freedom RM. Use of endovascular stents to increase pulmonary blood flow in pulmonary atresia with ventricular septal defect. *Am J Cardiol* 1992;70:411–412.

33a. Redington AN, Somerville J. Stenting aortopulmonary collaterals in complex pulmonary atresia. *Circulation* 1996;94:2479–2484.

34. Kumar S, Scagliotti D, Fisher EA, del Nido P. Surgical correction of pulmonary atresia with ventricular septal defect and no central pulmonary arteries. *Am J Cardiol* 1990;65:261–263.

35. Wilkinson JL, Ng YM, Iyer KS, Mee RBB. Morphologic and hemodynamic results of staged repair of pulmonary atresia with ventricular septal defect in the presence of hypoplastic pulmonary arteries and systemic-to-pulmonary collateral arteries. *Cardiol Young* 1993; 3:98–103.

36. Shanley CJ, Lupinetti FM, Shah NL, Beekman RH, Crowley DC, Bove EL. Primary unifocalization for the absence of intrapericardial pulmonary arteries in the neonate. *J Thorac Cardiovasc Surg* 1993;106:237–247.

37. Rudolph AM, Heymann MA, Fishman N, Lakier JB. Formalin infiltration of the ductus arteriosus. A method for palliation of infants with selected congenital cardiac lesions. *N Engl J Med* 1975;292:1263–1268.

38. Sawatari K, Imai Y, Kurosawa H, Isomatsu Y, Momma K. Staged operation for pulmonary atresia and ventricular septal defect with major aortopulmonary collateral arteries. New technique for complete unifocalization. *J Thorac Cardiovasc Surg* 1989;98:738–750.

39. McGoon DC, Baird DK, Davis GD. Surgical management of large bronchial collateral arteries with pulmonary stenosis or atresia. *Circulation* 1975;52:109–118.

40. McGoon MD, Fulton RE, Davis GD, Ritter DG, Neill CA, White RI Jr. Systemic collateral and pulmonary artery stenosis patients with congenital pulmonary valve atresia and ventricular septal defect. *Circulation* 1977;56: 473–479.

41. Kirklin JW, Bargeron LM, Pacifico AD. The enlargement

of small pulmonary arteries by preliminary palliative operations. *Circulation* 1977;56:612–617.

42. Hatem J, Sade RM, Upshur JK, Hohn AR. Maintaining patency of the ductus arteriosus for palliation of cyanotic cardiac malformations: The use of prostaglandin E1 and formaldehyde infiltration of the ductal wall. *Ann Surg* 1980;192:124–128.

43. Moulton AL. Formalin infiltration of the patent ductus arteriosus (letter). *J Thorac Cardiovasc Surg* 1989;98: 1150–1153.

44. Larson JE, Fleming WH, Sarafian LB, Rogler WC, Hofschire PJ, McManus BM. Combined prostaglandin therapy and ductal formalin infiltration in neonatal pulmonary oligemia. *J Thorac Cardiovasc Surg* 1985;90: 907–911.

45. Deanfield JE, Rees PG, Bull CM, De Leval M, Stark J, Macartney FJ, Taylor JFN. Formalin infiltration of ductus arteriosus in cyanotic congenital heart disease. *Br Heart J* 1981;45:573–576.

46. Gill CC, Moodie DS, McGoon DC. Staged surgical management of pulmonary atresia with diminutive pulmonary arteries. *J Thorac Cardiovasc Surg* 1977;73: 436–452.

47. Hofbeck M, Singer H. Pulmonary atresia with ventricular septal defect: Palliative operations in primarily inoperable cases. *Z Kardiol* 1983;72:622–632.

48. Puga FJ, Leoni FE, Julsrud PR, Mair DD. Complete repair of pulmonary atresia, ventricular septal defect, and severe peripheral arborization abnormalities of the central pulmonary arteries. Experience with preliminary unifocalization procedures in 38 patients. *J Thorac Cardiovasc Surg* 1989;98:1018–1029.

49. Barbero-Marcial M, Rizzo A, Lopes AAB, Bittencourt D, Junior JOA, Jatene AD. Correction of pulmonary atresia with ventricular septal defect in the absence of the pulmonary trunk and the central pulmonary arteries (so-called truncus type IV). *J Thorac Cardiovasc Surg* 1987; 94:911–918.

50. Watterson KG, Wilkinson JL, Karl TR; Mee RB. Very small pulmonary arteries: Central end-to-side shunt. *Ann Thorac Surg* 1991;52:1132–1137.

51. Iyer KS, Mee RBB. Staged repair of pulmonary atresia with ventricular septal defect and major systemic to pulmonary collateral arteries. *Ann Thorac Surg* 1991;51: 65–72.

52. Momma K, Takao A, Imai Y, Kurosawa H. Obstruction of the central pulmonary artery after shunt operations in patients with pulmonary atresia. *Br Heart J* 1987;57: 534–542.

53. Piehler JM, Danielson GK, McGoon DC, Wallace RB, Fulton RE, Mair DD. Management of pulmonary atresia with ventricular septal defect and hypoplastic pulmonary arteries by right ventricular outflow construction. *J Thorac Cardiovasc Surg* 1980;80:552–567.

54. Puga FJ, Uretzky G, McGoon DC. Establishment of right ventricle-hypoplastic pulmonary artery continuity without the use of extracorporeal circulation. *J Thorac Cardiovasc Surg* 1982;83:74–80.

55. Murphy DA, Sridhara KS, Nanton MA, Roy DL, Belcourt CL, Gillis DA. Surgical correction of pulmonary atresia with multiple large systemic-pulmonary collaterals. *Ann Thorac Surg* 1979;27:460–464.

56. Castaneda AR, Jonas RA, Mayer JE Jr, Hanley FJ. *Cardiac Surgery of the Neonate and Infant.* Toronto: WB Saunders; 1994, pp. 215–234.

56a. Reddy VM, Liddicoat JR, Hanley FL. Midline one-stage complete unifocalization and repair of pulmonary atresia with ventricular septal defect and major aortopulmonary collaterals. *J Thorac Cardiovasc Surg* 1995;109: 832–845.

57. Puga FJ, McGoon DC, Julsrud PR, Danielson GK, Mair DD. Complete repair of pulmonary atresia with nonconfluent pulmonary arteries. *Ann Thorac Surg* 1983;35: 36–44.

58. Rosenberg HG, Williams WG, Trusler GA, Higa T, Rabinovitch M. Structural composition of central pulmonary arteries. Growth potential after surgical shunts. *J Thorac Cardiovasc Surg* 1987;94:498–503.

59. Hofbeck M, Sunnegardh JT, Burrows PE, Moes CA, Lightfoot N, Williams WG, Trusler GA, Freedom RM. Analysis of survival in patients with pulmonic valve atresia and ventricular septal defect. *Am J Cardiol* 1991; 67:737–743.

59a. Dinarevic S, Redington A, Rigby M, Shinebourne EA. Outcome of pulmonary atresia and ventricular septal defect during infancy. *Pediatr Cardiol* 1995; 16:276–282.

60. Bull K, Somerville J, Spiegelhalter D. Presentation and attrition in complex pulmonary atresia. *J Am Coll Cardiol* 1995;25:491–499.

61. Sullivan ID, Wren C, Stark J, de Leval MR, Macartney FJ, Deanfield JE. Surgical unifocalization in pulmonary atresia and ventricular septal defect: A realistic goal? *Circulation* 1988;78(Suppl III):III-5-III-13.

62. Somerville J. Out of the blue and into the pink. Is it so rosy for the cardiologist? *Can J Cardiol* 1990;6:247–257.

63. Feldt RH, Liao P-K, Puga FJ. Clinical profile and natural history of pulmonary atresia and ventricular septal defect. *Prog Pediatr Cardiol* 1992;1:18–22.

64. Bertranou EG, Blackstone EH, Hazelrig JB, Turner ME Jr, Kirklin JW. Life expectancy without surgery in tetralogy of Fallot. *Am J Cardiol* 1978;42:458–466.

65. Ramsay JM, Macartney FJ, Haworth SG. Tetralogy of Fallot with major aortopulmonary collateral arteries. *Br Heart J* 1985;53:167–172.

66. Formigari R, Vairo U, de Zorzi A, Santoro G, Marino B. Prevalence of bilateral patent ductus arteriosus in patients with pulmonary valve atresia and asplenia syndrome. *Am J Cardiol* 1992;70:1219–1220.

67. Vitiello R, Moller JH, Marino B, Vairo U, Edwards JE, Titus JL. Pulmonary circulation in pulmonary atresia associated with the asplenia cardiac syndrome. *J Am Coll Cardiol* 1992;20:363–365.

68. Fisher EA, Thanopoulos BD, Eckner FAO, Hastreiter AR, Dubrow IW. Pulmonary atresia with obstructed ventricular septal defect. *Pediatr Cardiol* 1980;1:209–217

69. Martin RP; Radley-Smith R; Yacoub MH. Pulmonary atresia and aortic valve stenosis. *Int J Cardiol* 1987;16: 103–105.

70. Patel RG, Freedom RM, Bloom KR, Rowe RD. Truncal or aortic valve stenosis in functionally single arterial trunk. A clinical, hemodynamic and pathologic study of six cases. *Am J Cardiol* 1978;42:800–809.

71. Freedom RM, Olley PM, Coceani F, Rowe RD. The prostaglandin challenge. Test to unmask obstructed total anomalous pulmonary venous connection in asplenia syndrome. *Br Heart J* 1978;40:91–94.

72. Muster AJ, Paul MH, Nikaidoh H. Tetralogy of Fallot associated with total anomalous pulmonary venous drainage. *Chest* 1973;64:323–326.

72a. Lee ML, Wu MH, Lue HC. Infracardiac total anomalous pulmonary venous connection in tetralogy of Fallot with decreased pulmonary flow and masked pulmonary venous obstruction: Report of one case. *Int J Cardiol* 1994; 47:81–84.

73. Chiu I-S, Wang N-K, Wu M-H, Wu F-F, Hung C-R. Concealed pulmonary venous obstruction in right atrial isomerism with pulmonary outflow tract obstruction-surgical management following Blalock-Taussig shunt. *Cardiol Young* 1992;2:95–99.

74. Gersony WM. Obstruction to pulmonary venous return obscured by decreased pulmonary blood flow. *Chest* 1973;64:283.

75. Fyler DC. Report of the New England Regional Infant Cardiac Program. *Pediatrics* 1980;65(Suppl):376–461.

76. Ferencz C, Rubin JD, McCarter RJ, Brenner JI, Neill CA, Perry LW, Hepner SI, Downing JW. Congenital heart d1isease: Prevalence at livebirth. The Baltimore-Washington Infant Study. *Am J Epidemiol* 1985;121:31–36.

77. Congdon ED. Transformation of the aortic arch system during development of the human embryo. *Contrib Embryol* 1922;14:47–110.

78. Boyden EA. The time lag in the development of bronchial arteries. *Anat Rec* 1970;166:611–614.

79. DeRuiter MC, Gittenberger-de Groot A, Poelmann RE, VanIperen L, Mentink MMT. Development of the pharyngeal arch system related to the pulmonary and bronchial vessels in the avian embryo. With a concept on systemic-pulmonary collateral artery formation. *Circulation* 1993;87:1306–1319.

80. Huntington GS. The morphology of the pulmonary artery in mammalia. *Anat Rec* 1920;17:165–201.

81. Goldstein JD, Rabinovitch M, Van Praagh R, Reid L. Unusual vascular anomalies causing persistent pulmonary hypertension in a newborn. *Am J Cardiol* 1979;43: 962–967.

82. Nakajima Y, Nishibatake M, Ikeda K, Momma K, Takao A, Terai M. Abnormal development of fourth aortic arch derivatives in the pathogenesis of tetralogy of Fallot. *Pediatr Cardiol* 1990;11:69–71.

83. Kutsche LM, Van Mierop LHS. Pulmonary atresia with and without ventricular septal defect: A different etiology and pathogenesis for the atresia in the 2 types? *Am J Cardiol* 1983;51:932–935.

84. Bricker DL, King SM, Edwards JE. Anomalous aortic origin of the right and left pulmonary arteries in a normally septated truncus arteriosus. *Chest* 1975;68:591–595.

85. Beitzke A, Shinebourne EA. Single origin of right and left pulmonary arteries from ascending aorta, with main pulmonary artery from right ventricle. *Br Heart J* 1980; 43:363–365.

86. Freedom RM, Culham JAG, Moes CAF. *Angiocardiography of Congenital Heart Disease.* New York: Macmillan Publishing Co; 1984, pp. 195–210.

87. Aotsuka H, Nagai Y, Saito M, Matsumoto H, Nakamura T. Anomalous origin of both pulmonary arteries from the ascending aorta with a nonbranching main pulmonary artery arising from the right ventricle. *Pediatr Cardiol* 1990;11:156–158.

88. Momma K, Takao A, Ando M, Nakazawa M, Satomi G, Imai Y, Takanashi Y, Kurosawa H. Juxtaductal left pulmonary artery obstruction in pulmonary atresia. *Br Heart J* 1986;55:39–44.

89. Elzenga NJ, Gittenberger-de Groot AC. The ductus arteriosus and stenoses of the pulmonary arteries in pulmonary atresia. *Int J Cardiol* 1986;11:195–208.

90. Elzenga NJ, von Suylen RJ, Frohn-Mulder I, Essed CE, Bos E, Quaegebeur JM. Juxtaductal pulmonary artery coarctation. An underestimated cause of branch pulmonary artery stenosis in patients with pulmonary atresia or stenosis and a ventricular septal defect. *J Thorac Cardiovasc Surg* 1990;100:416–424.

90a. Waldman JD, Karp RB, Gittenberger-de Groot AC, Agarwala B, Glagov S. Spontaneous acquisition of discontinuous pulmonary arteries. *Ann Thorac Surg* 1996; 62:161–168.

91. Judeikin R, Rheuban KS, Carpenter MA. Ductal origin of the left pulmonary artery in severe tetralogy of Fallot: Problems in management. *Pediatr Cardiol* 1984; 5:323–326.

92. Freedom RM, Moes CAF, Pelech A, Smallhorn J, Rabinovitch M, Olley PM, Williams WG, Trusler GA, Rowe RD. Bilateral ductus arteriosus (or Remnant): An analysis of 27 patients. *Am J Cardiol* 1984;53:884–891.

92a. Law Y, Smallhorn JF, Adatia I. Echocardiographic delineation of anomalous origin of the right subclavian artery from the right pulmonary artery. *Cardiol Young*, (In press).

93. Anderson RH, Devine WA, del Nido P. The surgical anatomy of tetralogy of Fallot with pulmonary atresia rather than pulmonary stenosis. *J Card Surg* 1991; 6:41–59.

94. Rabinovitch M. Pathology and anatomy of pulmonary atresia and ventricular septal defect. *Prog Pediatr Cardiol* 1992;1:9–17.

95. Thiene G, Frescura C, Bortolotti U, Del Maschio A, Valente M. The systemic pulmonary circulation in pulmonary atresia with ventricular septal defect: Concept of reciprocal development of the fourth and sixth aortic arches. *Am Heart J* 1981;101:339–344.

96. Tobin CE. The bronchial arteries and their connections with other vessels in the human lung. *Surg Gynecol Obstet* 1952;95:741–750.

97. Haworth SG. The pulmonary circulation in congenital heart disease. *Herz* 1978;3:138–142.

98. Rabinovitch M, Herrera-DeLeon V, Castaneda AR, Reid L. Growth and development of the pulmonary vascular bed in patients with tetralogy of fallot with or without pulmonary atresia. *Circulation* 1981;64:1234–1249.

99. Stuckey D, Bowdler JD, Reye RD. Absent sixth aortic arch: A form of pulmonary atresia. *Br Heart J* 1968;30: 258–264.

100. Rossi M, Filho RR, Ho SY. Solitary arterial trunk with pulmonary atresia and arteries with supply to the left lung from both an arterial duct and systemic-pulmonary collateral arteries. *Int J Cardiol* 1988;20:145–148.

101. Schofield DE and Anderson RH. Common arterial trunk with pulmonary atresia. *Int J Cardiol* 1988;20:290–294.

102. Mocellin R, Krettek M, Buhlmeyer K. Special problems in pulmonary atresia with ventricular septal defect: Extreme hypoplasia of intra-pericardial pulmonary arteries and autofocal collateral vessels. *Eur J Cardiol* 1978; 8:503–513.

103. Penny DJ, Dua R, and Wilkinson JW. Solitary arterial trunk. *Cardiol Young* 1994;4:71–74.

104. Shore DF, Yen Ho S, Anderson RH, de Leval M, Lincoln C. Aortopulmonary septal defect coexisting with ventricular septal defect and pulmonary atresia. *Ann Thorac Surg* 1983;35:132–137.

105. Macartney F, Deverall P, Scott O. Haemodynamic characteristics of systemic arterial blood supply to the lungs. *Br Heart J* 1973;35:28–37.

106. Somerville J, Saravalli O, Ross D. Complex pulmonary atresia with congenital systemic collaterals. Classification and management. *Arch Mal Coeur* 1978;71: 322–328.

107. Macartney FJ, Haworth SG. The pulmonary blood supply in pulmonary atresia with ventricular septal defect. In: *Paediatric Cardiology*. Edinburgh: Churchill Livingstone; 1979, pp. 314–329.

108. Macartney FJ, Haworth SG. Pulmonary atresia with VSD: Investigation of pulmonary atresia with ventricular septal defect. In: Anderson RH, Macartney FJ, Shinebourne EA, Tynan M, eds. *Paediatric Cardiology*. Volume 5. Edinburgh: Churchill Livingstone; 1983, pp. 111–125.

109. Liao P-K, Edwards WD, Julsrud PR, Puga FJ, Danielson GK, Feldt RH. Pulmonary blood supply in patients with pulmonary atresia and ventricular septal defect. *J Am Coll Cardiol* 1985;6:1343–1350.

110. Krongrad E, Ritter DG, Kincaid OW. Aorticopulmonary tunnel: Angiographic recognition of pulmonary atresia and coronary artery-to-pulmonary artery fistula. *AJR* 1973;119:498–502.

111. Haworth SG, Macartney FJ. Growth and development of pulmonary circulation in pulmonary atresia with ventricular septal defect and major aortopulmonary collateral arteries. *Br Heart J* 1980;44:14–24.

112. Jefferson K, Rees S, Somerville J. Systemic arterial supply to the lungs in pulmonary atresia and its relation to pulmonary artery developement. *Br Heart J* 1972;34: 418–427.

113. Johnson RJ, Sauer U, Buhlmeyer K, Haworth SG. Hypoplasia of the intrapulmonary arteries in children with right ventricular outflow tract obstruction, ventricular septal defect, and major aortopulmonary collateral arteries. *Pediatr Cardiol* 1985;6:137–143.

114. Haworth SG, Macartney FJ. Pulmonary Atresia with VSD: The pulmonary blood supply. In: Anderson RH, Macartney FJ, Shinebourne EA, Tynan M, eds. *Paediatric Cardiology*. Volume 5. Edinburgh: Churchill Livingstone; 1983, pp. 102–110.

115. Haworth SG, Reid L. Quantitative strctural study of pulmonary circulation in the newborn with pulmonary atresia. *Thorax* 1977;32:129–133.

116. Frescura C, Talenti E, Pellegrino PA, Mazzucco A, Faggian G, Thiene G. Coexistence of ductal and systemic pulmonary arterial supply in pulmonary atresia with ventricular septal defect. *Am J Cardiol* 1984;53:348–349.

117. Daliento L, Stritoni P, Chioin R, Frescura C, Thiene G. Systemic-pulmonary arterial supply in pulmonary atresia with ventricular septal defect. *Chest* 1978;74: 685–687.

118. Marino B, Guccione P, Carotti A, De Zorzi A, Di Donato R, Marcelletti C. Ductus arteriosus in pulmonary atresia with and without ventricular septal defect. *Scand J Thorac Cardiovasc Surg* 1992;26:93–96.

119. Yen Ho S, Catani G, Seo J-W. Arterial supply to the lungs in tetralogy of Fallot with pulmonary atresia or critical stenosis. *Cardiol Young* 1992;2:65–72.

120. McCotter RE. On the occurrence of pulmonary arteries arising from the thoracic aorta. *Anat Rec* 1910; 4:291–297.

121. Dark JH, Pollock JCS. Coronary artery-pulmonary artery fistula in tetralogy of Fallot with pulmonary atresia. *Eur Heart J* 1985;6:714–716.

122. Suzuki K, Matsui M, Nakamura Y, Kurosawa H, Ogawa K, Hoshino K. [A case of coronary artery-pulmonary artery fistula in tetralogy of Fallot with pulmonary atresia and major aortopulmonary collateral arteries (MAPCA)]. *Nippon Kyobu Geka Gakkai Zasshi* 1992;40: 2252–2257.

122a. Yoshigi M, Momma K, Imai Y. Coronary artery-pulmonary artery fistula in pulmonary atresia: With ventricular septal defect. *Heart Vessels (Japan)* 1995;10: 163–166.

123. Pahl E, Fong L, Anderson RH, Park SC, Zuberbuhler JR. Fistulous communications between a solitary coronary

artery and the pulmonary arteries as the primary source of pulmonary blood supply in tetralogy of Fallot with pulmonary valve atresia. *Am J Cardiol* 1989;63:140–143.

124. Vigneswaran WT, Pollock JCS. Pulmonary atresia with ventricular septal defect and coronary artery fistula: A late presentation. *Br Heart J* 1988;59:387–388.

125. Solowiejczyk DE, Cooper MM, Barst RJ, Quaegebeur JM, Gersony WM. Pulmonary atresia and ventricular septal defect with coronary artery to pulmonary fistula: Case report and review of the literature. *Pediatr Cardiol* 1995; 16:90–94.

126. Anderson RH. Pulmonary atresia with ventricular septal defect and coronary artery fistula: A late presentation. *Br Heart J* 1988;60: 264–265.

127. Bogers AJJC, Rohmer J, Wolsky SAE, Quaegebeur JM, Huysman HA. Coronary artery fistula as source of pulmonary circulation in pulmonary atresia with ventricular septal defect. *Thorac Cardiovasc Surg* 1990;38: 30–32.

128. Macartney FJ, Scott O, Deverall PB. Haemodynamic and anatomical characteristics of pulmonary blood supply in pulmonary atresia with ventricular septal defect—including a case of persistent fifth aortic arch. *Br Heart J* 1974;36:1049–1060.

129. Yoo SJ, Moes CA, Burrows PE, Molossi S, Freedom RM. Pulmonary blood supply by a branch from the distal ascending aorta in pulmonary atresia with ventricular septal defect: Differential diagnosis of fifth aortic arch. *Pediatr Cardiol* 1993;14:230–233.

129a. Kishkurno S, Harada M, Tamura M, Ito T, Ogasawara M, Abe T, Takada G. Morphological change of the 5th aortic arch with tetralogy of Fallot and pulmonary atresia: echocardiographic and angiographic findings (letter). *Eur Heart J* 1995; 16:2010–2011.

130. Freedom RM, Silver M, Miyamura H. Tricuspid and pulmonary atresia with coarctation of the aorta: A rare combination possibly explained by persistence of the fifth aortic arch with a systemic-to-pulmonary arterial connection. *Int J Cardiol* 1989;24:241–245.

131. Gerlis LM, Dickinson DF, Wilson N, Gibbs JL. Persistent fifth aortic arch. A report of two new cases and review of the literature. *Int J Cardiol* 1987;16:185–192.

132. Gerlis LM, Ho S-Y, Anderson RH, Da Costa P. Persistent fifth aortic arch-a great pretender: Three new covert cases. *Int J Cardiol* 1989;23:239–247.

133. Hashimoto K, Kurosawa H, Tatara A. Total correction of tetralogy of Fallot with pulmonary atresia associated with an unusual aortopulmonary collateral artery. *Cardiol Young* 1993;3:75–77.

133a. Bhagwat AR, Pinto RJ, Sharma S. Tetralogy of Fallot with pulmonary atresia associated with aortopulmonary window and major aortopulmonary collaterals. *Cardiol Young* 1995;5:289–290.

134. Pfefferkorn JR, Loser H, Pech G, Toussaint R, Hilgenberg F. Absent pulmonary artery. A hint to its embryogenesis. *Pediatr Cardiol* 1982;3:283–286.

135. Presbitero P, Bull C, Haworth SG, De Leval MR. Absent or occult pulmonary artery. *Br Heart J* 1984;52:178–185.

136. Murray CA, Korns ME, Amplatz K, Edwards JE. Bilateral origin of pulmonary artery from homolateral ductus arteriosus. *Chest* 1970;57:310–317.

137. Milanesi O, Daliento L, Thiene G. Solitary aorta with bilateral ductal origin of non-confluent pulmonary arteries in pulmonary atresia with intact ventricular septum. *Int J Cardiol* 1990;29:90–92.

138. Todd EP, Lindsay WG, Edwards JE. Bilateral ductal origin of the pulmonary arteries. Systemic-pulmonary arterial anastomosis as first stage in planned total correction. *Circulation* 1976;54:834–836.

139. Stone FM, Amplatz K, Lucas RV Jr, Fukuda T, Edwards JE. Ventricular septal defect, solitary aortic trunk, and ductal origin of pulmonary arteries. *Am Heart J* 1976;92: 506–512.

140. Manhoff LJ Jr Howe JS. Absence of the pulmonary artery: A new classification for pulmonary arteries of anomalous origin. *AMA Arch Pathol* 1949;48:155–170.

141. Kearney MS. Total absence of the pulmonary artery with bilateral patent ductus arteriosus. *J Pathol* 1969;97: 729–731.

142. Lenox CC, Neches WH, Zuberbuhler JR, Park SC, Mathews RA, Siewers RD, Lerberg DG, Bahnson HT. Management of bilateral ductus arteriosus in complex cyanotic heart disease. *J Thorac Cardiovasc Surg* 1977;74: 607–613.

143. Kelsey JR Jr, Gilmore CE, Edwards JE. Bilateral ductus arteriosus representing persistence of each sixth aortic arch. *AMA Arch Pathol* 1953;55:154–161.

144. Hofschire PJ, Rodd EP, Varco RL, Kaplan EL, Edwards JE. Anomalous double blood supply to the lung. *Chest* 1976;69:439–441.

145. Fong LV, Anderson RH, Siewers RD, Trento A, Park SC. Anomalous origin of one pulmonary artery from the ascending aorta: A review of echocardiographic, catheter, and morphological features. *Br Heart J* 1989;62:389–395.

146. Gerlis LM, Yen Ho S, Smith A, Anderson RH. The site of origin of nonconfluent pulmonary arteries from a common arterial trunk or from the ascending aorta: Its morphological significance. *Am J Cardiovasc Pathol* 1990; 3:115–120.

147. Gerlis LM, MacGregor CC d'A, Yen Ho S. An anatomical study of 110 cases with deficiency of the aorticopulmonary septum with emphasis on the role of the arterial duct. *Cardiol Young* 1992;2:342–352.

148. Schulze-Neick I, Hausdorf G, Lange PE. Maldevelopment of conotruncal and aorto-pulmonary septum with absent left central pulmonary artery: Anatomical and clinical implications. *Br Heart J* 1994;71:89–91.

149. Danilowicz D, Ross J Jr. Pulmonary atresia without cyanosis. Report of two cases with ventricular septal defect and increased pulmonary blood flow. *Br Heart J* 1971;33:138–141.

150. Lacina SJ, Hamilton WT, Thilenius OG, Bharati S, Lev M, Arcilla RA. Angiographic evidence of absent ductus arteriosus in severe right ventricular outflow tract obstruction. *Pediatr Cardiol* 1983;4:5–11.

151. Freedom RM, Rabinovitch M. The angiography of the pulmonary circulation in patients with pulmonary atresia and ventricular septal defect. In: Tucker BL, Lindesmith GC, Takahashi M, eds. *Obstructive Lesions of the Right Heart.* Baltimore: University Park Press; 1984, pp. 191–216.

152. Jones RSW, Culham JAG, Freedom RM. Aortic vasa vasorum in cyanotic congenital heart disease. *Cathet Cardiovasc Diagn* 1979;5:145–150.

153. Bjork L. Anastomoses between the coronary and bronchial arteries. *Acta Radiol* 1966;4:93–98.

154. Bjork L. Angiographic demonstration of extracardial anastomoses to the coronary arteries. *Radiology* 1966; 87:274–277.

155. Doherty JU, Laskey WK, Wagner H, Stephenson LW, Rashkind WJ. Coronary-bronchial artery fistula with partial absence of a pulmonary artery: Association with partial anomalous pulmonary venous drainage. *J Am Coll Cardiol* 1983;2:369–373.

156. Cauldwell LW, Siekert RG, Lininger RE, Anson BJ. The bronchial arteries. An anatomic study of 150 human cadavers. *Surg Gynecol Obstet* 1948;86:395–412.

157. Burrows PE, Freedom RM, Rabinovitch M, Moes CAF. The investigation of abnormal pulmonary arteries in congenital heart disease. *Radiol Clin North Am* 1985;23: 689–717.

158. Gerlis LM, Ho SY, Anderson RH. Maldevelopment of conotruncal and aorto-pulmonary septum with absent left central pulmonary artery: Anatomical and clinical implications (letter). *Br Heart J* 1994;72:210–211.

159. Neye-Bock S, Fellows KE. Aortic arch interruption in infancy: Radio- and angiocardiographic features. *AJR* 1980;135:1011–1016.

160. Norwood WI, Stellin GJ. Aortic atresia with interrupted aortic arch. Reparative operation. *J Thorac Cardiovasc Surg* 1981;81:239–244.

161. Hessel EA II, Boyden EA, Stamm SJ, Sauvage LR. High systemic origin of the sole artery to the basal segments of the left lung: Findings, surgical treatment and embryologic interpretation. *Surgery* 1970;67:624–632.

162a. Haworth SG. Collateral arteries in pulmonary atresia with ventricular septal defect. A precarious blood supply. *Br Heart J* 1980;44:5–13.

162. Matsuda H, Kuratani T, Shimizaki Y, Kadoba K, Kobayashi J, Ohtake S, Nakayama M, Nakada T. Deposition of collagen in the alveolar wall of lungs from patients with tetralogy of Fallot and pulmonary atresia with major aortopulmonary collateral arteries-an ultrastructural study. *Cardiol Young* 1994;4:277–284.

163. Brown RT, Fellows KE. Cervical collateral arteries in pulmonary atresia with ventricular septal defect. *Am J Cardiol* 1988;62:1310–1311.

164. Metras DR, Kreitmann B, Tatou E, Riberi A, Wernert F. Tetralogy of Fallot with pulmonary atresia, coronary artery-pulmonary artery fistula, and origin of left pulmonary artery from descending aorta: Total correction in infancy (letter). *J Thorac Cardiovasc Surg* 1993;105: 186–188.

165. DeRuiter MC, Gittenberger-de Groot AC, Bogers AJJC, Elzenga NJ. The restricted surgical relevance of morphologic criteria to classify systemic-pulmonary collateral arteries in pulmonary atresia with ventricular septal defect. *J Thorac Cardiovasc Surg* 1994;108:692–699.

166. Faller K, Haworth SG, Taylor JFN, Macartney FJ. Duplicate sources of pulmonary blood supply in pulmonary atresia with ventricular septal defect. *Br Heart J* 1981;46: 263–268.

167. Haworth SG, Rees PG, Taylor JFN, Macartney FJ, de Leval M, Stark J. Pulmonary atresia with ventricular septal defect and major aortopulmonary collateral arteries. Effect of systemic-pulmonary anastomosis. *Br Heart J* 1981;45:133–141.

167a. Velasquez G, Nath PH, Castaneda-Zuniga WR, Amplatz K. Aberrant left subclavian artery in tetralogy of Fallot. *Am J Cardiol* 1980;45:811–818.

168. Husseini ZM, Slim MS, Kutayli FN, Hatem JN. Tetralogy of Fallot with double aortic arch: Successful staged repair. Case report and review of literature. *J Cardiovasc Surg* 1987;28:339–340.

169. Virdi IS, Keeton BR, Shore DF, Monro JL. Surgical management in tetralogy of Fallot and vascular ring. *Pediatr Cardiol* 1987;8: 131–134.

170. Nakajima Y, Satomi G, Kawamura T, Nishibatake M, Nakazawa M, Takao A. Right aortic arch with aberrant retroesophageal innominate artery: A report of 2 cases and review of the literature. *Int J Cardiol* 1993;38: 247–251.

171. Takahashi Y, Miyamura H, Kanazawa H, Watanabe H, Yamato Y, Sugawara M, Shinonaga M, Tatebe S, Takahashi M, Eguchi S. [Surgery of vascular rings associated with complex intracardiac anomaly]. *Kyobu Geka* 1992; 45:299–304.

172. Murdison KA, Weinberg PM. Tetralogy of Fallot with severe pulmonary valvar stenosis and pulmonary vascular sling (anomalous origin of the left pulmonary artery from the right pulmonary artery). *Pediatr Cardiol* 1991; 12:189–191.

173. Fujiwara K, Naito Y, Takagaki Y, Higashiue S, Takimoto M, Uemura S. [A case report of compression of right pulmonary artery and bronchus by aneurysmal dilated ascending aorta in tetralogy of Fallot—suspension of ascending aorta]. *Nippon Kyobu Geka Gakkai Zasshi* 1989; 37:374–378.

174. Gnanapragasam JP, Keeton BR, Fong LV. Double aortic arch, tetralogy of Fallot with pulmonary atresia and atrioventricular septal defect. *Clin Cardiol* 1991;14: 522–524.

174a. Markowitz RI, Fahey JT, Hellenbrand WE, Kopf GS, Rothstein P. Bronchial compression by a patent ductus arteriosus associated with pulmonary atresia. *Am J Radiol* 1985;144:535–540.

174b. McKay R, Stark J, de Leval M. Unusual vascular ring in infant with pulmonary atresia and ventricular septal defect. *Br Heart J* 1982;48:180–183.

175. Kerns SR, Glantz MG, Sabatelli FW, Hawkins IF Jr. Mediastinal mass and tracheal compression due to an aneurysm of a systemic-to-pulmonary collateral artery in a patient with pseudotruncus arteriosus. *Cardiovasc Intervent Radiol* 1994;17:158–160.

176. Gunthard J, Murdison KA, Wagner HR, Norwood WI Jr. Tetralogy of Fallot and coarctation of the aorta: A rare combination and its clinical implications. *Pediatr Cardiol* 1992;13:37–40.

177. Bullaboy CA, Derkac WM, Johnson DH, Jennings RB Jr. Tetralogy of Fallot and coarctation of the aorta: Successful repair in an infant. *Ann Thorac Surg* 1984;38: 400–401.

178. Korula RJ, Bais A, Lal N, Jairaj PS. Interrupted aortic arch with tetralogy of Fallot. A report of an unsuccessful surgically treated case. *J Cardiovasc Surg* 1991;32: 541–543.

179. Rey C, Coeurderoy A, Dupuis C. Coarctation de l'aorte et tetralogie de fallot. A propos de deux observations. *Arch Mal Coeur Vaiss* 1984;77:526–533.

180. Yoshigi M, Momma K, Imai Y. Tetralogy of Fallot and coarctation of the aorta. *Cardiol Young* 1994;4:75–78.

181. Shinebourne EA, Elseed AM. Relation between fetal flow patterns, coarctation of the aorta, and pulmonary blood flow. *Br Heart J* 1974;36:492–498.

182. Rudolph AM, Heymann MA, Spitznas U. Hemodynamic considerations in the development of narrowing of the aorta. *Am J Cardiol* 1972;30:514–525.

183. Olley PM, Coceani F, Bodach E. E-type prostaglandins. A new emergency therapy for certain cyanotic congenital heart malformations. *Circulation* 1976;53:728–731.

184. Freedom RM, Olley PM, Rowe RD. The angiocardiography and morphology of ductal-dependent congenital heart disease: Selected topics with reference to the clinical application of E-type Prostaglandins. In: Gallucci V, Bini RM, Thiene G. *Selected Topics in Cardiac Surgery.* Bologna: Casa Editrice Bologna; 1980, pp. 109–143.

185. Freed MD, Heymann MA, Lewis AB, Roehl SL, Kensey RC. Prostaglandin E_1 in infants with with ductus arteriosus-dependent congenital heart disease. *Circulation* 1981;64:899–905.

186. Cole RB, Abman S, Aziz KU, Bharati S, Lev M. Prolonged prostaglandin E1 infusion: Histologic effects on the patent ductus arteriosus. *Pediatrics.* 1981;67: 816–819.

187. Gittenberger-de Groot AC, Moulaert AJ, Harinck E, Becker AE. Histo-pathology of the ductus arteriosus after prostaglandin E1 administration in ductus dependent cardiac anomalies. *Br Heart J* 1978;40:215–220.

188. Park I-S, Nihill MR, Titus JL. Morphologic features of the ductus arteriosus after prostaglandin E1 administration for ductus-dependent congenital heart defects. *J Am Coll Cardiol* 1983;1:471–475.

189. Silver MM, Freedom RM, Silver MD, Olley PM. The morphology of the human ductus arteriosus: A reappraisal of its structure and closure with special reference to prostaglandin E₁ therapy. *Hum Pathol* 1981;12; 1123–1136.

190. Teixeira OHP, Carpenter B, MacMurray SB, Vlad P. Long-term prostaglandin E₁ therapy in congenital heart disease. *J Am Coll Cardiol* 1984;3:838–843.

191. Tsubata S, Hashimoto I, Ichida F, Miyazaki A, Okada T, Murakami A, Morita H, Fukahara K. Aneurysmal change of the ductus arteriosus after prostaglandin E1 administration for pulmonary atresia: Demonstration with magnetic resonance imaging. *Pediatr Cardiol* 1994;15:30–32.

192. Gibbs JL, Rothman MT, Rees MR, Parsons JM, Blackburn ME, Ruiz CE. Stenting of the arterial duct: A new approach to palliation for pulmonary atresia. *Br Heart J* 1992;67:240–245.

193. Abrams SE, Walsh KP. Arterial duct morphology with reference to angioplasty and stenting. *Int J Cardiol* 1993; 40:27–33.

194. Hausdorf G, Schulze-Neick I, Lange PE. Radiofrequency-assisted "reconstruction" of the right ventricular outflow tract in muscular pulmonary atresia with ventricular septal defect. *Br Heart J* 1993;69:343–346.

195. Haworth SG and Silove ED. Pulmonary arterial structure in pulmonary atresia after prostaglandin E2 administration. *Br Heart J* 1981;45:311–316.

196. Haworth SG, Sauer U, Buhlmeyer K. Effect of prostaglandin E1 on pulmonary circulation in pulmonary atresia. A quantitative morphometric study. *Br Heart J* 1980;43:306–314.

197. Pahl E, Muster AJ, Ilbawi MN, DeLeon SY. Tetralogy of Fallot with absent ductus arteriosus and absent collateral pulmonary circulation: Diagnostic and surgical implications during the neonatal period. *Pediatr Cardiol* 1988;9:45–49.

198. Anderson RH, Macartney FJ, Shinebourne EA, Tynan MJ, eds. *Paediatric Cardiology.* Edinburgh: Churchill Livingstone; 1987, pp. 799–827.

199. Hernandez RJ, Bank ER, Shaffer EM, Snider AR, Rosenthal A. Comparative evaluation of the pulmonary arteries in patients with right ventricular outflow tract obstructive lesions. *AJR* 1987;148:1189–1194.

200. Smyllie JH, Sutherland GR, Keeton BR. The Value of Doppler color flow mapping in determining pulmonary blood supply in infants with pulmonary atresia with ventricular septal defect. *J Am Coll Cardiol* 1989;14: 1759–1765.

201. Ueda K, Nojima K, Saito A, Nakano H, Yokota M, Muraoka R. Modified Blalock-Taussig shunt operation without cardiac catheterization: Two-dimensional echocardiographic preoperative assessment in cyanotic infants. *Am J Cardiol* 1986;54:1296–1299.

202. Huhta JC, Piehler JM, Tajik AJ, Hagler DJ, Mair DD, Julsrud PR, Seward JB. Two dimensional echocardiographic detection and measurement of the right pulmonary artery in pulmonary atresia-ventricular septal defect: Angiographic and surgical correlation. *Am J Cardiol* 1982;49:1235–1240.

203. Ma MH-M, Hwang J-J, Lin J-L, Shyu K-G, Chen W-J, Kuan P, Lien W-P. Detection of major aortopulmonary collateral arteries by trans-esophageal echocardiography in pulmonary atresia and ventricular septal defect. *Am Heart J* 1993;126:1227–1229.

204. Marino B, Corno A, Pasquini L, Guccione P, Grazia Carta M, Ballerini L, de Simone G, Marcelletti C. Indication for systemic-pulmonary artery shunts guided by two-dimensional echocardiography: Criteria for patient selection. *Ann Thorac Surg* 1987;44:495–498.

205. Marino B, Pasquini L, Guccione P, Giannico S, Bevilacqua M, Marcelletti C. Pulmonary atresia with ventricular septal defect. Selection of patients for systemic-to-pulmonary artery shunt based on echocardiography. *Chest* 1991;99:158–161.

206. Hagler DJ. Doppler color flow imaging and determination of pulmonary blood supply in infants with pulmonary atresia with ventricular septal defect. *J Am Coll Cardiol* 1989;14:1759–1765.

207. Acherman RJ, Smallhorn JF, Freedom RM. The echocardiographic assessment of the pulmonary blood supply in patients with pulmonary atresia and ventricular septal defect. *J Am Coll Cardiol* 1996; 28:1308–1313.

208. Calder AL, Chan NS, Clarkson PM, Kerr AR, Neutze JM. Progress of patients with pulmonary atresia after systemic to pulmonary arterial shunts. *Ann Thorac Surg* 1991;51:401–407.

209. Fermanis GG, Ekangaki AK, Salmon AP, Keeton BR, Shore DF, Lamb RK, Monro JL. Twelve year experience with the modified Blalock-Taussig shunt in neonates. *Eur J Cardiothorac Surg* 1992;6:586–589.

210. Hoffman JIE, Rudolph AM, Nadas AS, Gross RE. Pulmonic stenosis, ventricular septal defect and right ventricular pressure above systemic level. *Circulation* 1960; 22:405–411.

211. Bharati S, Lev M. *The Pathology of Congenital Heart Disease. A Personal Experience with More than 6,300 Congenitally Malformed Hearts.* Volume I. Armonk, NY: Futura Publishing Company, Inc; 1996, p. 390.

212. Neufeld HN, McGoon DC, DuShane JW, Edwards JE. Tetralogy of Fallot with anomalous tricuspid valve simulating pulmonary stenosis with intact septum. *Circulation* 1960;22:1083–1086.

213. Faggian G, Frescura C, Thiene G, Bortolotti U, Mazzucco A, Anderson RH. Accessory tricuspid valve tissue causing obstruction of the ventricular septal defect in tetralogy of Fallot. *Circulation* 1983;49:324–327.

214. Monterroso J, Fonseca MC, Cunha D, Ramalhao C. Tetralogy of Fallot with accessory tricuspid valve tissue obstructing the ventricular septal defect. The need of its early recognition by noninvasive methods. *Acta Cardiol* 1991;46:33–37.

215. Flanagan MF, Foran RB, Van Praagh R, Jonas R, Sanders SP. Tetralogy of Fallot with obstruction of the ventricular septal defect: Spectrum of echocardiographic findings. *J Am Coll Cardiol* 1988;11:386–395.

216. Glaser J, Rosenmann D, Balkin J, Zion MM. Acquired obstruction of the ventricular septal defect in tetralogy of Fallot. *Cardiology* 1989;76:309–311.

217. Johnson GL, O'Connor WN, Verble SM, Cottrill CM, Noonan JA. Ventricular septal defect with mobile tricuspid valve pouch mimicking tetralogy of Fallot. *Pediatr Cardiol* 1986;7:53–56.

218. Musewe NN, Smallhorn JF, Moes CAF, Freedom RM, Trusler GA. Echocardiographic evaluation of obstructive mechanism of tetralogy of Fallot with restrictive ventricular septal defect. *Am J Cardiol* 1988;61:664–668.

219. Dabizzi RP, Caprioli G, Aiazzi L. Distribution and anomalies of the coronary arteries in Tetralogy of Fallot. *Circulation* 1980;61:95–102.

220. Fellows KE, Freed MD, Keane JF, Van Praagh R, Bernhard W, Castenada AC. Results of routine preoperative coronary angiography in tetralogy of Fallot. *Circulation* 1975;51:561–566.

221. McManus BM, Waller BF, Jones M, Epstein SE, Roberts WC. The case for preoperative coronary angiography in patients with tetralogy of Fallot and other complex congenital heart disease. *Am Heart J* 1982;103:451–456.

222. Meng CC, Eckner FAO, Lev M. Coronary artery distribution in tetralogy of Fallot. *Arch Surg* 1965;90:363–396.

223. Berry JM Jr, Einzig S, Krabill KA, Bass JL. Evaluation of coronary artery anatomy in patients with tetralogy of Fallot by two-dimensional echocardiography. *Circulation* 1988;78:149–156.

224. White RI Jr, French RS, Castaneda A, Amplatz K. The nature and significance of anomalous coronary arteries in tetralogy of Fallot. *Am J Roentgen Radium Therapy Nuclear Med* 1972;114:350–354.

225. Shrivastava S, Mohan JC, Mukhopadhyay S, Rajani M, Tandon R. Coronary artery anomalies in tetralogy of Fallot. *Cardiovasc Intervent Radiol* 1987;10:215–218.

226. Humes RA, Driscoll DJ, Danielson GK, Puga FJ. Tetralogy of Fallot with anomalous origin of left anterior descending coronary artery. Surgical options. *J Thorac Cardiovasc Surg* 1987;94:784–787.

227. Carvalho JS, Silva CM, Rigby ML, Shinebourne EA. Angiographic diagnosis of anomalous coronary artery in tetralogy of Fallot. *Br Heart J* 1993;70:75–78.

228. O'Sullivan J, Bain H, Hunter S, Wren C. End-on aortogram: Improved identification of important coronary artery anomalies in tetralogy of Fallot. *Br Heart J* 1994;71:102–106.

229. Baker WP, Vogel JHK, Blount SG Jr. Coronary artery-right ventricular communication associated with pulmonary atresia and ventricular septal defect. *Circulation* 1967;35:923–927.

230. Kromann Hansen O, Hasenkam JM, Paulsen PK, Baandrup U. Tetralogy of Fallot associated with anomalous origin of the left coronary artery from the pulmonary artery, pulmonary artery hypoplasia and atrial septal defect. A case report. *Scand J Thorac Cardiovasc Surg* 1988;22:291–294.

231. Yamaguchi M, Tsukube T, Hosokawa Y, Ohashi H, Oshima Y. Pulmonary origin of left anterior descending coronary artery in tetralogy of Fallot. *Ann Thorac Surg* 1991;52:310–312.

232. Saxena A, Sharma S, Shrivastava S. Coronary arteriovenous fistula in tetralogy of Fallot: An unusual association. *Int J Cardiol* 1990;28:373–374.

233. Perez-Martinez VM, Burgueros M, Quero M, Perez Leon J, Hafer G. Aorticopulmonary window associated with tetralogy of Fallot. Report of one case and review of the literature. *Angiology* 1976;27:526–534.

234. Castaneda AR, Kirklin JW. Tetralogy of Fallot with aortico-pulmonary window. *J Thorac Cardiovasc Surg* 1977;74:467–468.

235. Sondheimer HM, Oliphant M, Schneider B, Kavey REW, Blackman MS, Parker FB. Computerized axial tomography of the chest for visualization of "absent" pulmonary arteries. *Circulation* 1982;65:1020–1025.

236. Canter CE, Gutierresz FR, Mirowitz SA, Martin EC, Hartmann AF Jr. Evaluation of pulmonary arterial morphology in cyanotic congenital heart disease by magnetic resonance imaging. *Am Heart J* 1989;118:347.

237. Rao PS. Pulmonary vein wedge angiography in visualization obstructed ipsilateral pulmonary artery. *Radiology* 1978;1:151–152.

238. Rao PS. Complications of pulmonary vein angiography. *Br Heart J* 1980;43:124.

239. Freedom RM, Pongiglione G, Williams WG, Trusler GA, Moes CAF, Rowe RD. Pulmonary vein wedge angiography. Indications, results, and surgical correlates in 25 patients. *Am J Cardiol* 1983;51:936–942.

240. Nihill MR, Mullins CE, McNamara DG. Visualization of the pulmonary arteries in pseudotruncus by pulmonary vein wedge angiography. *Circulation* 1978;58:140–147.

241. Hruda J, Julsrud PR. Diagnostic selective balloon occlusion technique in pulmonic valve atresia and ventricular septal defect. *Am J Cardiol* 1989;63:1408–1409.

242. Vincent RN, Hawkins LE, Pelech AN, Collins GF. Balloon occlusion aortography. *Can J Cardiol* 1987;3:52–59.

243. Fiddler GI, Partridge JB. Balloon occlusion angiography in critically ill neonates. *Cathet Cardiovasc Diagn* 1983;9:309–312.

244. Rao PS. Descending aortography with balloon inflation. A technique for evaluating the size of persistent ductus arteriosus in infants with large proximal left to right shunts. *Br Heart J* 1985;54:527–532.

245. Hardy C, Wong J, Young JN, McCray J. Balloon occlusion scintigraphy of aortopulmonary collaterals. *Pediatr Cardiol* 1994;15:241–245.

246. Keane JF, McFaul R, Fellows K, Lock J. Balloon occlusion angiography in infancy: Methods, uses and limitations. *Am J Cardiol* 1985;56:495–497.

247. Burgener FA, Gutierrez OH, Logsdon GA. Complications and hazards with angiographic occlusion balloon catheters. *Radiology* 1981;140:647–650.

248. Castaneda-Zuniga WR, Bass JL, Lock JE. Selective opacification of arteries with balloon-occlusion angiography. *Radiology* 1981;138:727–729.

249. Moll JN, Santos MA, Drumond C, Romao N, Murad M, Reis NB. Improved visualization of aortopulmonary collateral arteries by abdominal aortic compression during angiography. *Circulation* 1982;65:953–955.

250. Herraiz I, Bermudez-Canete B, Cazzaniga M, Merino G, Pena I, Diez Balda JI, Quero M. *Occlusion Aortography. Evaluation of Our Results with this Technique.* Abstracts of World Congress of Paediatric Cardiology. 1980, p. 174.

251. Levin DC, Baltaxe HA, Goldberg HP, Engle MA, Ebert PA, Sos TA, Levin AR. The importance of selective angiography of systemic arterial supply to the lungs in planning surgical correction of pseudotruncus arteriosus. *AJR* 1974;121:606–613.

252. Fulton RE, Davis GD. Congenital pulmonary atresia: Photographic subtraction as an aid in recognizing hypoplastic pulmonary arteries. *AJR* 1978;131:1003–1007.

252a. Chesler E, Beck W, Schrire V. Selective catheterization of pulmonary or bronchial arteries in the preoperative assessment of pseudotruncus arteriosus and truncus arteriosus Type IV. *Am J Cardiol* 1970;26:20–24.

253. Chesler E, Matisonn R, Beck W. The assessment of the arterial supply to the lung in pseudotruncus arteriosus and truncus arteriosus Type IV in relation to surgical repair. *Am Heart J* 1974;88:542–552.

254. Ishizawa E, Horiuchi T, Tadokoro M, Okada Y, Suzuki Y, Tanaka S, Takamiya M, Sato T, Kano I. Diagnosis and surgical treatment of "angiographically absent pul-

monary artery syndrome". *Tohoku J Exp Med* 1978;125: 1–9.

255. Mair DD and Julsrud PR. Diagnostic evaluation of pulmonary atresia and ventricular septal defect: Cardiac catheterization and angiography. *Prog Pediatr Cardiol* 1992;1:23–36.

256. Soto B, Pacifico AD, Luna RF, Bargeron LM Jr. A radiographic study of congenital pulmonary atresia with ventricular septal defect. *AJR* 1977;129:1027–1037.

257. Davis GD, Fulton RE, Ritter DG, Mair DD, McGoon DC. Congenital pulmonary atresia with ventricular septal defect: Angiographic and surgical correlates. *Radiology* 1978;128:133–144.

258. Shimazaki Y, Maehara T, Blackstone EH, Kirklin JW, Bargeron LM Jr. The structure of the pulmonary circulation in tetralogy of Fallot with pulmonary atresia. A quantitative cineangiographic study. *J Thorac Cardiovasc Surg* 1988;95:1048–1058.

259. Soto B, Kassner EG, Baxley WA. *Imaging of Cardiac Disorders. Volume 1: Congenital Disorders.* New York: Lippincott/Gower; 1992, pp. 169–171.

260. Yoo S-J, Choi Y-H. *Angiocardiograms in Congenital Heart Disease. Teaching File of Sejong Heart Institute.* Oxford: Oxford Medical Publications; 1991, pp. 111–126.

261. Soto B, Pacifico AD. *Angiocardiography in Congenital Heart Malformations.* Mt. Kisco, NY: Futura Publishing Company; 1990, pp. 449–491.

262. Amplatz K, Moller JH. *Radiology of Congenital Heart Disease.* St. Louis: Mosby Year-Book; 1993, pp. 583–598.

263. Freedom RM, Culham JAG, Moes CAF. *Angiocardiography of Congenital Heart Disease.* New York: McMillan Publishing Co; 1984, pp. 173–213.

264. Capelli H, Ross D, Somerville J. Aortic regurgitation in tetrad of Fallot and pulmonary atresia. *Am J Cardiol* 1982;49:1979–1981.

265. Marelli A, Perloff JK, Child JS, Laks H. Pulmonary atresia with ventricular septal defects in adults. *Circulation* 1994;89:243–251.

266. Bull K, Somerville J, Ty ED, Spiegelhalter D. Presentation and attrition in complex pulmonary atresia. *J Am Coll Cardiol* 1995;25:491–499.

267. Folliguet TA, Laborde F, Mace L, Dervanian P, Dibie A, Grinda J-M, Neveux J-Y. Aortic insufficiency associated with complex cardiac anomalies. *Cardiol Young* 1995; 5:125–131.

267a. Kito H, Yagihara T, Kawashima Y. Aortic valve replacement in tetralogy of Fallot and pulmonary atresia with major aortopulmonary collateral arteries. *Cardiol Young* 1994;4:298–300.

Chapter 22

The Absent Pulmonary Valve
Tetralogy of Fallot and Other Variants

Congenital absence of the pulmonary valve can occur in relative isolation,[1–16] but its best known association is with tetralogy of Fallot: so-called tetralogy of Fallot with absent pulmonary valve.[10,15,17–29] A completely absent pulmonary valve or just vestigial leaflets have been observed in a wide range of congenitally malformed hearts (Table 22-1). Please see specific chapters for the association between absent pulmonary valve and complex forms of congenital heart disease.

Congenital Absence of the Pulmonary Valve with an Intact Ventricular Septum

Congenital absence of the pulmonary valve with an intact ventricular septum is an unusual condition usually presenting in the newborn infant.[1–16,30] It is of interest that this condition profoundly volume loads the right ventricle, often producing fetal right heart failure (Figs. 22-1 and 22-2). The neonatal constellation usually includes a patent foramen ovale as well as a patent arterial duct. The presence of a patent arterial duct in the patient with a congenitally absent pulmonary valve and intact ventricular septum is a departure from its association with tetralogy of Fallot where absence of the patent arterial duct is characteristic. In another departure from the tetralogy variant, the branch pulmonary arteries usually do not assume aneurysmal proportions with tufting in the patient with congenitally absent pulmonary valve and intact ventricular septum and profound bronchial compression is thus not a conspicuous feature in the patient with an intact ventricular septum although occasionally this may occur (Table 22-2) (Figs. 22-1 and 22-2).[10]

Those findings leading to consideration of absent pulmonary valve with an intact ventricular septum in a neonate include right heart failure and cyanosis in a baby with a loud regurgitant diastolic murmur along the left sternal edge. The normalcy of the arterial pulses should focus clinical attention to the pulmonary root as opposed to a severely regurgitant truncal valve or aortic root (ie, aorto-left ventricular tunnel, etc.). Airway obstruction has been observed in an occasional patient with absent pulmonary valve with an intact ventricular septum. Echocardiographic reports of absent pulmonary valve in isolation have been published and the clinical condition of the patient and the echocardiographic assessment may determine the timing of the cardiac catheterization.

Angiocardiography of Congenital Absence of the Pulmonary Valve with an Intact Ventricular Septum

The cardinal features of this disorder reflect the disordered pulmonary valve and its impact on the neonatal right ventricle.[10,15] Thus, echocardiographic examination should have excluded a significant ventricular septal defect. A right ventriculogram in the frontal projection with craniocaudal tilt will define a very much enlarged right ventricle and a dilated main pulmonary trunk (Figs. 22-1 and 22-2). The dilation may extend to the proximal right and left pulmonary artery branches, but the angiographic appearance of the pulmonary arteries in this disorder is considerably different from that of the pulmonary arteries in patients with absent pulmonary valve complicating tetralogy of

From: Freedom RM, Mawson JB, Yoo SJ, Benson LN: *Congenital Heart Disease: Textbook of Angiocardiography.* Armonk NY, Futura Publishing Co., Inc. ©1997.

Table 22-1

Conditions Associated with Absent Pulmonary Valve

Atrial Septal Defect
Atrioventricular Septal Defect
Intact Ventricular Septum
Ebstein's Anomaly
Patent Arterial Duct
Tetralogy of Fallot
Transposition of the Great Arteries
Tricuspid Atresia and Intact Ventricular Septum
Uhl's Anomaly of the Right Ventricle
Ventricular Septal Defect
Others

Table 22-2

Condition/ Variable	*Patent Arterial Duct*	*Aneurysmal Branch Pulmonary Arteries*
Tetralogy with absent pulmonary valve	Usually Absent	Present
Absent pulmonary valve and intact ventricular septum	Present in the newborn. Not part of the pathogenesis	Conspicuous main pulmonary trunk, but not branches

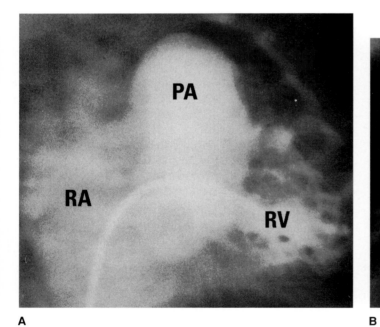

A

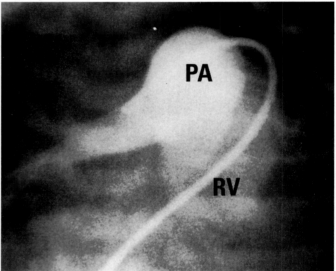

B

Fig. 22-1: Absent pulmonary valve and intact ventricular septum in a newborn infant with severe right heart failure.
A: This right ventriculogram demonstrates a moderately dilated main pulmonary artery and tricuspid regurgitation. **B:** The selective main pulmonary arteriogram shows the pulmonary regurgitation into the right ventricle; the branch pulmonary arteries do not show the massive dilatation with tufting so characteristic of tetralogy of Fallot and absent pulmonary valve.

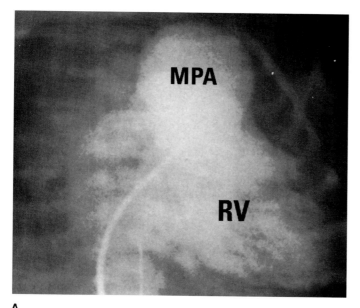

A

B

Fig. 22-2: Absent pulmonary valve and intact ventricular septum in another newborn infant with severe right heart failure.
A: The selective main pulmonary arteriogram shows the pulmonary regurgitation into the right ventricle. **B:** The left ventricle is "pancaked" by the dilated right ventricle as shown by this left ventriculogram in the long axial oblique.

Fallot. An injection of contrast in the pulmonary arteries may define some degree of pulmonary regurgitation, but how much is catheter induced? The levophase of either the right ventricular or pulmonary artery injection will opacify the left atrium and then there is often some degree of left-to-right atrial shunting as well. It has been unusual to observe significant pulmonary arterial branch stenoses in patients with this disorder. The right ventricle has been noted to be relatively smooth in appearance, consistent with Uhl's anomaly. A left ventricular angiocardiogram performed in the long axial oblique projection should exclude most ventricular septal defects. The left ventricle may seem "pancaked" by the much dilated right ventricle (Fig. 22-2). The aortic arch is left-sided, and in the neonate with this disorder the arterial duct or its remnant will be evident.

Tetralogy of Fallot with Absent Pulmonary Valve

Tetralogy of Fallot with absent pulmonary valve is also very uncommon, and data from the New England Regional Infant Cardiac Program suggests a prevalence of about 0.0065 per 1000 livebirths.[31] Like other conotruncal abnormalities, there is an association with the DiGeorge syndrome and deletion within chromosome 22.[32–33a] Tetralogy of Fallot with absent pulmonary valve produces the substrate for varying degrees of right ventricular outflow tract obstruction, pulmonary regurgitation because of a pulmonary valve annulus completely devoid or nearly so of valvar issue, and right-to-left ventricular shunting at ventricular level because of a large ventricular septal defect resulting from anterior displacement of the infundibular septum, a finding considered characteristic of tetralogy of Fallot. As some have emphasized as well is the relative hypoplasia of the pulmonary valve annulus. Some of these patients will have significant left-to-right shunting at the ventricular level because of only modest right ventricular outflow tract obstruction. What is so unusual about patients with tetralogy of Fallot and absent pulmonary valve is the aneurysmally dilated pulmonary arteries with their potential for compression of the major bronchi (Figs. 22-3 through 22-12). The etiologies for the profound dilatation of the pulmonary arteries were summarized by Emmanoulides in 1976 who suggested a relation between absence of the arterial duct and the massive dilatation of the pulmonary arteries.[20,34] Emmanoulides and colleagues suggested that absence of the arterial duct in fetal life may contribute to this aneurysmally dilated pulmonary arteries by preventing the main fetal outlet of the right ventricular output in the presence of the fetal pattern of pulmonary vascular resistance. Other factors contributing to the profoundly dilated pulmonary arteries include the ef-

(text continues on p. 603)

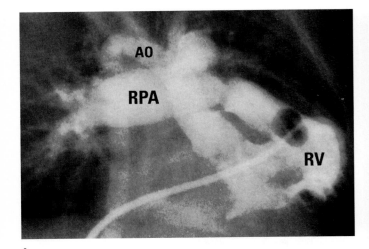

A

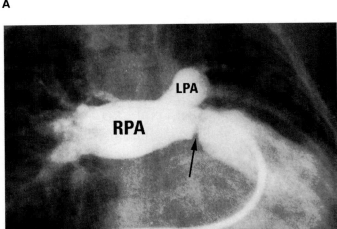

B

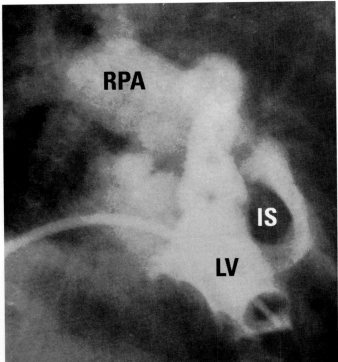

C

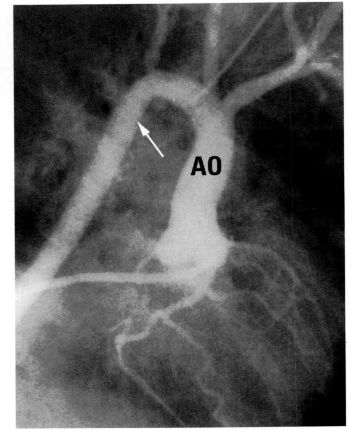

D

Fig. 22-3: Tetralogy of Fallot and absent pulmonary valve, right aortic arch, and absence of arterial duct.
A: Frontal right ventriculogram with craniocaudal tilt shows the aneurysmally dilated right pulmonary artery and right-to-left shunting at ventricular level opacifies the aorta. **B:** Selective injection of contrast into the proximal right pulmonary artery provides good definition of both right and left pulmonary arteries. **C:** The right axial oblique left ventriculogram shows the anteriorly deviated infundibular septum. **D:** The aortic arch is right sided and in this newborn there is no evidence of a right-sided arterial duct (arrow).

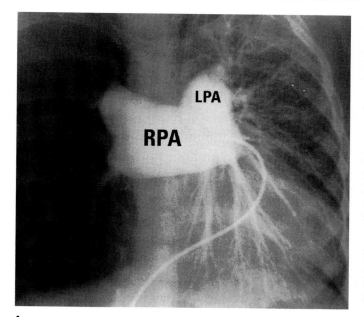

A

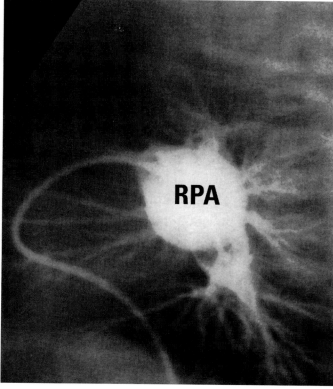

C

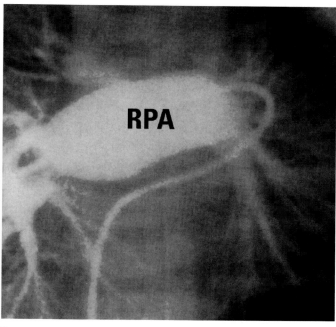

B

Fig. 22-4: The spectrum of pulmonary artery caliber and infundibular anatomy in patients with tetralogy of Fallot and absent pulmonary valve syndrome.
A: Massively dilated branches. **B and C:** Frontal and lateral pulmonary angiogram shows a much enlarged right pulmonary artery. *(figure continues)*

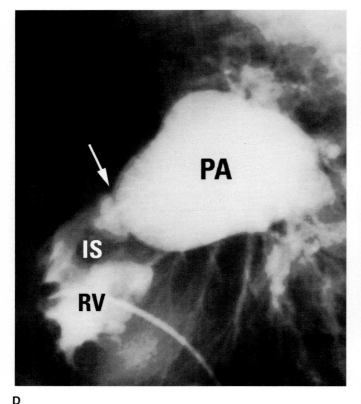

D

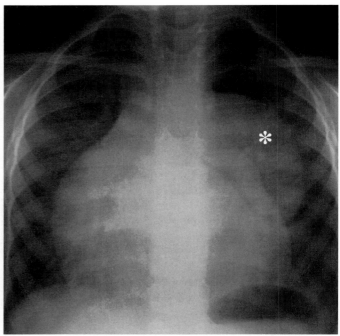

A

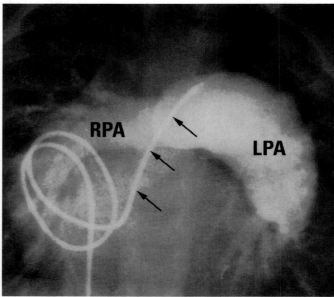

B

E

Fig. 22-4: *(continued)*
D: Lateral right ventriculogram shows the anteriorly deviated infundibular septum and the ridge-like tissue at the pulmonary valve ring (arrow). **E:** A mild form of tetralogy of Fallot and absent pulmonary valve syndrome with only mild anterior deviation of the infundibular septum and a thickened ridge of tissue at the pulmonary valve annulus (arrow).

Fig. 22-5: Aneurysmally dilated left pulmonary artery in an older child with tetralogy of Fallot and absent pulmonary valve syndrome.
A: Frontal chest radiograph shows moderate heart enlargement and a conspicuous left pulmonary artery (✱). **B:** Selective left pulmonary arteriogram shows the very much larger left pulmonary artery; the course of the right ventricular outflow tract as noted by the arrows indicates preferential flow into the left pulmonary artery.

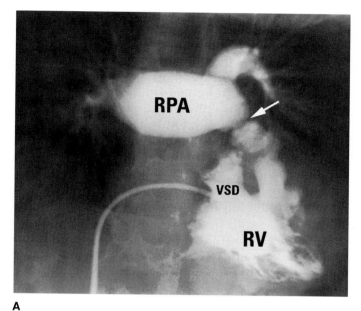

A

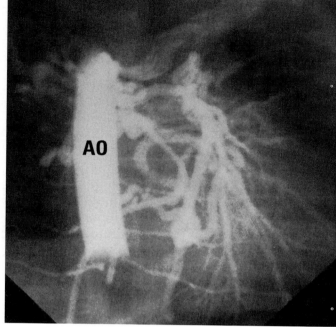

C

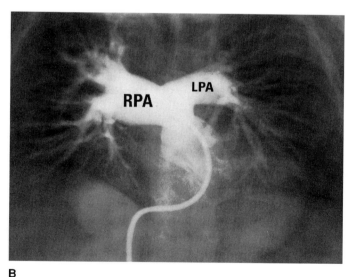

B

Fig. 22-6: Tetralogy of Fallot, absent pulmonary valve syndrome, and extensive aortopulmonary collaterals.
A: Frontal right ventriculogram shows anatomy typical of this syndrome and a ridge (arrow) at the pulmonary valve annulus. **B:** Selective injection into the pulmonary arteries with characteristic tufting. **C:** Balloon occlusion aortogram shows extensive direct aortopulmonary collaterals. *(figure continues)*

fects of pulmonary regurgitation with its impact on right ventricular stroke volume.[35] In discussing patients from the newborn to the older patient with this disorder, one of the recurrent themes is compression of the larger airways by the massively dilated pulmonary arteries, and the impact of a disordered airway on morbidity, mortality, and indeed surgical management has focused primarily on dealing with the pulsatile and aneurysmally dilated pulmonary arteries. Profound bronchial compression may result in massively hyperinflated lungs, and spontaneous pneumothorax has been observed in the critically-ill neonate or infant with this disorder. Rabinovitch and colleagues[36] some years ago suggested that not only were the larger bronchi compressed by the often huge mediastinal pulmonary arteries, but that abnormally branching pulmonary ar-

teries associated with an absent pulmonary valve resulted in compression of intrapulmonary bronchi. This finding could possibly explain why some patients do not demonstrate airway improvement after "successful" surgical repair of the cardiac malformation. Others have corroborated the abnormal branching pattern with its typical tufting pattern, but have not been able to document compression of intrapulmonary bronchi.[37] Nonetheless, the patient with profound bronchial compression poses a therapeutic dilemma and a number of surgical therapies have been derived, none completely satisfactory.[38-50] Because tracheobronchial cartilage matures over the first 6 to 9 months of life, some patients with relatively modest airway obstruction may demonstrate spontaneous improvement.[51-54] The respi-

(text continues on p. 608)

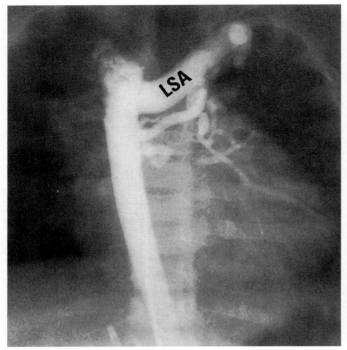

D

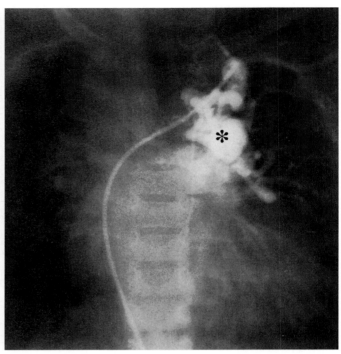

E

Fig. 22-6: *(continued)*
D and E: Selective injection into the left subclavian artery and collateral vessel (✽) originating from this vessel.

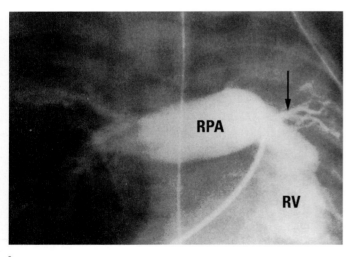

A

Fig. 22-7: Left pulmonary artery hypoplasia in a patient with tetralogy of Fallot, absent pulmonary valve syndrome, and some aortopulmonary collaterals.
A: Frontal right ventriculogram demonstrates typical right pulmonary artery and small left pulmonary artery (arrow). *(figure continues)*

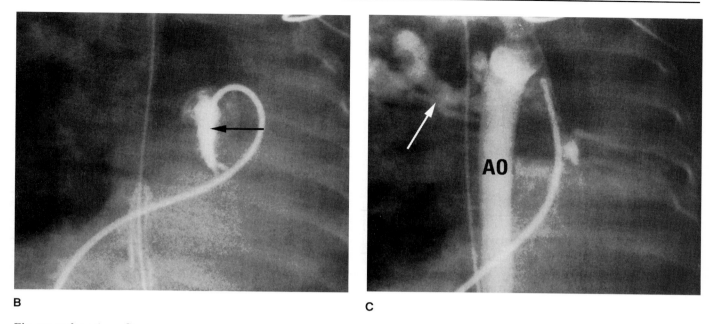

B   C

Fig. 22-7: *(continued)*
B: Selective injection in left pulmonary artery confirms its hypoplasia and abnormal arborization. **C:** Aortography shows right-sided collaterals.

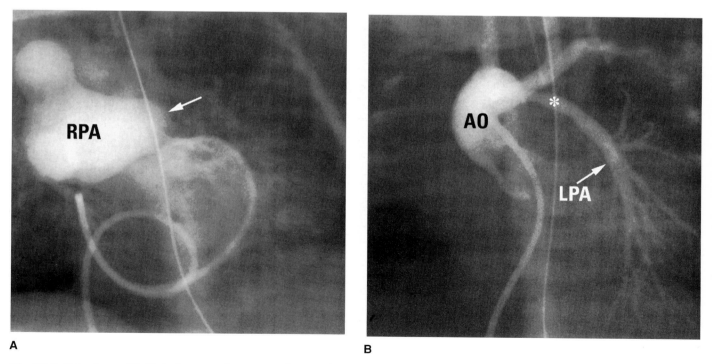

A   B

Fig. 22-8: Tetralogy of Fallot, absent pulmonary valve syndrome, right aortic arch and nonconfluent pulmonary arteries with ductal origin of left pulmonary artery.
A: Frontal injection in right pulmonary artery demonstrates massive dilatation of this vessel, but there is no left pulmonary artery (arrow). **B:** Aortography demonstrates ductal (✱) origin of left pulmonary artery. *(figure continues)*

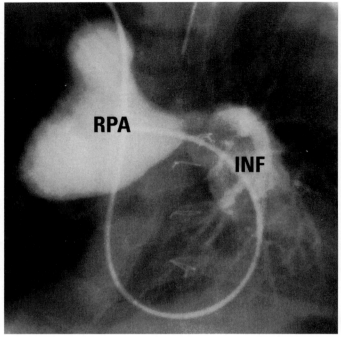

C

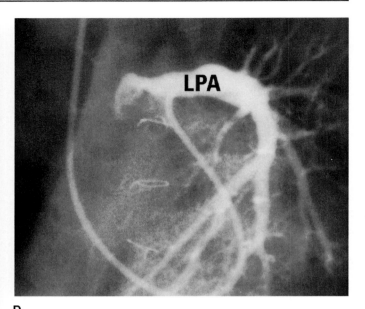

D

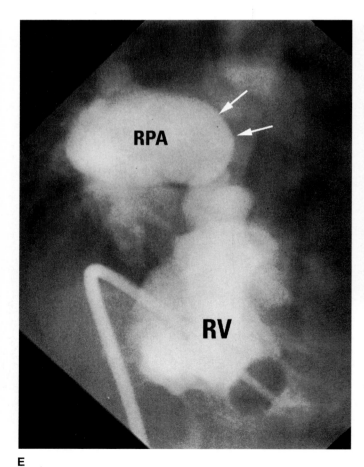

E

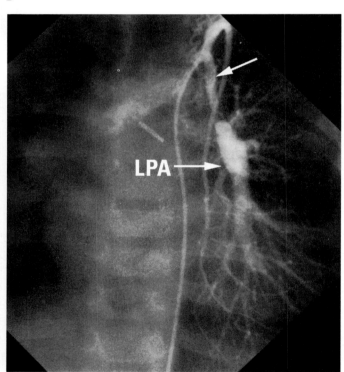

F

Fig. 22-8: *(continued)*
C: Infundibulum and right pulmonary artery after complete repair. **D:** The left pulmonary artery is still very small. **E and F:** A different patient with nonconfluent pulmonary arteries. **E:** Aneurysmal dilatation of right pulmonary artery is demonstrated in this right axial oblique right ventriculogram, but there is not a left pulmonary artery (arrows). **F:** The left pulmonary artery remains small after a modified Blalock-Taussig shunt (arrow). *(figure continues)*

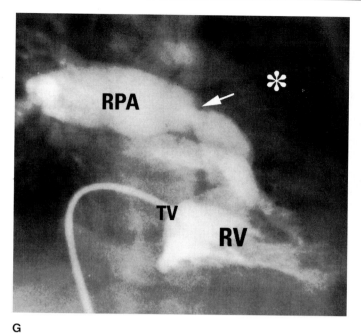

G

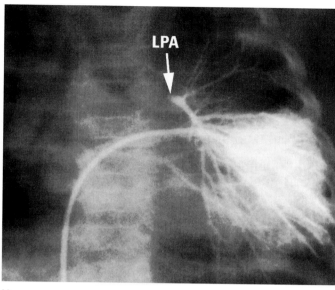

H

Fig. 22-8: *(continued)*
G and H: Yet another patient with nonconfluent pulmonary arteries. **G:** The frontal right ventriculogram shows the narrowed pulmonary valve ring (arrow) and the aneurysmally-dilated right pulmonary artery; no left pulmonary artery is seen (✳). **H.** The small left pulmonary artery is demonstrated only by left pulmonary vein wedge angiography as the arterial duct had closed, virtually isolating the left pulmonary artery.

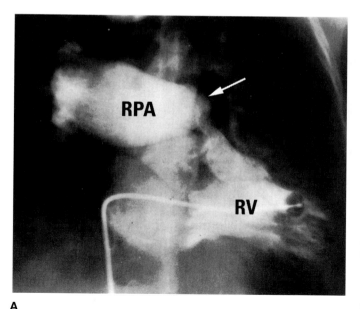

A

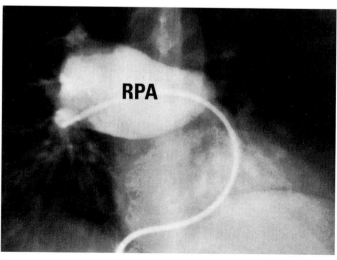

B

Fig. 22-9: Tetralogy of Fallot, absent pulmonary valve syndrome, and nonconfluent pulmonary arteries with aortic origin of left pulmonary artery.
A: Frontal injection in right ventricle demonstrates massive dilatation of this vessel, but there is no left pulmonary artery (arrow). **B:** Massive dilatation of the right pulmonary artery. *(figure continues)*

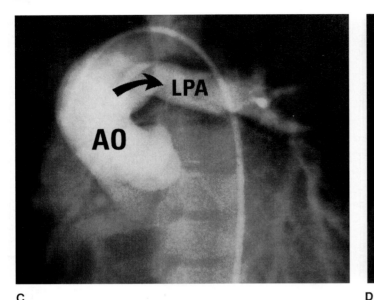

C

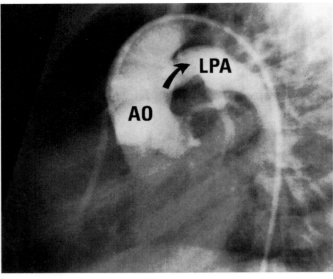

D

Fig. 22-9: *(continued)*
C and D: Frontal and lateral aortography demonstrates to advantage origin of left pulmonary artery from the ascending aorta (see Chapter 20, Fig. 20-13).

ratory findings may be particularly severe in the neonate and it may be the respiratory distress that brings these patients to medical attention.[55–61]

In the patient with tetralogy of Fallot with absent pulmonary valve, one branch pulmonary artery may exhibit more spectacular dilatation than the other. It has been suggested that the inclination of the right ventricular outflow tract towards the right pulmonary artery will produce greater dilatation of the right pulmonary artery, and vice versa (Figs. 22-3 through 22-6).[62] Not infrequently, the dilatation of both branch pulmonary arteries will be spectacular. Coarctation, stenosis, or hypoplasia of one pulmonary artery may also occur in the patient with tetralogy and absent pulmonary valve,[63–65] and the recognition of this observation will impact on angiocardiography (Fig. 22-7).

The pulmonary arteries in this condition, like "standard" tetralogy, or indeed pulmonary atresia and ventricular septal defect, may be nonconfluent (Figs. 22-8 and 22-9). One pulmonary artery, usually the left, may be "isolated," originating from a left-sided arterial duct (Fig. 22-8).[10,15,66–67b] The pulmonary artery with a ductal origin does not demonstrate the aneursymal dilatation of the contralateral pulmonary artery with its right ventricular origin. Calder and colleagues[63] and others have also reported nonconfluent pulmonary arteries in this condition, but with one pulmonary artery originating from the ascending aorta.[68–70] In the three patients in Calder's report with tetralogy of Fallot and absent pulmonary valve leaflets, the left pulmonary artery originated from the ascending aorta in two and the right pulmonary artery originated from the ascend-

ing aorta in the third (Fig. 22-9). We have studied several patients in whom the left pulmonary artery had a distal ductal origin, and two patients with origin of the left pulmonary artery from the ascending aorta (Figs. 22-8 and 22-9).

Aortopulmonary collaterals of variable size may coexist in the patient with tetralogy of Fallot and absent pulmonary valve (Figs. 22-6 and 22-7).[10] Often the collaterals are small and indirect. Less frequently, they are large, direct, and thus originating from the decending thoracic aorta entering the lung at the hilum, and clearly will complicate surgical management unless they are dealt with prior to repair. The laterality of the aortic arch and the frequency of abnormalities of coro-

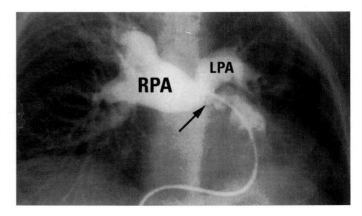

Fig. 22-10: **Appearance of pulmonary arteries after palliative pulmonary artery banding (arrow).**

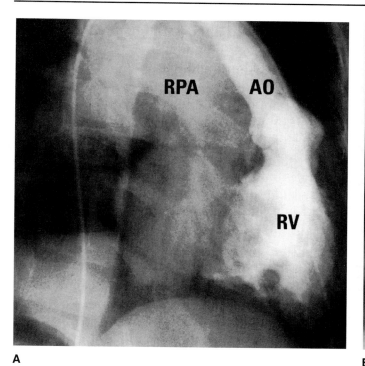

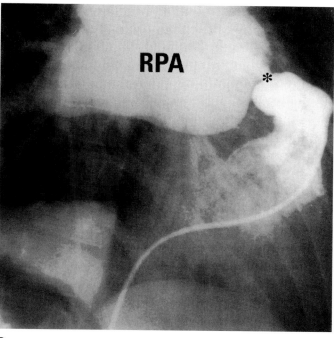

A

B

Fig. 22-11: Absent pulmonary valve syndrome in an older child with double-inlet right ventricle.
A: Right anterior oblique ventriculogram shows anteriorly positioned aorta, and aneurysmally dilated pulmonary artery. **B:** Infundibular injection shows the massively dilated right pulmonary artery and hypoplastic pulmonary valve ring (✱). This patient was successfully treated with a lateral tunnel Fontan.

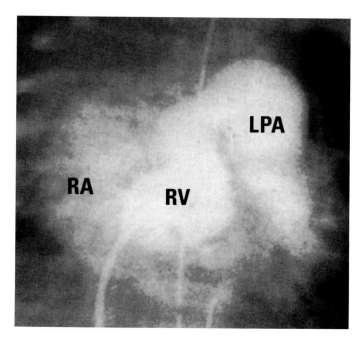

Fig. 22-12: Absent pulmonary valve and absent right pulmonary artery in an infant with dominant left form of atrioventricular septal defect.
Frontal ventriculogram in small right ventricle shows the aneurysmal left pulmonary artery.

nary arterial epicardial distribution is that of the usual expression of tetralogy of Fallot. The aortic arch is right-sided in about 30% of patients with tetralogy of Fallot and absent pulmonary valve. The left anterior descending coronary artery originates from the right coronary artery, thus crossing the right ventricular outflow tract in from 2% to 7% of these patients.

Echocardiographic Imaging

The echocardiographic features of tetralogy of Fallot with absent pulmonary valve have received considerable attention.[15,71–74] This condition has been recognized in the fetus as well.[75–77b]

Angiocardiographic Considerations

The considerations in the angiographic investigation of the patient with tetralogy of Fallot and absent pulmonary valve are similar in most respects to that of tetralogy of Fallot (Figs. 22-3 through 22-12).[10,15,20, 36,62,78] Right ventricular angiography with craniocaudal angulation will demonstrate the character of the right ventricular outflow tract and the pulmonary arteries. Because of the pulmonary regurgitation, the infundibulum rarely appears severely obstructive. There is often a discordant appearance between the hugely dilated pulmonary arteries and the hypoplastic pulmonary valve annulus. It is often desirable to perform a selective injection into the main pulmonary artery with craniocaudal angulation, and if there are any concerns about proximal left pulmonary artery stenosis, then about 30° left anterior oblique should also be used. The pulmonary valve annulus is often hypoplastic, but on occasion may have a nearly normal diameter. With a vestigial or absent pulmonary valve, the pulmonary valve annulus is not dilated, and this is seen as a ridge that demonstrates upward and backward movement during the cardiac cycle. As this ridge may be mistaken for a dysplastic valve leaflet, the aneurysmal dilatation of the mediastinal segment of the pulmonary artery is a sentinel finding of the tetralogy variant with absent pulmonary valve. Left ventricular angiocardiography in the long axial oblique injection should demonstrate the ventricular septal defect. Aortography in the aortic root should image the epicardial course of the coronary arteries and demonstrate the presence or absence of significant aortopulmonary collaterals. Unless the pulmonary arteries are nonconfluent, a patent arterial duct or its remnant is unlikely to be imaged by aortography. Aortography will be necessary to image an aortic origin of the left pulmonary artery (Fig. 22-9). One may image a thoracic coarctation that is rarely seen in the patient with tetralogy and absent pulmonary valve.[79] The absent pulmonary valve constellation may be seen in patients with double-inlet ventricle (Fig. 22-11), or atrioventricular septal defect (Fig. 22-12) among others.

The Peculiar Constellation of Absent Pulmonary Valve, Tricuspid Atresia, and Intact Ventricular Septum

The usual basis for tricuspid atresia is an absent right atrioventricular connection (see Chapter 39).[79a] Less commonly, the morphological basis for tricuspid atresia is an imperforate valve with tensor apparatus in the right ventricle (see Chapter 15) (Fig. 22-13). Subsequent to the original description of an imperforate tricuspid valve with congenital absence of the pulmonary valve and intact ventricular septum by Marin-Garcia and colleagues, a number of publications have defined the scope of this rare condition.[80–85] We and others have characterized the disproportionately thickened ventricular septum, demonstrating the right ventricular dysplasia and persistence of spongy-like, endothelial cell-lined myocardium (see also Chapter 27).[82,85] The ventricular septum is so hypertrophied in some of these patients that it simulates hypertrophic cardiomyopathy, a feature commented on in the original description by Marin-Garcia.[80] In our report of three patients with imperforate tricuspid valve with congenital absence of the pulmonary valve and intact ventricular septum, the ventricular septum was spectacularly thickened.[82] The

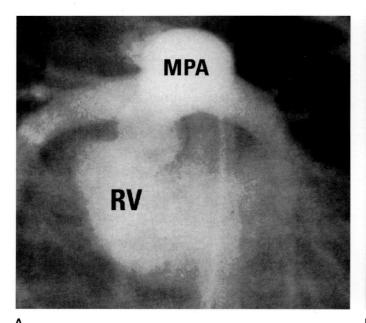

A

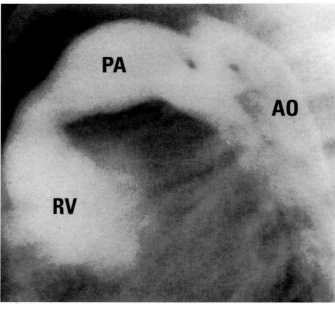

B

Fig. 22-13: Imperforate tricuspid valve, absent pulmonary valve, intact ventricular septum, and so-called spongy myocardium.
A and B: Frontal and lateral aortogram opposite arterial duct. Free pulmonary regurgitation shows a reasonably-formed right ventricle. *(figure continues)*

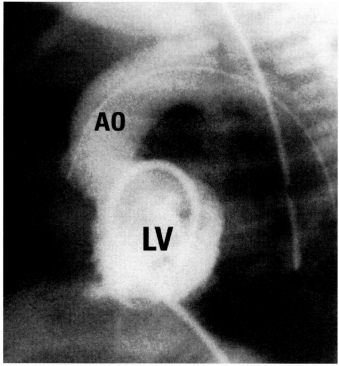

C

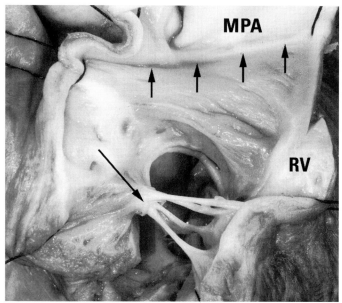

E

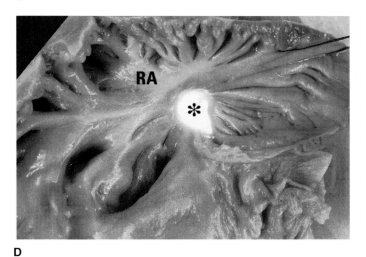

D

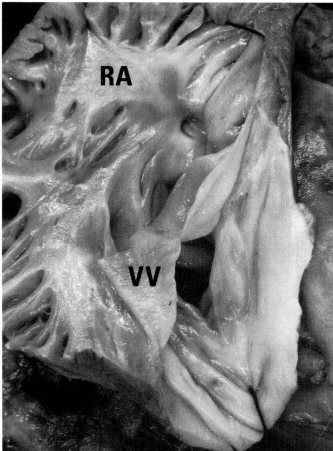

F

Fig. 22-13: *(continued)*
C: The left ventriculogram shows an intact ventricular septum. **D:** The transilluminated tricuspid valve (✳) when viewed from the right atrium. **E:** Appearance of imperforate tricuspid valve (single long black arrow) when viewed from the right ventricle; note the absent pulmonary valve leaflets (small black arrows). **F:** Persistence of right venous valve (VV) in one patient. *(figure continues)*

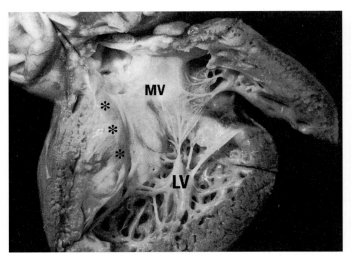

G

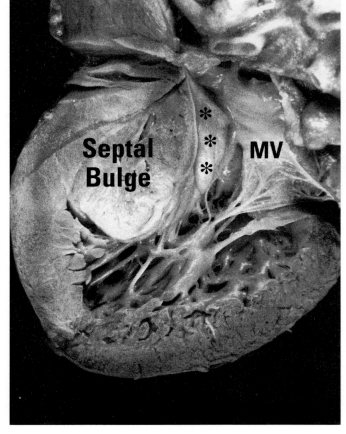

H

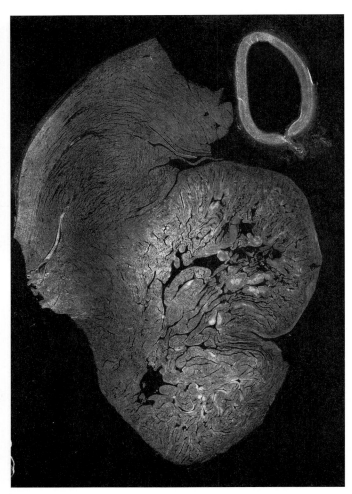

I

Fig. 22-13: *(continued)*
G and H: Peculiar septal bulge (✱) when viewed from the left ventricle. **I:** Whole-mount showing appearance of spongy myocardium.

coronary arteries in our patients had normal aortic origin. The more recently published experience of Mori and colleagues[86] has extended the clinical, gross, and microscopic findings in nine patients. The right coronary artery was absent in one of their patients, and in three patients the coronary arterial supply was characterized as scanty to the right ventricular free wall. The right ventricular free wall was fibrous and aneurysmal. The majority of patients presenting as symptomatic neonates have not survived palliation; this has been our experience as well as that of Mori and O'Connor and their respective colleagues.[85,86] The clinical experience of Forrest and colleagues[83] is more favorable, with all four patients in their report surviving surgical palliation. Indeed, one of their four patients successfully underwent a modified Fontan procedure.

Angiocardiography of Congenital Absence of the Pulmonary Valve, Imperforate Tricuspid Valve, and Intact Ventricular Septum

Left ventricular angiocardiography will demonstrate the intact ventricular septum, the left-sided aortic arch, and with filling of the patent arterial duct, dilated with prostaglandin, regurgitation across the unguarded pulmonary root into the blind right ventricle will be apparent (Fig. 22-13).[82] Right atriography is typical for tricuspid atresia, with obligatory right-to-left shunting at atrial level. Because of the observations of Mori and colleagues[86] regarding the abnormal coronary circulation, we would advocate imaging of the coronary arterial circulation.

References

1. Campeau LA, Ruble PE, Cooksey WB. Congenital absence of the pulmonary valve. *Circulation* 1957;15:397–404.
2. Chiemmongkoltip P, Replogle RL, Gonzalez-Lavin L, Arcilla RA. Congenital absence of the pulmonary valve with atrial septal defect surgically corrected with aortic homograft. *Chest* 1972;62:100–103.
3. Childers RW, Crea PC. Absence of the pulmonary valve. A case occurring in the Marfan syndrome. *Circulation* 1964;29:598–603.
4. D'Cruz IA, Lendrum BL, Novak G. Congenital absence of the pulmonary valve. *Am Heart J* 1964;68:728–740.
5. Ito T, Engle MA, Holswade GR. Congenital insufficiency of the pulmonic valve: A rare cause of neonatal heart failure. *Pediatrics* 1961;28:712–718.
6. Macartney FJ, Miller GAH. Congenital absence of the pulmonary valve. *Br Heart J* 1970;32:483–490.
7. Mainwaring RD, Lamberti JJ, Spicer RL. Management of absent pulmonary valve syndrome with patent ductus arteriosus. *J Card Surg* 1993;8:148–155.
8. Ozer S, Karademir S, Yurdakul Y, Bilgic A. Congenital absence of pulmonary valve leaflets with intact ventricular septum in a neonate. *Jpn Heart J* 1991;32:853–857.
9. Osman MZ, Meng CC, Girdnay BR. Congenital absence of the pulmonary valve: Report of eight cases with review of the literature. *AJR* 1969;106:58–69.
10. Pelech AN, Rabinovitch M, Freedom RM. The absent pulmonary valve: A consideration of tetralogy of fallot and other variants. In: Tucker BL, Lindesmith GG, Takahashi M, eds. *Obstructive Lesions of the Right Heart. The Third Clinical Conference on Congenital Heart Disease.* Baltimore: University Park Press; 1984, pp. 34–64.
11. Pouget JM, Kelly CE, Pilz CG. Congenital absence of the pulmonic valve: Report of a case in a 73-year-old man. *Am J Cardiol* 1967;19:732–734.
12. Smith RD, DuShane JW, Edwards JE. Congenital insufficiency of the pulmonary valve. Including a case of fetal cardiac failure. *Circulation* 1959;20:554–560.
13. Tanabe Y. Takahashi M. Kuwano H. Izumi T. Shibata A. Oda E. Long-term fate of isolated congenital absent pulmonary valve. *Am Heart J* 1992;124:526–529.
14. Zajtchuk T, Gonzales-Lavin L, Replogle RL. Pulmonary artery aneurysm associated with atrial septal defect and absent pulmonary valve. *J Thorac Cardiovasc Surg* 1973;65:699–701.
15. Freedom RM, Rabinovitch M. Tetralogy of Fallot with absent pulmonary valve. In: Freedom RM, Benson LN, Smallhorn JF, eds. *Neonatal Heart Disease.* London: Springer-Verlag; 1992, pp. 257–267.
16. Alpert BS, Moore HV. "Absent" pulmonary valve with atrial septal defect and patent ductus arteriosus. *Pediatr Cardiol* 1985;6:107–112.
17. Anderson RH, Macartney FJ, Shinebourne EA, Tynan M. *Paediatric Cardiology.* Edinburgh: Churchill Livingstone; 1987; pp. 765–798.
18. Durnin RW, Willner R, Virmani S, Lawrence T, Fyler DC. Pulmonary regurgitation with ventricular septal defect and pulmonic stenosis: Tetralogy of Fallot variant. *AJR* 1969;106:42–51.
19. Elliott LP, Shanklin DR, Schiebler GL. Congenital insufficiency of the pulmonary valve with a ventricular septal defect. *Dis Chest* 1962;42:534–540.
20. Emmanouilides GC, Thanopoulos B, Siassi B, Fishbein M. "Agenesis" of ductus arteriosus associated with the syndrome of tetralogy of Fallot and absent pulmonary valve. *Am J Cardiol* 1976;37:403–409.
21. Fischer DR, Neches WH, Beerman LB, Fricker FJ, Siewers RD, Lenox CC, Park SC. Tetralogy of Fallot with absent pulmonic valve: Analysis of 17 patients. *Am J Cardiol* 1984;53:1433–1437.
22. Keith JD, Rowe RD, Vlad P. *Heart Disease in Infancy and Childhood.* Third Edition. New York: Macmillan Publishing Company; 1978, pp. 3–13.
23. Miller RA, Lev M, Paul MH. Congenital absence of the pulmonary valve: The clinical syndrome of tetralogy of Fallot with pulmonary regurgitation. *Circulation* 1962;26:266–278.
24. Fyler DC. Tetralogy of Fallot. In: Fyler DC, ed. *Nadas' Pediatric Cardiology.* St. Louis: Mosby-Year Book Inc; 1992, pp. 471–492.
25. Nasrallah A, Williams RL, Nouri S. Absent pulmonary valve in tetralogy of Fallot: Clinical and angiographic considerations with review of the literature. *Bull Texas Heart Inst* 1974;1:392–399.
26. Pinsky WW, Nihill MR, Mullins CE, Harrison G, mcNamara DG. The absent pulmonary valve syndrome: Considerations of management. *Circulation* 1978;57:159–162.
27. Rowe RD, Freedom RM, Mehrizi A. *The Neonate with*

Congenital Heart Disease. New York: WB Saunders Co; 1981, pp. 301–308.

28. Rowe RD, Vlad PM, Keith JD. Atypical tetralogy of Fallot: A noncyanotic form with increased lung vascularity. *Circulation* 1955;12:230–238.

29. Ruttenberg HD, Carey LS, Adams Jr P, Edwards JE. Absence of the pulmonary valve in the tetralogy of Fallot. *AJR* 1964;91:500–510.

30. Nakayama-K, Okazaki-H. Eguchi-S. Long-term fate of isolated congenital absent pulmonary valve. *Am Heart J* 1992;124:526–529.

31. Fyler DC. Report of the New England Regional Infant Cardiac Program. *Pediatrics* 1980;65(Suppl):376–461.

32. Rose JS, Levin DC, Goldstein S, Laster W. Congenital absence of the pulmonary valve associated with congenital aplasia of the thymus (DiGeorge's syndrome). *AJR* 1974; 122:97–102.

33. Radford DJ, Thong YH. The association between immunodeficiency and congenital heart disease. *Pediatr Cardiol* 1988;9:103–108.

33a. Johnson MC, Strauss AW, Dowton SB, Spray TL, Huddleston CB, Wood MK, Slaugh RA, Watson MS. Deletion within chromosome 22 is common in patients with absent pulmonary valve syndrome. *Am J Cardiol* 1995;76: 66–69.

34. Thanopoulos B, Siassi B, Emmanouilides G. "Agenesis" of ductus arteriosus associated with the syndrome of tetralogy of Fallot and absent pulmonary valve. *Am J Cardiol* 1975;35:173–177.

35. Hiraishi S, Bargeron LM, Isabel-Jones JB, Emmanouilides GC, Friedman WF, Jarmakani JM. Ventricular and pulmonary artery volumes in patients with absent pulmonary valve. Factors affecting the natural course. *Circulation* 1983;67:183–190.

36. Rabinovitch M, Grady S, David I, Van Praagh R, Sauer U, Buhlmeyer K, Castaneda AR, Reid L. Compression of intrapulmonary bronchi by abnormally branching pulmonary arteries associated with absent pulmonary valves. *Am J Cardiol* 1982;50:804–812.

37. Milanesi O, Talenti E, Pellegrino PA, Thiene G.. Abnormal pulmonary artery branching in tetralogy of Fallot with "absent" pulmonary valve. *Int J Cardiol* 1984; 6:375–380.

38. Bove EL, Shaher RM, Alley R, McKneally M. Tetralogy of Fallot with absent pulmonary valve and aneurysm of the pulmonary artery: Report of two cases presenting as lung disease. *J Pediatr* 1972;81:339–343.

39. Byrne JP, Hawkins JA, Battiste CE, Khoury GH. Palliative procedures in tetralogy of Fallot with absent pulmonary valve: A new approach. *Ann Thorac Surg* 1982;33: 499–502.

40. Dunnigan A, Oldham HN, Benson DW. Absent pulmonary valve syndrome in infancy: Surgery reconsidered. *Am J Cardiol* 1981;48:117–122.

41. Ilbawi MN, Fedorchik J, Muster AJ, Idriss FS, DeLeon SY, Gidding SS, Paul MH. Surgical approach to severely symptomatic newborn infants with tetralogy of Fallot and absent pulmonary valve. *J Thorac Cardiovasc Surg* 1986; 91:584–589.

42. Ilbawi MN, Idriss FS, Muster AJ, Wessel HU, Paul MH, DeLeon SY. Tetralogy of Fallot with absent pulmonary valve. Should valve insertion be part of the intracardiac repair? *J Thorac Cardiovasc Surg* 1981;81:906–915.

43. Karl TR, Musumeci F, de Leval M, Pincott JR, Taylor JFN, Stark J. Surgical treatment of absent pulmonary valve syndrome. *J Thorac Cardiovasc Surg* 1986;91:590–597.

44. Layton CA, McDonald A, McDonald L, Towers M, Weaver J, Yacoub M. The syndrome of absent pulmonary valve.

Total correction with aortic valvular homografts. *J Thorac Cardiovasc Surg* 1972;63:800–808.

45. Litwin SB, Rosenthal A, Fellows K. Surgical management of young infants with tetralogy of Fallot, absence of the pulmonary valve, and respiratory distress. *J Thorac Cardiovasc Surg* 1973;65:552–558.

46. Opie JC, Sandor GGS, Ashmore PG, Patterson MWH. Successful palliation by pulmonary artery banding in absent pulmonary valve syndrome with aneurysmal pulmonary arteries. *J Thorac Cardiovasc Surg* 1983;85:125–128.

47. Stafford EG, Mair DD, McGoon DC, Danielson GK. Tetralogy of Fallot with absent pulmonary valve. Surgical considerations and results. *Circulation* 1973;47/48(Suppl III):III-24-III-30.

48. Stellin G, Jonas RA, Goh TH, Brawn WJ, Venables AW, Mee RBB. Surgical treatment of absent pulmonary valve syndrome in infants: Relief of bronchial obstruction. *Ann Thorac Surg* 1983;36:468–475.

49. Waldhausen JA, Friedman S, Nicodemus H, Miller WW, Rashkind W, Johnson J. Absence of the pulmonary valve in patients with tetralogy of Fallot: Surgical management. *J Thorac Cardiovasc Surg* 1969;57:669–674.

50. Watterson KG, Malm TK, Karl TR, Mee RB. Absent pulmonary valve syndrome: Operation in infants with airway obstruction. *Ann Thorac Surg* 1992;54:1116–1119.

51. Robotham JL, Freedom RM. Case report: Tetralogy of Fallot. *Clin Notes Respir Dis* 1978;17:15–16.

52. Olsen CR, DeKock MA, Colebatch HJH. Stability of airways during reflex bronchoconstriction. *J Appl Physiol* 1967;23:23–26.

53. Olsen CR, Stevens AE, McIlroy MB. Rigidity of tracheae and bronchi during muscular constriction. *J Appl Physiol* 1967;23:27–34.

54. Olsen CR, Stevens AE, Pride NB, Staub NC. Structural basis for decreased compressibility of constricted trachae and bronchi. *J Appl Physiol* 1967;23:35–39.

55. Backer CL, Ilbawi MN, Idriss FS, DeLeon SY. Vascular anomalies causing tracheoesophageal compression. Review of experience in children. *J Thorac Cardiovasc Surg* 1989;97:725–731.

55a. Godart F, Houyel L, Lacour-Gayet F, Serraf A, Sousa-Uva M, Bruniaux J, Petit J, Piot JD, Binet JP, Conte S, Planche C. Absent pulmonary valve syndrome; surgical treatment and considerations. *Ann Thorac Surg* 1996;62:136–142.

56. Borg SA, Young LW, Roghair GD. Congenital avalvular pulmonary artery and infantile lobar emphysema. *Radiology* 1975;125:412–421.

57. Cochran ST, Gyepes MT, Smith LE. Obstruction of the airways by the heart and pulmonary vessels in infants. *Pediatr Radiol* 1977;6:81–87.

58. Corno A, Picardo S, Ballerini L, Gugliantini P, Marcelletti C. Bronchial compression by dilated pulmonary artery. *J Thorac Cardiovasc Surg* 1985;90:706–710.

59. Fearon B, Shortreed R. Tracheobronchial compression by congenital cardiovascular anomalies in children: Syndrome of apnea. *Ann Otol Rhinol Laryngol* 1963;72: 949–969.

60. Pernot C, Hoeffel JC, Henry M, Worms AM, Stehlin H, Louis JP. Radiological patterns of congenital absence of the pulmonary valve in infants. *Radiology* 1972;102: 619–622.

61. Stanger P, Lucas RV Jr, Edwards JE. Anatomic factors causing respiratory distress in acyanotic congenital cardiac disease. *Pediatrics* 1969;43:760–769.

62. Lakier JB, Stanger P, Heymann MA, Hoffman JIE, Rudolph AM. Tetralogy of Fallot with absent pulmonary valve. Natural history and hemodynamic considerations. *Circulation* 1974;50:167–175.

63. Calder AL, Brandt PWT, Barratt-Boyes BG, Neutze JM. Variant of tetralogy of Fallot with absent pulmonary valve leaflets and origin of one pulmonary artery from the ascending aorta. *Am J Cardiol* 1980;46:106–116.

64. Dixon LM, Franklin RB, Gorczycz CA. Congenital unilateral absence of a pulmonary artery: A report of three cases. *Am J Cardiol* 1966;18:754–760.

65. Peter T, Harper R, Vohra J, Hunt D. Effect of coexistent coarctation of pulmonary trunk in natural history of complete absence of pulmonary valve with ventricular septal defect. *Br Heart J* 1975;37:978–981.

66. Anjos RT, Suzuki A, Yen Ho S. A rare case of tetralogy of Fallot with unusual blood supply to the left lung. *Int J Cardiol* 1989;24:363–366.

67. Presbitero P, Pedretti E, Orzan F, Malara D, Villani M, Ferrazi P, Crupi GC, Parenzan L. Absent pulmonary valve syndrome with associated anomalies of the pulmonary blood supply. *Int J Cardiol* 1984;6:587–596.

67a. Sreeram N, Smith A, Peart I. Fallot's tetralogy with absent pulmonary valve and anomalous origin of the left pulmonary artery. *Int J Cardiol* 1993;42:175–177.

67b. Pac A, Ozme S, Celiker A, Ozkutlu S. Absent pulmonary valve syndrome with agenesis of the left pulmonary artery. *Turk J Pediatr* 1994;36:249–253

68. Kawada S, Nagamine I, Nishikawa K. Successful surgical correction of a case of tetralogy of Fallot associated with an anomalous left pulmonary artery originating from aortic arch and absence of the pulmonary valve. *Shinzo* 1971;3:1073–1082.

68a. O'Blenes SB, Freedom RM, Coles JG. Tetralogy of Fallot with anomalous left anterior descending coronary artery: Repair without conduit. *Ann Thorac Surg* 1996;62:1186–1188.

69. Saxena A, Shrivastava S, Sharma S. Anomalous origin of the left pulmonary artery from the ascending aorta in a patient with tetralogy of Fallot and absent pulmonary valve. *Int J Cardiol* 1991;33:315–317.

70. Wyler F, Rutishauser M, Olafson A, Kaulmann HJ. Congenital absence of the pulmonary valve in tetralogy of Fallot and origin of the left pulmonary artery from the aortic arch. *AJR* 1970;110:505–508.

71. Cheatham JP, Latson LA, Gutgesell HP. Echocardiographic pulsed Doppler features of absent pulmonary valve syndrome in the neonate. *Am J Cardiol* 1982;49:1773–1777.

72. Ettedgui JA, Sharland GK, Chita SK, Cook A, Fagg N, Allan LD. Absent pulmonary valve syndrome with ventricular septal defect: Role of the arterial duct. *Am J Cardiol* 1990;66:233–234.

73. Buendia A, Attie F, Ovseyevitz J, Zghaib A, Zamora C, Zavaleta D, Vargas-Barron J, Richheimer R. Congenital absence of pulmonary valve leaflets. *Br Heart J* 1983;50:31–41.

74. Segni ED, Einzig S, Bass JL, Edwards JE. Congenital absence of pulmonary valve with tetralogy of Fallot: Diagnosis by 2–dimensional echocardiography. *Am J Cardiol* 1983;51:1798–1780.

75. Rein AJ, Singer R, Simcha A. Prenatal diagnosis of tetralogy of Fallot with absence of the leaflets of the pulmonary valve. *Int J Cardiol* 1992;34:211–213.

76. Fouron J-C, Sahn DJ, Bender R, Block R, Schneider H, Fromberger P, Hagen-Ansert S, Daily PO. Prenatal diagnosis and circulatory characteristics in tetralogy of Fallot with absent pulmonary valve. *Am J Cardiol* 1990;64:547–549.

77. Callan NA, Kan JS. Prenatal diagnosis of tetralogy of Fallot with absent pulmonary valve. *Am J Perinatol* 1991;8:15–17.

77a. Sameshima H, Nishibatake M, Ninomiya Y, Tokudome T. Antenatal diagnosis of tetralogy of Fallot with absent pulmonary valve accompanied by hydrops fetalis and polyhydramnios. *Fetal Diagn Ther* 1993;8:305–308.

77b. Rowland DG, Caserta T, Foy P, Wheller JJ, Allen HD. Congenital absence of the pulmonary valve with tetralogy of Fallot with associated aortic stenosis and patent ductus arteriosus: a prenatal diagnosis. *Am Heart J* 1996;132:1075–1077.

78. Freedom RM, Culham JAG, Moes CAF. *Angiocardiography of Congenital Heart Disease.* New York: Macmillan Publishing Company; 1984, pp. 214–221.

79. Hofbeck M, Rockelein G, Singer H, Rein J, Gittenberger-de Groot AC. Coarctation of the aorta in the syndrome of absent pulmonary valve with ventricular septal defect. *Pediatr Cardiol* 1990;11:159–163.

79a. Orie JD, Anderson C, Ettedgui JA, Zuberbuhler JR, Anderson RH. Echocardiographic-morphologic correlations in tricuspid atresia. *J Am Coll Cardiol* 1995;26:750–758.

80. Marin-Garcia J, Roca J, Blieden LC, Lucas Jr RV, Edwards JE. Congenital absence of the pulmonary valve associated with tricuspid atresia and intact ventricular septum. *Chest* 1973;64:658–661.

81. Cox JN, De Seigneux R, Bolens M, Haenni P, Bopp P, Bruins C. Tricuspid atresia, hypoplastic right ventricle, intact ventricular septum and congenital absence of the pulmonary valve. *Helv Paediatr Acta* 1975;30:389–398.

82. Freedom RM, Patel RG, Bloom KR, Duckworth JW, Silver MM, Dische R, Rowe RD. Congenital absence of the pulmonary valve, associated imperforate membrane type of tricuspid atresia, right ventricular tensor apparatus and intact ventricular septum: A curious developmental complex. *Eur J Cardiol* 1979;10:171–196.

83. Forrest P, Bini RM, Wilkinson JL, Arnold R, Wright JG, McKay R, Hamilton DI, Bargeron LM Jr, Pacifico AD. Congenital absence of the pulmonic valve and tricuspid atresia with intact ventricular septum. *Am J Cardiol* 1987;59:482–484.

84. Ando M, Satomi G, Takao A. Atresia of tricuspid or mitral orifice. Anatomic spectrum and morphologic hypothesis. In: Van Praagh R, Takao A, eds: *Etiology and Morphogenesis of Congenital Heart Disease.* Mt. Kisco, NY: Futura Publishing Company, Inc; 1980, pp. 421–487.

85. O'Connor WN, Cottrill CM, Marion MT, Noonan JA. Defective regional myocardial development and vascularization in one variant of tricuspid atresia-clinical and necropsy findings in three cases. *Cardiol Young* 1992;2:42–52.

86. Mori K, Ando M, Satomi M, Nakazawa M, Momma K, Takao A. Imperforate tricuspid valve with dysplasia of the right ventricular myocardium, pulmonary valve, and coronary artery: A clinicopathologic study of nine cases. *Pediatr Cardiol* 1992;13:24–29.

Chapter 23

Pulmonary Atresia and Intact Ventricular Septum

In its simplest form, pulmonary atresia and intact ventricular septum is a disorder characterized by complete membranous, and in many patients, muscular obstruction to the right ventricular outlet.[1-6] The pulmonary valve is imperforate, and in many patients right ventricular infundibular muscular atresia of variable extent or length is also present. (Figs. 23-1 and 23-2). The ventricular septum is intact. With rare exception, pulmonary blood flow in these patients is mediated by a patent arterial duct, and there is an obligatory right-to-left shunt at the atrial level.[7] But this definition does no justice to this disorder. It is similar to characterizing Da Vinci as "just a painter." Pulmonary atresia and intact ventricular septum is a profoundly complex disorder encompassing considerable morphological heterogeneity.[2-6,8-17] It is perhaps this tremendous diversity in structure that continues to confound surgical- and catheter-based therapy.[18-57] As we will develop in this chapter, the coronary artery abnormalities that are so important in many patients with pulmonary atresia and intact ventricular septum have evolved from pathological curiosity to that of signal importance to surgical management, and ultimately, prognosis. To place this heterogeneity of form and function into a clinical perspective, two of the most significant factors in patients with pulmonary atresia and intact ventricular septum correlating with a poor outcome, ie, ventriculocoronary connections with a right ventricular-dependent coronary circulation and those forms of pulmonary atresia and intact ventricular septum with a right ventricular/left ventricular pressure ratio <1, are mutually exclusive, and hearts with these features are at extreme ends of the continuum of this disorder.[2,4,8,11-13,18,33,58-64]

Prevalence

Pulmonary atresia and intact ventricular septum is an uncommon form of congenitally malformed heart, accounting for only about 3% of newborns with serious congenital heart disease.[65] Data published in the report from the New England Regional Infant Cardiac Program identified 75 patients with this disorder, accounting for 3.1% of all babies encompassed by this study.[66] The more recently completed Baltimore-Washington Infant Study found the prevalence for pulmonary atresia and intact ventricular septum as 0.083 per 1000 livebirths.[67] This lesion accounts for 0.71% of all patients seen with congenital heart disease at the Toronto Hospital for Sick Children and this experience has recently been extensively reviewed.[65] As one surveys cyanotic neonates with congenital heart disease, this disorder ranks third, after transposition of the great arteries and pulmonary atresia and ventricular septal defect.[68] There are a few reports of familial aggregation of this disorder, but we have not identified siblings with this disorder among more than 170 families with one affected child seen in our institution.[69] Fetal echocardiography provides a unique window to study the later phases of the fetal heart and to define specific types of heart predisposed to fetal death. There is increasing evidence that fetuses with florid tricuspid regurgitation may not fare well.[70-74a] Such fetuses are known to develop right-sided heart failure with pleural and pericardial effusions, ascites, pulmonary hypoplasia, and fetal death. Thus, fetal loss might be anticipated in a specific subset of patients with pulmonary atresia, intact ventricular septum, extremely severe tricuspid regurgitation, and a low-pressure right ventricle.

From: Freedom RM, Mawson JB, Yoo SJ, Benson LN: *Congenital Heart Disease: Textbook of Angiocardiography.* Armonk NY, Futura Publishing Co., Inc. ©1997.

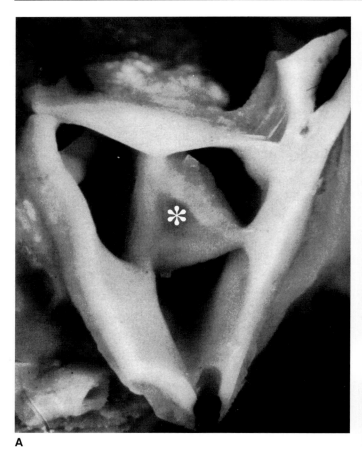

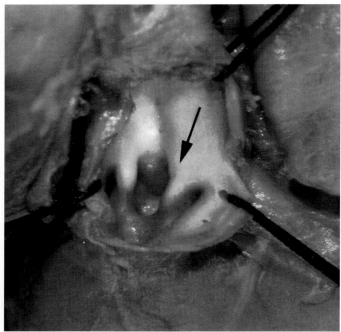

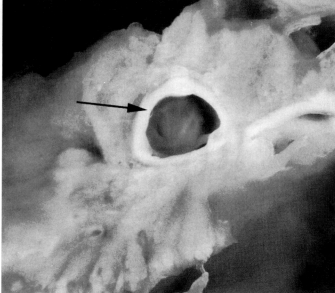

Fig. 23-1: Valvular nature of pulmonary atresia in patients with pulmonary atresia and intact ventricular septum.
A: Fused imperforate valve (✱) with obvious commissures and sinuses. **B:** An imperforate valve with more primitive features. **C:** The least well-formed pulmonary valve (arrow).

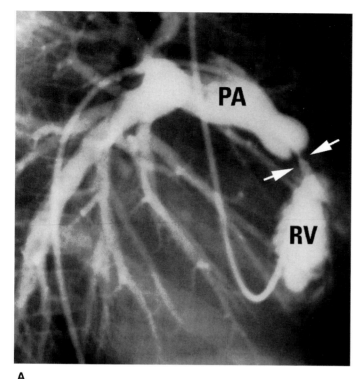

A

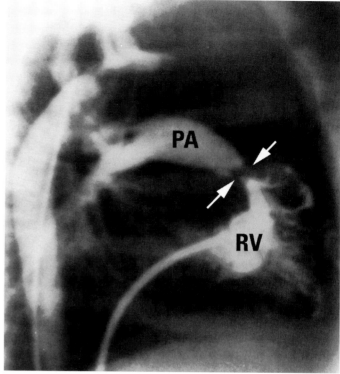

B

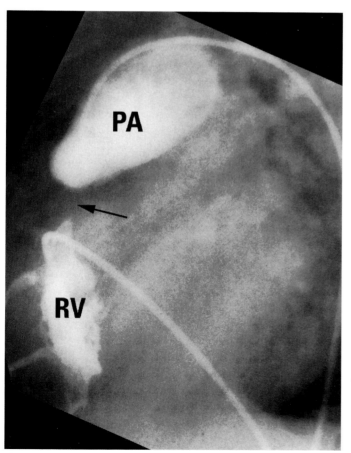

C

Fig. 23-2: Nature of infundibular atresia as demonstrated by double-catheter technique.[78]
A: Infundibular atresia just at imperforate valve plate with extreme proximal infundibular narrowing (arrows). **B:** Infundibular atresia (arrows) about 2–3 mm beneath imperforate pulmonary valve. **C:** Long-segment (arrow) infundibular atresia. The double-catheter technique uses simultaneous injection of contrast into the right ventricle and pulmonary artery.

Morphogenesis

Kutsche and Van Mierop[75] suggest that pulmonary atresia with ventricular septal defect occurs earlier in cardiac morphogenesis than pulmonary atresia and intact ventricular septum (see also Chapter 20). Their conclusion is based on an analysis of a number of morphological factors including the diameter of the pulmonary trunk, the morphology of the pulmonary valve, and the morphology and topography of the ductus arteriosus. Kutsche and Van Mierop[75] suggest that pulmonary atresia and ventricular septal defect occurs early in cardiac morphogenesis, at or shortly after partitioning of the truncoconal part of the heart, but before partitioning of the ventricular septum. Based on these morphological variables, they infer that pulmonary atresia and intact ventricular septum probably occurs after cardiac septation, speculating that this disorder might reflect a prenatal inflammatory disease rather than a congenital malformation. It is possible that their conclusions of the timing of the maturational arrest are correct for some forms of hearts with pulmonary atresia and intact ventricular septum, specifically those patients with pulmonary atresia, intact ventricular septum and a nearly normal-sized right ventricle, with an imperforate tricuspid pulmonary valve whose commissures are well formed, but completely fused. Indeed, there is evidence based on serial fetal echocardiographic studies that pulmonary atresia may be acquired in some patients, and these hearts tend to have better developed right ventricles. However, there is little data to support an inflammatory process as hearts with this disorder obtained from fetuses and from the immediate newborn have been studied histopathologically without providing any conclusive evidence of acute and subacute inflammation.[72,74] Furthermore, one would wonder whether those hearts with a diminutive right ventricle and ventriculocoronary artery connections represent an earlier insult than those with a well-formed right ventricle and a tricuspid, fused, imperforate valve. There is less certainty about the view advocated by Kutsche and Van Mierop[75] in those patients with pulmonary atresia and intact ventricular septum whose ventricles are minute, whose pulmonary valve is unicommissural and in whom there are extensive ventriculocoronary connections.

The Nature of Pulmonary Atresia

The morphological bases for pulmonary atresia in this disorder have been documented by Braunlin and colleagues,[76] and they have correlated the type of imperforate pulmonary valve with the nature of the right ventricle and its infundibulum (Fig. 23-1). As one might anticipate, in those patients with a well-formed infundibulum, the imperforate pulmonary valve ex-

hibits three semilunar cusps with complete fusion of the commissures forming a fused imperforate plate. In those patients with a very diminutive right ventricle and a severely narrowed or atretic infundibulum, the pulmonary valve is very primitive (Fig. 23-1C). The muscular nature of the infundibulum has received both morphological and clinical-angiocardiographic attention and the nature of those right ventricular muscle bundles contributing to the infundibular atresia have been described (Fig. 23-2).[77,78] With radiofrequency or laser interruption of the membranous and muscular forms of pulmonary atresia, these observations have perhaps gained more clinical relevance.[54–56,79]

The Pulmonary Circulation in Pulmonary Atresia and Intact Ventricular Septum

The pulmonary arteries are almost always confluent in patients with pulmonary atresia and intact ventricular septum (Fig. 23-3).[1–3,6,12,58,80,81] The pulmonary circulation in the overwhelming majority is maintained by a left-sided patent arterial duct, although very rarely by large direct aortopulmonary collaterals.[7a,7b] There is usually a main pulmonary trunk with imperforate continuity with the atretic pulmonary valve. This observation is of course germane to consideration of catheter-intervention in this disorder. While left pulmonary artery stenosis at the site of ductal insertion has been observed in these patients, it is our impression that this occurrence is less frequent than in patients with pulmonary atresia and ventricular septal defect (Fig. 23-4).[81–84] In this regard, Marino and colleagues[85] have provided data indicating that the arterial duct in patients with pulmonary atresia and intact ventricular septum constricts earlier than the arterial duct in patients with pulmonary atresia and ventricular septal defect. Rarely the pulmonary arteries in pulmonary atresia and intact ventricular septum are nonconfluent, each supported by its arterial duct.[7] Major aortopulmonary collaterals originating from the descending thoracic aorta have also been described as the source of pulmonary blood flow in these patients.[7a] This situation is very uncommon. A pulmonary sling has been observed in the patient with pulmonary atresia and intact ventricular septum.[86] The lungs may be underdeveloped in those babies with the largest hearts, and thus extremely severe tricuspid regurgitation.[70–74]

Segmental Analysis

The atrial situs is normal or solitus, the atrioventricular and ventriculoarterial connections are concordant, and the heart is left sided in more than 98% of hearts exhibiting pulmonary atresia and intact ventricular septum. Dextrocardia with solitus atria is infrequent as is pulmonary atresia and intact ventricular

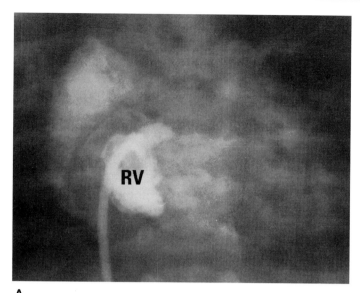

A

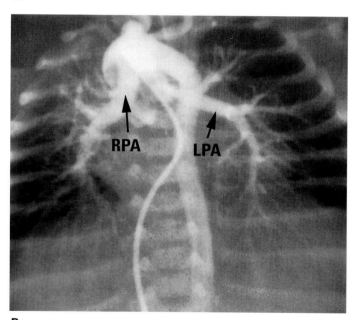

B

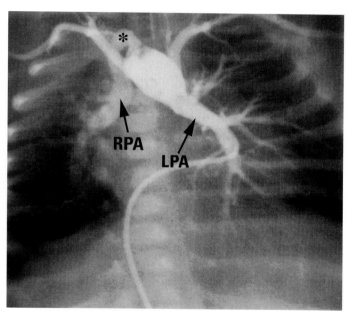

C

Fig. 23-3: Nonconfluent pulmonary arteries in pulmonary atresia and intact ventricular septum.
A: Frontal right ventriculogram shows a small right ventricle with an intact ventricular septum. **B and C:** Nonconfluent pulmonary arteries, each pulmonary artery mediated by an ipsilateral arterial duct. The right-sided arterial duct is evdent (✳) in Fig. 23-3B.

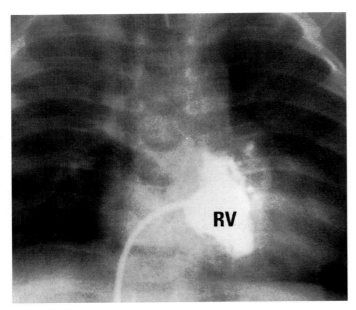

A

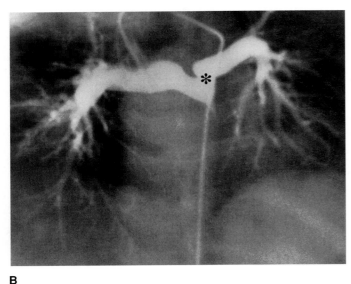

B

Fig. 23-4: Mild left pulmonary artery stenosis in pulmonary atresia and intact ventricular septum.
A: Frontal right ventriculogram shows a small right ventricle with an intact ventricular septum. **B:** The mild proximal left pulmonary stenosis is imaged via the right-sided arterial shunt.

septum with discordant atrioventricular and ventriculoarterial connections (see Chapter 36, Fig. 36-31).[87–89] The aortic arch is usually left sided.

The Tricuspid Valve in Pulmonary Atresia and Intact Ventricular Septum

As we and others have emphasized, the designation "pulmonary atresia and intact ventricular septum" denies significance to the right ventricular in-

let[2,4,6,8,11–14,17,49,53,58,63,90,91] and the inlet of the right ventricle with its tricuspid valve is often terribly abnormal and disordered. The tricuspid valve in some patients with this disorder is severely stenotic, while in others the tricuspid valve is massively regurgitant, with a very dilated annulus, at times virtually devoid of valvular tissue (Fig. 23-5).[2,4,8,14,16,17,49,58,59,60,63] In those patients with the most stenotic tricuspid valve, the annulus is obstructive, muscularized, and all components of the valve apparatus are abnormal with a thickened free-valve margin; thickened and shortened and attenuated chordae tendineae; and abnormal papillary muscles, including a parachute configuration. The massively regurgitant tricuspid valve shows a very dilated annulus. In this situation, the tricuspid valve demonstrates features of displacement and/or dysplasia, and a portion of the annulus may be unguarded. Ebstein's anomaly of the tricuspid valve has been found in about 10% of autopsied patients with pulmonary atresia and intact ventricular septum.[17] Displacement without dysplasia is virtually unknown in patients with Ebstein's anomaly complicating pulmonary atresia and intact ventricular septum.[8,62] An obstructive form of Ebstein's valve has been observed in some patients with pulmonary atresia and intact ventricular septum (see Chapter 14).[17,89,90]

Hanley and colleagues[33] have advocated the use of the so-called tricuspid Z-value as a measure of the normalized tricuspid valve diameter. This is the diameter of the tricuspid valve normalized to body surface area and based on the data of Rowlatt, Rimoldi, and Lev initially published in 1963.[92] The more negative the Z-value of the tricuspid valve, the smaller and more obstructive the tricuspid valve. The larger the Z-value of the tricuspid valve, the larger the tricuspid valve diameter, and the more severe the regurgitation. These authors showed that the Z-value was highly correlated with right ventricular cavity size; the more negative the Z-value, the smaller the right ventricle. This correlation was highly significant with the presence of ventriculocoronary connections as well. More recently, Drant and colleagues[92a] have provided data supporting the observation that infundibular diameter was a better predictor of a right ventricular-coronary communication than the Z-value of the tricuspid valve.

The Right Ventricle in Pulmonary Atresia and Intact Ventricular Septum

Numerous classifications or categorizations of the right ventricle have been made in this disorder, including attempts to capture its volume.[1,3,6,25,28,29,33,38,39,46,53,93–100] These classifications have evolved from a qualitative assessment of cavity size (from small to very large), to a semimorphological characterization of the ventricle in term of its morpho-

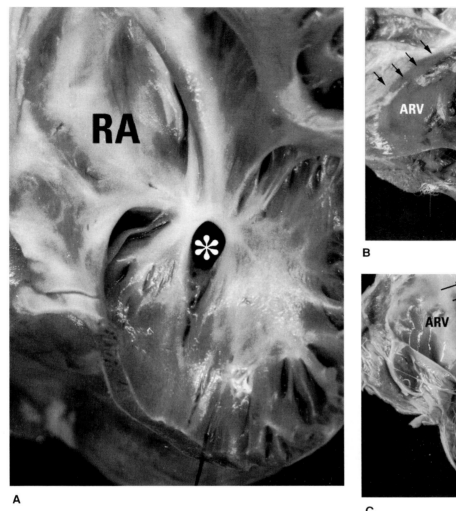

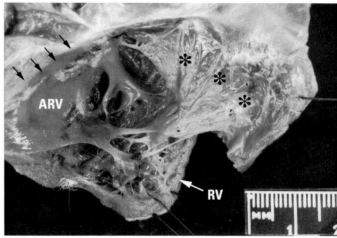

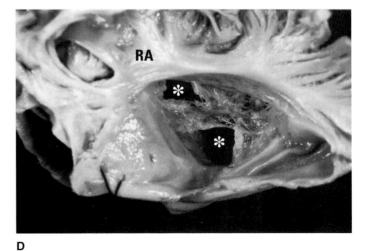

Fig. 23-5: The spectrum of the tricuspid valve in pulmonary atresia and intact ventricular septum.
A: View of the very hypoplastic and stenotic tricuspid valve (✱) from the right atrium. Arrows indicate annulus of the tricuspid valve; **B and C:** Massively regurgitant atrioventricular valves displaying both displacement and dysplasia (✱) (Ebstein's anomaly). Arrows indicate annulus of the tricuspid valve. **D:** An Ebstein deformity of the tricuspid valve with a double-orifice (✱).

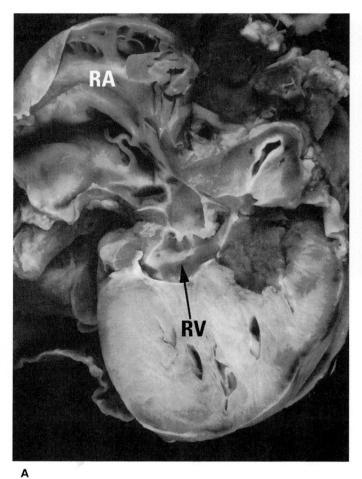

A

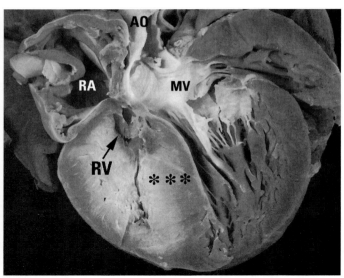

B

Fig. 23-6: The hypoplastic right ventricle in pulmonary atresia and intact ventricular septum.
A: Internal sagittal view of very hypoplastic right ventricle in a patient with pulmonary atresia and intact ventricular septum. **B:** Four-chamber view of heart from a patient with pulmonary atresia and intact ventricular septum. The right ventricle and its tricuspid valve are diminutive, with a much thickened interventricular septum. Note the ventricular septum (✱) bulges into the left ventricular outflow tract.

logical components (inlet, apical trabecular, and outlet zones), to semiquantitative assessment of the inlet-outlet dimensions (Figs. 23-6 through 23-9). Right ventricular volume determinations have also been reported, but whatever the methodology in these determinations, such techniques are challenged by the marked myocardial hypertrophy that attenuates the apical trabecula

and infundibulum. The right ventricle in some of these patients is very underdeveloped, seemingly formed only of an inlet portion. In others, the right ventricle has an inlet and trabecular portion, while in others the right ventricle is represented by inlet, apical trabecular, and infundibular components (Fig. 23-6). The degree of in-

(text continues on p. 627)

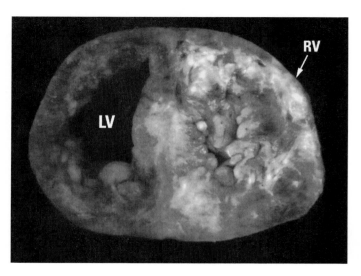

Fig. 23-7: The right ventricular cavity is compromised by muscular hypertrophy as shown by this cross section through both ventricles and the ventricular septum. The right ventricle is fibrotic with white patches.

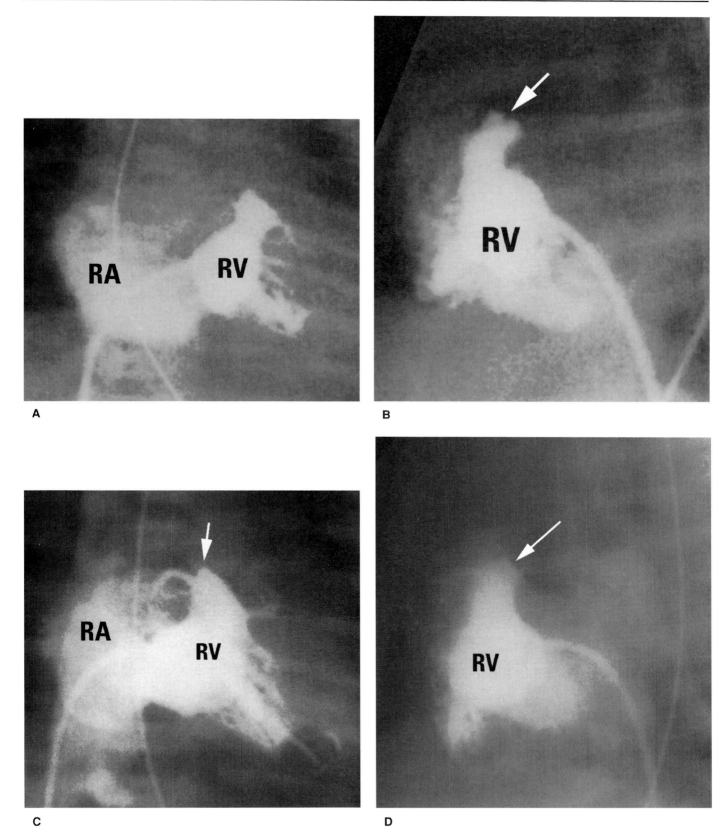

Fig. 23-8: Spectrum of right ventricular development among a cohort of patients with pulmonary atresia and intact ventricular septum, but without significant ventriculocoronary connections.
A and B: A small right ventricle with an imperforate valve with recognizable features (arrow). **C and D:** Better right ventricular development with an atretic valve. *(continued)*

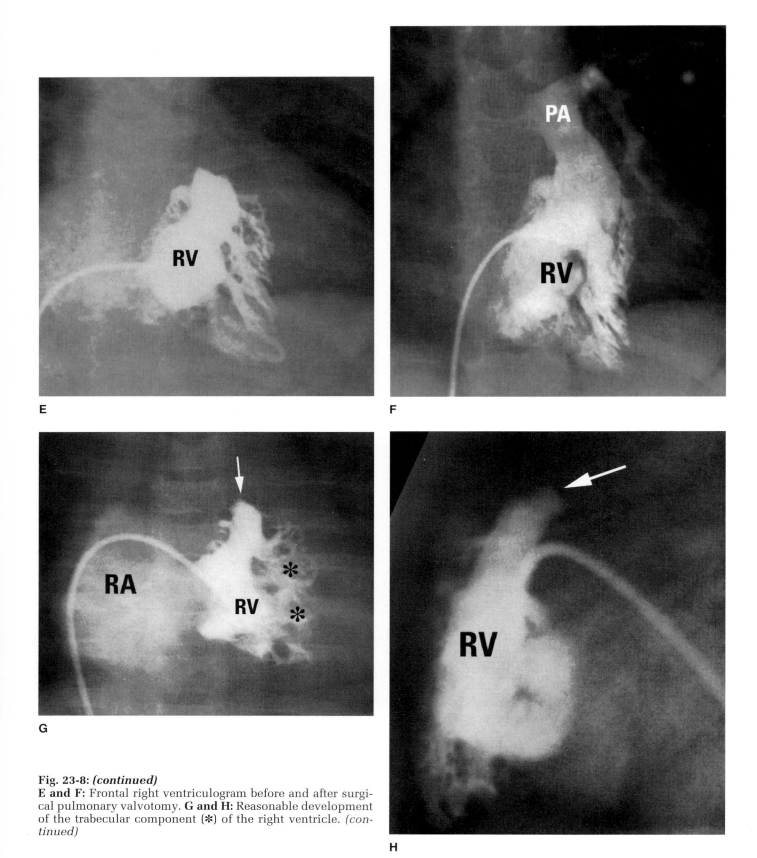

Fig. 23-8: *(continued)*
E and F: Frontal right ventriculogram before and after surgical pulmonary valvotomy. **G and H:** Reasonable development of the trabecular component (✳) of the right ventricle. *(continued)*

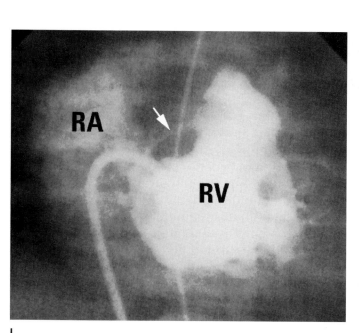

I

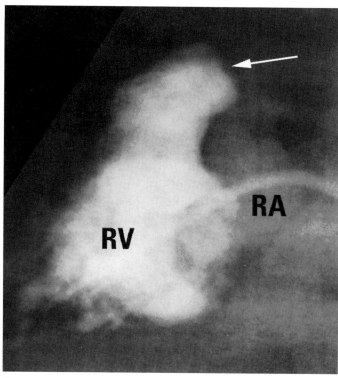

J

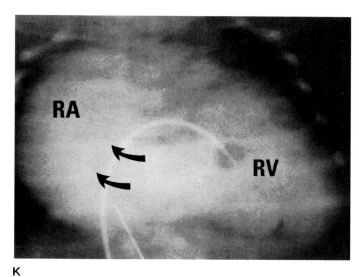

K

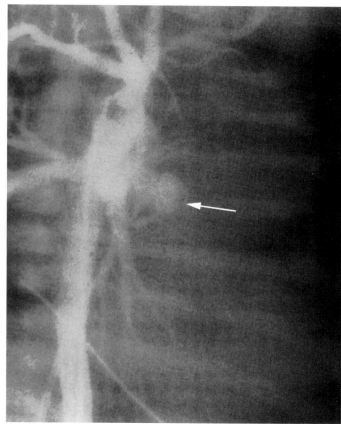

L

Fig. 23-8: *(continued)*
I and J: A very well-developed right ventricle with faint opacification of the right coronary artery (arrow in Fig. 23-8I). The infundibulum is well expanded (arrow). **K and L:** A very large right ventricle in the patient with florid tricuspid regurgitation and pulmonary atresia. Retrograde, prostaglandin-enhanced aortogram showing pooling of contrast in the imperforate pulmonary valve sinuses in Fig. 23-8L. *(continued)*

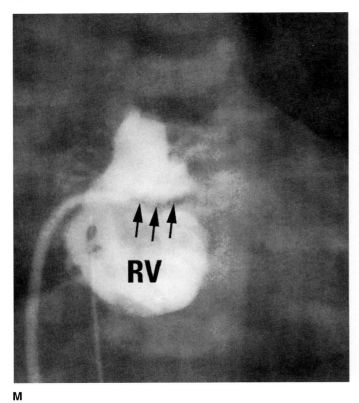

M

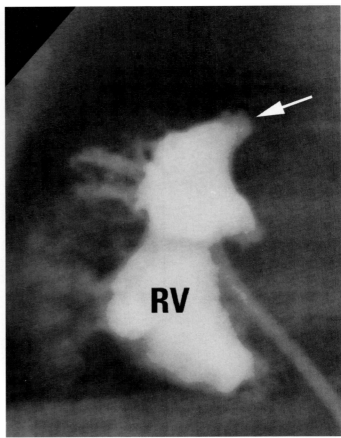

N

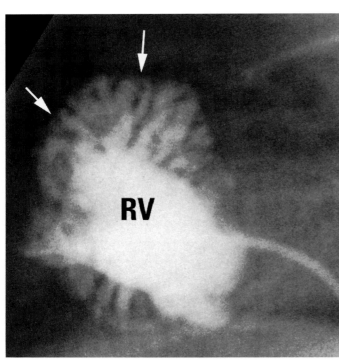

O

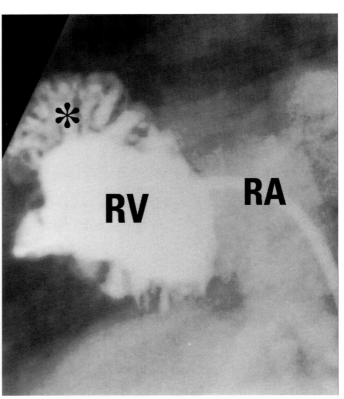

P

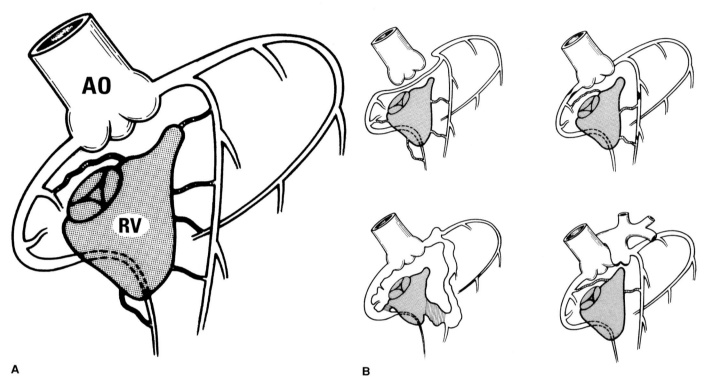

A

B

Fig. 23-9: Examples of ventriculocoronary connections in patients with pulmonary atresia and intact ventricular septum.
A: This diagram depicts a small right ventricle with extensive ventriculocoronary connections to both the right coronary artery and anterior descending coronary artery. **B:** These diagrams show various types of right ventricular-dependent coronary circulation in pulmonary atresia and intact ventricular septum. **Upper left panel:** Absent connections between coronary arteries and aorta. **Upper right panel:** Multiple connections with proximal right coronary artery narrowing and left anterior descending interruption. **Bottom left panel:** severe ectasia of both coronary arteries with coronary-cameral fistulae. **Bottom right panel:** Multiple ventriculocoronary connections with origin of left coronary artery from pulmonary artery. *(continued)*

Fig. 23-8: *(continued)*
M and N: Divided right ventricle almost devoid of apical trabeculations. A horizontal linear defect (arrows) divides the right ventricle into the superior infundibular chamber and the inferior body. This dividing tissue may be related to the tricuspid valve leaflet. **O and P:** The appearance of spongy myocardium (arrows or ✳) in two patients with pulmonary atresia and intact ventricular septum.

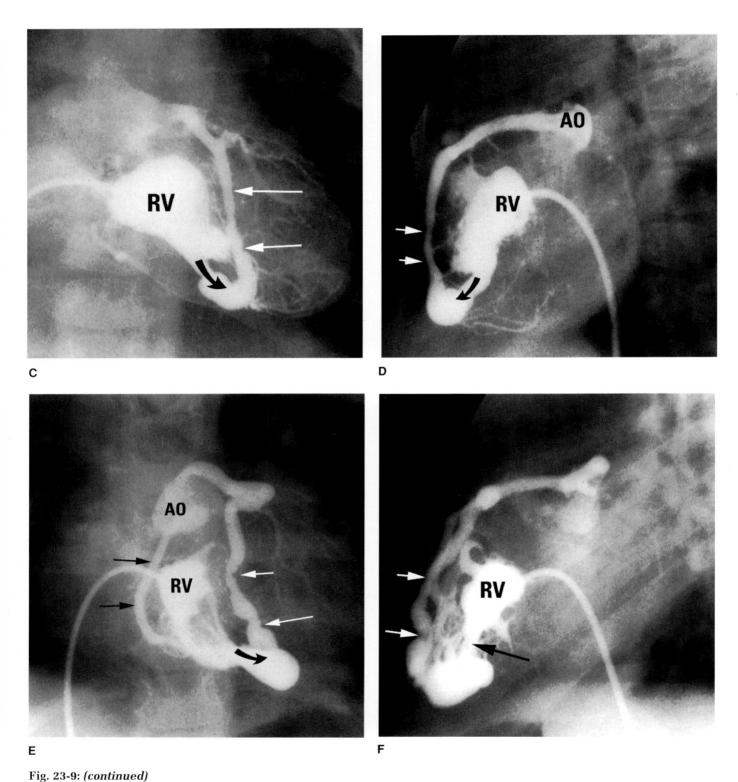

Fig. 23-9: *(continued)*
C and D: Frontal and lateral right ventriculograms show a small chamber without trabecular and infundibular components; the left anterior descending coronary artery (arrows) opacifies via the ventriculocoronary artery connection (curved arrow). Note the caliber changes in the left anterior descending coronary artery. **E and F:** Another patient with a very hypoplastic right ventricle seemingly formed of only an inlet component. From the right ventricular injection, the right coronary artery (black straight arrows) in Fig. 23-9E and anterior descending coronary artery (white arrows) opacify with obvious connection to the aortic root. Note again the caliber changes in the anterior descending coronary artery.

vestment of the components in any given patient may vary considerably, and muscular hypertrophy and overgrowth may obviate recognition of the trabecular and outlet portions of the right ventricle (Fig. 23-7).[6,10] Thus, there are some patients in whom all three components are clearly recognizable, but the right ventricle is still small, and the Z-value of the tricuspid valve will range from −2.5 to −4.5. In contrast, there are those patients with massive tricuspid regurgitation, a Z-value of +4.0 to +5.0, a much enlarged right ventricle, and very well expanded, inlet, trabecular, and infundibular components (Fig. 23-8).

The Coronary Circulation in Pulmonary Atresia and Intact Ventricular Septum

A remarkable evolution in our understanding of the coronary artery circulation in patients with pulmonary atresia and intact ventricular septum has occurred, and this has had profound effect on surgical management and outcome. Ventriculocoronary connections and myocardial sinusoids are an important aspect of this disorder.[10,11–13,15,16,18,31,33,39,52,53,58,98,101–129] Data published from the Congenital Heart Surgeons Study by Hanley and colleagues[33] indicated that of the 145 patients in whom this information was available (of a total of 171 neonates enrolled in the study), ventriculocoronary connections were observed in 45% (Fig. 23-9). Although these peculiar connections between the cavity of the right ventricle and the coronary arteries were observed at the autopsy table nearly 60 years ago, it is just slightly more than two decades since Freedom and Harrington[101,109,129] suggested that such connections might promote myocardial ischemia. A substantial literature has subsequently been published defining the character of the coronary arteries, their pathology, and the coronary circulation in these patients, and surgical strategies have been defined on the basis of the coronary circulation.[10,11–13,15,16,18,31,33,39,52,53,58,98,101–131] In the UK National Collaborative study of pulmonary atresia and intact ventricular septum, of 140 patients identified since 1991, the coronary arteries were considered normal in 58% and minor and major coronary artery fistulae were identified in 15% and 17%, respectively. Ten patients were recognized as having coronary artery stenosis.[131a] The median tricuspid Z-value for this cohort of patients was −1.6.

Kaufman and Anderson in 1963 commented on the frequent association between hearts with ventriculocoronary connections, and pulmonary atresia and intact ventricular septum, but no specific functionality was assigned to these peculiar communications.[115] The angiocardiographic features of the right ventricle and ventriculocoronary connections were documented in the New England Journal of Medicine in 1964.[132] Over the next two decades, an extensive literature documented the vast array of changes in the coronary arteries in patients with pulmonary atresia and intact ventricular septum.[10,11–13,15,16,18,31,33,39,52,53,58,98,101–131] The histopathologic alterations of those coronary arteries participating in the ventriculocoronary communications, a process not characterized by inflammation as once thought, but more appropriately as myointimal hyperplasia with a rich background of glycosoaminoglycans, has been amply documented (Fig. 23-10).[11,12,58,108,110,111,113,114,119,124] There is a wide spectrum of histopathologic lesions of both the extramural and intramural coronary arteries. These lesions range from mild degrees of intimal and medial thickening in which a continuous internal elastic lamina and normal lumen is present to a loss of normal arterial wall morphology with replacement of the arterial wall by fibrocellular tissue containing irregular, nonorganized elastin strands and severe stenosis or obliteration of the arterial lumen. Some have designated these changes "fibroelastosis" of the coronary arteries, but it is clear that the emphasis should be placed on myointimal hyperplasia.[133] Staining for glycosamino-glycans shows the prominence of ground substance formation by the activated smooth muscle cells, rather than reduplicated elastica and collagen that is characteristic of fibroelastosis. This pathological process results in profound distortion of the normal architecture, eventuating in endothelial irregularity, stenosis or interruption. These coronary arterial changes occur only in patients with ventriculocoronary connections, and by inference, with a hypertensive right ventricle. These alterations have not been observed in those patients with the massively enlarged heart with free tricuspid regurgitation, and a thinned right ventricle incapable of generating systemic pressures. Indeed, the presence of ventriculocoronary

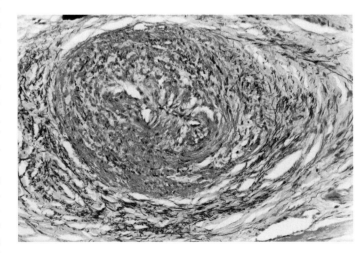

Fig. 23-10: **Virtual obliteration of coronary arterial lumen by myointimal hyperplasia with a rich background of glycosoaminoglycans.**

connections and the thin-walled, low-pressure right ventricle are mutually exclusive. We have speculated that the pathogenesis of these arterial lesions is predicated on the repeated and sustained injury to the coronary arterial intima from high-pressure right ventricular systolic turbulent blood flow mediated by the presence of the ventriculo-coronary connections.[124] Intra- or extramural coronary arteries remote from the ventriculocoronary connections do not demonstrate these arterial lesions nor do hearts *not* exhibiting ventriculocoronary connections. These lesions have been found in fetal hearts with pulmonary atresia and intact ventricular septum and in hearts of the immediate newborn.[124] The capillary distribution in the ventricles of hearts with pulmonary atresia and intact ventricular septum has been studied by Oosthoek and colleagues.[124a] Disarray and other disturbances of capillaries and myocytes were found in hearts with pulmonary atresia and intact ventricular septum, a hypoplastic right ventricle, and ventriculocoronary connections. They found that these changes were more extensive when coronary artery interruptions were present.[124a] These abnormalities of the coronary arteries are far more common in those babies with the smallest tricuspid valve, and by inference the most underdeveloped right ventricle.[33] But ventriculocoronary connections have been noted in the right ventricle of normal dimension, or nearly so (Fig. 23-11).

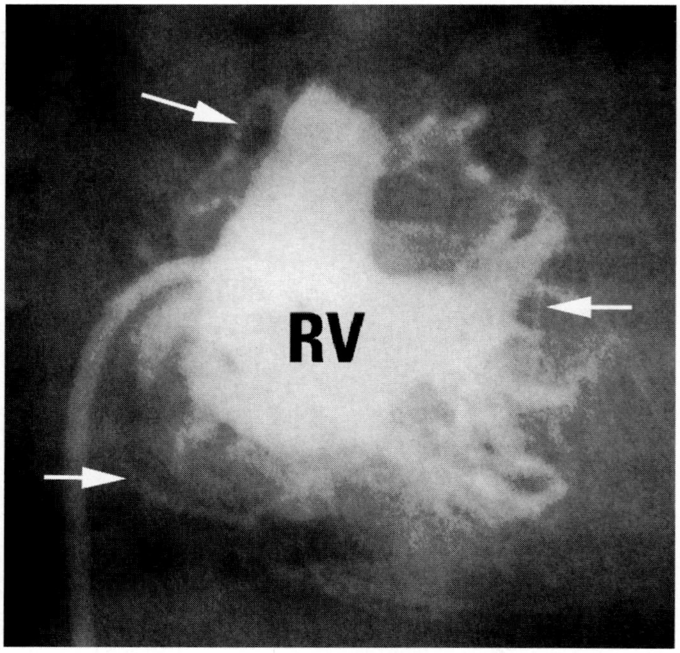

The abnormalities of coronary origin and distribution in patients with pulmonary atresia and intact ventricular septum embrace the same spectrum of those abnormalities as seen in patients with otherwise normal hearts, including abnormalities of origin, epicardial course, and number. A single coronary artery may originate from the aorta, or rarely from the pulmonary trunk.[117,123] But there are a number of congenital and acquired conditions of the coronary circulation specific to pulmonary atresia and intact ventricular septum that impact on surgical management. These include absence of proximal aortocoronary connection between one or both coronary arteries; coronary arterial stenosis or interruption; or a so-called coronary-cameral fistula with a major fistula between the right or left coronary artery and the right ventricle (Figs. 23-9 through 23-23).[10,11,12,31,53,58,89,100,107–114,116–118,120,122–128,130,131]

(text continues on p. 641)

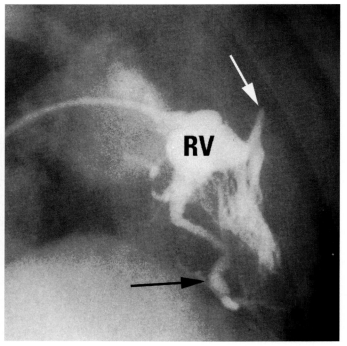

A

Fig. 23-11: Connections between the right ventricle and both coronary arteries were demonstrated by right ventriculography in this patient with a slightly small right ventricle and a tricuspid Z-value of −1.

Fig. 23-12: Absence of connection between the left coronary artery and the aortic root: a right ventricular-dependent coronary artery circulation.
A through C: Frames from shallow right anterior oblique right ventriculography. The right ventricle is small with a very narrowed infundibulum. Contrast enters a ventriculocoronary connection with subsequent opacification of the left coronary artery system; however, despite dense opacification of the entire left coronary artery system, the aortic root does not opacify, presumptive evidence of absence of connection between the left coronary artery and the aortic root. *(continued)*

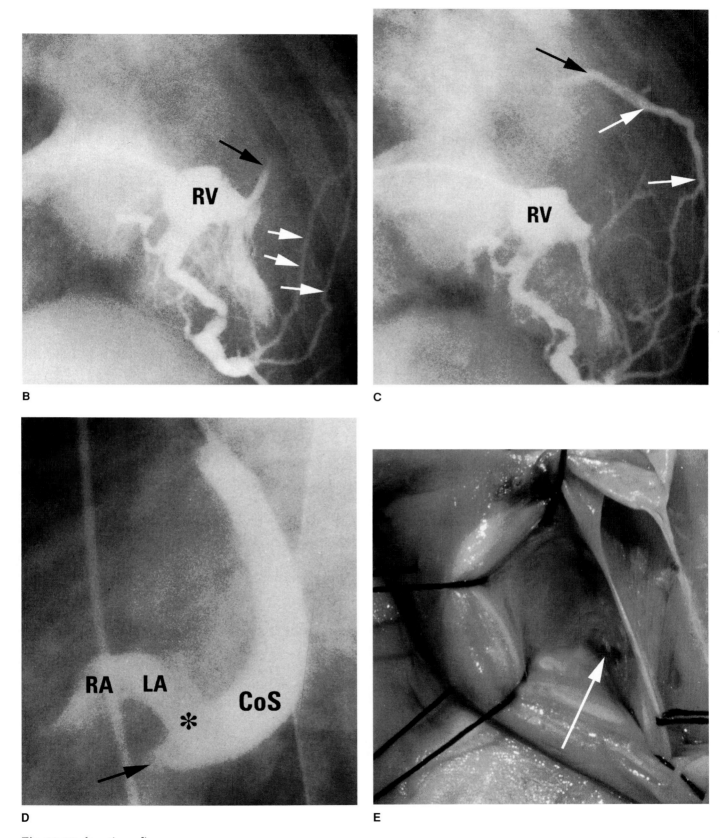

Fig. 23-12: *(continued)*
D: Coronary sinus ostial stenosis (arrow) was recognized as well. There is a fenestration (✱) in the wall between the coronary sinus and the left atrium. The right atrium is opacified by the shunt flow from the left atrium through the secundum atrial septal defect. **E:** Opened right atrium shows coronary sinus ostial stenosis (arrow) with an adjacent venous valve.

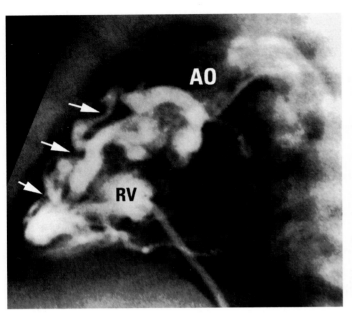

A

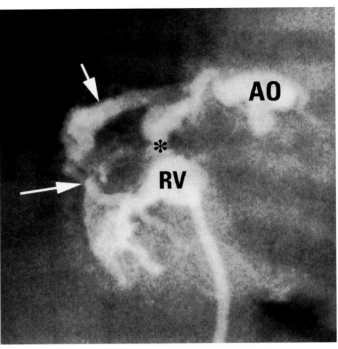

B

Fig. 23-13: Two patients with multiple levels of coronary artery stenosis and/or interruption, promoting a right ventricular-dependent coronary circulation.
A: Lateral right ventriculogram showing a most compromised coronary artery with multiple levels of coronary arterial stenosis and interruption (arrows). **B:** Near lateral right ventriculogram in another newborm with extensive caliber changes in the anterior descending coronary artery (arrows) and a stenotic ventriculocoronary fistula (✲).

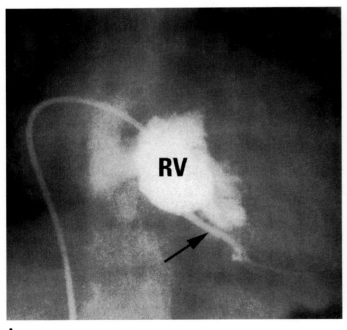

A

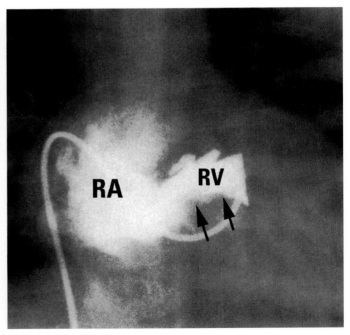

B

Fig. 23-14: A stenotic form of Ebstein's malformation of the tricuspid valve and pulmonary atresia and intact ventricular septum with ventriculocoronary artery communications without obvious stenosis or interruption.
A and B: These two frames of the frontal right ventriculography show the stenotic Ebstein's valve (arrows). **C:** Frontal right ventriculogram shows a hypoplastic chamber with opacification of a coronary artery. **D:** A later frame of Fig. 23-14C shows dense opacification of the entire left coronary artery system (arrows) without obvious obstruction.

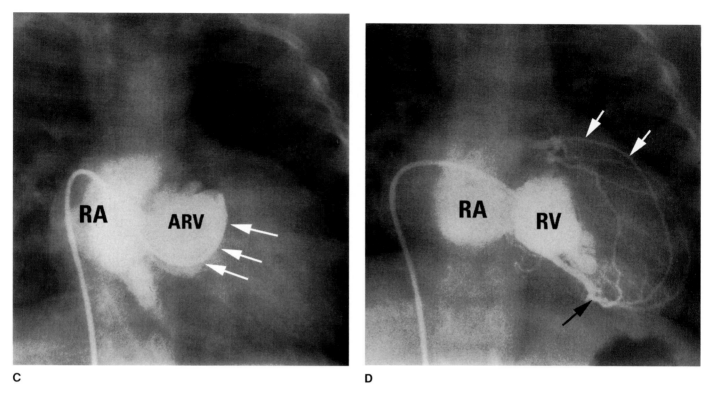

C   D

Fig. 23-14: *(continued)*

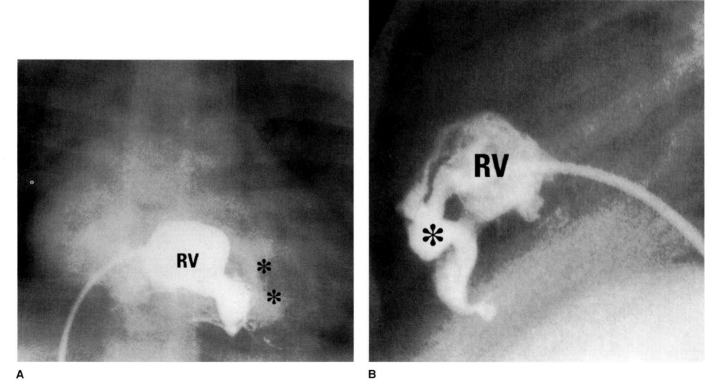

A   B

Fig. 23-15: A unipartite right ventricle with angiographic absence of apical trabecular and outlet components with a ventriculoarterial connection.
A: Frontal right ventriculogram shows a very small chamber devoid of apical trabeculations (✽). **B:** The ventriculoarterial connection is noted (✽) in the lateral projection.

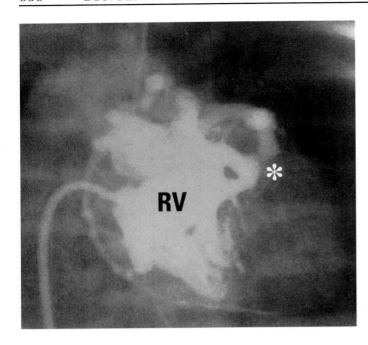

Fig. 23-16: Moderate right ventricular hypoplasia with a Z-value of −2.5. A complete interruption (✳) of the proximal left anterior descending coronary artery is seen.

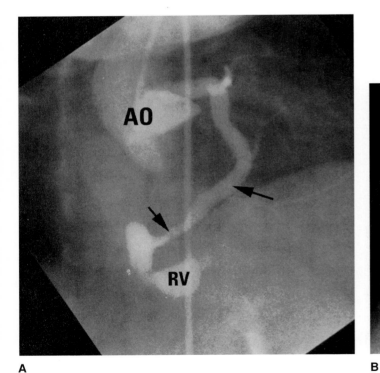

A

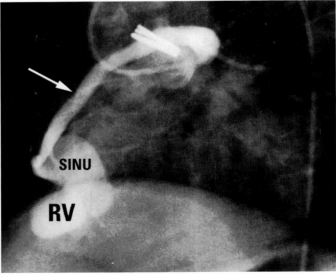

B

Fig. 23-17: A right ventricular-dependent coronary circulation with absence of connection between the right coronary artery and the root of the aorta. In addition, the left anterior descending coronary artery had a fistulous connection with the right ventricle and significant caliber changes (arrows).
A: Aortogram in right anterior oblique view shows a communication between left anterior descending coronary artery and the diminutive right ventricle. There are obvious caliber changes (arrows) in this coronary artery. Despite multiple injections in the aortic root and right aortic sinus, the right coronary artery was never opacified, suggestive evidence that the right coronary artery lacked a normal aortic connection. B: Selective left coronary angiogram shows similar features.

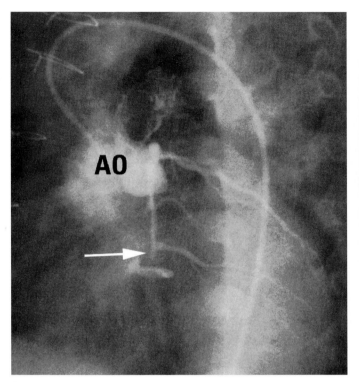

A

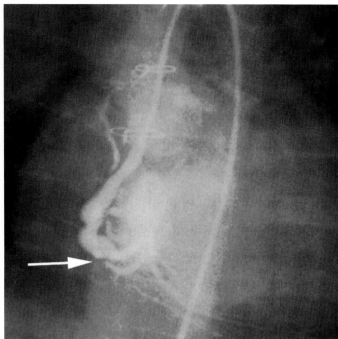

B

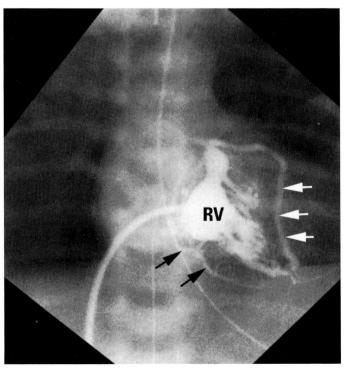

C

Fig. 23-18: A right ventricular-dependent coronary circulation with a left anterior descending coronary artery interruption and ectasia and obvious stenosis of the distal right coronary artery. Despite the egregious nature of the coronary arteries, this child remains well 6 years after a lateral tunnel Fontan.
A: Left anterior oblique aortogram shows an interruption (arrow) of the proximal left anterior descending coronary artery. **B:** Ectasia and caliber abnormalities (arrow) of the right coronary artery demonstrated by selective right coronary arteriography in frontal view. **C:** A different infant with dense opacification of both coronary arteries, but no opacification of the aortic root: does this indicate lack of proximal aortocoronary connections?

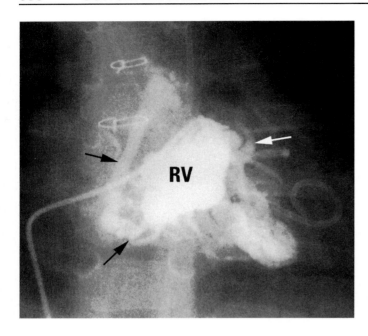

Fig. 23-19: Hypoplastic right ventricle and ventriculo-coronary communications to both coronary arteries.
Frontal right ventriculogram shows an anterior descending coronary artery interruption (white arrow) and caliber changes (black arrows) in the right coronary artery. These changes were interpreted as consistent with a right ventricular-dependent coronary artery circulation.

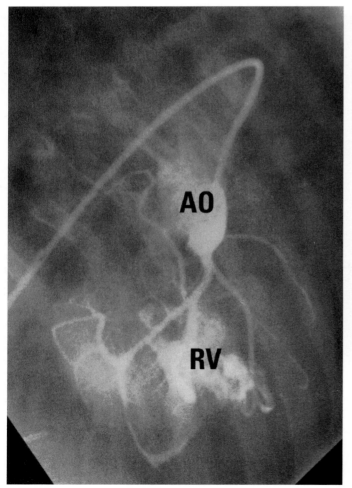

A

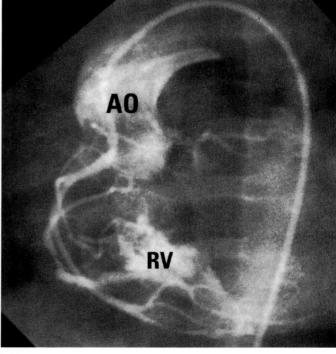

B

Fig. 23-20: A solitary fistulous communication between the right coronary artery and the right ventricle demonstrated by selective coronary arteriography in a 3-month-old infant.
A and B: Right and left anterior oblique views.

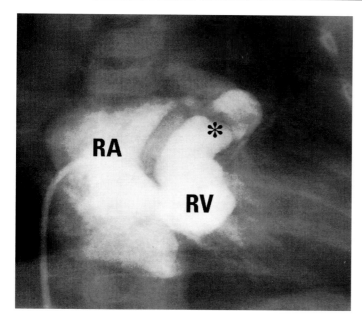

Fig. 23-21: A huge fistula from a small, smooth-chambered right ventricle connecting to the anterior descending coronary artery. This infant had a to-and-fro continuous murmur indicative of the bidirectional coronary-cameral flow, and vice-versa.

Frontal right ventriculogram shows the huge fistula (✻).

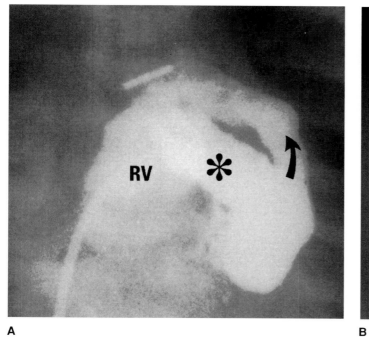

A

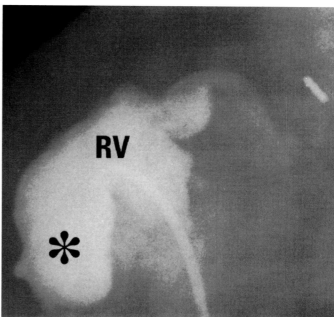

B

Fig. 23-22: A huge fistula between the right ventricle and anterior descending coronary artery in a baby with pulmonary atresia and intact ventricular septum.

A and B: Frontal and lateral right ventriculograms show the huge fistulous communication (✻). *(continued)*

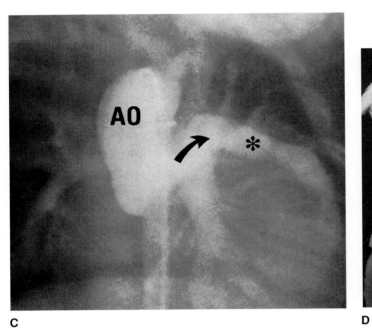

C

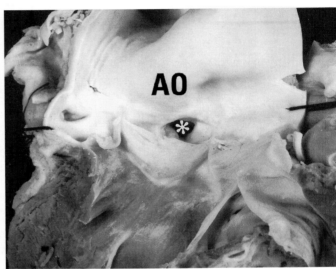

D

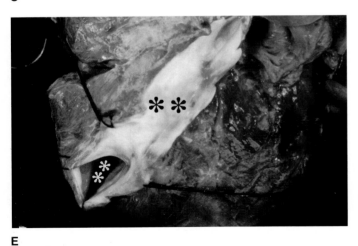

E

Fig. 23-22: *(continued)*
C: The aortogram shows the caliber of the proximal left coronary artery (✱). **D:** Internal view of aortic root shows the much enlarged left coronary artery ostium (✱). **E:** The very dilated anterior descending coronary artery (black ✱) communicates through a very large fistula (white ✱) with the right ventricle.

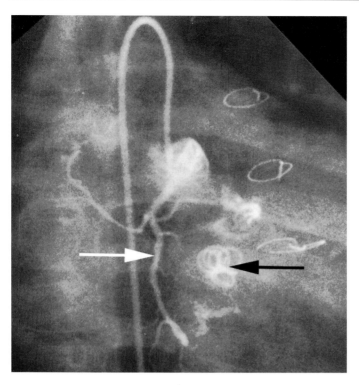

Fig. 23-23: Even after thromboexclusion of the right ventricle, coronary artery-right ventricular fistulous communications may persist. The coils (black arrow) are seen in the right ventricle as is the course of the right coronary artery (white arrow).

A Right Ventricular-Dependent Coronary Artery Circulation

As the characterization of the unusual coronary circulation in patients with pulmonary atresia and intact ventricular septum increased, it became evident that surgical outcomes were related to or determined at least in part by the involvement of the coronary arteries. Intrinsic to the awareness of ventriculocoronary connections in this disorder and their impact on the myocardium was the appreciation and development of the concept of a right ventricular-dependent coronary artery circulation.[10,11,12,31,53,58,89,100,107–114,116–118,120,122–128,130,131] In the normal circulation it is in large part the aortic diastolic pressure that is the driving pressure for coronary blood flow. Those factors reducing aortic diastolic pressure or shortening diastole will compromise coronary blood flow. The presence of ventriculocoronary artery connections may promote coronary artery stenosis and interruption and aortic diastolic pressure may not be sufficient to drive coronary blood flow when there are obstructive lesions within the coronary circulation (Figs. 23-9, 23-12, 23-13, 23-16, 23-17, and 23-18). Remembering that these babies are ill, tachycardiac, and often receiving prostaglandin and palliated with a sys-

temic-to-pulmonary artery shunt to augment pulmonary blood flow (both of these maneuvers will also reduce aortic diastolic pressure), in these situations retrograde coronary blood flow from the hypertensive right ventricle occurring during systole and mediated by the ventriculocoronary connections may be necessary for myocardial perfusion. Thus, in a coronary circulation that is wholly or in part right ventricular-dependent, it is both the blood that gets into the right ventricle and the systemic or above systolic right ventricular pressure that drives or mediates the coronary circulation in a retrograde fashion. Yet this process may lead to further coronary arterial distortions. The coronary circulation was considered wholly right ventricular-dependent in 9% of the 145 patients enrolled in the Congenital Heart Surgeons Study.[33] These data are very similar to that published from this institution in a series of papers addressing the coronary circulation.[11–13,18,19,53,58,89,108–110,124] The management corollary to this is clear: interference with blood flow into the right ventricle or reduction of right ventricular systolic pressure in those situations in which the coronary circulation is right ventricular-dependent could result in myocardial ischemia, infarction, and death. These observations were clearly substantiated in the Congenital Heart Surgeons multi-institutional study of pulmonary atresia and intact ventricular septum. One hundred seventy-one neonates with pulmonary atresia and intact ventricular septum were entered into a prospective, multi-institutional study between January 1, 1987 and January 1, 1991 under the aegis of the Congenital Heart Surgeons Study.[33] Multivariable analysis of their data showed that small diameter of the tricuspid valve, a coronary circulation that was severely right ventricular-dependent, birth weight, the date and type of initial surgical procedures were risk factors for time-related death. The data on the deleterious effects of ventriculocoronary connections and a right ventricular-dependent coronary circulation as defined in the publication of Hanley et al[33] is similar to the data published from Toronto in a series of publications.[11–13,18,19] Giglia and colleagues[98] from the Children's Hospital in Boston studying the influence of right heart size on outcome in patients with pulmonary atresia and intact ventricular septum have come to similar conclusions: "These results support our current hypothesis that coronary artery anatomy and not RV or TV hypoplasia predicts which patients with PA-IVS will do well after early RV decompression." While this study did not find a correlation between small right heart size and survival, the data of Giglia and colleagues[98] appropriately places the emphasis on the risk of right ventricular decompression on the nature of the coronary circulation. Mair and colleagues[98a] at the March 1995 American College of Cardiology meetings presented a patient with a normal-sized right ventricle and proximal interruption of the

Table 23-1

Coronary Artery Anomalies Contributing to a Right
Ventricular-Dependent Coronary Circulation

Absent Proximal Aortocoronary Connection(s)
Coronary Artery Interruption or Stenosis
Coronary-Cameral Fistula

left anterior descending coronary artery placed on a
Fontan-tract because of the right ventricular-dependent
coronary circulation. De Leval, Laks and colleagues and
others have constructed an aortic to right ventricular
shunt in patients with pulmonary atresia, an intact ventricular septum, and a right ventricular-dependent
coronary circulation in order to reverse myocardial ischemia.[98b–98d] Those patients with a massive coronary
artery-cameral (right ventricular) fistula are also right
ventricular-dependent. If the right ventricular pressure
is reduced, such patients will develop a fatal steal,
rapidly leading to coronary artery insufficiency, and
myocardial ischemia and/or infarction (Figs. 23-21 and
23-22).

Data from a number of institutions indicate that
those morphological/physiological variables most correlated with a poor outcome are: 1) a small diameter of
the tricuspid valve[98e]; 2) a coronary circulation that was
severely right-ventricular dependent (Table 23-1); and
3) a right ventricular:left ventricular pressure ratio <1.
This last factor is consistent with a globally disadvantaged right ventricle. The right ventricle is usually
thinned, and there is very severe tricuspid regurgitation. The functional disturbance of severe tricuspid regurgitation correlates with Ebstein's abnormality of the
tricuspid valve or severe tricuspid valve dysplasia.
Rarely, the tricuspid valve may be unguarded, or nearly
so.

Myocardial Abnormalities

The myocardium of patients with pulmonary atresia and intact ventricular septum demonstrates a wide
range of myocardial abnormalities.[10,11,15,58,105,
108,110,111,119,124,129,134–150] In view of the profound disturbances in the coronary circulation, it is not surprising that frank ischemia, fibrosis, infarction, and myocardial rupture have been identified in these patients.
In a provocative paper, Akiba and Becker[151] suggest
that disease of the left ventricle might be the limiting
factor for long-lasting successful surgical intervention.
They found in the eight hearts that they studied both
grossly and microscopically signs of acute myocardial
ischemia, and the volume density of interfiber collagen
showed high levels of normal in five hearts, but ex-

ceeded twice the standard deviation of normal in three
patients. The subendocardium was disproportionately
disadvantaged with higher levels of interfiber collagen
than the subepicardium. They suggest that the high levels of endomysial collagen is consistent with chronic ischemia in relation to left ventricular hypertrophy, and
that these abnormalities may render the left ventricle
less able to cope with a volume load, and thus the left
ventricle might be the limiting factor for long-lasting
successful surgical intervention. Other abnormalities
include myocardial disarray, the appearance of so-
called spongy myocardium, and ventricular endocardial fibroelastosis (see Chapter 27). In this regard, there
is a reasonably consistent inverse relationship between
ventricular endocardial fibroelastosis and extensive
ventriculo-coronary communications.[136,141,142] Perhaps
this observation is fundamental to the frequent finding
of ventriculocoronary connections in pulmonary atresia and intact ventricular septum: dense "sugar-coating" right ventricular endocardial sclerosis is uncommon. Conversely, dense "sugar-coating" left ventricular
endocardial sclerosis is common in those patients with
a hypoplastic left heart syndrome, but a perforate mitral
valve, and thus ventriculocoronary connections are less
frequent, and their pathology less extreme. There is certainly ample clinical and morphological evidence that
the left ventricle in patients with pulmonary atresia and
intact ventricular septum is abnormally hypertrophied
and noncompliant. The right ventricular myocardium
may be particularly thinned in those babies with severe
tricuspid regurgitation. These patients with a grossly
regurgitant tricuspid valve, dysplasia and displacement
of the tricuspid valve, do not have ventriculocoronary
connections.

Further Characterization of Hearts
with Pulmonary Atresia and Intact
Ventricular Septum

The heart may be only mildly enlarged, or in patients with extreme tricuspid regurgitation, tremendously enlarged, with a hugely dilated right atrium oc-
cupying much of the right hemithorax. In this latter
situation, the lungs may be compressed by the very
much enlarged heart, and the lungs may exhibit a varying degree of hypoplasia. Right atrial hypertrophy and
dilatation is influenced by restriction at atrial enlargement and the severity of tricuspid regurgitation. When
the heart is only mildly enlarged, the course of the anterior descending coronary artery in the anterior interventricular sulcus outlines a smaller than normal right
ventricle. The right atrium is usually somewhat enlarged, accounting for the cardiac enlargement. The
right ventricle may be profoundly thinned, and this
may be apparent even with the heart in situ.

Obvious clues that significant abnormalities of the

coronary artery circulation may be present just from external inspection of the heart. The coronary arteries may be obviously thickened and nodular, and rarely, the coronary artery(s) may be seen originating from the pulmonary trunk. So-called dimples may be observed on the epicardial surface of the heart, usually, but not exclusively, in association with the subepicardial coronary arteries.[152] Such dimples may be considered the external stigmata of ventriculocoronary connections, and may indicate the site of such connections.

The Great Veins, Atrial Septum, Coronary Sinus and Venous Valves

The superior and inferior caval veins usually terminate normally in the right atrium. Kauffman and Anderson[115] demonstrated more than 20 years ago the relation between persistent right venous valve, ventriculocoronary connections, and pulmonary atresia and intact ventricular septum. It is probably too simplistic, indeed incorrect, to speculate that a persistent venous valve is causal to right heart hypoplasia (see also Chapter 12). The coronary sinus usually terminates in the right atrium, although stenosis and atresia of the coronary sinus ostium has been observed, with decompression through an unroofed coronary sinus-left atrial fenestration (Fig. 23-12).[153]

Because of the obligatory right-to-left shunt at the atrial level, with very rare exception, there is either a defect of the foramen ovale or true secundum atrial septal defect. Premature closure of the ovale foramen has been observed in this disorder, usually with fetal death. Rarely, if the interatrial septum is intact or nearly so, alternative pathways for systemic venous return have been recognized, including coronary sinus-left atrial fenestration.[154] Septum primum may assume aneurysmal proportions in those patients with a restrictive atrial septal defect and herniation through the mitral valve has been documented.[155,156]

The left atrium usually receives the pulmonary veins in a normal fashion, although one or more pulmonary veins may connect anomalously to the systemic circulation. Akiba and Becker[151] in a recent discussion of the disease of the left ventricle in patients with pulmonary atresia and intact ventricular septum found that 4 of 8 hearts in their study showed short and almost dysplastic chords of the mitral valve, and 1 heart exhibited a small central cleft of the anterior mitral leaflet. The left ventricle may exhibit variable degrees of hypertrophy, especially in those patients surviving past infancy. Some years ago, Zuberbuhler and Anderson[6] called attention to a convexity of the outlet portion of the interventricular septum occurring in those patients with small and very hypertensive right ventricles. We and others have also noted this convexity of the ventricular septum in patients with the hypertensive form of pulmonary atresia and intact ventricular septum (Fig. 23-24 and 23-25).[151,157] This subaortic bulge has not been observed to promote left ventricular outflow tract obstruction prior to Fontan's operation. However,

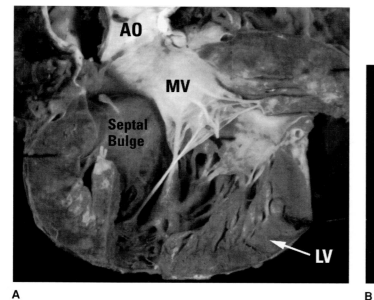
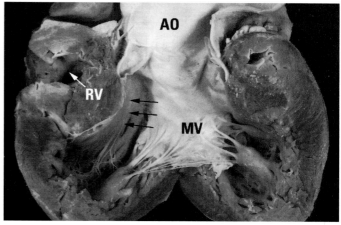

A　　　　　　　　　　　　　　　　　　　　　**B**

Fig. 23-24: **Convex septal bulge in two patients with pulmonary atresia and intact ventricular septum with unrelieved right ventricular hypertension. This septal convexity can contribute to fatal left ventricular outflow tract obstruction after reduction of the left ventricular end diastolic volume coincident with conversion to a Fontan circulation.**
A and B: Two patients with convex septal bulge (arrows) that has the potential for promoting left ventricular outflow tract obstruction after Fontan's operation.

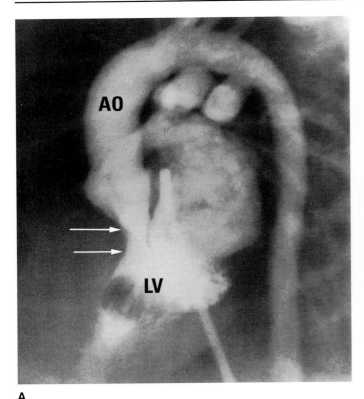

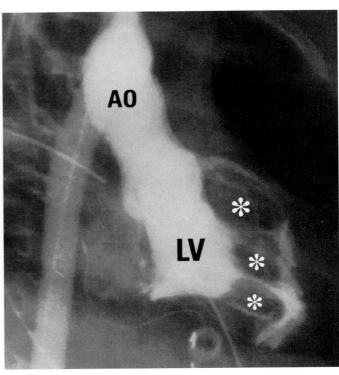

A   B

Fig. 23-25: Striking septal convexity in the patient with pulmonary atresia and intact ventricular septum with unrelieved right ventricular hypertension.
This long axial oblique left ventriculogram shows the septal bulge (arrows).

we have observed severe left ventricular outflow tract obstruction resulting in death occurring after Fontan's operation when there is an unfavorable change in the ratio between left ventricular mass/end-diastolic volume.[158] Aortic valve stenosis has also been well-described in patients with pulmonary atresia and intact ventricular septum, including the neonate with critical aortic stenosis, or the somewhat older child with severe aortic valve stenosis (Figs. 23-26 and 23-27).[159]

Imaging in Pulmonary Atresia and Intact Ventricular Septum

There is no doubt that the diagnosis of pulmonary atresia and intact ventricular septum can be made with cross sectional echocardiography.[160–169] We have previously demonstrated the efficacy of Doppler in the differentiation of functional from organic pulmonary atresia, a role once reserved for prostaglandin-enhanced retrograde aortography.[59,167,168] In those patients with the hypertensive and underdeveloped right ventricle, there are those who advocate cross-sectional echocardiography as the sole mode of imaging in the neonatal period.[164] We would take issue with this approach because so much of the treatment and thus prognosis rests with the definition of the coronary artery circulation.

There is now considerable data that the presence of ventriculocoronary connections and a right ventricular-dependent coronary circulation is highly correlated with a negative tricuspid valve Z-value: the smaller the Z-value, the smaller the tricuspid valve and the morphologically right ventricle and the greater the likelihood of a right ventricular-dependent coronary circulation. We and others have provided data that coronary arterial lesions can impact on the fetus and can progress after birth.[145,148,151] Thus we believe there is the necessity to define as accurately as possible the nature of the coronary artery circulation even in the newborn. This same conclusion about the need to precisely define the coronary arterial anatomy in neonates was reached in the retrospective review by Giglia et al[130] of the diagnosis and management of the right ventricular-dependent coronary artery circulation. Gentles and colleagues[131] have studied the influence of less extensive coronary anomalies in patients with pulmonary atresia and intact ventricular septum on left ventricular function undergoing right ventricular decompression. They found, using echocardiographic methodologies to assess global and regional left ventricular function and wall motion abnormalities, that regional left ventricular dysfunction was rare in patients without coronary artery abnormalities. In addition, they found mild to modest

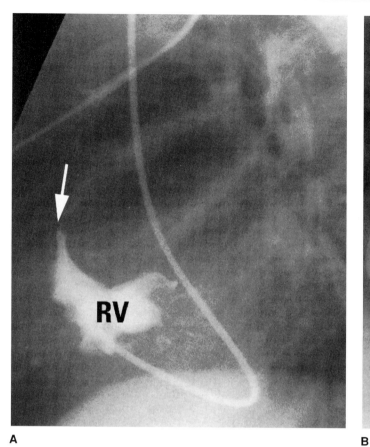

A

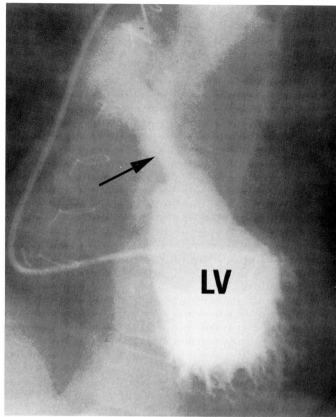

B

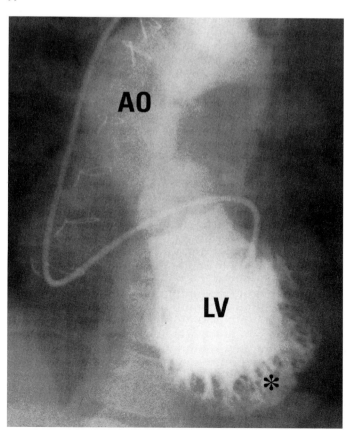

C

Fig. 23-26: Severe aortic stenosis and the appearance of spongy myocardium in the patient with pulmonary atresia and intact ventricular septum treated by surgical tricuspid valve excision.
A: Lateral right ventriculogram shows a very small ventricle with a narrowed infundibulum (arrow). **B and C:** Two frames from long axial oblique left ventriculography show the jetting of blood (arrow) through the stenotic aortic valve. **C:** A pattern of so-called spongy myocardium (✷) (see also Chapter 27).

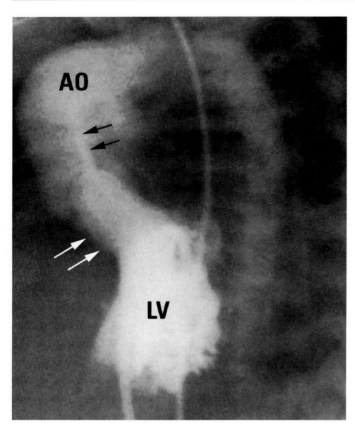

Fig. 23-27: Critical aortic stenosis in a newborn with pulmonary atresia and intact ventricular septum (same patient as shown in Fig. 23-8A and 23-8B).
Long axial oblique left ventriculogram shows the septal bulge (white arrows) and the jetting of contrast (black arrows) from the left ventricle into the dilated ascending aorta.

regional left ventricular dysfunction was common both before and after right ventricular decompression in those patients with less extensive coronary artery abnormalities.

Angiographic Imaging

The nature of the superior caval connections should be documented because certainly some patients will be placed on a one-ventricle or Fontan tract. Because staging towards a univentricular repair may require a bidirectional cavopulmonary connection, it is important to exclude a left superior caval vein connecting either to the coronary sinus or to the left atrium directly, and the size of the interconnecting brachiocephalic vein (see Chapter 12). We have observed stenosis and atresia of the ostium of the coronary sinus in patients with pulmonary atresia and intact ventricular septum (Fig. 23-12).[153] This is particularly germane to that unusual patient in whom coronary venous flow exits via the left superior vena cava.[170]

Selective right atriography rarely provides enough anatomic information to be justified (Fig. 23-28).[89] In those patients with just a miniscule tricuspid valve, opacification of the right ventricle may not occur. Right atriography will demonstrate a dilated right atrium, right-to-left shunting at atrial level with subsequent opacification of the left heart chambers, but again anatomic detail is lacking. Selective injection of contrast material into the morphologically right ventricle in frontal and lateral projections will demonstrate the size and form of this chamber, demonstrating as well the presence and degree of attenuation, or absence of the right ventricular infundibulum, as well as the severity of tricuspid regurgitation (Figs. 23-3, 23-4, 23-8, 23-9, 23-11, 23-12 through 23-14, and 23-19 through 23-22).[9,11,12,58,59,68,78,80,89,100,108,110,120,124,171,171a] Much of this information should be complemented by cross-sectional echocardiographic techniques. We had advocated some years ago a double-catheter technique to define the length of the atretic infundibulum (Fig. 23-2).[78] This was accomplished by simultaneous injection of contrast media into the right ventricle and pulmonary artery. Until the recent introduction of radiofrequency catheter ablation of the atretic pulmonary valve plate, this technique seemed to be of more academic than of practical application.

Right ventricular angiography will also demonstrate the presence or absence of ventriculocoronary connections, and whether the right, left, or both coro-

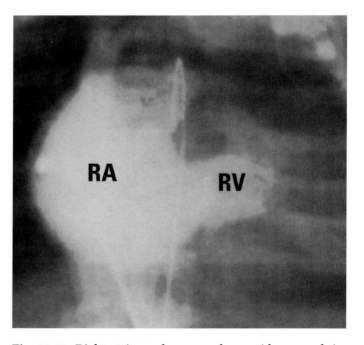

Fig. 23-28: Right atriography so rarely provides enough information about the form of the right ventricle and the nature of ventriculocoronary connections that this approach is rarely justified.

nary arteries are involved in these abnormal communications. In the assessment of right ventricular-coronary artery connections, it is important to determine that the coronary arteries, when they opacify from a right ventricular angiocardiogram, have a normal proximal connection to the aorta. Of those several egregious conditions contributing to a right ventricular-dependent coronary circulation, absent proximal connections between the aorta and one or both coronary arteries have been established both at the autopsy table as well as clinically. Rarely, the coronary artery will originate from the pulmonary trunk in the patient with pulmonary atresia and intact ventricular septum. As we stated earlier, even the newborn and young baby requires imaging of the coronary artery circulation. This can be achieved by ascending aortography, perhaps enhanced by the technique of balloon occlusion. Left ventriculography may provide gross information about the origin of the coronary arteries. More subtle, but important information, including caliber irregularities as well as frank stenosis or even interruption, may be missed on left ventricular angiography. In the older infant and child, selective coronary arteriography is necessary in those patients with ventriculocoronary connections.[172] Burrows from this institution (Hospital for Sick Children, Toronto) and Giglia from Boston and their respective colleagues have both demonstrated progressive changes in the coronary circulation.[131,172] Mild coronary arterial luminal irregularities have been observed to progress to frank coronary arterial stenosis, indicative that such changes are not static. We believe that in any patient in whom right ventricular decompression has not been achieved and in whom ventriculocoronary connections have been demonstrated by previous right ventricular angiocardiography that coronary arterial lesions may progress in severity possibly impacting on future management. Rarely, collateralization from the gastroepiploic artery to the coronary circulation will occur (B. Hanna, MD, Division of Cardiology, the Izaak Walton Killam Hospital, Halifax, Nova Scotia, unpublished observations). A hypertensive and underdeveloped right ventricle with ventriculocoronary connections is not specific just for pulmonary atresia and intact ventricular septum.

A hypertensive right ventricle with ventriculocoronary connections has been identified in a wide variety of congenitally malformed hearts (Table 23-2; see also Chapters 7, 26, 35, and 38).

It is important to distinguish anatomical from functional pulmonary atresia.[9,49,58–61,63,64,68,171,173] In the former the pulmonary valve is anatomically imperforate, whereas in the latter the lack of forward flow is due to poor right ventricular function in the face of high pulmonary artery pressure. Functional pulmonary atresia usually occurs in the setting of Ebstein's malformation of the tricuspid valve or with other abnormalities

Table 23-2

Hearts Exhibiting a Hypertensive, Underdeveloped, Right Ventricle with Ventriculocoronary Connections

Pulmonary Atresia and Intact Ventricular Septum
Double-Outlet Left Ventricle and Intact Ventricular Septum
Aortic Atresia, Transposition of the Great Arteries, and Intact Ventricular Septum
Truncus Arteriosus with Intact Ventricular Septum

promoting extreme tricuspid regurgitation (Figs. 23-8 and 23-29; see also Chapter 14, Fig. 14-18). In general, the pulmonary valve is morphologically normal, but functionally closed due to the associated poor right ventricular function and severe tricuspid valve regurgitation. Occasionally it is possible to have anatomic valve atresia with extreme tricuspid regurgitation and a low right ventricular pressure, hence the importance of differentiating the two conditions. With the use of Doppler echocardiography it is possible to do this by detecting systolic regurgitation of the pulmonary valve, which is caused by a jetting affect of the patent ductus arteriosus against the valve.[161,167,168] This is not observed in those cases with anatomical pulmonary valve atresia. Another technique is through the use of Doppler echocardiography during positive pressure ventilation, which transiently results in opening of the pulmonary valve and forward Doppler flow.[168]

For those patients placed on or considered for a one ventricle repair, it is important to define the hemodynamics and anatomy of the pulmonary circulation.[84] These considerations are important when the patient is considered for a bidirectional cavopulmonary connection. Left ventriculography will provide information about ventricular function, and in a rare patient, a small ventricular septal defect will be imaged.[174] Akagi and colleagues[175] from the Toronto Hospital for Sick Children have used left ventricular angiography to assess the influence of ventriculocoronary arterial connections on left ventricular performance and clinical course. Their data indicated that patients with significant ventriculocoronary artery connections and coronary arterial abnormalities had a higher incidence of wall motion abnormalities, probably reflecting ongoing ischemia, and that such patients were at risk for late death. In the older patient, aortic root angiography will demonstrate the coronary artery origin and distribution, as well as any structural and functional abnormalities of the aortic root.

Left ventricular angiography performed in the long axial oblique projection will, in those patients with the nondecompressed, hypertensive right ventricle, demonstrate the septal convexity that may contribute to

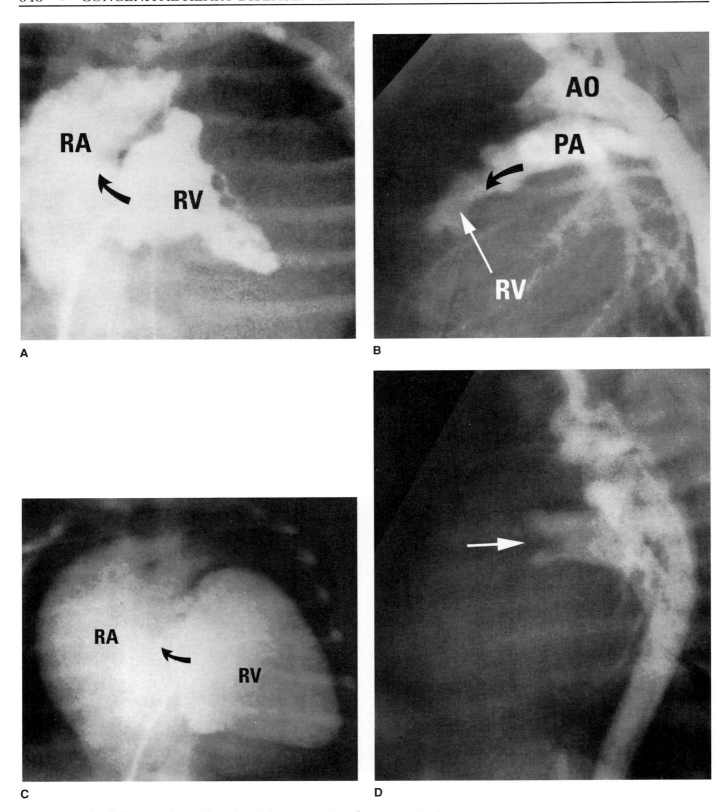

Fig. 23-29: The differentiation of functional from organic pulmonary atresia.
A and B: Frontal right ventriculogram does not show any forward pulmonary blood flow, but there is significant tricuspid re-gurgitation (arrow). **B:** Retrograde prostagandin-enhanced aortography shows regurgitation (black arrow) across the pulmonary valve into the right ventricular infundibulum, revealing the functional nature of the pulmonary atresia. **C and D:** A newborn with massive tricuspid regurgitation and organic pulmonary atresia. **C:** Massive tricuspid regurgitation (arrow) and no forward flow. **D:** The lack of regurgitation across the pulmonary valve (arrow) was interpreted as consistent with anatomic pulmonary atresia (this was confirmed at surgery). *(continued)*

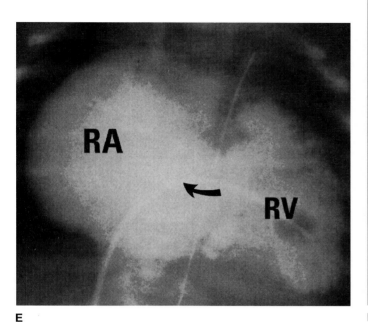

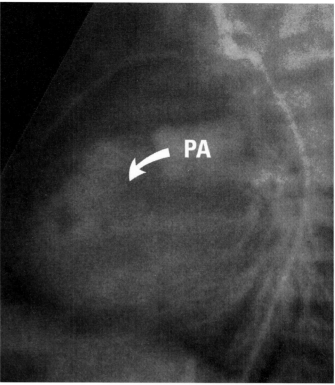

E

F

G

Fig. 23-29: *(continued)*
E and F: A newborn with severe tricuspid regurgitation (arrow) and functional pulmonary atresia. The frontal right ventriculogram shows severe tricuspid regurgitation. **F:** The functional nature of the pulmonary atresia was provided by retrograde prostaglandin-enhanced aortography. **G:** Another baby with Ebstein's anomaly of the tricuspid valve and pulmonary atresia.

fatal subaortic stenosis after Fontan's procedure (Figs. 23-24 through 23-27).[158] This angiogram should also provide information about the form and function of the left ventricle, gross definition of the coronary arteries and their aortic connection, the laterality of the aortic arch, and caliber of the arterial duct or patency of a surgically-created systemic-to-pulmonary artery anastomosis. A number of these patients with a right ventricular-dependent coronary circulation are successfully undergoing a fenestrated lateral tunnel Fontan, and it is

likely that these patients will require surveillance of their coronary arteries.[18,21,31,33,98a-98c,176]

The right ventricle may remain small after right ventricular outflow tract reconstruction and right ventricular hypoplasia and a small tricuspid valve may confound a biventricular repair (Fig. 23-30). We have also observed in one patient active endocarditis causing an inflammatory valvotomy and resulting in a perforation in the once imperforate pulmonary valve (Fig. 23-31).

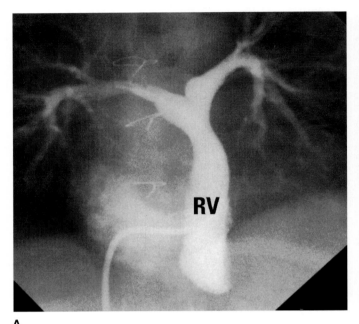

A

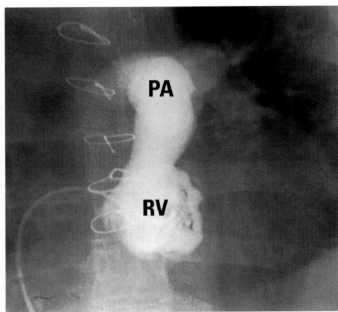

B

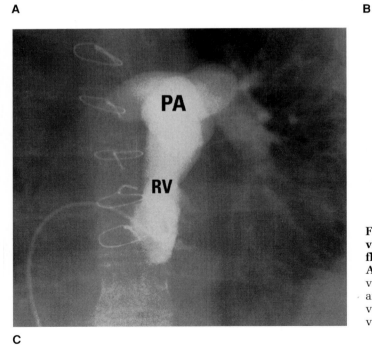

C

Fig. 23-30: Right ventricular hypoplasia reflecting lack of ventricular growth is still a reality after right ventricular outflow tract reconstruction.
A: Little growth in this right ventricle was achieved by right ventricular outflow tract reconstruction. **B and C:** Diastolic and systolic frames from a right ventriculogram after a right ventricular outflow tract patch demonstrating persistent right ventricular hypoplasia.

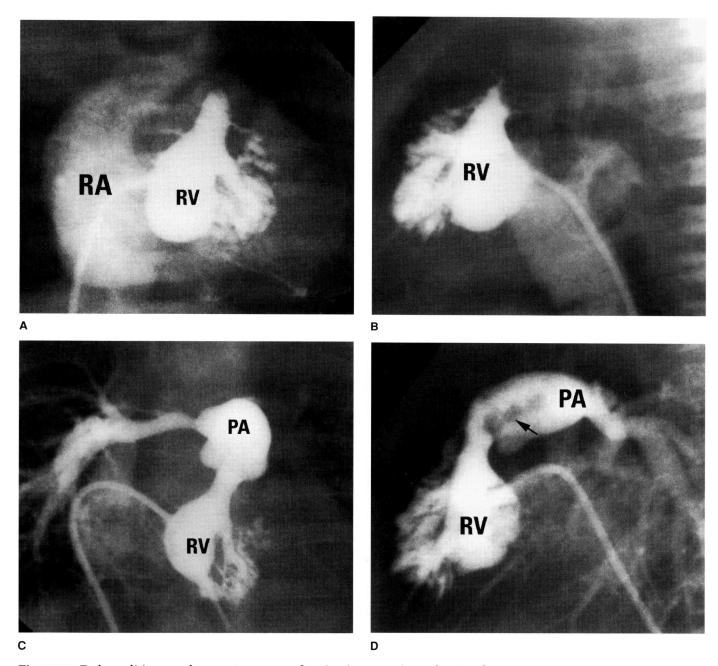

Fig. 23-31: Endocarditis caused a spontaneous perforation in a once imperforate valve.
A and B: The appearance of the right ventricle before endocarditis, but after performance of a right-sided Blalock-Taussig shunt. **C and D:** The pulmonary artery is now in perforate continuity with the right ventricle. **D:** In the lateral projection, a filling-defect (arrow) is visible, and in view of the history, a diagnosis of infective endocarditis with a pulmonary artery thrombus was made (and confirmed at surgery).

Trancatheter Intervention for Pulmonary Atresia and Inact Septum

Surgical algorithms in the management of patients with this condition have focused on the probability of achieving either a biventricular or a one ventricle repair. In patients with a right ventricle able to sustain most, if not all, of the systemic venous return, many centers advocate establishing continuity between the right ventricle and the main pulmonary artery segment with or without a systemic-to-pulmonary artery shunt depending on the calculated size of the ventricle. The ideal patient would have a tripartite right ventricle of near normal size with valvar pulmonary atresia and a well developed pulmonary arterial circulation. It is likely that the myocardial insult associated with ventriculotomy and reperfusion injury in the setting of pre-existing myocardial fiber disarray, diffuse fibrosis, and an abnormal coronary artery circulation may adversely affect the ultimate surgical outcome.[108–114,128,137, 151,172,175] This has encouraged some centers to comple-

ment the surgical algorithm with interventional catheterization techniques to achieve ventriculopulmonary continuity. Mechanical or thermal transcatheter perforation of the atretic pulmonary valve with subsequent balloon dilation has been suggested as an alternative to surgical valvotomy in selected patients.[18,55]

Mechanical perforation of the atretic pulmonary valve has been achieved but has the disadvantage of achieving a relatively uncontrolled perforation (Figs. 23-32 through 23-34). Thermal energy applied to the tip of a small wire has allowed for more controlled perforation of the atretic valve tissue and has been accomplished in several patients with good results in short term follow-up. This technique was first reported using excimer laser energy as the energy source.[54–56,177] However, laser therapy carries the disadvantages of increased risk to staff, the requirement for protective eyewear, limited portability, and considerable capital expense in the setting of an uncommon defect. Radiofrequency energy that can safely achieve well-de-

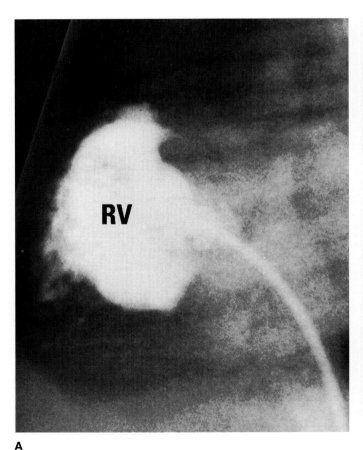

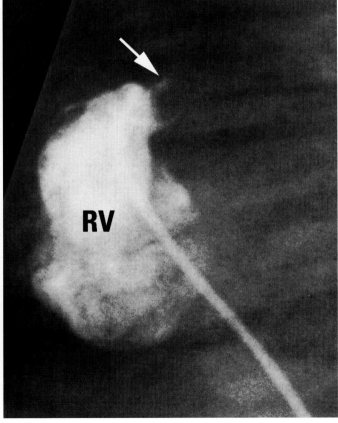

A   **B**

Fig. 23-32: Establishing the diagnosis of valvar atresia.
A: Right ventricular angiogram appears to demonstrate valvar pulmonary atresia. **B:** Selective injection using an endhole catheter positioned in the right ventricular outflow tract demonstrates forward flow from the right ventricle to the pulmonary artery illustrating the presence of severe valvar stenosis and not atresia. The valve was crossed with a hydrophilic wire for a conventional pulmonary valvotomy.

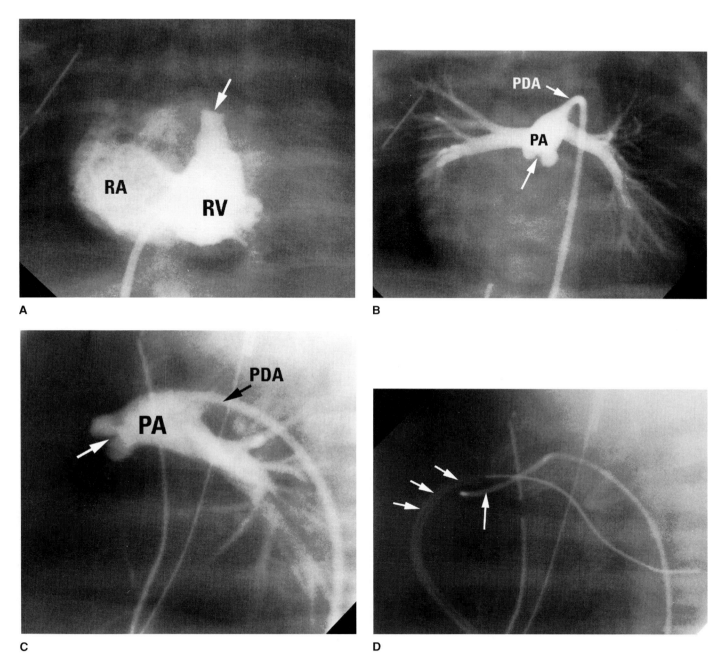

Fig. 23-33: Radiofreqency-assisted perforation of the atretic pulmonary valve demonstrating the technique.
A: Cranially tilted right ventricular angiogram demonstrating atresia of the pulmonary valve evidenced by a lack of forward flow to the pulmonary artery (arrow). **B and C:** Frontal and lateral angiogram of the pulmonary artery obtained by retrograde catheter introduced by traversing the PDA from the aorta demonstrating true valvar atresia with well developed sinuses. **D:** Judkins right coronary artery catheter introduced antegrade from the femoral vein to the RV outlet (three arrows). After an application of radiofrequency energy to the atretic valve, a wire has been advanced into the PA. The pulmonary valve sinus has been marked by a wire introduced retrograde through the ductus arteriosus (single arrow). *(continued)*

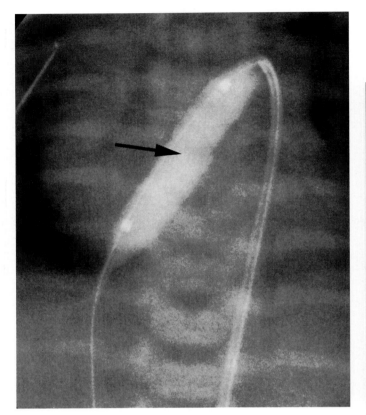

E

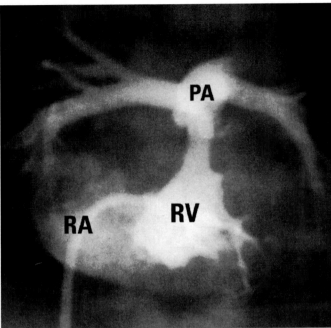

F

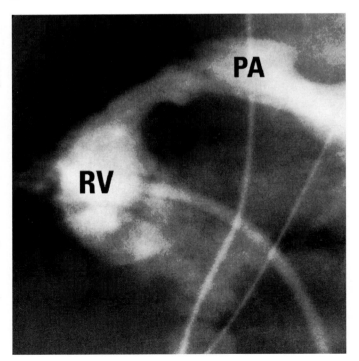

G

Fig. 23-33: *(continued)*
E: The wire is advanced from the RV, through the ductus arteriosus and into the descending aorta to allow a balloon (black arrow) to be introduced across the perforated pulmonary valve for valvotomy. **F and G:** After valvotomy, RV-PA continuity is clearly established with improvement in tricuspid incompetence.

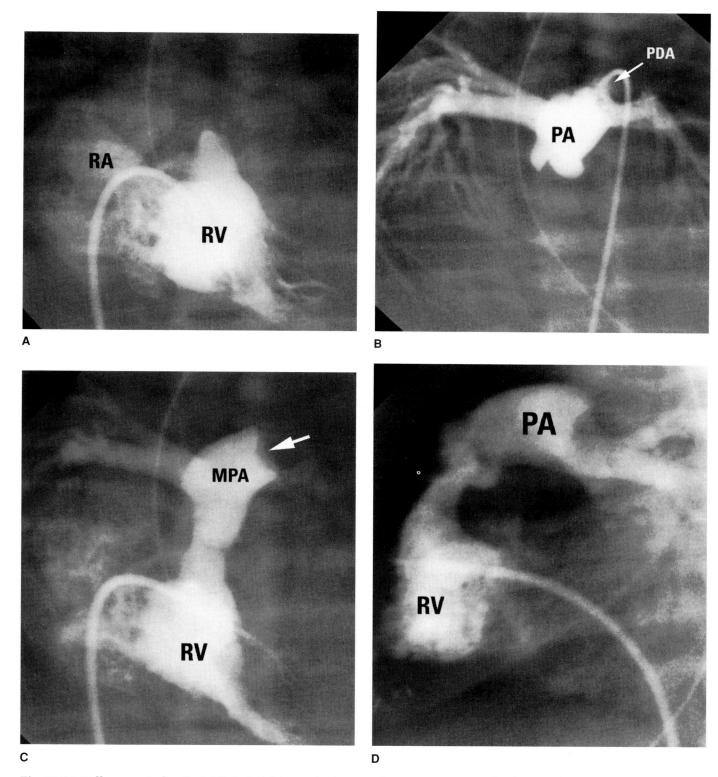

Fig. 23-34: Follow-up study of established right ventricular to pulmonary artery continuity in pulmonary atresia and intact ventricular septum.
A and B: Right ventricular angiogram in frontal projection and retrograde pulmonary arteriogram establishing the presence of valvar pulmonary atresia. **C and D:** Immediately after the procedure a right ventricular angiogram confirms a successful procedure. Note the presence of wash-in due to flow from the patent ductus arteriosus (arrow) and the dilated main pulmonary artery segment. *(continued)*

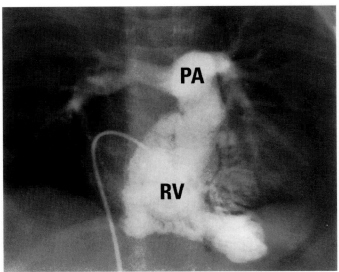

E

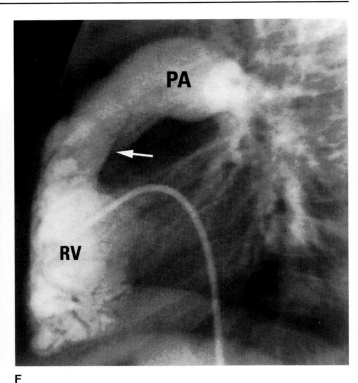

F

Fig. 23-34: *(continued)*
E and F: Repeat angiography 2 years later demonstrates persistent continuity, a thin pulmonary valve (arrow) and no subpulmonary obstruction. The right ventricle, however, remains heavily trabeculated.

fined lesions of coagulation necrosis is now widely applied in the treatment of many cardiac dysrhythmias. Utilization of this energy to perforate atretic valve tissue has the advantages of being considerably less expensive, more portable, and less hazardous to staff.

Initial results of radiofrequency assisted perforation of the atretic pulmonary valve have been encouraging, however, the current literature is confined to early results in small series due to the relative infrequency of the disease.[79,178,179] In addition, the technique has been recently applied in the setting of longer segment muscular pulmonary atresia.[79,180] While initial application will likely focus on patients destined for a biventricular circulation, application as a technique to decompress the right ventricle in an effort to improve long-term results for those patients on track for a total cavopulmonary connection remains a tantalizing

possibility. Such decompression may serve to reduce the potential for left ventricular outflow tract obstruction imposed by the interventricular septum displaced by the hypertensive right ventricle. Decompression may also result in regression of fistulous connections and improved aortocoronary myocardial perfusion may decrease the incidence of late coronary artery luminal abnormaities associated with high shear stress on the vessels imposed upon by the high-velocity systolic ventriculocornary flow perhaps reducing the incidence of ventricular wall motion abormalities. Future studies must focus on acute issues of safety and efficacy. While a percutaneous approach may avoid or delay the use of cardiopulmonary bypass in the newborn period it remains to be seen if it results in a decrease in neonatal or long-term morbidity or mortality.

References

1. Elliott LP, Adams PJ, Edwards JE. Pulmonary atresia with intact ventricular septum. *Br Heart J* 1963;25:489–501.
2. Anderson RH, Macartney FJ, Shinebourne EA, Tynan M. *Paediatric Cardiology.* Edinburgh: Churchill Livingstone; 1987, pp. 711–720.
3. Van Praagh R, Ando M, Van Praagh S, Senno A, Hougen TJ, Novak G, Hastreiter AR. Pulmonary atresia: Anatomic considerations. In: *The Child With Congenital Heart Disease After Surgery.* Mount Kisco, NY: Futura Publishing Company, Inc; 1976, pp. 103–135.
4. Bharati S, McAllister HAJ, Chiemmongkoltip P, Lev M. Congenital pulmonary atresia with tricuspid insufficiency: Morphologic study. *Am J Cardiol* 1977;40:70–75.
5. Bharati S, McAllister HAJ, Tatooles CJ, Miller RA, Weinberg MJ, Bucheleres HG, Lev M. Anatomic Variations in underdeveloped right ventricle related to tricuspid atresia and stenosis. *J Thorac Cardiovasc Surg* 1976;72:383–400.
6. Zuberbuhler JR, Anderson RH. Morphological variations

in pulmonary atresia with intact ventricular septum. *Br Heart J* 1979;41:281–288.

7. Milanesi O, Daliento L, Thiene G. Solitary aorta with bilateral ductal origin of non-confluent pulmonary arteries in pulmonary atresia with intact ventricular septum. *Int J Cardiol* 1990;29:90–92.

7a. Luciani GB, Swilley S, Starnes VA. Pulmonary atresia, intact ventricular septum, and major aortopulmonary collaterals: Morphogentic and surgical implications. *J Thorac Cardiovasc Surg* 1995;110:853–854.

8. Freedom RM, Dische MR, Rowe RD. The tricuspid valve in pulmonary atresia and intact ventricular septum. *Arch Pathol Lab Med* 1978;102:28–31.

9. Freedom RM, Moes CAF. The hypoplastic right heart complex. *Semin Roentgenol* 1985;20:169–183.

10. Anderson RH, Anderson C, Zuberbuhler JR. Further morphologic studies on hearts with pulmonary atresia and intact ventricular septum. *Cardiol Young* 1991;1:105–113.

11. Freedom RM, Wilson G, Trusler GA, Williams WG, Rowe RD. Pulmonary atresia and intact ventricular septum. A review of the anatomy, myocardium, and factors influencing right ventricular growth and guidelines for surgical intervention. *Scand J Thorac Cardiovasc Surg* 1983;17:1–28.

12. Freedom RM, Wilson GJ. The anatomic substrate of pulmonary atresia and intact ventricular septum. In: Tucker BL, Lindesmith GG, Takahashi M, eds. *Third Clinical Conference on Congenital Heart Disease. Obstructive Lesions of the Right Heart*. Baltimore: University Park Press; 1984, pp. 217–255.

13. Freedom RM. The morphological variations of pulmonary atresia with intact ventricular septum: Guidelines for surgical intervention. *Pediatr Cardiol* 1983;4:183–188.

14. Freedom RM, Perrin D. The tricuspid valve: Morphologic considerations. In: Freedom RM. *Pulmonary Atresia and Intact Ventricular Septum*. Mount Kisco, NY: Futura Publishing Company, Inc.; 1989, pp. 37–52.

15. Freedom RM, Perrin D. The right ventricle: Morphologic considerations. In: Freedom RM. *Pulmonary Atresia and Intact Ventricular Septum*. Mount Kisco, NY: Futura Publishing Company, Inc; 1989, pp. 53–74.

16. Kanjuh VI, Stevenson JE, Amplatz K, Edwards JE. Congenitally unguarded tricuspid orifice with coexistent pulmonary atresia. *Circulation* 1964;30:911–917.

17. Stellin G, Santini F, Thiene G, Bortolotti U, Daliento L, Milanesi O, Sorbara C, Mazzucco A, Casarotto D. Pulmonary atresia, intact ventricular septum, and Ebstein anomaly of the tricuspid valve. *J Thorac Cardiovasc Surg* 1993;106:255–261.

18. Coles JG, Freedom RM, Lightfoot NE, Dasmahapatra HK, Williams WG, Trusler GA, Burrows PE, Himansu K. Long-term results in neonates with pulmonary atresia and intact ventricular septum. *Ann Thorac Surg* 1989;47:213–237.

19. Lightfoot NE, Coles JG, Dasmahapatra HK, Williams EG, Chin K, Trusler GA, Freedom RM. Analysis of survival in patients with pulmonary atresia and intact ventricular septum treated surgically. *Int J Cardiol* 1989;24:159–164.

20. Fyler DC. *Nadas' Pediatric Cardiology*. Boston: Mosby-Year Book; 1992, pp. 557–576.

21. Alboliras ET, Julsrud PR, Danielson GK, Puga FJ, Schaff HV, McGoon DC, Hagler DJ, Edwards WD, Driscoll DJ. Definitive operation for pulmonary atresia with intact ventricular septum. Results in twenty patients. *J Thorac Cardiovasc Surg* 1987;93:454–464.

22. Amodeo A, Keeton BR, Sutherland GR, Monro JL. Pulmonary atresia with intact ventricular septum: Is neonatal repair advisable? *Eur J Cardiothorac Surg* 1991;5:17–21.

23. Battistessa SA, Jackson M, Hamilton DI, Patel RG, McKay R. Staged surgical management of pulmonary atresia with intact ventricular septum. *Cardiol Young* 1992;2:395–402.

24. Billingsley AM, Laks H, Boyce SW, George B, Santulli T, Williams RG. Definitive repair in patients with pulmonary atresia and intact ventricular septum. *J Thorac Cardiovasc Surg* 1989;97:746–754.

25. Bull C, Kostelka M, Sorensen K, de Leval M. Outcome measures for the neonatal management of pulmonary atresia with intact ventricular septum. *J Thorac Cardiovasc Surg* 1994;107:359–366.

26. Cobanoglu A, Metzdorff MT, Pinson CW, Grunkemeier GL, Sunderland CO, Starr A. Valvotomy for pulmonary atresia with intact ventricular septum. *J Thorac Cardiovasc Surg* 1985;89:482–490.

27. Coles J, Williams WG, Trusler GA, Lightfoot N, Freedom RM. Surgical considerations and outcome. In: Freedom RM. *Pulmonary Atresia and Intact Ventricular Septum*. Mt. Kisco, NY: Futura Publishing Company, Inc; 1989, pp. 249–257.

28. De Leval M, Bull C, Hopkins R, Rees P, Deanfield J, Taylor JFN, Gersony W, Stark J, Macartney FJ. Decision making in the definitive repair of the heart with a small right ventricle. *Circulation* 1985;72(Suppl II): 52–60.

29. De Leval M, Bull C, Stark J, Anderson RH, Taylor JFN, Macartney FJ. Pulmonary atresia and intact ventricular septum: Surgical management based on a revised classification. *Circulation* 1982;66:272–280.

30. Foker JE, Braunlin EA, St. Cyr JA, Hunter D, Molina JE, Moller JH, Ring WS. Management of pulmonary atresia with intact ventricular septum. *J Thorac Cardiovasc Surg* 1986;92:706–715.

31. Freeman JE, DeLeon SY, Lai S, Fisher EA, Ow P, Pifarre R. Right ventricle-to-aorta conduit in pulmonary atresia with intact ventricular septum and coronary sinusoids. *Ann Thorac Surg* 1993;56:1393–1395.

32. Giannico S. Successful balloon avulsion of tricuspid valve in a neonate with pulmonary atresia and intact ventricular septum. *J Thorac Cardiovasc Surg* 1988;96:488–489.

33. Hanley FL, Sade RM, Blackstone EH, Kirklin JW, Freedom RM, Nanda NC. Outcomes in neonatal pulmonary atresia with intact ventricular septum. *J Thorac Cardiovasc Surg* 1993;105:406–427.

34. Hawkins JA, Thorne JK, Boucek MM, Orsmond GS, Ruttenberg HD, Veasy LG, McGough EC. Early and late results in pulmonary atresia and intact ventricular septum. *J Thorac Cardiovasc Surg* 1990;100(4):492–497.

35. Joshi SV, Brawn WJ, Mee RBB. Pulmonary atresia with intact ventricular septum. *J Thorac Cardiovasc Surg* 1986;91:192–199.

36. Leung MP, Mok CK, Lee J, Lo RN, Cheung H, Chiu C. Management evolution of pulmonary atresia and intact ventricular septum. *Am J Cardiol* 1993;71:1331–1336.

37. Lewis AB, Wells W, Lindesmith GG. Evaluation and surgical treatment of pulmonary atresia and intact ventricular septum in infancy. *Circulation* 1983;67:1318–1323.

38. Lewis AB, Wells W, Lindesmith GG. Right ventricular growth potential in neonates with pulmonary atresia and intact ventricular septum. *J Thorac Cardiovasc Surg* 1986;91:835–840.

39. Mainwaring RD, Lamberti JJ. Pulmonary atresia with intact ventricular septum. Surgical approach based on ventricular size and coronary anatomy. *J Thorac Cardiovasc Surg* 1993;106:733–738.

40. McCaffrey FM, Leatherbury L, Moore HV. Pulmonary atresia and intact ventricular septum. Definitive repair in the neonatal period. *J Thorac Cardiovasc Surg* 1991; 102:617–623.

41. Milliken JC, Laks H, Hellenbrand H, George B, Chin A, Williams RG. Early and late results in the treatment of patients with pulmonary atresia and intact ventricular septum. *Circulation* 1985; 72(Suppl II):61–69.

42. Niederhuser U, Bauer EP, von Segesser LK, Carrel T, Laske A, Schonbeck M, Turina M. Pulmonary atresia and intact ventricular septum: Results and predictive factors of surgical treatment. *Thorac Cardiovasc Surg* 1992;40:130–134.

43. Pawade A, Capuani A, Penny DJ, Karl TR, Mee RB. Pulmonary atresia with intact ventricular septum: Surgical management based on right ventricular infundibulum. *J Card Surg* 1993;8:371–383.

43a. Pawade A, Karl T. Management strategy in neonates presenting with pulmonary atresia with intact ventricular septum. *Curr Opin Pediatr* 1994;6:600–605.

44. Rao PS. Comprehensive management of pulmonary atresia with intact ventricular septum. *Ann Thorac Surg* 1985;40:409–413.

45. Ruttenberg HD, Veasy LG, McGough E. Tricuspid valve removal for pulmonic atresia, intact ventricular septum and right ventricular coronary fistulae. *Circulation* 1985; 72(suppl):260.

46. Schmidt KG, Cloez J-L, Silverman NH. Changes of right ventricular size and function after valvotomy for pulmonary atresia or critical pulmonary stenosis and intact ventricular septum. *J Am Coll Cardiol* 1992;19: 1032–1037.

47. Shaddy RE, Sturtevant JE, Judd VE, McGough EC. Right ventricular growth after transventricular pulmonary valvotomy and central aortopulmonary shunt for pulmonary atresia and intact ventricular septum. *Circulation* 1990;82(Suppl IV):IV-157-IV-163.

48. Squitieri C, Di Carlo D, Giannico S, Marion B, Giamberti A, Marcelletti C. Tricuspid valve avulsion or excision for right ventricular decompression in pulmonary atresia with intact ventricular septum. *J Thorac Cardiovasc Surg* 1989;97:779–784.

49. Starnes VA, Pitlick PT, Bernstein D, Griffin ML, Choy M, Shumway NE. Ebstein's anomaly appearing in the neonate. A new surgical approach. *J Thorac Cardiovasc Surg* 1991;101:1082–1087.

50. Waldman JD, Lamberti JJ, Mathewson JW, George L. Surgical closure of the tricuspid valve for pulmonary atresia, intact ventricular septum, and right ventricle to coronary artery communications. *Pediatr Cardiol* 1984; 5:221–224.

50a. Waldman JD, Karp RB, Lamberti JJ, Sand ME, Ruschhaupt DG, Agarwala B. Tricuspid valve closure in pulmonary atresia and important RV-to-coronary artery connections. *Ann Thorac Surg* 1995;59:933–940.

51. Weldon CS, Hartmann AFJ, McKnight RC. Surgical Management of Hypoplastic Right Ventricle with Pulmonary Atresia or Critical Stenosis and Intact Ventricular Septum. *Ann Thorac Surg* 1984;37:12–24.

52. Williams WG, Burrows P, Freedom RM, Trusler GA, Coles JG, Moes CAF, Smallhorn JF. Thromboexclusion of the right ventricle in a subset of children with pulmonary atresia and intact ventricular septum. *J Thorac Cardiovasc Surg* 1991;101:222–229.

53. Freedom RM. How can something so small cause so much grief? Some thoughts about the underdeveloped right ventricle in pulmonary atresia and intact ventricular septum. *J Am Coll Cardiol* 1992;19:1038–1040.

54. Parsons JM, Rees MR, Gibbs JL. Percutaneous laser valvotomy with balloon dilatation of the pulmonary valve as primary treatment for pulmonary atresia. *Br Heart J* 1991;66:36–38.

55. Latson LA. Nonsurgical treatment of a neonate with pulmonary atresia and intact ventricular septum by transcatheter puncture and balloon dilation of the atretic valve membrane. *Am J Cardiol* 1991;68:277–279.

56. Rosenthal E, Qureshi SA, Chen KC, Martin RP, Skehan DJ, Jordan SC, Tynan M. Radiofrequency-assisted balloon dilatation in patients with pulmonary valve atresia and an intact ventricular septum. *Br Heart J* 1993;69: 347–351.

57. Vosa C, Arciprete P, Caianello G, Palma G. Pulmonary atresia with intact ventricular septum: Is it possible to improve survival? *Cardiol Young* 1992;2:391–394.

57a. Gentles TL, Keane JF, Jonas RA, Marx GE, Mayer JE Jr. Surgical alternatives to the Fontan procedure incorporating a hypoplastic right ventricle. *Circulation* 1994; 90(Part 2):II-1-II-6.

58. Freedom RM, Burrows PE, Smallhorn JF. Pulmonary atresia and intact ventricular septum. In: Freedom RM, Benson LN, Smallhorn JF, eds: *Neonatal Heart Disease.* London: Springer-Verlag; 1992, pp. 285–307.

59. Freedom RM, Culham G, Moes F, Olley PM, Rowe RD. Differentiation of functional and structural pulmonary atresia: Role of aortography. *Am J Cardiol* 1978;41: 914–920.

60. Haworth SG, Shinebourne EA, Miller GAH. Right-to-left interatrial shunting with right ventricular pressure. A puzzling haemodynamic picture associated with some rare congenital malformations of the right ventricle and tricuspid valve. *Br Heart J* 1975;37:386–391.

61. Schrire V, Sutin GJ, Barnard CN. Organic and Functional Pulmonary Atresia with Intact Ventricular Septum. *Am J Cardiol* 1961;8:100–108.

62. Becker AE, Becker MJ, Edwards JE. Pathologic spectrum of dysplasia of the tricuspid valve: Features in common with Ebstein's malformation. *Arch Pathol* 1971;91: 167–178.

63. Anderson RH, Silverman NH, Zuberbuhler JR. Congenitally unguarded tricuspid orifice: Its differentiation from Ebstein's malformation in association with pulmonary atresia and intact ventricular septum. *Pediatr Cardiol* 1990;11:86–90.

64. Berman WJ, Whitman V, Stanger P, Rudolph AM. Congenital tricuspid incompetence simulating pulmonary atresia with intact ventricular septum: A report of two cases. *Am Heart J* 1978;96:655–661.

65. Keith JD. Prevalence, incidence and epidemiology. In: Keith JD, Rowe RD, Vlad P, eds. *Heart Disease in Infancy and Childhood.* Third Edition. New York: MacMillan; 1978, pp. 3–13.

66. Fyler DC. Report of the New England Regional Infant Cardiac Program. *Pediatrics* 1980;65(Suppl):376–461.

67. Ferencz C, Rubin JD, McCarter RJ, Brenner JI, Neill CA, Perry LW, Hepner SI, Downing JW. Congenital heart disease: Prevalence at livebirth. The Baltimore-Washington Infant Study. *Am J Epidemiol* 1985;121:31–36.

68. Rowe RD, Freedom RM, Mehrizi A. *The Neonate with Congenital Heart Disease.* New York: WB Saunders Company; 1981, pp. 328–349.

69. Chitayat D, McIntosh N, Fouron J-C. Pulmonary atresia with intact ventricular septum and hypoplastic right heart in sibs: A single gene disorder? *Am J Med Genet* 1992;42:304–306.

70. Hornberger LK, Sahn DJ, Kleinman CS, Copel JA, Reed KL. Tricuspid valve disease with significant tricuspid

insufficiency in the fetus: Diagnosis and outcome. *J Am Coll Cardiol* 1991;17:167–173.

71. Roberson DA, Silverman NH. Ebstein's anomaly: Echocardiographic and clinical features in the fetus and neonate. *J Am Coll Cardiol* 1989;14:1300–1307.

72. Lang D, Oberhoffer R, Cook A, Sharland G, Allan L, Fagg N, Anderson RH. Pathologic spectrum of malformations of the tricuspid valve in prenatal and neonatal life. *J Am Coll Cardiol* 1991;17(5):1161–1167.

73. Allan LD, Crawford DC, Tynan MJ. Pulmonary atresia in prenatal life. *J Am Coll Cardiol* 1986;8:1131–1136.

74. Allan LD and Cook A. Pulmonary atresia with intact ventricular septum in the fetus. *Cardiol Young* 1992; 2:367–376.

74a. Hornberger LK, Benacerraf BR, Bromley BS, Spevak PJ, Sanders SP. Prenatal detection of severe right ventricular outflow tract obstruction: Pulmonary stenosis and pulmonary atresia. *J Ultrasound Med* 1994;13:743–750.

75. Kutsche LM, Van Mierop LHS. Pulmonary atresia with and without ventricular septal defect: A different etiology and pathogenesis for the atresia in the 2 types? *Am J Cardiol* 1983;51:932–935.

76. Braunlin EA, Formanek AG, Moller JH, Edwards JE. Angiopathological appearances of pulmonary valve in pulmonary atresia with intact ventricular septum. Interpretation of nature of right ventricle from pulmonary angiography. *Br Heart J* 1982;47:281–289.

77. Arom KV and Edwards JE. Relationship between right ventricular muscle bundles and pulmonary valve. Significance in pulmonary atresia with intact ventricular septum. *Circulation* 1976;54(Suppl 3):79–83.

78. Freedom RM, White RI Jr, Ho CS, Gingell RL, Hawker RE, Rowe RD. Evaluation of patients with pulmonary atresia and intact ventricular septum by double catheter technique. *Am J Cardiol* 1974;33:892–895.

79. Hausdorf G, Schultze-Neick I, Lange PE. Radiofrequency-assisted "reconstruction" of the right ventricular outflow tract in muscular pulmonary atresia with ventricular septal defet. *Br Heart J* 1993;69:343–346.

80. Braunlin EA. Pulmonary atresia and stenosis with hypoplastic right ventricle. In: Moller JH, Neal WA, eds. *Fetal, Neonatal, and Infant Cardiac Disease.* Norwalk, CT: Appleton and Lange; 1989, pp. 671–687.

81. Freedom RM, Rabinovitch M. The Angiography of the pulmonary circulation in patients with pulmonary atresia and ventricular septal defect. In: Tucker BL, Lindesmith GC, Takahashi M, eds. *Obstructive Lesions of the Right Heart.* Baltimore: University Park Press; 1984, pp. 191–216.

82. Momma K, Takao A, Ando M, Nakazawa M, Satomi G, Imai Y, Takanashi Y, Kurosawa H. Juxtaductal left pulmonary artery obstruction in pulmonary atresia. *Br Heart J* 1986;55:39–44.

83. Elzenga NJ, Gittenberger-de Groot AC. The ductus arteriosus and stenoses of the pulmonary arteries in pulmonary atresia. *Int J Cardiol* 1986;11:195–208.

84. Burrows PE, Freedom RM, Rabinovitch M, Moes CAF. The investigation of abnormal pulmonary arteries in congenital heart disease. *Radiol Clin North Am* 1985;23:689–717.

85. Marino B, Guccione P, Carotti A, De Zorzi A, Di Donato R, Marcelletti C. Ductus arteriosus in pulmonary atresia with and without ventricular septal defect. *Scand J Thorac Cardiovasc Surg* 1992;26:93–96.

86. Zenati M, del Nonno F, Marino B, di Carlo DC. Pulmonary atresia and intact ventricular septum associated with pulmonary artery sling (letter). *J Thorac Cardiovasc Surg* 1992;104:1755–1766.

87. Steeg CN, Ellis K, Bransilver B, Gersony W. Pulmonary atresia and intact ventricular septum complicating corrected transposition of the great vessels. *Am Heart J* 1971;82:382–386.

88. Shimizu T, Ando M, Takao A. Pulmonary atresia with intact ventricular septum and corrected transposition of the great arteries. *Br Heart J* 1981;45:471–474.

89. Freedom RM, Culham JAG, Moes CAF. *Angiocardiography of Congenital Heart Disease.* New York: Macmillan Publishing Company; 1984, pp. 221–253.

90. Huhta JC, Edwards WD, Tajik AJ, Mair DD, Puga FJ, Ritter DG. Pulmonary atresia with intact ventricular septum, Ebstein's anomaly of the hypoplastic tricuspid valve, and double-chamber right ventricle. *Mayo Clin Proc* 1982;57:515–519.

91. Bull C, De Leval M, Mercanti C, Macartney FJ, Anderson RH. Pulmonary atresia and intact ventricular septum: A revised classification. *Circulation* 1982;66:266–272.

92. Rowlatt JF, Rimoldi MJA, Lev M. The quantitative anatomy of the normal child's heart. *Pediatr Clin North Am* 1963;10:499–588.

92a. Drant SE, Allada V, Williams RG. Infundibular diameter predicts the presence of right ventricular-dependent coronary communications in pulmonary atresia and intact ventricular septum (abstract). *J Am Coll Cardiol* 1995;25:140A.

93. Davignon AL, Greenwold WE, DuShane JW, Edwards JE. Congenital pulmonary atresia with intact ventricular septum. Clinicopathologic correlation of two anatomic types. *Am Heart J* 1961;62:591–602.

94. Scognamiglio R, Daliento L, Razzolini R, Boffa GM, Pellegrino PA, Chioin R, Dalla Volta S. Pulmonary atresia with intact ventricular septum: A quantitative cineventriculographic study of the right and left ventricular function. *Pediatr Cardiol* 1986;7:183–187.

95. Shen C-T, Hung C-R, Chen C-M, Lue H-C. A new angiocardiographic classification of pulmonary atresia with intact ventricular septum. *Chinese J Cardiol* 1981; 1:77–86.

96. Daliento L, Scognamiglio R, Thiene G, Hegerty A, Yen Ho S, Caneve F, Anderson RH. Morphological and functional analysis of myocardial status in pulmonary atresia with intact ventricular septum-an angiographic, histologic and morphometric study. *Cardiol Young* 1992; 2:361–366.

97. Freedom RM, Finlay CD. Right ventricular growth potential in patients with pulmonary atresia and intact ventricular septum. In: Freedom RM. *Pulmonary Atresia and Intact Ventricular Septum.* Mount Kisco, NY: Futura Publishing Company; 1989, pp. 239–247.

98. Giglia TM, Jenkins KJ, Matitiau A, Mandell VS, Sanders SP, Mayer JE Jr, Lock JE. Influence of right heart size on outcome in pulmonary atresia with intact ventricular septum. *Circulation* 1993;88(part 1):2248–2256.

98a. Mair D, Danielson GK, Puga FJ. The Fontan procedure for pulmonary atresia and intact ventricular septum (PA and IVS): Operative and late results (abstract). *J Am Coll Cardiol* 1995;25:37A.

98b. Laks H, Gates RN, Grant PW, Drant S, Allada V, Harake B. Aortic to right ventricular shunt for pulmonary atresia and intact ventricular septum. *J Thorac Cardiovasc Surg* 1995;59:342–347.

98c. Freeman JE, DeLeon SY, Lai S, Fisher EA, Ow EP, Pifarre R. Right ventricle-to-aorta conduit in pulmonary atresia with intact ventricular septum and coronary sinusoids. *Ann Thorac Surg* 1993;56;1393–1394.

98d. De Leval M. Myocardial perfusion in congenital heart disease: Surgical implications. In: Marcelletti C, Anderson RH, Becker AE, Corno A, di Carlo D, Mazzera E, eds. *Paediatric Cardiology. Volume 6.* New York: Churchill Livingstone; 1986; pp. 97–107.

98e. Blackstone EH, Kirklin JW, Hanley FE. What proportion of neonates with pulmonary atresia and intact ventricular septum reach difinitive repair. *Circulation* 1996;94(suppl. 1):1–173.

99. Graham TPJ, Bender HW, Atwood GF, Page DL, Sell CGR. Increase in right ventricular volume following valvulotomy for pulmonary atresia or stenosis with intact ventricular septum. *Circulation* 1974;49/50(Suppl II):69–79.

100. Patel R, Freedom RM, Moes CAF, Bloom K, Olley PM, Williams WG, Trusler GA, Rowe RD. Right ventricular volume determinations in 18 patients with pulmonary atresia and intact ventricular septum. Analysis of factors influencing right ventricular growth. *Circulation* 1980; 61:428–440.

101. Grant RT. An unusual anomaly of the coronary vessels in the malformed heart of a child. *Heart* 1926;13: 273–283.

102. Guidici C, Becu L. Cardio-aortic fistula through anomalous coronary arteries. *Br Heart J* 1960;22:729–733.

103. Anselmi G, Munoz S, Blanco P, Carbonell L, Puigbo JJ. Anomalous coronary artery connecting with the right ventricle associated with pulmonary stenosis and atrial septal defect. *Am Heart J* 1961;62:406–414.

104. Williams RR, Kent GBJ, Edwards JE. Anomalous cardiac blood vessel communicating with the right ventricle. *Arch Pathol* 1951;52:480–487.

105. Cornell SH. Myocardial sinusoids in pulmonary valvular atresia. *Radiology* 1966;86:421–424.

106. Finegold MJ, Klein KM. Anastomotic coronary vessels in hypoplasia of the right ventricle. *Am Heart J* 1971;82: 678–683.

107. Calder AL, Co EE, Sage MD. Coronary arterial abnormalities in pulmonary atresia with intact ventricular septum. *Am J Cardiol* 1987;59:437–442.

108. Freedom RM, Benson L, Wilson GJ. The coronary circulation and myocardium in pulmonary and aortic atresia with an intact ventricular septum. In: Marcelletti C, Anderson RH, Becker AE, Corno A, di Dicarlo D, Mazzera E, eds. *Paediatric Cardiology.* Volume 6. Edinburgh: Churchill Livingstone; 1986, pp. 78–96.

109. Freedom RM, Harrington DP. Contribution of intra-myocardial sinusoids in pulmonary atresia and intact ventricular septum to a right-sided circular shunt. *Br Heart J* 1974;36:1061–1065.

110. Freedom RM, Benson LN, Trusler GA. Pulmonary atresia and intact ventricular septum: A consideration of the coronary circulation and ventriculo-coronary connections. *Ann Cardiac Surg* 1989;38–44.

111. Gittenberger-de Groot AC, Sauer U, Bindl L, Babic R, Essed CE, Buhlmeyer K. Competition of coronary arteries and ventriculo-coronary arterial communications in pulmonary atresia with intact ventricular septum. *Int J Cardiol* 1988;18:243–258.

112. Kasznica J, Ursell PC, Blanc WA, Gersony WM. Abnormalities of the coronary circulation in pulmonary atresia and intact ventricular septum. *Am Heart J* 1987;114: 1415–1420.

113. O'Connor WN, Cottrill CM, Johnson GL, Noonan JA, Todd EP. Pulmonary atresia with intact ventricular septum and ventriculocoronary communications: Surgical significance. *Circulation* 1982;65:805–809.

114. O'Connor WN, Stahr BJ, Cottrill CM, Todd EP, Noonan JA. Ventriculocoronary connections in hypoplastic right

115. Kauffman SL, Andersen DH. Persistent venous valves, mal-development of the right heart, and coronary artery-ventricular communications. *Am Heart J* 1963;66: 664–669.

116. Hamazaki M. Congenital coronary arterio-ventricular fistulae, associated with absence of proximal coronary artery from aorta. *Jpn Heart J* 1982;23:271–277.

116a. Dyamenahalli U, Hanna BD, Sharratt GP. Pulmonary atresia with intact ventricular septum: management of the coronary arterial anomalies. Cardiol Young 1997; 7:80–87.

117. Ho SY, De Carvalho J, Sheffield E. Anomalous origin of single coronary artery in association with pulmonary atresia. *Int J Cardiol* 1988;20:125–128.

118. Lenox CC, Briner J. Absent proximal coronary arteries associated with pulmonic atresia. *Am J Cardiol* 1972;30: 666–669.

119. Oppenheimer EH, Esterly JR. Some aspects of cardiac pathology in infancy and childhood. II. Unusual coronary endarteritis with congenital cardiac malformations. *Bull Johns Hopkins Hosp* 1966;19:343–354.

120. Sauer U, Bindl L, Pilossoff V, Hultzsch W, Buhlmeyer K, Gittenberger-de Groot AC, Deleval M, Sink JD. Pulmonary atresia with intact ventricular septum and right ventricle-coronary artery fistulae: Selection of patients for surgery. In: *Pediatric Cardiology.* New York: Springer-Verlag; 1986, pp. 568–578.

121. Sissman NJ, Abrams HL. Bidirectional shunting in a coronary artery-right ventricular fistula associated with pulmonary atresia and an intact ventricular septum. *Circulation* 1965;32:582–588.

122. Ueda K, Saito A, Nakano H, Hamazaki Y. Absence of proximal coronary arteries associated with pulmonary atresia. *Am Heart J* 1983;106:596–598.

123. Gerlis LM, Yen Ho S, Milo S. Three anomalies of the coronary arteries co-existing in a case of pulmonary atresia with intact ventricular septum. *Int J Cardiol* 1990;29:93–95.

124. Wilson GJ, Freedom RM, Koike K, Perrin D. The coronary arteries: Anatomy and histopathology. In: Freedom RM. *Pulmonary Atresia and Intact Ventricular Septum.* Mount Kisco, NY: Futura Publishing Company, Inc; 1989, pp. 75–88.

124a. Oosthoek PW, Moorman AFM, Sauer U, Gittenberger-de Groot AC. Capillary distribution in the ventricles of hearts with pulmonary atresia and intact ventricular septum. *Circulation* 1995;91:1790–1798.

125. Blackman MS, Schneider B, Sondheimer HM. Absent proximal left main coronary artery in association with pulmonary atresia. *Br Heart J* 1981;46:449–451.

126. Garcia OL, Gelbang H, Tamer DF, Fojaco RM. Exclusive origin of both coronary arteries from a hypoplastic right ventricle complicating an extreme tetralogy of Fallot: Lethal myocardial infarction following a palliative shunt. *Am Heart J* 1988;115:198–201.

127. Rigby ML, Salgado M, Silva C. Determinants for outcome of hypoplastic right ventricle with duct-dependent pulmonary blood flow presenting in the neonatal period. *Cardiol Young* 1992;2:377–381.

128. Van der Wal HJCM, Smith A, Becker AE, Wilkinson JL, Hamilton DI. Morphology of pulmonary atresia with intact ventricular septum in patients dying after operation. *Ann Thorac Surg* 1990;50:98–102.

129. Wearn JT, Mettier SR, Klumpp TG, Zschiesche LJ. The nature of the vascular communications between the coronary arteries and the chambers of the heart. *Am Heart J* 1933;9:143–164.

130. Gentles TL, Colan SD, Giglia TM, Mandell VS, Mayer JE, Sanders SP. Right ventricular decompression and left

ventricular function in pulmonary atresia with intact ventricular septum. The influence of less extensive coronary anomalies. *Circulation* 1993;88(part 2):183–188.

131. Giglia TM, Mandell VS, Connor AR, Mayer JE Jr, Lock JE. Diagnosis and management of right ventricular-dependent coronary circulation in pulmonary atresia with intact ventricular septum. *Circulation* 1992;86:1516–1528.

131a. Daubeney PEF, Delany DJ, Slavik Z, Anderson RH, Keeton BR, Webber SA. Pulmonary atresia with intact ventricular septum: Range of morphology in a population based study (abstract). *Circulation* 1995;92(Suppl I):1–126.

132. Lauer RM, Fink HP, Petry EL, Dunn MI, Diehl AM. Angiographic demonstration of intramyocardial sinusoids in pulmonary-valve atresia with intact ventricular septum and hypoplastic right ventricle. *N Engl J Med* 1964;271:68–72.

133. MacMahon HE, Dickinson PCT. Occlusive fibroelastosis of coronary arteries in the newborn. *Circulation* 1967;35:3–9.

134. Arcilla RA, Gasul BM. Congenital aplasia or marked hypoplasia of the myocardium of the right ventricle (Uhl's anomaly). *Pediatrics* 1961;58:381–388.

135. Becker AE, Caruso G. Myocardial disarray. A critical review. *Br Heart J* 1982;47:527–538.

136. Bryan C, Oppenheimer EH. Ventricular endocardial fibro-elastosis. Basis for its presence or absence in cases of pulmonic and aortic atresia. *Arch Pathol* 1969;87:82–86.

137. Bulkley BH, D'Amico B, Taylor AL. Extensive myocardial fiber disarray in aortic and pulmonary atresia: Relevance to hypertrophic cardiomyopathy. *Circulation* 1983;67:191–198.

138. Cornell SH. Myocardial sinusoids in pulmonary valvular atresia. *Radiology* 1966;86:421–424.

139. Cote M, Davignon A, Fouron J-C. Congenital hypoplasia of right ventricular myocardium (Uhl's anomaly) associated with pulmonary atresia in a newborn. *Am J Cardiol* 1973;31:658–661.

140. De Morais CF, Fiorelli AI, Marcial MB, Macruz R, Ebaid M, Lopes EA, Jatene AD. Infarto do miocardio e lesao coronaria em paciente portador de atresia pulmonar. *Rev Latina de Card Inf* 1985;1:201–206.

141. Dusek J, Ostadal B, Duskova M. Postnatal persistence of spongy myocardium with embryonic blood supply. *Arch Pathol* 1975;99:312–317.

142. Essed CE, Klein HW, Krediet P, Vorst EJ. Coronary and endocardial fibroelastosis of the ventricles in the hypoplastic left and right heart syndromes. *Virchows Arch A Path Anat and Histol* 1975;368:87–97.

143. Esterly JR, Oppenheimer EH. Some aspects of cardiac pathology in infancy and childhood. I. Neonatal myocardial necrosis. *Bull Johns Hopkins Hosp* 1966;119:191–199.

144. Freedom RM, Wilson GJ. Endomyocardial abnormalities. In: Freedom RM. *Pulmonary Atresia and Intact Ventricular Septum*. Mount Kisco, NY: Futura Publishing Company; 1989, pp. 89–99.

145. Fyfe DA, Edwards WD, Driscoll DJ. Myocardial ischemia in patients with pulmonary atresia and intact ventricular septum. *J Am Coll Cardiol* 1986;8:402–406.

146. Hausdorf G, Gravinghoff L, Keck EW. Effects of persisting myocardial sinusoids on left ventricular performance in pulmonary atresia with intact ventricular septum. *Eur Heart J* 1987;8:291–296.

147. Hubbard JF, Girod DA, Caldwell RL, Hurwitz RA, Ma-

hony LA, Waller BF. Right ventricular infarction with cardiac rupture in an infant with pulmonary atresia with intact ventricular septum. *J Am Coll Cardiol* 1983;2:363–368.

148. Koike K, Perrin D, Wilson GJ, Freedom RM. Myocardial ischemia and coronary arterial involvement in newborn babies less than one week old with pulmonary atresia and intact ventricular septum. In: Freedom RM. *Pulmonary Atresia and Intact Ventricular Septum*. Mount Kisco, NY: Futura Publishing Company, Inc; 1989, pp. 101–108.

149. Setzer E, Ermocilla R, Tonkin I, John E, Sansa M, Cassady G. Papillary muscle necrosis in a neonatal autopsy population: Incidence and associated clinical manifestations. *J Pediatr* 1980;96:289–294.

150. Uhl HMS. Previously undescribed congenital malformation of the heart: Almost total absence of the myocardium of the right ventricle. *Bull Hopkins Hosp* 1953;91:197–202.

151. Akiba T, Becker AE. Disease of the left ventricle in pulmonary atresia with intact ventricular septum. The limiting factor for long-lasting successful surgical intervention. *J Thorac Cardiovasc Surg* 1994;108:1–8.

152. Vigorita V. Epicardial nodules: A possible sign of coronary endarteritis with hypoplastic right heart syndrome. *Johns Hopkins Med J* 1978;142:215–217.

153. Freedom RM, Culham JAG, Rowe RD. Left atrial to coronary sinus fenestration. (Partially unroofed coronary sinus). Morphological and angiocardiographic observations. *Br Heart J* 1981;46:63–68.

154. Rose AG, Beckman CB, Edwards JE. Communication between coronary sinus and left atrium. *Br Heart J* 1974;36:182–185.

155. Sahn DJ, Allen HD, Anderson R, Goldberg SJ. Echocardiographic diagnosis of atrial septal aneurysm in an infant with hypoplastic right heart syndrome. *Chest* 1978;73:227–229.

156. Casta A. Atrial septal aneurysm herniation across the mitral valve orifice in pulmonary atresia. *Am Heart J* 1988;115:1136–1138.

157. Freedom RM. General morphologic considerations. In: Freedom RM. *Pulmonary Atresia and Intact Ventricular Septum*. Mount Kisco, NY: Futura Publishing Company, Inc; 1989, pp. 17–36.

158. Razzouk AJ, Freedom RM, Cohen AJ, Williams WG, Trusler GA, Coles JG, Burrows PE, Rebeyka I. The recognition, identification of morphological substrate, and treatment of subaortic stenosis after a Fontan operation: An analysis of 12 patients. *J Thorac Cardiovasc Surg* 1992;104:938–944.

159. Patel RG, Freedom RM, Bloom KR, Rowe RD. Truncal or Aortic Valve Stenosis in Functionally Single Arterial Trunk. *Am J Cardiol* 1978;42:800–809.

160. Hanseus K, Bjorkhem G, Lundstrom NR, Laurin S. Cross-sectional echocardiographic measurements of right ventricular size and growth in patients with pulmonary atresia and intact ventricular septum. *Pediatr Cardiol* 1991;12:135–142.

161. Musewe N, Smallhorn JF. Echocardiographic evaluation of pulmonary atresia with intact ventricular septum. In: Freedom RM. *Pulmonary Atresia and Intact Ventricular Septum*. Mount Kisco, NY: Futura Publishing Company, Inc; 1989, pp. 133–155.

162. Andrade JL, Serino W, de Laval M, Somerville J. Two-dimensional echocardiographic evaluation of tricuspid hypoplasia in pulmonary atresia. *Am J Cardiol* 1984;53:387–388.

163. Isaaz K, Cloez JL, Danchin N, Marcon F, Worms AM, Pernot C. Assessment of right ventricular outflow tract in children by two-dimensional echocardiography using a new subcostal view. *Am J Cardiol* 1985;56:539–545.

164. Leung MP, Mok C-K, Hui P-W. Echocardiographic assessment of neonates with pulmonary atresia and intact ventricular septum. *J Am Coll Cardiol* 1988;12:719–725.

165. Marino B, Ballerini L, Marcelletti C, Piva R, Pasquini L, Zacche C, Giannico S, De Simone G. Right oblique subxiphoid view for visualization of the right ventricle in congenital heart disease. *Am J Cardiol* 1984;54: 1064–1069.

166. Marino B, Franceschini E, Ballerini L, Marcelletti C, Thiene G. Anatomical-echocardiographic correlations in pulmonary atresia with intact ventricular septum. Use of subcostal cross-sectional views. *Int J Cardiol* 1986;11:103–109.

167. Smallhorn JF, Izukawa T, Benson L, Freedom RM. Noninvasive recognition of functional pulmonary atresia by echocardiography. *Am J Cardiol* 1984;54:925–926.

168. Silberbach GM, Ferrara B, Berry JM, Einzig S, Bass JL. Diagnosis of functional pulmonary atresia using hyperventilation and Doppler ultrasound. *Am J Cardiol* 1987; 59:709–711.

169. Sanders SP, Parness IA, Colan SD. Recognition of abnormal connections of coronary arteries with the use of color flow mapping. *J Am Coll Cardiol* 1989;13:922–926.

170. Yokota M, Kyoku I, Kitano M, Shimada I, Mizuhara H, Sakamoyo K, Nakano H, Hamazaki M. Atresia of the coronary sinus orifice. Fatal outcome after intraoperative division of the drainage left superior vena cava. *J Thorac Cardiovasc Surg* 1989;98:30–32.

171. Freedom RM. Angiocardiography of the right ventricle. In: Freedom RM. *Pulmonary Atresia and Intact Ventricular Septum*. Mount Kisco, NY: Futura Publishing Company, Inc; 1989, pp. 163–206.

171a. Guzzo D, Castellanos C, Castellanos L-M, de Rubens J, Calderon J, Attie F. Atresia pulmonar con septum interventricular intacto y anomalia de Ebstein de la valvula tricuspide. *Arch Inst Cardiol Mex* 1989;59:133–138.

172. Burrows PE, Freedom RM, Benson LN, Moes CAF. Coronary angiography of pulmonary atresia, hypoplastic right ventricle, and ventriculocoronary communications. *AJR* 1990;154:789–795.

173. Freedom RM, Olley PM, Rowe RD. The angiocardiography and morphology of ductal-dependent congenital heart disease: Selected topics with reference to the clinical application of E-type prostaglandins. In: Gallucci V, Bini RM, Thiene G, eds. *Selected Topics in Cardiac Surgery*. Bologna: Casa Editrice Bologna; 1980, pp. 109–143.

174. Sideris EB, Olley PM, Spooner E, Farina M, Foster E, Trusler GA, Shaher R. Left ventricular function and compliance in pulmonary atresia with intact ventricular septum. *J Thorac Cardiovasc Surg* 1982;84:192–199.

175. Akagi T, Benson LN, Williams WG, Trusler GA, Freedom RM. Ventriculo-coronary arterial connections in pulmonary atresia with intact ventricular septum, and their influences on ventricular performance and clinical course. *Am J Cardiol* 1993;72:586–590.

176. Najm H, Williams WG, Coles JG, Freedom RM, Rebeyka I. Pulmonary atresia with intact ventricular septum: Results of the Fontan procedure (abstract). *Circulation* 1995;92(Suppl 1):1–54.

177. Qureshi SA, Rosenthal E, Tynan M, Anjos R, Baker EJ. Transcatheter laser-assisted balloon pulmonary valve dilation in pulmonic valve atresia. *Am J Cardiol* 1991; 67:428–431.

178. Rosenthal E, Qureshi SA, Kakadekar AP, Anjos R, Baker EJ, Tynan M. Technique of percutaneous laser assisted valve dilatation for valvar atresia in congenital heart disease. *Br Heart J* 1993;69:556–562.

179. Redington AN, Cullen S, Rigby ML. Laser or radiofrequency pulmonary valvotomy in neonates with pulmonary atresia and intact ventricular septum-description of a new method avoiding arterial catheterization. *Cardiol Young* 1992;2:387–390.

180. Hausdorf G, Schneider M, Lange P. Catheter creation of an open outflow tract in previously atretic right ventricular outflow tract associated with ventricular septal defect. *Am J Cardiol* 1993;72:354–356.

Index